The Pioneers of NMR and Magnetic Resonance in Medicine

The Story of MRI

James Mattson and Merrill Simon

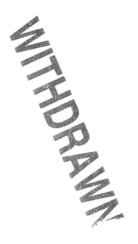

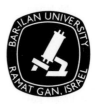

Bar-Ilan University Press

THE PIONEERS OF NMR AND
MAGNETIC RESONANCE IN MEDICINE: *THE STORY OF MRI*

Copyright © 1996 by Dean Books Company

Published by Bar-Ilan University Press
Published in the U.S.A. by Dean Books Co., P.O. Box 346, Jericho, NY 11753

The opinions expressed in this book are those of the authors.
Bar-Ilan University assumes no responsibility for the contents.

No part of this book may be reproduced in any manner without prior
written consent from Dean Books Company

Printed in the United States of America
All Rights Reserved by Dean Books Company

ISBN 09619243-1-4

The Pioneers of NMR and Magnetic Resonance in Medicine

The Story of MRI

James Mattson and Merrill Simon

The world that we have made as a result of the level of thinking we have done thus far creates problems we cannot solve at the same level at which we created them.

—ALBERT EINSTEIN

To my son, Rabbi Melech, his wife, Devorah, and my grandchildren.

To my daughter, Michal, her husband, Rabbi David, and my grandchildren.

—MERRILL SIMON

To my son, Kevin, his wife, Debbi, and to my son, Kyle.

—JAMES MATTSON

ABOUT THE AUTHORS

The Pioneers of NMR and Magnetic Resonance in Medicine is co-authored by Merrill Simon and James Mattson. The driving force behind the conception and completion of this landmark volume, Mr. Simon began working on the project nearly 10 years ago and soon thereafter began compiling documentary evidence regarding the development of magnetic resonance in medicine. The writer of this book, James Mattson, drew much of his material from primary sources, including interviews he conducted with NMR and MRI pioneers featured in this history.

MERRILL SIMON

As a healthcare consultant, Merrill Simon became involved with the state of Florida's 1991-92 cost-cutting healthcare reforms, building on his previous experience with non-doctor-owned MR imaging centers; he also contributed to the understanding of MR in relation to other diagnostic modalities in order to encourage the availability of MRI to primary care physicians.

Mr. Simon is an internationally recognized engineering and science writer. He holds a Bachelor of Science degree in electrical engineering from Purdue

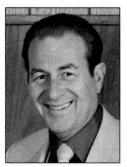

University and an MSEE with an emphasis in solid-state physics. Mr. Simon has taught electronics at the university level. He served as a semiconductor design engineer for IT&T and RCA. As a design engineer at IT&T, he pioneered the development of the newly implemented germanium power devices. As a design engineer at RCA, he designed and developed the first power rectifiers and silicon-controlled rectifiers. For 25 years, he was Vice President of Marketing Worldwide of Veeco Instruments/Lambda Electronics, a manufacturer of high technology semiconductor manufacturing equipment and power hybrids and sophisticated electronic power supplies, retiring at age 50. Mr. Simon served in Korea as a first lieutenant in the Signal Corps during the Korean War.

Merrill Simon is an expert on high technology and is currently a high-tech business consultant in Israel and in the United States. He has helped to establish R&D facilities and three high-tech factories in Israel for several U.S. firms.

A renowned authority and prolific writer on the Middle East and a multi-dimensional activist on behalf of the State of Israel, Mr. Simon is a popular lecturer and featured guest on television and radio talk shows. He was national political editor for the Los Angeles-based biweekly *Israel Today* and the *National Jewish Daily*. Mr. Simon has been a political advisor in Israel; an advisor to the Center for International Security, a Washington-based think tank; and a research associate at the Tel Aviv University Center for Strategic Studies. For the past 15 years he has served first as president and then chairman of the board of Mercaz Hatorah, an institute for rabbinic studies in Jerusalem. Mr. Simon, the author of seven books, maintains residences in Israel and the United States.

JAMES MATTSON

In 1969, James Mattson graduated from journalism school at the University of Wisconsin at Eau Claire and accepted employment in St. Paul, Minnesota as a technical writer for Univac, the pioneer computer man- 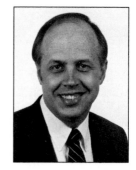 ufacturer. Twenty-six years later, he can look back on a career path that has taken him into such diverse assignments as touting the benefits of industrial tapes manufactured by Minnesota's 3M Company, writing video scripts for a national defense contractor to help train production workers on the screen-printing techniques needed for thick-film production of PC boards, as well as writing and producing publications to help educate physicians on the fast-growing field of magnetic resonance imaging. For eight of those years, in addition to his full-time employment, he edited and produced a 16-page magazine for the fellowship of churches in which his pastor-father ministered for more than four decades. Mattson's recruitment for that task occurred after he took a two-year hiatus from regular employment to attend a theological seminary.

Despite Mr. Mattson's diverse writing experience, this book represents his first foray into book publishing, a career path that he hopes to explore further in the future. "Particularly gratifying for me," he said, "has been the opportunity to speak directly with those pioneers who participated in the development of NMR and MRI. Researching the history of NMR has been fascinating. Like any history, it comes alive when you know more about its pioneers."

As a case in point, Mattson told of his 1986 move from Minnesota to New York. As the grandson of Swedish emigrants to the United States—his middle name is Einar—Mattson had always been conscious of the fact that, although he enjoyed American history and viewed its events as part of his personal heritage, his own ancestors had not lived in the U.S. for much of its past. After he and his wife, Mary Ellen, moved to Long Island, they learned from a genealogy buff in Mary Ellen's family that her ancestors had played an integral part in the founding of America. Ten generations back, her uncle, Richard Nicolls, was the first English governor of New Amsterdam, which he promptly renamed New York after securing the surrender of the Dutch. They also learned that his brother, Mary Ellen's direct ancestor, was an early settler of Southold, Long Island, just an hour's drive to the east. "Suddenly," said Mattson, "Long Island's Nicolls Road, which we passed daily while commuting, took on special significance."

A similar phenomenon takes place, Mattson observes, when we read the biographies of scientists. "Once we learn the stories of the scientists behind the science, the technology that we experience in our daily lives takes on new meaning. I trust that the readers of this book will find this to be true." ✍

TABLE OF CONTENTS

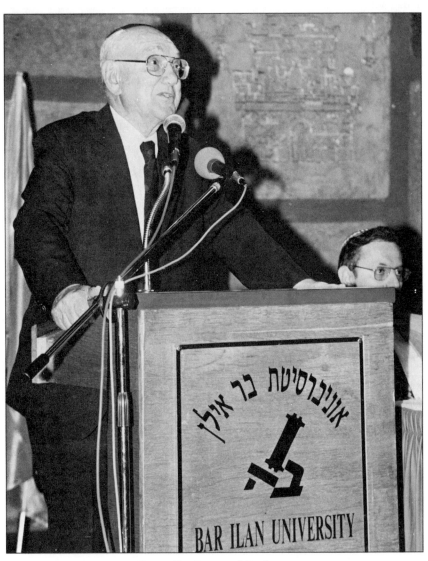

Chancellor Emanuel Rackman

FOREWORD

I<small>N</small> THIS, THE FORTIETH YEAR since its establishment, Bar-Ilan University in Israel has undertaken intensive research in what is called NMR, nuclear magnetic resonance. It has been favored by both the government of Israel and faithful patrons with the resources to do so. It also has staff eminently qualified for the purpose. It is therefore fitting and proper that Bar-Ilan University should publish this introductory volume as it undertakes to play an important role in this very promising sphere of scientific development. It is hoped that this volume will be only the first in a series of studies to advance both the theory of magnetic resonance and its applications. As Chancellor of the University, I am proud that it has taken this major step forward for the following reasons:

First, one great man who has been rightfully considered the father of the basic theory, Nobel laureate Isidor Rabi, is an honorary alumnus of Bar-Ilan. Indeed, ours was the only university in Israel that conferred upon him an honorary degree, and it was with leaders in our University with whom he maintained a long and intimate connection, both with his religious heritage and his mother tongue, Yiddish, as well as with the "songs his mother taught him." His biography and his theoretical and experimental contributions to NMR are contained in Chapter 1 of this book.

Second, as a creation of world Jewry and the young state of Israel, Bar-Ilan University is dedicated, in opposition to the forces of evil, to making science a blessing rather than a scourge that contributes to the possibility of speedy genocide. The nine biographies contained in this volume, which include six Nobel laureates and two Wolf Prize recipients, dramatize the tremendous positive potential science has for benefiting mankind and, by contrast, the great evil of those who would misuse science to destroy humanity. Much is owed the geniuses who fled Nazi Germany in the Hitler era. Who can fathom how many equally great men perished leaving humanity bereft of the contributions they might have made!

Third, Abraham Gelbart, the distinguished mathematician to whose memory this book is dedicated, was a major factor in Bar-Ilan's concentration on mathematics and science in the last decade. The founder of the Gelbart Institute for Mathematical Research, he solicited millions of dollars for research in chemistry, physics and the life sciences for the University as a whole. "He had a dream" for the University and he contributed mightily to its realization. This book is most appropriately dedicated to his memory.

And lastly, I trust this book shall serve to shed light on a controversy between two great contributors to MRI—Dr. Raymond Damadian and Dr. Paul Lauterbur—that such controversy is at most, in the words of Nobel laureates Nicolaas Bloembergen, Edward Purcell and Norman Ramsey, "an honest difference of opinion."

It gives me great pleasure in the autumn of my life and at the end of a score of years in the service of Bar-Ilan University to be involved with this historic project.

—EMANUEL RACKMAN
Chancellor, Bar-Ilan University

IN APPRECIATION

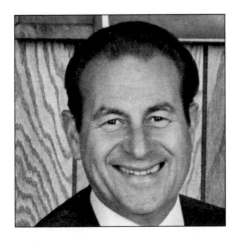

To my Dear Friend:

I am especially grateful to Rabbi Emanuel Rackman, Chancellor of Bar-Ilan University, for the example he has provided me, indeed provided all humanity, by his exceptional wisdom and his lifelong exercise of that wisdom in upholding justice and truth.

—MERRILL SIMON

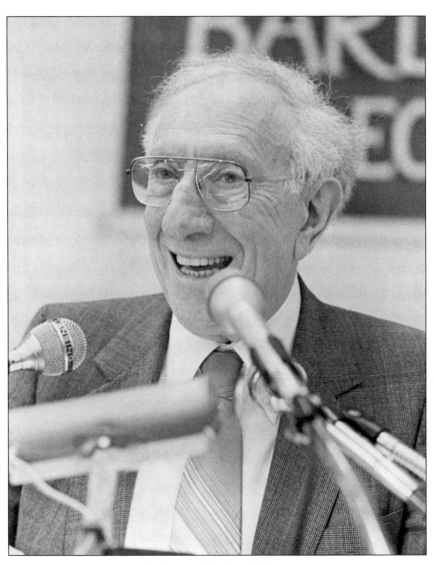

Professor Abraham Gelbart

IN FOND MEMORY

＊ ＊ ＊

Abraham Gelbart, better known as Abe, among friends and family, earned his PhD in mathematics at Massachusetts Institute of Technology in 1940. Following a faculty appointment at North Carolina State College (1940-1942), Professor Gelbart went to Brown University in 1942 as a research associate doing work for the United States Government. In 1943 he continued his government research at Langley Field, Virginia. Later that year, he went to Syracuse University, Syracuse, N.Y., where he spent the next 15 years as full professor of mathematics. As a mathematician, Professor Gelbart's interests were in methods of generalizing complex function theory, nonlinear partial differential equations, functions of complex variables, theory of pseudo-analytic functions, existence theorems in integral equations and fluid dynamics. However, for many years, he also applied his skills in the field of theoretical physics. He was a visiting lecturer at the Sorbonne in Paris (1949); visiting professor at the University of Southern California (1951); Fulbright Lecturer, Norway (1951-52); and was the editor of *Scripta Mathematica* for 20 years (1957-77).

In the period from 1947-1948 Professor Gelbart held a concurrent position as a member of the Institute for Advanced Study in Princeton, N.J. While there, Abe had the honor of working with some of the most brilliant scientists the world has ever known, including Paul Dirac (1933 Nobel Prize in physics, quantum mechanics), Niels Bohr (1922 Nobel Prize in physics, structure of the atom), and Albert Einstein (1921 Nobel Prize in physics, photoelectric effect).

At that time Professor Einstein was attempting to explain gravitation, electromagnetism and subatomic phenomena with just one set of laws, i.e. a unified field theory, but was faced with a daunting system of 64 simultaneous nonlinear partial differential equations in which, he believed, was embedded the solution he sought.

Gelbart and Einstein had become friendly and since Professor Gelbart's area of expertise was nonlinear partial differential equations, Einstein asked for Gelbart's assistance. Although they worked on the problem every day for months, they were unable to solve it. (To this day, Einstein's system of equations remains unsolved.)

In 1958, Professor Gelbart joined the distinguished faculty at Yeshiva University, first as director of the Institute of Mathematics and, subsequently, as the founding dean of the Belfer Graduate School of Science (1959-70). He was named Distinguished University Professor of Mathematics in 1968 and emeritus dean of Belfer Graduate School of Science in 1970. In 1972 Professor Gelbart received an honorary LLD from Dalhousie University, Halifax, Nova Scotia, Canada, his alma mater. From 1962 to 1968, concurrent with his position at Yeshiva, Abe was the director of mathematical sciences at the Office of Scientific Research, U.S. Air Force.

In 1977, because of Yeshiva's policy on retirement age, Professor Gelbart was forced to take what was to be the first of his three retirements. Clearly not the "retiring type," Professor Gelbart spent a couple of years at the Institute for Advanced Study in Princeton where he had worked with Einstein 30 years earlier. After he "retired from there," as he put it, he joined Bard College in New York in 1979.

Professor Gelbart had a very distinguished career at Bard. He received the Bard Medal in 1981 and was named a David Rose Distinguished Professor of Natural Science and Mathematics in 1982. It was a particularly special time for Professor Gelbart, because he succeeded in putting together an instantaneously successful lecture series—the Distinguished Scientists Lecture Series. The series would become extremely well-known in the scientific and academic communities simply because of the extraordinary caliber of guest speakers Abe was able to assemble from its very beginning. He recounted:

The very first speaker in the lecture series was Paul Dirac, a very close friend of mine from England. At the time that I accepted the position at Bard, Dirac was a house guest of mine. When he told me he would like to visit Bard, I asked him right then and there, "Why don't you come up to the college and give a lecture?" He agreed to come.

Now, keep in mind [Gelbart continued] that Bard was a relatively small college. When the president of the college, Leon Botstein, a real go-getter, was informed that the famous Dirac was coming, he sent mailgrams announcing the event to every university within a 200-mile radius! They came by the busloads—from Columbia, Harvard, from all over—just to see the great Dirac. No small wonder. Next to Einstein, in my estimation, Dirac was the greatest scientist of the 20th century. He held Newton's chair at Cambridge at the age of 25.

Since Bard College didn't have a hall large enough for everyone, they had to set up folding chairs in the student dining area and hall-ways along with loudspeakers to accommodate the overflow crowd. So it was that little Bard College had as distinguished a guest speak-er as one might expect to see only at Harvard or some other presti-gious university. I think the next speaker after Dirac [in the lecture series] was Isidor Rabi. As you can imagine, with speakers of this cal-iber kicking off the lecture series, any who were subsequently asked to be guest speakers were not inclined to refuse the invitation.

Some 50 Nobel laureates would speak at Abe's lecture series before his final retirement in 1992. Isidor Rabi agreed to speak in the lecture series for the same reason Dirac did. Gelbart was an old friend. Abe told an amusing story as to how the Rabi Chair of Physics at Columbia University came to be:

> David Rose, a friend of mine who happened to be a wealthy man, was very impressed with Rabi and asked that I introduce him to Rabi, which I did. Completely enamored with Rabi, David asked him if Columbia had done anything in his name. Rabi shrugged his shoulders as if to say, "What should be done in my name?" When Rabi told him that they hadn't, David said, "Well, they should!" I suggested that we meet with the president of Columbia to pursue the matter.
>
> When we met, David suggested to the president that Columbia should definitely do something in Rabi's name—at least establish a chair in his name. After some discussion, the president told us that a chair would cost about a million-and-a-quarter. David Rose respond-ed, "No problem." That's how the Rabi chair was established.

Professor Gelbart was an old and very dear friend of Rabbi Emanuel Rackman. He was committed to the mission of Bar-Ilan and was one of the university's strongest and most loyal supporters. In 1979, Abe became chairman of the International Research Institute for Mathematical

Sciences, which would later be renamed the Gelbart International Research Institute for Mathematical Sciences in his honor. Abe was named its honorary chairman. He also served as a trustee of Bar-Ilan University beginning in 1981. When asked about a Bar-Ilan chair in mathematics that was created in his name, Professor Gelbart, in his characteristic humility, replied, "Yes. That was also one of those David Rose things. He liked to go around establishing chairs in the name of other people. He did a few of those."

Having known and worked with so many accomplished scientists and having made significant contributions of his own, Professor Gelbart was a keen observer of the impact of scientific developments on a number of fields, including NMR and magnetic resonance in medicine,* the subject of this book. *(See Chapter 8, page 676, for Professor Gelbart's personal assessment of the contributions made by the two MRI pioneers featured in this book.)*

It is with great pleasure and pride that Bar-Ilan University publishes this fine work. And so it is only fitting that it be dedicated to someone who has blessed us with so much of the same.

✲ ✲ ✲

"If the dismissal of Jewish scientists means the annihilation of contemporary German science, then we shall do without science for a few years."
—Adolf Hitler, 1933

It was both my privilege and my pleasure to have spent many hours in discussion with my friend Abe Gelbart in my Tel Aviv apartment. What follows is my summary of some of Abe's thoughts and observations on the impact that Nazi Germany and Stalinist Russia have had on America and the establishment and growth of the State of Israel, a subject that has, over the years, been of great interest to both of us. In appreciation of Abe's astute insight on these matters, I am obliged, honored and delighted to record them here.

Following the turn of the century, colleges and universities across the United States and Europe taught only classical 19th-century physics. This was reflected by the fact that the entire range of weapons utilized in World War I and those developed prior to World War II were based on the principles of this "old physics."

Even the weapons systems utilized at the start of World War II by both the Allied and Axis powers, including airplanes, tanks, surface ships, artillery,

---

* Chapter 8, page 676.

mortars, submarines and explosives, were basically improvements or extensions of World War I weaponry. Outstanding among them was the war-time introduction of TNT (trinitrotoluene) by German-Jewish chemist Fritz Haber.

With the mass utilization and new-found tactical applications of these weapons, they were greatly improved as the war progressed. Although "old physics" applications, some significant new technologies did emerge. For example, early on in the war, both the Allied and Axis powers developed crude versions of radar. The Germans also made substantial advancements in rocketry.

At the same time that the "old physics" was being employed on the battlefields, brilliant young scientists working in isolated pockets in Europe, primarily in Germany, were in the process of theorizing the "new physics"—quantum mechanics and relativity. They included some of the finest scientific minds the world has ever known, Jewish and non-Jewish: Einstein, Heisenberg, Planck, Schrödinger, Bohr, Fermi and Dirac. Hitler would later categorize them, like he did everyone, into two groups— Aryans and non-Aryans (Jewish, half-Jewish, etc.). By Hitler's definition, a person with a Jewish great-grandparent was Jewish.

There were basically three waves of the "new physics" scientific thinkers. Although there were many of them, the greatest were:*

1. Early twentieth century: Max Planck (German, Aryan), Albert Einstein (German, Jewish, 1933), Ernest Rutherford (British, Aryan) and Niels Bohr (Danish, Jewish).

2. The 1920s: Werner Heisenberg (German, Aryan), Erwin Schrödinger (Austrian, Aryan, 1933), Paul Dirac (English, Aryan), Niels Bohr, Wolfgang Pauli (Swiss-Austrian, Jewish), Hans Bethe (German, Jewish, 1933) and James Franck (German, Jewish, 1933).

3. The 1930s: Hans Bethe, Lise Meitner (Austrian-Swedish, Jewish), Otto Hahn (German, Aryan), John von Neumann (Hungarian, Jewish, 1930), Eugene Wigner (Hungarian, Jewish, 1933), Edward Teller (Hungarian, Jewish, 1930), Leo Szilard (Hungarian, Jewish) and Enrico Fermi (Italian, Aryan, Jewish wife).

By the 1930s, the "new" physics was spreading throughout Europe. Not yet available to them in the American university system, interested

---

* The years shown in parentheses are those in which the scientists departed from their posts at German universities. Source: Katherine Sopka, *Quantum Physics in America: The Years Through 1935,* (New York: Tomash, 1988), 330.

young American physicists had no choice but to travel to Europe to learn more about it.

At the same time, Hitler was creating oppressive conditions in Germany, including the purging of its universities of Jews and any others he deemed undesirable. Naturally this caused no small amount of consternation in the scientific community. This was of little concern to Hitler, however. "If the dismissal of Jewish scientists means the annihilation of contemporary German science, then we shall do without science for a few years," Hitler told quantum physicist and Nobel laureate Max Planck in 1933. Hitler's oppression, coupled with attractive economic opportunities at American universities, resulted in the flight of a host of non-Aryan scientists to the United States, a mass transfer of precious "new physics" expertise from Europe to America.

At this time, the American scientific institutions had fine teams of experimental physicists and a profusion of equipment in their laboratories, especially powerful accelerating machines and other large-scale apparatus for the study of nuclear phenomena. What they lacked, however, was the theoretical depth that Europe's Jewish scientists could provide.

At the same time, the great European theoretical physicists had little contact with experimental work. Working alone, or in small groups, with limited resources even in the richest and most industrialized European nations, they would have had little chance of ever seeing their theories tested by experimentation.*

The emigration of European theorists to the United States resulted in an unprecedented, mutually-beneficial scientific match of experimental and theoretical genius in a single country—a country rich in scientific resources—a country that would eventually become Hitler's most formidable enemy. Ironically, the collaboration of these American and European scientists, unified in their desire to defeat their common enemies, would eventually lead to the demise of the very man who had unwittingly joined them together in the first place. The stage was set for the emergence of America as a first-rate scientific power and, together with her enormous industrial and agricultural production capacity, the eventual victory of the Allied forces.

Integral to the Allied victory was the initial invention of the magnetron prior to World War II by a Jewish physicist in the Soviet Union. It was

---

* Laura Fermi, *Illustrious Immigrants: The Intellectual Migration from Europe,* 1930-1941, 2nd Edition, (Chicago: The University of Chicago Press, 1971).

then built in England and later employed in microwave radar systems in America by Isidor Rabi, a Jewish immigrant from Europe. (Rabi, one of the pioneers profiled in this book, was a very close friend of Abe Gelbart.) The magnetron, basic to microwave radar, marked the beginning of the new physics. From 1942, Allied radar, superior to that of the Germans, turned the tides of war in their favor, giving them key victories in battles from the deserts of Africa to the submarine depths of the Atlantic. Towards the close of the War, Germany's "new physics" scientists developed the jet engine and the ultra-short-range jet, the M109.

While "new physics" radar may be the technology that won the war, it was atomic power that ended it. The European scientists played a decisive role in the development of atomic energy. Without their presence in America, it is doubtful that the Americans would have been able to develop the bomb on their own. This is especially pertinent in view of information offered by Danish-Jewish Niels Bohr to the Los Alamos atomic bomb team in 1943. Bohr told them that two years earlier, in mid-1941, German physicist Werner Heisenberg had told him that he was working on nuclear weapons that he thought could decide the outcome of the war. Bohr, at the time, was skeptical of Heisenberg's ideas because of the great technical difficulties that would have to be overcome.* The rest is history.

During World War II, the work of the Jewish immigrant scientists on the "new physics" resulted in the development of nuclear and advanced radar technology. After the war, the "new physics" has resulted in the development of solid-state physics, microwave spectroscopy, NMR in condensed matter, electro-optics and radio astronomy.

Abe Gelbart, eminently qualified to evaluate the role of European non-Aryan emigrations, did so with great excitement. He recognized that their emigration to the United States prior to and during World War II stripped Germany of its scientific preeminence, leaving it crippled for decades, and catapulted America to the world's greatest scientific power. He also saw that the emigration of persecuted Jews to the United States and Palestine would eventually result in the creation of Israel in 1948. Finally, he saw that the continuing emigration of Jews from the Soviet Union to Israel is turning Israel into the dominant economic and military power in the Middle East.

More specifically, Abe told how the State of Israel was created by seven catastrophes and eight *Aliyas* and how these catastrophes precipitated a series of massive Jewish emigrations:

---

* Jeremy Bernstein, "What did Heisenberg Tell Bohr about the Bomb?" *Scientific American* (May 1995), page 72.

1. In 1905, the pogrom in Kishinev resulted in large-scale emigration to the United States and also created the second *Aliya* (meaning "ascent" in Hebrew) to Palestine. The latter was the great *Aliya* of Russian-Jewish socialists that created Israel's Histadrut labor unions and the structural foundation of all the country's social institutions including the foundation for Kibbutzim (collective settlements). David Ben Gurion was the leader of this group. (The first *Aliya*, unlike the others that would follow, was not catastrophic. Rather, it was an ideological *Aliya* comprised of some of the greatest Jewish minds and talents of the time including Ben Yehuda, the "Father of the Hebrew Language.")

2. The second catastrophe was the Gravke *Aliya* from Poland in the 1920s. Gravke was the finance minister of Poland who exacted enormous taxes which severely oppressed Poland's Jewish population. This brought about a huge Polish-Jewish emigration to the United States and the third *Aliya* to Palestine. The latter created the Kibbutzim and the agricultural base for the Palestinian community.

3. The third catastrophe was Aryan laws and Hitler's persecution of the Jews in Germany in the 1930s, prior to the outbreak of World War II. Just as the German-Jewish emigration to the United States helped make America a leading scientific power, those who chose to go to Palestine (the fourth *Aliya*) and succeeded in getting there (the British "White Paper" severely limited the number of Jews that could enter legally), supplied the skills, the educated class and the money for creating the infrastructure for the establishment of the modern State of Israel in 1948. They established two great institutions, the Hebrew University and the Technion, as well as a juridical system, a thriving manufacturing base, an administrative structure and a banking system.

4. The fourth catastrophe was the Holocaust of World War II. Following the War, the bulk of Jewish emigrants went to the United States, Canada and Latin America. Those who went to Palestine comprised the fifth *Aliya* (1945-1949). (Prior to declaration of the State of Israel in 1948, the land was known as Palestine, the Jews were known as "Palestinians" and the Arabs were known as "Arabs." Upon declaration of the State of Israel, the land became "Israel," the Jews became "Israelis" and the Arabs became the "Palestinians.") Illegal immigrants provided manpower for the Jewish army, for the settlers of the new Kibbutzim that were being established and for expanding the existing Kibbutzim.

5. The fifth catastrophe took place when large numbers of Jews were expelled from the Arabic lands, such as Yemen, Tunisia, Morocco, Libya, Iraq, Syria and Egypt. They emigrated by entire communities, most to

Israel, but many to France. Those who went to Israel provided the pool of unskilled labor needed for the building of new towns and settlements scattered across the new nation's landscape. This was the sixth *Aliya*.

6. The sixth catastrophe was the 1967 Six Day War. Following Israel's victory, hundreds of thousands of educated and highly-skilled Jews of eastern Europe, Hungary and the Soviet Union were allowed to leave for Israel and the United States; most went to America. Many who arrived in Israel filled positions in universities, schools and hospitals. Engineers found work in Israel's growing number of factories, particularly those factories involved in military projects since Israel was aggressively working towards becoming less reliant on imported weapon systems. This was the seventh *Aliya*.

7. The seventh catastrophe, the 1990 collapse and subsequent dismantling of the Soviet Union, triggered the eighth *Aliya*. By the end of 1995, some 600,000 Jews will have reached Israel. This on-going *Aliya* is expected to reach a million by the year 2000, two million by the year 2010. College-educated in many fields, including medicine, science and engineering, these immigrants have significantly broadened the country's scientific, industrial and economic base. Israel's technological capability is witnessed by its development of a space program and the emergence of an advanced computer programming industry—the fastest-growing industry in Israel. Russian-Jewish immigrants are now flourishing in their new capitalistic environment. They have opened a huge commercial window into Eastern Europe, are bringing hundreds of millions of dollars into the country and are creating the greatest economic boom the country has ever seen. For example, Israel will soon become one of the world's largest producers of magnesium, an achievement directly attributable to the Russian-Jewish immigration.

Incidentally, it is the publicly-expressed hope of Jordan's Prince Hassan that by the year 2010 the combined GNP of all Arab nations will match Israel's current GNP—$85 billion at this writing.

In addition, the many extraordinary Russian-Jewish artists who have emigrated to Israel, including some of the world's finest musicians, have had an enormous positive effect on Israeli culture.

At present, Israel is the economic and military leader of the Middle East. If she is to maintain that status in future decades, it will be as a result of the continuing flow of immigrants from the former Soviet republics.

Abe Gelbart understood the great irony of the 20th century. From its beginning, the 20th century saw the rise of history's cruelest and most powerful dictatorships—Hitler's Germany and Stalin's Soviet Union—with Hitler dedicated to the world-wide extermination of Jewry, and

Stalin to the task of the spiritual extinction of his country's Jewish population. It saw these evil forces implement and carry out their planned
destruction. But before their eventual fall, the 20th century also saw them
unwittingly, accidentally and independently contribute to what each of
them would only despise—the creation of a Jewish state that is today the
leading economic and military power in the Middle East and the emergence of America as the only surviving superpower.

—MERRILL SIMON

✳ ✳ ✳

TRIBUTES TO ABRAHAM GELBART*

That Abe was a superb mathematician was not overlooked by his friend
Albert Einstein who asked Abe to ply his skills in partial differential
equations in a collaborative effort to arrive at the solution to Einstein's
unified field theory. Nor, by virtue of Abe's extraordinarily broad-based
knowledge and interest in science as well as his unique camaraderie with
many of the finest minds of the century including Isidor Rabi and Paul
Dirac, can we overlook Abe's determination of the key paths that led to
the development of MRI. This volume, *The Pioneers of NMR and Magnetic
Resonance in Medicine*, which recounts the achievements of the fields'
acknowledged pioneers, is a fitting tribute to Abe.

—ROSALYN S. YALOW
Nobel laureate, Physiology or Medicine, 1977
for the development of radioimmunoassays of peptide hormones

Abe was one of the most broadly knowledgeable people that I have ever
met. Not only was he a great mathematician, but he also had a tremendous grasp of quantum theory and of magnetic resonance phenomena
and the applications of NMR to medicine. We became good friends, discussing many subjects and evaluating many ideas with particular interest in the applications of high technology. In a world filled with problems,
Abe, one of its greatest optimists, saw solutions.

—MELVIN (MEL) SCHWARTZ
Nobel laureate, Physics, 1988
for the neutrino beam method and the demonstration of the doublet
structure of the leptons through the discovery of the muon neutrino

---

* Some tributes have been condensed for brevity.

While Abe was a mathematician, I was very impressed with his enthusiasm for science, particularly his keen interest in nuclear magnetic resonance and lasers in which I have specialized. It is most appropriate that this volume, a thorough and scholarly tracing of the lives, aspirations and accomplishments of the "pioneers" of NMR and MR, be dedicated to him.

—NICOLAAS BLOEMBERGEN
Nobel laureate, Physics, 1981
for contributions to the development of laser spectroscopy

Abe's passion and love for mathematics, research and teaching flowed powerfully into his broader commitment to an appreciation of all fields of science. He had an almost 17th-century optimism about the power of science to make the world a more civilized place, and he had the faith that the art of mathematics could make it more beautiful.

—ARTHUR KORNBERG
Nobel laureate, Physiology or Medicine, 1959
for his work in contributing to an understanding of the
enzymatic synthesis of deoxyribonucleic acid (DNA)

Abe had a deep and abiding interest in the education of young students, particularly those with an interest in the sciences. Both of us were mathematicians with a broad interest in the physical and life sciences. We were convinced that mathematics had the potential to play a major, even essential, role in the development of the natural sciences. Abe was a visionary and a dreamer, a unique and gifted man.

—HERBERT A. HAUPTMAN
Nobel laureate, Chemistry, 1985
for the development of direct methods for
the determination of crystal structures

—Tribute compiled by Merrill Simon and Mona Gelbart

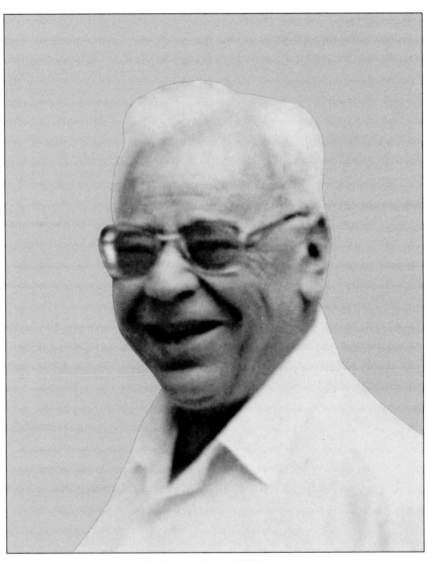

Professor Henry Wallman

FOR THE PAST TEN YEARS it has been both my burden and my passion to trace the discovery and development of nuclear magnetic resonance (NMR) and magnetic resonance (MR) in medicine—a journey on which I've embarked for a number of personal reasons. As an engineer, I have found the technical aspects and scientific impact of the subject matter to be extremely important and fascinating. As an author, I wanted to actually meet the pioneers behind their great discoveries—to hear their stories at a personal level. As a devoted Jew, ever haunted by the Holocaust, I wanted to trace the impact of World War II and the Nazis' plan for the "final solution to the Jewish problem" on the lives of the then young European pioneers, Jews and non-Jews alike. And finally, as a man of conscience who, in the course of attempting to accurately attribute "credit to whom credit is due" in this subject area, has repeatedly come across sometimes gross inaccuracies and confusion, I wanted to, once and for all, finally set the record straight.

My inspiration for doing just that was my good friend and mentor, Professor Henry Wallman. In my quest to determine the true pioneering contributors to NMR and MR in medicine, it was Professor Wallman who encouraged me to settle for nothing less than the truth; his influence on this work cannot be over-emphasized. Accordingly, it is both my privilege and my obligation to profile a very special man to whom I shall always be indebted.

Henry Wallman, born in Brooklyn, New York in 1915, earned his PhD in mathematics from Princeton University at just 22 years of age. He joined the University of North Carolina and then the University of Wisconsin as an assistant professor of mathematics. Following the Japanese bombing of Pearl Harbor, Professor Wallman was summoned to the Radiation Laboratory at Massachusetts Institute of Technology (MIT) where he would join other prominent scientists, including physicists Isidor Rabi and Edward Purcell (both profiled in this book), to work on the development of radar. Professor Wallman's specific task was to supervise the development of radar receivers. It has been said that although it was the atom bomb that ended the war, it was radar that won it.

During this time Professor Wallman made several lasting theoretical and experimental contributions to microwave technology. Particularly innovative was his work in broad-band and low-noise amplifiers. One of the latter, the Wallman-cascode, would be found in essentially every television receiver made following the War.

Professor Wallman joined MIT as Professor of Mathematics in 1946. In 1948, he was invited to be Guest Professor at the Chalmers University of Technology in Gothenburg, Sweden, for the purpose of developing the field of radar in Sweden, which had been cut off from advances in that field because it had not participated in the War. Professor Wallman and his family adjusted well to life in Sweden and, therefore, accepted the invitation to extend their stay. The entire family became Swedish citizens in 1954.

In his early years at Chalmers, Professor Wallman spent much time developing "electronic mathematics machines" for the rapid solution of differential and integral equations. He worked on the problem of interference-plagued radio communication associated with electrically-driven trains and on the choice of a system to be used in the development of the Swedish radio broadcasting network.

An accident in 1954, which resulted in a broken wrist, dramatically changed the direction of Professor Wallman's research. The hospital treatment in connection with the reposition of the fracture aroused his curiosity as to why X-rays could not be used to monitor the medical procedure continuously. The answer he was given was that it was impossible since the radiation dosage to the medical personnel would be too high. This led to his design and construction of an X-ray television system which was placed in service at the Sahlgren Hospital in Gothenburg in the fall of 1955. It was used in X-ray diagnosis, X-ray therapy and surgical procedures. Professor Wallman devoted more and more of his time to the applications of electronics to medicine, working on, among other problems, electronic subtraction, the intensive care of newborn infants, especially premature babies, and the treatment of scoliosis.

In 1966, Professor Wallman was a J.F.K. Visiting Professor at the Weizmann Institute in Rehovot, Israel. In 1967, the Swedish Ministry of Education created the position of Professor of Medical Electronics for him. At the same time, he became professor in the medical faculty of the University of Gothenburg as well as at the Chalmers University of Technology. Professor Wallman was a member of the Royal Swedish Academy of Sciences and the Royal Swedish Academy of Engineering Sciences. He was awarded an Honorary Doctorate in medicine by the Faculty of Medicine of the University of Gothenburg and was a recipient of the Chalmers University of Technology Medal of Merit.

Professor Wallman retired in 1980 and, at the age of 65, took up residence in the Jewish quarter of the old city of Jerusalem. He died on November 30, 1992.

It is quite unique that a mathematical abstraction and a technical innovation be named after the same person, for few have the rare ability to transform the beauty of mathematics into the practical reality of engineering.

Professor Wallman was such a person. To the abstract world of mathematics, the professor left "Wallman Spaces," "Wallman Rings" and "Wallman Compactifications" in the field of topology; and to the world of technology he left the "Wallman-cascode." In Sweden, Professor Wallman was known as the "Father of Medical Electronics."

Professor Wallman was a meticulous man; a man of the greatest integrity—qualities recognized by all who knew him either professionally or personally. I had the privilege of meeting with Professor Wallman on 18 separate visits to Israel and spent hours and hours with him discussing NMR and MR. He, like I, had followed and carefully researched the development of MRI* and was concerned that each pioneer be given proper recognition for his achievements. *(See Chapter 8, pages 612 and 676, for Professor Wallman's personal assessment of the contributions made by the two MRI pioneers featured in this book.)* Professor Wallman was pleased to play an advisory role in this project, for it would be a work based on truth and fairness, a work of integrity—the hallmark of everything he stood for.

The death of beloved Professor Wallman has been a great loss for me, as it has been for his devoted family, other friends, the Jewish community, the scientific community, even the world which has, through Professor Wallman's loving kindness and contributions, become a better place. For his friendship, assistance, help, encouragement and inspiration I shall forever be grateful.

—MERRILL SIMON

---

* Chapter 8, pages 612 and 676.

ACKNOWLEDGEMENTS

I wish to show my appreciation to all the thousands of healthcare workers and medical doctors, the many hundreds of scientists and a score or more of Nobel laureates whom I have interviewed over a 10-year period.

I wish to extend my profound gratitude to my wife, **Amalia,** who continues her loving support with understanding and patience, while supporting my efforts on behalf of the Jewish people and the State of Israel; my dearest friend, **Yosi,** whose career, education and interests parallel and complement my own; and my secretary, **Joan Gannett,** for coordinating and preparing materials for this as well as my seven books.

— MERRILL SIMON

✍ ✍ ✍

I wish to thank **Mary Ellen,** my wife, best friend and business partner, for her loving patience and support throughout the duration of this project as well as for her invaluable editing. Her incisive objectivity, tempered with sensitivity, served frequently to sharpen those passages in which I thought I had achieved perfection and to get rid of those extraneous "gems" to which I was unjustifiably loyal.

I wish to thank the following for their willingness to participate in the project by granting personal interviews, for reviewing their chapters and providing valuable suggestions and for granting approval to their completed chapters: **Professor Norman F. Ramsey,** Harvard University; **Professor Edward M. Purcell,** Harvard University; **Professor Nicolaas Bloembergen,** Harvard University; **Professor Erwin L. Hahn,** University of California, Berkeley; and **Dr. Raymond V. Damadian,** FONAR Corporation. Special thanks to **Professor Ramsey** for reviewing the Rabi chapter and **Professor Hahn** for reviewing the Bloch chapter.

I wish to thank **Helen Rabi,** wife of the late Isidor I. Rabi, for permission to quote from her husband's interview with Barbara Land and **Dr. Lore Bloch,** wife of the late Felix Bloch, for taking the time to read Chapter Four and to offer suggestions for its improvement.

I wish to thank the following organizations and individuals for their prompt and courteous response to my requests while conducting the research for this book during the past three years:

American Institute of Physics: R. Joseph Anderson, head of the Niels Bohr Library; Douglas Egan, Niels Bohr Library; and Tracey Keifer, Library Assistant, AIP Emilio Segrè Visual Archives; **Purdue University Special Collections Library:** Helen Q. Schroyer, Head Librarian; **Balch Institute for Ethnic Studies,** Philadelphia: Mrs. Schwartz; **Case Western Reserve University:** Nora Blackmun; **Ellis Island Restoration Commission:** Brian G. Andersson; **Harvard University Archives:** James McCarthy; **MIT Museum:** Michael Yates; **Time-Life:** Debbie Kuhn; **AP/Wide World Photos:** Joanna Bruno; **Museum of the City of New York; Stanford University Special Collections, Stanford Libraries:** Patricia White and Linda Long; **University of Illinois:** Robert Dinkelberger; **Brooklyn Historical Society; Columbia University, Columbiana Collection:** Hollee Haswell; **Columbia University; Oral History Research Office:** Bernard Crystal; **British Newspaper Library; New York Public Library; Grand Rapids Public Library,** Grand Rapids, Minnesota; as well as libraries at the following institutions: University of Wisconsin, Milwaukee; University of Minnesota, Minneapolis; University of Minnesota, Duluth; Gustavus Adolphus College, St. Peter, Minnesota; St. Olaf College, Northfield, Minnesota; State University of New York, Stony Brook; St. Cloud State University, St. Cloud, Minnesota; and Itasca Community College, Grand Rapids, Minnesota.

Finally, I wish to thank **Merrill Simon** for first conceiving the idea for this book, for the extensive groundwork he laid for it years before I became involved in the project, for making the key contacts needed to bring it about and for his continuing efforts to make the book a reality.

— JAMES MATTSON

To a physicist, the 20th century begins in 1895, with Wilhelm Roentgen's unexpected discovery of X-rays.

—Steven Weinberg

Magnetic resonance imaging has the potential of totally replacing computed tomography. If history was rewritten, and CT invented after MRI, nobody would bother to pursue CT.

—Philip Drew

FROM X-RAYS TO MRI

One Hundred Years After the Discovery of X-Rays,
Magnetic Resonance Scanning and Imaging Promise to
Make Roentgen's Rays Obsolete in Medicine

On NOVEMBER 5, 1895, Wilhelm Roentgen, head of the department of physics at the University of Würzburg in Bavaria, adjusted the thin, black cardboard he had fashioned around a Crookes' vacuum discharge tube, darkened his laboratory, and prepared to observe again a phenomenon that fascinated him, the faint mysterious luminescence created in certain chemicals when exposed to radiation from the tube. Ironically, the cardboard Roentgen used to block the light competing with the gentle, eerie glow of the chemicals would disclose to him the invisible existence of an even more amazing phenomenon. As Roentgen activated the tube and waited for the glow to be generated, his attention was arrested by a light where none should exist, on a sheet of paper well-shielded from the tube by the cardboard. True, the paper was coated with barium platinocyanide, one of the luminiscent substances he had been studying, but the pathway from the tube to the paper was clearly blocked by the cardboard.

His excitement aroused, Roentgen worked quickly to discover the source of the mysterious light and found that it was indeed the tube. When he turned it off, the paper stopped glowing; when he turned it on, the glow returned. Whatever was causing the light, however, gave off no visible light itself. Other scientists had been using Crookes tubes in laboratories for more than 30 years and some had even noticed the fluorescence that they generated—Sir William Crookes himself had noticed that photographic plates became fogged near his cathode-ray tubes—but no one had followed up the phenomenon before.

For seven weeks after making his discovery, Roentgen kept his secret from the world while he experimented feverishly to find the nature of what he called X-rays. He found that they travel in straight lines, cannot be refracted or reflected, and that they do not respond to electric or magnetic fields.

Finally, on December 28, 1895, he submitted his first paper in which he announced his dramatic discovery and revealed its unusual properties.

The world was enthralled and no one was more excited by X-rays than physicists. They rushed to confirm Roentgen's findings and, in the next year alone, a thousand papers were published on the phenomenon. In New York, Columbia faculty member Michael Pupin, a physicist and electrical engineer from Hungary, was one of the first to duplicate Roentgen's results. He later wrote, "No other discovery within my lifetime had ever aroused the interest of the world as did the discovery of the X-rays. Every physicist dropped his own research problems and rushed headlong into the research. . . ."

"To a physicist," Nobel Prize laureate Steven Weinberg has written, "the 20th century begins in 1895, with Wilhelm Roentgen's unexpected discovery of X-rays."

Commercial interests quickly became involved. Thomas Alva Edison heard of Roentgen's discovery, rushed to test various chemicals for reaction to the rays, found that calcium tungstate crystals fluoresced beautifully, and made off immediately for the Patent Office. Unaware of the safety hazards, others also rushed to exploit the phenomenon that Roentgen had demonstrated shortly after introducing his rays to the world, their remarkable, magic-like ability to reveal bony structures in the human body without resorting to surgery.

There was no dismissing the medical benefits of X-rays. In spite of their radiation hazards, X-rays contributed tremendously to the rise in the level of health care that took place in the 20th century. Roentgen's discovery, for which he was made an honorary doctor of medicine by the University of Würzburg in 1896 and awarded the first Nobel Prize in physics in 1901, ushered in not only a new era in physics, but a new era in medicine that allowed physicians to observe the inside of the human body without surgery.

One hundred years later, the century that began for physicists and physicians with the introduction of X-rays is ending with the growing prominence of another diagnostic tool made possible by another physical phenomenon—nuclear magnetic resonance—the initial discovery of which would not take place until four decades after Roentgen's discovery.

Louis Pasteur is said to have observed that "good fortune favors the prepared mind." Science is often in the position of waiting, sometimes unnecessarily it seems, for such a mind. Wilhelm Roentgen is one example of such a "prepared mind," Raymond Damadian is another.

In the case of X-rays, the Crookes tube was around for more than 30 years before Roentgen became engrossed by the phenomenon of luminescence induced by these electron discharge tubes and, in the process, discovered X-rays. Similarly, in the case of MRI, 25 years elapsed between the discovery of NMR in condensed matter by Purcell and Bloch and the discovery by Raymond Damadian, a medical doctor, that different biological tissues exhibit different relaxation rates and that cancerous tissues exhibit unusually prolonged relaxation times. As a result of his discovery, Damadian immediately envisioned the possibility of a new diagnostic modality and perceived in the ubiquitous table-top NMR spectrometer a miniature precursor for his vision of a whole-body NMR scanner.

On Weinberg's shifted time line in which the 20th century began with Roentgen's discovery of X-rays in 1895, I.I. Rabi invented the molecular beam magnetic resonance method 42 years into the century and Edward Purcell discovered nuclear magnetic resonance in condensed matter just a little over a month past the century's midpoint, followed a few weeks later by Felix Bloch. (Purcell's published announcement was submitted to the publisher just four days less than a half-century after Roentgen's.)

A quarter century after the discoveries by Purcell and Bloch, Damadian found that nuclear magnetic resonance could be used to detect disease in biological tissue and proposed that NMR could be used as an "external probe for the internal detection of cancer." Today, another quarter century later, as the 20th century is about to meet the 21st and nearly 100 years after Roentgen's spectacular discovery, X-ray-based diagnostic modalities—from chest X-rays to CAT scans to X-ray mammograms—are destined for obsolescence while MRI, still in its developmental adolescence, is the modality of choice for a preponderant list of clinical applications that continues to grow.

Fifteen years after Damadian exhibited the first commercial NMR scanner to the world at the annual meeting of the American Roentgen Ray Society in April of 1980 and later that fall at the annual meeting of the Radiological Society of North America (RSNA), both gatherings have changed dramatically in both technical content and in products exhibited.

Back then, the reigning modality of radiology was computed axial tomography. Although greatly advanced beyond plain film radiography, CAT scans, also known as CT, still used harmful X-rays and were limited in their portrayal of soft tissue. For many of the radiologists roaming through the technical exhibits of the RSNA in 1980, just a few weeks after Ronald Reagan was elected president of the United States for the first time, magnetic resonance imaging wasn't even in their vocabulry. Eight annual RSNA meetings later, the world of radiology was vastly different. Reagan was still the president of the United States, winding up the last few months of his second term, but magnetic resonance was no longer a curiosity, no longer on the fringe of diagnostic radiology. By 1988, those who had initially remained loyal to CT over MRI were quietly studying scientific posters featuring the latest case studies declaring the superior benefits of MRI over CT and attending courses to learn the difference between T_1 and T_2. Instead of one MRI exhibitor, there were more than a dozen marketing MR scanners.

It had been an amazing eight years. When President Reagan came into office, MRI was in its infancy. Before he left office, he awarded the National Medal of Technology to two of the people featured in this book—Dr. Raymond Damadian and Dr. Paul Lauterbur—for their "independent contributions in conceiving and developing the application of magnetic resonance technology to medical uses, including whole-body scanning and diagnostic imaging." Magnetic resonance had come into its own and was well on its way to fulfilling the prediction of radiological consultant Dr. Philip Drew when he stated in 1987: "Magnetic resonance imaging has the potential of totally replacing computed tomography. If history was rewritten, and CT invented after MRI, nobody would bother to pursue CT."

The nine pioneers selected for this book have been chosen because of the significance of their contributions—the critical mass they provided, you might say—in moving magnetic resonance to where it is today. There were others who came close to equalling their contributions, in some cases even preceding them, but who fell short either in the conception or the implementation of their idea.

Cornelis Gorter is perhaps the best example. In 1936, one year before Rabi's successful use of magnetic resonance in molecular beams, Gorter tried unsuccessfully to detect nuclear magnetic resonance in lithium (^{7}Li) using lithium chloride and in hydrogen (^{1}H) using aluminum potassium alum. And in 1942, three years before Purcell and Bloch were successful in finding NMR in the hydrogen of paraffin and water, Gorter and his collaborator, L.J.F. Broer, again reported unsuccessful attempts to observe NMR in lithium chloride and potassium fluoride. Gorter even gave a speech about these and other ill-fated scientific efforts he made—he also had many successes—when he received the Fritz London Award in 1960, later reprinted in *Physics Today* as "Bad Luck in Attempts to Make Scientific Discoveries."

In the early 1950s, Robert Gabillard in Paris and, in the U.S., Herman Carr and Edward Purcell at Harvard, independently superimposed magnetic field gradients onto the main field to achieve spatial localization, but it was Paul Lauterbur who combined that approach with a technique known as "back projection," which had just recently been used in the development of CAT scanning, to provide a method for pictorially visualizing the tissue relaxation differences uncovered by Damadian.

And then there's Henry Torrey who, in 1945, along with Robert Pound, had helped Edward Purcell discover NMR in condensed matter. He preempted Erwin Hahn in 1949 with his more comprehensive report on transient nutations, also called the Rabi flop, and might have found spin echoes and free induction decay in the process had his RF pulses been shorter and less periodic. Instead, it was Erwin Hahn, frustrated by some strange, unwanted blips, who discovered both echoes and FIDs.

And there were others who, like Damadian, found it interesting to look for signals from biological tissue. In fact, two other pioneers featured in this book, Edward Purcell and Norman Ramsey, sneaked, as Erwin Hahn tells the story, into the Harvard cyclotron magnet and subjected themselves to the proton continuous-wave Larmor frequency but experienced no apparent negative effects. Hahn also points out that he and his former student, Sven Hartmann, tried the same experiment with the intent of observing the gross proton FID from the head. "Unfortunately," he said, "because of the short T_2 and lack of enthusiasm for engineering a better non-adiabatic cut-off, we saw no signal."

Or there is Erik Odeblad, cited by some as a precursor to Damadian for discovering the abnormal NMR signal emitted by cancer. He himself, however, has acknowledged that, although he did do some work in measuring radio frequency absorption in cancer tissue, he did not use nuclear magnetic resonance. He credits Damadian with the original work in that area.

And there were J.R. Singer, J.A. Jackson and others who came close to the target by looking at blood flow. But again, it was Damadian's vital idea to use NMR to differentiate between normal and diseased tissue that provided the impetus for the clinical development of NMR.

And on it goes. The history of science is replete with nearly-identical discoveries—like the discovery of NMR in condensed matter by Edward Purcell and Felix Bloch, for example—that occur independently and almost simultaneously, as though Nature, unable to contain its latest never-before-revealed secret, giddily shares it with two or three.

Countless others not mentioned in this book have contributed to the science and technology of magnetic resonance, and neither the science nor the industry would be where they are today without their important contributions. It is the purpose of this book, however, to feature those pioneers of NMR and MRI who set out first on the unmarked path and who opened up horizons never seen before. ■

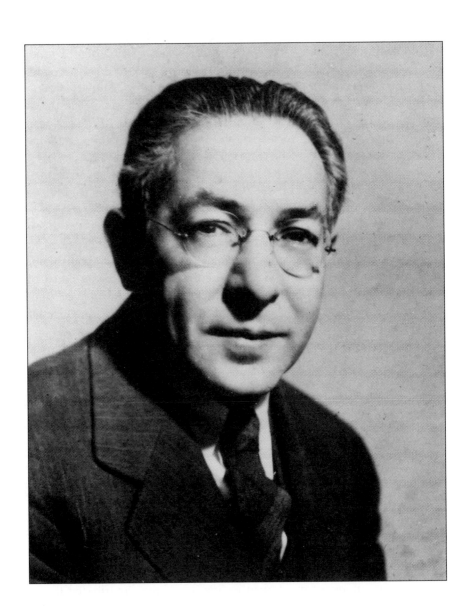

CHAPTER

1

ISIDOR I. RABI

Discoverer of Nuclear Magnetic Resonance in Molecular Beams

"I BEGAN MY CONSCIOUS LIFE at the very beginning of this century, and have tried to be a 20th-century man," Professor I.I. Rabi told students at California's Claremont College in 1960. "Perhaps that ambition dictated the choice of my life work in science."[1]

Rabi was just two-and-a-half years old when Germany's Max Planck fired what could be called the first shot in physics' Quantum Revolution with his announcement to the German Physical Society in late 1900 that radiant energy can be emitted by matter only in discontinuous bundles called quanta, and that the size of these quanta are governed by a universal constant h, thereafter known as Planck's constant.

If Planck's quanta and constant represented the first shot directed toward the fortress of classical physics, certainly other events had warned of at least a coming shake-up. In 1896, just a few months after Roentgen's discovery in Germany of the X-ray, Henri Becquerel in France discovered radioactivity. That same year, Pieter Zeeman of Holland discovered that the band of yellow light diffracted from sodium became broader when placed in a magnetic field, an indication that the magnetic field was actually splitting the spectral lines. And in 1897 J.J. Thomson in England discovered the first atomic particle, the electron.

Although Rabi was too young to participate in the first wave of development in quantum theory and more than two decades would pass before he would begin his own study of the new physics, he was ready to participate fully in the development and propagation of the second wave ushered in by de Broglie, Heisenberg, Schrödinger and Dirac.

Contemporaneous with Werner Heisenberg, Wolfgang Pauli and Paul A.M. Dirac—they were all born within a four-year time span—Rabi would play a key role in transporting the Quantum Revolution to the shores of

America and then, during the 1930s and 1940s, would add to its ongoing scientific and technological impact with, among other contributions: 1) the discovery of magnetic resonance in molecular beams;[2] 2) co-origination of a new area of spectroscopy known as radiofrequency spectroscopy;[3] 3) co-discovery of the electric quadrupole moment of the deuteron;[4] 4) co-discovery of a discrepancy between theory and experiment in the hyperfine separation of atomic hydrogen which drew attention to the possibility of an anomaly in the magnetic moment of the electron[5] (shown to be real a few months later in a Nobel Prize-winning experiment by Polykarp Kusch and Henry Foley); and 5) co-discovery with W.W. Havens and L.J. Rainwater of the first experimental evidence of interaction between the neutron and the electron[6] (confirmed later by Enrico Fermi who had earlier sought for such evidence and had not detected it).

To isolate the atomic and molecular phenomena he investigated in his laboratory at Columbia University, most of Rabi's scientific experiments took place in a physical vacuum, free of most external influences, but Rabi himself could never be accused of operating in a vacuum. His insights—both scientific and philosophical—were products of his openness to input from a wide variety of outside sources.

He was an atomic scientist, but he was also political scientist, historian and arts aficionado who enjoyed Broadway plays, operas and literature. He served his country as a consultant to the scientific director of the Manhattan Project, but few have exerted more energy in seeking to control the awesome power of the atom. He sought diligently after knowledge, but he was not so short-sighted as to sacrifice wisdom on its altar. "What we are really looking for," he once said, "is wisdom. Our great accumulation of knowledge needs the added quality of wisdom. . . . Wisdom is inseparable from knowledge; it is knowledge plus a quality which is within the human being. Without it, knowledge is dry, almost unfit for human consumption, and dangerous to application."[7]

To Make a Living

He was born Israel Isaac Rabi on July 29, 1898, the only son of David and Sheindel Rabi, in the town of Rymanow, in the region of Galicia, once the northeasternmost province of the old Austro-Hungarian empire. Today, after two world wars and subsequent border changes, Rabi's birthplace in the foothills of the Carpathian Mountains is located in the southern tip of Poland, about 12 miles from Slovakia and 50 miles from the western border of Ukraine. His father, David Robert Rabi had been born about 23 years earlier on January 1, 1875 in Jablonica, Austria—now

Jablonica, Slovakia; his mother Sheindel (Teig) Rabi—listed as Jennie in the 1920 U.S. Census—was born in 1878 in Rubonoff, Austria, making her about 20 when Israel was born.

On July 21, 1899, eight days before Israel's first birthday, David Rabi emigrated to the United States by way of Hamburg, Germany. Poor, unskilled and with no formal education to prepare him for a specific trade or occupation,* David Rabi's plan, typical of many immigrants, was to earn enough money to bring his wife and child over as soon as possible.

It may have taken longer than David Rabi expected to accumulate the money for "Jennie" and Israel. Years later, I.I. Rabi didn't know exactly when he and his mother followed his father to the United States—he told one interviewer that it was just a few months afterward[8] and another that it must have been about 1900, or thereabouts.[9] "I have no recollection of it . . . and I have no precise dates," he said. "The family just didn't keep that kind of record."[10]

According to the U.S. Census Bureau, however, young Israel and his mother came to the United States in 1902.[11] Most likely, they came sometime in the first four months of 1902, when he was about three-and-a-half years of age, as his sister Gertrude was born in January of 1903.

"[My family] came directly to New York," Rabi said, "It was a period of great immigration."[12] Indeed, it was. Nearly 250 years after the first Jewish immigrants arrived in 1654 in what is now New York City[13]—then called New Amsterdam—1902 saw more than 58,000 Jewish immigrants arrive in that busy port.[14] Many of them, like the Rabis, were from Galicia in Austria-Hungary. And many of them, also like the Rabis, chose to go no further.

After being reunited, David and Jennie Rabi and their young son settled on Manhattan's Lower East Side, less than four miles from where Jennie and Israel disembarked on Ellis Island.†

---

* This is not to say he was uneducated. Even poor Orthodox Jews in the Eastern European Jewish communities known as *shtetls* were diligently educated in the commandments of Scripture starting as early as age three. To be "a good Jew," it was necessary to obey the commandments of Scripture. To obey the commands, one must know them. To know them, one must study them. Furthermore, study itself was commanded by God. Thus, it has been written of David Rabi: "He had been educated to be a good Jew, but not to make a good living."
—Quote by John Rigden, *Rabi: Scientist and Citizen*, (New York: Basic Books, 1987), 17.

† In 1899, David Rabi probably disembarked at the Barge Office, a landing at Lower Manhattan's Battery Park where immigrants were processed for two-and-a-half years following an 1897 Ellis Island fire that destroyed nearly all of its buildings.
—"Ellis Island History," *Ellis Island & Statue of Liberty*, (San Francisco: American Park Network, 1993), 30-31.

At the turn of the century, New York City was already a bustling metropolis, but quite different in appearance from what it would be just a few decades later. A 1902 view of the city would show an island tightly packed with multi-story buildings, but without the skyscrapers associated with modern-day Manhattan. The first steel-skeletoned buildings had not appeared until the early 1890s and one of the earliest skyscrapers, the Flatiron Building, was just being completed the year Rabi and his mother arrived. Still standing today at the triangle intersection of Broadway, Fifth Avenue and 23rd Street, it was for a time the world's tallest at 300 feet—short by today's standards.

Only four years before their arrival, Brooklyn had voted, along with the rest of the present-day boroughs, to become part of New York City, a decision that would stimulate dramatic growth in the decades to come, especially as it became better connected to Manhattan by bridges and tunnels, but as of 1902 the Brooklyn Bridge, completed 19 years earlier, was still the only bridge available for crossing the East River. The second bridge to connect Brooklyn and Manhattan, the Williamsburg, was under construction but would not open until the following year. The Rabi dwelling at 98 Willett Street* was situated just off its Delancey Street approach.

The Lower East Side of Manhattan had once been home to wealthy merchants and ship captains, but by the 1840s many of its fine, single-family homes had given way to cramped tenements designed to accommodate in minimum space for maximum profit the waves of immigrants who had begun flooding into the area. First came the Irish in the 1840s, then the Germans, and then, starting in the 1880s and crescendoing until the early years of the 20th century, Jews from Russia and Eastern Europe.

Unlike Jewish refugees from Russia, the Rabis did not come to the United States to escape persecution. "[My parents] lived quite freely in the Jewish community of Rymanow," said Rabi. "They had no resentment against Emperor Franz Josef. He was apparently well liked. The real problem was how to make a living, and my father, who had no skills, finally had to emigrate."[15]

It was fortunate they came when they did. About 68 years after leaving Rymanow, and about 23 years after the Holocaust that wiped out millions of European Jews, Professor Rabi returned to his childhood home for the

---

* Although this address differs slightly from the one transcribed from a Rabi interview (97 Willard Street) and the one given by John Rigden in his biography of Rabi (91 Willett Street), it is the one shown on David Rabi's Original Declaration of Intention to become a U.S. citizen, filed December 12, 1905. David Rabi became a citizen on February 24, 1914.

first time, where he was hosted by the town's mayor. Most of the evidence of his Jewish heritage was gone. "There may have been a Jew left, I don't know," said Rabi. "I asked to see the Jewish cemetery. We got into a car and drove along this very bad road until we came upon a beautiful field." The only evidence that it was a cemetery was an occasional stone protruding slightly above the surface of the soil. At one time, the cemetery had been much larger than the town's Catholic cemetery, which was still intact, but all of the stones marking Jewish graves had been leveled during the war.[16]

Almost totally Jewish in 1902, the Lower East Side of Manhattan was divided into a mosaic of Jewish subcultures, an international microcosm reflecting the population's national and regional origins in Europe. For the Rabis, the New World version of Galicia bordered on Hamilton Fish Park, at the corner of Willett and Stanton. (Today the portion of Willett Street where the Rabis lived from 1902 to 1907 is gone, and another massive housing project called Samuel Gompers Houses has taken its place, ironically immortalizing in a new generation of multiple dwellings the famous leader of the American Federation of Labor, once a resident of the area.)

It has been observed that "the influx [of immigrants to the Lower East Side] produced conditions common to all slums—overcrowding, poverty, lack of privacy, crime, sweatshops, and suffering."[17] The Rabi family would experience all of these, yet years later I.I. Rabi would recall the area and the experience with fond memories and "real affection."

"I remember a very cheerful happy childhood there on the sidewalks of New York," he said. In spite of the fact that his family had little money and that they lived in what Rabi also regarded as a slum, he had no feeling of being underprivileged. "We knew that we were poor, but we did not consider ourselves underprivileged. We were just poor."[18]

Home was a two-room tenement flat shared by six occupants: David and Jennie, Israel, his little sister Gertrude, and two boarders. One room served as kitchen, dining room and living room as well as bedroom for the boarders; the other room, windowless, was just large enough for a bed.[19] The bathroom was a toilet in the backyard shared by everyone in the building. The Rabi dwelling was probably very similar to a barrack building described by Pulitzer Prize-winning author Oscar Handlin. Built during the 1850s, the building described by Handlin was located only about six blocks from where the Rabis lived.

Five stories in height, it stretched back one hundred and fifty feet from the street between two tight alleys (one nine, the other seven feet wide). Onto the more spacious alley opened twelve doors through each of which passed the ten families that lived within, two on each floor in identical two-room apartments (one room, 9 x 14; one bedroom, 9 x 6). Here, without interior plumbing or heat were the homes of five hundred people. . . . Certainly the flats were small and overcrowded. . . . [they] shrank still further when shared by more than one family or when they sheltered lodgers, as did more than half those in New York at the end of the century.[20]

Home wasn't the only place that was overcrowded. According to Rabi, the area was densely populated and filled with kids, "something happening all the time." If there was such a thing as a right to privacy, nobody knew about it. "In the summer time," he said, "people sat outside. Everyone knew everyone else's business. It was a little exciting because of street gangs and otherwise."[21] Probably included among the "otherwise" were the saloons and prostitutes. "There were lots of prostitutes and saloons—every intersection had three or four saloons. And, of course, there were a lot of synagogues. There were no Christians living there then."[22]

Sin and synagogues. Both had their place on the Lower East Side. For Orthodox Jews like David and Jennie Rabi, you avoided the first by being faithful to the second. The Sabbath was the highlight of the week. Just as the Sabbath brought the joy of the future into the Eastern European *shtetl*,[23] so the Sabbath could bring joy to Orthodox Jews living in less-than-ideal surroundings on Manhattan's Lower East Side.

[My parents, said Rabi] had a very strong Orthodox, Chassidic, fundamentalist tradition, which they carried on in New York. I was raised on that, and heard all the stories that go with it—all the stories about evil spirits and devils and, of course, on the other side, God and the Founding Fathers, so to speak. For those people, God was present all the time. In conversation, not a paragraph—hardly a sentence—would go by without a reference to God. The Orthodox Hebrew religion requires a lot of doing; there is a lot of ritual, so that you're pretty busy at it. It isn't just going to the synagogue on Saturdays and holidays. Indeed, if you have the time, if you don't have to make a living, you go there every day—three times a day, as a matter of fact. You're kept pretty busy with prayers and with the learning that accompanies them. It is not a superficial kind of culture.[24]

The Rabis did have to make a living, however, and that too kept them busy. Since David Rabi had no particular skills to offer, he had to settle for menial jobs—as a night watchman, as a tender of coal in a cellar, as an ice man, and finally, as a factory worker manufacturing women's blouses in a sweatshop. Eventually, by working hard, by being thrifty and by borrowing, he was able to open a small grocery store.

Early each morning, David would open the store to get whatever morning trade there was before leaving for his job at the sweatshop. After a long day at work, during which Jennie attended to any customers that came in, he would return to the store again in the evening in hope of gleaning a few more sales before heading home. But the Rabis felt fortunate. In a time when there were few economic safety nets, there was nothing worse than being without a job.

> People always worried about being out of a job [said Rabi]. That was the big problem. Nobody worried about working long hours. That was a sort of blessing, to have the opportunity to work these long hours. . . . There was no question that we were pretty cheerful about it, and the Lord was with us all the time, in the sense that hope was around the corner because the Lord was watching you. . . . In that way, we had a pretty optimistic outlook.[25]

"My father was a very mild man," said Rabi, "who never had very much to say. He'd sit and listen, a very fair man, a natural gentleman, but he didn't have the drive that my mother had. He was a very, very hardworking man. I have never seen anybody that worked as hard as he did during his life." Rabi's mother, "a very remarkable woman," he noted, "was really the motor force, the guiding force of the family."[26]

In spite of the hard work, the Rabi family still found time to enjoy life. Relatives from both sides of the family were also in the neighborhood and when they got together there would be singing and story telling. "We used to have pretty jolly times," said Rabi. The singing ranged from sentimental songs then being sung in New York's theater and music halls to religious hymns passed on from centuries past. The stories, on the other hand, tended toward the hair-raising. Coming as they did from Eastern Europe's Carpathian Mountains, just to the north of Transylvania, Rabi's relatives were well aware of Count Dracula and other stories that would keep young children awake at night.

> I was full of tales of the supernatural. The whole world was under the direct supervision of the Almighty, and tales of supernatural events and ghosts, every kind of thing which is so well described in

Dracula, so that I was absolutely full of that when I was a child, completely afraid of the dark. I'd say my prayers for no other reason than that I was really scared.[27]

Asked if there was any particular experience in those early days that turned his mind toward science, Rabi replied, "Yes, a very profound one."

One time, I was walking along and looked down the street—looked right down the street, which faced east. The moon was just rising. And it scared hell out of me! Absolutely scared the hell out of me!

Another profound experience that I had revolved around the first verses of Genesis. They were very moving to me as a kid. The whole idea of the creation—the mystery and the philosophy of it. It sank in on me, and it's something I still feel.[28]

Although Rabi didn't start public school until he was eight years old because of frequent illnesses—"In that congested region I caught them all," he said—he actually started school much earlier. Somewhere around the age of three or four, his parents started him in synagogue school, where he learned to recognize Hebrew characters. Although he never learned Hebrew, he did learn to read Yiddish* at a very early age and read it a great deal which, he said, "was a great concern to my mother who would much have preferred to have had me outside playing with the boys, rather than immersed in a book."[29]

His extensive reading in Yiddish books and Bible stories did have its social benefits, however. "Because I was very small," said Rabi, "I needed protection. I had it because I was so good at telling Bible stories. I'd keep them fascinated—the big boys. I was kind of a mascot because of my Bible stories."[30]

It was public school that changed Israel to Isidor. When Jennie enrolled him and was asked for his name, she replied, "Izzy," a term of endearment he had acquired at home. The school administrator assumed "Izzy"

---

* Even though the Lower East Side was divided into Jewish sub-cultures, Yiddish provided a common language. A medieval German dialect integrated with certain Hebrew elements, Yiddish was able to absorb the regional variations of its users and yet be understandable to anyone who knew it. "Whoever knows Yiddish can understand the Yiddish of anyone else," it has been said, "even though some of the words may be incomprehensible."
  —Jeremy Bernstein, "Profiles: Physicist–I," *New Yorker*, 13 October 1975, 48.

was a variant of Isidor and thus was Rabi's name forever changed, a mistake he never corrected. From then on, the I.I. in Rabi's name stood for Isidor Isaac rather than Israel Isaac.[31] (As an adult, he was often just called Rabi.)

Public School (P.S.) 22 where Rabi attended still faces the Columbia Street side of Hamilton Fish Park, as it did when Rabi went there. (The park was built in 1900, two years before Rabi's arrival.) The street name seems significant somehow. For more than 60 years of his life, he would be associated with another Columbia—Columbia University—located on Manhattan's Upper West Side.

Crisis of Faith

Five years after Rabi and his mother came to the United States, it was clear that the family grocery store was not proving to be a financial success and in the Panic of 1907, as the nation entered a deep depression, both the family and the store moved to the Brownsville section of Brooklyn. Six miles southeast of their former neighborhood, Brownsville was easily accessible via the new Williamsburg Bridge. Although a present-day Long Island commuter would view the area as just out of the City, as Manhattan is called, Rabi described it as the "far reaches" of Brooklyn, "quite the opposite," he said, "of where we had lived. It was semi-rural. There were chickens and goats in the streets. I used to go in the morning to a farmer to buy milk."[32]

Even though it meant a longer commute, David Rabi didn't give up his job at the blouse-making factory in Manhattan. As they had done on the Lower East Side, he took care of the store in the morning and evening, while Jennie took care of it during the day, but now, instead of a two-room flat in a large tenement, the Rabis shared a three-family house. Located at 481 Hopkinson Avenue,* the Rabi portion of the building included the store and three rooms in back.

It was about a year after their move to Brooklyn that Rabi, then about 10 years of age, discovered the local branch of the Brooklyn Public Library, located on Dumont Avenue. Also known as the Brownsville Children's Library, it was built like so many others across the United States through the philanthropy of steelmaker Andrew Carnegie. Young Rabi started reading in the children's section, going alphabetically from

---

* Address based on David Rabi's Petition for Naturalization, No. 10792, filed October 25, 1913 with the District Court of the Eastern District of New York.

author to author, starting with Alcott and working down through Trowbridge. After devouring those books, the next shelf he came to was science. Alphabetically, astronomy came first, so that's where he started reading. What he discovered next—the Copernican system—was for him a brand-new revelation that contradicted the information he had received from his very orthodox parents who believed the earth was flat. "I still have the feeling of wonder and revelation when I think of the solar system and the laws that govern it,"[33] Rabi said.

Seen through the filter of his new world view, the moon he had seen hovering at the east end of that Manhattan street was now part of an ordered astronomical system and was no longer terrifying. The cosmological change of perspective immediately changed Rabi's theological perspective.

> There is certainly a contradiction between [the Copernican theory] and what I was told as a child—that the earth is flat and that there is a big fish, the Leviathan, which surrounds it, which has its own tail in its mouth, and which will be eaten on the Day of Judgment by the good Orthodox Jews while the others will get nothing. It's a bit of a jump from there to the Copernican system. Besides, when you are Orthodox, you say prayers for the new moon. When you have the astronomical explanation, the rising of the moon becomes a sort of non-event.[34]

Rabi's theological conclusions, in turn, affected him and his family sociologically. Typical of many immigrant parents and their offspring, the potential for diverging world views to develop between Rabi and his parents was already present, even without Copernicus. While young Rabi was attending public school, speaking English in the streets, and absorbing massive quantities of new ideas, David and Jennie, feeling very insecure with their English, continued speaking Yiddish—Polish when they didn't want their children to understand.

One of the new ideas gathering momentum at the time was socialism. The Panic of 1907 had people scared, and socialism, which was just beginning to come to America, seemed to offer answers. "There were tremendous discussions of that," said Rabi, "and of course the socialistic position at that time was very anti-religious."[35]

One of the books Rabi read during this period was Jack London's *The Iron Heel*, which Rabi said was "a sort of poor man's introduction to the materialistic interpretation of history, the Marxist theory of value, things of that sort. I became very interested in it, and for about two years I used to go to the local Socialist Club most every night, and watch them play chess and other things." By the time Rabi was in his last year of elementary school, he had become, he said, "a very convinced Socialist."[36]

After two years of going to the Socialist Club, not once having anyone speak to him, and meanwhile growing increasingly disillusioned with their ability to run the country if they were successful in gaining power, he changed his mind and decided it was an entirely impractical idea.

When it came time for Rabi's *bar mitzvah*, the Jewish rite of passage for 13-year-old boys where they are accepted into the congregation of men and called upon to deliver a talk at the synagogue based on the Torah, God's Law, he was not willing to participate. To him, the Torah was no longer truth, and he was unwilling to take part in what he thought was superstition. Finally, they compromised. Instead of a bar mitzvah in the synagogue, they would have it at home, and instead of a talk on the Torah, he could give a talk on whatever he wanted. His topic? "How the Electric Light Works." "I look back on it now," Rabi said, "and when I consider the sorrows I brought on them, it horrifies me."[37]

> When I think about it, for my family it was rather tragic [said Rabi], because there was nothing they could do. I was the firstborn, the only son. And I could outtalk them. They hadn't read about Copernicus. So we reached a sort of *modus vivendi* where at home I conformed to everything. I didn't try to persuade them of anything else. They would have really suffered from that. And they didn't ask very much about what I did outside. So I was a good son in that respect. I tried to help with the holidays—to make them joyful occasions. I have a great respect and a great feeling for these things. It's part of a culture, a way of life, an outlook. Sometimes I feel I shouldn't have dropped it so completely—I'm talking about the way of life. There's no question that basically, somewhere way down, I'm an Orthodox Jew. In fact, to this very day, if you ask for my religion, I say 'Orthodox Hebrew'—in the sense that the church I'm not attending is that one. If I were to go to a church, that's the one I would go to. That's the one I failed. It doesn't mean I'm something else.[38]

By this time, Rabi had learned about other things than the Copernican theory on the science shelf at the public library. He had also read about electricity, telegraphs and telephones. From a boy whose father was a junkman, he acquired wire, which he and his friends strung across the streets to make telegraphs. He even made a little money on the side by installing electric bells and alarm systems.

Nearly three decades would pass before Rabi, then a faculty member at Columbia University, would publish along with his associates, Norman Ramsey, Jerome Kellogg and Jerrold Zacharias, a paper in *Physical Review*[39] in which they announced the first application of radiofrequency spectroscopy using "ordinary radio waves," but Rabi first got his start in radio in Brooklyn when it was still called "wireless." When his father was able to purchase the building that included their home and store, Rabi immediately put up a big antenna. "It was a point of pride," he said, "to get the news not from the newspaper but . . . from ships."[40] It is also noteworthy that Rabi's first scientific paper, describing the making of a condenser, was published by Hugo Gernsback in *Modern Electrics* when Rabi was still in elementary school.[41]

His parents neither encouraged him nor discouraged him in these pursuits, even when his home-based radio station took up a major wall in the living room.

> I was a very formidable kid [said Rabi]. There was nothing much they could do about it, when I was set on doing this. Besides, I was an only son, and an only son in a Jewish family is in a very special position. Anyway, I was very formidable. Did [my mother] mind it? No, I don't think she did, actually. I don't think she did.[42]

Although Rabi spent a great deal of time alone reading, he was not what you would call a loner. Whether it was stringing wire across Brooklyn streets or starting a chess club, Rabi "always had an organization," he said. "In whatever I was interested in, I would generate interest in others."[43]

When it came time to graduate from elementary school and select the high school he would be attending for the next four years, Rabi chose Manual Training High School. The school had once been located at Court and Livingstone, but sometime around 1904 a new building was constructed at Seventh Avenue and Fourth Street, a couple blocks west of Brooklyn's Prospect Park.

Rabi thought it was about three miles to the school from his house on Hopkinson Avenue, but it appears, according to a city map, to have been closer to five miles. "If one walked," he said, "it was a very interesting experience, usually quite dangerous, in a way, because of the hostile groups one passes through. The structure of New York is well known by the neighborhoods, their characteristics, and kids going through are entering hostile territory."[44]

As its name implied, the school offered a full curriculum in shopwork, but that wasn't the main reason Rabi chose the school. His parents wanted him to continue his Hebrew studies—at a yeshiva preferably. But Rabi, having grown up in a neighborhood that was 100 percent Jewish, vetoed that idea and selected instead a high school in which relatively few Jews were enrolled.

> I went there purposely. Normally, I should have gone to Boys High—that was the school. All the very smart Jewish kids went to it. But I had been raised in an environment where we didn't see anything but Jews. My elementary school was just full of Jews, with maybe here and there a few gentiles who had, as it were, crossed district lines. I wanted to get away from that. I had very definite notions of being an American in a broader sense. I had read a great deal of history, and I wanted to be part of the greater thing, so I went to Manual Training.
>
> I had four years of shopwork—woodworking, cabinetmaking, printing, and various kinds of mechanical work. I did that sort of thing at home with wireless telegraphy and model airplanes. But the great advantage of going to a second-rate school was that I didn't have to do more than 10 minutes of homework a day.[45]

Rabi had been accused of being undisciplined before, by his father, who told him, "It's not that you're irreligious—you're lazy."[46] You couldn't chalk off his lack of diligence entirely to laziness, however, as he energetically pursued those things in which he took personal interest. He continued, for example, devouring books at the local library, reading, in particular, biographies, including biographies of scientists, history books of all kinds, as well as fiction. One of his favorite fiction writers was James Fenimore Cooper.

He also read fairly advanced science books, including Charles Steinmetz' *Electricity*, which he read, he said, "not with understanding, but just out of the sheer pleasure in reading that sort of thing. I'd read it almost as a regular novel, not really trying hard to understand and work it out, but absorbing a lot of it in the same sense in which a child absorbs the language."[47]

For Rabi, the world was a very interesting place during his high school years from 1912 to 1916. He enjoyed politics and was absorbed by the

1912 election when Theodore Roosevelt ran for president under the third-party Bull Moose banner, splitting the Republican vote and giving the election to Woodrow Wilson. When the First World War started in 1914, Rabi couldn't wait for school to open so he could discuss the dramatic events with his classmates. "When I got there," he said, "to my great disappointment, none of them knew anything about it. They weren't interested. But I used to read about it with great interest and followed all the advances and movements of the armies."[48]

In spite of devoting less than 10 minutes a day to homework, Rabi ended up with a very high score on the comparative performance scale set up by the New York State Board of Regents, somewhere in the top 10, as he recalled, which earned him a scholarship to Cornell University, but overall, he viewed his high school career negatively, both intellectually and socially.

> I really didn't get much more out of it than going to class. I had one or two good teachers, but they were not great men in any way. I got to see another part of the world, because there were very few Jewish people in that school. It was very important to me to see the others, and I was very much surprised that some of them did very well. But there was no social connection really built up. I never got to be friendly with any of the non-Jewish boys, not one. I talked with them some. We weren't unfriendly, [but] I wasn't in any of their homes or vice versa. In that sense there was, I think, in my case and the case of all the people I knew, segregation. It wasn't the best school.[49]

In spite of Manual Training High School's emphasis on workshop courses, Rabi was able to take enough math and science to earn credits all the way into his junior year at Cornell. The school was strongest in chemistry, so that's where Rabi concentrated. Although his physics teacher had a PhD, the only teacher in the school with a doctorate, Rabi classified him as one of his worst teachers. "In fact, all my life I never got good instruction in physics," he claimed.

"Our math teacher was marvelous."[50] It was Rabi's math teacher who influenced his decision to attend Cornell, but not because of Cornell's math program. The math teacher, who was also the football coach, had prevailed upon Rabi and one of his friends to sell tickets for their school's football games and had rewarded them with complimentary tickets. As a result, Rabi became interested in football at a time when Cornell happened to be prominent in the sport with an All-American quarterback named Charlie Barrett. Since Cornell also placed a greater emphasis on science and engineering than other schools did, had a "liberal attitude about it, a sense of freedom and novelty," was out in Western New York's James Fenimore Cooper country, and put out a good humor magazine, "it seemed like a nice place to go,"[51] said Rabi. He would later conclude that, for him, choosing Cornell "was a very great mistake."[52]

> I missed a great deal by doing that, because many of the people I met later on, I would have met earlier in life. People who were very stimulating and who influenced me a great deal, I probably would have met earlier on if I'd stayed in New York, instead of spending three years in that isolated little town of Ithaca.[53]

However, there was one man at Cornell, a fellow student, who did stand out in Rabi's mind.

> In my freshman year, a man who had tremendous influence on me was a fellow by the name of Philip Subkow, a tall, thin, gangling chap who was fantastically well read, and I found a real kindred spirit in him. He was, I thought, more well read than I, but I must have had many things which he didn't have because we were intimate almost immediately. It was at an entirely different level than with the others, in a very sophisticated and scientific and literary way.[54]

Subkow introduced Rabi to the quantum and Planck's constant. He had apparently heard about it from "a nut," Rabi said, "who wrote very widely and was very well known, an inventor by the name of [Albert Cushing] Crehore."[55] Although this "mysterious constant h," as Rabi referred to it, had been revealed to the German Physical Society by Max Planck about 16 years earlier, it was known to very few people at that time in the United States, said Rabi, even at the highest scientific levels. Unfortunately, Subkow disappeared after the first term. Rabi never heard from him or about him again, but as far as he was concerned, until he met J. Robert Oppenheimer a decade later, Subkow's breadth, interest and quickness of mind was the greatest he had encountered.[56]

As for physics at Cornell, said Rabi, it was, as in high school, very badly taught.

> The essence of physics never came through to me; it seemed to me to be the sort of thing where you measured the resistance of copper to another decimal point. Nothing duller than a physics teaching lab-

oratory, nothing. Chemistry, on the other hand, was very interesting; there were things to do. You could experiment and so on, which appealed to my research instinct.[57]

Although Rabi started out majoring, as did many physicists during that period, in electrical engineering, he chose it largely by default. He knew he wanted to study science, and he knew he wanted to study the fundamental structure of matter; he just didn't know the name of that science. Because his roommates were taking chemistry, he decided to study chemistry as well as electrical engineering, taking as many as 25 credits at a time, a schedule, he pointed out, which would not be permitted today. He eventually graduated with a degree—Bachelor of Chemistry—which is not conferred today. It's as obsolete, he said, as Chrysler's DeSoto.

It is noteworthy that in the 1920 U.S. Census, which was probably responded to by Rabi's parents, his occupation is listed as "engineer."[58] The fact that he was no longer pursuing a career in electrical engineering had apparently not been communicated to his family, an oversight that can probably be explained by the fact that, at least as far as Rabi was concerned, it was all the same to them.

I think I was the first man in the family who had ever gone to college and they certainly had no idea of science whatsoever. They would have been happy if I'd gone in for medicine or for the rabbinate, but as far as this was concerned, it was *terra incognita* with them and they had no views on it whatsoever.[59]

Rabi's degree truly was a bachelor of chemistry, he said, in that he took no courses outside of mathematics, physics and chemistry, except for freshman English, until his last year, when he took an elective course in philosophy. Again, he took the same approach he used in high school. Study minimally, a few minutes a day, on courses in which he was enrolled. Use the rest of the time to read and reflect in other areas.

I had made up my mind actually that I would never read in a subject in which I was taking a course. So if I was taking a course in qualitative analysis, I might be reading Freud. I did an immense amount of reading. So in a strange way, without taking courses, I got myself a liberal education. Indeed, if one doesn't try to get high grades, as I didn't, one has a lot of time in college, even if you take a heavy schedule, as I did. I was graduated in three years easily.[60]

He earned good grades, but he didn't study for the purpose of grades. He didn't know exactly how he did grade-wise in college, although he figured he was in the top quarter of his class. He recalled working for an A once, just to win a bet. His interest in the history of a subject often gave him a more comprehensive view of the material, an asset when it came time to take exams.

> Many times, I would walk up to the exam with some classmate, and say, "Well, I will review you for the exam. I'll ask you questions," and he would give me the answers he'd studied. I'd go in, take the exam, and get 20 percent more than he did. Because he was so full of it he couldn't see the woods for the trees. Just because of my more relaxed approach, and the historical, more synoptic view, I got much more pleasure out of the thing than the others did, and I didn't have to do much work.[61]

Looking back on his college career later, Rabi regretted that he had not taken courses in the other areas that interested him, such as history and economics, courses taught by "great historians" such as Carl Becker, who had just started his nearly-30-year career at Cornell in 1917.

> In a certain sense, my life was a narrow one. But there was the whole world of books. The library was nice and acceptable, and it was in a nice location. . . . I never got to know any of [my teachers]. I never joined any club or organization or fraternity. I took long walks. I didn't know any girls. I was a very shy kid.[62]

Because of the war in Europe, Rabi was inducted into the Students' Army Training Corps (SATC). Although military training was a standard part of a student's life at Cornell, this was different. This training was conducted with full military discipline and the students lived in barracks. When the Armistice came at the end of the war, an officer inspecting the barracks caught Rabi reading about the Armistice instead of the assigned military regulations. When he inquired whether Rabi knew his infantry drill regulations backwards, Rabi replied, "No, sir," and ended up with 10 days of KP. "It gave me a permanent distaste for military life," said Rabi, "which has sustained me ever since."[63]

The experience probably influenced the advice Rabi would give Robert Oppenheimer, scientific director at Los Alamos, more than two decades later. In establishing the Manhattan Project, General Groves and the

Manhattan District wanted Oppenheimer and the rest of the scientists involved in atomic bomb development to operate under military rules and wear military uniforms. Oppenheimer was about to cave in to their demands, but Rabi and Robert Bacher strongly advised him against it, saying it would compromise their scientific freedom. Oppenheimer took their advice and, although the scientists did live and work in a military environment at Los Alamos, they did so as civilians.

Before graduating from Cornell, Rabi was required to do a senior research project in chemistry. He had read somewhere about a suboxide of magnesium that was first noticed in 1866. He was able, using electrolysis and more modern methods such as single potentials, to find it again and to substantiate that the black substance he obtained was indeed a suboxide of magnesium. Shortly before finishing his project, however, he discovered that a few years before, a man had gotten his doctorate at Cornell for showing that this material did not exist.

"But I had it," said Rabi. When he wrote up the paper and gave it to his professor for publication, the department refused to publish it. Seven years later, his work was repeated by an Englishman and published. "That made me angry," said Rabi, "because I'd done this piece of work which I thought was pretty good. . . . It was clear to me that this wasn't a good place to do [research], only I didn't know of a better place."[64]

Back to Brooklyn

For the next three years, Rabi floundered. He didn't go on to graduate school because he didn't know what it really was—"It was never made clear to me"—and besides, he said, in 1919 "the whole world was stirring—very great events—it didn't seem right to stay up there in this out-of-the-way school."[65]

Unfortunately, it wasn't a good time to look for a job, certainly not a good time for a Jew to look for a job, although his grades were definitely acceptable. "I wasn't offered any jobs," he said, "while the non-Jewish boys were all snapped up by various chemical companies."[66]

Did he think anti-Semitism was, in many cases, behind the apparent disparity, he was asked. "In all cases," he responded, "not in many but in all cases. There were just no exceptions that I knew of, and also there were just no jobs within the university. It was an entirely different situation [at that time]. So it was clear to me that somehow or other, if I wanted to pursue my interests, I would have to make money some other way; that's the way it looked."[67]

After graduation, Rabi moved back home to live with his parents who, by then, had moved to the Eastern Parkway section of Brooklyn. "As a result of the war, as prices went up . . . they managed to actually make some money," said Rabi. "Then there was a real estate boom. My father bought some real estate and that went up, so altogether they were in much more comfortable circumstances. . . . I never had much hesitancy about taking money from the family. If they had it, they were very glad to give it."[68]

Rabi did get a job, however, as an analytical chemist for Lederle Laboratories located, as he recalled, on 36th Street in Manhattan, where he analyzed things like mothers' milk and furniture polish. While there, he met Benedict Cassen, a "most extraordinary young fellow," then in his late teens, who told Rabi "all sorts of things" he hadn't picked up at college, including Maxwell's theory and quantum theory. "He didn't know too much," said Rabi, "just suggestions—elements of mathematics that I hadn't studied."[69] It was probably because of Cassen, Rabi said, that he kept going to the New York Public Library during this doldrums period in his life, a practice that kept him exposed to science even though he was not actively engaged in study and research. The laboratory job didn't last long, only a few months—"I really wasn't too good at it. I wasn't interested. I would say I was more fired than left," he said.[70]

> I was drifting. I had this job, then another job. . . . I spent some time in a business which was a sort of private banking business, discounting accounts receivable. That didn't last long, either. Several years went by when I did practically nothing.[71]

He was joined in his non-productivity by three friends who were in the same boat: Maurice Finkelstein, Benjamin Ginzburg, and Joseph Lapin. "We were all more or less not doing anything very much,"[72] Rabi said. Rabi's parents never once asked him what he was doing about his job situation. "It's the most extraordinary thing," said Rabi. "I have never seen anything like it. They showed complete faith . . . and love."[73]

After three years of this, he and his friends were ready for a change. "It was Ginzburg who broke the spell," Rabi recalled. "He simply said, 'It's time to quit horsing around.' "[74] Rabi agreed. "This won't do," he told himself. "It's either now or never. You're 25; you've been doing your reading but you're not getting anything."[75]

Nearly simultaneously, the four of them decided to go back to school. Finkelstein entered Harvard law school. Ginzburg also went to Harvard, where he earned a PhD in philosophy. Lapin entered medical school. Rabi returned to remote Ithaca and Cornell University.

Back to Cornell

Three years after leaving Cornell, Rabi returned there to do graduate work in physical chemistry. He had taken all the courses he could in chemistry, however, so he thought he would study physics and concoct his own version of physical chemistry—"You see, I was that kind of person,"[76] he said. This time, he had no scholarship to finance his studies and he was unable to get an assistantship in either chemistry or physics, so his parents paid his way.

Because Rabi had been away from school for over three years and the physics courses he had taken before at Cornell had, in his estimation, laid a poor foundation, he found that he had to work very diligently to handle the intermediate and advanced physics courses with which he was now confronted. Fortunately, by this time, he said, he knew "a little something" about the subject from the self-directed reading he had done and, in spite of the increased work load, he came to realize that "the part of chemistry I liked was called physics."

> If somebody had pointed that out to me before, it would have saved me many, many years. I was charmed by Gauss' theorem, circuit theory, maximum-minimum effects, and that sort of thing. I took an enormous number of courses. I took electricity and magnetism, statistical mechanics, some mathematics courses, both advanced calculus and calculus of variations, something they called 'modern physics.'[77]

For the first time, Rabi found it necessary to develop disciplined study habits.

> I set myself an extraordinary schedule, which I've never done since, because I'm not a systematic person. But I had a program which I wrote down, which started from the time I got up every morning to the time I went to bed, from 8 o'clock in the morning or whatever it was, till midnight—something for every hour, every minute, lunch and so on, which I carried out for about six or seven months. I knew if I broke it once, I'd never go back to it. One Sunday they persuaded me to go out for a walk with a group, and I never got back to it.[78]

Although Rabi's intensive pattern of self-discipline had been broken, his objective had been accomplished. "I broke the back of the thing," said Rabi. "I was on the road to physics."[79]

Rabi did not achieve an outstanding record as a student during that intensive catch-up year, nevertheless he applied in March of 1923 for a fellowship for the following academic year, 1923-24. In spite of a strong letter of recommendation by Professor A.W. Browne,[80] the person he listed as a reference on his application, he was denied the fellowship. So he decided to leave Cornell after attending the summer session and transfer to Columbia University in New York City. He cited two reasons for making the change: 1) Cost—Columbia was much closer to home—and 2) Helen Newmark.

Helen had come to Ithaca to attend the summer session at Cornell. "It was a place people came to spend their summer vacations," said Rabi, "and maybe take a course." According to Helen, when she arrived at the train station in Ithaca, Rabi was there along with others to greet a popular guy by the name of Harry who was on the same train. But when she stepped off the train, "[Rabi] stepped forward," she said, "picked up my bag, said to somebody else, 'Take it up the hill; we're going to walk.' " Coincidentally, Rabi's mother had dispatched his sister, Gertrude, to Ithaca about the same time to see how it was with her brother. When she saw Helen and the look in her brother's eyes, she later commented to her mother, "Mama, you're going to have a beautiful daughter-in-law."[81]

When Helen went back at the end of the summer session to attend Hunter College that fall, Rabi also went back to New York and registered at Columbia. Years later, Helen Rabi stated that when Rabi decided to follow her back to New York and go to Columbia, it was "about the most fortunate thing that ever happened to him."[82] She did not indicate whether she meant scientifically or otherwise.

Columbia University

After one year of graduate school in Ithaca, Rabi was back in New York City and back at his parents' home in Brooklyn, but for the first time, at the age of 25, he was officially registered in physics. Although it wasn't apparent from his first semester at Columbia, he had finally found his niche. He registered for four courses that fall, and he received a "P" for pass in two of them, he withdrew from the third, and he was given an I for "incomplete inthe fourth.[83] He probably had too many irons in the fire. On top of his academic load, he and Helen Newmark's brother started a newspaper that fall called *The Brownsville Bulletin*. The paper folded after one year.

The following spring, however, Rabi reached a turning point when he met a professor from the College of the City of New York who encouraged him to apply for a teaching assistantship at the school. He did so and was hired as a part-time tutor in physics at CCNY at an annual salary of $800. Although the tutoring job was time intensive, requiring him to teach 16 hours a week during the day and later 25 hours a week, both day and night, it didn't seem to Rabi that he was working hard. He even found time to attend the opera. With his financial concerns lessened, he could also focus more energy on his studies at Columbia. "That changed everything," said Rabi. "I didn't have to worry and I dropped the other stuff, moved into a dormitory; I was on the road and had full time, so to speak, to devote to [physics] without the other necessary distractions."[84]

Rabi found the atmosphere at Columbia much more to his liking than what he had experienced at Cornell. It wasn't that Columbia's faculty was better than Cornell's, he said, but Cornell had encouraged a laxness in its students by not requiring course examinations and by not requiring them to take advanced courses. As a result, the advanced courses were not given and the students regarded the ones that were given as "just mathematics."

"The faculty at Columbia at that time was not overpowering," said Rabi, "but they kept a pretty high standard in the courses which were taught, so that one got the tools of a subject very well."[85] There was one faculty member at Columbia in particular, Professor A.P. Wills, who was a firm believer in solid training and who insisted that everybody had to take a course in the partial differential equations of physics, "basic stuff," said Rabi, "that one should have but which one really didn't get at Cornell."[86]

Rabi pointed to this time, when he was studying physics at Columbia and tutoring at City College, as the real starting point of his life as a scientist. In a sense, he had floundered, not just during the three years between 1919 and 1922 when he had been out of school and unemployed, but ever since his days as a boy in Brooklyn. He had been disappointed with his choice of a high school, but made the best of it. He had been disappointed with his choice of undergraduate school, but had completed it anyway, in spite of being socially disconnected and stuck in the isolation, as he saw it, of Ithaca. Now finally, he had become connected, challenged and inspired. "I was self-supporting, I saw where I was going," he said. He felt like he was in charge of his own destiny and it reminded him of his childhood back in Brooklyn.

Now again I was getting around to doing things I had done as a little boy, when I organized a group. Here I organized a group to study modern physics that the faculty didn't teach. We would have seminars just amongst our students, which would be attended by professors from other institutions. It was an enormously wonderful time. On Sunday, seminar started at 11 o'clock here [at Columbia and would continue] until 11 o'clock at night. We'd adjourn to a Chinese restaurant. I met four or five people this way, all of whom became men of considerable distinction.[87]

The students in the seminar group included: Ralph de Laer Kronig, who would later make significant contributions to theoretical physics in Holland including, independently of Samuel Goudsmit and George Uhlenbeck, the discovery of spin in electrons; Mark Zemansky, who became a well-known professor at City College and physics textbook author; Francis Bitter, who became a professor of physics at MIT and a highly-regarded authority on magnetism; and S.C. Wang, whose contributions to applied quantum mechanics would have significance in spectroscopy. There were also about four full professors from New York University who attended the Rabi-organized seminars, including Wheeler Loomis who would later chair the physics department at the University of Illinois and serve as recruitment director for MITs Radiation Laboratory during World War II.

Nearly 40 years later, as Rabi looked back to this period, the excitement and energy he felt were still fresh in his mind.

I was enormously full of ideas about certain things. Just speculations and ideas. My mind kept churning . . . all the time . . . all sorts of problems, all sorts of tricks, all sorts of inventions, all sorts of questions.

We were all at about the same stage. Nobody knew more than anybody else. . . . Since then, I'm a believer in students learning from one another, even though they may not know very much, because that's where they develop their own bents. I found the whole thing . . . very interesting—the library, the reading, the thinking, the talking. I found it, in that sense, a very stimulating place.[88]

Less stimulating was the prospect looming before Rabi that it would soon be time to get on with the research for his PhD dissertation. It wasn't that he didn't enjoy research. Research was what had attracted him first to chemistry and then to physics. Often, however, a dissertation seems to be more of a hurdle placed in one's path just to meet an academic requirement than it is an opportunity for personal development, and so it was for Rabi. Just then, as far as Rabi was concerned, what was really interesting was what was happening in physics in Europe.

Eight years had passed since Rabi's freshman year at Cornell when Philip Subkow first introduced him to the quantum and Planck's constant. It had been old news even then—nearly 16 years old, in fact—when Rabi first heard about it, but old news is new news to one who hasn't heard it before. In 1919, Benedict Cassen at Lederle Laboratories had filled him in further on quantum theory, whetting his appetite to keep abreast of current developments in science.

Unfortunately for American science, there was a lot of physics that had developed during the first two decades of the century in Europe which was not yet known in the United States. For example, it wasn't until Rabi's graduate year at Cornell that he first "really" heard, he said, about the quantum theory more definitely, and even then he picked up that information from a book he read on the side. It was not part of any formal course offering.

> In lectures that I gave a little later [said Rabi], I would often say that I came, essentially, from an underdeveloped country as far as science was concerned. Just as in most underdeveloped countries, there were a few great men, but an undergraduate in America would never see them and could not be influenced by them.[89]

With America lagging behind in physics and Rabi just becoming aware of developments in Europe's new physics, there was a great deal of "old" news in 1925 for him to assimilate. More than a dozen years after Max Planck introduced his constant h, Niels Bohr of Denmark, intrigued by the fact that hydrogen emitted spectral light only at certain frequencies, theorized an atomic structure in 1913 that looked like a classically-determined solar system, but with an important difference. Although Bohr's model had electrons revolving around the nucleus like a miniature Copernican system, they were restricted in total energy to only certain discrete, quantized values. The total value of the atom, in turn, Bohr postulated, dictated that an atom's electrons could move only in certain discrete, quantized orbits. Thus an electron could emit or absorb spectral light only at certain frequencies, dependent on whether it was going from a higher-energy level to a lower-energy one, or vice versa.

In the decade that followed Bohr's atomic model, other European physicists such as Arnold Sommerfeld, Peter Debye and Max Born had posited additional theories, creating a somewhat leaky but better-than-nothing umbrella which is now referred to as the old quantum theory. In the early 1920s, although he was intrigued by the questions that were being discussed, Rabi wasn't willing to take Bohr's theory on atomic structure as the final word on the matter. "I was very far from convinced about quantum theory,"[90] he said. "I thought the old quantum theory was stupid."[91]

Whereas Bohr talked in terms of quantum transitions between energy levels, Arnold Sommerfeld of Munich, Germany began speaking, in 1916, of space quantization or spatial orientations of electrons to explain what was called the Zeeman effect. In 1896, two years before Rabi was born, a Dutchman by the name of Pieter Zeeman had performed a spectroscopic experiment that had earned him the Nobel Prize in 1902, the same year young Rabi emigrated to the United States. Although visible-light spectroscopy had been around for quite a while at that point and scientists were aware that each element had its own spectroscopic signature, somewhat analogous to today's bar codes with their unique patterns of bars and spaces, Zeeman wondered what would happen to the spectroscopic light pattern of a material placed in a magnetic field. To find out, he placed a Bunsen burner in a strong magnetic field and observed the spectral band of yellow light emitted by sodium. He found that the usual single band had split into multiple bands, making the total yellow portion of the spectrum broader than normal.

What caused the splitting? Arnold Sommerfeld theorized that the dual, quantized energy states of Bohr's model were, in the presence of a strong magnetic field, being split into additional energy states. Since there were two original energy states—a higher one and a lower one—in the original mode, the subdivided energy states would also have dual energy levels, thus explaining the additional spectral lines created.

But why? Sommerfeld further theorized that, although the electrons in the relatively weak magnetic field of the earth were randomly oriented, when placed in a strong magnetic field they were suddenly given a powerful incentive to orient themselves to the magnetic field—and only certain, quantized orientations were allowed. Space quantization, it was called.

If space quantization reflected physical reality, that would explain the Zeeman effect. But did it reflect reality? In 1921 and 1922, Otto Stern in Frankfurt, Germany came up with a way to test Sommerfeld's theory, using molecular beams, about the same time Rabi entered graduate school at Cornell University. The basic idea of a molecular beam—first demonstrated by L. Dunoyer in 1911—was to vaporize an element by heating it in a furnace and then allowing atoms or molecules to escape through a narrow slit located at one end of the furnace adjacent to a vacuum chamber. As the atoms or molecules entered the chamber, they were collimated into a narrow beam of isolated, non-colliding particles via a series of apertures and directed toward the opposite end of the vacuum chamber where they could be detected by a flat piece of cold glass that caused the heated molecules or atoms to condense and be deposited for post-flight analysis.

As mentioned previously, Pieter Zeeman had found, 25 years earlier, that sodium's single band of yellow spectral light split into multiple, narrow bands when placed in a strong magnetic field. Now, Otto Stern and his collaborator, Walther Gerlach, added a strong magnetic field to a molecular beam—actually, in this case, a beam of silver atoms—and found that they were deposited on the beam detector in two distinct and separate bands. The pattern was not what they had expected.

Midway through the normal flight path of the beam, Stern had placed a C-shaped electromagnet, positioned in such a way that a beam of silver atoms traveling along and between its north and south poles would encounter, perpendicular to the beam's direction of motion, a strong, non-uniform magnetic field acting upon the magnetic moments of the atoms in the beam. How would the external field affect the individual magnetic moments? The answer they expected, based on classical physics, was that their degree of reorientation would be determined by their initial orientation. In other words, they expected that as the randomly oriented atoms encountered the magnetic field, those atoms whose moments tended toward parallel orientation with the external field would be attracted toward the south pole of the external magnet, those that tended toward anti-parallel orientation with the external field would be repelled or pushed toward the north pole of the external field, and those that were basically at right angles to the field would proceed to the destination unaffected. Under that scenario, the magnetic field would tend to widen the narrow beam, because of the reorientations, resulting in a fairly solid smear of silver being deposited in the center of the detector and decreasing in density toward the edge of the beam.

That's not what happened. The silver atoms did initially enter the chamber randomly oriented, as expected, but when they encountered the magnetic field, they were apparently given only two choices, either parallel or antiparallel, either Beamlet 1 or Beamlet 2. No other options were allowed. And apparently all the moments complied, as two distinct arc-ing bands of silver were deposited on the detector glass with nothing in between. Where the heaviest deposit should have accumulated, according to conventional understanding, there was nothing!

It's noteworthy, incidentally, that these two ways of looking at quantum effects—Bohr's quantum transitions between energy levels and Sommerfeld's space quantization—would foreshadow the two approaches to magnetic resonance taken by Rabi and his associates at Columbia University nearly two decades later as well as the nearly-simultaneous, but independent discoveries of NMR in condensed matter in late 1945 and early 1946. Rabi and his collaborators would use both approaches. Edward Purcell would focus on quantum transitions between energy levels and Felix Bloch on physical reorienting of magnetic moments.

What it all meant in 1922 wasn't yet clear, but one thing was as clear to Rabi as the two distinct smears—there was definitely something to this quantum stuff, after all. Bohr didn't have all the answers, nor did Sommerfeld, nor did Born. But they were on to something, and Rabi knew he needed to give the new physics more attention.

> What finished me really was when I read the Stern-Gerlach experiment; that was it, because I thought, "Well, I'm a pretty smart guy; I can make models and so on, imagine things, but this is something quite different. This comes out of space and it's quantized—nothing interior." So I began to take it very seriously and to study books like Sommerfeld['s *Atombau und Spektrallinien*[92] and] Born's [*Vorlesungen Über*] *Atommechanik*.[93-94]

The old quantum theory, said Rabi, was largely a collection of ad hoc special rules that could not be applied across the board. There were exceptions to these rules and whenever new, previously-unnavigated waters were entered, the physicist had to continually refer back to classical physics for guidance and permission to proceed.

> It was a theory [said Rabi] with which one could have great success if one had sensitive insight, so to speak, into the nature of things, intuitive insight, because the correspondence principle which was devised [to correlate classical theory with quantum theory] was merely a general guide. Any number of assumptions had to be made to get from one place to another. . . . On the other hand, it was a tremendous challenge, most fascinating, and tantalizing. It was such a break with the past, and yet it was not frozen. Obviously, the theo-

ry was awaiting other ideas and, as such, was just the sort of thing that a young fellow would get interested in. . . . It was always strange and wonderful when it was put down in the textbooks, because it was quite non-understandable, if I wanted to understand it logically, although it had been written as if one should understand it logically. . . . [There was] this feeling of possibility, this feeling of puzzlement, in a certain sense, of frustration—but possibility—in these wonderful revolutionary thoughts which cropped up all the time, and which had to be used to explain different properties of atomic structure and the nature of light, and the nature of matter.[95]

It was no wonder that it was difficult for Rabi to get down to the nitty-gritty details of researching and writing his doctoral thesis. From elementary school all the way through graduate school, he had done what was needed to meet academic requirements, but had been most inspired by the things he read and discovered on his own. It wasn't any different now. And then, just as Rabi was about to get into his thesis, there came the second wave of quantum theory—the new quantum theory—with papers by de Broglie, Debye, Heisenberg and Schrödinger.

Here, all at once, there seemed to be the possibility of a really consistent, logical, although very strange neo-physics. A whole new set of laws. There were very definite ways of doing things. There didn't seem to be any ad hoc explanations. One after another, things which had defied reasonable explanation before just fell into place.[96]

As with the first wave of quantum theory, the second wave also came largely from Europe and you learned about it by reading the European scientific journals, not the American ones. Rabi would later tell of arriving in 1927 at the University of Göttingen, of looking around in the library and finding no current issues of *Physical Review* on the shelf. It seems they valued the leading American physics journal so little that, to save postage, they would wait until the end of the year and order the previous 12 issues all at once. "We were not highly regarded," said Rabi, "nor was there any thought that America would amount to anything as far as physics was concerned."[97] Ten years later, *Physical Review* would be the leading physics journal in the world, a reflection of the dramatic rise of American physics during that period.[98]

In 1924, no professor at Columbia was able to adequately direct a student in the writing of a thesis on the new physics, so Rabi chose what he thought was the next best option. Since Professor Bergen Davis was doing work with X-rays, which had been discovered in 1895 and which had helped usher in the new physics, Rabi tried to enlist him as his mentor. Davis refused, "very fortunately," said Rabi, "and I went with Professor Wills, who took me on."[99]

Wills suggested that Rabi measure the magnetic susceptibility of alkali gases. Magnetic susceptibility is the degree to which a material takes on magnetic properties when placed in a magnetic field. The more Rabi considered the suggestion, the less he wanted to take on the project.

> These alkalis in gaseous, vapor form are very corrosive, and measuring the susceptibility of the gas in itself is a very difficult proposition. The more I thought about it, the less I liked it. Finally, I came to Professor Wills, after thinking about it for a month or so, and said I didn't want to do it. I didn't think I was good enough to do it. That's the only way I knew how to say it. But privately, I felt it was a very bad thing to try to do for a dissertation.
>
> He said he was disappointed and would give the problem to somebody else, but he had no other problem for me. Fortunately, this left me on my own.[100]

To himself, Rabi said, "*Moichel!*" [Good riddance.] The sentiment applied to the preparation of his dissertation as well as its selection. "I didn't get any help from [Wills]," he said. "Nor did I want any. The last thing in the world I wanted when I was doing my dissertation was for somebody to help me."[101]

Although selecting and doing his own research was a personal preference of Rabi's, a few years later he would apply the same standard to doctoral candidates under his tutelage who called themselves theoretical physicists. Those who chose theory over experiment also had to prove the merit of their claim by choosing their own dissertation topic. As Norman Ramsey, a physicist who has excelled in both categories, expressed it:

> Rabi's theory on training theoretical physicists was to tell a young man when he arrived that if he was brilliant enough to be a theoretical physicist that he was bright enough to find his own problem. He told him to go ahead and find his own problem and solve it and when he got finished to come back and tell Rabi. This was a technique in training theoretical physicists that eliminated most of them.

Most of the potential theorists who arrived left Columbia, but the ones that survived turned out to be extremely good. [Julian] Schwinger is the best example.[102]

As it was, Rabi saw the dichotomy between theoretical physics and experimental physics as somewhat arbitrary, and would respond when pressed to say whether he was a theoretical physicist or an experimental physicist that he was neither, "just a physicist," he would reply.

> I just don't believe in the bifurcation [between theorist and experi-menter, he said]. During the '30s, [Leo] Szilard used to come to my office almost every other day with an idea for an experiment for me to do, and I determined that I would never do an experiment that Szilard suggested. Why shouldn't I have my own fun? I said, "Now look here, Leo; I will get you all the apparatus you need; I will get you an assistant, space and everything you want. Do this experiment. It's a beautiful thought." But of course he wouldn't, and a lot of things he suggested were later done by others.
>
> It's a special Columbia knack. Our experimental people didn't need any theorists to help them and I always stood strongly against employ-ing a theorist just because he might be useful to experimenters. . . . I brought Willis Lamb, a pure theorist, an Oppenheimer student, and he got the Nobel Prize for experiments. . . . Ever since then, I've said, "What sort of physicists are you anyway, if you have to go to a theo-rist to tell you what to do in some places and after you've done it, to have to go to the theorist to tell you what you've done?"[103]

Rabi has also said, however, that he was "absolutely fascinated" by theoretical physics and that he might not have done an experimental dis-sertation had there been any theoretical physicists at Columbia.[104]

His selection of a dissertation came in the fall of 1924 after he attended a seminar by Nobel laureate William Lawrence Bragg of England who had just completed measuring the electric susceptibility of a group of crystals called the Tutton salts. Although they were very similar in crys-talline structure, these salts, which include nickel-ammonium, sulphate-hydrate and potassium-sulphate hexahydrate, had surprisingly different electrical properties. So it occurred to Rabi that he should investigate their magnetic susceptibility.

This was similar to Wills' thesis suggestion from the standpoint that both experiments were measuring magnetic susceptibility, but quite different as far as experimental procedures were concerned since the first was a gas and the second was a crystal. But that didn't mean Rabi had chosen an easy experiment. It was a "very, very difficult experiment," he said, requiring all the skill of "a good watchmaker."[105] It also required the patience of a saint.

The method Rabi planned to use had been invented by a German, Woldemar Voigt, in the late 19th century. First, because the crystal had to be in pure form, it had to be grown from a seed crystal. Second, after a crystal of sufficient size was obtained, it had to be cleaved into three sections, each section displaying a facet that was oriented differently than the other two in relation to the crystal's internal structure. This part of the experiment required painstaking care, not only the skill of a good watchmaker but the technique of a diamond cutter. Finally, each section, suspended from a torsion balance, was lowered into the gap between the poles of an electromagnet. The magnetic susceptibility was determined by calculating the difference in balance readings when the magnet was turned off and when it was turned on.[106]

If Rabi had the required watchmaking and diamond-cutting skills, he didn't have the patience, but he would face that later. The first part of the experiment—growing the crystals—was easy. Make a solution of the material you want to crystallize, suspend a small seed of that crystal in the solution, and leave the laboratory. That's it. With time, and no further attention, the crystal seed grows by accretion into a large crystal, identical in structure and cleavage patterns to the seed.

That part was no problem; for that Rabi had patience. He was still teaching at City College of New York, he was doing a lot of reading on the latest physics developments in Europe, and besides, he could use the time to attend the Broadway plays and the Metropolitan operas he enjoyed so much. Periodically, he would check his crystals, see that they were doing OK, and get back to his other priorities.

Eventually, of course, the crystals were large enough, the time he had allotted for this part of the research was almost gone, and he had to get on with the real work of the experiment. That meant he would soon have to get down to the difficult task of cutting and grinding the crystals, a task for which he had no equipment, a task which, as he recalled, looked "pretty tedious."[107]

That's when he fortuitously came upon James Clerk Maxwell's *Treatise on Electricity and Magnetism,* published in 1873. Suddenly, because of what he read, Rabi found the motivation to get on with his research. Physicist Jeremy Bernstein describes the event as follows:

Rabi's eye was caught by a passage that discussed the force of a non-uniform magnetic field on a body immersed in a medium—a fluid with a magnetic salt dissolved in it. . . . If a medium has a certain magnetic susceptibility, he read, and if one immerses in the medium an object that itself has a magnetic susceptibility, then the object's effective magnetic susceptibility is altered by its being in the medium. If the medium has a greater susceptibility, then the immersed object will move in a certain direction in a non-uniform magnetic field; if the medium has a smaller susceptibility, the object will move in the opposite direction; and if the susceptibilities are the same, there will be no motion. This was all Rabi needed to know.[108]

In addition to requiring less equipment than the former method, equipment he didn't have, the method Rabi invented had two major advantages over the older Voigt method: a savings in labor and a significant increase in accuracy. As for the difference in labor, the Voigt method required cleaving a particular crystal along each of its three axes; the Rabi method required no cutting of the crystal. And although the Rabi method required two comparison steps to arrive at the magnetic susceptibility for a particular crystalline axis instead of the one direct measurement used by Voigt, the new method had a certain finesse that the older one lacked. Rabi described it as "just sheer magic!"[109]

Here's how it worked: A crystal, attached with shellac to a glass fiber (to avoid the useless, non-measurable twisting you would get from a string) and suspended from a torsion balance, was lowered into a glass tube containing a saturated solution which Rabi knew would not dissolve the crystal and positioned in place between the two poles of an electromagnet.

Rabi knew from Maxwell that if he increased or decreased the magnetic susceptibility of the solution until it matched that of the crystal, the effect of the magnet upon the crystal would be nullified and that no movement of the crystal would occur when the magnet was turned on or off. So if the crystal moved one direction when the power was turned on, he knew the solution had a lower magnetic susceptibility than the crystal and he would add magnetic salt to the solution. If, on the other hand, the crystal moved in the other direction when power was applied, he knew the solution had a higher magnetic susceptibility than the crystal and he would decrease the concentration of salt. When no movement occurred, he knew he had achieved near-perfect magnetic equilibrium between the solution and the crystal and he could proceed to the final step in the experiment, which was to compare the magnetic susceptibility of the solution with the magnetic susceptibility of water, which was already known.

Because Rabi knew there was a direct relationship between a liquid's weight in a magnetic field and its magnetic susceptibility, all he needed to do was extract some of the solution from the tube with a pipette, individually weigh it and an equal amount of water in a magnetic field, determine the weight ratio between them, and calculate accordingly the solution's magnetic susceptibility. Whatever it was, so it was for the crystal!

The method was so simple, elegant and precise that six weeks after he began the project, Rabi had his dissertation completed. Entitled "On the Principal Magnetic Susceptibilities of Crystals,"[110] he sent it to *Physical Review* for publication on July 16, 1926, just 13 days short of his 28th birthday. On July 17, 1926, he married Helen Newmark.

Europe

Those who follow the history of physics, particularly in this century, will recognize the period from 1925 to 1927 as key years in the development of the new quantum theory, or quantum mechanics, as it is also called. About a year after Prince Louis de Broglie of France introduced his stunning concept that material particles, like radiation, have dual personalities—both wave and particle—Werner Heisenberg, then of Göttingen University in Germany, ushered in a new generation of quantum theory with his matrix mechanics in 1925. Less than a year later, in 1926, an Austrian physicist, Erwin Schrödinger, then teaching at the University of Zürich in Switzerland introduced a wave equation and theory called wave mechanics that gave substance to de Broglie's theory. Though Heisenberg's and Schrödinger's papers were not immediately recognized as equivalent—Schrödinger's mathematical approach was much more user-friendly—Schrödinger published a paper a short time later that revealed their essential equivalency.

Also in 1926, Paul A.M. Dirac, a physicist from England, introduced his own general version of quantum mechanics and, a short time later, was able to tie all three approaches into one integrated theory. Heisenberg was awarded the 1932 Nobel Prize in physics (received in 1933); Schrödinger and Dirac shared the 1933 Nobel Prize.

In 1927, Heisenberg once again shook the physics world when he put forth his Uncertainty Principle in which he stated that "we cannot know, as a matter of principle, the present in all its details." Slightly analogous to the charge that television coverage of news events affects the events themselves, the Uncertainty Principle said that any attempt to measure reality at the quantum level of physics will affect the reality itself.

With all these new developments in quantum theory taking place on the Continent, it's no wonder that Rabi had a difficult time keeping his mind on his dissertation in the early part of 1926. "One just couldn't wait for the magazines [from Europe]," he said. "Each issue brought very new and exciting things. So I was just dying to get over to Europe and see these people and be where these things were happening."[111]

He would have to wait nearly one year. That fall he and postdoctoral fellow Ralph de L. Kronig sent off a paper in which they had applied the Schrödinger equation (purely for the joy of understanding and using the method) to the physics of a symmetrical spinning top,[112] a paper which would have long-term usefulness in textbooks for correlating classical physics to quantum physics. In developing the theory for it, Rabi and Kronig ran into an impasse in the form of a differential equation that they could not solve, nor could they find anyone else that could help them solve it. Rabi, however, "just happened" to come across the same equation while leafing through the works, purely for his own pleasure, of Karl Gustav Jakob Jacobi, the eminent 19th-century German mathematician. Jacobi had solved the same equation a century earlier in a different context. With Jacobi's help, the paper was published in the February 1927 issue of *Physical Review*.

In 1926, Rabi and Helen moved in with Helen's parents in the Washington Heights area of New York. Also that year, the physics department at Columbia moved from Fayerweather Hall to Pupin Hall, the building that would be Rabi's academic home for most of the remainder of his life.

Early in 1927, Rabi took the formal oral examination for his doctoral degree. Although all the other requirements for the degree had been completed earlier, he waited to take his oral exam until reprints of his dissertation, published in the January 1927 issue of *Physical Review,* were available to submit to the department.

Rabi's European opportunity came soon afterward. A month after sending off his dissertation, Rabi applied for one of the two Cutting Fellowships that were awarded annually and a Barnard Fellowship. The Cutting Fellowship was the most lucrative, but he didn't get it. He was, however, offered a nine-month Barnard Fellowship worth $1500, but he would have to pay his own travel expenses. Rabi took it and asked for a leave of absence from his teaching position at CCNY. When it was denied, he resigned. "I don't think I was very popular over there," he said, "so I had to resign, which was a very serious step, for jobs were very, very hard to find."[113] For Rabi, turning down the Barnard Fellowship just to keep his job at CCNY wasn't an option.

> It was the kind of thing where I'd made up my mind that I lived only once, and I was not going to do anything I didn't want to do. I was not going to lead a humdrum existence, which I would have done if I'd stayed on at City College. I made up my mind to go to Europe and study with the great masters, because before that I'd never run into a first-class mind anywhere.[114]

As soon as the academic term ended, Dr. I.I. Rabi sailed for Europe from New York in July of 1927 on "the old Majestic"[115] with a good friend of his, Rene Carrier. Then a student of mathematics and physics, Carrier would later became a professor of history at Barnard College. Helen Rabi would come later and meet Rabi in London. Traveling in tourist class to save money—it was really steerage, said Rabi—they landed in Cherbourg, France, took a train first to Paris and, from there, Rabi took a train directly to Zürich where he planned to study with Erwin Schrödinger.

Schrödinger didn't know Rabi was planning to study with him, however, and he had resigned his position as professor at the University of Zürich and was about to leave for Germany to succeed Max Planck as director of the Theoretical Institute of Berlin. Rabi only stayed in Zürich for two weeks, but in those two weeks he began lifelong friendships with J.A. Stratton, who later became president of Massachusetts Institute of Technology, and Linus Pauling, who would someday be a famous chemist and Nobel laureate.

Rabi went to Germany next to work with Arnold Sommerfeld at the University of Munich. Sommerfeld didn't know Rabi was coming, either. Rabi used what would become his *modus operandi* during his sojourn in Europe. Soon after arriving in a city, he would proceed as soon as possible to the university or institution at which he planned to work, and introduce himself by saying, "I'm Rabi. I've come to work here."

"I didn't plan these things," said Rabi, "and I never wrote beforehand that I was coming to any of these places. In each case, I was simply beautifully received. I'd get a key to the place. That's all there was to it."[116]

"I was very well received by Professor Sommerfeld,"[117] said Rabi. After accepting Rabi's request to work at the University, Sommerfeld showed him around, and introduced him to other visitors and students, including graduate students Rudolf Peierls and Hans Bethe. At Munich, Rabi met two more Americans who would become long-time friends: Edward Condon of the University of California, Berkeley and H.P. Robertson of the California Institute of Technology.

"I worked on some problem or other," said Rabi. "I think I was chiefly interested then in trying to calculate the magnetic susceptibility of the hydrogen molecule. But we bummed around, Ed Condon, Bob Robertson, and I. We had a really nice time that summer."[118]

Rabi stayed in Munich only about two months, until the term was completed. He was still looking for his niche, and Munich hadn't provided it. Although he had great respect for Sommerfeld as an effective communicator of physics, he didn't provide the stimulus Rabi felt he needed. "Sommerfeld was a wonderful man," Rabi once said, "very slow witted, beautiful lectures, grand lectures—slow witted so that by the time he understood it, everybody else did."[119]

From Munich, Rabi went to London, both to meet his wife and to attend the annual meeting of the British Association for the Advancement of Science, held in Leeds, England from August 31 to September 27. Rabi's mentor at Columbia, Professor Wills, had written him, encouraging him to attend the conference if at all possible because of the quality of the papers that would be presented and the scientific eminence of the presenters—in particular, Peter Debye and Werner Heisenberg.[120]

From England, the Rabis went to what was considered at the time the Mecca of physics, Copenhagen and Niels Bohr's Institute for Theoretical Physics. Rabi presented his usual credentials—"I'm Rabi. I've come to work here"—and was received kindly by Bohr who, very graciously, Rabi said, told him what he was working on rather than asking what Rabi was working on. Unfortunately—at least that's what Rabi thought at the time—Bohr was tired and unwilling to take on any additional load, so he arranged for Rabi and Yoshio Nishina, a Japanese physicist who had been at Copenhagen for a number of years and who would later bring modern physics to Japan, to go to Hamburg, Germany and work with Wolfgang Pauli.

"I very much regretted leaving Copenhagen," said Rabi, "because there's no question it has been the inspiration for many, many scientists."[121] Working with Pauli in Hamburg was certainly an honor, albeit a frightening one—Felix Bloch, who would later share that honor, admitted being afraid of Pauli[122]—but Copenhagen was considered the place to be. Although Rabi wasn't able to accomplish as much as he wanted in the brief time he was in Denmark—he was still trying to compute the magnetic susceptibility of a hydrogen molecule—he had enjoyed the food, the scenery, and the Institute. It had provided a stimulating atmosphere in which, said Rabi, you "wouldn't dare to be trivial. Somehow or other . . . you had the feeling if you stayed there you had to think of really significant things."[123] Later, however, Rabi would decide that getting "kicked out"[124] of Copenhagen was one of the best things that ever happened to him.

For one thing, he was able to escape the *Kopenhagener Geist*, the Spirit of Copenhagen, an approach to physics that Rabi saw as constrictive. Supported by Heisenberg's Uncertainty Principle, the idea that at the atomic level attempted measurements of reality change reality, and Bohr's Principle of Complementarity, the concept that there were always two complementary and mutually exclusive ways of looking at a physical phenomenon, Rabi felt that the Spirit of Copenhagen's tendency to impose limitations on the kinds of questions one should ask also tended to stop discussion. "In that sense," he said, "I'm glad that I was not permitted to stay, because I might have been charmed into it and have forgone my natural rhythm."[125]

Another reason Rabi was glad he left Copenhagen was that Hamburg, he discovered later, would prove to be a rendezvous with destiny. Five years earlier, in 1922, it had been a molecular beam experiment by Otto Stern and Walther Gerlach in Frankfurt, Germany that had convinced Rabi that quantum theory was, in fact, connected to physical reality. And now, as Rabi and his wife, Helen, were enroute to Hamburg, he had no idea that he would soon be working with Otto Stern—a fellow Galician—and molecular beams. "It's fantastic how a man's fate is determined in this way," Rabi said. "I went to Pauli and I didn't know that Stern was there."[126]

Hamburg

On July 21, 1899, 28 years before Dr. and Mrs. I.I. Rabi arrived in Hamburg, David Rabi boarded a ship called the *Pennsylvania** moored at the same German port, watched as families of other emigrants embraced and said tearful goodbyes, and then saw the banks of the Elbe River grow further apart as the vessel headed toward the North Sea and America. Behind him, back in Rymanow, already more than 250 miles distant, were his young wife and his infant son, Israel, soon to have his first birthday. Ahead were a host of unknowns. What would America be

---

* Based on information contained in David Rabi's Original Declaration of Intention to become a U.S. citizen, filed December 12, 1905.

like? Where would he work? Where would he live? How soon could he bring his wife and child?

Eventually, those and many more questions were answered, the family was reunited, and they had survived, even thrived, in their adopted country. They had escaped the tenements of the Lower East Side, had become American citizens in 1914, had purchased their own store building in Brooklyn, had begun making money in real estate, and, very important to them, had been able to provide their children with good educations.

As a result, when David Rabi's son Isidor came to Hamburg in 1927, he was asking different questions than his father would have asked 28 years earlier. Although he was not rich, he was well educated, he was there on a fellowship, and he had been sent to work with one of the world's greatest physicists, Wolfgang Pauli, on the recommendation of another legendary physicist, Niels Bohr.

David Rabi had gone through Hamburg on his way to America where he hoped "to make a living" and was filled with questions about survival. His son, Isidor, was in Hamburg on a different quest. He was filled with 'otherworldly' questions about the basic structure of matter. For him, making a living was necessary, but secondary.

> I have never thought of physics as a profession, and in that sense I think I'm a gentleman as far as science is concerned. I never thought of doing it for a living. I didn't care what I did for a living. Science was something I would follow and admire. And enjoy.... Some said, "It's fun." I always hated the idea that it was "fun." I know other ways to have fun. Physics has a much deeper emotional quality for me than that.... Physics is an otherworldly thing. It requires a taste for things unseen, even unheard of—a high degree of abstraction and a sort of profound innate philosophy. These faculties die off somehow when you grow up.... At a certain age, the children just become adults and are no longer very deeply interested in anything, except in the process of making a living and in sex and power. Money. Otherwise, they're not terribly interested. Profound curiosity happens when they are young. I think physicists are the Peter Pans of the human race.[127]

Economically, America had been good to the Rabis, but there was still one hurdle over which they had little control, anti-Semitism. Rabi had encountered it when he graduated from Cornell; the non-Jewish students who excelled in their studies were hired quickly by the chemical companies and Jewish students were not. Even in 1927, although he had his doctorate and a post-doctoral fellowship that was bringing him in contact with the top physicists in the world, Rabi had little hope that he'd be able to find a job in physics after his Barnard Fellowship expired in June 1928. As far as Rabi's expectations were concerned, when his fellowship money ran out, his short-lived career in physics would also end.

> I had no hope of getting a job. It seemed to me that it would be very difficult to get one. Anti-Semitism was unbelievably rife in the universities and elsewhere. I thought I would go back to New York and see what would happen and maybe, if worst came to worst, join my father in real estate. I didn't feel terrible about it; I had wanted to know physics, and I had had a tremendous experience.[128]

In Hamburg, because everything had been pre-arranged by Niels Bohr, Rabi was able to dispense with his usual method of showing up unannounced and Wolfgang Pauli, seen by many as arrogant and rude, was actually civil and friendly. In fact, Rabi felt Pauli had a very kind nature, although he recognized that Pauli probably responded to him the way he did because Rabi had unwittingly got in the first blow.

> We were talking about something, and I wanted to disagree, but my German wasn't very good, so I said, *"Das ist Unsinn"*—"That is nonsense." One didn't say that to Pauli—he kept walking around afterward saying, *"Unsinn? Unsinn?"* Later, it turned out that the disagreement was purely linguistic— the similarity of "p" and "pi." In German, "pi" is pronounced like "p." It was a misunderstanding. But he never attacked me the way he did some of the others. We got along very well.[129]

In 1927, Pauli was "at the height of his powers," said Rabi, "a very young man, younger than I am by two years, but of tremendous international reputation. He was one of these prodigies; at the age of 19, as a student, he had written the definitive work on relativity."[130] (It is said that when Einstein read the article, which was published in *Encyclopadie der Mathematischen Wissenschaft*, he felt that perhaps Pauli knew more about relativity than he himself did.)[131]

Rabi felt that, in Hamburg, he really had, for the first time in his life, "very intimate contact with very superior minds." Besides Pauli, there

was Otto Stern, who Rabi rated as "one of the great experimental physi-
cists of this century," as well as Professor Wilhelm Lenz, formulator of
Lenz' law, Walter Gordon, with whom Rabi struck up "a very great
friendship," Scottish physicist Ronald Frazer, and American physicist
John Taylor, a chemist from Urbana, Illinois who was working with Otto
Stern in molecular beams.[132]

In Hamburg, for the first time since coming to Europe, Rabi had found
his niche. Here was the concentration of fine minds he had been looking
for. Here was the stimulating give-and-take atmosphere that energized
him, free of the restrictive Spirit of Copenhagen. "Some environments are
inhibiting," said Rabi, "some environments are liberating. And for me the
environment there in Hamburg with those people was very liberating."[133]

Every day, the group of people mentioned above, joined frequently by
a steady stream of notables such as Bohr, Born, Dirac, Eddington,
Ehrenfest, Langmuir and others who came by to visit Pauli and Stern,
would eat lunch together and talk politics and physics, two topics that
were always of special interest to Rabi.

> Not only did I learn German, but I got a tremendous insight into
> German politics, academic politics, but above all, their discussions of
> physics were of a depth and range which I had not encountered
> before, and I considered that a great part of whatever education and
> taste I have in physics was formed around that period, with these
> very informal discussions at this luncheon table in Hamburg.[134]

Rabi also found that, except for Arnold Sommerfeld, Pauli was not a
respecter of persons. Rabi noted that Pauli always treated his mentor
Sommerfeld with respect, but would display his "extraordinary arro-
gance" to anyone, including Niels Bohr. No one was immune.

> I could have killed [Pauli]. I invited [R.D. Richtmyer, a former pro-
> fessor of Rabi's at Cornell] to join us at this luncheon table. Richtmyer
> at the time must have been, I suppose, about 50, maybe more, and
> Pauli was about 27, 28. Well, we arrived there, and Richtmyer want-
> ed to meet these great people, and I wanted them to meet him. He
> was a very important man in American physics, and indeed I was
> hoping he'd get me a job some time. Pauli arrived, and I started,
> "Pauli, *Ich möchte vorstal . . .*" (Mr. Pauli, I'd like to introduce . . .)
> He held up his hand and said, "First, I'll order." He took a long
> time in ordering his lunch. Then he put his hand down and said with

a smile, "So!" You can see how I felt. I'd brought this very important man, and to have him treated in this way by this youngster! But that's the way he was.[135]

Although Rabi was assigned to do theoretical work with Pauli,* he was keeping in touch with work done in Stern's molecular-beam laboratory through his English-speaking friends, Ronald Frazer and John Taylor. For the three of them, it was a nice break from talking German all day. Furthermore, because space quantization had made such an impression on Rabi and he had read the molecular-beam papers very carefully, he was able to help them with the theory.

It was from working with Frazer and Taylor that Rabi had an idea for overcoming the difficulty of measuring inhomogeneous fields which he suggested to Stern. It would be the first of many molecular-beam ideas Rabi would have in the next decade, culminating in the molecular-beam magnetic resonance method in 1937.

Although Stern had been the first to experimentally verify Sommerfeld's space quantization theory by intercepting an atomic beam with a magnetic field, the accuracy of his results had been limited. First, the deflections were small and their measurement therefore somewhat subjective. The splitting of the main beam into two beamlets was impressive but approximate. Although there was a definite separation of the beamlets, it was difficult to accurately determine the relative distributions of the atoms deposited on the beam detector. Second, since the magnetic field was non-uniform, you had to know the distribution of non-uniformity to measure its effect, and it was nearly impossible to calibrate the magnet accurately. It was the old GIGO principle at work: Garbage In, Garbage Out.

As Rabi considered in his mind's eye a beam traveling through the working chamber of the apparatus, he made a mental analogy between a molecular beam and a beam of light. More than 260 years earlier, Sir Isaac Newton had discovered that a narrow beam of visible light diffracted through a prism was not only separated into its component colors but was also spread out in an output spectrum that was much wider than the incoming beam. Perhaps the same idea could be applied to molecular beams. Would it be possible to achieve an effect with molecular beams similar to the one caused by a prism on light beams by positioning a *uni-*

---

* Rabi and Nishina were working on a paper on the scattering absorption of X-rays, which they published in the obscure *Deutsche Physikalische Gesellschaft.*

form magnetic field at an angle to the beam? A uniform magnetic field could be accurately calibrated, ensuring more accurate results, plus the beam would be collected over a wider area, improving one's ability to determine its distribution. "It was very much," said Rabi, "like the refraction of light."

> A molecular beam entering in this way will be diffracted in a number of branches; if the spin is a half it will be two branches, like double refraction. . . . This seemed to be a way of evaluating the magnetic moment of the atom, of the beam, without a difficult measurement of the gradients of the field. The beam itself would integrate. I made this suggestion to Otto Stern, who at first did not care for the idea but became enthusiastic and invited me to do the experiment.[136]

Here one sees why Rabi felt that the Spirit of Copenhagen, had he been exposed to it longer, could have affected his "natural rhythm." By not asking certain questions about atomic reality, one might overlook an experimental technique which would reveal that reality. Throughout his career, Rabi preferred visualizing effects. As one of his later collaborators, Polykarp Kusch, would say, "[Rabi] appears to ride around on the electrons within an atom or asks the question, 'If I were an electron, what would I do?' "[137]

Otto Stern told Rabi to give his idea a try and see if it came out the way he visualized it. First, of course, Rabi had to build the apparatus, a task for which he had no experience. Here John Taylor performed an invaluable service. "I learned my experimental technique really from him," said Rabi. He was "an extraordinarily gifted experimentalist" and "a wonderful person."[138]

Since Rabi had an obligation to Pauli and, at the same time, felt he couldn't afford to turn down an honor bestowed by Otto Stern, he chose to do both.

> I rode two horses, so to speak. I read and spent my time with the theoretical physicists. That's the way I expected my career to be. But I worked with this experiment. That's something I'd been doing previously at Columbia, too. I was doing an experimental dissertation, but reading theory and talking theory all the time, publishing these theoretical papers. So this was very much in line with my inclination, which has always been to be a physicist rather than a specialized particular kind, theoretical, nuclear, high energy, atomic or whatever.[139]

Within a year the molecular-beam apparatus was finished and it worked very well, said Rabi. The experiment was done with potassium atoms, and the separation of the beams, he said, was very good, "a fair step beyond the methods previously used." The rate at which the two Americans—Rabi and Taylor—completed their experiments made a "very great impression," said Rabi, on the Germans who worked in a more deliberate way.

The daily schedule of the Germans, he said, was very rigid; open at 7, close at 7. The Americans rebelled and instituted their own flexible scheduling. They might come in later, about 11 in the morning, for example, but then work until 2 or 3 o'clock the next morning. As a result, they wasted less time in daily adjustment of the apparatus and had more time available to collect their experimental data. "Research apparatus," Rabi pointed out, "is not like an engineered piece of equipment. It's put together for a specific purpose, and it's put together so that it just barely holds."[140]

Often, late in the evening, around 10 p.m., their wives would come to the laboratory and make toast, and they'd all sing. "It was a very, very happy time," said Rabi, "but we got things done at a rate which astonished the Germans."[141] In fact, he said, Stern was so impressed that he decided he would have to adopt this *Amerikanishe arbeiten methoden* (American work method).[142]

Because of Professor Stern's great reputation and the tendency to credit anything done in Hamburg to him, he very graciously suggested to Rabi that Rabi send a letter to the editor of *Nature*, an English-language publication, announcing his results, before sending his paper to the German publication *Zeitschrift für Physik,* so there would be no question that it was Rabi's experiment and not Stern's. The letter published in *Nature* was entitled "Refraction of Beams of Molecules," the article published in German was *"Zur Methode der Ablenkung von Molekularstrahlen"* (On a Method of Deflecting Molecular Beams). Both were published in early 1929.[143] Although Rabi's one-year Barnard Fellowship had expired in June of 1928, Stern had been able to arrange an International Education Board Fellowship, provided by the Rockefeller Foundation in Europe, to continue his work into 1929.

After completing his molecular-beam experiment with Stern, Rabi went to Leipzig during the first week of 1929 to work with Werner Heisenberg, which came as a surprise to Heisenberg. Once again, Rabi had employed his show-up-at-the-door-unannounced routine. Although Heisenberg welcomed him and Rabi enjoyed the camaraderie of Leipzig while it lasted—Robert Oppenheimer and Edward Teller were also there at the time—it didn't last very long, as Heisenberg was scheduled to begin a lecture tour in the United States beginning March 1.

Rabi's final months in Europe, from March through July, were spent in Zürich. After Rabi had left Hamburg, Pauli had been elevated from an assistant professor at the University of Hamburg to professor of physics at the Federal Institute of Technology, or ETH in Zürich (in the chair formerly held by Albert Einstein and Peter Debye). Once again, Rabi enjoyed the stimulating environment that accompanied Pauli wherever he went. In addition to Pauli, Rabi was able to spend time talking physics with Paul Dirac, Enrico Fermi, Walter Heitler, Fritz London, Wheeler Loomis, Robert Oppenheimer, Rudolf Peierls, John Slater, Leo Szilard, Eugene Wigner and John von Neumann.[144]

Felix Bloch was also at the ETH during part of the time Rabi spent at that institution. In the fall of 1928, shortly before Rabi arrived in Leipzig, Bloch had just finished his doctoral dissertation under Heisenberg and had left Leipzig to work with Pauli at the ETH. In March 1929, Rabi came to Zürich to work with Pauli and both Rabi and Bloch were there until Rabi's return to the United States in July of 1929. Bloch, another pioneer of NMR, would later have close association with Rabi in the United States.

Although Rabi had been unable to spend very much time with Heisenberg in Leipzig, it had been time well spent. Shortly after arriving in the United States, Heisenberg visited Columbia University and was told that they were looking for a theoretical physicist to teach quantum mechanics. Heisenberg recommended Rabi. So on March 26, 1929, about four months before leaving for the United States, Rabi received a cable from Columbia University offering him a lectureship at $3,000 a year, an amount that seemed to Rabi "large beyond dreams of avarice"[145] and an opportunity beyond anything he had even hoped.

Anti-Semitism, at its peak in the United States during the 1920s and '30s, had taught Rabi to limit his professional aspirations. A poll taken during that period found that 53 percent of Americans thought that Jews were "different," and their actions indicated that they thought the difference, whatever it was, was worthy of discrimination. Employment ads blatantly declared that Jews were unwanted as employees. Hotels and resorts declared that they accepted gentiles only. No wonder then that Columbia's offer came as such a surprise to Rabi. Not only did it mean he wouldn't have to go into the real estate business with his father, it also meant he would be paid for doing what he loved.

Helen Rabi left Europe for the United States in April 1929, more than three months earlier than Rabi, because she was pregnant and wanted to avoid traveling toward the end of her pregnancy. Rabi returned to the United States at the end of July. As it turned out, their first daughter, Nancy, was born just as Rabi assumed his new position at Columbia. "My daughter was born on September 24, 1929." said Rabi. "I combined my first lecture and my first daughter."[146] The stock market crashed October 29. Had Rabi returned from Europe a year later, he would have been caught by the Great Depression and would have been out of luck, he said, as there just weren't any jobs after that—"for rich, poor, Jew or gentile."[147] As far as Rabi knew, he was the first Jewish member of the Columbia Physics Department.[148]

Bridge Building

Because of the imminent arrival of their baby, the Rabis felt it was unwise to immediately set up housekeeping on their own, so they again lived with Helen's parents, sharing expenses and rent in the Washington Heights area of Manhattan, just north of the eastern approach to the George Washington Bridge, then under construction. Begun in 1927 and completed in 1931, the George Washington Bridge at the time it was built was nearly twice as long as any suspension span previously constructed.

Once again, Rabi was living in the shadow of a major New York City suspension bridge. When the Williamsburg opened in 1903 near his home on Willett Street, Rabi was five years old. When the George Washington opened near his home in Washington Heights, he was 33. The first bridge helped the Rabi family escape the tenements of the Lower East Side and enabled young Rabi to discover the Copernican system in the "far reaches" of Brooklyn. The second bridge would link the island of Manhattan with the state of New Jersey and the rest of America and would bring Rabi, now an evangelist for the new quantum physics, into contact with physicists, politicians, and military leaders across the "far reaches" of the United States.

Bridges serve as apt symbols of the kind of influence Rabi would have on physics in the years to come. Although Rabi would not participate in the Quantum Revolution in the same foundational way that Planck, Bohr, de Broglie, Heisenberg, Schrödinger and Dirac did, he would play a key role in bridging a gap as wide as the Atlantic Ocean, the chasm that still existed between physics in Europe and physics in the United States. The Rabi Tree, a graphic device created in 1958 for the Office of Naval Research by the Arthur D. Little Company to depict the far-reaching effects of basic research, also illustrates how effective Rabi was in propagating the new physics in America.

It wasn't really until after he returned to the United States that Rabi realized how much those two years in Europe had meant to him. Not only had he gained knowledge, he had also gained perspective and self-confidence.

In the United States, we had very few scientists who had made important contributions, very few of the original creators. So although I had learned a great deal of physics in the United States, it was in a certain sense provincial. I could say that I had memorized the *libretto* but didn't have the music. It was [in Europe] you could see the people who were really creating the great ideas, and the manner in which they operated. I have had the belief that science is much more an oral tradition than is commonly supposed, and that it goes on from teacher to student, and is a great deal the function of the environment. . . .

I began to understand what my own capacities might be. Measuring myself against the German students and even some of the great men that I've named, I found that I also had a contribution to make, and that I could . . . think for myself. I did not have to defer to authorities. In that sense, it freed me of inhibitions which I think many Americans had at that time—freed me of the provincialism which was prevalent.

Most of all, I learned to understand quantum mechanics in . . . a more profound way than I would have gotten just by reading the papers and books alone. I was able, I think, to transmit that same understanding and feeling, very often intuitive, to my students in subsequent years.[149]

His time in Europe had provided a two-fold benefit, however. Not only had the experience increased his appreciation for European science; it had also given him a greater appreciation for his own science education and for science in the United States in general.

It was chiefly in Europe that I learned to appreciate the great virtues of America because, before I left, I was particularly sensitive about the faults. . . . One began to realize the great potential strength of the United States in science, which was not manifest at that time, but we began to appreciate the hidden strength of the nature of our institutions.

I know that in my discussions in Europe, I got to be known as a chauvinist, because although I was very much aware of our deficiencies, what they criticized very often were not our deficiencies but our virtues. They didn't understand, and perhaps don't to this day, what this country is all about, because although it looks simple on the surface, it is rather subtle.[150]

Still, there was no question that the United States had been lagging behind Europe when it came to science. For Rabi and his American colleagues abroad, it was an embarrassment they intended to correct.

Together with some of my friends that I met there, like Ed Condon and Bob Roberts and Oppenheimer and others, [we] decided that it was humiliating to have a situation where it was necessary for an American to go to Europe . . . to get a higher education in science, in physics. We decided that we would put a stop to that—that we would raise the level of American physics so that this would no longer be necessary. So I think in that sense, this group of us who were in Germany at that time, and came back, and founded our own schools in various places, had an enormous influence in the development of science in the United States.[151]

The Rabi School

The next 10 years, from 1930 to 1940, would be the most productive of Rabi's personal research career. Once again, he would be filling the role of organizer and inspirational leader, a role he had first found so natural back on the streets of Brooklyn and which he had again exhibited in the mid-1920s while a graduate student at Columbia.

Although Rabi was hired as a lecturer, the lowest academic rank there was at Columbia and a position often given the heaviest teaching load, Rabi was given a very light load, only two hours a week in contrast with full professors who were teaching as much as 14 hours a week. This was due to the foresight of George Pegram, who had hired Rabi for the express purpose of bringing the new quantum mechanics to Columbia and who recognized that teaching the new physics from the original sources—textbooks were not yet available—would be a formidable task. "G.B. Pegram, the dean of the Columbia School of Mines, Engineering and Chemistry, had great faith in me," said Rabi.[152]

In preparing for his first course, statistical mechanics, Rabi worked from early morning until late at night, and "was so well prepared by the time each lecture came," he said, "that the students understood practically nothing, because I spoke to them as one expert to another."[153] Although he eventually changed his methods, he said, and learned a great deal on how to teach, his classroom teaching would continue to receive mixed reviews.

Judged on the basis of organization and lecture style, he was at best mediocre—"dreadful" and "awful" were two terms that came to mind by a couple of his more famous students. If judged, on the other hand, on the basis of instilling in students an appetite to learn more about the subject and to think more deeply about it, he would have to be judged as a very effective teacher.

Norman Ramsey, who became a Nobel laureate in 1989, found Rabi's courses "extremely enlightening," his mathematics "fine," his organization "really pretty dreadful." "He'd get stuck in the middle," he said. "He was working it out from scratch."[154]

Leon Lederman, who took classes from Rabi in the 1950s and became a Nobel laureate in 1988, said Rabi's lectures were bad, but his teaching was successful. "There was a sort of electricity in the air. After a confused lecture, we'd rush to the library, open the journals and books, and try to dope out what in the world he had said."[155] William Nierenberg, who worked with both Rabi and Ramsey and later became director of the Scripps Oceanographic Institute, rated Rabi's lectures as "awful," but his availability to talk with students as "great." "He would take the time. He had full patience to work with his students. A couple of us would come to see him after class; if it was an hour, or two hours, he would stay."[156]

Whether Rabi, who rated Niels Bohr as "acoustically, the world's poorest lecturer"[157] and Wolfgang Pauli as "one of the poorest lecturers in existence,"[158] saw himself in the same category is unclear but he did recognize his ability to instill enthusiasm for physics in both students and professors alike. "I think I made life interesting from the scientific point of view. . . . We just had a great time, the students and I. We worked every day of the year with the exception of three or four days: New Year's Day and Christmas Day and so on. It was just real fun."[159]

Rabi was hired by Pegram to provide a theoretical component in quantum mechanics for the department, but was given latitude to do either theory or experiments "as my ideas came to me,"[160] he said. Although he soon began tilting his work more and more toward experiments, that didn't mean he abandoned theory. On the contrary, he maintained a balance between the two which has been described as "quite different from what one ordinarily would expect of an experimentalist. Although he spent the necessary time in his laboratory to ensure the success of an experiment, he spent most of his time on theory, leaving the technical details of the experiments to his assistants."[161]

The fact of the matter is, that's the way both Rabi and his assistants wanted it. "We wouldn't let him touch the apparatus," said Jerrold Zacharias.[162] Rabi himself admitted he had "no experimental technique whatever. The first time I picked up a galvanometer, I broke the suspension."[163] Norman Ramsey said that although Rabi was very active on the ideas for experiments, he was "completely uninterested in details."

> In other words, [said Ramsey,] he really was the stimulating and guiding force. When things were going well and you were getting interesting data, he was right there on top of the experiment helping with the interpretation. But when there were leaks in the apparatus, he just disappeared. In fact, during the construction he did virtually no work himself in the form of building the apparatus.[164]

Initially, the theoretical ideas that came to Rabi were in the field of solid-state physics, an area he had started to pursue under Heisenberg back in Leipzig. In fact, it was because Heisenberg had been impressed with Rabi's insights in solid-state physics that he had recommended him for the position at Columbia. Although Rabi recognized the great importance of the field, and that some of the ideas he had "were quite good," he found that he just wasn't interested in solid state.

"Since I was not getting theoretical ideas which I found interesting enough to fully absorb my drive, so to speak," he said, "I therefore resolved to turn back to my experimental experience, and do some experiments."[165] Although Rabi did write papers after that which were theoretical in nature, he never did get back to doing solely theoretical work and, in fact, influenced many of his students to wear both hats—theorist and experimentalist.

Rabi did not find it necessary to follow the typical "publish or perish" pattern. Because of his positive influence on the department in general, he was promoted to assistant professor after one year (1930), given a raise after the second year (1931), and promoted to associate professor at the end of three years (1932). While changing rank, he was also changing streets. After moving out of his in-laws' apartment in Washington Heights, Rabi moved his family every year for several years—first to Claremont Avenue near Columbia University, then to 113th Street, then to 118th Street, then to 120th Street. Although the apartments improved in accommodations with each move, the rent remained the same for each of them—$75 a month—evidence, said Rabi, of the effect the Depression was having throughout the city. Rabi, on the other hand, continued receiving steady promotions and pay increases throughout the period so that by the 1936-37 academic year, he was a full professor.

Nuclear Spins

In 1930, I.I. Rabi of Columbia University and Gregory Breit of New York University began a weekly joint seminar between the two institutions. In the process of coordinating the seminar, Rabi and Breit found they had mutual interests ranging over a broad area of physics. "We had a great many fascinating discussions," said Rabi, "and many of the ideas which have since come up in physics were first touched upon by us in our discussions, before, during and after these seminars."[166] One topic that kept attracting their attention was the magnetic properties of the atomic nucleus.

A layperson may tend to think of "nuclear physics" as synonymous with "atomic physics," but in fact the nucleus of the atom was not discovered until 1911, much later than the discovery of the atom, and it wasn't until 1924 that Wolfgang Pauli postulated, on the basis of hyperfine splittings in spectral lines, that an atomic nucleus, like the atom itself, has a spin and therefore a magnetic moment.

In seeking to test Arnold Sommerfeld's theory of space quantization, Stern and Gerlach had, in 1922, used a non-uniform magnetic field to split a beam of silver atoms into two beamlets, based on the magnetic moments of the atoms in the beam and the fact that silver has two possible spin states or orientations, parallel and anti-parallel. In the years that followed, Stern and his collaborators in Hamburg had further refined their method so that they were able to determine not only the number of orientations atoms of certain elements could assume but also, within limits, the magnetic moments of several atoms. The degree of limitation was imposed by how accurately the magnetic field was calibrated and by how accurately one could determine the average velocity with which individual atoms traveled through the magnetic field. Both of these limitations had been dealt with by Stern in arriving at fairly accurate measurements of atomic magnetic moments.

Determining the magnetic properties of an atom, however, was one thing; determining the magnetic properties of an atom's nucleus quite another as nuclear magnetic moments are about 2,000 times smaller than atomic magnetic moments. (In 1931, Rabi and Breit did not know about a major nuclear component, the neutron, which would be discovered the following year by James Chadwick of Cambridge University. One or more neutrons help comprise the atomic nucleus of every atom except hydrogen. Although neutrons have no electrical charge, they do have a magnetic moment, an attribute that would soon capture the imagination of another NMR pioneer, Felix Bloch.)

Theoretically, atomic spectroscopy with its hyperfine spectral lines could provide information about the magnetic properties of the nucleus, but when used on sodium, the technique had been found wanting. Rigden points out[167] that a 1928 paper[168] on "the rotational structure of the blue-green [spectral] bands of Na_2 [sodium]" by Wheeler Loomis and R.W. Wood concluded that the spin of that atom's nucleus had to be "extraordinarily large." In contrast, however, a 1931 paper[169] by Harold Urey at Columbia concluded that "the spin of the [sodium] nucleus is probably 5/2 or less." If the spin of sodium had been 5/2, that would have meant that the nucleus of a sodium atom could be found precessing in a magnetic field in one of six space-quantized orientations with components along the magnetic field of 5/2, 3/2, 1/2, -1/2, -3/2, and -5/2.

The wide disparity between the Loomis and Urey papers attracted Rabi and Breit and in a letter to the editor of *Physical Review* dated November 10, 1931,[170] they suggested atomic beams as another way of determining the nuclear spins of atoms and provided a classic formula that would be used by Rabi and his collaborators in the years to come to calculate both nuclear spin magnitudes and magnetic moments.

The opening lines of their letter stated: "Hyperfine structures of spectral lines and alternating intensities of band spectra constitute at present the only available means of determining angular momenta of atomic nuclei. We wish to point out another means of finding nuclear spins."[171] Building on the foundation of the famous Stern-Gerlach experiment, Rabi and Breit proceeded to show theoretically how the strength of the external magnetic field would affect the internal magnetic coupling between an atom's nucleus and its electrons. If an atomic beam passed through a weak magnetic field, they said, it would deflect the beam into a different number of beamlets than if it passed through a strong field. In a weak field, the internal coupling would remain intact, relatively unaffected by the external field. In a strong field, the internal coupling would be overpowered and the electrons would be primarily coupled to the external field.

It was implied that the formula combined with a properly designed atomic beam apparatus should be able to provide the nuclear spin of an atom. The Breit-Rabi letter ended with the statement, "The nuclear spins of Cs [cesium] and Rb [rubidium] are at present being investigated with this method by one of us (I.I.R.)."[172]

At this point, although he had together with Breit developed the theory for determining nuclear spins using molecular beams, Rabi had not proven it experimentally. Just as Stern and Gerlach had made Sommerfeld's space quantization theory come alive with molecular beams, Rabi wanted to prove to himself that the theory was based on reality. As he expressed it, "I wanted to be sure, in the most primitive way, of convincing myself that there was such a thing as nuclear spin. Not that I doubted it deeply, but I wanted to be sure, since I intended to devote a good deal of time, years, to the subject."[173]

By this time, Victor Cohen, Rabi's first graduate student, had completed building Columbia University's first atomic/molecular beam apparatus and beams of alkali metals were wending their way from the vaporizing oven to the beam detector. In the coming months, Rabi and Cohen analyzed a number of atoms, including cesium and sodium. Rabi never published the cesium results—he never got around to it—although he did report them at the December 1931 meeting of the American Physical Society.[174]

As for sodium, Rabi could have published the nuclear spin of sodium from his experiments much earlier than he did—he and Cohen reported them in 1933—but the calculations required to compute them didn't appeal to his innate self-described "laziness." Reminiscent of his doctoral dissertation where he just couldn't bring himself to measure magnetic susceptibilities in the traditional way, Rabi failed to publish any of the results they obtained between 1931 and 1933. He was waiting to think of a better way that gave the results more directly, procrastination that paid off handsomely. Had he had modern computers to calculate and plot the graphs formed by his data points, Rabi said, "I would never have gotten my Nobel Prize. . . . Dull work like that is not my forte."[175]

What he came up with was a new design for his apparatus that would provide separated beams—not separated beams giving atomic answers from which you had to extrapolate nuclear answers, but separated beams which gave nuclear information directly. The hindsight provided by the space of just a few years would reveal this decision as a critical one on the road to magnetic resonance.

At the oven end of their new apparatus, Rabi and Cohen started with the basic Stern-Gerlach beam separator, an inhomogeneous strong-field magnet that divided the incoming beam into two beamlets. Had they stopped there, they would have gotten the two smears caused by space quantization that first convinced Rabi a decade earlier of the merits of the quantum theory. But this was now just the starting point. Next in line, for one of the two beamlets, came a weak inhomogeneous field oriented opposite to the first one which was intended to act more delicately than the first, separating the half-beam into its atomic and nuclear components based on the merits of the Breit-Rabi theory. To negate much of the velocity differential between particles in this beamlet, the field was positioned in the opposite direction from the first field.

At this point in the apparatus, a roadblock was inserted. Only the split beamlets formed by the weak field were allowed, by means of a slit, to continue on toward the beam detector. The unused half of the main beam came to a sudden, premature stop.

Finally, another strong field was inserted to return the now-refined beamlets to the center of the apparatus for detection. According to the formula, if the nuclear spin were designated as "I," the number of beamlets hitting the detector area should total $2I + 1$.

Late one night, Cohen tested the completed apparatus for the first time. With the oven heated to the proper temperature for vaporizing sodium and with the working chamber at a good vacuum, he was ready to check the target area of the apparatus with the improved beam detector the Rabi team had devised. Instead of a cold glass plate that provided evidence of a beam with a visual smear, they had now developed a method that used a cold wire which heated up when it was impinged by a beam, and thus measured the strength of the beam "ballistically," as Rabi described it.[176]

As Cohen moved the detector wire across the target area, the signal rose and then fell as the wire entered a beamlet on one side and then exited on the other. One peak. He kept moving the wire. Another peak, another beamlet. And another, and another. Four peaks in all, four beamlets. According to the formula $2I + 1$, if 4 was the result, the value of I was three halves (3/2). As Cohen headed for home in the early hours of that morning in 1933, he looked at the other passengers riding in his subway car and thought: "I know something that none of you know. I am the only one in the world who knows that the nuclear spin of sodium is 3/2."[177]

Rabi compared the emotion he felt upon viewing the successful sodium experiment to that of a religious experience.

The world was young and I was young and the experiment was beautiful. It satisfied everything I wanted to see. There was an artistry in it or whatever it is called. . . . It just charmed me. These atoms in spatially quantized states, analyze them in one field, turn your focus back, and there it is. Count them! It was wonderful. There

I really, I really believed in the spin, there are the states, count them! Each one, I suppose, seeks God in his own way.[178]

For Rabi, who had come from an Orthodox Jewish background, there was one God and in Rabi's view good physics brought one nearer to Him:

The world was a creation of His, and therefore it must have a meaning and a coherency. When I chose physics, I was no longer practicing the Jewish religion, but the basic attitudes and feelings have remained with me. Somewhere way down, I'm an Orthodox Jew.

To choose physics in the first place requires a certain direction of interest. In my case it was something that goes to my background, and that is religious in origin. Not religion in a secular way, but religion as the inspirer of a way of looking at things. Choosing physics means, in some way, you're not going to choose trivialities. The whole idea of God, that's real class . . . real drama. When you're doing good physics, you're wrestling with the Champ. You have one life to do it in, you don't want to waste it.[179]

"Wrestling with the Champ." Isidor Isaac Rabi, who was born Israel Isaac Rabi, knew the story from the Scriptures about Jacob's wrestling match with God. It was probably one that he had told, maybe embellished, to the big boys who had protected him back on Manhattan's Lower East Side. Jacob had hung on to his heavenly visitor all night long, refusing to let go until God blessed him, and finally, God had complied with his request. At the same time, He gave Jacob a new name, Israel, which meant "a prince of God."[180] If there was one story from the Scriptures that Rabi knew—and he knew many—it was the story about the origin of his name. "When you're doing good physics, you're wrestling with the Champ." Rabi and Cohen had done good physics with the sodium experiment. In Rabi's terms, that meant he was getting "nearer to God."

Between 1933 and 1937, Rabi and his collaborators continued to compel countless beams of atoms and molecules to divulge their nuclear secrets. Twenty-seven years after Rabi and Cohen found the nuclear spin of sodium, Rabi told students at Claremont College in California:

Most new insights come only after a superabundant accumulation of facts have removed the blindness which prevented us from seeing what later comes to be regarded as the obvious.[181]

The quote is reminiscent of a quotation by another scientist, Edwin Land of Polaroid Corporation, who is said to have observed that "every creative act is the result of a sudden cessation of stupidity." Land and Rabi would both serve as science advisors to the president of the United States.

Nuclear Magnetic Moments: Their Magnitude

The next question Rabi wanted answered was: How can the apparatus be configured to reveal not just the spin of a nucleus but its magnetic moment as well? To do that would require more than counting signal peaks with a wire beam detector.

Rabi had ideas for finding the answer, some of which were already beginning to be incorporated in an experiment he was doing with Victor Cohen to analyze the magnetic properties of cesium. To further implement the ideas he had been mulling over, Rabi enlisted the help of a graduate student, Sidney Millman, suggesting that he set up for his dissertation experiment a molecular beam to determine the nuclear spin and magnetic moment of potassium. Millman readily agreed, although in the end his doctoral dissertation was done using lithium.

To accomplish the objective, Rabi had come up with another apparatus modification that involved what is called the "zero-moment" method. The new method, if successful, would provide both a measurement of the nuclear spin and the magnetic moment. The nuclear spin measurement would be direct, using a different approach than the sodium experiment, and measurement of the nuclear magnetic moment would be indirect, but more accurate than anything previously available.

It is noteworthy that, although quite different in technique, there was a principle involved in the zero-moment method that carried over from Rabi's own doctoral dissertation. In that experiment, Rabi had derived the magnetic susceptibility of certain crystals by immersing them in a doctored-up solution that equaled the magnetic susceptibility of the crystal. By determining the magnetic susceptibility of the solution and comparing it, based on its weight, with the known magnetic susceptibility of water, he was able to determine the magnetic susceptibility of both the solution and the crystal. In other words, by eliminating the *effective* magnetic susceptibility of the crystal, he was able to determine the *actual* magnetic susceptibility of the crystal.

The Breit-Rabi theory had revealed that if you adjusted a deflecting field in a molecular beam apparatus to certain values, you could eliminate the effective nuclear magnetic moment of the atoms traveling through the field. Just as in his magnetic susceptibility experiment where he didn't change the actual magnetic susceptibility of the crystal, Rabi would not be changing the actual nuclear magnetic moments of the atoms in the beam. He would just make their effect non-existent, the achievement of which in a deflecting field would be signified by an undeflected beam.

The problem with making such a deflecting field work, of course, was one they had struggled with before, namely accuracy of calibration plus adjustability. Although the nuclear magnetic moment could be determined with this experiment, it would require calculation based on theory, less desirable than a more direct determination. Here Jerrold Zacharias, a postdoctoral fellow working with Rabi, came up with the answer—an electromagnetic deflecting field. If carefully constructed, you could precisely control the calibration of the field as well as its strength, and the strength of the nuclear magnetic moment could be calculated in a more straightforward, non-theoretical manner.

The experiment was started with everything on and operating, except for the deflecting field, which was off. The beam of atoms was streaming through the apparatus, striking the beam detector at full strength. As the deflecting field was then turned on and slowly increased in strength, some of the space-quantized spins were deflected, causing a decrease in signal—a peak—at the beam detector. Again, as in the sodium experiment, the peaks were counted and the magnitude of lithium's nuclear spin was determined. With the precise information provided by the electromagnetic field, the nuclear magnetic moment could be calculated fairly simply. When the experiment worked, it provided the most accurate data of any method used prior to the magnetic resonance method.

Another method developed during this period was the refocusing technique, which had first been used on the sodium experiment. One of the inherent unknowns in molecular and atomic beams is the velocity of individual atoms or molecules. Since their velocities are different, the time they spend traveling through a magnetic field is different and, as a result, the size of their deflections are affected accordingly; either more (if traveling at a lower velocity) or less (if traveling at a higher velocity).

In a sense, the solution for this problem was borrowed from Rabi's magnetic susceptibility experiment as well. If you can't control the velocity of an individual atom, eliminate its effect. That's what the refocusing method did with two deflecting fields. Deflecting-field A would cause the atoms to be deflected in one direction, but the problem was still there. The atoms were still traveling at differing speeds and spending differing times in the field. Had a beam detector been inserted at the end of Field A, the same problem would be evident. The answer was to follow up Field A with another deflecting field, Field B, which deflected the beams in the opposite direction, bringing them back to their original target, but eliminating the effect of multiple velocities.

While Cohen and Millman were working with Rabi on the fifth floor of Pupin Hall on the alkalis, cesium, rubidium and potassium, Jerome Kellogg and Jerrold Zacharias had begun working with Rabi and the hydrogens on the 10th floor. In Germany, Stern had devised an experiment that measured the magnetic moment of the proton and had found an unexpected result—"remarkable"[182] is how Rabi described it. Instead of being close to the theoretical value of one nuclear magneton, it was almost three times as large. Likewise, Stern had found the magnetic moment of the deuteron to be less than expected.

Compelled to confirm these findings for himself, Rabi found that the proton's magnetic moment, according to his team's measurements, although similar to Stern's, was even larger, about three-and-a-quarter nuclear magnetons (3.25 ± 10 percent) and that the value for the deuteron's moment was very low, about three-fourths of a Bohr magneton (0.77 ± 0.2).[183-185]

As Rabi's methods evolved, from the deflection method to the zero-moment method to refocusing, the beams streaming through his team's apparatuses were compelled to yield more and more information about their magnetic properties. Soon, with the advent of magnetic resonance, they would come to reveal their closely-held information to the experimenters even more accurately.

Nuclear Magnetic Moments: Their Sign

Determining the sign, positive or negative, of a nuclear magnetic moment was one of the last hurdles encountered by the Rabi team before development of the magnetic resonance method. The sign of a magnetic moment is affected by two variables. If the space-quantized direction of the spin matches the direction of the magnetic moment, the sign of the moment is positive. If the space-quantized direction of the spin is opposed to the direction of the magnetic moment, the sign of the moment is negative.

It was this known fact that instigated Rabi's thinking about an experiment Otto Stern had done in 1932 and 1933, before leaving Germany, in which he had wondered what would happen if you suddenly changed the direction of a magnetic field in mid-course for an atom traveling through a beam apparatus. Would the atom suddenly change its space-quantized orientation? Could it be "forced" to leave its pre-determined orientation or would it insist on staying with its pre-programmed flight plan? Stern and his collaborators found that, yes, they could change an atom's orientation if they changed the field direction quickly enough.

As Rabi thought about this phenomenon, he saw he could use it in an experiment for determining the signs of nuclear magnetic moments. He put his thoughts down in a theoretical paper entitled "On the Process of Space Quantization" that he submitted to *Physical Review* and which they received on December 23, 1935.[186] The paper opened by referring to the Stern experiments conducted about three years earlier, but called attention to the fact that Stern, et al. had not considered the effect of nuclear spin, a shortcoming Rabi would eliminate in an upcoming experiment.

The Rabi team had come up with the "T-field" which would be inserted between deflecting Field A and deflecting Field B. Treelike in its design, with two branches and a trunk, the configuration was designed so that a beam particle would enter the "T" from the top, moving against the magnetic field, and exit through the bottom, but now moving with the magnetic field. The magnetic field itself would not change direction, but the juxtaposition of the two fields would make it "appear" to the particle that it would suddenly have to respond to changing magnetic conditions. To a particle in the beam, not only would the magnetic direction appear to be changing, it would also appear to rotate.

At this point, Rabi designed the apparatus so that he could change the rate of rotation of the upcoming field (from the particle's perspective) to match the precession rate of the particle (its Larmor frequency). When the match was close, Rabi knew, the magnetic moment could be made to tip or flop from one orientation to another. Meanwhile, Rabi's collaborators, Jerome Kellogg and Jerrold Zacharias, added another beam-selecting feature to the apparatus that made it possible to infer the sign even more directly.

The T-field experiment worked as planned and the Rabi team was now standing on the threshold of achieving magnetic resonance.

Magnetic Resonance

Just one more important step remained before opening the curtains on magnetic resonance. In 1937, Rabi completed another paper for *Physical Review* that was entitled "Space Quantization in a Gyrating Magnetic Field."[187] It was submitted in February of that year and published in April. Combining theory with the results of his T-field experiments, Rabi pointed out that the critical factor in making the beam particle reorient when it anticipated what appeared to be a gyrating field up ahead was the frequency of that rotation, and the closeness of that frequency with the frequency of the atom's magnetic moment. If the frequencies were close to each other or right on, the probability that reorientation would occur would be large. On the other hand, if the frequencies were quite divergent from one another, there was little chance that reorientation would occur.

With this paper, the stage was set for magnetic resonance, but the curtain still remained closed. In fact, it remained closed for at least seven more months. The reasons? First, so much was happening right then that the Rabi team just didn't get around to implementing the theory experimentally. Secondly, as Norman Ramsey points out, Rabi didn't immediately recognize its full potential. Although the resonance equation used in the paper would become the basis for all subsequent magnetic and electric resonance experiments, the form of the equation "obscured the resonant nature of the result," wrote Ramsey, "and Rabi failed to see it immediately."[188]

There were two important differences between the T-field apparatus and the magnetic resonance apparatus that would follow. Otherwise, they were nearly identical. Those differences were: 1) a third field, Field C, electromagnetic for adjustability as well as homogeneous, which was inserted between Field A and Field B and 2) an oscillator, which could create via a tunable radio frequency, a much smaller magnetic field perpendicular to Field C.

It wasn't long after Rabi submitted his paper, noted Ramsey, that Rabi and Zacharias discussed the possibility of using "an oscillator to produce a magnetic field that truly rotated with time instead of simulating one with the motion of particles." Ramsey added, however, that they were "so fully occupied with their highly successful research programs that they gave this idea no further thought."[189] Or at least they gave it no further thought until Dutch physicist Cornelis J. Gorter [pronounced Horter], then at the University of Groningen in the Netherlands, visited Rabi at Columbia in September of 1937.

Gorter had tried to detect nuclear magnetic resonance in solid matter by nuclear resonance heating of the sample just the previous year, but had been unsuccessful. It's not clear why his method hadn't worked although it has generally been ascribed to either the sample or to shortcomings in the actual technique. As other early pioneers in both NMR and MRI can attest, when you don't know exactly what to expect or what variables have to be working in what combination, getting a signal can be "iffy." When Gorter saw Rabi's sophisticated molecular beam apparatuses, however, he quickly saw their potential for magnetic resonance and soon mentioned the magic word "oscillator" to Rabi.

From Gorter's perspective, Rabi had already been experiencing substantial success in coaxing isolated atoms traveling in beams to reveal their secrets, so the chances were good that using the magnetic resonance variable would be successful. Furthermore, since Gorter's unsuccessful attempt, Rabi had published an article that provided a strong, theoretical basis for its success.

For Rabi, who had been busily enjoying the string of successes made with so-called "conventional" manipulation—although those methods were all innovative as well—Gorter's suggestion suddenly added a time pressure he hadn't been feeling for awhile. As Rabi recounted that, he noted that: 1) there was a backlog of other work to finish, 2) he was enjoying the elegant simplicity and results he was getting with the T-field apparatus, and 3) "There was this very happy condition that nobody was competing with us. It was such a wonderful period."[190]

Now it was clear that someone might soon be competing with them and Rabi almost immediately gave the word to dismantle Millman's apparatus on the fifth floor and to reassemble it in the arrangement described above, removing the T-field and replacing it with the C-field and tunable oscillator, and to do likewise with the molecular hydrogen apparatus on the tenth floor.

Within a relatively short period of time, the modifications were made on the less-complex fifth-floor apparatus and the collaborators involved were ready for the first beam to make its way from oven to detector. This was a molecular beam experiment. Although they* were going to be looking for the magnetic moment of the atomic nucleus of lithium, they were using a beam of lithium chloride molecules.

After adjusting a collimating slit (located in the center of the C-field) to register a good signal at the beam detector, Millman began adjusting the other variables. He turned on the B-field, thereby deflecting the beam away from the detector, and then he turned on the A-field, refocusing the beam back onto the detector so that, once again, the beam detector was registering a full-strength beam.

---

* Of the six collaborators participating in these early magnetic resonance experiments, three of them—Rabi, Ramsey and Kusch—would eventually receive Nobel Prizes, all for separate achievements.

There are two ways of achieving magnetic resonance, either: 1) adjust the magnet strength and leave the oscillator at a preset frequency, or 2) preset the magnet strength and adjust the oscillator frequency. They were using the first method. (The second method is the basis for radiofrequency spectroscopy, which would also be pioneered in the same laboratory within a few months, and which is described in the next chapter featuring Norman Ramsey, who was the first to actually conduct the experiment.)

Millman first set the frequency of the oscillator to 3.518 million cycles per second (3.518×10^6 Hertz). Then he began adjusting the amperage for the C-field. Starting at 110 amperes, he increased the current slowly with a rheostat—111, 112, 113. No change. At 114 amperes, the level dropped significantly; at 115, more yet; at 116, the signal bottomed out. At 117, the signal began returning; 118, more signal; 119, a full strength signal; at 120, no further changes. The experiment had worked.[191] They had achieved magnetic resonance. From here, a simple calculation would provide a very precise measurement of lithium's magnetic moment.

What had happened was that as they approached optimum resonance at 115 amperes, the atoms of lithium under the influence of the C-field nearly matched the Larmor frequency for lithium at that field strength and also nearly matched the frequency of the oscillator. (As mentioned before, Millman had been analyzing the magnetic properties of lithium using the other methods, so the team knew they should be in the "ballpark" with the combination of magnet amperage and oscillator frequency they had selected as starting points for the experiment.) At near resonance, many atoms were reoriented, causing them to be defocused away from the beam detector by the B-field deflecting magnet. At 116 amperes, the match between the two frequencies was nearly perfect, and almost all of the atoms were deflected away from the detector. As the amperage was increased further, leaving the resonance "sweet spot," fewer atoms were deflected and the signal began to return; eventually to full strength as the beam was completely restored.

If the first sodium, non-resonance experiment had brought I.I. Rabi "nearer to God," as he expressed it, the magnetic resonance method had brought him even closer. Seven years later, he would receive the Nobel Prize for his accomplishment.

Rabi, Zacharias, Millman and Kusch published the results of that first magnetic resonance experiment in a letter to the editor of *Physical Review* dated January 31, 1938. The letter opened with the statement, "It is the purpose of this note to describe an experiment in which nuclear magnetic moment [sic] is measured very directly. The method is capable of very high precision and extension to a large number and variety of nuclei."[192] The letter ended with a statement that a full account of the experiment would be provided when the homogeneous field was recalibrated. (The more complete description arrived at *Physical Review* about a year later on January 20, 1939.[193] In the meantime, the team was also publishing the results of its new radiofrequency spectroscopy methods which had revealed that the deuteron had an electric quadrupole moment.)[194]

A footnote added to the end of the first article acknowledged the important contribution Gorter had made to the discovery: "We are very much indebted to Dr. Gorter who, when visiting our laboratory in September 1937, drew our attention to his stimulating experiments in which he attempted to measure nuclear moments by observing the rise in temperature of solids placed in a constant magnetic field on which an oscillating field was superimposed."[195]

Added to the same footnote was the statement, "Dr. F. Bloch has independently worked out similar ideas but for another purpose (unpublished)."[196] Out at Stanford, Bloch had also come up with magnetic resonance. Although he would not use it experimentally for more than another year, he had worked out the details of magnetic resonance using an approach very similar to Rabi's which he would use in his quest to determine the magnetic moment of the neutron. Later, after the war, Bloch and another war-time colleague of Rabi's, Edward Purcell, would take magnetic resonance a step further, to discover the NMR signal in condensed matter.

Although Rabi had detected magnetic resonance from atomic nuclei only in isolated molecules streaming through an air-evacuated chamber, he knew that the same phenomenon was present, even though it might be difficult to detect, in condensed matter as diverse as human tissue and steel. On December 29, 1939, at a meeting of the American Association for the Advancement of Science in Columbus, Ohio, Drs. Rabi, Kusch and Millman, according to a report in the *New York Post*, said that all atoms, whether part of the heart tissue of man or a piece of steel, constantly emit radio waves which can be detected and measured. The article bore the headline, "We're All Radio Stations, Columbia Scientists Report." Even the death of an animal organism, the article went on to say, does not mean the stopping of this activity, since the atoms which form part of the living cell continue to emit radiation after the organism as a whole has ceased to function.[197]

One area of science that Dr. Rabi took little interest in during his early years of voracious reading was biology, he told science historian Thomas

Kuhn—"Somehow I never cottoned to biology, never remembered reading biology," he said—but he did recognize in 1939 that the atoms of biological tissue would emit the same kind of signals he and his associates
had detected with radiofrequency spectroscopy.[198]

He did not at that time realize that those tiny broadcasting stations
within living tissue could be tuned in to announce whether or not they
were diseased. That revelation would come from a medical doctor by the
name of Raymond Damadian, but it would not come for another 31 years.

The Winds of War

As the Rabi teams at Columbia were making their discoveries throughout the 1930s, Adolf Hitler was enacting steps in his plan to take over
Europe. During the five years he had been in power, he had acted swiftly to enact his political and social agenda: 1) Jews had become targets of
persecution and were being sent to concentration camps where, eventually, millions would lose their lives; 2) the Saarland, governed by the
League of Nations following World War I, had been reincorporated by
Germany following a 1935 plebiscite; 3) the Rhineland, a demilitarized
zone established by the Allies after World War I, was taken back and
occupied; 4) two months after Rabi submitted his Nobel Prize-winning
findings about magnetic resonance to *Physical Review*, Hitler annexed
Austria; 5) in September of that year he demanded the Sudetanland portion of Czechoslovakia, was not refused, and was thereby emboldened in
early 1939 to dissolve Czechoslovakia altogether; 6) six months later, in
September 1939, Hitler declared war on Poland and thereby initiated
World War II, bringing France and Britain directly into the fray.

During roughly the same period that these events were occurring in
Europe, Rabi was taking a sabbatical for the 1938-39 academic year, with
much of that period spent at the Institute for Advanced Study in
Princeton, New Jersey. By that time, many of the Jewish scientists
expelled from Germany's universities with Hitler's rise to power in 1933
had found their way to the United States. Among the early ones to leave
Germany, even before Hitler was appointed chancellor in January of
1933, was Albert Einstein, who took a position at the Institute for
Advanced Study and, soon afterward, renounced his German citizenship.

At Princeton, Rabi was able to spend some time with Einstein and, in
particular, recalled an evening with the great physicist.

There was one evening after a concert when we all went back to his
house. Einstein brought out a bottle of lovely cognac. He didn't

drink. His secretary didn't drink. Nobody drank except me. So I drank the cognac, and the more I drank, the mellower I got. But then everybody else did, too. It was very interesting. At one point, Helen Dukas, Einstein's secretary, brought out Einstein's report cards. It turned out [contrary to some legends] that he had been a pretty good student.[199]

By the time Einstein met Rabi, Einstein had led an exodus of more than 200 scientists from Europe to the United States, was warning that Hitler had much larger designs than Germany, and was concerned that his adopted country not stand by and let Hitler take over all of Europe. Rabi, too, was concerned and was wondering what he could do to help stop Hitler. "I really felt I ought to do something. And later, with the fall of France [in May 1940], I became desperate to get into the war." His chance would come later that same year.[200]

Our entry into the war seemed to me to be inevitable. I cast about to find some way in which I could be useful to our forthcoming war effort or at least could help the British in their dire straits. Opportunity came in late summer when Dr. DuBridge was asked by Karl Compton, then president of MIT, to organize a group to work on microwave radar, a new field which had been opened by the British a short time before.

Early in November of 1940, I joined Lee DuBridge and about 30 others—mostly nuclear physicists or atomic physicists as they are now called—to organize this new laboratory in a space which MIT made available to us. Little did I realize then that it would be five years before I would return to Columbia and to a new world.[201]

During those five years, Rabi would serve initially as head of the Radiation Laboratory's research division (Division 4) and then as the "Rad Lab's" associate director under DuBridge. But he would also serve as a consultant to J. Robert Oppenheimer at Los Alamos.

As a citizen and patriot of the United States and as a human being distressed by Hitler's expansionism, Rabi gave the war his best effort, including development of the atomic bomb, although that wasn't his personal choice for a weapon. For him, it was too indiscriminating.

I was strongly opposed to bombing ever since 1931 when I saw those pictures of the Japanese bombing that suburb of Shanghai. You drop a bomb and it falls on the just and the unjust. There is no escape from it. The prudent man can't escape, [nor] the honest man. . . . During the war with Germany, we [in the Rad Lab] certainly helped to develop devices for bombing, . . . but this was a real enemy and a serious matter. But atomic bombing just carried the principle one step further and I didn't like it then and I don't now. I think it's terrible.[202]

Compared to the work he was doing at the Radiation Laboratory, which he knew was accomplishing its objectives, Rabi felt the chances of developing an atomic bomb were rather uncertain, and not necessarily the best place to deploy much-needed human and financial resources. In mid-July of 1945, however, it was clear that what was once "iffy" was now a terrible reality as he viewed the first test of the new device in a remote desert north of Alamogordo, New Mexico.

At first, the announcer said: "Thirty seconds"—"Ten seconds"— and we were lying there, very tense, in the early dawn, and there were just a few streaks of gold in the east; you could see your neighbor very dimly. Those ten seconds were the longest ten seconds that I ever experienced. Suddenly, there was an enormous flash of light, the brightest light I have ever seen or that I think anyone else has ever seen. It blasted; it pounced; it bored its way into you. It was a vision which was seen with more than the eye. It was seen to last forever. You would wish it would stop; altogether it lasted about two seconds. Finally it was over, diminishing, and we looked toward the place where the bomb had been; there was an enormous ball of fire which grew and grew and it rolled as it grew; it went up into the air, in yellow flashes and into scarlet and green. It looked menacing. It seemed to come toward one.[203]

Rabi was both thrilled and chilled—thrilled by the successful test that marked the completion of a massive scientific undertaking and chilled as he considered their creation's awful potential.

At first I was thrilled [upon viewing the successful test]. It was a vision. Then, a few minutes afterward, I had gooseflesh all over me when I realized what this meant for the future of humanity. Up until then, humanity was, after all, a limited factor in the evolution and process of nature. The vast oceans, lakes and rivers, the atmosphere, were not very much affected by the existence of mankind. The new powers represented a threat not only to mankind but to all forms of life: the seas and the air. One could foresee that nothing was immune from the tremendous powers of these new forces. My own concern was to join in any efforts to contain these dangers.[204]

In 1983, at the 40th anniversary of Los Alamos, Rabi expressed sorrow in a television interview with Bill Moyers that the place still existed. "Many of the first Los Alamos scientists thought atomic weapons would be banned after the war. They had, after all, been present at the creation."

The realization that such would not be the case, Rabi told Moyers, "has determined my subsequent career. We bent ourselves to eliminate this. From then on, that was my interest."[205]

Before the war [Rabi told students in a 1960 speech], I used to tell my friends and students that the history of a physicist's life is very simple. He was born; he became interested in physics in some way either through reading or through the personal influence of a teacher or a lecturer; he wrote his thesis and received his PhD degree; he died. The rest and the essential part of his biography could be read only in the scientific journals, in which were described his own work and the work of his students and colleagues. It was an eminently satisfactory life, to my mind the only serious occupation for a gentleman.

This has all changed, at least for some of us. . . . All groups of our population were greatly affected by the war, but except for the military, there is hardly a professional group whose existence was more upset by the demands of the time than the scientists—especially the physicists.[206]

Within months after the end of World War II, Rabi and Robert Oppenheimer held discussions which eventually resulted in the Acheson-Lilienthal-Baruch proposal to the United Nations by the United States for international control of atomic energy. "One of Rabi's greatest disappointments," noted Norman Ramsey, "was that this forward looking plan, after initial favorable consideration, was never adopted by the United Nations."[207]

It was only after the war that Rabi came to the conclusion that the United States was left with "a power that no nation on earth should have,"[208] although he did feel, as of 1949, that it was only through the atomic bombing of Japan that an unconditional surrender was brought about. That year he made a trip to Japan on a fact-finding mission about the state of Japanese science and reported that most Japanese scientists he had spoken to while on that trip did not seem to be sullen or resentful against the United States and had been glad to see the fall of the military clique. They were, however, fearful that the Soviet Union would develop their own atomic weapons, which did occur soon afterward.[209]

At the national level, Rabi was a member of the General Advisory Committee for the Atomic Energy Commission, and voted, along with Enrico Fermi, against a crash program to develop the hydrogen bomb. He also conceived and helped organize the first International Conference on the Peaceful Uses of Atomic Energy and, from then on, was a regular participant in their deliberations.

I.I. Rabi, Nobel Laureate

It was a call from a Mr. Johnson, representing a Swedish newspaper, that first informed Rabi with any degree of certainty that he was being awarded the 1944 Nobel Prize in physics. With the world engaged in a global war, no prizes had been awarded since 1939, but with the end of the conflict almost in sight, the Royal Swedish Academy of Sciences had chosen to select two Nobel laureates in physics simultaneously—Otto Stern, the physicist who had first inspired Rabi about quantum mechanics with his demonstration of space quantization, was being awarded the prize for 1943, and Isidor I. Rabi was being awarded the 1944 prize.

It was still too dangerous to convene the award ceremony in Stockholm, so the prize was given to Rabi in New York at the Waldorf-Astoria by Nicholas Murray Butler, president of Columbia University and 1931 recipient of the Nobel Peace Prize. According to a December 11, 1944 article in the *New York Times*, it was the first time since the award of the prizes began in 1901 that the prize had not been presented in Stockholm, and the first time it had not been presented by the King of Sweden. Crown Prince Gustaf Adolf of Sweden did address the gathering by shortwave radio, however, and Crown Princess Martha of Norway was present on the dais. In a lecture broadcast from Stockholm on December 10, 1944, Professor Erik Hulthén of Stockholm recapped the scientific phenomenon of magnetic resonance and then concluded: "Rabi literally established radio relations with the most subtle particles of matter, with the world of the electron and of the atomic nucleus."[210]

Rabi was 46 when he won the prize. Jeremy Bernstein asked him whether he felt winning it at that relatively young age could be harmful to a scientific career afterwards:

Yes [Rabi replied]. There are many examples. I think it can be a very useful thing to have, but it subjects the individual to enormous pressures. . . . The Nobel Prize does have this strong public appeal. There is some romance attached to it. It's like winning a huge lottery, except that you don't exactly compete—apart from the fact that once you enter one of the professions involved, you are, in a certain sense, competing all the time. It puts the winner on a sort of pedestal, because of the great public attention and prestige and also the prestige among one's colleagues. So that unless you are very competitive you aren't likely to function with the same vigor afterward. You know, it's like the lady from Boston who said, "Why should I travel when I'm already here?"[211]

Although Rabi's metamorphosis from active scientist to statesman was facilitated by his selection as a Nobel Prize winner in 1944, the change was neither immediate nor complete. The war effort would continue to occupy his attention for a major portion of the next year, although the development activity at the Radiation Laboratory would quickly wind down. Even during this transition period, Rabi showed a prescient awareness of the post-war needs of the nation by heading up an effort to recap for the scientific community what he and his fellow scientists at the Rad Lab had learned in their more than four years of intensive effort to defeat the enemy technologically. In the fall of 1944, Rabi initiated a publishing project that, according to him, was "the biggest thing since the Septuagint."[212] The Radiation Laboratory Series, 28 volumes in all, published by McGraw-Hill, would serve a dual purpose, as Rabi envisioned it.

In the summer of '44, it was clear to me that the war was over in the sense of our developing new radar equipment. Yet I realized that we had amassed so much knowledge that unless we put it down in the form of books, then, after the war, there would only be one group who would know all this technology—the Bell Telephone Laboratories. Furthermore, remembering the First World War, there would be Senate investigations on how we spent all this money. With the books, we'd have something to show for it.[213]

As soon as the war was over and it was possible to return to the "civilian" life of an academician, Rabi directed the rebuilding of the physics department at Columbia University, a department that had been decimated in the five years Rabi had been gone. In a sense, it was the second time he built the department, in that it was through Rabi's work at Columbia during the 1930s that the school had achieved much of its prominence. It would be a tougher task to accomplish the second time around.

Back in the 1930s, when research money was scarce, it had been easier to attract and keep a top-flight scientific team. Now that research money was becoming much more abundant, the recruiting job was becoming much more difficult, according to Rabi.

> I set out to bring in some senior people. Nobody came. I was offering people jobs at five thousand dollars a year more than my own salary, and I had the Nobel Prize—and yet I was being turned down. I never understood it. . . . Finally, I decided that we would have to begin by developing our own young people and bringing in other young people. I felt that what I could do was to make sure they would have facilities that otherwise they might not have. New fields were opening up, like the study of elementary particles—the mesons, and so on. So I got money from the Navy to build what was then a large accelerator. I knew that if we had such a facility we would attract young people who wanted to work in the new areas. . . . My own research efforts were a small proportion of the whole thing. But we became a great physics department once again.[214]

Although Rabi's own research efforts were now a smaller slice of the physics pie at Columbia, they were by no means insignificant. During the short period Rabi had been with Niels Bohr at Copenhagen in 1927, he had noticed that the stimulating scientific environment was one in which you "wouldn't dare to be trivial. Somehow or other . . . you had the feeling if you stayed there you had to think of really significant things."[215] It may well be, however, that neither Rabi's training at Columbia University nor his association with Niels Bohr should be credited with his ability to get to the heart of the matter. According to one account, Rabi was inspired in his early studies by his mother, Sheindel Rabi, who always asked him upon his arrival at home from school, "Did you ask any good questions today?"[216] Rabi's ability to ask good questions and his aversion to things trivial had served him well ever since his days as a graduate student at Columbia when he had found a better way to measure the magnetic susceptibility of a crystal, and after the war, in spite of his Nobel Prize, there was no evidence that those instincts had deserted him.

Before the end of the war, Rabi and Norman Ramsey had discussed what they might explore experimentally when they got back to their academic environment and they had agreed that measuring the hyperfine separation in atomic hydrogen against its theoretically predicted value should be a leading candidate.

After returning to Columbia, Rabi and Ramsey were able to reconstruct some of their old molecular-beam equipment—much of which had been destroyed or lost in the interim—and to analyze the response of molecules and atoms to various magnetic stimuli as they wended their way from oven to detector. With one of the old apparatuses, William Nierenberg and Ramsey measured the radiofrequency spectra of alkali halides. During the same period, Rabi and Ramsey and two of their graduate students, John Nafe and Edward Nelson, began preparations to look for the hyperfine interaction in atomic hydrogen.

In fact, they had invented what Ramsey described as a "very, very good experiment"[217] that was about to reveal whether reality reflected theory when, unfortunately for Ramsey, he gave up his part in those experiments to become the head of the physics department at the fledgling Brookhaven National Laboratory on a half-time basis. (At the same time the Columbia physics department was being rebuilt, Rabi and Ramsey had also played a key role in the founding of the new laboratory. See Chapter 2.)

"It was an extremely important experiment," said Ramsey. "The anomaly of the magnetic moment of the electron might even be Rabi's most important experiment,"[218] he said.

With Ramsey spending a significant portion of his time on Long Island, Rabi, Nafe and Nelson made the dramatic discovery which Ramsey later summarized as follows:

> With his students John Nafe and Edward Nelson, Rabi successfully applied the magnetic resonance method to atomic hydrogen and discovered that the hyperfine separation due to the interaction between the magnetic moments of the proton and electron was slightly different from the theoretical expectation. This was the first indication that the magnetic moment of the electron was different from the expected Dirac value, an observation later confirmed by Kusch's direct measurements of the electron magnetic moment. This experimental anomalous magnetic moment was the principal stimulus for the development of relativistic quantum electrodynamics, the first successful quantum field theory.[219]

For his direct measurement of the electron magnetic moment later that year (1947), Polykarp Kusch would receive the 1955 Nobel Prize in physics. The Rabi-Nafe-Nelson experiment would also stimulate Julian Schwinger into finding a theoretical explanation for the anomaly, for which he shared the 1965 Nobel Prize.

Also in 1947, in his first departure from molecular beams since bringing them to Columbia in 1931, Rabi made another key discovery, the first experimental evidence of the interaction between the electron and the neutron.[220] Enrico Fermi at the University of Chicago had attempted, independently, to discover the same effect, but had concluded that there was none. Rabi, together with his Columbia colleagues William Havens and James Rainwater, found that when they directed a beam of neutrons through a piece of lead there was a small effect as some of the neutrons collided with the heavy lead nuclei. Fermi later confirmed their findings.

If Rabi had followed further the experimental path he had set off on with Havens and Rainwater, he would have been on the leading edge of the explosion in particle physics that followed, but it was not to be. Although Rabi would continue his involvement with experiments until 1960 and would continue guiding the efforts of numerous PhD candidates—he actually mentored more PhD candidates after the war than before—he would not pursue his love for physics with the intensity he once had shown.

Like Moses, whose attention had been arrested by a burning bush in the desert, and had felt compelled to deliver his people from Egypt, Rabi's attention had been arrested by a sight in the deserts of New Mexico that compelled him for the rest of his life to raise his voice in a call for wisdom and prudence as a safeguard against the hostile use of atomic energy.

Rabi had been born into a century that would see unparalleled scientific achievement, and unparalleled war. He participated and excelled in the former and when his nation called upon his expertise to help defeat Nazism and imperialism, was willing to participate in the latter. But he also believed, in spite of the atrocities he had seen against his own people, the Jews, that mankind was meant to accomplish greater things and to that end he dedicated the last 43 years of his life.

I.I. Rabi, Speaking His Mind

Rabi was never afraid to share his wisdom and personal opinions with others, whether they wanted to hear it or not. He also wasn't into being "politically correct."

On Basic Science: In 1959, he told a symposium on basic research that scientists should be "odd balls" and "curious types," not unlike writers and painters. In particular, he warned scientists against "going suburban."

"What happens when a scientist goes suburban?" he queried. "He gets in at 8:30 a.m. by carpool. Then he has to quit at 4:30 to make his carpool back home, so he can work on his garden and a little on his leaky cesspool.

"Then he has some friends over in the evening for talk and they talk about what? Carpools and cesspools."

"I can't imagine Picasso arriving at work by his carpool," said Rabi, "painting furiously for a few hours, quitting about 4:30 to return home by carpool to work on his garden or cesspool."

Rabi preferred the term "pure science" to basic science. These intellectual oddballs, he said, often prefer not to have their work applied, and quoted a mathematician who once gave a toast, "Here's to pure mathematics. May it never find an application."

Although Rabi had rather closely-trimmed hair, he also warned scientists not to go for the Madison Avenue look that he had noticed some scientists adopting in 1959. "I don't go for these disguises," he said. "Once you put on the clothes and cut the hair, you begin acting the part."[221]

On Knowing When to Retire: Upon retiring from teaching in 1967 after a 40-year career at Columbia, Dr. Rabi said, "I don't believe in boring people. When you're too old to go on, your best friends won't tell you, and there's nothing worse than an elder statesman of science.

"Besides, physics is a young man's game. Newton and most of the few really great physicists made their important discoveries while still in their 20s. You have to be very smart to be a physicist. Older men are wiser, but the young ones are smarter."[222]

On Teaching Science Biographically: Rabi felt that educators should teach science humanistically, in relation to the great personalities who have affected it, and not as an isolated scheme "with an assorted bag of tricks."

While political history is taught "blow by blow," he said, there are "no really great historians" of science recording the present revolution in science in jargonless prose. He regretted, he said, that while even minor literary figures have volumes of biography written about them, the scientist remains "an invisible man."[223]

On the Need for More People Choosing Science as a Career:
"Enormous numbers of people go into science," Rabi said in 1985. "If they were all good, it would be enough. But so many people go into law—now people who go into law are not dumb, at least not visibly dumb. It's such a waste of human talent, all these MBA's. It's a hell of a way to provide a basis for a powerful country."[224]

On the Need for More Powerful Bombs: During testimony in defense of J. Robert Oppenheimer during the 1954 hearings on whether to suspend Oppenheimer's security clearance, Rabi said, "We have an A-bomb—a whole series of them. What more do you want? Mermaids?" Sharply critical of Edward Teller's testimony against Oppenheimer, Rabi said, "It was brilliantly thought out to meet the needs of those twerps on the [Atomic Energy Commission] board."[225]

On Columbia versus Cornell: "The idea of going to school with a lot of green grass is nonsense. You have the rest of your life to look at green grass. If you really want to enter into civilization, you get it at Columbia better than anywhere else. The whole culture of the United States—or what passes for culture: literature, drama, science, art, the creative intellectual element—is to be found in New York [City]. People who study here can never become provincial. I know. I was at Cornell and at Columbia. It was certainly much pleasanter living on campus in Ithaca, but what you see, after awhile, you more and more tend to imitate—the trees, the cows . . ."[226]

On Politics: "We could use intelligent people in politics. Just the whole idea of electing Jimmy Carter, or Reagan, or Nixon . . . I used to go around lecturing, and I'd say, 'Look at those people—Kennedy and Nixon. What is it about those two people that fits them to be president of the United States apart from the desire to be president?' Neither was an outstanding scholar, but each was determined to be the president. Carter and his wife decided he wants to be president. They bought a pair of walking shoes, and as they say in Yiddish, *'gleichen der welt'*—'just like that.' In history you blow in so sweetly; it comes out so sour."[227]

On Educational Standards: "If you set high standards, students will meet them. The New York City high schools were very good 'til the liberals caught hold of them—the kind of people who say, 'The kids won't be happy if you flunk them.' . . . How can a person understand science if half the high schools in the United States don't even have a physics course? . . . Sputnik made an enormous difference. For a time there was great improvement in American education. And now the United States has declined in 10 years as much as England declined in 50. We can't compete industrially. Scientifically it's not right, either, but forget it. Without natural resources, the Japanese can sell steel more cheaply than we can."[228]

On Anti-Semitism: Asked whether he had ever encountered anti-Semitism, Rabi took care to distinguish between cause and effect: "Once I stepped on the academic ladder, I just skyrocketed. But I had disappointments. I don't know whether they were due to anti-Semitism or not. You know, you don't get a fellowship; you see other people getting jobs that you don't get. It's hard to tell whether people just don't like you as a person or don't like you as a Jew. As far as I'm concerned, I prefer to think they just don't like me."[229]

I.I. Rabi: World Citizen, National Treasure

Although Rabi continued to be directly involved in physics experiments up until 1960 and retained an active interest in the field up until the time of his death on January 11, 1988, his attention after the war turned more and more to the role of advisor, consultant and advocate for sanity in the arms race. In addition to being a member of the General Advisory Committee for the Atomic Energy Commission and a founder of the International Conference on the Peaceful Uses of Atomic Energy, Rabi was a member of the U.S. delegation to the General Conference of UNESCO, a member of the U.S. delegation to NATO's Science Committee, and a member of the United Nations Science Committee. He also held positions on science committees of the International Atomic Energy Agency and the Arms Control and Disarmament Agency.

In addition to his key role in the founding of Brookhaven National Laboratory on Long Island, and his long-time stint as a trustee of that institution, Rabi also served as president of Associated Universities, Inc., the organization overseeing Brookhaven and the National Radio Astronomy Observatory. He was also instrumental in the establishment of the European Center for Nuclear Research (CERN) in Geneva, Switzerland.

Nationally, it was the result of Rabi's advice to his friend, President Dwight D. Eisenhower, a former president of Columbia University, that the President's Science Advisory Committee was elevated in importance and became a direct liaison between the president and the scientific community. The establishment of the Office of Special Assistant to the President for Science and Technology was also a Rabi suggestion enacted by President Eisenhower.

For his scientific achievements and humanitarian efforts, Rabi was the recipient of many awards in addition to the 1944 Nobel Prize in physics, including: the Elliot Cresson Medal of the Franklin Institute (1942), the U.S. Medal of Merit (1948), Britain's King's Medal (1948), the Barnard Medal (1960), the Priestley Memorial Medal of Dickinson College (1964), the Niels Bohr International Gold Medal (1967), the Atoms for Peace Award (1967), the Michael T. Pupin Medal of Columbia (1981), the Oersted Medal of the American Association of Physics Teachers (1982), the Franklin D. Roosevelt Four Freedoms Medal (1985), the Public Welfare Medal of the National Academy of Sciences (1985), the New York City Award for Science and Technology (1985), and the Vannevar Bush Award of the National Science Board (1986).

In addition to awards and medals, Rabi was the recipient of 20 honorary degrees, including degrees from Bar-Ilan University in Israel and the Jewish Theological Seminary in New York City. In Israel, he was also a member of the board of governors of Weizmann Institute of Science and a member of the board of trustees for Hebrew University in Jerusalem. In New York, he was a member of the board of trustees for Mount Sinai Hospital. In addition to serving as president of the American Physical Society, Rabi was a member of the National Academy of Sciences and the American Philosophical Society, an officer in the French Legion of Honor, and Commander of the Order of the Southern Cross of Brazil.

I.I. Rabi: Loyal and Honored Columbian

As evidenced by his comparison of Cornell and Columbia Universities, Rabi was fiercely loyal to the school from which he had received his PhD degree and where he had served as a faculty member for so many years. Although he was not blind to its faults, he was a strong voice in pointing out its strengths. In a time when anti-Semitism had been particularly apparent in the United States, Columbia University had chosen to select him as a lecturer and Rabi never forgot that.

Perhaps, in part, that loyalty accounted for his reaction when student radicals took over Columbia for a time in 1970 and brought everything to a halt. By that time, Rabi was retired and off the school's payroll, but was still seen regularly at his old office and laboratory. Loyalty to Columbia, however, was probably only partly responsible for his reaction, as a letter written to the editor of the *New York Times* by a visiting scholar of linguistics suggested so eloquently. The writer began by quoting from an earlier news report which described Professor Rabi being blocked from his laboratory, the same laboratory in which he had made his great scientific discoveries, "by a group of young men with arms linked across the door."

"Dr. Rabi tried to argue with them unsuccessfully. Exasperated, tears in his eyes, he tapped his cane on the granite step and said: 'What you are doing is wrong, and you are crazy. You are blocking my way. Do you want to fight with me? Would you fight with me?' "

Why the tears in his eyes? queried the letter writer, who then responded to his own question.

Why, indeed? Does Dr. Rabi's memory reach back further than the empty minds of the smiling student onlookers?
I can only surmise, but perhaps he was thinking of other times, other places, some long ago and far away—when distinguished professors in great universities were not permitted to enter their classrooms or their laboratories, when the light of learning went out for much of mankind, when elite groups (often dedicated to the point of dying for their goals) preached their catechisms and made "demands." And so many were spectators—and were amused.[230]

Fortunately, the takeover was not permanent and the light of learning continued shining at Columbia. Seven years later, both the man and the building were honored by that institution.

The physics department had moved into the newly-built Pupin Hall in 1926. Named for Columbia physicist Michael I. Pupin, a major scientific figure whose research and inventions helped make possible long-distance telephone calls, the 13-story, red-brick building had opened formally in 1927, the same year that Rabi received his PhD degree. It has been said that more physics history may have been made in that building at Broadway and 120th Street than in any other single building in the United States. In 1965, the building was designated a national landmark.

As of 1977, the 50th anniversary of the building's formal opening, 14 Nobel laureates had either taught or studied in the building and eight of them had done their Nobel Prize-winning work there. Scientists working there had discovered heavy hydrogen, invented the maser (forerunner to the laser), devised experiments that clarified significantly an understanding of the structural basis of elementary particles and nuclei, and disproved parity conservation, previously considered "fundamental."

In announcing a two-day symposium honoring the occasion, organizer Samuel Devons said, "In many ways, Dr. Rabi, the Pupin building and the rise of American physics are inseparably linked."[231] During that event, Columbia President William J. McGill announced plans to establish a professorship in Dr. Rabi's name, a position designed to have a university-wide role in bringing "mature areas of study and investigation, including law, government, international affairs, journalism and other disciplines where scientific considerations are prominent and scientific knowledge is essential."[232]

The cross-fertilization emphasis was an obvious reflection of Dr. Rabi himself who often decried the separation between science and the general culture:

Why should not the professor of physics be expected to refresh himself every seven years, as in a sabbatical, by taking a course in aesthetics of comparative literature, or in the Greek drama? Why shouldn't the professor of medieval philosophy or the professor of ancient history take a course in modern physics and become acquainted with the profound thoughts underlying relativity and quantum mechanics? By taking in one another's wash, we might all become cleaner and more wholesome. . . .

Only by the fusion of science and the humanities can we hope to reach the wisdom appropriate to our day and generation. The scientist must learn to teach science in the spirit of wisdom, and in the light of the history of human thought and human effort, rather than as the geography of a universe uninhabited by mankind. Our colleagues in the non-scientific faculties must understand that if their teachings ignore the great scientific tradition and its accomplishments, however eloquent and elegant their words, they will lose meaning for this generation and will be barren of fruit.[233]

The two-day symposium at Columbia was not the first time the school had recognized the merits of Rabi's theme nor the first time he had been singularly honored for his contributions to the institution.

Although Rabi had been a Higgins Professor of Physics from 1950 to 1964, a special honor in its own right, he was appointed in 1964 as a University Professor at Columbia, a position which enabled him to teach courses without reference to departmental boundaries. (He was the first to be given that title in the University's then 210-year history. Only three may hold that title at any one time.) In 1967, upon his retirement from Columbia, Rabi was named University Professor Emeritus.

But there were yet more honors that Columbia would bestow on its beloved professor. In 1979, a Rabi Visiting Professorship was established, funded by the Sloan Foundation. For academic year 1983-84, the honor was given to Jeremy Bernstein, the physicist-historian who was both an academician and a long-time staff member of *The New Yorker*.

In 1980, Rabi received an honor that normally is bestowed on scholars one-fourth his age, a Phi Beta Kappa key. As an undergraduate at Cornell earning a bachelor's degree in chemistry, they didn't bestow Phi Beta Kappas, he explained, as it was considered more a professional program. In announcing the award, Ward Dennis, dean of the School of General Studies, said: "We felt it was time that someone made up for that long-standing omission in the distinguished record of so great and so loved a Columbia teacher."[234]

In 1985 came the greatest Columbia-bestowed honor of all, the Isidor Isaac Rabi Chair in Physics, which came about through Rabi's long-time friendship with Abraham Gelbart, the co-developer of the theory of pseudo-analytic functions.

In 1982, Bar-Ilan University in Israel had established the Abraham Gelbart Chair in honor of the noted Jewish mathematician, funded by David and Rosalie Rose, and in 1990, renamed its International Research Institute in Math and Sciences the Gelbart International Research Institute in Math and Sciences.

Although David Rose, the same person who had funded the Gelbart Chair at Bar-Ilan was very impressed with Rabi and wanted to meet him.

"So I introduced him to Rabi," recalled Gelbart, "and he was very enamored of him. He then asked Rabi whether Columbia had done anything in his name. And Rabi sort of shrugged his shoulders as if to say, 'I don't know. What should have been done in my name?'

"So David Rose said, 'Well, did they establish a chair in your name?' And Rabi said, 'No.' So he said, 'Well, they should.' "

At that point, Gelbart suggested that they meet with the president of Columbia University and talk it over. When Rose told him that a chair should be established for Rabi, the president said, "It will cost about a million and a quarter," to which David Rose responded, "No problem."[235]

The Isidor Isaac Rabi Chair in Physics was established in 1985 and is presently held by Nobel laureate and Columbia alumnus Melvin

Schwartz who resigned his position at Brookhaven National Laboratory
in 1994 to accept the permanent, tenured position.

In a *New York Times* article announcing the Rabi Chair, author James
Gleick wrote, "Columbia University's trustees had one great honor left to
give I.I. Rabi, and they gave it yesterday, announcing the creation of an
Isidor Isaac Rabi chair in physics.

> Columbia has named few professorships for its scholars in their
> lifetimes. Dr. Rabi, its first University Professor, the Nobel Prize win-
> ner who created its renowned postwar physics department, was rec-
> ognized at the age of 87 for a rare combination of achievements in
> pure science and public service.
>
> "I.I. Rabi is a brilliant jewel in Columbia's crown," said Columbia's
> president, Michael I. Sovern. "He is one of the truly extraordinary
> scientists of our century, a wise and humane man who has been and
> remains a beacon for nuclear sanity in our threatened world. We are
> exceptionally proud to create a professorship in the name of this wor-
> thy man."[236]

Afterward, when asked for a statement about the honor, Rabi responded, "I'm pleased, of course, but there's always another side—to have this
named chair, you really ought to be dead. It may be a case of over-
survival." Recalling how it had all begun, the former immigrant from
Rymanow and one-time resident of the turn-of-the-century slums on
Manhattan's Lower East Side said, "It was only by accident that I discovered the kind of chemistry I liked was called physics. Physics addresses
the problem of what is." As he had said many times before, he added,
"It's the only game for a gentleman."[237]

He had played the game like no one else in this century. "I've tried to
be a 20th-century man," he had told the students at Claremont in 1960,
linking that ambition to his choice of an occupation in science. It's interesting to note that in 1981, on the occasion of being awarded the Michael
T. Pupin Medal at Columbia, Rabi was described as "the outstanding
American scientist of the century."[238] The citation which accompanied the
medal read as follows:

> You have set the standards of excellence for generations of scien-
> tists, not only here at Columbia, but throughout the United States
> and the world. Your ground-breaking work in atomic physics which
> led to the 1944 Nobel Prize brought honor and respectability to the

entire American scientific community, and provided the basis for the flowering of research in physics, chemistry and biology—a flowering that continues to this very day. Many scientific advances have been made, and many great prizes awarded, because of your personal commitment to research and your sustained devotion to the welfare and prestige of science.

As a public servant you have changed the world. Your name is well known in Los Alamos, in Vienna, in Jerusalem, in NATO and UNESCO; you have lent your efforts and your insights to every agency and organization concerned with the growth of science and its appropriate management . . . you have been responsible for many presidential decisions on the practical uses of science, and for many international conferences on the peaceful uses of atomic energy.[239]

When Rabi received the Pupin Medal at the age of 82, he stated that he was working on an autobiography entitled *Celebrations* because, he said, "I've been so fortunate that every misfortune has turned into a good thing." As a case in point, he said, "I was a graduate student at Cornell, but I didn't get a fellowship, so I had to come to Columbia."[240] ∎

REFERENCE NOTES:

1. I.I. Rabi, *My Life and Times as a Physicist*, (Claremont, CA: Claremont College, 1960), 39.
2. I.I. Rabi, J.R. Zacharias, S. Millman, P. Kusch, "A new method of measuring nuclear magnetic moment," *Physical Review* **53**, (1938), 318.
3. J.M.B. Kellogg, I.I. Rabi, N.F. Ramsey, and J.R. Zacharias, "The magnetic moments of the proton and the deuteron: the radiofrequency spectrum of H_2 in various magnetic fields," *Physical Review* **56**, (1939), 728.
4. J.M.B. Kellogg, I.I. Rabi, N.F. Ramsey, and J.R. Zacharias, "An electrical quadrupole moment of the deuteron," *Physical Review* **55**, (1939), 318.
5. J.E. Nafe, E.B. Nelson, and I.I. Rabi, "The hyperfine structure of atomic hydrogen and deuterium," *Physical Review* **71**, (1947), 914-915.
6. W.W. Havens, Jr., I.I. Rabi, and L.J. Rainwater, "Interaction of neutrons with electrons in lead," *Physical Review* **72**, (1947), 636.
7. Rabi, *My Life and Times as a Physicist*, 44.
8. Jeremy Bernstein, "Profiles: physicist-I," *The New Yorker*, 13 October 1975, 47.
9. I.I. Rabi, interview by Barbara Land, 12 November 1962, transcript, Columbia Oral History, Columbia University, New York, 1.
10. Ibid.
11. Department of Commerce, Bureau of the Census, Fourteenth Census of the United States: 1920, Borough of Brooklyn, Enumeration District No. 1504, Sheet 11, enumerated January 8, 1920.
12. I.I. Rabi, interview by Land, 1.
13. *The World Almanac and Book of Facts, 1991*, (New York: Pharos Books, 1990), 439.
14. *American Jewish Yearbook, 1899*, Jewish Publication Society, American Jewish Committee; information provided by Balch Institute for Ethnic Studies, Philadelphia, PA.
15. Bernstein, "Profiles: physicist-I," 47.
16. I.I. Rabi, interview by Edwin Newman, December 1972, transcript, William E. Weiner Oral History Library, New York, 4-5; quoted by Rigden in *Rabi: Scientist and Citizen*, 18.
17. Michael S. Durham, *The Smithsonian Guide to Historic America, The Mid-Atlantic States*, (New York: Stewart, Tabori & Chang, 1989), 46.
18. I.I. Rabi, interview by Land, 31.
19. Rigden, *Rabi: Scientist and Citizen*, 20.
20. Oscar Handlin, *The Uprooted*, Second Edition (Boston: Little, Brown & Company, 1972), 132-133, 135.
21. I.I. Rabi, interview by Land, 31.
22. Bernstein, "Profiles: physicist-I," 48.
23. Mark Zborowski and Elizabeth Herzog, *Life Is With People*, (New York: Schocken Books, 1952), 37.
24. Bernstein, "Profiles: physicist-I," 48.
25. I.I. Rabi, interview by Land, 34-35.
26. Ibid., 35.
27. Ibid., 33.
28. Bernstein, "Profiles: physicist-I," 49.
29. I.I. Rabi, interview by Thomas S. Kuhn, 8 December 1963, transcript, Niels Bohr Library, American Institute of Physics, College Park, MD, 1.
30. I.I. Rabi, interview by Land, 3.
31. Rigden, *Rabi: Scientist and Citizen*, 20.
32. I.I. Rabi, interview by Land, 3.
33. Ibid., 5.
34. Bernstein, "Profiles: physicist-I," 50.
35. I.I. Rabi, interview by Land, 36.

36. Ibid., 39.

37. I.I. Rabi, interview by Stephen White, 11 February 1980, transcript, Rabi private collection, 20; quoted by Rigden in *Rabi: Scientist and Citizen*, 28.

38. Bernstein, "Profiles: physicist-I," 50.

39. J.M.B. Kellogg, I.I. Rabi, N.F. Ramsey, and J.R. Zacharias, "The magnetic moments of the proton and the deuteron: the radiofrequency spectrum of H_2 in various magnetic fields," *Physical Review* **56**, (1939), 728.

40. I.I. Rabi, interview by Land, 7.

41. Bernstein, "Profiles: physicist-I," 53.

42. I.I. Rabi, interview by Land, 7.

43. I.I. Rabi, interview by Kuhn, 2.

44. I.I. Rabi, interview by Land, 8.

45. Bernstein, "Profiles: physicist-I," 53-54.

46. Ibid., 50.

47. I.I. Rabi, interview by Land, 42-43.

48. Ibid., 44.

49. Ibid., 41.

50. Bernstein, "Profiles: physicist-I," 54.

51. Ibid.

52. I.I. Rabi, interview by Kuhn, 4.

53. I.I. Rabi, interview by Land, 46.

54. Ibid., 47.

55. I.I. Rabi, interview by Kuhn, 2.

56. I.I. Rabi, interview by Land, 47.

57. I.I. Rabi, interview by Kuhn, 1-2.

58. Department of Commerce, Bureau of the Census, Enumeration District No. 1504, Sheet 11, enumerated January 8, 1920.

59. I.I. Rabi, interview by Kuhn, 3.

60. I.I. Rabi, interview by Land, 10-11.

61. Ibid., 12-13.

62. Ibid., 13, 47-48.

63. Ibid., 14-15.

64. Ibid., 50.

65. Ibid., 15.

66. Bernstein, "Profiles: physicist-I," 54.

67. I.I. Rabi, interview by Kuhn, 5.

68. I.I. Rabi, interview by Land, 16.

69. I.I. Rabi, interview by Kuhn, 6.

70. Rigden, *Rabi: Scientist and Citizen*, 33.

71. I.I. Rabi, interview by Land, 50, 16.

72. Ibid., 17.

73. Rigden, *Rabi: Scientist and Citizen*, 34.

74. Ibid.

75. I.I. Rabi, interview by Kuhn, 6.

76. I.I. Rabi, interview by Land, 17.

77. I.I. Rabi, interview by Kuhn, 6-7.

78. I.I. Rabi, interview by Land, 18.

79. I.I. Rabi, interview by Kuhn, 7.

80. Rigden, *Rabi: Scientist and Citizen*, 37.

81. Ibid.

82. Ibid.

83. Ibid.

84. I.I. Rabi, interview by Kuhn, 9.

85. I.I. Rabi, interview by Land, 54.

86. I.I. Rabi, interview by Kuhn, 8.

87. I.I. Rabi, interview by Land, 21.

88. Ibid., 53-54.

89. Bernstein, "Profiles: physicist-I," 54.

90. I.I. Rabi, interview by Kuhn, 10.

91. Bernstein, "Profiles: physicist-I," 78.

92. Arnold Sommerfeld, *Atombau und Spektrallinien*, 1st ed., (Vieweg: Braunschweig, 1919).

93. Max Born, *Vorlesungen über Atommechanik*, (Berlin: Springer, 1925).

94. I.I. Rabi, interview by Kuhn, 10.

95. I.I. Rabi, interview by Land, 58-59.

96. Ibid., 63.

97. I.I. Rabi, interview by Kuhn, 29.

98. I.I. Rabi, interview by Land, 107.

99. Ibid., 54.

100. Ibid., 54-55.

101. Bernstein, "Profiles: physicist-I," 58.

102. Norman F. Ramsey, interview by Joan Safford, July 1960, transcript, Niels Bohr Library, American Institute of Physics, College Park, MD, 25.

103. I.I. Rabi, interview by Kuhn, 35.

104. I.I. Rabi, interview by Land, 56.

105. Bernstein, "Profiles: physicist-I," 60.

106. Rigden, *Rabi: Scientist and Citizen*, 41.

107. Bernstein, "Profiles: physicist-I," 60.

108. Ibid.

109. I.I. Rabi, interview by Kuhn, 12.

110. I.I. Rabi, "On the principal magnetic susceptibilities of crystals," *Physical Review* **29**, (1927), 174-185.

111. I.I. Rabi, interview by Land, 63.

112. R. de L. Kronig and I.I. Rabi, *Physical Review* **29**, (1927), 262.

113. I.I. Rabi, interview by Land, 24.

114. Ibid.

115. Ibid., 70.

116. Ibid., 26.

117. Ibid., 73.

118. I.I. Rabi, interview by Kuhn, 21.

119. Ibid., 29.

120. Rigden, *Rabi: Scientist and Citizen*, 57.

121. I.I. Rabi, interview by Land, 79.

122. I.I. Rabi, interview by Kuhn, 26.

123. Ibid., 28.

124. Ibid., 21.

125. I.I. Rabi, interview by Land, 81.

126. I.I. Rabi, interview by Kuhn, 21.

127. Bernstein, "Profiles: physicist-I," 53; "Profiles: Physicist-II,"*The New Yorker*, 20 October 1975, 58.

128. Bernstein, "Profiles: physicist-I," 85.

129. Ibid.

130. I.I. Rabi, interview by Land, 83.

131. Henry A. Boorse, Lloyd Motz, and Jefferson Hane Weaver, *The Atomic Scientists: A Biographical History*, (New York: John Wiley & Sons, 1989), 253.

132. I.I. Rabi, interview by Land, 84-85.
133. Ibid., 97.
134. Ibid., 85.
135. Ibid., 88-89.
136. Ibid., 93.
137. Rigden, *Rabi: Scientist and Citizen*, 86.
138. I.I. Rabi, interview by Land, 28.
139. Ibid., 90.
140. Ibid., 95.
141. Ibid., 29.
142. Rigden, *Rabi: Scientist and Citizen*, 64.
143. I.I. Rabi, "Refraction of beams of molecules," *Nature* **123** (1929), 163-164; I.I. Rabi, "Zur methode der ablenkung von molekularstrahlen," *Zeitschrift für Physik* **54,** (1929), 190-197.
144. Rigden, *Rabi: Scientist and Citizen*, 66.
145. I.I. Rabi, interview by Land, 103.
146. Ibid.
147. Bernstein, "Profiles: physicist-I," 85.
148. Ibid., 95.
149. I.I. Rabi, interview by Land, 97, 106-107.
150. Ibid., 105-106.
151. Ibid., 107-108.
152. Bernstein, "Profiles: physicist-I," 95.
153. I.I. Rabi, interview by Land, 110.
154. Norman F. Ramsey, interview by Safford, 25.
155. Rigden, *Rabi: Scientist and Citizen*, 71.
156. Ibid., 72.
157. I.I. Rabi, interview by Land, 79.
158. Ibid., 102.
159. I.I. Rabi, interview by Kuhn, 35-36.
160. I.I. Rabi, interview by Land, 104.
161. Boorse, Motz, and Weaver, *The Atomic Scientists: A Biographical History*, 387.
162. Rigden, *Rabi: Scientist and Citizen*, 116.
163. Bernstein, "Profiles: physicist-I," 60.
164. Norman F. Ramsey, interview by Safford, 24.
165. I.I. Rabi, interview by Land, 112.
166. Ibid., 116-117.
167. Rigden, *Rabi: Scientist and Citizen*, 79.
168. F.W. Loomis and R.W. Wood, "The Rotational Structure of the Blue-Green Bands of Na_2," *Physical Review* **32,** (1928), 223-36.
169. Harold Urey, "The alternating intensities of Na_2 bands," *Physical Review* **38,** (1931), 1074-75.
170. G. Breit and I.I. Rabi, "The measurement of nuclear spin," *Physical Review* **38,** (1931), 2082-83.
171. Ibid., 2082.
172. Ibid., 2083.
173. I.I. Rabi, interview by Land, 123.
174. Rigden, *Rabi: Scientist and Citizen*, 80.
175. I.I. Rabi, interview by Kuhn, 26.
176. I.I. Rabi, interview by Land, 126.
177. Rigden, *Rabi: Scientist and Citizen*, 82.
178. Ibid., 88.
179. Ibid., 80.

180. Genesis 32:28.

181. Rabi, *My Life and Times as a Physicist*, 28.

182. I.I. Rabi, interview by Land, 126.

183. Ibid., 129.

184. I.I. Rabi, J.M.B. Kellogg, and J.R. Zacharias, "The magnetic moment of the proton," *Physical Review* **46**, (1934), 157-163.

185. I.I. Rabi, J.M.B. Kellogg, and J.R. Zacharias, "The magnetic moment of the deuton," *Physical Review* **46**, (1934), 163-165.

186. I.I. Rabi, "On the process of space quantization," *Physical Review* **49**, (1936), 324-328.

187. I.I. Rabi, "Space quantization in a gyrating magnetic field," *Physical Review* **51**, (1937), 652-654.

188. N.F. Ramsey, "Early magnetic resonance experiments: roots and offshoots," *Physics Today*, October 1993, 40.

189. Ibid., 41.

190. Rigden, *Rabi: Scientist and Citizen*, 96.

191. Ibid., 97-98.

192. I.I. Rabi, J.R. Zacharias, S. Millman, P. Kusch, "A new method of measuring nuclear magnetic moment," *Physical Review* **53**, (1938), 318.

193. I.I. Rabi, S. Millman, P. Kusch, J.R. Zacharias, "The molecular beam resonance method for measuring nuclear magnetic moments: the magnetic moments of $_3Li^6$, $_3Li^7$ and $_9F^{19}$," *Physical Review* **55**, (1939), 526-535.

194. J.M.B. Kellogg, I.I. Rabi, N.F. Ramsey, and J.M.B. Kellogg, "An electrical quadrupole moment of the deuteron," *Physical Review* **55**, (1939), 318.

195. I.I. Rabi, J.R. Zacharias, S. Millman, P. Kusch, "A new method of measuring nuclear magnetic moment," *Physical Review* **53**, (1938), 318.

196. Ibid.

197. "We're all radio stations, Columbia scientists report," *New York Post*, 29 December 1939.

198. I.I. Rabi, interview by Kuhn, 2.

199. Bernstein, "Profiles: physicist-I," 109.

200. Ibid.

201. Rabi, *My Life and Times as a Physicist*, 3.

202. Rigden, *Rabi: Scientist and Citizen*, 152.

203. Bernstein, "Profiles: physicist-II," 54.

204. Ibid., 58.

205. I.I. Rabi, television interview with Bill Moyers, 26 June 1983.

206. Rabi, *My Life and Times as a Physicist*, 2-3.

207. N.F. Ramsey, "I.I. Rabi," *Physics Today*, October 1988, 84.

208. "A tribute to one of Columbia's great teachers," *Time*, 26 May 1967.

209. "Says Japanese scientists don't resent bombs' use," *Herald Tribune*, 13 January 1949.

210. Niels H. de V. Heathcote, *Nobel Prize Winners in Physics*, 1901-1950, (New York: Henry Schuman, 1953), 410.

211. Bernstein, "Profiles: physicist-II," 56.

212. Rigden, *Rabi: Scientist and Citizen*, 164.

213. Ibid.

214. Bernstein, "Profiles: physicist-II," 63-64.

215. I.I. Rabi, interview by Kuhn, 28.

216. "Portrait of a man of science," *Columbia University Quarterly*, Summer 1963.

217. Norman Ramsey, interview by James Mattson, 13 May 1994.

218. Ibid.

219. Ramsey, "I.I. Rabi," *Physics Today*, October 1988, 84.

220. W.W. Havens, Jr., I.I. Rabi, and L.J. Rainwater, "Interaction of neutrons with electrons in lead," *Physical Review* **72**, (1947), 636.

221. Earl Ubell, "Be 'odd ball,' Dr. Rabi says to scientists," *Herald Tribune*, 16 May 1959.

222. John Leo, "I.I. Rabi teaches last class after 40 years at Columbia," *New York Times*, 18 June 1967.

223. "Humanistic scientist," *New York Times*, 28 October 1964.

224. James Gleick, "Columbia lauds Rabi as its 'brilliant jewel'," *New York Times*, 21 November 1985.

225. Estelle Gilson, "A profile in candor: I.I. Rabi," *Columbia Magazine*, April 1984, 25.

226. Ibid., 27.

227. Ibid., 28.

228. Ibid.

229. Ibid., 29.

230. Paul K. Benedict, letter to the editor, *New York Times*, published 15 May 1970.

231. Press release, Office of Public Information, Columbia University, 28 October 1977.

232. Ibid.

233. Rabi, *My Life and Times as a Physicist*, 54-55.

234. Press release, Office of Public Information, Columbia University, 8 May 1980.

235. Abraham Gelbart, interview by James Mattson, 7 June 1994.

236. Gleick, "Columbia lauds Rabi as its 'brilliant jewel'," 21 November 1985.

237. Ibid.

238. Rabi, *My Life and Times as a Physicist*, 39.

239. Press release announcing Rabi as recipient of Pupin Medal, Office of Public Information, Columbia University, 20 March 1981.

240. Albin Krebs and Robert McG. Thomas, Jr., "Dr. Rabi receives Pupin Medal for service to nation," *New York Times*, April 1, 1981.

There is nothing that nuclear spins will not do for you, as long as you treat them as human beings.

—Erwin L. Hahn

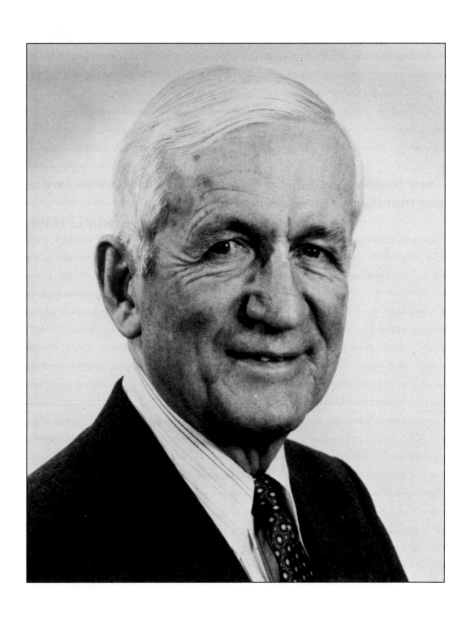

NORMAN F. RAMSEY

Pioneer of Magnetic Resonance Spectroscopy and
Originator of the First Successful Chemical Shift Theory

To REVIEW the career of Norman F. Ramsey is to review the role of a
key scientific figure in some of the most significant front-page news of the
20th century, including:

1) The development of radar as an effective military tool against
Germany and Japan in World War II (Ramsey was in charge of develop-
ment of 3-centimeter radar from 1940 to 1942 at the MIT Radiation
Laboratory, technology that played a major role in the Allied victory);

2) the development of atomic bombs (Ramsey was head of the delivery
group responsible for converting what were basically experimental pro-
totypes into deliverable weapons);

3) the McCarthy hearings in the early years of the Cold War that fueled
fears of Communist infiltration of government, entertainment and academia (Ramsey supported Professor Wendell Furry of Harvard, accused of
spying by Senator Joseph McCarthy because of Furry's association with
Communist groups in the 1930s; Ramsey was one of the first, on television's "Meet the Press," to publicly point out the evils of a national para-
noia that denied due process of law);

4) the 1954 hearing by the Atomic Energy Commission to determine
whether J. Robert Oppenheimer's security clearance should be revoked
because of his alleged association with Communist organizations (both
Ramsey and I.I. Rabi were key witnesses in support of the former scientific director of the Manhattan Project); and

5) as recently as 1982, the lingering controversy surrounding the assassination of President John F. Kennedy and the conclusions of the Warren
Commission (a panel of distinguished scientists headed by Ramsey
showed the invalidity of claimed acoustic evidence for a second gunman
on the basis of a Dallas police transmission received at headquarters, pre-

sumably from a police-motorcycle microphone left on during the shooting).[1-2]

To review Ramsey's career is also to review, however, the significant contributions of a scientist which did not initially appear on the front page of a daily newspaper, but rather in the relatively obscure pages of scientific journals. Only later would their far-reaching ramifications become more apparent to the general public with:

1) The development of the atomic clock, which has improved the accuracy of time-keeping a million-fold in 50 years, brought us such spectacular space achievements as the Voyager "close-up" of Neptune, changed the internationally-accepted definition of the second, and made possible the development of the Global Positioning System, and;

2) the development of radiofrequency spectroscopy and chemical-shift theory which, after revolutionizing chemical analysis a few decades ago, were vital components in the development of magnetic resonance scanning as a tool for medical diagnosis, the capabilities of which have only begun to be exploited.

The Nobel committee awarded Norman Ramsey the 1989 Nobel Prize in physics specifically for his invention of the separated oscillatory fields method and the atomic hydrogen maser, but the 1990 Britannica Book of the Year noted that "for many observers," Ramsey's invitation to appear before the Swedish Academy of Science in Stockholm "was as much a recognition of his lifetime contribution to science as an acknowledgment of any particular achievement."[3] And, indeed, it could be argued that other of his accomplishments were likewise worthy of the prize:

1) In 1939, he shared in the discovery of the deuteron's electric quadrupole moment, ranked by Nobel laureate Hans Bethe as one of the top three developments to come along in the early years of nuclear physics.[4] The quadrupole moment implied the existence of a previously-unknown nuclear tensor force between the neutron and the proton, a force which Ramsey and his associates were able to measure.

2) In a series of publications in 1950 and 1951, Ramsey developed the first successful theory of the chemical shift observed experimentally with NMR techniques. Chemical shifts in NMR have revolutionized chemical analysis.

3) Based on experiments with Robert Pound and Edward Purcell, Ramsey developed the theory of thermodynamics at negative absolute temperatures[5] and discovered that, as he expressed it, "one of the most popular statements of the Second Law of Thermodynamics is incorrect when one recognizes the existence of thermodynamic systems at negative absolute temperatures."[6]

4) Seven years before Tsung Dao Lee, Chen Ning Yang, Chien-Shiung Wu and others disproved the law of conservation of parity in 1957, for which Lee and Yang were awarded the Nobel Prize the same year, Norman Ramsey and Edward Purcell wrote the first paper questioning the parity assumption and showing the lack of experimental evidence for that assumption.[7] Ramsey, in collaboration with others, discovered in 1980 the first parity non-conserving spin rotation for a neutron passing through solid materials and measured this rotation in tin, lead and lanthanum.[8]

5) Similarly, seven years before Christenson, Cronin, Fitch and Turlay disproved time reversal (T) symmetry in 1964, for which Cronin and Fitch were awarded the Nobel Prize in 1980, Norman Ramsey and J.D. Jackson published papers, independently of each other, pointing out that T symmetry was also an assumption that required an experimental basis and that a search for a neutron electric dipole moment would provide such a test.[9-10] Although Ramsey has searched since 1949 for the neutron's electric dipole moment and has never found it, he has succeeded over a 30-year period in establishing successively lower limits for its value, lowering it from an initial value of 10^{-15} e cm to $(-3 \pm 5) \times 10^{-26}$ e cm.

Ramsey also succeeded in significantly increasing the accuracy of the measurement of the magnetic moment of the neutron. Fifty years after Felix Bloch and Luis Alvarez measured it with magnetic resonance at -1.93 ± 0.02 absolute nuclear magnetons, Norman Ramsey noted in his Nobel lecture that he and his associates had been able to add six additional digits to the right of the decimal point, establishing it at $-1.91304275 \pm 0.00000045$ nuclear magnetons.[11-14]

6) In addition to all of the above, Ramsey and his collaborators have measured and provided theories for a large number of nuclear and magnetic properties including nuclear and rotational magnetic moments, spin-spin magnetic interactions, spin-rotational interactions, nuclear electric quadrupole moments, scalar electron coupled spin-spin interactions, the dependence of nuclear magnetic shielding upon molecular orientation and the dependence of molecular diamagnetic susceptibilities on molecular orientation. As of 1994, his bibliography of professional publications, going back to 1938, totaled 386 and was still growing.[15]

Son of a Mathematician and a General

Had you been in Washington, D.C. on August 15, 1915, the day Norman Foster Ramsey, Jr. was born, and predicted that, based on his mother's and father's occupations, he would someday be involved in mathematics and military operations, you would not have been far off the mark. Like his mother, one of the future physicist's strengths would be mathematics, and although he would never wear the uniform of a soldier like his father, an Army general, he would be an active scientific combatant in World War II a full year before the bombing of Pearl Harbor brought the United States officially into the war, and for the last three years of that conflict, Ramsey would find his services needed by the U.S. Secretary of War.

Ramsey's mother, Minna (Bauer) Ramsey, a daughter of German immigrants, was once a mathematics instructor at the University of Kansas and his father, descended from Scottish refugees, was a West Point graduate and an officer in the Army Ordnance Corps. "My father's frequently changing assignments," Ramsey wrote in the autobiographical sketch he provided the Nobel Foundation, "took us from Washington, D.C. to Topeka, Kansas, to Paris, France, to Picatinny Arsenal near Dover, New Jersey, and to Fort Leavenworth, Kansas. With two of the moves I skipped a grade and, encouraged by my supportive parents and teachers, I graduated from high school with a high academic record at the age of 15."[16] Young Norman was able to skip grades each time the family moved west, where the schools lagged somewhat behind Eastern schools.

It was after he began attending the public high school in Fort Leavenworth, Kansas that Ramsey recalls first getting more interested in science, although at the time he didn't realize physics was a career option. In the 1920s, chemistry and engineering were the two main science options.

As president and valedictorian of his graduating class, Ramsey was awarded a scholarship to the University of Kansas, but decided not to use it when his father was transferred back East, this time to Governor's Island, almost in the shadow of the Statue of Liberty in New York City's busy harbor.

His parents had always planned that he would attend the United States Military Academy at West Point since he was the son of an Army officer, but at age 15, Ramsey was too young. He was also too young, according to official rules, to enter Massachusetts Institute of Technology. He found out later that the rules were not always strictly enforced, and although he would have been 16 by the time he matriculated, only a year less than the requirement, his parents felt that rules are rules and if they said you had to be 17 to enter, you had to be 17.

Ramsey decided the only alternative was to bide his time and enter a New York preparatory school, until a perceptive administrator at the prep school told him he would probably be bored at his institution and recommended instead he apply to Columbia University.

Columbia University

Ramsey hadn't even considered Columbia, though he remembered seeing an announcement on his high-school bulletin board that the New York City college was looking for graduates from the Midwest to improve their geographic diversity. (He found out later that, with his academic record, he would have been a "complete pushover" to win a scholarship.) He had once attended, when he was about eight, a football game pitting Columbia against a greatly-superior West Point—Columbia was badly beaten—but beyond that, he knew little about the school. Nevertheless, he applied to Columbia with the idea that it would be a temporary home for just one year. It turned out to be his academic home on an intermittent basis for more than 10 of the next 16 years and the institution from which he would receive one of his two bachelor degrees as well as his PhD.

Typical of many physicists educated during this period, Norman Ramsey initially planned to major in engineering, until he became unhappy with the excessive emphasis on engineering's handbooks and tables. That's when he switched to mathematics, and started accumulating a strong minor in physics.

Although his parents were "perfectly well off,"[17] and could have provided his entire educational support, Ramsey was able to supply a significant portion of his own support during each of his undergraduate years by winning Columbia's annual mathematics contest with its $300 prize money. In his senior year, he was awarded a teaching assistantship in mathematics, a position that normally went only to graduate students.

At the time he entered Columbia in 1931—less than two years after the stock market crash in October of 1929—the United States was in the throes of the Great Depression, but Ramsey's family was spared from much of it because of his father's occupation.

School teachers and Army officers [said Ramsey] both have the characteristic that their prosperity is another person's depression, in that their salaries tend to go up slowly in an inflation period and down slowly in a deflation period. So, as far as my family was personally concerned, except for some stocks my parents had invested in which diminished, we were in fine shape. This was an abnormal situation. The average person in school was very much affected by [the Depression].[18]

Ramsey was affected by the pain others were experiencing during that period. "It had a big effect on me. I worried quite a lot about things at that time, even though I personally was not in financial trouble. Many of my friends were, and that bothered me."[19]

Typical of many colleges in the early 1930s, a large number of students at Columbia University were disillusioned with capitalism, an economic system that, to them, appeared to have failed. They were looking for alternative answers and many thought the answer was communism.

> The most active political group at Columbia [said Ramsey] was the so-called Social Problems Club. We all suspected at the time that a fair fraction of the members were members of the Communist Party, and actually, subsequently, this has proved to be the case. They were on the whole very bright people; I always had a high regard for them.
>
> With the Depression, I think it was quite understandable. The people who, perhaps more than most, were willing to follow their consciences and what looked like the rational course were probably the ones nearest the Left group. . . . And I think a fair fraction of the students who didn't do something like that just didn't have the nerve to follow the logic of their argument. So I always respected them, although I'm glad I didn't happen to join.[20]

Two decades later, the pragmatic wisdom of that decision would become clearer with the start of the Cold War and the rise of McCarthyism. On "Meet the Press," Ramsey would be one of the first to publicly point out the "real evils done by the McCarthy Committee,"[21] a stand that might well have drawn the attention of McCarthy's intimidating searchlight had Ramsey's record not been above reproach. (McCarthy, in fact, was so impressed with Ramsey's performance on the nationally-televised program that he tried to hire him as his director of publicity at a higher salary than he was getting as a professor at Harvard, an offer Ramsey did not seriously entertain.)[22]

In the early 1930s, however, long before the lines of the Cold War were drawn between East and West, with capitalism reeling groggily against the ropes as the Depression deepened and with communism romanticized as the inevitable economic victor, Ramsey, like many during that period, listened sympathetically to political speeches in Manhattan's Union Square and tried to compare capitalism, with its weaknesses exposed by the Depression, to communism which was, as yet, unproven.

I think the most misleading thing at that time [said Ramsey], which really is the reason to a fair degree that their popularity was high, was that most of us got talked into making a rather unfair comparison; namely a comparison of the situation as it was then in the United States with the situation as they hoped it would be in Russia at a future time. Well, this isn't quite fair. . . . Of course, there was a good argument for not doing that. They could argue that the Russian system was a very new one, and [to compare the two systems according to the same measure] wasn't fair.[23]

With fear and anger providing the fuel, a heated debate was all that was sometimes needed to touch off an explosion of emotion and the police department would respond by sending in the riot squad.

It was perfectly obvious that we were in a depression [said Ramsey], particularly in New York City. There were lots of people looking for work and asking for handouts, and a fair amount of political discussion ending sometimes in a fight or violent rioting. . . . The New York Riot Squad was fairly developed. It was part of the education I acquired.[24]

Like I.I. Rabi, Ramsey's future PhD mentor and colleague, who had seriously considered the claims of socialists during the first decade of the 20th century and then lost interest when he found their claims impractical, Ramsey considered the merits of communism in the 1930s and then rejected them when he found the system incapable of delivering on its promises. As a result of their honest searches, both men were instilled with a lifelong sense of justice that would make them unwilling to stand by when others who had made their own search were later presumed guilty of disloyalty to their country, in spite of evidence to the contrary.*

---

* In 1953, Wendell Furry, a physics professor at Harvard, was called before the Velde Committee and later before a McCarthy hearing to defend himself against charges that he had supplied secret information to Communist spies. Eventually, although he was cited for contempt of Congress, the case was thrown out of court.

A year later, Robert Oppenheimer, who had been the scientific director of atomic bomb development during World War II and was later a member of the General Advisory Committee of the Atomic Energy Commission, had his security clearance revoked when proponents of a crash development program for a hydrogen bomb associated his opposition to the H-bomb with his past associations with known Communists.

As recently as April 26, 1994, when a best-selling book written by a former Soviet spy appeared to offer evidence incriminating J. Robert Oppenheimer, Enrico Fermi and Niels Bohr of giving classified information to the Soviet Union about U.S. atomic bomb development in the 1940s, Ramsey again felt constrained to refute what he saw as an unfair, poorly documented and error-riddled attack. The charges, made by a person who "had every reason to exaggerate his accomplishments as a spy" were "incompatible," said Ramsey, "with my knowledge of these great men."[25]

By the time Ramsey was ready to graduate from Columbia, he had come to realize, as Rabi had discovered a dozen years earlier, that the parts of chemistry he liked were the parts that were really physics[26] and that physics was a subject you could go into rather than one you used only as an adjunct to other pursuits. It was his penchant for mathematics, however, that opened the door to a Kellett Fellowship at Cambridge University in England.

Although the Kellett Fellowship was intended for students of letters, the mathematics department at Columbia, said Ramsey, "persuaded the group of people administrating the fellowships that alphas, betas and gammas were included in letters."[27] Once Ramsey's foot was in the door for the scholarship, he negotiated one more change by saying he would accept the fellowship obtained for him by the mathematics department, provided he could change from mathematics to physics. Permission was granted and Ramsey sailed for England in 1935 to begin work toward his second bachelor's degree.

Cambridge University

At Cambridge, Ramsey would have the opportunity to see and hear some of the greatest names in physics. Although the golden period of the famous Cavendish Laboratory founded by Scottish physicist James Clerk Maxwell was about to end—many of its top-notch physicists left within a year or so of Ramsey's departure—it was still flush with legendary physicists including its retired director J.J. Thomson (discoverer of the electron), its then-current director Lord Ernest Rutherford (discoverer of the nucleus), James Chadwick (discoverer of the neutron), as well as John Cockroft, Arthur Eddington, Max Born, R.H. Fowler, Edward Bullard, Maurice Goldhaber, P.I. Dee, Francis Aston, Paul A.M. Dirac, Norman Feather, Sir Edward Appleton and H.M. Lewis. "I knew Cockroft fairly well," Ramsey said, "and R.H. Fowler."[28]

He was instructed by all of them, including Max Born, formerly of Göttingen University, one of the first in the exodus of Jewish scientists from Hitler's Germany. J.J. Thomson, though retired at age 79, was still teaching a class and was usually quite interesting, said Ramsey. Rutherford, on the other hand, did not initially impress Ramsey. In fact, as a mathematician, Ramsey was "really rather appalled," he said, when he took Rutherford's course on the constitution of matter and found that the famous physicist had trouble with his mathematics.

> One of the saddest sights I've ever witnessed in a lecture was Rutherford deriving Rutherford's Scattering Law, because he got completely fouled up in the math, and he finally ended up by telling us to go home and work it out for ourselves.* In fact, my impression at the end of the year was that Rutherford was indeed typical of a British Lord but not very typical of a great physicist.[29]

That impression took a 180-degree turn the following summer when Ramsey had occasion to refer to his Rutherford notes and found them "fascinating," that they contained, in fact, "lots of very useful information." He was so impressed, in fact, that he went back to the same lecture series the following year. This time, when Rutherford again stumbled through the Rutherford Scattering Law creating just as much of a mathematical shambles as he had the previous year, Ramsey was no longer paying attention to the legend's mathematical errors but was focusing instead on the wonderful insights he was providing into physics. Instead of it being one of the worst courses he had ever taken, concluded Ramsey, "I found it to be just about the best course I'd ever taken. . . . The difference was that the second year I was concentrating on physics rather than mathematics."[30]

Rutherford, said Ramsey, would raise a number of very interesting questions in his course, very fundamental questions such as why electrons whirled around protons and not the other way around or, why shouldn't there be an electron cloud? What was the evidence against it? When Rutherford attended seminars, he would always ask the most questions, 90 percent of which, to Ramsey, seemed "utterly stupid, with perfectly obvious answers. But there was a remaining 10 percent," said Ramsey, "which were extremely profound, very good, very much to the

---

* Physicist George Gamow points out in *Thirty Years that Shook Physics* that "the great experimentalist Lord Rutherford was so poor in mathematics that the famous Rutherford formula for alpha-particle scattering was derived for him by a young mathematician, R.H. Fowler," Rutherford's son-in-law, with whom Norman Ramsey, we have seen, was "fairly well" acquainted.
— George Gamow, *Thirty Years That Shook Physics*, (Garden City, NY: Doubleday & Co., 1966), 140.

point, and such that they would frequently start the investigation off in a new direction."[31]

When balanced against one another, Ramsey decided, Rutherford's insights into physics far outweighed Rutherford's struggle with mathematics. "He was a very stimulating fellow," said Ramsey, "and I think I really began to grow up in physics when I realized that just an ability to make a formal mathematical derivation was not the criterion of being a good physicist."[32]

James Chadwick, a protégé of Rutherford's who had discovered the neutron in 1932, which earned him a Nobel Prize in physics the year Ramsey arrived at Cambridge, said of Rutherford that his ultimate distinction was his "genius to be astonished."[33]

It was appropriate that Ramsey would find Rutherford to be of special significance as a teacher. In 1938, 27 years after Rutherford's discovery of the nucleus and just months after his death, it was Norman Ramsey who began recording the first magnetic resonance data ever gathered from the nucleus of deuterium—otherwise known as the deuteron—that would reveal that it had an electric quadrupole moment. Had he lived, Lord Rutherford would once again have been astonished.

According to author Richard Rhodes, "Rutherford trained no fewer than 11 Nobel Prize winners during his life, an unsurpassed record."[34] That was as of 1988. In 1989, Norman Ramsey received his Nobel Prize, raising the number of Nobel laureates trained by Rutherford to at least 12. Ironically, Rutherford, though a physicist of the highest order, received his own 1908 Nobel Prize, not in physics but in chemistry, for his discovery that radioactive elements change or "transmute" into other elements.

Back to Columbia

The two years Ramsey spent at Cambridge confirmed his decision to focus on physics instead of mathematics. Upon graduating from Cambridge, he had two offers from Columbia University to consider, either an instructorship in the mathematics department or a teaching assistantship in the physics department at half the salary. He took the lower-paid position in physics, where his research time would be spent on molecular beams working with Professor Isidor I. Rabi (Rabi had just become a full professor, eight years after beginning at Columbia as a lecturer.) Ramsey's interest in beams had been sparked by an essay he had written on the topic for Maurice Goldhaber, his tutor at Cambridge.

[He] asked me to write a report on nuclear magnetic moments and spins. Well, there were only two places that did these measurements; one was Otto Stern's lab in Hamburg and Rabi's laboratory at Columbia. And I was very impressed by Rabi's work, partly because not only was he doing very, very good work but his work was very closely related with theory and I originally had been a mathematician. I had used my time at Cambridge doing both mathematics and physics. And I was very interested in quantum mechanics, and this was a case where quantum mechanics entered in very vigorously so I said I wanted to work with him.[35]

Rabi had been working with beams ever since a two-year, fellowship-sponsored working tour of Europe's physics centers had brought him in contact in 1927 with Otto Stern, the great molecular beamist, at the University of Hamburg in Germany. While at Hamburg, Rabi had come up with an important modification to the Stern method in which he used a uniform magnetic field to deflect a molecular beam, positioned at an oblique angle to the molecules' line of flight. The advantage was ease of calibration and increased accuracy in measuring deflection.

That experiment was the first of many variations that Rabi would perform in the years that followed. In fact, by the time Ramsey contacted Rabi in the summer of 1937 about the possibility of working with him, Rabi had concluded, prematurely, that he had just about milked the method for all it was worth as far as new discoveries were concerned and thought that Ramsey could better spend his PhD research time on something with more potential. Although the intervening years had been very fruitful and many wonderful methods had been developed and discoveries made, from now on, Rabi thought, it was likely to be a case of diminishing returns. "It shows how things change," said Ramsey.

Little did Rabi know that in the space of about two months he would be directing a molecular beam experiment that would earn him a Nobel Prize and little did Ramsey know that he would soon be writing the first PhD thesis ever on nuclear magnetic resonance.

Magnetic Resonance

In the 10 years between his first meeting with Otto Stern in Hamburg and his first meeting with Norman Ramsey at Columbia,* Rabi and his

---

* Although Ramsey had taken physics courses as an undergraduate student at Columbia, he had never taken any courses taught by Rabi.

collaborators had guided the flights of countless streams of isolated atoms and molecules through the airless space of molecular beam chambers, influencing their paths with a variety of magnetic fields—both uniform and non-uniform—deflecting them, refocusing them, and in other ways manipulating them to reveal their mysterious quantized personalities.

In the process, the Rabi team had developed ingenious methods that enabled them to: 1) isolate and measure nuclear magnetic moments which are approximately 2,000 times smaller than the atomic magnetic moments of which they are a part; 2) determine the magnitude of nuclear spins; 3) eliminate the accuracy-reducing effect of beam particles traveling through the apparatus at differing velocities; 4) improve the accuracy of their experimental results from a factor of 10 percent uncertainty down to 3 percent; and 5) observe the reorientation or "flopping" of atomic spins as they traveled through magnetic fields that appeared, from the perspective of the spins, to change direction.

In early 1937, the Rabi team was poised on the threshold of discovering nuclear magnetic resonance in molecular beams, but had not made the apparatus changes that would make it a reality. In 1936, a modification they had made to their apparatus called a "T-field" was flopping atomic spins from one orientation to another and in April 1937 Rabi had published a fundamental paper[36] that presented the theory upon which NMR and a host of related developments, including masers, lasers, and atomic clocks, would be based. Because of Rabi's interest in measuring spins and their signs by observing flopping orientations, he didn't fully realize the powerful potential of resonance. A calculation in his paper was based on the assumption that atoms were streaming through the apparatus at a single, averaged velocity, and with averaged velocities, said Ramsey, "it wasn't particularly apparent that there should be a sharp resonance."[37]

Meanwhile, circumstances, pressing and otherwise, delayed experimental implementation of the theory until September 1937 when the Dutch physicist, Cornelis Gorter, returning to Holland from a summer seminar in Ann Arbor, Michigan, stopped by Rabi's Pupin Hall laboratories at Columbia. In Holland, Gorter had attempted to observe NMR by measuring thermal changes at the point of resonance, but had been unsuccessful. When he came to Columbia, however, and saw Rabi's apparatuses, he recognized that if Rabi replaced the magnetic field that gyrated in space (the T-field) with a magnetic field that oscillated with time, he would probably achieve magnetic resonance.

In 1966, when he was given the Fritz London Award for his many scientific achievements, Gorter recalled his 1937 stop-off at Columbia:

On the way home—by Greyhound bus and ship—I visited Columbia University. One of Rabi's collaborators showed me the details of the various atomic beam apparatuses. Seeing the set-up in which the beam passed through a magnetic field, the direction of which rotated in space so that the sign and approximate magnitude of the magnetic moments of the nuclei could be evaluated, I realized that replacing this magnetic field [Rabi's T-field] by a constant plus a transverse radiofrequency field would make the apparatus immediately suitable for the observation of nuclear magnetic resonance.[38]

That's when Gorter mentioned the key word, oscillator, to Rabi. Gorter left for Holland thinking Rabi was unconvinced, but apparently his mention of the word 'oscillator' had not been taken as lightly as he thought. The following Monday, both of Rabi's laboratory groups—the fifth-floor group and the 10th-floor group—began modifying their apparatuses to incorporate what would become the magnetic resonance method.

It wasn't that Gorter's idea was totally new to Rabi; it served more as a trigger. As Ramsey has written:

Some time [after publication of the 1937 paper in which he provided the theoretical foundation for magnetic resonance], Rabi and his collaborator Jerrold Zacharias casually discussed the possibility of using an oscillator to produce a magnetic field that truly rotated with time instead of simulating one with the motion of particles. But they were so fully occupied with their highly successful research programs that they gave this idea no further thought. . . . In the course of his discussions with Gorter, Rabi came to appreciate fully how much sharper his resonances would be if the frequencies were generated by an oscillator, because each atom or molecule would see the same frequency. . . . He immediately redirected the laboratory research program.[39]

Within a short time, Rabi and his collaborators on the project—Jerrold Zacharias, Sidney Millman, and Polykarp Kusch—along with other physicists, were watching an ammeter and a beam detector gauge as a ribbon of lithium chloride molecules wended its way through the reconfigured apparatus that now comprised four magnetic fields. Field A, the first field through which the molecules traveled, and Field B, the last field they encountered before hitting the detector, were deflecting fields which offset one another and nullified the unwanted effect of molecules traveling through the chamber at different speeds. Between Field A and Field B was the new field, Field C, a homogenous field created by an adjustable-current electromagnet that took the place of the T-field formerly used to reorient nuclear spins. And in the center of Field C was a fourth field, the R field, positioned transversely to Field C, through which all molecules in the beam would have to pass. The R field was created by a radiofrequency oscillator which, like the electromagnet, was also operator adjustable.

The idea behind the new arrangement was that, by initially setting the oscillator to a frequency that matched the known Larmor frequency of the atoms—the frequency displayed by the atoms at a particular magnetic field strength—and then by slowly changing the field strength by varying the current of the electromagnet through a limited range, there should be a point in that range at which the Larmor frequency of the atoms streaming through the C-field would match or be in resonance with the frequency of the oscillating field, causing them to absorb energy, and to "flop" from one spatial orientation to another. When that happened, it was reasoned, the molecules should be thrown off course, thereby missing the detector where they would normally arrive, resulting in loss of signal.

That was the plan and, as Sidney Millman turned the rheostat controlling the current of the C-field's electromagnet, every eye watched for the anticipated signal loss. They started the experiment by setting the frequency of the oscillating field to 3.518 million cycles per second, near the range of the anticipated Larmor frequency for lithium atoms, and setting the current for the electromagnet at 110 amperes. As anticipated, the detector plate was still being hit by a full-strength beam of lithium chloride molecules.

Slowly, the current was turned up one amp at a time. When the current reached 115 amperes, the signal began to drop off, indicating that some of the spins had absorbed energy, had flopped to a new orientation, and were now being thrown off course as a result. As the current was increased further to 116 and then 117 amperes, the signal dropped off completely.

As they continued to raise the amperage, to 118, 119 and 120, the signal returned to full strength, indicating that the Larmor frequency of the atoms was no longer in resonance with the frequency of the oscillator, that the lithium spins were no longer flopping to new orientations and being thrown off course, and that the strength of the beam was back to what it was at the beginning of the experiment.

There was no doubt about it. The experiment had worked flawlessly, just the way they had hoped. Not only had the phenomenon of nuclear magnetic resonance been clearly confirmed, but physicists would now be able to determine the nuclear magnetic moments of various elements with greater accuracy than ever before.

Suddenly, molecular beams were front-and-center again in the minds of Rabi and his collaborators. One of those collaborators, fresh from two years at Cambridge, was 22-year-old Norman F. Ramsey, Jr. who would have "the great good fortune," as Ramsey expressed it in his Nobel lecture 52 years later, "to be the only graduate student to work with Rabi and his colleagues"[40] in the development of magnetic resonance.

Ramsey was at Columbia in September 1937 when Gorter came through on his way back to Holland. In fact, he was the Rabi collaborator mentioned by Gorter who showed him around the laboratory.

In regard to the subsequent switchover to magnetic resonance, Gorter's view was that, although his contribution, from which he derived "some pride," was acknowledged by Rabi in his initial letter to the editor of *Physical Review*, Gorter felt his idea had been "somewhat undervalued."[41]

Ramsey's view is that Rabi had developed the theory to such a point in his 1937 paper on gyrating fields that "all anybody had to do was essentially say 'oscillator' and it was there. It's a combination of the two [perspectives]," Ramsey added, "but I think it is very clear that Rabi's 1937 paper has [the foundation for magnetic resonance] in it."[42]

As to Gorter's impression of Rabi's interest or lack of it, Ramsey has said, "It's not at all surprising that two people may have a different point of view on the same conversation."[43]

Radiofrequency Spectroscopy

For a number of years, the Rabi team had been doing its work on the fifth and tenth floors of Pupin Hall. In the latter part of 1937, Victor Cohen, Sidney Millman, Polykarp Kusch, Jerrold Zacharias, and graduate student Don Hamilton were on the fifth floor, along with Rabi, working with beams of alkali metals and other non-gaseous atomic elements. On the tenth floor, Kellogg worked with Zacharias and Rabi, where they had independently confirmed, prior to their first magnetic resonance experiment, that the magnetic moment of the proton was approximately three times larger than originally thought. Because of his theoretical and mathematical abilities, Norman Ramsey was put to work, like Zacharias, on both floors.

After Gorter's visit in September of 1937, modifications were begun on both the fifth- and tenth-floor apparatuses with the expectation that the fifth-floor apparatus would be completed first. (The fifth-floor apparatus was of simpler design because it would be used to study easily-detectable molecules like lithium fluoride, whereas the tenth-floor apparatus would be used to study the more interesting, but harder-to-detect H_2 molecules.) Soon after successfully using the magnetic resonance method on a beam of lithium chloride, Millman, Kusch and Zacharias, led by Rabi, used the same apparatus to accurately determine the magnetic moments of other alkali metals, achieving measurements with uncertainties of less than 1 percent.

Rabi's first magnetic resonance experiment, submitted to *Physical Review* on January 31, 1938,[44] as well as the magnetic resonance experiments conducted with other alkali metals, all had a common feature. When the intensity of the beam was plotted on a line graph against the magnetic force of the C-field, the line would start out at 100 percent beam intensity, would drop away to nearly nothing as the strength of the C-field was increased, thereby satisfying the resonance condition, and then would return to full intensity as the magnet strength was further increased. They called the lines formed by these plots 'resonance curves' and Rabi and his collaborators thought they would find only resonance curves representing interaction between magnetic moments and the external field. Ramsey, the only student at that time in Rabi's 10th-floor magnetic resonance laboratory, would soon find evidence to the contrary.

The other three researchers in that laboratory were all instructors or professors. Kellogg, a graduate of the University of Iowa, had come to Columbia as a physics instructor and had also chosen to work in Rabi's laboratory. Zacharias had obtained his PhD from Columbia but, because he was Jewish, was unable to get a job there. (Although Rabi, also Jewish, had gotten a job at Columbia, he was, said Zacharias, "an unusual case."[45]) When Zacharias was hired to a full-time position at Hunter College—they "needed an exhibit Jew,"[46] he said—he continued to work 30 to 40 hours a week, unpaid, at Rabi's Columbia University laboratories.

Ramsey's first experiment at Columbia and corresponding paper, "On the Magnetic Moments of Neon and Argon," published with Jerome Kellogg in *Physical Review* in 1938,[47] was based on work done before the invention of the magnetic resonance method. His next seven papers, however, all on the hydrogens, as well as his doctoral thesis, did make use of magnetic resonance.[48-54] It was during this period, from 1938 until his departure for Washington, D.C. as a Carnegie Institution Fellow in 1940, that Ramsey would contribute greatly to the science of NMR by introducing, for the first time, the analytical power of radiofrequency spectroscopy.

The science of spectroscopy began in 1666 when Sir Isaac Newton observed that visible white light separated into a continuum—a spectrum—of brilliant multi-colored light when diffracted through a triangular piece of glass called a prism.

An 18th-century Scottish physicist by the name of Thomas Melvill made spectroscopy useful for chemical analysis when he mixed various chemical salts with alcohol, lit them with a flame, and by studying the light of the flame diffracted through a prism, was able to observe that different mixtures exhibited different band combinations, or spectra.

With the advent of the prism spectrascope in 1859, the science became more quantitative. By projecting prismatic light through a narrow slit onto ruled scales, and later photographic film, one could measure the spacing of the projected light bands and calculate their distinctive frequencies. Somewhat analogous to the way bar codes are used today to identify products with their unique combination of lines and spaces, spectra could identify chemicals on film with their unique combination of exposed and unexposed bands. In fact, by 1868, visible-light spectroscopy had evolved to such a level that "helium was discovered in the chromosphere of the sun . . . as a series of unusual spectral lines twenty-three years before it was discovered mixed into uranium ore on earth."[55]

Spectroscopy had also played a major role in the Quantum Revolution. The question it raised for Niels Bohr, for example—Why do hydrogen atoms emit a unique spectral light?—led him to conclude that hydrogen electrons exist only in discrete, quantized energy states and that energy in the form of light is emitted only at discrete frequencies, unique to hydrogen, when electrons make a quantum transition from a higher energy state to a lower one. Wolfgang Pauli, seeking to understand why bright spectral lines actually consisted of several, closely-spaced lines, deduced that these "hyperfine splittings" occur because the nucleus of the atom has a spin and therefore a magnetic moment.

In other words, the science of spectroscopy has been, from its birth, the use of frequency measurement for the purpose of identifying materials and their unique properties. Radiofrequency spectroscopy, which works with frequencies in the lower-frequency end of the microwave portion of the spectrum and the higher-frequency end of the radio-wave portion, began in 1938 when PhD candidate Norman Ramsey found that, by varying the amplitude of an oscillator, he could induce molecules to disclose secrets about their structure and interactions that had never before been revealed.

By the summer of 1938, Kellogg, Zacharias and Ramsey were plotting graphs based on magnetic resonance data taken from beams of molecular hydrogen (H_2), heavy hydrogen or deuterium (D_2), and mixed hydrogen (HD). The only one of the three molecules that seemed to fit the pattern they had seen on the fifth floor was HD. Its two resonance curves were what they had expected, one for the proton's magnetic moment and one for the deuteron's magnetic moment, although the resonance curve for the deuteron did not fall off to zero as rapidly as expected. The results seemed sufficiently satisfactory, however, for them to announce the proton magnetic moment to be 2.780 nuclear magnetons and the deuteron moment to be 0.853 nuclear magnetons, with an uncertainty of just 0.7 percent.[56]

When Norman Ramsey began trying to sort out the data he was getting for molecular hydrogen (H_2), however, it didn't conform at all to the pattern the team had been expecting.

> At the time we did the experiments [said Ramsey], our dominant thoughts . . . our expectations, all our discussions were as if we were measuring a nuclear magnetic moment. The model was a precessing top within a magnetic field and since the proton had a single magnetic moment, we were very much expecting to see a single, sharp resonance. . . . We were very upset by our first H_2 result. We had gotten this great experiment going and all we had to do was to get one beautiful resonance . . . and all we saw was a bunch of junk.[57]

The graph they plotted from the offending data was "so bad," said Ramsey, "I don't know anywhere that it is preserved."[58] However, since he needed a topic for his PhD dissertation, it fell to his lot to sort through and try to make sense of the apparently useless junk he and his associates had been collecting.

> There was always a problem at Columbia [Ramsey explained]. They had a rule at that time that any PhD thesis could only have one author. Therefore, one of the the problems in having PhD people was to find a somewhat uninteresting topic for the PhD candidate which he could take as his own and publish. So it was decided that the uninteresting topic for me should be to study this mess.[59]

He would have to study it on his own. Rabi would be gone for much of that summer to California, where he would be lecturing at Stanford University at the invitation of Felix Bloch, who had emigrated to the United States from Switzerland three years before. While he was gone, Ramsey could start working on his PhD thesis while Kellogg and Zacharias began constructing the next round of apparatus they would need to achieve higher resolution and more accurate results.

"It was basically one hard summer," said Ramsey. "I was working alone."[60] As he began testing various approaches to the messy problem facing him, he found that if he lowered the amplitude of the oscillating magnetic field, the poorly-defined mess they had originally plotted began to form a definite pattern of multiple resonance curves.

> Unfortunately [said Ramsey], I dropped the amplitude in too-small steps. I would drop it a factor of two and when I found it was much better, another factor of two. I should have done it in factors of 10 and it would have gone a little faster. It took about two days to get one of those curves, because each point was taken very slowly. At low enough oscillating field amplitude it became apparent that there were several resonances, as in a spectrum.[61]

In fact, Ramsey found five or six resonance curves, depending on how he counted them; one of the curves seemed to have a double-dip pattern.

> This was really the first case of line spectra [said Ramsey]. We should have anticipated that there would have been spectra, but we didn't. You know, you don't do that when you're looking for things. All we thought we were doing was looking for magnetic moments, so that should be one line, and instead of that, we had a combination.[62] . . . At this point, it began to become clear that we were studying spectroscopy, not just magnetic moments.[63]

The six-peak spectrum that Ramsey and the rest of the Rabi team had viewed after modifying the apparatus for their H_2 experiment was, said Ramsey, the "first instance of multiple line spectroscopy with coherent electromagnetic radiation, a characteristic of subsequent radiofrequency, microwave and laser spectroscopy."[64]

He also did similar studies that summer with deuterium. There, too, distinct patterns began emerging as he plotted his data. "Initially," said Ramsey, "there appeared to be a single, nice isolated peak, but when I studied it with a little more care over that summer, it became apparent that there were really subsidiary resonances in the background there, too."[65]

By the end of that summer, Kellogg and Zacharias had completed construction of the new, high-resolution apparatus, enabling the tenth-floor group to redo the molecular hydrogen and heavy hydrogen experiments. Now when they beamed molecular hydrogen through the new vacuum chamber and replotted the data, they found six sharp peaks instead of five single resonance curves and one double-dip curve. For deuterium, they confirmed the presence of one very marked resonance curve and several subsidiary ones. "At this point," said Ramsey, "it was quite clear that we were studying radiofrequency spectroscopy."[66]

The old, lower-resolution apparatus had worked fine for ascertaining flopping spins in molecules with a single magnetic moment, but it was pushing its design limits when they tried to make sense of data where the resonance condition was satisfied six or more times because of subtle, internal influences.

After modifying the apparatus, the peaks became more defined and the team came to realize that molecular hydrogen with its two protons had two magnetic moments and that these magnetic moments, in turn, related not only to the external fields imposed upon them by the experimenters, but also to the complex internal magnetic influences imposed upon them by their own molecular structure.

It was as if the researchers suddenly had the opportunity to learn much more about these molecules than they had at first thought the molecules were willing to tell them. It was like calling a telephone number and expecting one response to a standard query from one member of a family and finding instead that you've been connected to a party line and that you are eavesdropping on conversations that reveal closely-guarded secrets between two or more family members. With careful listening and analysis of these interactions, the Columbia researchers could learn much more than they had expected to learn. The multiple resonances they were seeing reflected not only the interactions they had expected between the magnetic moments and the external field but also the internal interactions within the molecule. The spacings of the resonance curves measured the energies of these interactions.

They had asked molecular hydrogen for a single magnetic moment and were informed by its two protons that, because of their own inter-dynamics as well as their interaction with the external field, they had two different magnetic moments. In addition, the team was also getting feedback from interaction between the protons and the rotational magnetic moment of the molecule itself. (The rotational magnetic moment of a molecule is produced by its tumbling action in the high vacuum of the molecular-beam apparatus.) Altogether, the resonant condition was being satisfied at six different frequencies.

Using the analogy of a radio receiver—actually, they were using a radiofrequency oscillator which they built themselves from instructions in the *Radio Amateur's Handbook*—the Rabi team was finding that the station they were expecting to find at one frequency actually offered a variety of information that was simultaneously available at different frequencies. As they varied the frequency, they pulled in additional information.

And that brings up a fundamental change that took place in how the Rabi experiments were performed. In the original magnetic resonance experiment, the Rabi team had set the frequency of the oscillator at 3.518 million cycles per second and left that setting unchanged as they varied the strength of the electromagnetic field from 110 amperes up to 121 amperes. But when the Rabi group modified their apparatus in 1938, they also modified their technique. Now when they did their experiments, they preset the current of the electromagnet at a certain amperage and left it there for the entire experiment while they varied the frequency of the radiofrequency oscillator. Although it was a minor change in technique, it was a major change in concept. The power of the new method for raising new questions—and giving clues to some of the answers—would soon be evident.

Paper No. 7 in Ramsey's list of scientific publications, entitled "The Magnetic Moments of the Proton and the Deuteron," co-authored by Kellogg, Rabi and Zacharias, includes the subtitle, "The Radiofrequency Spectrum of H_2 in Various Magnetic Fields."[67] The subtitle was inserted as a compromise. "We had a bit of an argument on titles, which should be the main title, which should be the subtitle." said Ramsey.[68] He wanted the phrase "radiofrequency spectroscopy" in the main title. Rabi, who still preferred the conceptual perspective of flopping magnetic moments to that of quantum transitions, argued against using the phrase.

But Ramsey, who had done the measurements and, along with Kellogg and Zacharias, had correlated the theory to the actual numbers, was no longer thinking only of magnetic moments. He had discovered multiple spectral lines when he began reducing the amplitude of the oscillating field, and he could no longer settle for the conceptual and quantitative limitations imposed by flopping moments.

Now when he turned on the apparatus, he was overhearing inter- and intra-molecular conversations that he couldn't resist. Now the plotted line graphs were spectra instead of resonance curves and the peaks and valleys represented quantum transitions. Now he was doing radiofrequency spectroscopy, a new field of science that would occupy much of his scientific career, with far-reaching impact.

How much resistance was there on Rabi's part to the use of the phrase "radiofrequency spectroscopy?" "Oh, not too bad," Ramsey said. "I think putting in the subtitle made both of us happy. Basically, we had several important things we wanted emphasized. I mean the magnetic moment of the proton was important. So was the deuteron quadrupole moment."[69]

The Electric Quadrupole Moment of the Deuteron

The team's discovery of the deuteron quadrupole moment came about as a result of further high-resolution analysis of the spectral pattern that Ramsey had initially obtained for deuterium with its one isolated peak and several subsidiary ones. The high-resolution equipment completed by the end of that momentous summer had, in turn, made those peaks more defined.

Because the nucleus of deuterium, called a deuteron, contains one proton and one neutron, the group had expected the deuteron to have a magnetic moment, but they were seeing seven spectral lines, one large dominant peak flanked on each side by three small peaks, and more widely separated than would have been expected according to existing theory.

The evidence soon started pointing to the possibility that the deuteron, in addition to its magnetic dipole moment, had an electric quadrupole moment. Perhaps, they speculated, instead of the deuteron being a perfect sphere that rotated about its axis like a spinning basketball, it was actually an elongated sphere shaped somewhat like a football—the technical term is prolate spheroid—that rotated about its primary axis in a wobbly spiral.

When Rabi, Ramsey, Zacharias, and Kellogg reanalyzed the data and the theory in light of this idea, it made sense and their conclusions were announced in a letter dated January 15, 1939 from J.M.B. Kellogg, I.I. Rabi, N.F. Ramsey, Jr. and J.R. Zacharias to the editor of *Physical Review*.[70]

Ramsey said that it was probably Rabi who first came up with the possibility of a quadrupole moment, although he remembered it as basically a joint conclusion arrived at by discussion. "I do have," said Ramsey, "a handwritten letter from a very early time that I wrote to Rabi at Stanford [during the summer of 1938] . . . in which I reported little wiggles that I said could indeed be due to a deuteron quadrupole moment, but I suspect that Rabi knew of the possibility of quadrupole moments before I did."[71]

An 18-page paper, the last one in the Rabi hydrogen series and Ramsey's eighth in a two-year period, published in the April 18, 1940 issue of *Physical Review*,[72] explained the significance of their discovery. "The implication of the quadrupole moment," they wrote in the second paper, "is that the forces between proton and neutron in the deuteron are not 'central.' " Up until then, it had been assumed that the forces acting between atomic-level protons and neutrons were of the same nature as those "central" forces which act at a celestial level along an imaginary line between the centers of heavenly bodies.

It was a major discovery, one that would change a basic assumption of physicists. Nobel laureate Hans Bethe, 30 years later, would rank it among the top three developments that came along in the early years of nuclear physics.[73] (This paper and six others co-authored by Ramsey in the coming years dealing with the quadrupolar interactions of the deuteron also dealt with the strength of this neutron-proton "tensor force." Later in his career, after he and his physicist colleagues had returned to academic pursuits following World War II, Ramsey would set a limit to a possible long range non-magnetic tensor force acting between two protons at long range.)[74-76]

Had the initial plan for Ramsey's PhD thesis been followed, he may well have received the Nobel Prize in physics decades earlier, if not for introducing radiofrequency or magnetic resonance spectroscopy, perhaps for the electric quadrupole moment of the deuteron which followed soon after. When the rest of the Rabi team realized that they had stumbled onto the quadrupolar moment of the deuteron while performing spectroscopic analysis of deuterium, it was decided that this was really a larger finding than was anticipated when Ramsey was given his PhD assignment to investigate the "fuzz" he was finding in the diatomic hydrogens of H_2 and D_2. Since they had shared in the setup of the new apparatus, it was agreed they would share in the discovery of the electric quadrupole moment of the deuteron and Ramsey would have to find another topic for his PhD thesis.

Although he had already done much of the development of the quadrupolar theory, Ramsey was philosophical about it:

Well, that was obviously a much more important discovery than any of the others, and since we'd built the apparatus together we also pooled on that and published that together. Since four of us had done that work together [Kellogg, Zacharias, and myself, under Rabi's supervision], it seemed to all of us, including myself, it would have been very unfair for me to cop the principal thing . . . as a thesis topic. . . . I would have gotten more fame earlier if I had insisted on holding on to it, but I think it was perfectly fair.[77]

Ramsey would take for his PhD thesis the study of the radiofrequency spectrum associated with the rotational magnetic moment of the molecule. "As part of the exchange," said Ramsey, "Zacharias and Kellogg took some of the data for my PhD thesis while I was down taking the written exam. It was a very happy sort of interchange."[78]

Of the committee Ramsey faced for his final PhD examination, all but one had either received or would receive a Nobel Prize. Among them were Isidor Rabi, who four years later would receive the Nobel Prize for observing magnetic resonance in molecular beams; Harold Urey, 1934 laureate in chemistry for his co-discovery of deuterium; Willis Lamb, 1955 laureate for discoveries on the structure of the atomic hydrogen spectrum; Polykarp Kusch, 1955 laureate for determining the magnetic moment of the electron; and Enrico Fermi, 1938 laureate for discovering new radioactive elements beyond uranium.

"It was an extremely strong department at the time," said Ramsey, "but I didn't realize it when I was there; then I chiefly saw deficiencies in the department and the poor lectures some people gave. Most of them had not yet really done their best work . . . but in actual practice it was probably about the best in the country at the time."[79]

War in Europe

Enrico Fermi would not have been on Ramsey's PhD exam committee had it not been for the rapidly-deteriorating situation in Europe. In September of 1938, the same month Britain's Neville Chamberlain had appeased Hitler by agreeing to a dismemberment of Czechoslovakia, Fermi, then living in Italy, saw the handwriting on the wall when Italian anti-Semitic laws were put into effect. Because his wife was Jewish, he immediately wrote four American universities seeking a position and received offers from five, including one from Columbia that he confidentially accepted.[80]

The following month, after being told by Niels Bohr on a trip to Copenhagen that he was likely to receive the 1938 Nobel Prize in physics—a departure from the usual rules of secrecy—Fermi began making plans for getting his wife and family to safety.[81]

On the morning of November 10, Laura Fermi received a telephone call advising her that her husband could expect a call from Stockholm that evening at six o'clock. When the phone rang at nearly the appointed hour, they thought it was the official Nobel notification, but instead it was Ginestra Amaldi, wife of Italian physicist Edoardo Amaldi, asking if they had heard the latest news. Laura Fermi in her book, *Atoms in the Family*, recalled what they heard when they turned on the radio:

> Hard, emphatic, pitiless, the commentator's voice read the second set of racial laws. The laws issued that day limited the activities and the civil status of the Jews. Their children were excluded from public schools. Jewish teachers were dismissed. Jewish lawyers, physicians, and other professionals could practice for Jewish clients only. Many Jewish firms were dissolved. "Aryan" servants were not allowed to work for Jews or to live in their homes. Jews were to be deprived of full citizenship rights, and their passports would be withdrawn.[82]

Richard Rhodes, in writing of that evening, speculated that they might also have heard the news of a vast pogrom that had taken place in Germany the previous night, *Kristallnacht*, the night of glass, in which thousands of windows had been broken, synagogues burned, businesses destroyed, and families taken from their homes and beaten. At least 100 people had died and some 30,000 Jewish men—especially wealthy ones—had been sent off to concentration camps at Buchenwald, Dachau and Sachsenhausen, to be released only if they accepted emigration from Germany as paupers.[83]

The Nobel call from Stockholm came through shortly after the radio broadcast. Fermi was being awarded the Nobel Prize in physics "for his demonstrations of the existence of new radioactive elements produced by neutron irradiation, and for his related discovery of nuclear reactions brought about by slow neutrons."[84]

Using the Nobel Foundation's December 10 award ceremony as a pretense for requesting visas, a request politically difficult for the government to reject, the Fermis were granted permission to travel to Stockholm. (Enrico Fermi had been able to keep his wife's passport clear of restrictions.) Instead of returning to Italy, however, they traveled west to New York City and Columbia University.

Fermi arrived at Columbia about midway through Ramsey's first year as a graduate student at the school. Contrasted with Rabi, whose course organization Ramsey has described as "pretty dreadful" even though the content was "extremely enlightening,"[85] Fermi was, according to Ramsey, "an absolutely superb lecturer. His courses and written work," he said, "both were logically arranged, beautifully and clearly presented. He always had an easily understandable way of presenting things; no matter how hard the idea, he could make it clear.[86]

Two weeks after the Fermi family docked in New York, Niels Bohr also disembarked there, enroute to Princeton as a visiting professor, bringing with him news of the recent discovery of nuclear fission.[87] Achieved by chemists Otto Hahn and Fritz Strassmann at the Kaiser Wilhelm Institute for Chemistry in Berlin and interpreted theoretically by Lise Meitner and Otto Robert Frisch in Sweden, physicists with Jewish ancestry who had fled Hitler's Germany, fission was immediately duplicated and confirmed in laboratories across the United States, including those at Columbia.

Although the phenomenon had actually happened on numerous occasions in the years preceding 1938, scientists had assumed that they were producing hybrid, "transuranic" elements with properties similar to other elements rather than actually creating lighter elements by splitting heavier ones.

> These transuranic elements [said Ramsey] were found to have supposedly the properties of lanthanum and other things. Well, they were lanthanum. They didn't have the properties of it; they were it. All that was required in nuclear physics at that time was the one word, even the suggestion. It didn't have to have experimental evidence. I think that if anyone had even asked Fermi the question, or asked me the question, "Is there any chance that this could have been not a transuranic element but a splitting of uranium?" we would suddenly have said, "Why, yes, of course. How reasonable."[88]

Ramsey didn't know it then, but the discovery of fission would have a greater impact on his life than he could ever have suspected when he first heard of it, although "everyone," he said, "more or less simultaneously recognized that since fission was both initiated by neutrons and that it, in turn, produced neutrons that there was a chance (though I think at that time it was thought to be a very small chance) that it might be a source of nuclear energy."[89] Although Fermi* immediately began experiments to see whether it could produce enough neutrons to support a self-sustaining reaction, "the likelihood of it," said Ramsey, "was by no means clear at that time."[90]

When Fermi arrived in the United States, Ramsey was, like most Americans, still relatively unaffected by events in Europe and, looking west, the possibility of a U.S. war with Japan in the Pacific also seemed rather remote. Although Japan had become imperialistic and had invaded and conquered large areas of Manchuria and China, inducing the U.S. government to freeze Japanese assets in the United States and to impose an embargo of goods that might bolster Japan's military strength, a direct conflict with Japan was, for most Americans, incomprehensible.

After completing his PhD requirements in the first half of 1939, Ramsey moved to Washington, D.C. as a Carnegie Institution Fellow. In the year that followed, he would study neutron-proton and proton-helium scattering and co-author three papers, one of them written in collaboration with the other recipient of a Carnegie Institution Fellowship that year, post-doctoral fellow James A. Van Allen,[91] for whom the Van Allen radiation belt would later be named.

The following spring, on June 3, 1940, 24-year-old Norman Ramsey, now officially a Doctor of Philosophy, married Elinor Jameson of Brooklyn, New York, and a few months later, in September, the newlyweds moved cross-country to the Midwest where he had accepted a position as an associate, one level below instructor, at the University of Illinois at Urbana-Champaign. As far as he and his wife were concerned, said Ramsey, they expected to spend the rest of their lives there, but that

---

* Given Ramsey's long-term association with Fermi (from his arrival at Columbia in early 1939 until his death from cancer in 1954) and his personal observation of Fermi's "lifetime reputation for honesty and reliability," it is understandable that Ramsey was angered by the recent publication of the book *Special Tasks* in which a former Soviet spy from the Stalin era impugned Fermi's integrity.

"Enrico Fermi [Ramsey said at a press conference sponsored by the American Physical Society] was a truly great scientist of the highest scientific and moral integrity who contributed unselfishly to the welfare of our country. He was a deeply loyal naturalized citizen who often expressed his joy at being welcomed here. As a citizen by birth, I find it embarrassing to be called upon now to defend the reputation and honor of this wonderful man."

Ramsey was not alone in his reaction to the book. Pulitzer-Prize winning author Richard Rhodes labeled the spy's claims as "gumshoe braggadocio," and Edward Teller, advocate of the hydrogen bomb, discounted the credibility of Fermi's accuser on the basis that Fermi "clearly opposed the Stalinist nightmare."

—Quoted in *Time* magazine, May 23, 1994, p. 63.

was not to be. After just a few weeks in Illinois, he was recruited by Ernest Lawrence to work on a relatively new technology, soon to be known as radar, at a newly-created institution called the Radiation Laboratory at another Cambridge, this one in Massachusetts.

The Radiation Laboratory

A conference on Applied Nuclear Physics held October 28-31, 1940 at MIT had two agendas, one published and one hidden.

The published agenda, typical of most scientific conferences, offered an opportunity for participants to give papers, to hear about and discuss the latest developments in physics, and to get together with old friends.

The hidden agenda was to inform a small, select group of attendees, who had received special invitations by phone, of government-sponsored plans to establish a laboratory for the development of microwave radar on the campus of MIT.[92]

Formed under the auspices of the National Defense Research Committee (NDRC), the microwave project would be a joint effort with the British, who had just brought to the United States a new device called the cavity magnetron. Although radar had been in existence for some time and, in fact, had already proven its usefulness against the German Luftwaffe in the Battle of Britain, this new device, developed by John Randall and Harry Boot at the University of Birmingham, greatly increased its radiating power. Much work remained to be done, however, to reap the many military benefits made possible by the device and, because of the pressing priorities of war, they turned to their American allies for assistance.

Norman Ramsey had not received one of the special invitations, but his ex-mentor from Columbia University, I.I. Rabi, was there, as was Ramsey's new boss, F. Wheeler Loomis, the head of the physics department at the University of Illinois. In that meeting, said Ramsey, there was a "fair urging"[93] that he be recruited for the project and it wasn't long before E.O. Lawrence contacted him about returning east, this time to Massachusetts. Soon after, Norman Ramsey was one of the first half-dozen scientists to arrive in Cambridge—his badge number at the Radiation Laboratory was 14—and the first 10 or so were issued to the Microwave Committee that oversaw the project. Elinor Ramsey was the first wife connected with the project to arrive from out of town.[94]

At this point, it wasn't clear that the new laboratory, which did not have a name, would end up as a semi-permanent establishment. Initial expectations, in fact, were that the participants, after becoming educated on radar and the project's objectives, would return to their own institutions after three months or so to carry out specific assignments. It soon became apparent, however, that this would not be the most effective way to operate and the members of the project, initially appointed as consultants to the NDRC, realized that they would probably be in Cambridge for the duration of the war in Europe that, by now, was threatening to become a world war.[95]

"When it came time to name the laboratory," said Ramsey, "we had a vigorous discussion, thinking of all sorts of names."[96] They didn't want to call it a radio location laboratory because that would tip off any German spies as to the nature of the valuable information with which they were working. Then it occurred to them that if they named it Radiation Laboratory they would simultaneously achieve several objectives: 1) It would be technically correct, since they were working with electromagnetic radiation, 2) it would honor the esteemed E.O. Lawrence, who had spearheaded the recruitment of the first dozen or so scientists to the Cambridge laboratory, and 3) since Lawrence's laboratory was doing nuclear physics, it might even mislead the Germans into thinking that they were doing "something impractical like trying to develop a nuclear bomb. We thought it was a really clever idea," said Ramsey, "a fine smoke screen to make the Germans think that instead of our working on something really important and practical like radar, that we were wasting our time on something completely impractical and useless like an atomic bomb." He added, "We were delighted to have the false word leak out that this was what we were working on."[97]

As further evidence that radar was then seen as more important to the war effort than an atomic bomb, Ramsey points out that well into 1941, he had a long conversation with Enrico Fermi's chief assistant, Herbert Anderson of Columbia, who felt he was wasting his time working on nuclear reactor development and wanted to get into "something practical, like radar."[98] In fact, even the chairman of the NDRC's chemistry and explosives division was unaware of "the remote possibility of a bomb" until March 1941.[99]

The immediate objective of the "Rad Lab," as it soon came to be called, was to further refine the 10-centimeter magnetron provided by the British and to incorporate it into a working radar system. Within a couple months of the arrival of the first scientists at Cambridge, the group was able to detect echoes of radar signals beamed at downtown Boston buildings and to overcome the immediate hurdle of designing a system that could send and receive radar signals on the same antenna, a task especially challenging since the transmission signals were millions of times stronger than the returning echoes. Not long after that achievement, they were able to pick up echoes bouncing off airplanes at the Boston airport as well as submerged submarines operating off the Connecticut coast.

As soon as the team was able to overcome some of these immediate challenges, they were able to become further specialized in their efforts and to begin focusing on longer-term challenges, such as increasing the detection and object recognition powers of their systems by reducing wavelengths from 10 centimeters down to 3 centimeters. Norman Ramsey was put in charge of the Advanced Development Group which was working on what seemed at the time as "more futuristic things," namely 3-centimeter radar. "We had the feeling," said Ramsey, "that, to a certain extent, we were preparing to fight World War III, rather than World War II."[100] Later, however, that wavelength was used extensively in World War II and wavelengths would be reduced even further, down to 1 centimeter, with an auxiliary development program at Columbia University that began initially in 1942 with the molecular-beam team of Kellogg, Kusch and Millman.

During the first year or two of the Rad Lab's existence, when radar was yet largely unproven, the Army and Navy had to be convinced of its usefulness. "After that," said Ramsey, "due to the combination of some of the earlier successes of the Laboratory and the presence of a real war to contend with [following the Japanese bombing of Pearl Harbor in December, 1941], the reverse was true. The Army and Navy from then on were pretty much beating a path to our door."[101]

Expert Consultant to the Secretary of War

The Army Air Force, however, as the Air Force was then designated, was not yet convinced. So in the fall of 1942, with 3-centimeter radar largely developed and well on its way to implementation in the field, 27-year-old Norman Ramsey was named Expert Consultant to the Secretary of War and transferred to Washington, D.C. to assist 74-year-old Secretary of War Henry Stimson, "officially," said Ramsey, "to work in his office for the purpose of helping out with getting radar into the services and particularly into the Air Force."[102]

The Air Force was chiefly interested in strategic bombing, said Ramsey, and not so much in air-ground support. They were "fairly vigorously committed," he said, "to 'pickle-barrel bombing.' "

It was argued that any Air Force plane could drop a bomb from 20,000 feet into such a small target that it was optimistically called a pickle barrel. The bombing was actually done pretty nicely with the visual bomb sights under practice conditions, but rarely under combat. As a result of this faith in precision bombing, the Air Force essentially said that unless one could say the bomb would fall within 50 to 100 feet of its target, it wasn't worth using radar equipment, even though in actual practice they were not bombing with anywhere near that precision.[103]

In Washington, Ramsey was under Dr. E.L. Bowles in the Secretary of War's office but was assigned to the directorate of military requirements, whose purpose was to specify what kind of airplanes the Army should have and how they should be equipped. "I worked there almost, I'm afraid, as a sort of salesman,"[104] said Ramsey.

His "sales" tactics took a three-pronged approach. The first objective was to have an operating unit in the Air Force that actually used radar and used it effectively. This was done by establishing the first microwave radar anti-submarine search-and-attack group at Norfolk, Virginia. Named in honor of Colonel Wright, the head of the group, the so-called Wright project, said Ramsey, focused on the German submarines which were then operating fairly vigorously off the coast of the United States. Because submarines at that time had to surface at night to charge their batteries, they soon found themselves vulnerable to these radar-equipped planes.

Although the Air Force was used to projecting long-range requirements for aircraft and weapons, they were not used to that kind of planning for radar. Here, Ramsey served as a valuable aide in helping to establish a guide to the radar systems currently available and in predicting the capabilities that could be expected in the future. Once the requirements were published, they began to give procurement officers an excuse, said Ramsey, for buying radar systems. Up until then, they had lacked authority to buy radar as it was not yet a designated military requirement.

Perhaps the most effective role Ramsey played in "selling" the Air Force on radar, however, was assisting in the procurement planning process. Although budgeting was not one of his official functions, said Ramsey, he remembered one Friday afternoon when an officer from the Materiel Division came to him for help; he had been given the assignment of having a three-year budget plan prepared by the next Monday for the Air Force's procurement of radar and he didn't have the vaguest notion of what it should be.

So . . . we spent all day Saturday and Sunday [said Ramsey] making budget estimates. I used the list of military requirements I'd gotten through my own office and a list I had of the possible radars. We
also had a list of how many airplanes there were going to be, and
then we sort of said, very informally, "Well, if there are going to be x
numbers of B-29s, half of them ought to have this kind of radar, and
half another kind of radar." We necessarily did this in a very arbitrary
fashion. Then we looked and decided maybe this was a little bit too
many, so we would reduce it, or maybe we would up it. Then we
would decide, "Well, there ought to be some additional equipment
such as a tail warning device on some airplanes."

In this fashion, we ended up with some quite arbitrary numbers.
When these were totaled up, the whole sum came to about two billion dollars worth of radar. The officer then submitted this preliminary budget through channels and I was given to understand that
eventually it was approved with only minor modifications. It was the
basis for most of the money that the Air Force had from that point on
to actually procure radar during the war.[105]

Three years later, two U.S. B-29 bombers would be guided to their fateful rendezvous with history over the Japanese cities of Hiroshima and
Nagasaki with 3-centimeter radar developed at the Radiation Laboratory
under Ramsey's direction and installed as a result of his weekend exercise in budget making.

Ramsey had been "impressed" upon coming to Washington, he said,
with the number of people [in government organizations] who were
"very conscientious, very hard working, and who only make a negative
contribution—who only serve as bottlenecks."[106] He determined that he
would not be one of them.

He was "rather shocked," therefore, after being in Washington only
about a year, to find himself sounding a cautionary note when Lee
DuBridge and others came down from the Rad Lab to talk about their latest creations. "I found myself saying in a conference, yes, I was sure it
was wonderful equipment but did they realize how difficult it was to get
a program started and to get planes assigned? And I suddenly said,
'Where have I heard that before?' Oh, yes, it was one of those civil-
servant bottlenecks. It's time I move out."[107]

About the same time Ramsey came to the conclusion that it was time
for him to move on, he was invited by J. Robert Oppenheimer to a
meeting at the National Academy of Sciences where "[Oppenheimer]

began talking some," said Ramsey, "about what was happening at Los Alamos and the state of affairs on atomic weapons, which was quite exciting. He did a superb job. He was the best recruiter and salesman I've ever seen."[108]

The first time Ramsey had ever seen Oppenheimer was a few days after he married Elinor, on what Ramsey refers to as their three-person honeymoon. After an initial four-day honeymoon by themselves, Norman and Elinor Ramsey were joined by Jerrold Zacharias, Ramsey's former molecular-beam associate at Columbia, who drove them to a meeting of the American Physical Society in Seattle where Zacharias and Ramsey had been invited to give papers on their discovery of the deuteron's electric quadrupole moment. Ramsey saw "quite a bit of Oppie"[109] in Seattle and then, when the meeting was over, the three of them together with Oppenheimer traveled down the coast to Berkeley, California where they stayed at Oppenheimer's home.

The trip was "just delightful," said Ramsey. "[Oppenheimer] was a wonderful conversationalist and a real pleasure to meet. He was very impressive and, at that time, with my being a fairly young physicist, I probably didn't hold my own too well in conversation with him."[110]

Unfortunately, Oppenheimer had invited more people to spend the night than he had beds—"this was before he had attempted to become a better administrator," said Ramsey—and the newlyweds were assigned a single bed on the porch separated from Zacharias' bed only by a thin, removable wall. "We could poke the wall and communicate to Zacharias who was so near," said Ramsey, "that not only were the three of us on our honeymoon but almost in the same bed." Elinor Ramsey ended up cooking for the whole household. "She never cooked for so many people in her life,"[111] he said.

Between 1940 and 1943, except for an occasional meeting where they greeted each other briefly, Ramsey and Oppenheimer had not talked with each other. "By this time," said Ramsey, "he had changed considerably. He was still the same Oppenheimer, but his hair was a little more under control and he was proving to be an excellent administrator in building up the lab [at Los Alamos]."[112]

On this trip to Washington, Oppenheimer and Robert Bacher were recruiting two people: Kenneth Bainbridge and Norman Ramsey. In addition to giving the prospects information about what was happening at Los Alamos and telling them how he hoped they could each contribute to the project, Oppenheimer told them about the first nuclear chain reaction, produced by fission of the uranium isotope U-235, on December 2, 1942 at the University of Chicago by Enrico Fermi.* Although nearly a year had passed since Fermi and his colleagues at Chicago had demonstrated the first self-sustaining nuclear chain reaction, this was the first time Ramsey had heard of it.

Over lunch at the Watergate Restaurant—the restaurant was later replaced by a famous office building that played an important role in the political fortunes of President Richard Nixon—Oppenheimer told the prospective recruits about the living conditions at Los Alamos, which he made, said Ramsey, sound quite attractive. Bainbridge, who enjoyed fishing, was particularly concerned about opportunities for pursuing that interest at Los Alamos, and Oppenheimer enthusiastically assured him that, yes, there were streams and lakes, even the Rio Grande, in the vicinity. Because it was wartime, however, and gas was being rationed, Bainbridge pressed the topic further. Could these fishing spots be reached fairly easily by bicycle? To which Oppenheimer immediately replied affirmatively; you could get to the Rio Grande by bicycle in not more than 10 to 15 minutes, he said. He waited a few minutes, however, before telling Bainbridge that, because Los Alamos was about 2,000 feet higher in elevation than the Rio Grande, what was a 10- to 15-minute descent by bicycle would require at least two hours on the return trip.[113]

At the end of the day, when Oppenheimer asked him for his reaction about coming to Los Alamos, Ramsey told him he would come. "He did a beautifully effective job in persuading people to come to Los Alamos," Ramsey said, "indeed, he persuaded all of us on the spot."[114]

Since Ramsey was working for Bowles in the Secretary of War's office, Oppenheimer told him that the request for his services could be expected to come through the appropriate channels and not to say anything about their discussions. Since General Groves, the commanding general of the Manhattan District, had higher priority than anyone else, Oppenheimer told Ramsey, there would be no problem in getting the transfer approved.

In the meantime, Oppenheimer wanted Ramsey to conduct some ballistics tests on the side at the Dahlgren Proving Grounds in Silver Spring, Maryland, just to make sure that the bomb designs they were considering

---

* After Ramsey's departure from Columbia in 1939, Fermi had joined forces with Leo Szilard, the actual inventor of the nuclear chain reaction, as well as Herbert Anderson and Walter Zinn to develop a self-sustaining uranium reactor. Other groups meanwhile were also working toward the same objective, including groups at Princeton and the University of Chicago. In early 1942, it was decided that these three groups should combine their efforts at the University of Chicago.

would drop correctly with the right end up instead of head over heels. That work, Oppenheimer figured, shouldn't require more than one afternoon every other week, and probably after no more than two such afternoons were completed in this fashion, Ramsey's release would have come through.

Oppenheimer was correct about Grove's status, said Ramsey, but he underestimated the power of Bowles. When Grove's request for Ramsey's services was submitted to Secretary of War Stimson who, in turn, routed it to Bowles for approval, Bowles responded that Ramsey's services were too important to be spared right then. Of course, in the middle of World War II, the Secretary of War was a busy man and therefore didn't get Bowles' response immediately. When he did come across it, he routed it on to Groves who resubmitted his request. This pattern was repeated three or four times, as Ramsey recalled, and before the power struggle was resolved, nearly half a year had elapsed.

Oppie was initially recruiting me around March [said Ramsey].* I still hadn't heard through channels by the following August, by which time I was in the embarrassing position that the preliminary Los Alamos tests I was starting at Dahlgren Proving Grounds, instead of taking half an hour every other week, were taking about a day or two a week . . . a fair fraction of my time.[115]

The standoff was finally resolved when Bowles asked Ramsey what he wanted to do. "I think I startled him," said Ramsey, "by saying I really thought I should go out to Los Alamos."[116]

As a face-saving move, it was decided that Ramsey would remain a member of Bowles' office as an expert consultant to Secretary of War Stimson but would be assigned to Los Alamos where, in addition to his

---

* Oppenheimer and a small team of aides arrived at Los Alamos in mid-March followed by the first contingent of scientists and their families in the next month. Los Alamos essentially began its scientific operation in April 1943 with a series of introductory lectures given by Robert Serber of Berkeley. Serber was one of nine "luminaries," as Oppenheimer referred to them, who had spent the previous summer at Berkeley behind locked doors studying the technical challenges of developing an atomic bomb. The group included, in addition to Oppenheimer and Serber, Felix Bloch, Hans Bethe, Edward Teller, John Van Vleck, Emil Konopinski and two unnamed post-doctoral fellows.
— Richard Rhodes, *The Making of the Atomic Bomb* (New York: Simon and Schuster, 1988), 416.

other duties, he could act as a sort of watchdog for the interests of Stimson and Bowles.*

Oppenheimer shrewdly took advantage of this arrangement several times in the years that followed. When Groves would drag his feet on a request that Oppenheimer considered important, on at least two occasions, according to Ramsey, Oppenheimer called him in and said, 'Look, is it all right if I quote you as saying that you will feel obliged to report this fact as an expert consultant to the Secretary of War unless we do so and so?' and I said, 'Sure.' In both cases, we got what we wanted, so I never did have to give a direct report in this fashion."[117]

Los Alamos

In the fall of 1943, Norman and Elinor Ramsey left Washington, D.C. and moved west to Los Alamos, New Mexico. Although Oppenheimer, with strong urging from Rabi, had insisted that the scientists connected with the Manhattan Project remain civilians, it was clearly evident to the scientists and their wives that Los Alamos was a high-security military post, complete with uniformed guards, Army vehicles, and drab, one-color Army-type housing. Upon arriving at the 7,000-foot-high mesa, the Ramseys, however, had the good fortune of moving into a beautifully refurbished dormitory, which had been part of a ranch school that had occupied the property prior to the military. They shared the building with the Kenneth Bainbridges and the Lyman Parrotts.

For the wives of the scientists, Los Alamos was a mixed blessing. For example, said Ramsey, "it was probably easier to get meat in the commissary at Los Alamos than it was to get meat at a grocery store in the town in which you would otherwise have been living." On the down side, however, there was censorship of all outgoing mail since tight security was required. "This is one of the things that was very conspicuous to

---

* An interesting sidenote to this story was told in 1987 by Henry H. Barschall, then a professor of physics at the University of Wisconsin in Madison. Forty-five years earlier, then a recently naturalized immigrant from Germany teaching at the University of Kansas, Barschall was being recruited to work at Los Alamos because of his expertise in fission. Barschall's chancellor at the University of Kansas, however, was unwilling to release him, even when pressured by Dr. James B. Conant, head of the National Defense Research Council. Conant thereupon recommended that he contact General Groves to personally request the Secretary of War to intervene in asking for his release. "We have adopted this extreme approach," the personnel director at Los Alamos wrote to Barschall, "in the case of only one other man." That man, Barschall found out later from General Groves, was Norman Ramsey.
— Henry H. Barschall, "Reminiscenses of the early days of fission," *Physics Today*, June 1987, 30.

the wives," said Ramsey. "If you took any pictures, they had to be sent to a place where essentially they were developed by the censors and the censors did a bad job of development. As a result, a fair number of us who had never before—or since—developed our own pictures had to undertake doing this at Los Alamos in the hope of not having the pictures just completely ruined."[118]

Although General Groves was an Army engineer, he had been granted, as the head of the Manhattan District, unique authority which enabled him to operate, to a large extent, independently of the Army and its highly-developed division of labor. As a result, said Ramsey, Groves didn't have too much to do with other Army officers except in getting certain equipment from them, getting airplanes assigned, ordering practice bombs, and the like. As the military overseer of the scientific work, he did have a lot to do, however, with Oppenheimer and, because of Ramsey's assignment as head of the Delivery Group charged with delivering the bombs to their eventual targets, Groves also had a "fair amount"[119] to do with Ramsey. Operating under Admiral William S. ("Deke") Parson's divisional control, the Delivery Group was responsible for converting what was, so far, just an experimental device into a usable bomb.

When Ramsey first arrived at Los Alamos, the scientists were still primarily working on development of the original bomb design. In this design, a major portion of the bomb was comprised of a gun assembly in which the fissionable material was partly contained in the muzzle end of the gun. As Ramsey explained it, "The gun would then be fired so that the two pieces would be shot together, and there would be a super-critical amount of material and the explosion would follow. This was initially thought to be the only way of doing the job."[120]

Around the time Ramsey arrived, however, work had also begun on a spherical design that used implosion to achieve the required compression. In this design, the fissionable material—plutonium 239—was positioned at the center of the sphere like a small pit in the center of a large fruit. Upon detonation, an outer shell of high-explosives designed to focus the blast toward the center of the sphere compressed a tamper of natural uranium inward toward the focal point, forcing the start of a chain reaction and capturing any neutrons tempted to escape outward, thus achieving a more complete chain reaction while using less material. Conserving material was an important objective because U.S. production of uranium and plutonium was still minimal.

"Had we known," said Ramsey, "as much about the difficulties when the idea was first proposed as we knew a year and a half later, I think we never would have pursued it because it would have looked too impossible."[121] A major hurdle was to design the bomb with such perfect symmetry that, when imploded, equal pressure would be centered on the core from all sides, without developing unwanted jets to relieve the pressure. That hurdle was overcome, however, and it was even discovered that a sustained chain reaction could be achieved with less compression than originally thought necessary. Eventually, the decision was made to use both designs and Ramsey's group had to come up with systems capable of delivering both types of bombs to their targets.

The gun assembly type, initially dubbed Tall Man because of its length—it required the length of both bomb bays in a B-29 plus the section in between—was eventually renamed Little Boy when a new design requiring a much shorter gun assembly was created. This was the design used at Hiroshima. The implosion type, dubbed Fat Man because of its spherical shape, was used at Nagasaki. The names Tall Man and Fat Man were originally selected as code names suggestive of President Roosevelt and Prime Minister Churchill so that anyone overhearing phone discussions would be led to think they might be discussing the preparation of an airplane to take the two Allied leaders to a meeting somewhere.[122]

Before the bombs could be delivered, a number of additional design challenges had to be overcome. For one, the spherical shape of Little Boy had to be made ballistically stable by adding various amounts of flaring, tailfins and drag plates to make it fall without tumbling and upsetting the electronics. A number of tests were conducted over a dry lake at Muroc Army Air Force Base in California using radar to check the ballistic characteristics of bombs dropped from 30,000 feet.

The B-29 had to be modified with special bomb hooks needed to hold the bomb securely in place for delivery to its destination but trustworthy to release the bomb on command. After dropping a dummy bomb in flight onto the closed doors of a bomb bay, a bomb release adapted from a mechanism used for towing gliders was modified for the job, but then abandoned in favor of a stronger hook that was being used in the British Lancaster bomber.

The most effective altitude for detonation of an atomic bomb in order to impact the greatest area was initially determined to be more than 1,000 feet. To assure detonation of the bombs at this altitude, radar technology again was used, this time radar altimeters that measured the distance from bomb to ground, initiating detonation at the appointed altitude.

Because of the obvious need for reliability, back-up systems were installed. Instead of one radar altimeter, four were used. If more than one of the four disagreed that the appointed altitude had been reached, the bomb would not be detonated. And since the altimeters had been designed for flight rather than for the vibrations of free fall, they also required modifications.

Although there weren't many scientists who liked General Groves, said Ramsey, "one thing for which I will really give him very great credit is that he did . . . stick his neck out further than almost anyone else I have seen. And really, he did back up the scientists very well."

We asked for an awfully lot of expensive and difficult-to-obtain equipment [Ramsey said]. If we made a convincing case to [Groves], he was willing to go a very long way to get it. In a certain sense, if the whole project had proved to be a complete and utter fiasco, the man to suffer the most probably would have been Groves. He would have been the victim of the many subsequent congressional investigations as to why he had squandered two billion dollars on a useless project.

Certainly he supported me well when we needed a B-29 early in the game, when there were only half-a-dozen B-29s in the U.S. and they were extremely hard to get. Once we convinced him that we needed it, he went to town and fought with the chiefs of the Air Force and did whatever was required to get it. This was his virtue. His principal fault as an administrator was that he could be rather irritating to the scientists that worked under him.[123]

Even though security was tight, with so much traffic coming and going to such an isolated place, many people knew something was going on but they didn't know what.

Most of the physicists [said Ramsey] knew there was the possibility of an atomic bomb and that a lot of people were out there in New Mexico. . . . That there was a theoretical possibility of making an atomic bomb was known in the published literature by everybody in advance. The fact that it really was looking feasible in detail and the fact that the work had progressed that far was certainly very new information.[124]

Residents in the surrounding area knew that something was happening. In testing the implosion device, forest fires were sometimes set in the Los Alamos area by flying pieces of hot metal. Eventually, said Ramsey, a large region of the woods was deliberately burned off to prevent uncontrolled fires. As a result, he said, the rumor quickly spread around nearby Santa Fe that "it worked." What "it" was wasn't known, but whatever it was, it was working.[125]

Because the wives of many of the physicists at Los Alamos worked in the technical area, many of them were aware of the place's purpose. The Ramseys, however, had a new baby when they arrived at Los Alamos, making it impractical for Elinor to take employment. "As a result," said Ramsey, "she did not know what we were working on until President Truman publicly announced it. I think I was unusually conscientious," he continued. "I think she was one of the few wives who really didn't know what I was working on."[126]

Trinity and Tinian

The first atomic bomb test took place at Alamogordo, New Mexico on July 16, 1945. Laura Fermi, who was at Los Alamos with her husband Enrico, wrote 25 years later: "The word 'Alamogordo' sounds alien to me, as it must sound to all persons who were in Los Alamos toward the end of the war. The big test was then an also-big secret, and Alamogordo, where it was to take place, was never mentioned. We heard only about 'Trinity.' "[127]

The code name Trinity had been given to both the test and the test site by Oppenheimer who said it was inspired by the poetry of John Donne in which he prays, "Batter my heart, three person'd God."[128] Oppenheimer compared the dual role of the bomb as both an instrument of death as well as a deterrent to war to the complementary relationship between death and resurrection as seen by Donne in another of his poems entitled "Hymne to God My God, in My Sickness."

For Norman Ramsey, Trinity meant that it would soon be time to implement all the plans that had been put in place since his arrival at Los Alamos nearly two years earlier. Although he did some supervisory work at Trinity, he was chiefly there, he said, as an observer so that he and his delivery group would be prepared for any contingency that might arise once they and their nuclear cargo were relocated on Tinian, the Pacific island from which the bombing runs over Japan would take off.

My big activity during my last two weeks at Los Alamos was getting the final arrangements for going overseas. . . . The things I'd had to produce were already being produced and other people were installing them, and my principal concern was to watch all the operations, particularly the assembly operations, to note any trouble they had and how they got out of it because we would presumably have the same trouble at Tinian. So during the whole job of assembly at Trinity my job was to stand slightly off to the side with a pencil and paper and note every operation and particularly every difficulty. By the time the bomb was all put together and stowed in the tower, I was more or less a free observer. . . . Frankly, we just stayed on to see what happened.[129]

The Trinity test site, which was actually about 60 miles northwest of the city of Alamogordo, New Mexico, was about 150 miles due south of Los Alamos. Located in the northern part of what was then known as the Alamogordo Bombing Range and now known as the White Sands Missile Range, it was a flat, high-altitude desert valley flanked on the west by the Rio Grande, about 30 miles away, and on the east, rising another 4,000 feet above their arid surroundings, by the hilly Sierra Oscura Mountains. Known as the Jornada del Muerto, the Journey of Death, the valley seemed hospitable only to rattlesnakes, scorpions, tarantulas and the like.

Although two types of atomic bombs had been designed—the gun type, using uranium 235, and the implosion type, using plutonium 239— and both would be used on Japan, only the implosion version, the spherical Fat Man model, would be pre-tested using nuclear components. If an atomic bomb worked at all, it was reasoned, Little Boy with its U-235 gun mechanism was most likely to succeed, and if the least-likely-to-succeed bomb passed the test, you could probably forego testing its counterpart. And besides, with only one U-235 bomb in the entire U.S. nuclear arsenal in July of 1945, it needed to be saved for the real thing.

More than a year before the Trinity test, Kenneth Bainbridge had selected the site for its desolate flatness, its distance from Los Alamos—close enough to be logistically feasible, far enough not to be obviously connected—and its constancy of weather. But a week before the target date of Monday, July 16, picked by General Groves to coincide with the meeting of Truman and Stalin at Potsdam, the weather had turned unstable. A test time of 0400 on Monday, set on Sunday the 15th, had to be postponed just two hours before it was to occur because of thunderstorms and 30 mile-per-hour winds. Clearing was predicted, however, between 0500 and 0600, and this time, the revised schedule of 0530 held.

As the countdown began, Ramsey was with a group of about a dozen observers that included I.I. Rabi, who was next to him, Kenneth Greisen and Enrico Fermi. Everybody, said Ramsey, was fairly jittery and excited, everyone, that is, except Greisen. He was a calm, laid-back fellow who had been given the delicate, risky and very stressful task of assembling the high explosives used in detonating the bomb and now, as they waited those final minutes, he was dozing.

"About five minutes or so before the bomb was to be set off," said Ramsey, "Rabi turned disgustedly to Greisen and said, 'Aren't you going to get excited at all?' Greisen said he could see no reason to get excited about it. Rabi said, 'You tell me when you get excited.' He said, 'Okay,' and went back for his snooze. When [the countdown] got to something like minus 15 seconds, Ken Greisen nudged Rabi and said, 'Rabi, I'm excited.' "[130]

Physicists like to speak of orders of magnitude, and on July 16, 1945, the laboratory that Rabi and Ramsey shared with the other scientists in the desert of Southern New Mexico and the test they would observe were of an entirely different order of magnitude than the first magnetic resonance experiment they had viewed together nearly eight years earlier in Pupin Hall at Columbia. Here, the distance from their observation point to the apparatus was more than five-and-a-half miles instead of a few feet. And no man-made experiment had ever before yielded in power what the experts at Los Alamos were predicting for this test—an explosion equal to 18,000 tons of TNT. Ramsey, as a small boy living at Picatinny Arsenal in New Jersey, had probably viewed a larger explosion than any of the other observers gathered at Trinity when 500 tons of TNT had been detonated by lightning about a mile from their house, but this would be at least 36 times stronger and, visually, even more dramatic.

"One of those who was admittedly excited about the bomb but still fairly calm, and doing a very intelligent experiment," said Ramsey, "was Fermi. He was dropping pieces of paper when the shock wave came along to see how much the paper was carried by the shock which would then provide a first-hand estimate of the magnitude of the shock."[131]

Rabi won the betting pool on how large the shock would be. He went with the official prediction of 18,000 tons of TNT. Actually, he didn't have much choice. That was the only bet left when he arrived at the site just a few days before the test. Richard Rhodes states that Norman Ramsey bet a "cynical zero,"[132] but mathematician Ramsey saw his selection as "a fairly intelligent bet."

> I'd bet on zero tons of TNT because any failure would come in this category, plus this was a problem best measured in generations of neutrons. The first 80 percent or more of the generations all corresponded to zero tons, and the rest of the energies all come in the last few generations. So all sorts of failures would come in my category, but I lost. . . . Practically everybody bet under.[133]

The observers had been issued welders' glasses and told to look in the opposite direction, away from the blast, a precaution that Ramsey thought was going too far, but he followed instructions, fearful that if he didn't, he might not see anything at all.

My memories are clearest about the visual part of the explosion. In some ways the most astonishing thing to me was that looking in the opposite direction, through these welders' glasses, the hills miles away were brilliantly lighted. You could look more in the bomb direction only gradually, at the fastest rate you dared come around, because the brightness of the light . . . my recollection is of a very blue-white light. I'm not sure when I had the welders' glasses on and when I looked at the distance without them, but compared to what you usually think of an explosion or fire the light was intensely bright and white. Eventually, it turned redder. By the time we took the glasses off and looked more directly, it was the very nasty looking, well-known fireball which is much nastier to see [in reality] than it is in a movie. This fireball then went up into a mushroom cloud. I don't know if we were anticipating quite as big a cloud effect. After that, there was a good deal of worry about where the cloud was drifting.[134]

They stayed around the test site until noon or so, as Ramsey recalled, and sometime that afternoon, he drove Rabi and Oppenheimer back to Los Alamos. Oppenheimer had driven his own car down to Trinity, but Rabi and others were concerned that he might be too jittery to drive back. They took a slight detour on the return trip through a more scenic route in an attempt to calm their nerves.

I remember, [said Ramsey], the thing I was most struck with was knowing this whole thing depended upon squeezing a small sphere of plutonium. I just couldn't get over the fact that indeed that little sphere got squeezed so hard and produced, from that very small amount, that very huge result. That kept coming back into my mind. All I could think of was this little sphere being squeezed and releasing all this energy while it was still squeezed to such a small size.[135]

Even though Ramsey was a trained scientific observer, some of what he had seen just a few hours earlier was beyond his recollection.

An intriguing thing illustrates the problem of observation in the presence of something major of this kind: During the shot I had a very clear impression of all the visual portions of it. I have absolutely no memory of any direct sound or any shock wave coming from the bomb. I remember one exception, which was purely visual. You could see the indications of the shock wave running over the ground, due to both dust being stirred up by it and possibly even the slight effect of the compression on the index of refraction. Also I can remember hearing the sound of the explosion echoing from the hills for what seemed to be minutes later . . . certainly for a long period of time we heard echo reverberations. On the other hand, I have no memory whatsoever of any noise when the sound wave got to me or any feel of the shock wave. If I had to give sworn evidence, solely on the basis of myself, as to whether the direct shot produced a noise, I would have to say, "I don't know, other than to know that at some period later there were echoes."[136]

The next day, Norman Ramsey left for Tinian Island, about 1600 miles southeast of Japan in the Pacific, to supervise, over the next three weeks, the delivery of the two atomic bombs.

Columbia and Brookhaven

When it became evident that the end of the war was imminent, Norman Ramsey sent Elinor a telegram from Tinian Island urging her to immediately reserve a moving van for sometime in October. Knowing that personnel could leave Los Alamos only when a round trip could be scheduled for moving vans, he feared a mass exodus of scientists could delay a move back east and a return to 'civilian' life for as much as a year. Unbeknownst to Ramsey, however, at his remote outpost in the Pacific, Oppenheimer had requested that scientific personnel remain at Los Alamos to provide a smooth transition between wartime and peacetime use of the mountaintop laboratory. "In his persuasion he was, as usual, successful," said Ramsey, "and practically everybody was staying until January or so."[137] As a result, Norman and Elinor Ramsey were one of the first couples in the scientific community at Los Alamos to head down the mountain for home.

Home was now New York. When Ramsey moved from Cambridge, Massachusetts to Washington in 1942, he also made an official transition from the University of Illinois, where he was on leave of absence, to Columbia University, where he would also be on leave of absence for the duration of the war. Now after three years of being on the faculty of

Columbia University in absentia, he was "anxious," he said, "to get back to peacetime research. It had been a long, long war as far as my research went."[138]

In 1944, Rabi and Ramsey had spent an evening together in Cambridge, Massachusetts talking about the direction their research should take after the war. Two ideas had been discussed at length. One was to use the potent measuring power of magnetic resonance and radiofrequency spectroscopy, first utilized by the Rabi team in 1938, to test a fundamental theory of quantum mechanics that predicted hyperfine separations in the spectral lines of atomic hydrogen. Another was to attempt to observe nuclear magnetic resonance transitions by their effects on the oscillator. When they made some initial calculations on what kind of signal-to-noise ratios they could expect, it looked very promising and both men became enthusiastic about the prospects. When they both recalled, however, that this approach was similar to the one used by Cornelis Gorter in the second of two ill-fated attempts to discover NMR in solids, they decided against it.[139]

In 1942, in a Holland occupied by Nazi Germany, not the best conditions for conducting research, C.J. Gorter and I.J.F. Broer had tried to detect nuclear magnetic resonance in powders of lithium chloride and potassium fluoride by observing its effects on the frequency of a self-excited oscillator as the applied magnetic field was moved through the anticipated point of resonance.[140] They saw some "irreproducible irregularities"[141] in the frequency, according to Gorter, but the results of the experiment were negative. The source of the problem in both of Gorter's experiments has never been definitively determined—some felt the sample was too pure, although Nicolaas Bloembergen was able some years later to measure relaxation times in the identical sample. Anyway, the prospect of achieving the same negative results put a damper on Idea Two for Rabi and Ramsey and tipped the balances in favor of the first idea, atomic beam experiments, although both ideas would eventually prove to have merit.

About a month after Ramsey returned to the laboratories at Columbia, two research teams operating independently—Edward M. Purcell, Henry C. Torrey, and Robert V. Pound at Harvard and Felix Bloch, William W. Hansen, and Martin Packard at Stanford—proved the basic merit of the Gorter-Broer experiment when they observed nuclear magnetic resonance in condensed matter,[142] or what Bloch called "nuclear induction."*

---

* The first published use of the phrase "nuclear magnetic resonance" appeared in Gorter's 1942 paper, a term he attributed to I.I. Rabi.

Although the Purcell and Bloch methods varied in their focus and approach, both methods detected resonance transitions by their effects on the radiofrequency system.

Getting back to research for Ramsey and Rabi wasn't as simple as just switching on the old apparatuses and picking up where the pre-war Rabi teams had left off. Rabi's laboratories on the fifth and tenth floors of Pupin Hall that had been used before the war for basic research with molecular and atomic beams had been reallocated during the war for applied research on radar and vacuum tubes and for the diffusion process used to separate isotopes for the Manhattan Project. Thus, much of the previous laboratory equipment and apparatus had either been thrown out or taken up to the attic. By searching through wastebaskets and piles of junk, however, Ramsey was able to find a few precious items that would have taken months to rebuild and, within a relatively short period, to resume his research.

He began where he had left off six years earlier at Columbia, with radiofrequency spectroscopy. As a quick scan of Ramsey papers published in 1946 and 1947 readily reveals, he continued to be fascinated by nuclear interactions within molecules. Working with William Nierenberg, his first graduate student, and S.B. Brody, Ramsey studied nuclear moments of the bromine isotopes, magnetic resonance spectra of the sodium halides, and nuclear quadrupole interactions.[143-146]

Following through on their 1944 discussion, Rabi and Ramsey together started two other students, John Nafe and Edward Nelson, on a fundamental experiment to measure accurately the hyperfine separation theoretically predicted for atomic hydrogen. This experiment was completed by Rabi, Nafe and Nelson and led to the first indication of an anomalous magnetic moment of the electron.[147] This anomaly started Julian Schwinger on his theoretical explanation[148] for which he shared the 1965 Nobel Prize in physics. The hyperfine studies also stimulated Polykarp Kusch in 1947 to make a direct measurement of the anomalous magnetic moment of the electron[149] for which he received the 1955 Nobel Prize in physics.*

During this same period, Ramsey and Rabi were working to obtain a nuclear reactor for universities in the New York area. The spoils of war had

---

* Dutch physicists Samuel A. Goudsmit and George E. Uhlenbeck were the first to propose, in 1925, that the electron has its own intrinsic magnetic moment. Goudsmit would later succeed Norman Ramsey as director of the physics department at Brookhaven National Laboratory.

left the University of Chicago with a "very nice reactor" and the University of California with a "nice high energy accelerator," said Ramsey, and "we really began worrying about what we should do in this connection."[150]

Rabi and I really felt—sometimes you do things for not always the best of motives and I would say this was one of them. We were rather jealous of the University of Chicago and felt we had even been a little done in by Karl Compton who was a professor at Chicago and also, at one stage, head of the uranium [chain reaction] project. Basically, before the war, we had at Columbia Enrico Fermi, who did the first work on nuclear reactor development there, and then when Compton became head of that division of NDRC, he decided all that work should be transferred to Chicago. So Chicago ended up at the end of the war with Fermi and with the Argonne Lab and we in the East had nothing in that direction. So we felt we really should try to get something going and did indeed.[151]

Recognizing that it would be more efficient to share the resource with other universities and less draining on their own departmental energies, Rabi and Ramsey, together with representatives from other institutions in the New York area formed an ad hoc committee called the Initiatory University Group to explore available options. The option they agreed upon was that they should apply for funding to the Manhattan District, still headed by General Groves (its successor agency, the Atomic Energy Commission had not yet been established).

Ramsey was appointed Executive Secretary, which meant, said Ramsey, that "I was stuck with having to write all the letters and with carrying on most of the activities."[152] In the meantime, Jerrold Zacharias and others at MIT got word of what their academic neighbors to the south were doing and they joined with Harvard to submit their own proposal to the Manhattan District for a similar laboratory to be built in the Cambridge, Massachusetts area.

By then, the Atomic Energy Act had already been passed setting up the structure for the Atomic Energy Commission. As a lame-duck director of a lame-duck agency, General Groves felt he should not saddle the new AEC with two laboratories in the same general region, and told the two competing groups to come up with one laboratory they could share.

The result, after a long search and tough bargaining between the two groups, was Brookhaven National Laboratory on Long Island, formed under the auspices of Associated Universities, Inc. (AUI), a consortium formed by nine New England and Mid-Atlantic institutions from as far south as Johns Hopkins, as far west as Rochester, and as far north as Harvard and MIT. Ramsey was appointed as the chairman of the physics department at Brookhaven in 1946, a position he held simultaneously with that of professor of physics at Columbia.

"I moved out to Bayport, Long Island," said Ramsey, "which was part way between the two places. In theory, I was teaching classes at Columbia something like Tuesdays, Thursdays and Saturdays, and I was going to Brookhaven to do physics research and head the physics department there Mondays, Wednesdays and Fridays."[153]

During that period, Ramsey hired a "fair fraction"[154] of the new Brookhaven staff and helped set in motion the development of Brookhaven's cosmotron, the first multi-billion-electron-volt machine ever built (rated at 3-billion-electron volts, notated as 3 GeV). One of the people hired by Ramsey was Maurice Goldhaber, his former tutor at Cambridge University in the mid-1930s, who later became director of Brookhaven National Laboratory.

Although Ramsey was "really very happy"[155] with his dual-role arrangement, a rough ride six months later on the Long Island Railroad convinced him to accept a very attractive offer from Harvard for a professorship that he had initially refused.

I thought I would effectively use my time on the train for study [Ramsey said]. I was at that time trying to understand Wigner's book on group theory, which was then available only in German. But with the combination of the German language, the subject of group theory, and the Long Island Railroad—on which I was trying to do the studying—it seemed to me I wasn't getting very far. So I changed my mind, called [Professor John] Van Vleck and asked if the offer at Harvard was still open.[156]

Ramsey had also come to the conclusion that he was caught in a kind of 'Catch-22' situation. The advantage of running a large laboratory like Brookhaven was that he had a large number of people working for him. Whenever he had a good research idea to pursue, he had access to both equipment and manpower to get the problem solved quickly. The disadvantage was that, with such a large organization and its accompanying administrative duties, he didn't have the time to think up the bright ideas to pursue in the first place. "So I convinced myself," said Ramsey, "that for my purposes and for the kind of basic research I wanted to do, running a small group—a dozen or so—of graduate students, people directly doing research with me, was just right. Running a big department, either there [at Brookhaven] or at a university was, for me, just wrong."[157]

Harvard Professor

In the summer of 1947, Dr. Ramsey left Columbia University and Brookhaven National Laboratory for Harvard University. He continued, however, as a consultant to Brookhaven and would later serve as a trustee representing Harvard on the board of Associated Universities, Inc.

He arrived at Harvard at a time when the basement of its Lyman Laboratory of Physics was a beehive of activity. Like other institutions around the country during the post-war period, Harvard's graduate school classes were filled with gifted students who had had to postpone their educational pursuits during World War II and were well motivated to get on with their lives and careers.

In late 1945, Purcell, Torrey and Pound had successfully detected nuclear magnetic resonance absorption in condensed matter and now, just a year-and-a-half later, graduate students that included Nicolaas Bloembergen, George Pake and Charles Slichter formed the vanguard of NMR greats that would follow in coming years, many of whom would be mentored by Norman Ramsey. Over the years, the number of students mentored by him would grow to a lifetime career total of 84.

Most of the initial papers published by Ramsey after moving to Harvard were authored solely by him, reflecting both a lag effect in the mentoring process as well as the fact that, for several years, he was very busy building Harvard's second cyclotron and setting up a molecular beam laboratory.

The first two papers Ramsey published at Harvard reported on his investigations of large quadrupole interactions using radiofrequency spectroscopy.[158-159] His third paper announced an invention that would result in his 1989 Nobel Prize.[160]

Separated Oscillatory Fields

From the beginning of his research career, Ramsey had been preoccupied with measurements, an obsession that continues to the present day. Perhaps a natural result of his mathematical bent, it was also influenced by his association with Dr. I.I. Rabi.

I fully echo Dr. Rabi's views that there is much to be said for precision measurements [Ramsey told a conference in 1982]. Out of them

them come unexpected things. At one time we thought that there would be no interest in clocks if they were more accurate than a part in 10^7, and now it is quite clear that each time we make a step forward, there is a small revolution. Now many highly accurate measurements are reduced to the measurement of a frequency because frequencies can be measured so well. Precision measurements of almost all quantities now remind me of my mother's story of a doctor who could cure only one disease—stomach ache—but he became a great doctor because he also knew how to reduce all other diseases to a stomach ache.[161]

It can't be said that Norman Ramsey is a one-theme physicist, but it is true that, by paying attention to the twin themes of time and frequency measurement throughout his career, his experimental and theoretical work has yielded a bounty of advancements in science and technology, an abundance that likely would have been diminished had he lost sight of his central focus.

His invention of the separated oscillatory fields method is a case in point. As he told the Swedish Academy of Science in 1989, when he was awarded his Nobel Prize, the method came about because he was "looking for a way to make more accurate measurements than were possible with the Rabi [magnetic resonance spectroscopy] method."[162]

In the process of developing his molecular-beam laboratory at Harvard in 1949, Ramsey was looking for a way to improve the accuracy of the H_2 and D_2 interactions they had first measured with the Rabi apparatus back in 1938-39. One way he knew to do it was to lengthen the apparatus and thereby lengthen the amount of time that individual molecules would be subjected to its magnetic field. "I was going to make a molecular-beam apparatus 10 times better than any previous by making it 10 times longer," said Ramsey. Trouble was, the idea had already been tested at Columbia and been found wanting because of inhomogeneities in the magnetic field. Instead of getting narrower spectral peaks, they got broader peaks. Although Ramsey kept building his apparatus, he hadn't figured out how to get around the problem. "I thought I knew how to do it," he said, "but it wasn't working very well, so I was worried."[163]

It so happened that he was teaching a course at the time on physical optics and was talking about the Michelson stellar interferometer. Nearly 15 years earlier, P.I. Dee, one of Ramsey's professors at Cambridge University, described how the Michelson device worked. If two stars giving lots of light are poorly resolved by a large telescope and you want to separate them, Dee had said, you can double the resolution by painting over the middle of the telescope with black paint and leaving just two narrow slits at the edge.

While describing this phenomenon to his optics class, Ramsey had thought to himself that since the middle of the glass is covered over with black paint, it must not depend on the quality of the glass in that region.

Of course, to make a Michelson stellar interferometer you don't actually take a 200-inch telescope and paint it black [said Ramsey]. You just make two slits at a distance. And I sort of had a feeling: "Isn't there some way I could do the same thing with our magnetic resonance experiment?" Well, this was the idea but I didn't know quite what "the same thing" was.[164]

"That took another week or two of stewing, but that was the triggering idea," said Ramsey, which led him to the idea of having two oscillating fields, driven phase-coherently by the same oscillator, one at the entrance of the homogeneous C-field and the other at the exit with a region between them that was free of rotation. The new method, combined with better means of taking data and the realization that there were certain advantages to using lower magnetic fields than they had used previously, improved accuracy not 10-fold, but 100-fold.[165]

Atomic Clocks and the Atomic Hydrogen Maser

Ramsey's separated oscillatory field method was well adapted to increasing the precision of atomic clocks. In the cesium based atomic clock, for example, which has an accuracy of 10^{-13}, the method led to the international redefinition of the second (equal to 9,192,631,770 periods of the cesium atom).

The separated oscillatory fields idea also led to the other achievement for which Ramsey was cited by the Nobel Committee—the atomic hydrogen maser. In the latter case, he was looking for a way to obtain greater accuracy in atomic beam experiments. On the basis of the principle mentioned above—the longer the atoms are in the apparatus the greater the accuracy of the measurement—Ramsey was looking for a way to keep cesium atoms from leaving the resonance area so quickly.

This time, instead of merely increasing the length of their flight and adding a second oscillating field, he came up with the idea of making the atoms stay around for awhile after encountering the first oscillating field by directing them into a storage container coated with Teflon where they would "bounce around for a period of time"[166] before eventually emerging to pass through the second oscillatory field. His PhD student at the time, Daniel Kleppner, undertook construction of the storage box as his thesis project and the experiment was called a broken atomic beam.

The experiment was partially successful; a separated oscillatory field pattern for an atomic hyperfine transition was obtained, but it was weak and, after a few wall collisions, it disappeared. After refining the experiment, however, and changing from cesium to atomic hydrogen, Ramsey and his collaborators, Kleppner and H.M. Goldenberg, developed the first atomic hydrogen maser which, in turn, has resulted in an atomic clock with the greatest stability of all. With a stability of 10^{-15} over a period of several hours, the atomic hydrogen maser has been used for the Voyager mission to Neptune as well as the recently-instituted Global Positioning System, or GPS.

In a recent article in *Physics Today*, Daniel Kleppner, now Lester Wolfe Professor of Physics and associate director of the Research Laboratory of Electronics at MIT, reflected on his association with Dr. Ramsey during that period and the resulting achievement. Making a case for the importance of basic research, he wrote:

> I entered Harvard as a graduate student just when Norman Ramsey had hit upon an idea for making a better atomic clock—a clock that might be accurate enough to show the gravitational red shift—by storing atoms in a "bottle." The result of our research was the hydrogen maser. . . . As an atomic clock, the hydrogen maser paid off in numerous unexpected ways. . . . However, the most spectacular payoff from atomic clocks is the GPS. . . . By interpreting the arrival times, the receiver [which can be the size of a hand-held calculator] determines latitude, longitude and altitude with an uncertainty that can be as small as 10 meters.[167]

The Search for the Missing Electric Dipole Moment

In 1947, as the new resident expert on molecular beams at Harvard, Ramsey was asked to teach a course on molecular beams and Edward Purcell decided to sit in on it. "It was great," Ramsey said, "to have Ed in the course and his presence led to many stimulating discussions. But whenever I was giving a proof that I did not fully understand, I could count on Ed asking an astute question that would reveal my ignorance."[168]

For that reason, a few days before he was to give the then-standard parity proof that nuclei could not have electric dipole moments, Ramsey began anticipating the possibility that Purcell might ask him in class for the experimental evidence for parity symmetry in nuclear forces, as contrasted to electromagnetic forces.

According to basic laws of physics, molecules, atoms and nuclei behave symmetrically. As one author has explained it:

> Nature does not care whether observers look at it directly or in a mirror. An experiment conducted in a mirror world should be the same as one conducted in our world. As a result of Emmy Noether's mathematical breakthrough during World War I, the laws of parity and symmetry had already explained much about molecules, atoms and nuclei. So why not inside the nucleus, too?[169]

When Ramsey began looking for the evidence, however, he found none, so "on the military principle," he said, "that if one is about to be attacked he should counter attack, I asked Ed if he knew of any evidence but he could provide none, either."[170]

Now that they were both on the same side of the problem, Ramsey and Purcell became seriously interested in the matter and began analyzing what experiments they could design that might prove or disprove the assumption. After examining a number of possibilities, they concluded that a search for a neutron electric dipole moment would be a "relatively sensitive test of parity conservation."[171]

Their first test, conducted by their graduate student, James Smith, at the Oak Ridge reactor in Tennessee failed to find an electric dipole moment, but they were able to lower its experimental limit by a factor of 1,000. Thus began what would become a search by Ramsey for more than 40 years for the elusive moment (if it exists). He still hasn't found it, although he has succeeded in further lowering of the experimental limit.

Seven years after Ramsey and Purcell published their paper reporting their question of the assumption,[172] Professors Lee and Yang of Columbia University published a paper in 1957 in which they questioned the assumption of parity for the weak force within the nucleus and suggested other experiments that might be conducted to resolve the question. Ironically, Lee and Yang referenced a 1957 paper by Smith, Purcell and Ramsey[173] as the principal evidence supporting the parity assumption—it was actually part of their ongoing effort to test the assumption—and failed to refer to Ramsey and Purcell's much-earlier paper in which they had questioned the assumption and suggested searching for the electric dipole moment of the neutron as a possible test.

In fact, "despite the negative result of our first search for an electric dipole moment," said Ramsey, "one consequence of our early arguments about parity was that I became quite comfortable with the idea of parity non-conservation."[174] In 1956, he became "enthusiastic" about searching for a parity violation in the weak force that might be observable in beta decay of cobalt 60 and suggested his idea to Frank Yang in two follow-up letters. Unfortunately for Ramsey, just as the project was about to get underway at Oak Ridge with collaborator Louis Roberts, it was pre-empted by a fission discovery at Oak Ridge that the facility's advisory group felt should be exploited first. As a result, the experiment was delayed for a year.

Meanwhile, before Lee and Yang's article was even published, Professor Chien-Shiung Wu of Columbia in collaboration with Ernest Ambler and others from the National Bureau of Standards succeeded in conducting an experiment that disproved the assumption by monitoring beta decay in cobalt, the same isotope Ramsey planned to use.

That same year, in what is probably record time between the achievement and Nobel recognition, Professors Lee and Yang received the 1957 Nobel Prize in physics for their paper questioning the assumption of parity. Professor Chien-Shiung Wu later received the first Wolf Prize from the state of Israel for her experimental proof.

Also in 1957, Ramsey published a paper[175] in which he pointed out that, just as parity conservation was an assumption that should be proven experimentally, so should time reversal symmetry be experimentally proven. Many years later, he learned that Jackson, et al. had published independently a paper that made the same point. Seven years later, Cronin and Fitch discovered experimentally a violation of time reversal symmetry, for which they received the Nobel Prize in 1980. Again, the early papers by Ramsey and Jackson were, by that time, all but forgotten.

Assistant Secretary-General for NATO

In February of 1958, Norman Ramsey, then 42 years old, was appointed as Science Advisor (later called Assistant Secretary General) to Paul-Henri Spaak, Secretary General of the North Atlantic Treaty Organization (NATO) for the purpose of advising the free-world alliance on better means for international cooperation in scientific research. Headquartered in Paris where Ramsey had once lived for a time as a boy, the position had been newly created in December of the previous year, about two months after the Soviet-made Sputnik first began orbiting the earth.

"I must admit," Ramsey told an interviewer four years later, "I did not even read this news as it came out, but a month or two later, [Detlev] Bronk, then president of the National Academy of Sciences, asked if it would be all right if he came up that afternoon to talk to me here [at Harvard].

"Well, my feeling," Ramsey continued, "is that it's bad enough if the president of the National Academy of Sciences wants you to come down to see him. It probably means you're going to be stuck for a time-consuming job. But if he wants to come to see you, it's even worse. This proved to be the case."[176]

Although Ramsey was not anxious to leave his research at Harvard and engage in an ill-defined position, he nevertheless recognized the benefits of getting cooperation started and agreed to take the job for a year. At first he wondered if that would be enough, but then he remembered his war-time experience with civil-service "bottlenecks" in Washington and decided that one year might be better than two. Ramsey made one other stipulation before accepting the job; that after he completed the assignment he would have a clear conscience in turning down other requests to serve on government committees for a few years until he was able to catch up on the time he would lose in Paris.

At the time of the appointment, Robert Doty, writer for the *New York Times*, wrote that little definition had been provided about the new position but that it appeared likely that Ramsey's principal problem would be to define the areas in which NATO, then an alliance of 15 member nations, could "effectively move into the scientific field, currently hedged about with secrecy restrictions. There was some speculation," he continued, "that one of the advisor's functions might be to serve as a clearing house and switching point for national research programs—to let the right hand know what the left was doing and keep them from doing the same jobs."

With tongue in cheek, Doty nevertheless thought that such a task would be a formidable one: "Until he took the NATO assignment," he wrote, "Dr. Ramsey had nothing more complicated with which to deal than the internal structure of atomic nuclei, the perfection of atomic clocks with an error of one in ten billion and supervisory work on the Harvard-Massachusetts Institute of Technology six billion-volt electron accelerator."[177]

Ramsey was on leave from Harvard for the year-and-a-half that he held the NATO job. Looking back in 1962 on what had been accomplished during his tenure in Paris, he said: "I think that on the whole it really worked out remarkably well. We had no clear, defined functions at all. I would say it was probably an advantage that it wasn't clear what we should do."[178]

Rather than start another paperwork bureaucracy, Ramsey hoped to use his year on the job to choose a few objectives that would really improve cooperation in scientific research and to begin just thinking about the longer-term ones. To help him in the task, he was blessed, he pointed out, with a Science Committee that, in most cases, was made up of effective scientists, not just administrators. The U.S. representative was Ramsey's PhD mentor and long-time colleague, Professor I.I. Rabi of Columbia.

One of their first objectives was to establish a fellowship exchange program for training of science students in different countries. Another was to establish a fund for supporting summer science institutes. These have grown from an initial two in theoretical physics to more than 150 in all fields of science. A third major objective, achieved on Ramsey's last day in office, was to fund cooperative research grants. As for reducing duplication in defense research, Ramsey found that the best way to improve that situation was just to bring together the directors of defense research for each of the countries. Many of them had never met before.

Chemical Shifts

Physicist Felix Bloch once commented that "when chemists get into a field it's time to get out,"[179] but when physicist Norman Ramsey formulated the theoretical foundation for chemical shifts, he opened the field of NMR to alert chemists who saw it as a powerful tool for chemical analysis.

In 1938, while a graduate student at Columbia, Ramsey had found that by presetting the amperage of the external field and by adjusting the oscillator frequency of the R-field—the basis for radiofrequency spectroscopy—he could discover much more about hydrogen than just the magnetic moment of its proton; he could learn a great deal about its localized, interactive environment.

Ten years later, soon after his arrival at Harvard, Ramsey began formulating the theory for what he described as "chemical effects" even before reports of their existence experimentally were published. Similar to his experience with magnetic resonance spectroscopy, in which he was able to learn about the interactive environment of atoms and molecules by "listening in" on their localized magnetic relationships, Ramsey theorized on the basis of what he had learned about interactive relationships from MR spectroscopy that different chemical bonds caused protons to resonate at different frequencies because of the unique shielding effect produced by the molecule's electrons. As Edward Purcell explained it in his 1952 Nobel lecture:

> The magnetic field at an atomic nucleus differs slightly from the field externally applied because of the shielding effect of the electron cloud around the nucleus. In different molecules the atom's electron configuration will differ slightly, reflecting differences in the chemical bond. The resulting resonance shifts have been called 'chemical shifts.' They are only a nuisance to the experimenter interested in exact ratios of magnetic moments. But they are interesting to the physical chemist because they reveal something about the electrons that partake in the chemical bond.[180]

The most famous example of this phenomenon, also mentioned by Purcell in his Nobel lecture, was discovered by Arnold, Dharmatti and Packard in 1951 from their radiospectral analysis of ethyl alcohol. Although the protons making up the molecule are all chemically equivalent and, if isolated, would resonate at the same frequency, instead, because of their unique chemical bonds, each of the three groups of protons making up the molecule resonates at slightly different frequencies, producing three spectral lines, each shifted from "normal" and producing a spectral line combination that serves as ethyl alcohol's "fingerprint."

Willis Lamb, a colleague of I.I. Rabi at Columbia, had published in 1940 the theory for magnetic shielding as it applied to single atoms. Ramsey was then at Carnegie Institution in Washington. Since there was no equivalent theory for molecules, Lamb's theory for atoms was also applied to molecules which, for atoms with many electrons, was a fair approximation.

In 1949, however, the same year in which he developed the separated oscillatory fields method for molecular beams, Ramsey published a paper which noted that, for atoms with few electrons, such an approximation was not valid and that, furthermore, even in atoms of many electrons, the approximation was insufficient to explain molecular shielding. In that paper and in a series of theoretical follow-up papers,[181-184] Ramsey published general formulas for calculating these magnetic shieldings or "chemical shifts"—Ramsey called them "chemical effects" at the time—in different molecules. He also pointed out in these papers that, for the same nucleus, the shielding could be different in different molecules and provided formulas to account for these differences.

At about the same time, these shifts began to be noticed experimentally in NMR by a number of researchers. In Holland, where he had just finished the dissertation for his PhD degree at Leiden University, Nicolaas Bloembergen, in what may well be the first experimental evidence of a chemical shift, found a large shift in a $CuSO_4 \cdot 5H_2O$ crystal he had grown.[185] Soon afterward, in 1950, Warren Proctor, F.C. Yu, W.C. Dickinson[186-187] and, subsequently, many others found chemical shifting in the range of a few hundredths of a percent in NMR frequencies when the same nucleus was combined with different chemical compounds. Also in 1950, Bloembergen and Dickinson[188] observed that, when paramagnetic atoms were added to liquid samples to reduce relaxation times, NMR resonance frequencies were shifted and that the magnitudes of these shifts were proportional to the concentrations of the ions.

Although Ramsey's original theory could account for cases in which the temperature shift was small compared to the chemical shift, it did not adequately explain the Packard-Dharmatti-Arnold observation of the relatively-large temperature shift for hydrogen in ethyl alcohol, mentioned earlier. A modification of the general theory in a 1951 paper by Ramsey and U. Liddel,[189] however, taking into account molecular association in liquid alcohol and its change with temperature did account for the Packard, et al. results.

A 1952 paper by Norman Ramsey and Edward Purcell,[190] in response to a different frequency shift discovered experimentally by Gutowsky, McCall, Slichter and McNeill[191] as well as by Erwin Hahn and D.E. Maxwell,[192] accounted for a shift which could not be explained by any previously-known interaction. Ramsey and Purcell attributed it to an electron-coupled nuclear spin-spin interaction. Such an interaction, they said, could arise from each nucleus interacting magnetically with the electron spin of its own atom. Later, Ramsey developed the theory quantitatively both for the observed interaction as well as anticipated anisotropic interactions.[193] Subsequent measurements with deuterium agreed with the theory.

Cyclotrons, Accelerators and Fermilab

As mentioned earlier, Professor Ramsey's decision to resign in 1947 as director of the physics department at Brookhaven National Laboratory was precipitated by two primary factors: 1) His plan to divide his time between Columbia University and Brookhaven was frustrated by a rough rail bed that made his ride on the Long Island Railroad unproductive. 2) The benefits of having access to manpower and a state-of-the-art research facility to conduct experiments were offset by the administrative responsibilities that limited the time he had available to develop new ideas. As a result of his rough ride on the LIRR and the lack of time for research, Ramsey changed his mind about the position at Harvard he had turned down a few weeks earlier, and moved to Massachusetts.

It appears that Ramsey must have stacked his inner arguments in Harvard's favor because his departure from Brookhaven neither marked his departure from doing "big physics" nor from administrating big departments. In fact, soon after arriving at Harvard, because of Ramsey's major role in founding Brookhaven, Professor Kenneth Bainbridge appointed Ramsey the chairman of Harvard's nuclear physics committee and gave him the responsibility of developing and overseeing construction of Harvard's second cyclotron.

Ten years earlier, Edward Purcell and others under the direction of Professor Kenneth Bainbridge had designed and built the first Harvard cyclotron. In 1947, the school's second cyclotron was under development, this time under the direction of Bainbridge and Robert Wilson. (Wilson would later become the first director of the Enrico Fermi National Laboratory, or Fermilab, the world's largest nuclear accelerator, located in Northern Illinois.) About the time Ramsey arrived at Harvard, Wilson left for a new position at Cornell University in Ithaca, New York. Soon afterward, Bainbridge asked Ramsey to take major responsibility for getting the cyclotron built and operating. In addition, Ramsey was setting up his new molecular-beam laboratory.

Soon after construction of the cyclotron was completed, a significant percentage of Ramsey's research time began to be given to "high-energy" physics as well as to "low-energy" molecular beams. It should be noted, however, that this was not a new course embarked upon by Ramsey at this point. As early as 1940, although it would hardly rate as "high-energy" physics by today's standards—"At that time," said Ramsey, "high energy was defined as 1 MeV"[194]—Ramsey had published papers as a post-doctoral fellow at the Carnegie Institution (co-authored with Van Allen, Salant and Heydenburg) that were clearly pointing in that direction.* Even more clearly, Ramsey's career path began to alternate between low- and high-energy physics when he accepted the chairmanship of the physics department at Brookhaven.

His move to Brookhaven was part of a calculated plan to get Polykarp Kusch back to Columbia from Bell Laboratories after the war. To overcome the reservations of the rest of the physics department at Columbia, who felt they already had too many people in the field of molecular beams, Ramsey agreed to take the chairmanship at Brookhaven and to devote half of his time and research to high-energy and nuclear physics at the Long Island facility, thus opening the door for Kusch at Columbia.

Although the ploy worked, and Kusch was rehired by Columbia, the bad news for Ramsey was that he may have maneuvered himself right out of making a fundamental discovery.

> In one sense, I probably did myself in a little bit because Rabi and I had invented a very, very good experiment, namely looking for the hyperfine interaction in atomic hydrogen. We knew the magnetic moment of the proton, we knew the magnetic moment of the electron, and knew we should be able to calculate exactly the result. Would it be what theory said it should be? Everything should have been exact. Well, that was one of the experiments I gave up. As it turned out, it wasn't exact. It was a very fundamental, basic discovery that led to what we call quantum electrodynamics (QED), that and the Lamb shift, two key discoveries. So you do yourself in occasionally.[195]

Ramsey's interest in high-energy physics would continue throughout his career. A cursory scan of Ramsey's publications reveals numerous high-energy experiments conducted by him and his associates, both colleagues and graduate students. From the late 1940s to the early 1960s, these experiments were conducted at both Harvard and Brookhaven.

In the early 1960s, Ramsey was appointed chairman of a joint Harvard-MIT committee to head up the design and construction of his third "high-energy" physics machine, a six-billion-electron volt (6 GeV) accelerator that the two Cambridge, Massachusetts schools would share.

---

* A 1976 textbook identifies 1947 as the beginning point for high-energy physics as a distinct branch of physics. Incidentally, the book was co-authored by Mark Zemansky, one of I.I. Rabi's fellow graduate students at Columbia University in the late 1920s.

By 1962, Brookhaven's first cosmotron which Ramsey had helped plan, rated at 3 GeV, had proven itself a "smashing" success and had been replaced by a 33 GeV accelerator. And the first accelerator built by the European Organization for Nuclear Research (CERN), a 600 MeV machine, had been replaced by a 30 GeV accelerator. "The agreement between design expectations and performances for these two accelerators [the new Brookhaven and CERN machines]," noted Ramsey, "encouraged designers to believe that much larger and less conservatively designed accelerators were feasible."[196]

As a result, by late 1962, more than a dozen proposals were before the Atomic Energy Commission, requesting approval for accelerators ranging from 10 to 1,000 GeV. To help sort out these requests and to assess the nation's future needs in high-energy accelerator physics, a joint panel was appointed in late 1962 by the President's Science Advisory Committee and the General Advisory Committee of the Atomic Energy Commission, with Norman Ramsey as its chairman.

About six months later, the Ramsey Panel recommended: 1) prompt construction of a 200 GeV proton accelerator by Berkeley's Lawrence Radiation Laboratory, 2) construction of colliding-beams storage rings at Brookhaven, 3) design studies at Brookhaven for a proton accelerator in the 600 to 1,000 GeV range, 4) construction of a high-intensity 12.5 GeV proton accelerator by the Midwest Universities Research Association (MURA) "without permitting this to delay the steps toward higher energy," and 5) development and construction of electron-positron colliding-beams storage rings at Stanford.

It was also recommended by the Ramsey Panel that the administrative structure of the larger installations should provide national representation to ensure equal access by qualified scientists. A subsequent review committee of accelerator users, also appointed by the President's Science Advisory Committee, concurred with all of the Ramsey Panel recommendations including the importance of providing representation by outside groups in laboratory management.

Shortly after, however, a significant portion of the plan went back to the drawing board when President Lyndon Johnson refused to support the MURA portion of the proposal and when disagreement arose between the management of the Lawrence Radiation Laboratory and its advisors concerning the extent to which management of its new accelerator should include national representation.

As a result of these new circumstances, the Atomic Energy Commission invited all 50 states to submit proposals for alternative sites. Forty-eight states responded with 125 proposals. After reducing the list of 125 down to 85, the AEC turned it over to a panel of the National Academy of Sciences, headed by Emanuel Piore, who was asked to select the six best sites. In early 1966, the Piore panel announced their selection of six sites in California, Colorado, Illinois, Michigan, New York and Wisconsin.

Over a year earlier, however, when the site selection issue was just being opened, Frederick Seitz, president of the National Academy of Sciences, called 25 university presidents together to express his belief that whatever site was selected, it should be administered by a national organization. At this meeting, held on January 17, 1965, it was decided to establish a new organization, Universities Research Association, Inc., which would offer its services to the Atomic Energy Commission as the managing agency for the proposed accelerator, wherever it might be located.

Although the AEC was careful to avoid any formal relationship with URA until after site selection was completed and asked the URA staff not to express their personal site preferences, URA's Board of Trustees used the intervening period to develop plans that enabled them to "hit the ground running" as soon as site determination was made. In July of 1966, Professor Norman Ramsey was elected president of an organization that did not yet have an officially recognized role.

Because of the intense competition between the top six contenders and the "real threat," said Ramsey, "that the accelerator might never exist [once final site selection was made] since the disappointed regions could easily kill the project by their protests . . . I arranged to speak to all Users Meetings to point out that it would be easy for any regional group to prevent the accelerator from going to the selected site, but it would be impossible to get it transfered to another region."[197]

Ramsey was able to talk with each User Meeting except the one at Berkeley before site selection was made and in each, because he was speaking about a "what if" situation, his message was welcomed. That was not the case with Berkeley. On December 16, 1966, before Ramsey could speak to the Berkeley group, it was announced that the new laboratory would be located on a 6,800-acre plot in Northern Illinois. When Ramsey arrived, "disappointment in Berkeley was at its peak," he said, "and the audience was inevitably unfriendly."[198]

The underground accelerator at the new Fermi National Accelerator Laboratory, or Fermilab as it is also called, would be four miles in circumference and would go into operation in 1972. "For the next 16 years," Ramsey wrote in his Nobel autobiography, "I was on leave half time from

Harvard as president of Universities Research Association which exercised its management responsibilities for the construction and operation of the Fermilab accelerator through two outstanding laboratory directors, Robert R. Wilson and Leon Lederman."[199]

The Fermilab accelerator [said Ramsey] has been a great success. It cost less than the originally budgeted $250 million; it now produces 800 GeV instead of the originally planned 200 (which makes it the world's highest energy accelerator); and it has been modified to provide colliding beams which greatly increases the effective energy in the center of mass system. A number of important experiments have been done with it, including the discovery of the upsilon particle, which provided the first experimental evidence for the b-quark.[200]

With the recent scuttling by the U.S. Congress (October 1993) of the Superconducting Supercollider (SSC) project in Waxahachie, Texas—an accelerator 54 miles in circumference designed to collide beams of protons together at 40-trillion-electron volts (40 TeV, or 40 tera-electron volts)—Fermilab will keep its status as the largest accelerator in the world at 800 GeV (with plans to reach 1 TeV, equal to 1000 GeV) for at least a few more years.* Congress' decision had lengthened the effective life of the accelerator he has championed since 1966, but Ramsey the scientist wasn't gloating.

It's expensive, so you can really worry, 'Should you do it?' But it's a terrible mistake cancelling it now. A fair amount has already been spent. It will cost a fair amount to close it down, and the science was very exciting. It was scientifically a very good project. I would say this differs very much from, say, the much more expensive space lab which has rather minimal science. The science [planned for the SSC] was really very important and very good. There's no question about that. I don't think cutting it off at this stage saves all that amount of money because there is very strong urging now for the United States to participate very vigorously in the CERN lower-energy machine which isn't going to be nearly as good. I think they will eventually need to follow it up with a bigger one some years later and it will probably cost more in the long run.[201]

---

* CERN in Europe will soon decide whether to proceed with its own version, called the Large Hadron Collider, or LHC.

Researcher, Teacher, Family Man

A tribute to Professor I.I. Rabi by Norman Ramsey in the *European Journal of Physics* following his mentor's death includes the following statement: "Some scientists make their greatest contribution through their own personal research while others are best remembered for their general wisdom and their influence on others. A few including Rabi excel in both respects."[202]

The same could be said of Professor Norman Ramsey, who has always placed high value on his association with his graduate students. In compiling a overview of his career objectives and accomplishments, Ramsey wrote:

> A large part of my life has been spent doing research, mostly in collaboration with graduate students. My association with the students has been close and friendly. At any one period of time, if I were asked to name my 20 closest and best friends, about 10 of them would have been my then-current graduate students.
>
> Our relations were much more those of joint collaborators than of professor and student. I encouraged them to be as independent and creative as possible. Many of the ideas for our joint work came from the students. Although I discussed with them our work every few days, they carried out their research quite independently. In general, when we did not agree on the best course of action but both were satisfactory, we usually followed the students' preference since they would be doing most of the work. All of us took full responsibility for safety and the reliability of our results. Inevitably, mistakes were made, but that would also have happened if I had made all the decisions. In my opinion, giving the students much freedom prepared them better for later becoming independent, creative scientists. Fortunately, we had excellent graduate students at Harvard who could take full advantage of the freedoms offered.[203]

In recognition of his many accomplishments, Norman Ramsey has received many awards and accolades. Presently Higgins Professor of Physics at Harvard, he has also been a Guggenheim Fellow, was the George Eastman Professor at Oxford University in 1973-74 and visiting professor at Middlebury, Mount Holyoke and Williams Colleges and at Virginia, Colorado, Chicago and Michigan Universities. He was chairman of the Physics Section of the American Association for the Advancement of Science, 1977-78, and president of the American

Physical Society, 1978-79. From 1966-81, he was president of Universities Research Association, which operates the Fermi National Accelerator Laboratory in Batavia, Illinois. He was a trustee of the Carnegie Endowment for International Peace and of Rockefeller University. From 1980 to 1986, he was chairman of the Board of Governors of the American Institute of Physics and, from 1985 to 1988, he was president of the national Phi Beta Kappa Society.

Ramsey has received the Presidential Certificate of Merit, the E.O. Lawrence Award, the Davisson-Germer Prize, the Columbia Award for Excellence in Science, the IEEE Centennial Medal, the IEEE Medal of Honor, the Monie Ferst Award, the Rabi Prize, the Rumford Premium, the Compton Medal, the Oersted Medal, the Pupin Medal, the Einstein Award, the National Medal of Science and the Erice Science for Peace Prize.

Ramsey is a member of the American Physical Society, the Institute of Electrical and Electronics Engineers, the American Philosophical Society, the American Academy of Arts and Sciences and the National Academy of Sciences, and is a foreign associate of the French Academy of Sciences.

As for the Nobel Prize that he might have gotten decades earlier had he followed the trail of his original PhD thesis and found, on his own, the electric quadrupole moment of the deuteron, Ramsey has put any such disappointments behind him:

> I could have worried at one stage . . . Rabi's [1944] prize was to a fair degree stimulated by the discovery of the quadrupole moment of the deuteron. Maybe I had a chance then, but it has been much better for me that it happened this way, to get it later on my own.[204]

In fact, he has particular admiration for those who have been bypassed in their first shot at the Nobel Prize and have not allowed the loss to keep them from making additional contributions. He mentioned two of them in particular—Felix Bloch and Luis Alvarez—in a recent issue of *Physics Today* in which he reviewed the early history of magnetic resonance:

> In 1940 Luis W. Alvarez and Felix Bloch applied a similar magnetic resonance method [similar to that of Rabi's] to a beam of neutrons to measure the neutron's magnetic moment. Because their paper appeared three years after the first magnetic resonance papers from Rabi's laboratory, their technique is usually presumed to be an adaptation of Rabi's method. I later learned from Alvarez, however, that

Bloch thought of his method before he had seen Rabi's papers. Bloch and Alvarez must have been greatly disappointed to discover that their resonance idea had been published earlier. But instead of allowing disappointment to blight their careers, they went on to other research, each man independently earning a Nobel Prize.[205]

As to his own Nobel Prize, Ramsey is glad he received it when he did.

I consider myself very lucky to have not gotten it any earlier. I mean I'm delighted to have gotten it, and when I got the prize, several of my friends congratulated me and said, 'It's too bad you didn't get it much earlier.' My response was, 'I got it two weeks too early,' because I was just leaving for a visiting professorship at Michigan. The announcement came out and I was really very swamped right during that particular period.

I think I've gotten most of the benefits and few of the harms. The benefits for me have been large. I've kept really much more actively involved in physics as a result. When I'm invited to go to an active research institution to give a series of lectures, when I'm there I learn about what they are doing and I have discussions which inspire me to do a lot of thinking. Most of my more recent papers are real consequences of things that probably did emerge from that. I had one published in *Physical Review* a month or so ago, which is an outgrowth of such a meeting.

Now it has prevented my retirement in the normal sense of retirement. My wife sometimes points out that I haven't retired yet, which is true as far as time is concerned.[206]

Ramsey officially retired from Harvard in 1986, but he remains very active in physics. Although he opposes the federal rule that forbids age as the basis for establishing mandatory retirement and is glad he came under the rule that mandated retirement from the university at age 66, he is thankful that he still has an office at Harvard. "I think my retirement is good for the University," he said. "It gives them another slot. It means that I can do what I want to do. There are several things I'm glad I don't have to do. I don't have to grade exams. I don't have to give exams."[207]

Since his retirement, Ramsey has been a research fellow at the Joint Institute for Laboratory Astrophysics at the University of Colorado and periodically still revisits JILA as an Adjunct Research Fellow. Later, he was a visiting professor at the University of Chicago, Williams College and the

University of Michigan. In addition, he continues writing and doing theoretical calculations in his Harvard office and is also continuing his neutron experiments in Grenoble, France. Although evidence of the neutron's electric dipole moment has eluded him, he continues to be, characteristically, an optimist about his search. As he told an audience in 1992:

> After 43 years of searching for, but not finding, a neutron electric dipole moment, I suppose I should be discouraged and believe that no particle dipole moment will ever be discovered and the search should be abandoned. On the contrary, I am now quite optimistic about the field. . . . My greatest reason for optimism . . . is the number and variety of promising experimental searches now being carried on by excellent physicists. For most of the past 43 years, the searches for electric dipole moments have been lonely ones with at most one or two groups looking primarily at one particle, the neutron. Now there are promising experiments with atoms, electrons and protons as well. I sincerely hope that someone hits the jackpot soon. I am extremely eager to learn the answer, but at age 76 I cannot wait another 43 years unless there is a way to achieve real time reversal for biological clocks.[208]

Although such a clock has not yet been made, Ramsey continues making the most of conventional, non-atomic clocks, packing a great deal of activity into each day.

Throughout his busy career, Dr. Ramsey has placed a high priority on his family relationships. After his wife, Elinor, died in 1983, he married Ellie Welch of Brookline, Massachusetts and they now have a combined family of seven children and a growing group of grandchildren. In his "free time" he enjoys downhill and cross-country skiing, hiking, bicycling and trekking as well as musical and cultural events. And to keep himself in top physical shape, he always tries to take the stairs instead of the elevator.

Since Ramsey no longer teaches classes at Harvard, the writer asked him if he misses it. As he hurried down the steps outside Lyman Laboratory of Physics, Ramsey replied, "I'm teaching now more than ever. It's just that now I'm teaching everywhere else."[209] Everywhere else includes a great deal of travel in foreign countries, where he continues to share his knowledge and enthusiasm about physics with others. ■

REFERENCE NOTES:

1. Report of the Committee on Ballistic Acoustics, National Research Council (John F. Kennedy Assassination); N.F. Ramsey, chmn., (Washington, DC: Nat'l. Academy Press, 1982).

2. N.F. Ramsey, et al., "Reexamination of acoustic evidence in the Kennedy assassination," *Science* **218** (1982), 127.

3. *1990 Britannica Book of the Year* (Chicago: Encyclopedia Britannica, Inc., 1990), 98.

4. Hans Bethe, quoted by John Rigden in *Rabi: Scientist and Citizen* (New York: Basic Books, Inc., 1987), 113; from interview by Charles Weiner and Jagdish Mehra, 27-28 October 1966, transcript, Niels Bohr Library, American Institute of Physics, College Park, MD.

5. N.F. Ramsey, "Thermodynamics and statistical mechanics at negative absolute temperatures,"*Physical Review* **103,** (1956), 20.

6. N.F. Ramsey, "Students, research and publications," (1938-1993), unpublished, 14.

7. E.M. Purcell and N.F. Ramsey, "On the possibility of electric dipole moments for elementary paraticles and nuclei," *Physical Review* **78,** (1950), 807.

8. M. Forte, B.R. Heckel, N.F. Ramsey, K. Green and G.L. Greene, "First measurement of parity-nonconserving neutron spin rotation," *Physical Review Letters* **45** (1980), 2088.

9. J.D. Jackson, S.B. Treiman and H.Wyld, Jr., *Physical Review* **106,** (1957), 517.

10. N.F. Ramsey, "Time reversal, charge conjugation, magnetic pole conjugation, and parity," *Physical Review* **109** (1958), 225.

11. G.L. Green, N.F. Ramsey, W. Mampe, J.M. Pendlebury, K. Smith, W.B. Dress, P.D. Miller and P. Perrin, "Measurement of the neutron magnetic moment,"*Physical Review,* **D20** (1979), 2139.

12. R.V. Reid and M.L. Vaida, *Physical Review* **A7,** (1973), 1841.

13. E.R. Cohen and B. Taylor, *Reviews of Modern Physics* **59,** (1987), 1121.

14. N.F. Ramsey, "Experiments with separated oscillatory fields and hydrogen masers," Nobel Lecture, December 8, 1989, *Les Prix Nobel 1989,* Nobel Foundation (Stockholm: Norstedts Tryckeri, 1990), 79.

15. N.F. Ramsey, "Students, Research and Publications," (unpublished).

16 N.F. Ramsey, autobiographical sketch, *Les Prix Nobel 1989,* Nobel Foundation, (Stockholm: Norstedts Tryckeri, 1990), 59.

17. N.F. Ramsey, interview by Joan Safford, July 1960, transcript, Niels Bohr Library, American Institute of Physics, College Park, MD, 8.

18. Ibid., 6.

19. N.F. Ramsey, interview by James Mattson, February 1994.

20. N.F. Ramsey, interview by Safford, 4-5.

21. Ibid., 246.

22. Ibid., 249-250.

23. Ibid., 5.

24. Ibid., 7.

25. N.F. Ramsey, "Statement regarding the book *Special Tasks,*" American Physical Society Press Conference, April 26, 1994.

26. N.F. Ramsey, interview by Safford, 8.

27. Ibid.

28. Ibid., 16.

29. Ibid., 14.

30. Ibid., 15.

31. Ibid., 15-16.

32. Ibid., 15.

33. Richard Rhodes, *The Making of the Atomic Bomb* (New York: Simon and Schuster, 1988), 36.

34. Ibid., 66.

35. N.F. Ramsey, interview by Mattson, 15 December 1993.

36. I.I. Rabi, "Space quantization in a gyrating magnetic field," *Physical Review* **51**, (1937), 652-654.

37. N.F. Ramsey, interview by Mattson, 15 December 1993.

38. C.J. Gorter, "Bad luck in attempts to make scientific discoveries," *Physics Today*, January 1967, 78.

39. N.F. Ramsey, "Early magnetic resonance experiments: roots and offshoots," *Physics Today*, October 1993, 41.

40. N.F. Ramsey, "Experiments with separated oscillatory fields and hydrogen masers," Nobel Lecture, December 8, 1989, *Les Prix Nobel 1989*, Nobel Foundation (Stockholm: Norstedts Tryckeri, 1990), 65.

41. C.J. Gorter, "Bad luck in attempts to make scientific discoveries," *Physics Today*, January 1967, 78.

42. N.F. Ramsey, interview by Mattson, 15 December 1993.

43. N.F. Ramsey, interview by Mattson, February 1994.

44. I.I. Rabi, J.R. Zacharias, S. Millman, and P. Kusch, "A new method of measuring nuclear magnetic moment," *Physical Review* **53**, (1938), 318.

45. Rigden, *Rabi: Scientist and Citizen*, 104.

46. Ibid.

47. J.M.B. Kellogg and N.F. Ramsey, "On the magnetic moments of neon and argon," *Physical Review* **53**, (1938), 331.

48. J.M.B. Kellogg, I.I. Rabi, N.F. Ramsey, and J.R. Zacharias, "On the magnetic moments of the proton and the deuteron," *Physical Review* **55**, (1939), 595.

49. J.M.B. Kellogg, I.I. Rabi, N.F. Ramsey, and J.R. Zacharias, "An electrical quadrupole moment of the deuteron," *Physical Review* **55**, (1939), 318.

50. I.I. Rabi, J.R. Zacharias, N.F. Ramsey, and J.M.B. Kellogg, "Magnetic resonance experiments on H_2 and D_2 molecules," *Physical Review* **55**, (1939), 595.

51. N.F. Ramsey, "Rotational magnetic moment measurements on H_2 and D_2 molecules," *Physical Review* **55**, (1939), 595.

52. J.M.B. Kellogg, I.I. Rabi, N.F. Ramsey, and J.R. Zacharias, "The radiofrequency spectrum of the HD Molecules in magnetic fields," *Physical Review* **56**, (1939), 213.

53. J.M.B. Kellogg, I.I. Rabi, N.F. Ramsey, and J.R. Zacharias, "The magnetic moments of the proton and the deuteron. the radiofrequency spectrum of H_2 in various magnetic fields," *Physical Review* **56**, (1939), 728.

54. J.M.B. Kellogg, I.I. Rabi, N.F. Ramsey, and J.R. Zacharias, "An electrical quadrupole moment of the deuteron. The radiofrequency spectra of HD and D_2 molecules in a magnetic field," *Physical Review* **57**, (1940), 677-695.

55. Rhodes, *The Making of the Atomic Bomb*, 72.

56. J.M.B. Kellogg, I.I. Rabi, N.F. Ramsey, and J.R. Zacharias, "On the magnetic moments of the proton and the deuteron," *Physical Review* **55**, (1939), 595.

57. Rigden, *Rabi: Scientist and Citizen*, 121, from interview of Norman Ramsey by John Rigden, 18 March 1982.

58. N.F. Ramsey, Proceedings of the Fourteenth Annual Precise Time and Time Interval (PTTI) Applications and Planning Meeting, NASA Goddard Space Flight Center, Greenbelt, MD, Nov. 30-Dec. 2, 1982, NASA Conference Publication 2265, 635.

59. N.F. Ramsey, interview by James Mattson, 15 December 1993.

60 Ibid.

61. N.F. Ramsey, Proceedings of the Fourteenth Annual Precise Time and Time Interval (PTTI) Applications and Planning Meeting, 636.

62. N.F. Ramsey, interview by James Mattson, 15 December 1993.

63. N.F. Ramsey, Proceedings of the Fourteenth Annual Precise Time and Time Interval (PTTI) Applications and Planning Meeting, 636.

64. N.F. Ramsey, "Students, research and publications," (unpublished), 5.

65. Ibid.

66. Ibid.

67. KJ.M.B. Kellogg, I.I. Rabi, N.F. Ramsey, and J.R. Zacharias, "The magnetic moments of the proton and the deuteron. the radiofrequency spectrum of H_2 in various magnetic fields," *Physical Review* **56,** (1939), 728.

68. N.F. Ramsey, interview by Mattson, 15 December 1993.

69. Ibid.

70. J.M.B. Kellogg, I.I. Rabi, N.F. Ramsey, and J.R. Zacharias, "An electrical quadrupole moment of the deuteron," *Physical Review,* **55,** (1939), 318.

71. N.F. Ramsey, interview by Mattson, February 1994.

72. J.M.B. Kellogg, I.I. Rabi, N.F. Ramsey, and J.R. Zacharias, "An electrical quadrupole moment of the deuteron. The radiofrequency spectra of HD and D_2 molecules in a magnetic field," *Physical Review* **57,** (1940), 677.

73. Rigden, *Rabi: Scientist and Citizen,* 113-114.

74. N.F. Ramsey, "Long range proton-proton tensor force," *Physical Review* **85,** (1952), 937.

75. N.F. Ramsey, "Molecular beam magnetic resonance studies of HD and D_2," *Physical Review* **A4,** (1971), 1945.

76. N.F. Ramsey, "The tensor force between two protons at long range," *Physica* **96A,** (1979), 285.

77. N.F. Ramsey, interview by Mattson, 15 December 1993.

78. Ibid.

79. N.F. Ramsey, interview by Safford, 23.

80. Rhodes, *The Making of the Atomic Bomb,* 242.

81. Roger H. Stuewer, "Bringing the news of fission to America," *Physics Today,* October 1985, 49-50.

82. Laura Fermi, *Atoms in the Family,* (Chicago: University of Chicago Press, 1954), 123; quoted by Rhodes, *The Making of the Atomic Bomb,* 249.

83. Rhodes, *The Making of the Atomic Bomb,* 249.

84. *The Who's Who of Nobel Prize Winners* (Phoenix: Oryx Press, 1986), 163.

85. N.F. Ramsey, interview by Safford, 25

86. Ibid., 25-26.

87. Stuewer, "Bringing the news of fission to America," 49-50.

88. N.F. Ramsey, interview by Safford, 32.

89. N.F. Ramsey, interview by Mattson, February 1994.

90. N.F. Ramsey, interview by Safford, 33.

91. J.A. Van Allen and N.F. Ramsey, "A technique of counting high energy protons in the presence of fast neutrons," *Physical Review* **57,** (1940), 1069.

92. Rigden, *Rabi: Scientist and Citizen,* 131-132.

93. N.F. Ramsey, interview by Paul Henriksen, 24 June 1982, untranscribed tape, Niels Bohr Library, American Institute of Physics, College Park, MD.

94. Ibid.

95. Ibid.

96. N.F. Ramsey, interview by Safford, 36.

97. Ibid.

98. Ibid., 37.

99. Rhodes, *The Making of the Atomic Bomb,* 359.

100. N.F. Ramsey, interview by Mattson, 15 December 1993.

101. N.F. Ramsey, interview by Safford, 45.

102. Ibid., 50-51.

103. Ibid., 50.

104. Ibid., 51.

105. Ibid., 53-54.

106. Ibid., 54.

107. Ibid., 58.

108. Ibid., 59.

109. Ibid., 130.

110. Ibid.

111. Ibid., 131.

112. Ibid., 132.

113. Ibid., 61.

114. Ibid., 133.

115. Ibid., 63.

116. Ibid.

117. Ibid., 64.

118. Ibid., 71.

119. Ibid., 66.

120. Ibid., 80.

121. Ibid., 81.

122. Ibid., 83.

123. Ibid., 69-70.

124. Ibid., 92-93.

125. Ibid., 92.

126. Ibid., 93.

127. Laura Fermi, "Bombs or reactors?" *Bulletin of the Atomic Scientists,* June 1970, 28.

128. Rhodes, *The Making of the Atomic Bomb,* 572.

129. N.F. Ramsey, interview by Safford, 120-121.

130. Ibid., 123.

131. Ibid., 124.

132. Rhodes, *The Making of the Atomic Bomb,* 656.

133. Ibid., 124.

134. Ibid., 124-125.

135. N.F. Ramsey, interview by Safford, 126-127.

136. Ibid., 129.

137. Ibid., 188.

138. Ibid., 189.

139. N.F. Ramsey, "Origins of magnetic resonance," (unpublished), 7.

140. Ibid., 4.

141. Gorter, "Bad luck in attempts to make scientific discoveries," 79.

142. F. Bloch. W.W. Hansen, and M.E. Packard, "Nuclear induction," *Physical Review* **69**, (1946), 127.

143. S.B. Brody, W.A. Nierenberg, and N.F. Ramsey, "Nuclear moments of the bromine isotopes," *Physical Review* **72**, (1947), 258.

144. W.A. Nierenberg, N.F. Ramsey, S.B. Brody, "Measurements of nuclear quadrupole moment interactions," *Physical Review* **70**, (1946), 773.

145. W.A. Nierenberg, N.F. Ramsey, S.B. Brody, "Measurements of nuclear quadrupole interactions," *Physical Review* **71**, (1947), 466.

146. W.A. Nierenberg and N.F. Ramsey, "The radiofrequency spectra of the sodium halides," *Physical Review* **72**, (1947), 1075.

147. J.E. Nafe, E.B. Nelson, and I.I. Rabi, "The hyperfine structure of atomic hydrogen and deuterium," *Physical Review* **71**, (1947), 914-915; *Physical Review* **73**, (1948), 718; *Physical Review* **75**, (1949), 1194; *Physical Review* **76**, (1949), 1859.

148. J. Schwinger, *Physical Review* **73**, (1948), 416 and *Physical Review* **76**, (1949), 790.

149. P. Kusch and H.M. Foley, *Physical Review* **72**, (1948), 1256 and *Physical Review* **74**, (1948), 250.

150. N.F. Ramsey, interview by Safford, 194.

151. N.F. Ramsey, interview by Mattson, December 15, 1993.

152. N.F. Ramsey, interview by Safford, 194.

153. Ibid., 199-200.

154. Ibid., 200.

155. Ibid.

156. N.F. Ramsey, interview by Paul Forman, 12 July 1983, Niels Bohr Library, American Institute of Physics, 2.

157. N.F. Ramsey, interview by Safford, 201.

158. N.F. Ramsey, "Large quadrupole interactions in nuclear radiofrequency spectra," *Physical Review* **73**, (1948), 1243.

159. N.F. Ramsey, "Effect of large quadrupole interactions on nuclear radiofrequency spectra at twice Larmor frequency," *Physical Review* **74**, (1948), 286.

160. N.F. Ramsey, "New molecular beam magnetic resonance method," *Physical Review* **75**, (1949), 1326.

161. Ramsey, Proceedings of the Fourteenth Annual Precise Time and Time Interval (PTTI) Applications and Planning Meeting, 639.

162. Ramsey, "Experiments with separated oscillatory fields and hydrogen masers," 65.

163. N.F. Ramsey, interview by Mattson, 15 December 1993.

164. N.F. Ramsey, interview by Forman, 4.

165. Ibid., 5.

166. Ramsey, "Experiments with separated oscillatory fields and hydrogen masers," 76.

167. Daniel Kleppner, "Where I stand," *Physics Today*, January 1994, 9.

168. Ramsey, "Earliest criticisms of assumed P and T symmetries," Time Reversal: Arthur Rich Memorial Symposium, American Institute of Physics Conference Proceedings **270**, (1992), 179.

169. Sharon Bertsch McGrayne, *Nobel Prize Women in Science,* (New York: Carol Publishing Group, 1993), 272.

170. Ramsey, "Earliest criticisms of assumed P and T symmetries," 180.

171. Ibid.

172. E.M. Purcell and N.F. Ramsey, "On the possibility of electric dipole moments for elementary particles and nuclei," 807.

173. J.H. Smith, E.M. Purcell and N.F. Ramsey, "Experimental limit to the electric dipole moment of the neutron," *Physical Review* **108**, (1957), 120.

174. Ramsey, "Earliest criticisms of assumed P and T symmetries," 181.

175. N.F. Ramsey, *Physical Review* **109**, (1958), 225.

176. N.F. Ramsey, interview by Safford, 342.

177. Robert C. Doty, "U.S. physicist to get NATO science post," *New York Times*, Thursday, February 6, 1958.

178. N.F. Ramsey, interview by Safford, 343.

179. Anatole Abragam, *Time Reversal, An Autobiography,* (New York: Oxford University Press, 1989), 215.

180. E.M. Purcell, "Research in Nuclear Magnetism," Nobel Lecture, December 11, 1952, *Les Prix Nobel 1952,* Nobelstiftelsen, (Stockholm: Imprimerie Royale, 1952), 97-109.

181. N.F. Ramsey, "The internal diamagnetic field correction in measurements of the proton magnetic moment, *Physical Review* **77**, (1950), 567.

182. N.F. Ramsey, "Magnetic shielding of nuclei in molecules," *Physical Review* **78**, (1950), 699.

183. N.F. Ramsey, "Dependence of magnetic shielding of nuclei upon molecular orientation," *Physical Review* **83**, (1951), 540.

184. N.F. Ramsey, "Chemical effects in nuclear magnetic resonance and in diamagnetic susceptibility," *Physical Review* **86**, (1952), 243.

185. N. Bloembergen, abstract, *Physical Review* **75,** (1949), 1326.

186. W.G. Proctor and F.C. Yu, *Physical Review* **77**, (1950), 717.

187. W.C. Dickinson, *Physical Review* **77**, (1950), 736 and *Physical Review* **78**, (1950), 339.

188. N. Bloembergen and W.C. Dickinson, *Physical Review* **79**, (1950), 179.

189. U. Liddel and N.F. Ramsey, "Temperature dependent magnetic shielding in ethyl alcohol," *Journal of Chemical Physics* **19**, (1951), 1608.

190. N.F. Ramsey and E.M. Purcell, "Interactions between nuclear spins in molecules," *Physical Review* **85**, (1952), 143.

191. H. Gutowsky, McCall, C. Slichter, and McNeill, *Physical Review* **82**, (1951), 748 and *Physical Review* **84**, (1951), 589 and 1246.

192. E.L. Hahn and D.E. Maxwell, *Physical Review* **84**, (1951), 1246 and *Physical Review* **88**, (1952), 1070.

193. N.F. Ramsey, "Electron coupled interactions between nuclear spins in molecules," *Physical Review* **91**, (1953), 303.

194. N.F. Ramsey, interview by Paul Henriksen, (untranscribed).

195. N.F. Ramsey, interview by Mattson, December 15, 1993.

196. N.F. Ramsey, "The early history of URA and Fermilab: viewpoint of a URA president (1966-1981)," 1987 Annual Report, Fermilab.

197. Ibid.

198. Ibid.

199. N.F. Ramsey, autobiographical sketch, 65.

200. N.F. Ramsey, letter to James Mattson, March 6, 1994.

201. N.F. Ramsey, interview by Mattson, December 15, 1993.

202. N.F. Ramsey, "Grand schools of physics: the Rabi school," *European Journal of Physics* **11**, (1990), 137.

203. N.F. Ramsey, "Students, research and publications," (unpublished), 2-3.

204. N.F. Ramsey, interview by Mattson, 15 December 1993.

205. Ramsey, "Early magnetic resonance experiments: roots and offshoots," 42.

206. N.F. Ramsey, interview by Mattson, 15 December 1993.

207. Ibid.

208. Ramsey, "Earliest criticisms of assumed P and T symmetries," 179.

209. N.F. Ramsey, interview by Mattson, 15 December 1993.

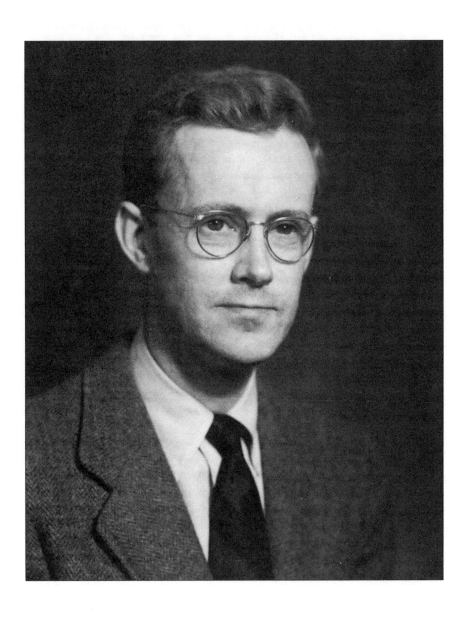

3

EDWARD M. PURCELL

Discoverer of NMR Signal in Condensed Matter
by Observing Energy Absorption

ACCORDING TO SIGNS planted at the edge of town, Taylorville, Illinois, population 11,133, is: 1) "A Great Place to Live," 2) winner of the "1989 Governor's Home Town Award," and 3) "the home of the 1944 Illinois state basketball champions, 45 and 0 in one season, the greatest basketball achievement in Illinois high school basketball."

Although no local booster sign acknowledges it, and his name doesn't ring a bell for the clerk at the Main Street bookstore on the town's central square—"If you asked me about romance novels, I could help you"—Taylorville is also the boyhood home of Edward Mills Purcell, co-winner of the 1952 Nobel Prize in physics for discovering the NMR signal in condensed matter.

It's possible that the town's memory may have served it better if Purcell's family had remained in Taylorville or if he had discovered something the average person on Taylorville's Main Street could understand and appreciate in 1952, but there is no question that the experiment that Dr. Purcell and his colleagues, Robert V. Pound and Henry C. Torrey, conducted in December of 1945 has made a positive impact on the lives of millions on Main Streets all around the world, including many from Taylorville.

The Road from Taylorville

Illinois State Highway 48 heading southwest into Taylorville from Decatur lies straight and flat, running parallel to the railroad and cutting through land that, on the surface, yields an annual bounty of corn, oats and soybeans and, below the surface, coal. Working 400 to 600 feet underground, the miners of Christian County continue to extract their living, as their fathers did, from a six-foot-thick layer of bituminous blackness that spans much of Central and Southern Illinois, the largest such reserves in the United States.[1]

Perpendicularly intersecting Highway 48 at Taylorville is State Highway 29. Follow it 25 miles to the northwest and you arrive at Springfield, the state's capital, where Abraham Lincoln, its most famous resident, once practiced law. Follow it southeast and you're taking the same route that 14-year-old Edward Purcell and his family took when they moved 60 miles from Taylorville to Mattoon, Illinois (present population 18,441) between his sophomore and junior years of high school. Although he adapted to his new environment and was elected senior-class president at Mattoon a year later, Purcell's affection for Taylorville would never leave. Forty-one years after his family's move, he recalled the emotions he felt when they left.

> As I grow older, my memories of Taylorville grow more vivid rather than less. . . . It was a wonderful time and place to grow up. As we drove toward Pana on our way to Mattoon in the heat of the 1927 summer, I was gravely depressed by the thought that I was leaving the best part of the world behind and, in a way, it was true.[2]

Although 25 years would pass between young Purcell's move from Taylorville until his trip to Stockholm to receive the Nobel Prize, Taylorville was proud to claim him as their own. When its daily newspaper, the *Breeze Courier*, ran the standard press release on Thursday, November 6, 1952 announcing that year's list of Nobel Prize winners, the editor changed the lead paragraph to bring the story's significance home to his readers.

> One of Taylorville's sons has been awarded the Nobel Prize in physics. Dr. Edward Mills Purcell, 40, was born in this city in 1912. His father, Edward [E.A.] Purcell, was head of the local telephone office for many years and was later transferred to Mattoon. Once again, this city has gained national prominence and is proud of producing such a distinguished man.[3]

That week had been a particularly busy one for the editor. The previous Saturday, President Truman's campaign train had made Taylorville one of its last whistlestops before Tuesday's election. Truman's reelection efforts had proven no match, however, against a war hero like Eisenhower and Wednesday's banner headline announced, IKE SWEEPS INTO WHITE HOUSE.

Even in November of 1952, seven years after Purcell's discovery of nuclear magnetic resonance in condensed matter, the potential benefits of NMR were still largely unrecognized. Another decade would pass before the usefulness of NMR spectroscopy would be appreciated by the rank and file of chemists. Even more distant was the revolution in medical diagnostics that would come about because of a discovery by a medical doctor that NMR could be used to differentiate between biological tissues—both diseased and normal—on the basis of their T_1 and T_2 relaxation rates and the idea of a physical chemistry professor to portray those signals in the form of images.

With this in mind, the failure in 1952 of *Boston Herald* reporter John Lynch to appreciate the potential of NMR after hearing Purcell describe his 1945 experiment is certainly understandable:

> [Professor Purcell's] discovery won't revolutionize industry or help the housewife, but it does provide physicists a precision tool for measuring very precisely the magnetic properties of nuclei—the hearts of atoms.
>
> Dr. Purcell did his best today to explain to newspapermen just what his prize-winning research consisted of, but it turned out to be a lot simpler to pepper him with such questions as what he planned to do with his half-share of the [$33,000]* Nobel Prize, and whether he had yet made arrangements to go to Stockholm, Sweden to accept it Dec. 10.[4]

Although Lynch attempted to relay Purcell's description of the experiment to his readers—and he did capture its essential elements—he had little confidence they would comprehend what he wrote:

> This pot was filled with paraffin, and the whole thing was placed between the poles of a big electromagnet in the frame extension back of Harvard's Lyman Laboratory of Physics. Then radio waves were directed into the resonator—radio waves around the 30 megacycle

---

* The amount was incorrectly stated as $44,000 in Lynch's newspaper article. According to another report in *The Boston Herald* on the same day, the cash part of the prize was 171,134 crowns (*kroner*), equal at the time to $33,037. This amount agrees closely with later statements of both Purcell and Bloch. The cash award for a Nobel Prize is split when there are multiple recipients.

frequency—and the frequency at which greatest absorption of the radio waves occurred was carefully measured.

(All this is roughly what the man said; we don't expect it to mean very much to you.)

At this point . . . well, anyway . . . it's a pretty important thing in the scientific field, and it shows what a fellow can do in his spare time.[5]

Telephones and Nice Diagrams

Biographical sketches characterize Edward Mills Purcell as "U.S. physicist," "physics educator" and "co-winner Nobel Prize in physics, 1952," but they are, like poorly-lit photographs, incomplete portraits of a complex, multi-faceted person.

The older of two boys in the Purcell family, Edward was interested in both the sciences and the humanities. His interest in science was encouraged in part by his father's occupation as manager of the local telephone exchange in Taylorville and later as general manager of the Illinois Southeastern Telephone Company in Mattoon.

> The telephone office, as we called it [said Purcell], was a place where all the switchboards and technical equipment was. In the basement were discarded sections of cable and wire, and I could bring home items like that from the telephone office. It was my source of wire and lead. If you got an old hunk of telephone cable, you could melt the lead sheath and take the paper insulation off the wire, and you had the makings for a lot of things.[6]

The magnetos of the old crank telephones were also a handy source of components for experiments.

> You could always get plenty of the bell-ringing generators . . . which consisted of a series of horseshoe magnets making the stator field and a rotating armature that was wound with what seemed like a mile of number 39 wire. These made good shocking machines, if nothing else, if vigorously cranked.[7]

Perhaps even more significant than Purcell's access to cast-off phone equipment, however, was his access to the *Bell System Technical Journal.* Illinois Southeastern was not part of the Bell System, but the company maintained all the phone lines in the area for American Telephone and

Telegraph and thus received the journal. Although the publications weren't avidly read by the linemen, they inspired young Edward. He held onto the journals and, even in college, found himself going back to them.

> They were fascinating [said Purcell] because for the first time I saw technical articles obviously elegantly edited and prepared and illustrated, full of mathematics that was well beyond my understanding. It was a glimpse into some kind of wonderful world where electricity and mathematics and engineering and nice diagrams all came together.[8]

Elizabeth Mills Purcell, Edward's mother, probably had the greatest influence on his interest in literature and the humanities. A graduate of Vassar College in Poughkeepsie, New York, she had grown up in Decatur, Illinois, the big city of Purcell's childhood, and was teaching Latin at Taylorville High School at the time of her marriage in 1910 to Edward A. Purcell. "Our house had many books in it," recalled Purcell. "Literature and books were a familiar part of my childhood, and also I spent a good deal of time in the public library."[9] That influence would be evident during Purcell's undergraduate years when he served as editor of his college literary magazine and won awards for creative writing while majoring in electrical engineering.

Both parents passed on to Edward their interest in and respect for teaching. His father, who had grown up on a farm near Taylorville, had also taught for a time in a one-room country school.

Attic and Basement Physics at Purdue

In 1929, the year Purcell started college, Purdue University was 60 years old with an enrollment of 4,223. (Its 1993 enrollment was 35,161, not including regional campuses.) Situated on a hill overlooking the Wabash River and the business district of West Lafayette, Indiana, Purdue was founded seven years after the federal Land Grant Act of 1862 which provided for public land sales to benefit agricultural education. By 1929, in addition to its agricultural program, the school was well-known for its solid engineering programs. Purcell chose electrical engineering because, as he once told a reporter for *The Harvard Crimson*, he did not know what physics really was.[10]

> I thought I wanted to be an electrical engineer, and the idea of being a physicist at that point just wasn't an image that one had to

consider somehow. You see, in the '20s the idea of chemistry as a science was extremely well publicized and popular, so the young scientist of—shall we say 1928—you'd think of him as a chemist holding up his test tube and sighting through it or something. And that was the result of the experience and history of World War I where the United States had to develop its chemical industry practically from scratch because German industry had previously supplied all that. . . . But [I had] no idea of what it would mean to be a physicist. The subject I knew about—but being a physicist—I don't remember considering that at that time as something you could be.

In fact, I've sometimes remarked that to me, at that time, the name Steinmetz was more familiar and exciting than the name Einstein, because Steinmetz was the famous electrical engineer at General Electric . . . this hunchback with a cigar who was reputed to know the four-place logarithm table by heart, and could be called with some justice the "father of AC."[11] *

"I really by intellectual taste," Purcell has said, "am almost as much of an engineer as a physicist. Much of what I've done in experimental physics, especially the work that came out of the Radiation Lab [during World War II], was engineering in style, and I've always found applications of physics in that field interesting and tempting."[12]

It is only fairly recently that, in retrospect, Purcell has noted a fairly close connection between his AC training and his work in NMR.

---

* Multiple claims have been made for the development of AC (alternating current). Although AC was being used as early as the 1870s, Nikola Tesla and Charles Steinmetz are generally given credit for its practical development. (In Europe, Gaulard and Gibbs produced the first alternating-current transformer; in the United States, a system designed by Elihu Thomson was powering arc lights in 1878.) Tesla conceived his polyphase induction, split-phase induction and polyphase synchronous AC motors in 1882 while in Europe and was issued 40 U.S. patents on them in 1891. In the 1890s, Steinmetz invented and received numerous patents for what General Electric called a "monocyclic" AC system.

According to Grolier Academic American Encyclopedia: "Over the course of nearly 25 years [Steinmetz] developed and refined a mathematical method for making AC calculations. By publishing and explaining his method, [he] made it possible for the average electrical engineer to understand and make use of alternating current. His work thus fulfilled the efforts of Nikola Tesla to establish the employment of alternating rather than direct current in electric power systems.

—Margaret Cheney, Tesla: Man Out of Time, (New York: Dell Publishing), 24, 42; On-Line Edition, Grolier Electronic Publishing, 1993.

I learned about AC generators and transformers and about the representation of AC amplitudes by complex algebra. Indeed, the 'monocyclic' system of Steinmetz (see footnote) has a close analogue resembling NMR. It could be argued that Steinmetz made the first contribution to magnetic resonance theory by developing the tools for analysis of AC circuits. The algebra we were learning as engineers is exactly the same algebra we had to use for NMR.[13]

Noting that numerous American physicists of his generation were trained as undergraduates in electrical engineering,[14] Purcell pointed out that electrical engineering during those years was quite different from the way it is taught today.

That electrical engineering was a very old-fashioned kind from the present viewpoint. I know two ways to wind armatures and things of that sort, which most of my physicist colleagues don't. Since I spent most of my life as an experimental physicist dealing one way or another with magnets and practical power supplies, in my generation electrical engineering was not too bad a preparation for physics.[15]

Actually, in 1929, the year Purcell started at Purdue, the school didn't even offer a major in physics, and the introductory course that was offered did little to entice a student into further pursuit of the subject. Taught by a Professor Ferry, a lecturer of notorious dullness who had written a small book on gyroscopes, the course made little permanent impact on Purcell. He said he remembered almost nothing from it, although he blamed himself for not really understanding the device.[16]

Had he known the direction his research would take him a decade and a half later, he might have paid more attention. The spinning top—and the spinning gyroscope—provide helpful insights from a classical physics perspective into the forces at work in the quantum-mechanical precessing proton. In fact, two years before Purcell entered Purdue, I.I. Rabi and Ralph de L. Kronig had published a paper that applied the Schrödinger equation to the physics of a symmetrical spinning top.[17]

Physics at Purdue experienced a tremendous boost in 1930 when Karl Lark-Horovitz became head of the physics department. A broadly-trained Viennese physicist, Lark-Horovitz had held research fellowships in Canada and the United States before coming to Purdue as professor of physics in 1928. By 1930, in addition to becoming head of the physics department and the director of the school's physical science laboratory, he had begun teaching modern physics and having graduate students.

Although it could be difficult working for "the Lark," said Purcell— "[he] ran the physics department on the European style: a pyramid with the professor at the top and everybody down below taking orders"—it was largely through his influence that the physics program at Purdue was developed and that Purcell began turning his attention to the subject.

Lark-Horovitz's influence soon extended beyond Purdue. In addition to the active role he personally played in the great explosion of quantum physics that occurred around that period, "his coming to Purdue," said Purcell, "was important for American physics in other ways. Over the years, he brought many important and productive European physicists to this country and to Purdue."[18]

"He was a remarkable man," Purcell continued. "And Betty Lark—she was a remarkable person herself." (After the marriage of Karl Horovitz and Betty Lark, they combined their last names, thus creating the hyphenated Lark-Horovitz.) "They loved music and the arts and they were sort of a little island of Middle European culture there in Central Indiana. I have a marvelous picture of him, complete with spats, taken at that time," Purcell said. "Imagine wearing spats at Purdue."

It wasn't just Lark-Horovitz's fashion statements that set him apart. At a time when anti-Semitism was still keeping many Jews off university faculties and in a place where political conservatism was the norm, Lark-Horovitz was both Jewish and politically liberal. "Yet he managed to hold his own in that setting,"[19] said Purcell.

Scientifically, Lark-Horovitz's interests would lead him more and more in the direction of what would come to be known as solid-state physics.

> He was interested generally in crystals [said Purcell], the physics of crystals and later on he developed the very well known and very important solid-state research laboratory that did work on semiconductors during World War II. . . . The trouble with the Lark was that he was slow to write things up and publish them. I think perhaps he didn't get as much credit as he might have for his work on germanium in the middle '40s prior to the transistor.[20]

In addition to the effect Lark-Horovitz had on the department, what first drew Purcell's attention to physics during his junior year at Purdue was a course offering independent study.

No one had ever signed up for that course before, but they let me sign up for it, and my immediate supervisor was a professor named Walerstein to whom I owe a tremendous amount. He was a real physicist. I think the first job he gave me was up in the attic of the physics building where there was a Rowland grating and a mount that had not been used for a long, long time. I was supposed to set it up and get it going and adjust it and everything all on my own and examine some spectra. Then he had some other things for me to do up in the attic, including making an electrometer to measure the half-life of something . . . I was really hooked at that point.[21]

The Rowland grating, a concave diffraction grating invented by Henry A. Rowland in the 1880s, facilitated accurate spectroscopy measurements by spreading visible light into its full spectrum. In doing so, it eliminated the need for the additional lenses and mirrors associated with spectrophotometers. The machine Rowland invented to make the gratings, which he called a 'dividing engine,' was capable of engraving as many as 20,000 lines per inch on concave mirrored surfaces. (Contrast that with the 300 dots per inch typical of many laser printers.) A personal friend of James Clerk Maxwell, Herman Ludwig Helmholtz and Thomas Alva Edison, Rowland was the first professor of physics at Johns Hopkins University. After installing his machine in the sub-basement of the physical laboratory at Johns Hopkins to minimize temperature fluctuations and to reduce vibrations from street traffic, he was eventually able to rule up to 800 lines per millimeter at an accuracy of better than 1/4000th of a millimeter![22] He sold his gratings at cost to various institutions including, apparently, Purdue University.

Rowland also sold one of his gratings to the University of Leiden in Holland where a young *privatdozent** by the name of Pieter Zeeman used it to achieve the Zeeman effect in 1896, the phenomenon whereby a spectral band of light emitted by an element is split into multiple, narrow bands when placed in a magnetic field.

Three years after the discovery of the Zeeman effect, the American Physical Society was formed† in 1899 by 38 physicists who gathered at

---

* Title given to a non-salaried university teacher or tutor who is paid for his or her services by a small fee paid by the students; not considered a faculty position.

† The journal, *Physical Review,* founded in 1893 by Edward Nichols and initially published "for Cornell University" would start being published in 1903 "with the cooperation of the American Physical Society."

Columbia's Fayerweather Hall, the same building where I.I. Rabi would begin his graduate work at Columbia in 1923. At that meeting, Henry Rowland was named the society's president. He was also named a foreign member of the Royal Society of London that same year.

Edward Purcell would succeed Rowland in both distinctions. Thirty-eight years after first using a Rowland grating at Purdue, Purcell would be elected president of the American Physical Society in 1970 and, in 1988, a foreign member of the Royal Society of London.

It is significant that Purcell was given a spectroscopy assignment so early in his physics career. Had he been assigned a more mundane task, who knows if he would have been "hooked" by physics—it was I.I. Rabi, after all, who said that there is nothing duller than a physics teaching laboratory.[23] The task also hinted of things to come. Fourteen years later, Purcell's discovery of NMR in a solid would usher in NMR spectroscopy* of condensed matter, opening up new vistas for chemical analysis and medical diagnosis.

In his senior year at Purdue, Purcell went from the attic of the physics building to the basement where electron and X-ray diffraction experiments were being done. Assigned to work with H.J. Yearian, a graduate student who was finishing up his thesis on electron diffraction, Purcell was allowed to conduct diffraction experiments with beryllium oxide and other substances using a 20-kilovolt electron diffraction camera Yearian had made.

Although the basement of the physics building was an exciting place to do physics, it also reflected the economic hard times with which people were coping in the early 1930s.

People were living down there in the cellar [said Purcell], sleeping on cots in the research rooms, because it was the Depression and some of the graduate students had nowhere else to live. I'd come in the morning and find them shaving. Yearian was very nice to me, tolerated my mistakes and taught me a great deal. That was such an exciting time. I'd never really developed a photographic emulsion

---

* As Norman Ramsey has pointed out, Rabi is credited by C.J. Gorter in a 1942 paper with coining the term "nuclear magnetic resonance" although the acronym NMR is largely restricted in usage to magnetic resonance methods used in condensed matter. Radiofrequency or magnetic resonance spectroscopy would become known, for purposes of differentiation, as NMR spectroscopy when used in non-molecular beam environments.
—N.F. Ramsey, "Origins of magnetic resonance," 1993, unpublished manuscript, 4, 33; C.J. Gorter and I.J.F. Broer, *Physica* **9**, (1942), 591.

before. Cameras had never been my hobby. I'd never done anything like that. And the first photographic emulsion I ever developed, when I turned on the light in the dark room, I had Debye-Scherrer rings on it from electron diffraction—and that was only five years after electron diffraction had been discovered. So it really was right in the forefront. For an undergraduate, to be encouraged to do that at that time was fantastic.[24]

Purcell normally worked for the telephone company in Mattoon during the summers, but he stayed on at Purdue the summer following his senior year to help compile a paper which he read that fall at a meeting of the American Physical Society in Cincinnati.[25] Purcell's first two scientific publications, in fact, the first dealing with electron diffraction from vacuum-sublimated layers[26] and the second describing a method for making these extremely thin films,[27] were the result of work done at Purdue.

Regarding the second paper, Purcell pointed out that "part of the game was to get a film of the material thin enough to be clearly transparent to electrons. Nowadays," he said in 1977, "it's not much of a problem. But Lark-Horovitz had an idea about how to do that, on which he put me to work."[28]

In addition to requiring extremely thin film, electron diffraction experiments called for film that was free of distortion and able to withstand repeated usage. The prevailing method at the time was to deposit the material to be investigated on "purest rocksalt." After deposition was completed, the supporting base of rocksalt would be dissolved in water, leaving a layer of film floating on the surface of the saltwater solution. The problem frequently encountered, however, was that these thin films were very fragile and subject to breaking, either when lifting the film from the liquid surface or during the drying process.

Lark-Horovitz's idea was to evaporate the material to be made into film onto a substrate such as camphor or napthalene which evaporates directly to a gas at room temperature. By depositing film onto these materials at very cold temperatures, and then placing the entire assembly in a vacuum chamber while allowing the temperature to rise, the underlying base would sublime (evaporate), leaving only the deposited film. Actually, it wasn't quite that simple. "Ordinarily, if you evaporated onto anything," Purcell pointed out, "the surface tension when the substrate melted would tear a film. So I spent a long time figuring a way to evaporate copper onto napthalene, or mothballs."[29] In fact, the "only interesting thing to me in memory about doing that paper," said Purcell, "was learning to polish mothballs,"[30] referring to his technique of preparing a surface for film deposition by flattening camphor or napthalene to a smooth, flat finish with a hot glass rod.

By the time the paper was submitted for publication to *Review of Scientific Instruments* in September 1935, the technique had been used to make thin films from 16 different substances for use in electron diffraction experiments. By then, Purcell had spent a year as a foreign exchange student in Germany and had returned to the United States to start his graduate work at Harvard.

In both cases, Karl Lark-Horovitz played an important role in securing scholarships for Purcell. "There's no question," Purcell said, "that I owe Lark-Horovitz a great deal. It was he who really helped me go on as a physicist by helping me get a scholarship [in Karlsruhe, Germany] that I had for a year after Purdue. . . . I'm sure that his recommendation was what made that go through."[31]

By the time he graduated from Purdue in 1933 with a Bachelor of Science in Electrical Engineering (B.S.E.E.), it was clear that Purcell was actually headed for a career in physics. Although economics may have played a partial role in Purcell's decision not to pursue an engineering career, he didn't recall that as the primary factor.

> It was, of course, the Depression, and whether I could have gotten a job as an electrical engineer anyway is doubtful. I don't remember that being the overriding reason, somehow. I can't remember worrying about it. By then I really wanted to go on in physics, and I'd really been fired up by those experiences.[32]

1933 to 1940

At the end of the summer of 1933, Edward Purcell left Purdue University, said goodbye to his parents in Mattoon, and headed east across the Atlantic to his next educational venue as an exchange student at the *Technische Hochschule* (TH) in Karlsruhe, Germany.

Located just a few miles from the banks of the Rhine River at the northern edge of the Black Forest, the city of Karlsruhe was founded when Karl Wilhelm, margrave of Baden-Durlach, built a castle near his hunting lodge, which had been known as *Karlsruhe,* or Karl's Retreat. Eventually, the tower of the castle became the focal point of a city laid out in the shape of a fan. By the time Purcell was there in 1933, Karlsruhe was a large city with considerable industry.

The Karlsruhe TH, also known as the Institute of Technology or the Polytechnic, had an auspicious past* and former teachers at the school, which was founded in 1825, included Heinrich Hertz, the discoverer of radio waves, and Fritz Haber, a Nobel Prize-winner in chemistry for developing a method for extracting nitrogen from the air to make ammonia.

It was fitting that Purcell should attend the same school where Hertz first produced electromagnetic waves as Purcell would be the first to use radio waves to stimulate the atomic nuclei of condensed matter to reveal their magnetic characteristics and, just a few years later, would be the first, in collaboration with Harold Ewen, to detect in outer space the unique frequency of radio waves emitted by atomic hydrogen. In 1933, however, Purcell was only "dimly aware," as he put it, of Heinrich Hertz's accomplishments. "I was not as aware as I should have been, in retrospect,"[33] he said.

With quantum mechanics then at the cutting edge of physics, Purcell would have preferred being assigned to the University of Munich. That's where Arnold Sommerfeld, one of physics' most renowned lecturers and the mentor of Werner Heisenberg, continued to attract a devoted following. In 1928, when Sommerfeld had been in the United States as part of an around-the-world lecture tour, Purcell was just finishing high school and the closest Sommerfeld had come to Purdue was a visit he made to the University of Minnesota. Now that Purcell was in Germany, preparing for a career in physics, the closest he could come to hearing Sommerfeld was to suggest to Beth Busser, another exchange student he had met on the ship while crossing the Atlantic, that she try to hear Sommerfeld, since she had been

---

* In 1860, the city of Karlsruhe had been the site of what has been said to be "one of the most important congresses in the history of chemistry."[34] Conceived by the renowned chemist August Kekulé of the University of Ghent and presided over by Professor Carl Weltzien of the Karlsruhe TH, the Karlsruhe Congress was, in fact, the first international conference on chemistry.[35]

A major objective of the conference was to resolve the then thorny question of whether atoms of the same chemical element could combine to form molecules as espoused by the Italian chemist Amadeo Avogadro or whether molecules could only be formed by chemical bonds between atoms of different elements, the position held by John Dalton. Although the question was not satisfactorily resolved at the congress, a chemist in attendance, Lothar Meyer, became convinced of the Avogadro position through a brochure distributed at the conference by Stanislas Cannizzaro, and became an avid proponent of it. He later discovered the system of the elements that we now call the periodic table.[36]

assigned to Munich. Although her field of study was German literature, she did take Purcell's suggestion, went to hear Sommerfeld, and
took notes on his lectures.[37] Four years later, Beth Busser and Edward
Purcell were married.

The student exchange program with Germany, operated under the auspices of the Institute of International Education, was a particularly active
one in the early 1930s, with many German students coming to the United
States for a year and vice versa, but in 1933 things were beginning to
change very quickly in Europe, and not for the better.

"Hitler had already come into power a few months before," said
Purcell, "so through the course of the year I had very few friends among
the German students, who were already—most of them—caught up in
the [Nazi] movement. My friends [in Germany] were from other
European countries who had come to study engineering."[38]

Just a few months before Purcell arrived in the country, Felix Bloch,
who would later share the Nobel Prize in physics with Purcell, had left
his position at the University of Leipzig because of the rapidly deterio-
rating attitude toward Jews and returned to his home in Switzerland.
Soon afterward, a civil service law enacted on April 7, 1933 had accomplished its intended purpose of ridding Germany's state-supported
schools of Jewish professors and others seen as undesirable by the
Nazis. One of those temporarily suspended under the new law was a
physics professor at Karlsruhe TH by the name of Walter Weizel who
had just written a volume on band spectra in the *Handbuch Der
Experimentalphysik.*

As Beyerchen points out in *Scientists Under Hitler*: "It seems clear that
the government policy was to place everyone potentially affected by the
Civil Service Law on leave, and then sort out the exemptions later."[39]
Although Weizel was not Jewish, his political activities during his student days were seen as unacceptable by the Nazis and he was removed
from his teaching post just as Purcell arrived at Karlsruhe.

Weizel's suspension didn't keep him entirely away from the students,
however, as Purcell and a number of others visited him in his apartment.
After his case was reconsidered, he was finally allowed to teach in the
second semester and was rated by Purcell as an excellent and inspiring
teacher. "Weizel gave beautiful lectures on thermodynamics and statistical mechanics," he said, "from which I learned a lot."[40]

A few years later, when Weizel, who was a theoretical physicist, left for
a new position at Bonn, he was not replaced at Karlsruhe since theoretical physics was regarded by the Nazi-favored "Aryan physicists" as an

influence of the Jewish spirit. Instead, his duties were absorbed by Alfons Bühl, a more "politically correct" physicist[41] (from the Nazi viewpoint) who once spelled out his views on Jews in no uncertain terms:

> This exceedingly mathematical treatment of physical problems had undoubtedly arisen from the Jewish spirit. The Jew has accepted this numerical, this calculational, as a special achievement of physics everywhere he has concerned himself with physics. And just as he otherwise—as in business—always has only the numerical, the credit and debit calculation before his eyes, so it must be designated as a typically racial characteristic even in physics that he places mathematical formulation in the foreground.[42]

Weizel would spend the rest of his academic career in Bonn where Purcell would visit him after the war.

Although Purcell was aware of anti-Semitism spreading throughout Germany when he was there, he was unaware of the extent of its virulence nor of its repercussions within the scientific community.

> My experience as a student in Karlsruhe in '33 and '34 was exactly at the point where, inside the German Physical Society, there was a struggle between the so-called Aryan physicists, on one hand, and the traditional physicists, including the ones with famous names like Planck and Sommerfeld, for control of the research physics in Germany. I was there as an innocent kid from Purdue at just that moment [but] I didn't even know this struggle was going on. I could have found out more if I had tried to, but I was so busy trying to learn a new language that I simply wasn't aware. Those of us who were American exchange students were intensely interested in what was going on in the political arena at the time.[43]

Purcell did remember attending a meeting of the German Physical Society in Freiburg in the early spring of 1934. "Everybody was sitting around and laughing about the neutrino idea," he said. "I remember sitting around a table drinking beer and the senior physicists joking about the neutrino."[44]

Proposed by Wolfgang Pauli in 1930 to account for energy that seemed to disappear with beta decay, the neutrino—not to be discovered experimentally until 1956—had been named by Enrico Fermi. "Little neutral one," it meant in Italian. Shortly before the meeting Purcell attended in

Germany, Fermi had developed a comprehensive theory about beta decay, including the idea that "electrons (or neutrinos) can be created and can disappear."[45] Soon afterward, Fermi began bombarding atomic nuclei with neutrons in the search for artificial radioactivity and creating what he called 'transuranic elements.' It later became evident that he was on the threshold of nuclear fission and, indeed, had unknowingly crossed it.

Because tuition was free, and Purcell could take any courses he desired, he took several from professors recognized for their elegant lecture style just to hear them speak the language, including one on art history and another on the history of the Upper Rhine Valley. He also did a fair amount of traveling while in Germany because of the reduced fares available to students, including a skiing trip to Austria, where Germans were, for a time, forbidden to travel.[46]

Purcell returned to the United States in 1934, the same year that Felix Bloch emigrated to America to take up his new position at Stanford University. After writing two or three places, Purcell was granted, with help from Karl Lark-Horovitz, a free-tuition scholarship to Harvard University—worth about $400, as he recalled. He has been a resident of Cambridge, Massachusetts ever since.[47]

Magnetic Cooling

In 1936, 24-year-old Edward Purcell reached what he called a "very important chapter" in his physics education. It came in the form of a course on electric and magnetic susceptibilities taught at Harvard by Professor John H. Van Vleck. Van Vleck had come to Harvard two years earlier from the University of Wisconsin where he had written a well-known book on the subject.[48] About 40 years later, Van Vleck would receive the Nobel Prize in physics—in 1977—for his role in the development of the quantum theory of magnetism.

Both the course and the book would contribute a great deal to Purcell's knowledge of quantum mechanics. "Many people," he said, "have learned a lot of quantum mechanics from Van's book."[49] Also contributing to Purcell's education in quantum theory that fall was Malcolm Hebb, a theoretical physics student who had switched from the University of Wisconsin to Harvard at the same time Van Vleck had changed schools. According to Purcell, Hebb "already knew a good deal of theory, which I did not."[50]

With a teacher-student ratio of 1 to 2, and with the other student contributing in the way of theory, Purcell received great benefit from the course, although he always wondered how the school handled the preparation of the exams. In those days, he said, exams at Harvard were typeset and printed with a serial number. "I guess Malcolm had #01 and I had #02," he said. "I don't know how they stopped the presses quickly enough."[51]

For their assigned problem for the term, the two students were to consider the theoretical aspects of cooling by adiabatic demagnetization which, at the time, was a rather new development in low-temperature physics then being investigated experimentally at Oxford University in England and at the University of Leiden in the Netherlands. In 1926, Peter Debye at the ETH in Zürich had published a paper proposing the method.[52] Essentially, it involved lowering the entropic energy of a paramagnetic salt, the energy otherwise unavailable for doing work, by subjecting it to a strong magnetic field while keeping it in contact with a bath of liquid helium. In the process, some of the entropic energy would be emitted in the form of heat. Next, with the sample thermally isolated and the magnetic field reduced to zero, an adiabatic change—a change in volume or pressure without loss or gain of heat—would occur which would enable the temperature of the sample to fall even further; hence, the name "cooling by adiabatic demagnetization."

Experiments conducted in the mid-1930s had confirmed Debye's prediction and temperatures of just a few hundredths of a degree above absolute zero had been reached. The paper published by Hebb and Purcell sought to explain certain anomalies in specific heats and magnetic susceptibilities that experimenters had noted at temperatures below 1 degree Kelvin.*

Although the class lasted only one semester, the two students worked on the term paper for more than a year. Hebb focused on adiabatic cooling with regard to cesium-titanium alum and Purcell with regard to iron-ammonium alum, two substances with which experimenters had been working. Their results were eventually published as a joint paper[53] in *Physical Review* along with a companion paper on the topic[54] by Professor Van Vleck. In looking back at the experience 40 years later, Purcell said:

---

* *Specific heat* is the ratio between the amount of heat required to raise the temperature of a unit mass of a substance one degree and the amount of heat required to raise the temperature of the same mass of water one degree. *Magnetic susceptibility* is the ratio of a substance's response to a magnetic field compared to the response of an equal mass of water to the same magnetic field.

This was a real turning point in my development as a physicist. I didn't contribute too much to the work. I really didn't understand extremely well what was going on in the calculations I was doing. But Malcolm did, and of course "Van" understood it with crystal clarity. Our paper was the first substantial theoretical paper on magnetic cooling and was widely referred to later by people working in that field. . . . And of course, as always, Van treated you as if you understood what was going on as well as he did, and he continues to speak to me about that paper as if I understood what I had been doing. . . . At any rate, this was an introduction to some physics that I was going to have to come back to again and again in my later work in nuclear magnetic resonance.[55]

It is noteworthy that the research Purcell considers "a very important chapter" and a "turning point" in his physics development was a course on magnetic susceptibilities, taken just before he began working on his PhD dissertation. Ten years earlier, I.I. Rabi had earned his PhD at Columbia with a dissertation entitled "On the Principal Magnetic Susceptibilities of Crystals."[56] Though separated in their educational process by a span of 10 years, at this key point in their academic careers both Rabi and Purcell were attracted by the mysterious power of the magnet.

As to Purcell's comment that this paper provided him with an introduction to some physics he would later use in NMR, the theory involved in explaining magnetic cooling required an understanding of angular momentum and spatial orientation, spin-spin coupling, crystalline structure, and magnetic dipolar interactions, all of which would have direct applications in Purcell's later work—from his first NMR experiment in 1945 to his group's work with crystals in the late 1940s to his 1952 work with Ramsey in explaining a special kind of chemical shift. This paper, like the first ones he had done with Karl Lark-Horovitz, also reveals the attention to detail, clarity and good writing that are typical of all of Purcell's publications and demonstrates why he had initially been attracted many years earlier by the *Bell System Technical Journal* "where electricity and mathematics and engineering and nice diagrams all came together."[57]

The class on magnetic cooling was also significant for Purcell in that, through Van Vleck, he became acquainted that year with Ralph H. Fowler. The son-in-law of Ernest Rutherford, discoverer of the atom's nucleus, Fowler had derived the mathematics for Rutherford's famous alpha-particle Scattering Law. "For the first time," said Purcell, "I found myself with a senior European physicist who had some slight interest in what we were doing. It was a step in my getting acquainted with the world of physics." Fowler was more than slightly interested in the subject of magnetic cooling. He and the Russian physicist, Peter Kapitza, had served as co-editors of a series of monographs that included Van Vleck's book on electric and magnetic susceptibilities. In 1936, Fowler had published *Statistical Mechanics*,[58] which Purcell and Hebb had quoted from in their paper. Reprinted 30 years later, Fowler's book continues to influence modern thermodynamics.

Purcell's Spherical-Condenser Spectrograph

From 1936 to 1938, in addition to his paper on magnetic cooling, Purcell was devoting major portions of his time to working as a teaching assistant, searching for a suitable dissertation topic—he had a couple of false starts—and conducting the research for his dissertation. His first thesis topic, suggested by Professor Chaffee, involved measuring the AC impedance—as a function of frequency—of condenser plates placed in a magnetic field and exposed to a gas discharge. Chaffee thought there might be some kind of anomaly at the cyclotron frequency, said Purcell, "what we would now call the cyclotron frequency of the ions." If there was such an anomaly, it was reasoned, perhaps it could be used as a mass spectrograph.[59]

The first mass spectrograph had been invented in 1919 by Francis W. Aston of Cambridge University. Inspired by the way Ernest Rutherford's positive-ray discharge tube used parallel magnetic and electrostatic fields to separate beams of ionized nuclei into their atomic components, Aston made a machine that also comprised an electrostatic field and a magnetic field, but which produced much more accurate results. It was called a mass spectrograph in that it sorted atomic isotopes according to their mass much as an optical spectrograph sorts light according to its frequencies.

Purcell began his project by making a coil for the magnetic field, but after doing some of the initial calculations, he went back to Chaffee and convinced him the idea wouldn't work. "Well, it just shows you," said Purcell. "Actually, the calculations were correct, but not completely relevant, and I feel quite sure that if I or anyone else had gone on energetically with that idea experimentally at that time, he would have discovered the trick he needed to make it work."[60] He would also have been well launched, Purcell noted, in the field now called plasma physics.[61]

"A mass spectrograph, [similar to the one] Chaffee was dreaming about," said Purcell, "was in a few years described and published by someone named John Hipple at the U.S. Bureau of Standards."[62]

Purcell's second dissertation topic, looking for beta ray tracks in photographic emulsions, was suggested by Professor Kenneth Bainbridge. It, too, wasn't very fruitful. "This time, instead of calculating myself out of it," said Purcell, "I spent quite a little time actually looking for the beta ray tracks and didn't see any. And in retrospect, it's clear that I should not have seen any; that with the emulsions at the state of perfection they had reached then, you could not yet see a minimum ionizing track."[63]

Bainbridge's next suggestion, looking at the focusing of charged particles in a spherical condenser, was more tempting. Like the first idea, the topic finally chosen for Purcell's dissertation would result in a variation on the mass spectrograph—this one for focusing electrons. In fact, Aston had mentioned in his landmark 1919 paper[64] that the possibility existed of using a portion of a spherical condenser as an energy analyzer and had pointed out, Purcell noted in his dissertation, that "particles of the proper energy entering the condenser in the proper direction would follow great circles and be united on the axis of the figure."[65] The fact that these particles would be refocused 180 degrees after beginning their circular travel was not brought out, however, by Aston, and the purpose of Purcell's dissertation was to prove, both theoretically and experimentally, that they could indeed be refocused.

Earlier studies had shown that it was possible to do this deflection and refocusing with a cylindrical condenser, but such a device was essentially two-dimensional in its operation, which was "analogous," said Purcell, "to optical systems composed of prisms and cylindrical lenses."[66] Refocusing particles with a spherical condenser, on the other hand, was a three-dimensional task.

I did a little calculating on that [said Purcell]—it looked very interesting. I set out to build an electron model, so to speak, to show that electrons would be focused by such a device, and to make it actually run. Again, it isn't clear why building it was a useful exercise except to get a PhD thesis; there was nothing dubious about the equation of motion for the electron in the electrostatic field. Nevertheless, it was a great experience to try and make this thing, which I finally succeeded in doing. It wasn't good for anything as it stood. That is, I was just focusing ordinary thermionic electrons to show that it would work. I wasn't measuring anything that needed to be measured. On the other hand, in working out the theory I did discover an interesting general property of the spherical electrostatic analyzer—the equivalent of which was known as Barber's rule for magnetic sector focusing.[67]

"Working out the theory for focusing electrons in a classical Coulomb field, where the trajectory is a portion of a Kepler ellipse, I made a very minor discovery," Purcell told the writer. "Conjugate foci are separated by a trajectory passing through the center. This had been known in two dimensions as 'Barber's rule.' It turned out to hold in spherical geometry, also."[68]

After developing the theory—including the necessary relativistic corrections—that supported what he called his "spherical-condenser spectrograph,"[69] Purcell set out to build the device. "It should be remembered," wrote Purcell in his dissertation, "that an analyzer of this type is really 'many spectrographs in parallel.' "[70]

The inner, working portion of the analyzer consisted of two spun-copper spheres of different radiuses, one approximately 6-3/4 inches in diameter, the other about 8 inches in diameter. When assembled, the smaller one was nested within the larger and both, if viewed as globes of the earth, were cut off at approximately 65 degrees north and south latitudes for mounting on grounded guard diaphragms that Purcell described as "heavier, pie-pan shaped plates."[71] The partial globes were positioned in such a way on the plates—which were inverted to one another—so that the 1-1/4 inch cavity between the globes coincided with the angled walls of the plates. A slit cut into the wall of the plates, continuous around their circumference except for a few short sections which were left uncut for structural integrity, provided entrance and exit paths for the electrons. The entire inner assembly was supported by the walls of the "glass envelope" by rigid insulating material called lavite. (See Figure 1.)

The axis of the analyzer was positioned in alignment with the earth's magnetic field and care was taken, wrote Purcell, to avoid other magnetic disturbances. At the input end of the spectrograph, accelerating electrodes provided an "entirely satisfactory"[72] source of electrons which were collected at the opposite end by a Faraday cage that carried a small fluorescent screen. The analyzer was operated with the cathode about 2000 volts below ground, reported Purcell, and with the inner and outer spheres at about 300 volts above and below ground, respectively.

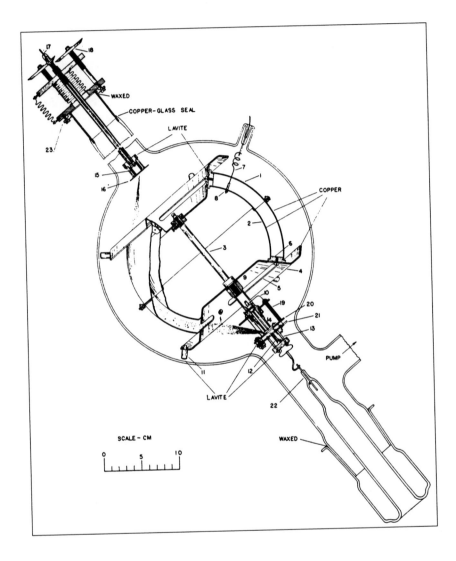

Figure 1. Cross-Sectional View of Purcell's
Spherical-Condenser Spectrograph (1938)

What Purcell called the "glass envelope" of the analyzer turned out to be somewhat of a problem. Although the results he obtained were sufficient to confirm that his theory was accurate, the device did not focus the electrons down to a single point as desired. After some experimentation, he was convinced that the deviation was caused by the condenser itself. Made from a large 11-litre flask blown specifically for the project, the sphere was cut along its equator and then resealed after internal assembly was completed, a technique somewhat analogous, said Purcell, to building a ship in a bottle. "One look at the drawing [Figure 1] and you can see the complications,"[73] he said.

Although the central glass bulb turned out to be not perfectly spherical, it was a deficiency that Purcell blamed on the design itself rather than on the glass blower. The project was "remarkable," said Purcell, "in the challenge it presented to our glass blower, Mr. H.W. Leighton. It required a real *tour de force* of glass blowing and anything that suggested it may not have been spherical was not the fault of the glass blower. Without him, I couldn't have done this thesis at all."[74] In concluding his thesis, Purcell noted that "a disadvantage of the complete three-dimensional spectrograph is its inherent difficulty of construction. However, it is believed that in the light of experience," he continued optimistically, "a considerably better design than the present one can be evolved."[75]

As a general conclusion, Purcell pointed out that the primary merit of the spherical condenser spectrograph was that it provided, because of its three-dimensional design, a very large aperture for any desired resolving power. From that experiment, said Purcell, "I learned a lot of practical things in high-vacuum electronics."[76]

"The astonishing thing," he said, "was that [the idea] actually was used about 30 years later as a spectrograph for slow electrons. I think somebody was actually selling a spectrograph based on that."[77]

Purcell submitted his paper, entitled "The Focusing of Charged Particles by a Spherical Condenser," to *Physical Review* in early August 1938. To place the time into its chronological context, Norman Ramsey was working at Columbia University that summer with molecular hydrogen and taking the first steps in opening up the new field of radiofrequency spectroscopy, in collaboration with I.I. Rabi, Jerome Kellogg and Jerrold Zacharias.[78] Rabi was on sabbatical, dividing his time between the Institute for Advanced Studies in Princeton, New Jersey and a four-week summer lecture series he was conducting at Stanford University at Felix Bloch's invitation.

In Germany, two chemists, Otto Hahn and Fritz Strassmann, would discover nuclear fission in a few months, while two of their former colleagues, Jewish physicists Lise Meitner and Otto Frisch, exiled in Sweden and Denmark respectively to escape Adolf Hitler, would determine that such a feat was theoretically possible.

In Italy, Benito Mussolini was about to imitate Hitler and take his first steps in severely limiting the civil rights of Jews. A few months later, Enrico Fermi and his family would emigrate from Italy to the United States by way of Stockholm, Sweden where he was awarded the Nobel Prize in physics.

In Eastern Europe, Hitler had already annexed Austria and was about to further test the limits of world opinion by threatening to invade Czechoslovakia. With acquiescence from Britain and France, he would encounter little resistance from Czechoslovakia itself. While the rest of the world sat by as stunned spectators, contemplating Hitler's first bold acts of expansionism and brutality and hoping his appetite for conquest had been satisfied, the little man with the strange mustache continued setting the stage for all-out war and annihilation of the Jews while, in the Pacific theater, Japan was taking its own aggressive steps toward empire.

Edward Purcell, like many other physicists in the United States and Britain, would soon find himself fighting the Second World War on both fronts with a relatively new weapon called radar. Without that weapon and the many refinements that physicists like Rabi, Ramsey and Purcell brought to it, World War II may well have come to a different conclusion.

After receiving his PhD in 1938, Purcell stayed on at Harvard as an instructor of physics. In addition to his teaching responsibilities, he helped design Harvard's first cyclotron, completed in 1939, working primarily on the magnet power supply and controls, experience that would also stand him in good stead about six years later when he would again become involved with the study of magnetic fields.

The Physicists' War

Whereas World War I was called the chemists' war, World War II came to be known as the physicists' war.[79] This second conflict was not only engaged in by soldiers on the islands of Okinawa, the beaches of Normandy and the deserts of North Africa; it was also fought by thousands of physicists near the banks of the Charles River in Cambridge, Massachusetts and on a 7200-foot-high mesa formed by an extinct volcano in Northern New Mexico called Los Alamos.

What comes to mind for most people regarding the physics of World War II is the Manhattan Project and the birth of the nuclear age in weapons when atomic bombs were dropped on the Japanese cities of Hiroshima and Nagasaki. And indeed, at the remote Los Alamos site, 80 miles from Santa Fe, where the bombs Fat Man and Little Boy were developed, it has been said that "one could sometimes see as many as eight Nobel laureates dining at once."[80]

Less known to many, but more important as far as the outcome of the war was concerned, was the radar and microwave development going on at MIT's Radiation Laboratory and at Harvard's Radio Research Laboratory (RRL). Kevles wrote: "Physicists in the war could respect the conviction of the Rad Lab staff, some of whom eventually worked on the Manhattan Project: The atom bomb only ended the war. Radar won it."[81] Professor Purcell is uncomfortable with such an all-encompassing claim—"I've never said that and I won't say that"[82]—but he does agree that radar played a decisive role in the Battle of the Atlantic by substantially reducing the threat of German submarines.

Although radar was in use prior to World War II, its utility was greatly expanded with the invention of the resonant cavity magnetron by British physicists at the University of Birmingham in late 1939.* Whereas earlier radar sets almost all operated in the VHF range—below 200 MHz and often with wavelengths of one to two meters—the magnetron made it possible to operate at much higher power and in the microwave portion of the spectrum, at a wavelength of only 10 centimeters. Not only did this make it possible to reduce the size of the antenna, it also provided greater accuracy, better reso-

---

* "In the ultimate development of radar," it has been noted, "Great Britain is usually given credit; but in many ways the device was an Anglo-American child. In 1921, an electronic tube called the magnetron had been invented by an American, Dr. Albert W. Hall. A greatly improved form was developed in Britain in 1939 by Dr. John T. Randall and Dr. Henry A.H. Boot. World War II radar used the magnetron as the high power pulse transmitter and the klystron tube as the low power, local oscillator in the receiver."

The article from which the above quotation is taken also points out that the klystron resulted from the combined efforts of W.W. Hansen, Russell Varian and Sigurd Varian. Hansen's design of a cavity resonator in the mid-1930s called a rhumbatron became the basic microwave amplifier for the klystron. W.W. Hansen would later be one of Felix Bloch's collaborators in his 1946 nuclear induction (NMR) experiment.

—Frederick A. Fender, "Stuffed clouds," *San Francisco*, December 1964, 66. From Department of Special Collections, Stanford University Libraries.

lution and object discrimination, and less interference from atmospheric noise.

To gain these benefits, however, a host of technical problems had to be overcome and it was Britain's willingness to share their new technology with their American allies in exchange for U.S. help in developing it into a practical military tool that led to the establishment of the Radiation Laboratory in the fall of 1940.

One of the first to become part of the Radiation Lab effort was Professor Isidor Isaac Rabi of Columbia University. Just three years after his landmark molecular beam-plus-magnetic resonance experiment, Rabi put aside the experiments that had demanded his complete attention for seven years, seven days a week, and volunteered his services to Lee DuBridge, the Rad Lab's newly-appointed director. Eventually, when the structure became more formalized, Rabi would become the head of Division 4, the Research Division, as well as the associate director of the laboratory.[83]

His first task, however, a full year before the bombing of Pearl Harbor that drew America directly into the war, was to recruit the best and the brightest of America's physicists to participate in the quest to defeat Germany technologically. Among the first 40 scientists—a figure which mushroomed to 4,000 by the end of the war— was Edward Purcell of Harvard, recommended for the task by his former mentor, Kenneth Bainbridge. Bainbridge would eventually become the operational chief of the first atomic test explosion at Alamogordo, New Mexico. Except for one week he spent as a transmission line expert at Los Alamos shortly before the Alamogordo test, Purcell would spend the next five years at the Rad Lab, on leave from Harvard.

Unlike the atomic bomb, which was subject to moral questions about its development and use, there was never any question about the need for developing radar. "Everybody, so far as I know," said Purcell, "completely accepted the proposition that it was a matter of desperate urgency to beat Hitler. In retrospect one might say the firebombing of Dresden was as great a human catastrophe—indirectly assisted by radar—as you could imagine. But at the time no one would have really raised that [question]. The situation was too desperate. Hitler was about to win."[84]

That radar development was critical to the war effort would be brought home dramatically to Purcell on a trip he made in the summer of 1942 to England with Rabi to talk with their counterparts in British radar. Although less than a year had gone by since the official U.S. entry in the war, German submarines had already exacted a heavy toll.

It was at the headquarters of RAF Coastal Command that we saw [said Purcell] . . . the big map of the Atlantic with a pin stuck in for every sunken ship. Along the coast of the United States, from Maine down to Florida, there was scarcely room for another pin.[85]

By that time, two years of intense research and development at the Radiation Lab was beginning to produce results. By mid-1943, the threat of Germany's U-boats to Allied shipping had been greatly diminished, a dramatic change from even a few months earlier.

In the first 20 days of March 1943, 97 Allied ships had been torpedoed and sunk by Hitler's U-boats, at a staggering loss of more than half-a-million tons. At that rate, there was little chance that a trans-Atlantic convoy designated ONS.5, which left the Azores two months later, in early May, would make it across intact. It didn't. Twelve merchant ships in that convoy were sunk by U-boats, but the tables had begun to turn as seven U-boats were also destroyed.

By the end of May, 33 U-boats had been destroyed, while Allied losses had sharply decreased. At that point, Germany's Grand Admiral Karl Doenitz pulled his submarine forces back, but not before a total of 237 U-boats were destroyed. When asked by Hitler for an explanation, Doenitz admitted: "It was 10 cm radar . . . which caused all the German losses."[86] (Perhaps he didn't dare tell Hitler the whole truth. By 1943, 3 cm wavelengths were common for much of the radar used by the Allies.) Soon afterward, British intelligence intercepted a message from the Führer to his U-boat crews passing on Doenitz's analysis: Germany's losses were due, explained Hitler, to "a single technical invention of our enemies."[87]

The importance of radar to Allied victory in the war is given further credence by the following statistics provided by Vannevar Bush, head of the National Defense Research Committee during the war:

Between September 1939 and May 1943, a period of 44 months, the Allies had destroyed 192 U-boats. In the three months of May, June and July, 1943, the Allies destroyed 100 more. Even more dramatically, early in the war, 40 Allied ships were sunk for every German submarine destroyed. With radar and other defensive methods, the ratio was reduced to less than one Allied ship per one German submarine.[88]

Playing a key role in this and subsequent Radiation Lab successes, evidenced on both land and sea, was Edward Purcell. After Norman

Ramsey, the first leader of the Fundamental Development Group (Group 41), left for Washington, DC in 1942, Purcell became the head of that group, which was part of Division 4, Rabi's Research Division. (Other groups in Division 4 were: Propagation, Group 42, headed by D.E. Kerr; Theory, Group 43, headed by George Uhlenbeck; Experimental Systems, Group 44, headed by J.L. Lawson; and Special Dielectrics, Group 45, headed by O. Halpern.)

Young Julian Schwinger, then in his early 20s and part of George Uhlenbeck's Theory Group, would work on wave guide theory and other aspects of radar at night after the other employees had gone home for the evening, which may explain why he is missing from a group photo taken during the daytime for a commemorative Rad Lab employee publication.[89] Twice a week, Schwinger would come in during the day and lecture on his latest findings, after which, as I.I. Rabi has pointed out, people like Edward Purcell and Robert Dicke [who was also in the Fundamental Developments Group] "would invent things like mad."[90]

Purcell: Absorbed with Absorption

John Rigden points out in a paper entitled "Quantum States and Precession: The Two Discoveries of NMR," that both Edward Purcell and Felix Bloch were products of their background and that their differing approaches to finding the NMR signals of hydrogen in paraffin (Purcell) and water (Bloch) were almost "foreordained" by their experiences both before and during the war.[91]

The phenomenon of nuclear magnetic resonance can be viewed from two different viewpoints, both essentially equivalent, but requiring a mental shifting of gears as you go from one perspective to the other.

The *dynamical* approach, as Rigden calls it, the one used by Bloch, draws more heavily upon the classical physics principles of precession, torques and electromagnetic induction and focuses on the spatial reorientation of magnetic moments with respect to an external magnetic field. The *spectroscopic* approach, the one used by Purcell, is preoccupied with quantum-mechanical transitions of nuclear spins from one discrete energy level to another as they absorb energy from an oscillating magnetic field.

Although Rabi had used both approaches in his magnetic resonance experiments between 1937 and 1940, he and his 'post-docs' and graduate student assistants at Columbia had moved from an initial focus on "flopping" magnetic moments (Bloch's perspective) to an emphasis on quantum transitions or radiofrequency spectroscopy (Purcell's perspective).*

For Purcell, the spectroscopic approach was a natural outgrowth of his conversations with members of Rabi's team and, perhaps even more significantly, a "water problem" encountered by the Rad Lab scientists.

Early on, developers of radar recognized the desirability of increasing frequencies—and shortening wavelengths—in order to reduce the size of antennas and to increase target definition. So even as scientists at the Rad Lab were struggling to overcome the technical hurdles raised by Britain's new resonant cavity magnetron and its 10-centimeter wavelengths, they began working to shorten wavelengths even further—first to 3 centimeters, and then to 1 centimeter. Each reduction in wavelength raised a concomitant set of challenges. Higher-frequency, higher-intensity radar not only required development of new magnetrons; it also required smaller waveguides† to transmit the waves.

As George Pake** recalled, who designed and tested a component for a 3-centimeter airborne radar set for Westinghouse toward the end of the

---

* "Rabi," Rigden points out, "publicly welcomed the new radiofrequency spectroscopy and reveled in the spectroscopic mode of thinking, and was the author of thoroughly spectroscopic papers. Privately, however, the situation was different. When asked the point at which he switched from thinking in terms of flopping moments [which Rigden noted has more vivid imagery] to thinking in terms of [the more abstract] quantum transitions, his answer was immediate and direct: 'Never switched. My thinking of this is, always has been, physical.' "
—John Rigden, *Rabi: Scientist and Citizen*, (New York: Basic Books, 1986), 123.

† "Electrical power is delivered to a pop-up toaster (and other applications) by a simple two-wire cord," Rigden explains. "Wires will not work for microwaves. Hollow, metal conduits, called waveguides, are required; and waveguide components had to be invented in order to shuttle microwave power from one part of the radar system to another."
—Rigden, 123.

** From 1946 to 1948, George E. Pake was a PhD student of Professor Purcell and a colleague of Nicolaas Bloembergen, who was doing the research for his PhD dissertation at the time. Between 1961 and 1981, Pake's paper entitled "Nuclear resonance absorption in hydrated crystals," [*J. Chem. Physics* **16**, (1948), 327], based on his doctoral thesis, was cited 435 times in the work of other scientists. In 1951, at age 27, Pake was made the head of the physics department at Washington University in St. Louis. Five years later, in 1956, he became a colleague of Felix Bloch in the physics department at Stanford University. In 1962, he returned to Washington University as provost and executive vice chancellor, a position he held for eight years until his appointment as head of Xerox Corporation's Palo Alto Research Center (PARC) in 1970. He retired in 1986 as Xerox group vice president for corporate research, but remained active in the field of physics and as head of the Institute for Research on Learning. During the Lyndon Johnson administration, Pake was a colleague of his former mentor, Edward Purcell, on the President's Science Advisory Committee.

war, waveguides for transmitting 3-centimeter wavelengths were approximately two-and-a-half inches wide and three-quarters of an inch thick, whereas waveguides for 1-centimeter radar measured only about a half-inch by a quarter-inch.

Improving waveguide designs, however, wasn't the only challenge. Unfortunately—at least from their perspective at the time—the Rad Lab physicists eventually settled on what seemed a "convenient" wavelength of 1.25 centimeters, a decision that Lee DuBridge, Director of the Rad Lab, would later describe as "a curious piece of bad luck."[92] Instead of seeing marked improvement, the physicists observed rather mediocre results. Not only was the range disappointing, but a problem developed that, according to Pake, "really began to drive the people at the Rad Lab nuts. . . . Sometimes the waves got almost no reflection back at all."[93]

It was John Van Vleck, Purcell's former professor and colleague from Harvard, then working at Harvard's Radio Research Laboratory, who provided an explanation. The Rad Lab's selection of 1.25 centimeters as the wavelength of convenience had placed them, very inconveniently, almost squarely on top of a water vapor absorption band centered at approximately 1.3 centimeters. As Pake explained:

> There is a molecular motion inside water-vapor molecules that occurs just at the frequency corresponding to that one-and-a-quarter centimeter wavelength. The reason that the new radar set was performing with considerable lack of dependability was that sometimes—on a humid day or if it was raining—there was just too much moisture in the air and all the radar energy was absorbed in the [water] molecules and nothing reached the airplane or came back to the receiver.
>
> That explanation immediately set forth thought processes, and you can see that Purcell's thinking and Torrey's and Pound's as they designed their equipment was heavily influenced by their understanding of this phenomenon of water vapor absorption of radar waves. . . . And that probably led them to think about doing this experiment in bulk matter to try to detect the absorption by the nuclei in a magnetic field.[94]

"Struck With the Idea"

By early 1945, it was becoming clear to the physicists at MIT's Radiation Laboratory and Harvard's Radio Research Laboratory that they would soon be able to return to physics as they knew it before 1941.

And yet, in a sense, it could not be physics as they knew it before because of the unique environments into which many of them had been thrust five years earlier.

The Rad Lab and the RRL had not only done their job in helping to reverse the initial advantages held by Germany and Japan; they had provided an educational and creative environment that would be a launching platform for much of the science that would take place in the last half of the century.

"To sort of rehabilitate us in physics,"[95] said Purcell, Rabi arranged to have weekly lectures at the Rad Lab for the thousands of physicists who would soon be leaving the unique environs of war-time MIT and heading back to their normal academic environments. Since Wolfgang Pauli was then at the Institute for Advanced Study in Princeton, Rabi got him to come up every other week to give a lecture. Rabi should have known better, as he was already aware that Pauli was, as Rabi expressed it, "one of the poorest lecturers in existence."[96]

"At the first lecture," said Purcell, "an enormous lecture room was packed with people to hear Pauli. It was almost totally non-understandable to most people, including me. At Pauli's next lecture, attendance had shrunk by about a factor of four, and we still didn't get much out of it."[97] That's when Rabi arranged for Julian Schwinger to give a bi-weekly lecture on pre-war developments in physics.

That was just marvelous [said Purcell]. Schwinger, [then 27 years old] reviewed the recent developments, pre-war developments in physics, going back to the '30s—where things had gone, what were the puzzles. So gradually the attendance at Julian's lecture went up and Pauli's went down. I remember the lecture when Julian was talking about the quadrupole moment of the deuteron and all that it implied, and how you measured it. That was really exciting—the quadrupole moment having been determined by Ramsey and Rabi and Kellogg and Zacharias just before the outbreak of the war. But that helped us to get back into real physics. We learned to do something more than merely apply the tricks that we had learned.[98]

Like many others at MIT's Radiation Laboratory who hoped that they would soon be able to "study war no more," Edward Purcell was thinking about his future research options and found his thoughts returning to the work Rabi and his associates at Columbia had done with magnetic resonance in molecular beams.

Came the end of the war and we were all thinking about what shall we do when we go back and start doing physics. In the course of knocking around with [the Rabi] people, I had learned enough about what they had done in molecular beams to begin thinking about what can we do in the way of resonance with what we've learned. And it was out of that kind of talk that I was struck with the idea for what turned into nuclear magnetic resonance.[99]

It was that idea—a way to make the atomic nuclei of solid, condensed material reveal their magnetic moments using magnetic resonance—that Purcell discussed over lunch with two of his colleagues from the Rad Lab, Henry Torrey and Robert Pound. According to a 1952 profile of Purcell in *The Harvard Crimson*, in the course of their conversation Purcell mentioned to Pound and Torrey "the idea he was mulling over" for measuring these magnetic moments, made possible by the fact that atomic nuclei act like small, rapidly-spinning bar magnets. "The only difficulty to be solved," Purcell told Crimson reporter David Rogers, "was that no one knew whether the extremely feeble effect of these magnets in ordinary substances could be detected."[100]

Until Purcell, Torrey and Pound did their NMR experiment with condensed matter just before Christmas of 1945, no one had successfully experimentally analyzed the internal atomic structure of matter without first changing it into another form.[101]

Professor I.I. Rabi of Columbia University had used the principle of magnetic resonance to determine in January of 1938 the nuclear magnetic moment of lithium (^{7}Li), but he had found it necessary to first vaporize molecules of lithium chloride before sending them caroming through a series of magnetic fields that included, midway through their airless flight, a strong, uniform field superimposed by a smaller, oscillating field.[102] That particular "molecular-beam" experiment—the first to use magnetic resonance—earned Rabi the Nobel Prize in 1944.

Purcell's idea, on the other hand, was to make the atomic nuclei of solid, condensed material reveal their magnetic moments while leaving the material itself—in Purcell's experiment, a two-pound chunk of paraffin purchased from a neighborhood grocery store—structurally undisturbed.

The approach they would use would be strongly influenced both by their discussions with the scientists from Columbia, who had been involved in radiofrequency spectroscopy before the war, as well as by their experience during the war at the Rad Lab with the "water problem"—molecules of water vapor of a certain frequency absorbing radar energy transmitted at the same frequency—and the resulting loss of signal they had experienced.

On the other hand, although both Rabi's 1937 experiment and Purcell's proposed 1945 experiment were based on nuclear magnetic resonance, the methods they used would be quite different from one another. Although both apparatuses used a strong external magnetic field combined with a much weaker oscillating field, the technique used to make hydrogen protons in a lump of paraffin disclose their magnetic moments would have to be, understandably, quite different from that used to make the nuclei of lithium in a tenuous beam of vaporized lithium chloride disclose theirs.

Since all three men—Purcell, Torrey and Pound—were still officially employed by the Radiation Lab, much of their time on the NMR experiment would have to be spent on the side, in the evenings and on weekends. The equipment for the experiment, Purcell said, also had to be scrounged up from "here and there:"

> I went around MIT trying to borrow a magnet from somebody, a big magnet . . . so we could try it there [near the Rad Lab] and I didn't have any luck. So I came back and talked to [Harvard physicist] Curry Street, and he invited us to use his big old cosmic-ray magnet which was out in the shed [behind Lyman Laboratory.] So I didn't ask anybody else's permission. I came back and got the shop to make us some new pole pieces, and we borrowed some stuff here and there. We borrowed our signal generator from the Psych Acoustic Lab of Smitty Stevens. I don't know that it ever got back to him. And some of the apparatus was made in the Radiation Lab shops. Bob Pound got the cavity made down there. They didn't have much to do—things were kind of closing up. And we did the experiment right here [at Harvard] on nights and weekends.[103]

In 1937, the "cosmic-ray magnet" mentioned by Purcell had provided Professor Street and Assistant Professor E.C. Stevenson with cloud-chamber evidence of a new particle that came to be known as the muon. The yoke of the magnet was rescued from a cast-off generator from the Boston Street Railways.

Much of the electronics for the experiment was developed by Robert Pound who had been, said Purcell, one of the "key people" at the Rad Lab when it came to sorting out signals from noise:

Bob's crucial contribution in our first nuclear magnetic resonance work with Torrey and me was his understanding of amplifier noise. Young as he was, he was as good as there was at the practical business of noise figures and inputs and receivers, which he had been working on under [Jerrold] Zacharias [head of the division of receiver technology at the Radiation Laboratory].[104]

George Pake, who came to know Robert Pound during his days at Harvard from 1946 to 1948, was also impressed with his expertise:

Pound was the real electronics wizard of those three guys. . . . He's done great science, been involved in these pioneering experiments and he also did some great experiments later on testing the general theory of relativity.

He became a full professor at Harvard even though he never had a PhD. He's my favorite example that you don't need a PhD to be a great scientist. The fact is that those experiments he did, any of the several he did, could easily—if he had wanted to get a PhD—have served as the centerpiece of a PhD thesis that would have been outstanding. Everybody knew how good he was.[105]

Torrey, as a graduate student under Rabi prior to the war, had worked with Sidney Millman and Jerrold Zacharias in determining the signs of the nuclear magnetic moments for the alkali metals prior to Rabi's inauguration of the magnetic resonance method.

The three young physicists set to work, every spare moment. "Unknowingly," Rogers stated, "they were working against time, for 3,000 miles away Bloch was constructing a similar experiment."[106]

The circuit comprising the various components gathered by the team was called a bridge. On one side of the bridge circuit, hooked up to the Psych Lab's signal generator, was the bootlegged resonant cavity containing two pounds of hydrogen-rich paraffin. (It was picked up by Purcell at the First National store between Harvard and his home.)[107] Oscillating at 30 MHz, the cavity would create a magnetic field that would circulate around its center post, perpendicular at all points to the main external field. The cavity assembly containing the paraffin was then placed between the new pole pieces of Street's magnet.

On the other side of the bridge, also hooked up to the signal generator, were an attenuator and phase shifters. The two-sided circuit was inductively coupled to a receiver, or ammeter.

With the signal generator driving both sides of the circuit at a fixed frequency, and with both sides initially balanced as to output, the idea was to watch for and measure a change in transmitted signal[110] from the paraffin side of the circuit containing the hydrogen protons. A change in transmitted signal from that side would indicate that, as the Larmor frequency was approached and then passed, the protons were absorbing energy and taking quantum leaps to the higher energy level, resulting in an imbalance that, as George Pake described it in a 1950 article, could be "amplified and detected by the receiver, and . . . placed on the vertical plates of an oscilloscope."[108] The electronic teeter-totter used in the experiment would clearly indicate if there was a "heavier" signal on one side of the circuit compared to the other and how much of a difference there was.

But there was a big unknown. How long would it take to reach thermal equilibrium? Hydrogen nuclei, like other nuclei, behave like tiny bar magnets which tend to align with a stronger magnetic field. Because of magnetic interactions between them, they are randomly oriented when spinning in the relatively-weak magnetic field of the earth. When exposed to a strong magnetic field, however, such as those used in NMR, the atomic nuclei or "protons" (in the case of hydrogen) "line up," precessing in a direction either with the external field (parallel) or against the field (antiparallel). Slightly more line up with the field than against it. In fact, a 1954 paper by Purcell[109] would reveal that, typically, for every million moments that line up with the field, there are 999,993 moments that line up against it. Those lining up parallel to the external field are at a lower energy level than those lining up opposite to the field.

The time required for this population redistribution of protons to take place is variously called the "longitudinal," "thermal," or "spin-lattice" relaxation time. When they were conducting their first experiments, the Purcell team did not know how long it would take for this thermal equilibrium to occur, a prerequisite condition if the goal of the experiment itself was to be achieved—the absorption of energy by lower-energy protons that would induce them to temporarily become higher-energy protons. If they responded as the team hoped they would, the teeter-totter would be temporarily unbalanced at some point, observable on the ammeter.

A paper by Ivar Waller, a Swedish theoretical physicist, written in the 1930s on electron spin relaxation in crystals,[110] suggested that it could take quite a lengthy period of time for thermal equilibrium to occur. When Torrey made his calculations for the Purcell experiment, based on Waller's theory, it appeared that the relaxation time required could be anywhere from a few hours to many hours.[111]

In the middle of their preparations, Rabi told the Purcell team of an attempt—a failed attempt—by Cornelius Gorter, three years earlier in Holland, to detect an NMR signal in condensed matter, and Rabi was unable to offer Purcell much encouragement. Although the experiment had been conducted in less-than-ideal conditions during the war, the method Gorter had used appeared valid. Theoretically, it should have worked. Although it was true that Gorter and Broer had looked for the signal through energy dispersion rather than absorption in lithium chloride and potassium fluoride, if Gorter had tried and failed—after all, it was Gorter who had suggested that Rabi try magnetic resonance with an oscillating field and it had worked—why go down that road again?

Although it was disheartening to find that someone else had already tried and failed to find nuclear magnetic resonance in a solid, the Purcell team pressed on with their preparations. For one thing, according to Torrey's calculations the nuclear spin relaxation time was on the order of a few hours or less, probably about an hour. In spite of Gorter's results, it should work. For another thing, work had already proceeded to such a point that to stop then without conducting their own test of the theory . . . well, that was not a pleasant option to consider, either.[112]

If At First You Don't Succeed

A newspaper clipping, published around the time of Purcell's 1945 NMR experiment, read in part:

> Purcell, Pound and Torrey stayed in their workshop until four o'clock one December morning. When they left to go home through a blinding snowstorm, they had completed their preparations. . . . Several days passed before they had any spare time. . . . One Saturday morning Purcell went into the shed, warmed the equipment, and waited for the others. . . . They threw the switches. The experiment worked.[113]

Parts of that account are true. Pound and Purcell both remember that there was a snowstorm on the first day and Purcell did go in earlier than the others a few days later—though it was actually much earlier than implied by the story—and the final phase of the experiment did take place on a Saturday, December 15. But that's about it. The rest of the story is largely inaccurate, including the implication that the experiment worked the first time.

Although the following account, written by Purcell in early 1994 and reviewed by Robert Pound, may differ somewhat from the traditional legend, Purcell said it "comes as close as we can (on one page) to 'how it really was.'"

In our first full trials with everything running smoothly and the bridge balanced, we swept the magnet current, which was controlled by the field rheostat on the generator, through a range of values chosen to bracket the current in amperes that would produce, according to our calculations, the axial magnetic field strength for resonance, H_0. We found no trace of a signal, only thermal noise of the expected intensity. The axial field had been on during the search, but only for short periods.

There remained the possibility that relaxation was really very slow so that thermal equilibrium had never been reached. With that in mind as we laid plans for another experiment two days later, we decided to 'pre-soak' the paraffin in a strong field for at least 10 hours before searching for resonance with a suitably weak radiofrequency field. As the motor-generator could not be left unattended, this cost Purcell a wakeful night before our next experiments began on Saturday, December 15.

That afternoon the three of us gathered, still hopeful, in the shed. Maintaining a strong axial field to preserve whatever polarization might have developed overnight, we repeatedly searched as before, and found nothing. Gloomily, we reviewed our apparatus and procedure, turning up no obvious flaw. We resolved to try every extreme before switching off—including the highest current it was possible to draw from the generator. That current should have raised the axial magnetic field distinctly higher than the resonance value H_0. But with the generator at its limit, while our water-cooled magnet coils got hotter, there was still no noticeable deflection in the meter on the bridge—until we started *decreasing* the magnet current. Then the meter briefly deflected to show a clear imbalance, the signal we were looking for!

It appeared that the field had been too strong for resonance at the maximum current and had passed through B_0 on its way down. Actually, we had not previously tested at this high magnetic-field strength. The reason was a fault in our earlier magnet calibration; we had underestimated the saturation (decrease in permeability) of the magnet iron at the highest field strength.

Once this was understood, we found we could move up or down through a narrow band of absorption. The behavior was beautifully reproducible. It became evident that the relaxation time, which we now call T_1, was more like seconds than hours. That permitted a greater amplitude of the transverse RF field, improving signal-to-noise. Before we went home, further experiments had removed any doubt that we were observing nuclear magnetic resonance absorption in paraffin. Our mood was elation, slightly sobered by the thought of how close we had been to missing it.[114]

They had allowed up to 10 hours for thermal equilibrium to be established. Instead, it turned out that, in paraffin, the relaxation time is actually 10^{-4} seconds. "So I had the magnet on," Purcell said, "exactly 10^8 times longer than necessary."[115]

Leon Lederman, who shared the Nobel Prize in physics in 1988 for his work on subatomic particles called neutrinos, has described the feelings of a scientist making such a discovery:

Physicists today feel the same emotions that scientists have felt for centuries. The life of a physicist is filled with anxiety, pain, hardship, tension, attacks of hopelessness, depression and discouragement. But these are punctuated by flashes of exhilaration, laughter, joy and exultation. These epiphanies come at unpredictable times. Often they are generated simply by the sudden understanding of something new and important, something beautiful, that someone else has revealed. However, if you are mortal, like most of the scientists I know, the far sweeter moments come when you yourself discover some new fact about the universe. It's astonishing how often this happens at 3 a.m., when you are alone in the lab and you have learned something profound, and you realize that not one of the other five billion people on earth knows what you know. Or so you hope. You will, of course, hasten to tell them as soon as possible. This is known as "publishing."[116]

There were fewer billions of people on the planet on Christmas Eve, 1945 when the editors of *Physical Review* received the Purcell team's announcement to the world of their discovery, a world that was still taking a deep, prolonged breath following the trauma of World War II. Entitled "Resonance Absorption by Nuclear Magnetic Moments in a Solid," the essence of their findings was summarized in the first two sentences of their letter:

In the well-known magnetic resonance method for the determination of nuclear magnetic moments by molecular beams, transitions are induced between energy levels which correspond to different orientations of the nuclear spin [sic] in a strong, constant, applied magnetic field. We have observed the absorption of radiofrequency energy, due to such transitions, in a *solid* material (paraffin) containing protons.[117]

Next they briefly described their theoretical assumptions and their concerns about the time required to reach thermal equilibrium:

In this case there are two levels, the separation of which corresponds to a frequency, v, near 30 megacycles/sec., at the magnetic field strength, H, used in our experiment, according to the relation $hv=2\mu H$. Although the difference in population of the two levels is very slight at room temperature ($hv/kT \sim 10^{-5}$), the number of nuclei taking part is so large that a measurable effect is to be expected providing thermal equilibrium can be established. If one assumes that the only local fields of importance are caused by the moments of neighboring nuclei, one can show that the imaginary part of the magnetic permeability, at resonance, should be of the order hv/kT. The absence from this expression of the nuclear moment and the internuclear distance is explained by the fact that the influence of these factors upon absorption cross section per nucleus and density of nuclei is just canceled by their influence on the width of the observed resonance.

A crucial question concerns the time required for the establishment of thermal equilibrium between spins and lattice. A difference in the population of the two levels is a prerequisite for the observed absorption, because of the relation between absorption and stimulated emission. Moreover, unless the relaxation time is very short the absorption of energy from the radiofrequency field will equalize the population of the levels, more or less rapidly, depending on the strength of this r-f field. In the expectation of a long relaxation time (several hours), we chose to use so weak an oscillating field that the absorption would persist for hours regardless of the relaxation time, once thermal equilibrium had been established.[118]

Midway through their nine-paragraph letter, the Purcell team described their apparatus, procedure, and experimental results.

A resonant cavity was made in the form of a short section of coaxial line loaded heavily by the capacity of an end plate. It was adjusted to resonate at about 30 mc/sec. Input and output coupling loops were provided. The inductive part of the cavity was filled with 850 cm^3 of paraffin, which remained at room temperature throughout the experiment. The resonator was placed in the gap of the large cosmic-ray magnet in the Research Laboratory of Physics, at Harvard. Radiofrequency power was introduced into the cavity at a level of 10^{-11} watts. . . . The cavity output was balanced in phase and amplitude against another portion of the signal generator output. Any residual signal, after amplification and detection, was indicated by a microammeter.

With the r-f circuit balanced the strong magnetic field was slowly varied. An extremely sharp resonance absorption was observed. At the peak of the absorption the deflection of the output meter was roughly 20 times the magnitude of fluctuations due to noise, frequency, instability, etc.

Resonance occurred at a field of 7100 oersteds, and a frequency of 29.8 mc/sec., according to our rather rough calibration of the field and frequency, and the value of the proton magnetic moment inferred from the above numbers, 2.75 nuclear magnetons, agrees satisfactorily with the accepted value, 2.7896, established by the molecular beam method.[119]

Next, they provided a short analysis of how the results were affected by their equipment, and how the method could be refined in the future:

The full width of the resonance, at half value, is about 10 oersteds, which may be caused in part by inhomogeneities in the magnetic field which were known to be of this order. The width due to local fields from neighboring nuclei had been estimated at about 4 oersteds.

The relaxation time was apparently shorter than the time (~one minute) required to bring the field up to the resonance value. The types of spin-lattice coupling suggested by I. Waller fail by a factor of several hundred to account for a time so short.

The method can be refined in both sensitivity and precision. In particular, it appears feasible to increase the sensitivity by a factor of several hundred through a change in detection technique. The method seems applicable to the precise measurement of magnetic moments (strictly, gyromagnetic ratios) of most moderately abundant nuclei. It provides a way to investigate the interesting question of spin-lattice coupling. Incidentally, as the apparatus required is rather simple, the method should be useful for standardization of magnetic fields. An extension of the method in which the r-f field has a rotating component should make possible the determination of the sign of the moment.[120]

Finally, Purcell, Torrey and Pound offered their speculations as to why Gorter and Broer had failed in their 1942 attempt to detect nuclear magnetic resonance in solid matter:

> The effect here described was sought previously by Gorter and Broer, whose experiments are described in a paper which came to our attention during the course of this work. Actually, they looked for dispersion, rather than absorption, in LiCl and KF. Their negative result is perhaps to be attributed to one of the following circumstances: (a) the applied oscillating field may have been so strong, and the relaxation time so long, that thermal equilibrium was destroyed before the effect could be observed—(b) at the low temperature required to make the change in permeability easily detectable by their procedure, the relaxation time may have been so long that thermal equilibrium was never established.[121]

"Bob, Henry and I have always taken pride in that letter for the wealth of concise information we put in it," commented Purcell. "An important feature of the PTP paper," he pointed out, "is its references, in which we acknowledge prior work."[122] Three references were cited in the letter: 1) I.I. Rabi, J.R. Zacharias, S. Millman, and P. Kusch, "A new method of measuring magnetic moments," *Physical Review* **53**, (1938), 318; 2) C.J. Gorter and L.J.F. Broer, "Negative result of an attempt to observe nuclear magnetic resonance in solids," *Physica* **9**, (1942), 591; 3) I. Waller, "Über die magnetisierung von paramagnetischen kristallen in wechselfeldern," *Zeitschrift für Physik* **79**, (1932), 370.

Why Gorter failed to achieve the desired results in 1942 has never been definitively determined. In addition to the conclusions of the Purcell team mentioned above, it was also thought that the sample may have been too pure—that was the reason Gorter accepted for a time—but that conclusion fell by the wayside when Nicolaas Bloembergen, years later, looked for the effect using the identical crystal sample used by Gorter and was able to obtain a resonance. Bloembergen himself has concluded that, although Gorter was "early on and deserves a lot of credit," the reason he didn't see what he was looking for in 1942 was the result of two factors: 1) "He wasn't a good enough experimenter," and 2) he was using "very primitive" electronic equipment.[123]

In the short interval between their experiment and the publication of its results, the Purcell team could, as described by Lederman, take satisfaction from the fact that they, at that moment, were the only ones who knew for sure that the nuclei of condensed matter could be made to reveal their magnetic moments just as the nuclei of isolated atoms and molecules in molecular beams had revealed theirs to Professor Rabi and his team.

After publishing the results of their experiment, however, the team couldn't revel long in the assumption that no one else had been on the same hunt at the same time. It turned out that Felix Bloch was right on their heels and would announce just a few weeks later the path that he had followed in successfully arriving at the same destination.[124]

Because the path Bloch used was so different from that taken by Purcell, it wasn't immediately apparent to either team that they had arrived at the same destination. As was mentioned earlier, the approach of the Purcell team had been based on quantum transitions, which evoke different mental images than those evoked by physical reorientations of atomic nuclei, the Bloch approach. As a result, it took the two teams a little while before they realized they had discovered the same thing.

> I remember [said Purcell] that the first actual personal contact between our two groups came when Bill Hansen came east a couple of months later—he frequently came to the Radiation Lab anyway—and we talked to him. We were talking at cross purposes for about 15 minutes before each of us understood the other's experiment in his own terms.[125]

Bloch, who first heard from Otto Stern that a similar experiment to his had been done by a group at Harvard, recalled years later that although he "didn't quite know what it was [that the Purcell group had done], . . . it was clear to me that it was in principle the same idea."[126]

His recollection is tempered somewhat, however, by that of Martin Packard, who informed John Rigden that, although it was "quite clear to us that it was the same phenomenon" approached from "a different experimental viewpoint," that it was also true that prior to Bloch's meeting with Purcell at an April meeting of the American Physical Society in Cambridge, "[Bloch] could not accept the fact that the results were equivalent."[127]

Arriving at the same destination via different routes does not mean, of course, that one of the roads is unnecessary. Both approaches—Purcell's resonance absorption and Bloch's nuclear induction—would be essential to a comprehensive understanding of the science of NMR, both its initial application in revolutionizing chemical analysis, and its eventual use in revolutionizing medical diagnostics.

The Two Experimenters

On the surface, there was little that Edward Purcell and Felix Bloch had in common.

Purcell, growing up on the plains of Midwestern America, sang in the boys choir of Taylorville's Presbyterian church ("from which the uncompromising Professor Rickaby extracted better music than most of us were capable of before or have been since"), played basketball in the Boy Scouts under famed local leader Boyd Dappert, played tennis and swam at Manners Park, and attended summer Chatauqua events held in a tent.[128]

After attending Purdue University for his undergraduate work and Harvard for his advanced degrees, Purcell began his career in 1936 as a teaching assistant, receiving his PhD in 1938. Professionally, however, Purcell had little opportunity to make a name for himself before 1940. Then age 28, his theoretical and experimental skills, though recognized by his colleagues at Harvard, were not yet well-recognized elsewhere, although World War II and the MIT "Rad Lab" would do much to change that.

Bloch, on the other hand, was born in Zürich and had grown up Jewish in a Europe heading toward Hitler and Nazism. In 1912, the year Edward Purcell was born in the flat lands of central Illinois, seven-year-old Felix—the name means "lucky"—went skiing for the first time in the mountains of his native Switzerland.[129]

After enrolling in Zürich's Federal Institute of Technology, also known on the basis of its German name as the ETH, Bloch had the good fortune of studying under several eminent physicists, including Hermann Weyl, Erwin Schrödinger, Peter Debye, and Werner Heisenberg. Under Heisenberg's mentorship, Bloch had written a doctoral thesis that had established him as a brilliant theorist and which still provides the basis for studying electron conduction in metals.

After emigrating to the United States in 1934 because of the looming threat of Hitler, Bloch had further strengthened his reputation by proposing a method for determining the magnetic moment of the neutron and in 1939, with Luis Alvarez, had modified his method using magnetic resonance to significantly increase its accuracy.

Although the microwave science developed during World War II would have a significant impact on the post-war research of both Purcell and Bloch, Purcell, as the younger of the two and still early in his professional career, would be influenced to a greater extent by the unique environment in which he worked for five years.

What I learned [at the Rad Lab, said Purcell] helped my own career in physics. I really consider myself extremely lucky, and I mean lucky, to have been able to profit personally from what I had to do there at the Radiation Lab. Not only did I learn a whole new armament, acquire a whole new kit of research tools—microwave technology, transmission lines, signal-to-noise theory, just a lot of different things, all of which were going to prove to be useful one way or another—but perhaps the most important thing was being thrown together in a working relationship with a number of physicists from other places; in particular, physicists from Rabi's laboratory at Columbia . . . and, of course, Rabi himself with whom I was very closely associated through all that time, Rabi being the head of the division to whom I reported.[130]

Other physicists from Rabi's Columbia University laboratory with whom Purcell worked closely included Norman Ramsey, Jerrold Zacharias, Jerome Kellogg, Polykarp Kusch and, of particular importance as far as his own 1945 experiment was concerned, Henry Torrey.

Apart from their divergent backgrounds, the personalities of Purcell and Bloch were also quite dissimilar. George Pake, who was mentored by Purcell at Harvard and was later a colleague of Bloch's at Stanford, knew both of them well.

Purcell was a very modest person. You know, some great scientists tend to have great egos. They know they're good. Ed was always too modest. He never thought of himself as doing the important things that he was doing or being the great scientist that he was. Bloch was a very successful European theoretical physicist . . . and he knew he was good. He enjoyed being center stage.

And I have the impression that Ed, while he could handle being center stage, never really enjoyed it that much.[131]

Which goes to show that impressions can be misleading. When informed of Pake's perception that he "never really enjoyed it that much," Professor Purcell borrowed a line from Captain Corcoran's song in Gilbert and Sullivan's musical, *HMS Pinafore,* "What, never? . . . well, hardly ever," and then added, "I enjoyed it plenty."[132]

In setting the record straight, Purcell only adds credibility to the words of another friend of his, Anatole Abragam. In writing his autobiography, published in 1989, Abragam observed:

> As a physicist and a human being Ed Purcell is perhaps the man I admire the most. I have never met anyone more profoundly authentic, more detached from the wish to appear other than he is.[133]

With regard to those who occupy center stage, sometimes the one onstage is unaware of who is in the audience. It is interesting, for example, to compare Bloch's and Purcell's recollections of an event that took place in late 1944, when both of them attended a party celebrating Rabi's Nobel Prize at the Rabi home in Cambridge—not in regard to the event itself, but rather in their recollection of each other.

Bloch didn't remember seeing Purcell at the party. As far as Bloch was concerned, he never met Purcell until the spring of 1946 when he traveled east to present his NMR findings at a meeting of the American Physical Society in Cambridge. Charles Weiner, who interviewed Bloch in 1968, asked him, "Had you known Purcell at all before?" Bloch responded, "No, I'd never met him before." Weiner restated his question again, "At none of these laboratories or meetings?" Again, Bloch responded, "No, strangely enough, not. He was at the Radiation Laboratory, I believe, in Cambridge, but we never met. I met him later."[134]

Purcell, on the other hand, recalled very clearly seeing Bloch at the party. He even remembered the humorous duet that Felix Bloch sang with Dutch physicist George Uhlenbeck as they reminded the attendees of Rabi's early association with Otto Stern, who received the 1943 Nobel Prize in physics at the same time Rabi received the 1944 prize.

> Twinkle, twinkle Otto Stern;
> How did Rabi so much learn?[135]

Purcell agreed with Bloch, however, that they had not personally met one another until 1946, after both of their original NMR experiments had been completed.[136]

Like beauty, of course, modesty is in the eyes of the beholder, and to his colleagues at Stanford—Marvin Chodorow, Arthur Schawlow, and J. Dirk Walecka—Bloch was also modest.

Despite the extraordinary gifts that Felix gave to the world, he remained a basically modest person all his life. We do not mean quietly modest, for he held strong opinions and was usually outspoken in expressing them. No one had any doubt about what Felix was saying or where he stood on any issue. He enjoyed a good intellectual fight, and together with his colleagues at Stanford there were often many sparks flying. He had tremendous self-confidence . . .[137]

Purcell also agreed with this assessment and said that it was "very well put. My relations with Felix," he noted, "remained thoroughly cordial from 1946 on. An hour after the Nobel announcement in 1952 I received this telegram:

I think it's swell for Ed Purcell
To share the shock with Felix Bloch.[138]

He continued, "And so it remained as our friendship developed. Especially memorable: our trip together (by ship) to Holland in 1950 for the historic NMR meeting and, in 1957, my summer semester at Stanford at Felix's invitation."[139]

The historic NMR meeting mentioned by Purcell would be harkened back to time and time again by those who were in on "the ground floor" of NMR. Abragam referred to this "important conference on radiofrequency spectroscopy . . . attended by all the stars of the field" as the place where he discovered NMR. "Having become a specialist on ESR in Oxford, I wanted to familiarize myself with NMR, to which the Harvard physics department was a shrine, and the beauty of which I had discovered in a few conversations with Ed Purcell at the Amsterdam Conference of 1950."[140]

"In my dotage, as an after-dinner speaker," Abragam wrote in his 1989 autobiography, "I always get some laughs out of the following beginning:"

I discovered NMR in 1950. To those of you who think that it was Bloch and Purcell four years earlier, I must explain that I say this the way people might say "I discovered sex at thirty-five." This is actually how old I was when I discovered it—I mean NMR.[141]

Although Purcell and Bloch may have differed in style, both men were careful to give credit where credit was due. When asked by the *Harvard*

Crimson reporter why he won the Nobel prize, Purcell replied, "I guess it's because I suggested the original experiment but I think it's only fair," he continued, "to say that the original experiment could not have been done without any one of the three of us [Purcell, Torrey and Pound]."[142] Felix Bloch was also careful to credit the contributions made by his collaborators, W.W. Hansen and Martin Packard, as well as others who had laid the foundation for his work.[143]

Both Purcell and Bloch appreciated the importance of effective teaching. Dr. George Pake, who later became head of the physics department at Washington University in St. Louis and head of research for Xerox Corporation, recalled the honor he felt when asked by Purcell to take his place in front of Purcell's class:

> Once or twice, while I was finishing up my work for Purcell, he would ask me to teach his class. And that was a big honor to be asked . . . also sort of daunting because I knew I couldn't teach as well as he did. He was a superb teacher. He was very considerate of his students. He spent a lot of time with us. He was a real father figure to us. And he was such a brilliant physicist.[144]

Anatole Abragam, in recalling his own teaching career, wrote: "I discovered, why be falsely modest, that I was an excellent teacher, that I liked to teach, and that (to repeat a phrase of E.M. Purcell, the discoverer of NMR, which I shall make mine): 'Anything I understand I can explain.' "[145]

Expanding on the quotation cited by Abragam, Purcell said, "Felix [Bloch] shared with me at least one attribute of the born teacher: When you understand something, you can hardly wait to explain it to someone else!"[146]

In spite of his stature as a physicist, Purcell, like Bloch, has done most of his teaching in undergraduate courses and, like Abragam, is proud of his teaching. "I am proud of being an effective and original teacher of undergraduates," he said. "I am especially proud of my Electricity and Magnetism book in the Berkeley Series, and delighted when students praise it."[147]

"I just have taken a lot of satisfaction in having written what I think is a good book," he said. "Really," he continued, "it was one of the memorable experiences of my life,"[148] which in itself is a memorable statement from one who has won the Nobel Prize, advised three United States presidents, received the National Medal of Science from President Carter (1980), been named Harvard's first Gerhard Gade University Professor (now Professor Emeritus), served as president of the American Physical Society (1970), and been elected a foreign member of the Royal Society of London (1988), among numerous other honors.

One of those other honors, the Oersted Medal, awarded to Purcell in 1968 by the American Association of Physics Teachers, is of special significance to him because it specifically recognizes that quality in which he has taken personal pride—excellence in teaching. Although he is proud of creatively teaching physics to undergraduates, they are not the only ones who have gained insight into the world of physics from his teaching. In addition to the classes he taught at Harvard from 1936 to 1983, and the two editions of the Berkeley college textbook he has written on electricity and magnetism, Purcell was also "intensely involved," he said, as a member of the Physical Science Study Committee (PSSC) that created a new high-school physics course in the 1950s. As a result of the program, Purcell lectured on inertia and inertial mass to thousands of high-school physics students by way of film.[149]

> PSSC [said Purcell] was one of the many times in my life when I have been enlisted under the banner of Jerrold Zacharias.* In most of those times, I was glad afterwards that I was, and this was certainly the case in PSSC. We wanted to do something about the teaching of physics in high schools, and whether we did any good in the end or how much good we did is still a matter for debate, but we certainly loosened the situation up. I had a lot of fun. In a way, it was a forerunner of the Berkeley physics course, in the conception of which Zacharias also took part.[150]

It is interesting to note that Dr. Raymond Damadian, the medical doctor who discovered that diseased tissues have prolonged relaxation rates and thus extended NMR to medical diagnosis, has also testified to the excellence of Purcell's teaching. In 1963, as a post-doctoral fellow researching cell metabolism in the department of biophysics at Harvard Medical School, Damadian decided to audit Purcell's introductory course on quantum mechanics. He found the class interesting and thought-provoking and Purcell "an excellent teacher:"

---

* Jerrold Zacharias was an instructor at Hunter College in the 1930s at the same time that he worked, unpaid, as a collaborator in molecular-beam experiments with I.I. Rabi at Columbia University. During the war, Zacharias worked on radar development at the MIT Radiation Laboratory and, after the war, accepted a faculty position at MIT.

He was the sort of teacher [said Damadian] who could take a classroom of students confused by the abstractions of a modern subject in physics and with a few phrases turn the lights on for the entire class.

I remember one specific example. The class was introduced to the concept of the blackbody radiator, which can easily startle a beginning student.

The next day Dr. Purcell arrived in class with a very large cardboard box, about four feet tall and two feet wide, and placed it on the lecture bench for the benefit of the class. The face of the box facing the class contained a hole cut in the box about the diameter of a silver dollar, so that the class could easily see into the dark interior of the box. Painted directly above the hole was an equal-sized disc that Dr. Purcell said he had painted with the darkest black paint he could find. One look at the box convinced all observers that the hole in the cavity radiator was far blacker than the comparison disc applied with paint, and engraved indelibly on the student's mind the significance of blackbody radiation.

As a researcher at Harvard at the time I was taking the course, I happened to have as my research assistant Margaret Ramsey, who was Norman Ramsey's daughter. I described Dr. Purcell's delightful demonstration after I returned to the laboratory from class. The next day when she arrived at the lab, she remarked that she had reported Dr. Purcell's demonstration of the blackbody radiation to her father. Dr. Ramsey responded to her by saying, "I have been teaching that course for years. Why didn't I think of that [demonstration]?"[151]

It was in that same course that Purcell planted a seed in the mind of Damadian that would eventually culminate in the extension of NMR spectroscopy to NMR scanning for medical diagnosis.

One day, as part of some now-forgotten discussion [Sonny Kleinfield wrote in his book on the invention of MR scanning], Purcell drew an NMR spectrum on the board. Intrigued, Damadian recognized that such a device might be helpful in the sodium-pump work he was doing in [Arthur] Solomon's lab, though he wasn't sure exactly how it might be useful. Damadian approached Solomon later in the day and asked him if they could use nuclear magnetic resonance—he didn't actually know it was called that at the time— and Solomon said that he was sorry but the machines were too expensive.[152]

From A Lump of Paraffin to Interstellar Space

When Purcell made his Nobel Prize-winning NMR discovery in December 1945, he was 33 years old; 40 when he received the prize. In the intervening years, he and his colleagues continued the research set in motion by the original experiment.

Henry C. Torrey, who had been on leave from Rutgers University for the duration of the war to work at the Radiation Laboratory, returned to Rutgers shortly after the December experiment where he continued his own experiments, making significant contributions to NMR theory.

Pound would also go on to make additional major contributions to physics, both in NMR and later in Mössbauer and gamma ray spectroscopy:

> Pound opened up a new field of electric quadrupole physics [said Purcell] using NMR with crystals. He also greatly improved the electronics of the device he had developed for the original experiment. Soon the 'Pound Box' was in every laboratory. Pound would also become famous for his beautiful experimental confirmation of Einstein's prediction of the effect of gravity on light. A truly fundamental experiment which NMR was not.[153]

Purcell and Pound together with an incoming PhD candidate from Holland, Nicolaas Bloembergen, soon began the process of extending the original experiment to other substances, focusing on the relaxation times for a wide variety of liquids at various temperatures and conditions, while the Bloch team concentrated primarily on determining the magnetic moments of various substances.

Other students and colleagues of Purcell's joined him in conducting the host of experiments that naturally follow on the heels of an experimental breakthrough. Joining in the follow-up experimentation was PhD candidate George E. Pake. After receiving his doctorate under Purcell's mentorship in 1948, Pake, in turn, helped spread the gospel of NMR to Washington University in St. Louis and, through his pedagogical writings, to a generation of waiting physicists and chemists.[154] Others who co-published articles on NMR with Purcell—besides Bloembergen and Pound—during this follow-up period included R.M. Brown,[155] J.H. Gardner,[156] H.S. Gutowsky, G.B. Kistiakowsky,[157] H.Y. Carr,[158] F. Reif, G.B. Benedek, G.B. Field,[159] Norman F. Ramsey and J.H. Smith.[160]

Of Purcell's own scientific publications, about 80 in all, he attributes about 30 to NMR-related research. The balance, not counting research done before 1945, are largely related to his interests in astrophysics and biophysics.[161] One of these papers, in which he and his collaborator, Harold I. Ewen, announced their discovery of 21-centimeter-wavelength radiation from atomic hydrogen, opened up the field of radio spectroscopy within radio astronomy.

Although several scientists, including Thomas Edison, had searched unsuccessfully for extraterrestrial radio waves in the late 1800s, they were not detected until 1931 when Karl G. Jansky of Bell Telephone Laboratories, in searching for the source of interference to shortwave radio transmissions, accidentally discovered cosmic radiation. Eight years later, Grote Reber, a young radio engineer, built the first reflector radio telescope at Wheaton, Illinois with which he was able to map radio emissions from the Milky Way galaxy, and obtain evidence for discrete radio sources, though for a time the significance of his work went unrecognized.

Following World War II and the development of more sophisticated radio receivers, radio astronomy enjoyed rapid growth, especially in Britain and Australia. During this period, astronomers discovered the first discrete radio sources and were able to identify them with distant stars and galaxies.[162]

But it wasn't until 1951, when Edward Purcell and his graduate student, Harold I. "Doc" Ewen, first picked up emissions of 21-centimeter-wavelength radiation from atomic hydrogen with a rather crude antenna aimed into the distant heavens that radio spectroscopy of interstellar space was born. Even then, other spectral lines were not discovered for another 12 years, until 1963, when radiation from the hydroxyl molecule was identified.[163] This was followed by a flood of spectral-line discoveries in the 1960s and '70s.

When Ewen, a PhD candidate in physics, initially came to Purcell for a thesis topic, he had been thinking about doing something with microwaves, said Purcell, "to detect or measure something in the upper atmosphere," but exactly what he wasn't sure. An astronomy buff who taught celestial navigation to naval air cadets during the war, Ewen was "already technically pretty adept," said Purcell, but "we didn't see anything particularly exciting" as far as upper atmosphere prospects were concerned.

They were still discussing ideas, in fact, when Ewen went off to one of his astronomy meetings. When he came back, he told Purcell that "somebody was talking about this hydrogen hyperfine line, whether you could detect it.'[164]

At the time, neither of them knew who had predicted such a line, although they soon found out that it was a Dutch astrophysicist, Hendrick C. van de Hulst. In 1944, van de Hulst, then a young astronomy student at the University of Leiden, proposed that "it might be possible to detect radio emissions from hydrogen atoms spread thinly through interstellar space."[165]

That such radiation existed was based solidly on quantum mechanics and spectroscopy. Visual-light spectroscopy had led Niels Bohr to theorize that the reason hydrogen atoms emit a unique spectral light is because hydrogen electrons exist only in discrete, quantized energy states and that when quantum transitions are made from one energy level to another, energy is emitted at discrete frequencies. In the 1920s, Wolfgang Pauli had explained the phenomenon of "hyperfine splittings"—bright spectral lines that actually consisted of several, closely-spaced lines—by theorizing that the nucleus of the atom has a spin and, therefore, a magnetic moment.

Van de Hulst theorized that interaction in interstellar space between the spin of the hydrogen atom's electron and the spin of its nucleus, or proton, would emit energy in the form of radio waves that might be detectable. He knew that a hydrogen atom in space can exist in only one of two energy states—either a lower energy state in which the single electron and the single proton are spinning in opposite directions or a slightly-higher energy state in which the particles are spinning in the same direction. When they are parallel, spinning in the same direction, the spin of the electron has the potential for flipping and spinning opposite to the nucleus, at the same time dropping to a lower energy state and releasing a photon that carries off the "lost" energy. The wavelength of this photon, predicted van de Hulst, is 21 centimeters (8.3 inches), equivalent to a frequency of 1,420 MHz.[166]

Van de Hulst's prediction was not well publicized, however, because of the German occupation of Holland and when word did get out more generally after the war, "few astronomers took it seriously, because it seemed likely that the hydrogen signal would be extremely faint."[167]

That would qualify as an definite understatement. Although interstellar atomic hydrogen is thought to be the most common element by far in interstellar space, accounting for about one percent of the total galactic mass in the Milky Way galaxy (up to as much as 30 percent in other galaxies), collecting emissions from these great "clouds" of hydrogen for spectroscopic analysis represented a great deal of optimism by Ewen and Purcell:

The amount of radiation from interstellar hydrogen falling on the entire surface of the earth is less than 10 watts. The amount of this energy that can be collected by a radio telescope is an extremely small fraction in which the numerator is the area of the telescope's collecting surface and the denominator is the area of the earth: about 5×10^{15} square feet.[168]

Furthermore, unlike the 1945 NMR experiment in which Purcell, Torrey and Pound were able to influence the detection of energy absorption by magnetically controlling the environment of a two-pound lump of wax, the protons of which were passively precessing in the shed behind Lyman Laboratory, Purcell and Ewen had no control over the vast reaches of interstellar space. It's true, they didn't have to worry about how long it would take to reach thermal equilibrium, but they did have to worry about how well their receiver could "hear."

They didn't know for sure how sensitive their equipment would have to be to detect the hydrogen emissions, but Purcell and Ewen decided they had a "fighting chance" and Ewen had his thesis topic. Purcell warned Ewen, however, that he was faced with a tough thesis problem. "If you don't find the line," said Purcell, "you're going to have to put in a hell of a lot of work to establish the limits. If you find it, of course, then it's great, it's fine. But if you don't detect it . . . "[169]

Although there was adequate funding available for Purcell's other projects, this one, reminiscent of Purcell's original NMR experiment, had to be done on a shoestring. In addition to some support from the physics lab, Purcell and Ewen received $500 from the American Academy of Arts and Sciences which they used to construct an antenna in the form of a copper-lined plywood horn.

Purcell credits Ewen for having "great nerve to look for [the hydrogen line]" and for doing "a superb job of building and testing the receiver." In acknowledging their "fortunate circumstances" in finding the line, Purcell points out, however, that "we went at it right. We used the simplest possible antenna but one which was good for the job. And Doc's receiver was really very good. It was probably as good a receiver of that type as existed in the world at the time he did the experiment."[170] Again, although Robert Pound's name wasn't on the paper announcing the results of the experiment, he did have a direct influence on its success by sharing his expertise about receivers with Harold Ewen.[171]

Purcell and Ewen performed their experiment March 25, 1951. "Luckily," said Purcell, they found the radiation they were looking for. "The original detection was such," he said, "that if it had been even five times weaker, we probably wouldn't have seen it. It was just barely there."[172]

Coincidentally, at the same time Purcell and Ewen were conducting their experiment, Dr. van de Hulst was a visiting professor at Harvard while, back in Holland, his own team was working to confirm his prediction. Although they had constructed a more elaborate experiment than Ewen and Purcell which, Purcell said, "enabled them to get better results when they finally got it," the Dutch team had to settle for coming in second. Set back about a week or so by a fire in their antenna, the van de Hulst team heard about the successful Harvard experiment by cable from van de Hulst, after viewing the Purcell-Ewen experiment for himself.[173]

Recognizing the priority of van de Hulst in making the prediction, Purcell asked the editors of *Nature* to postpone publication of their experiment until results were in from the University of Leiden and from a similar experiment in Australia. (Purcell had written Joseph Pawsey in Australia about his experiment. Although the Australians at the time were leading experts in radio astronomy, they had not thought of looking for the 21-centimeter radiation. When notified by Purcell about the Harvard experiment, it "didn't take them very long," Purcell said, "to throw together a 21-centimeter receiver for one of their antennas" and to achieve similar results.) Thus it was that all three documents—the Harvard letter from Harold Ewen and Edward Purcell, the Leiden letter from Jan Oort and C.A. Muller, and a cable from Joseph Pawsey in Australia—were published side-by-side in *Nature*.[174-176]

The discovery of the 21-centimeter line opened up intensive study of galactic structure in the years that followed. Within a few years of the Purcell-Ewen discovery, two radio telescopes at the 21-centimeter band were built at Harvard. In Holland, the late Professor Jan Oort, leader of the Dutch 21-centimeter project and renowned the world over as the authority on galactic structure, used the 21-centimeter line to study the galaxy for 40 years.[177]

Oort [Purcell noted] is the grand old man of galactic astrophysics, and right away he saw it as a tool for learning something about the structure of the galaxy. I don't think they recognized perhaps immediately the trick of using the Doppler shift to locate the hydrogen they were looking at, but that came very soon. It was clear that once you could [detect the 21-centimeter line], you could learn a lot.[178]

The Doppler shift phenomenon, mentioned above by Purcell, allows radio astronomers to determine the velocity with which clouds of hydrogen are either approaching the earth or receding from it. Since hydrogen's 21-centimeter line is a very sharp one, emitting radiation at one precise wavelength, any difference in measured wavelength from that standard—either shortening or lengthening—indicates that the hydrogen cloud is either moving toward the earth (resulting in a shorter wavelength) or away from the earth (resulting in a longer wavelength). The amount of change from the standard frequency easily translates into velocity.

In addition, by scanning frequencies around the 21-centimeter line and identifying wavelengths of strong radiation intensity versus wavelengths of weak intensity, scientists are able to determine relative concentrations of atomic interstellar hydrogen.[179]

Recordings from within our own galaxy have shown that hydrogen is concentrated in the spiral arms of the Milky Way. Even more significant, the 21-centimeter line has made it possible to map the location of hydrogen in distant regions of our galaxy as well as in other galaxies where stars are obscured by interstellar dust which blocks visible light but lets hydrogen radio waves pass through.[180]

Work on Negative Absolute Temperatures
Helps Open Door to Maser and Laser

About the time that Purcell became involved with tuning in to radio broadcasts of interstellar hydrogen, he and Robert Pound began investigating the possibility of achieving what was considered to be thermodynamically impossible—negative absolute temperatures. Before long their colleague, Norman Ramsey, also became involved in the intriguing possibility that, under certain rather unique conditions, negative absolute temperatures were indeed physically achievable.

It wasn't the first time that Purcell had questioned the so-called conventional wisdom. As described in more detail in Chapter 2, seven years before Tsung Dao Lee, Chen Ning Yang, Chien-Shiung Wu and others disproved the law of conservation of parity in 1957, for which Lee and Yang were awarded the Nobel Prize the same year, Edward Purcell and Norman Ramsey wrote the first paper questioning the parity assumption and showing the lack of experimental evidence for that assumption.[181]

As described in Chapter 2, the question had come up in the first place because Purcell was going to be sitting in on one of Ramsey's classes on molecular beams in which Ramsey would be providing the standard parity-based proof that nuclei do not have electric dipole moments. To avoid being caught off guard in class by an incisive question from Purcell—specifically, what experimental evidence was there for the existence of parity symmetry in nuclear forces—Ramsey asked Purcell beforehand if he knew of any such evidence. Purcell didn't. As a result of their discussion and subsequent collaboration in a paper on the topic, Ramsey began what would become a 40-year-plus search for the neutron's electric dipole moment, evidence which, if he found it, would disprove the parity assumption. Of course, by 1957, the assumption was proven invalid both theoretically and experimentally, anyway, by the people mentioned above, but by that time Ramsey was intent on finding the electric dipole moment of the neutron for its own sake, if it was there.[182]

The negative absolute temperature question was raised initially in Purcell's mind in response to work done by Robert Pound in the late 1940s in which he discovered nuclear quadrupole resonance in crystals.

I had been thinking a little about the spin temperature [said Purcell] and had just noted with amusement that if I had inverted levels, I could describe it with a negative temperature, that the thermodynamic relation between entropy ds and dq/t was perfectly valid for negative temperature, and that everything would go through formally with no particular trouble. And, in fact, I had started to write it up as a communication for the *American Journal of Physics*, thinking of it purely as kind of an amusing pedagogical point.

Then Bob came up one day with this crystal that had a five-minute relaxation time, the longest spin-lattice relaxation time we'd ever seen. So I said, "Look, Bob, if we've got this, why don't we just do it? Just for fun, let's invert the spins and show that they behave as if they were at negative temperature." So we devised an experiment to do that and it behaved just the way we thought it would. Then people started taking it a little more seriously, and when we began talking about it, we found that it really bothered people. Well, we wrote up our little letter[183] about the spins in the crystal sample and pointed out that it could be said to be at a negative temperature. Some people, especially chemists, were terribly bothered by that—old-line thermodynamicists.[184]

The Purcell-Pound letter to *Physical Review* was soon followed by a Ramsey-Pound letter[185] that discussed performing audiofrequency spectroscopy via resonant heating of the nuclear spin system. Perhaps not much more would have come of the idea for awhile had Norman Ramsey not been scheduled for a sabbatical year several years later at Oxford University and been encouraged to write up a theoretical paper on the topic by Sir Francis Simon.

Simon, earlier known as Franz Simon, was an outstanding Jewish physicist who had exchanged Hitler's Germany in 1933 for Oxford's Clarendon Laboratory through the beneficence of physicist Frederick Lindemann (Lord Cherwell), the laboratory's director. In 1937, his work had been cited by Purcell in his paper on magnetic cooling.[186] In 1940, Simon, who had written to his friend Max Born a few months before the Battle of Britain that he wanted to use his "whole force in the struggle for this country," was able to show his gratitude by devising a method for separating isotopes using "ordinary" gaseous diffusion that was adaptable to mass production. The method later proved useful as part of the overall U235 production program devised by the Manhattan Project.[187]

Simon would also verify experimentally the Third Law of Thermodynamics and, under his leadership, Oxford would become one of the leading low-temperature research centers in the world. (He is probably the only person to hold both the Iron Cross of Imperial Germany and a knighthood of the British Empire.)

Simon had been intrigued by the negative temperature idea from the start, although he had not initially, according to Ramsey, been able to accept its conclusions.[188] Nevertheless, unlike many of his colleagues, Simon was not offended by the idea's novelty. In fact, according to Purcell, "he enjoyed it very much and he kept urging Norman to write it up. So Norman, while he was at Oxford," said Purcell, "started writing up an article on negative temperature,[189] which he published."[190]

In writing this report [said Ramsey], I was surprised to discover that one of the most popular statements of the Second Law of Thermodynamics is incorrect when one recognizes the existence of thermodynamic systems at negative absolute temperatures. I showed how that statement of the Second Law could be modified to be valid at all temperatures. Although most lasers and masers are not in sufficient equilibrium to be properly describable by a temperature, the thermodynamic systems that approximate them are at negative absolute temperatures.[191]

I would regard our introduction of negative temperature as just one of the ideas and papers opening the door on that whole world of masers and lasers [said Purcell]. The idea of the inverted population was, of course, basic to it and that when you had the population inverted, it was an emitter, not an absorber. This whole sort of complex of ideas was knocking around. It was the general idea, I would say, of people thinking about what happens if I have an inverted population so that I have more in the upper state than in the lower state. How does the radiation interact? I have stimulated emission that exceeds the absorption, put it that way. Now, if I make the stimulated emission exceed the absorption and then use it to make itself a bootstrap, I have a laser.[192]

At the time [said Purcell], the negative temperature effect and its demonstration by Pound and myself were considered a curiosity by most physicists, but now there has been a steady growth, I think, in the recognition that that idea and the experiment that exemplified that idea was one of many important steps that led to the laser. It's important that that not get lost in the miscellany of magnetic resonance effects. It is the foundation in some points of view. The actual thermodynamics is complicated and subtle enough so that if anybody tells you that this [negative temperature] equation is the laser, you reject it, but it still is part of it.

There was a period there of just two or three years where things were coming together, including the physics of an inverted population, hyperfine emission and things. It was all sort of getting ready to blow up with the laser when they had more contributions—Townes, of course, and my own colleague, Nico Bloembergen. The door really opened there for a big surge of invention. Norman Ramsey, Pound and me were sitting at the center of one part of that piece of puzzle.[193]

Although Purcell would not become known for masers and lasers, two of his close colleagues at Harvard—Nicolaas Bloembergen and Norman Ramsey—would make major contributions to the field: Bloembergen with his three-level pumping system for a solid-state maser which would later be incorporated into the laser, and Ramsey with an atomic hydrogen maser that would find application, perhaps most notably, in a highly-stable atomic clock. All of which just goes to show what can come of an "amusing pedagogical point."

The Nobel Prize

On December 10, 1952,* exactly 56 years to the day after the death of Alfred Nobel, Edward Purcell, Felix Bloch and the rest of the 1952 Nobel laureates were in Stockholm, Sweden together with members of the Swedish royal family and prime minister, ambassadors from the United States, Great Britain and France.

On that occasion, Professor Hulthén, a member of the Nobel Committee for Physics, traced the development of man's knowledge and use of magnetism from its use in compasses by the ancient Chinese and medieval Norsemen to its first scientific analysis in *De Magnete* by Sir William Gilbert, physician to Queen Elizabeth I in 1600 A.D., to its subsequent classification into ferromagnetics, paramagnetics, diamagnetics and finally, to a new category, nuclear magnetics.

After a further brief review of nuclear magnetism as revealed by the work of Rabi, Gorter, Purcell and Bloch, Hulthén addressed his comments next to Professor Purcell, which are here quoted in full:

Professor Purcell. As far as I have been able to follow your activities since you stopped working at the great Radiation Laboratory at MIT at the end of the War, and up to your development of the excellent method of nuclear resonance absorption for which you have been awarded your Nobel Prize, you have happily realized man's old dream of beating the sword into a plowshare. Your wide experience in electronics and the deep interest you early showed in paramagnetic phenomena may thus conceivably have contributed to the invention of your method, which through its extraordinary sensitiveness gives us a deep insight into the constitution of crystals and fluids, and the interactions, so-called relaxations, between the tiniest particles of matter.

In part with this method, and in part without it, you and your collaborators have made a number of important discoveries, among which I would like particularly to stress the three following:

Your method for studying nuclear magnetic resonance in a weak magnetic field produced according to the solenoid method, which is of great value for the absolute determination of nuclear magnetic moments.

---

* Nobel Prize ceremonies are held on the same date every year, the anniversary of Alfred Nobel's death in 1896.

In the very interesting experiment which you performed together with Dr. Pound, you have produced with paramagnetic resonance the rather unique situation in which the state of the atomic nucleus corresponds to negative temperatures in the absolute-temperature scale.

Finally, as a quite spectacular discovery I may mention your observation with Dr. Ewen in 1951 of a line in the galactic radiospectrum caused by atomic hydrogen, an important contribution to radio astronomy.

Please accept our congratulations, and receive your Nobel Prize from the hands of His Majesty.[194]

In his Nobel lecture, Purcell briefly and eloquently described the effect of the experiment on his own personal appreciation of nature, and then quickly got down to what it all meant scientifically:

Professor Bloch has told you how one can detect the precession of the magnetic nuclei in a drop of water. Commonplace as such experiments have become in our laboratories, I have not yet lost a feeling of wonder, and of delight, that this delicate motion should reside in all the ordinary things around us, revealing itself only to him who looks for it. I remember, in the winter of our first experiments, just seven years ago, looking on snow with new eyes. There the snow lay around my doorstep—great heaps of protons quietly precessing in the earth's magnetic field. To see the world for a moment as something rich and strange is the private reward of many a discovery. But I'm afraid it has little bearing on the sober question we, as physicists, must ask ourselves: What can we learn from all this about the structure of matter?[195]

At a banquet held on the same day as the awards ceremony, Harold Cramer, a member of the Royal Swedish Academy of Sciences, summed up the unique achievements of Purcell and Bloch:

You have opened the road to new insight into the micro-world of nuclear physics. Each atom is like a subtle and refined instrument, playing its own faint, magnetic melody, inaudible to human ears. By your methods, this music has been made perceptible, and the characteristic melody of an atom can be used as an identification signal. This is not only an achievement of high intellectual beauty—

it also places an analytic method of the highest value in the hands of scientists.[196]

Those words were said in 1952. Had the Honorable Harold Cramer been able to look ahead at that moment even a quarter of a century, he would have been amazed at just how much value—chemically with NMR spectroscopy, medically with NMR scanning and imaging, and in many other areas of technology, such as masers and lasers—the Purcell-Bloch NMR achievements would engender.

Science Advisor to Presidents

As one who had served his country well as the winds of war in Europe became the global conflagration of World War II, Edward Purcell was a natural candidate for re-enlistment as those winds changed direction and became the icy blasts of the Cold War. From approximately 1950 to 1970, he was frequently called upon as a technical consultant and active participant in government-sponsored projects. "Those of us who were involved in these projects," said Purcell, "were ones who had been more or less continually involved since World War II in military technology and things like that. So it was natural for us to keep in the game."[197]

Almost immediately after the war, Purcell was pressed into service by Lee DuBridge, the director of the Rad Lab, to help in setting up a science advisory board for the U.S. Air Force. "That was my initiation into the government advising activities that took a good deal of my time in later years," said Purcell, "I was a member of the Air Force Science Advisory Board for quite a long time."[198] Led by the famous fluid dynamicist, Theodor von Karman, one of the early tasks of the board was to help the Air Force prepare for the future by trying to predict what that future might hold from a scientific and technological perspective.

Purcell attributed this close working relationship between the military and the scientific community to the rapport and confidence that had been built during the war years.

The scientific people evolved during World War II entirely new relationships with military people, one of mutual confidence and understanding of the problems and working together, so that the Radiation Lab finally put itself in a very strong position with respect to scientific undertakings with the military for military purposes. It wouldn't do anything just on order. It had to know the whole purpose and would attack the problem in the large but insisted on being in on that whole. The British had developed in the same way, in complete contrast to what happened in Germany, where the scientists were never really trusted by the military or the government at all.[199]

In 1950, Purcell was recruited by his friend and colleague from Radiation Lab days, Jerrold Zacharias, to participate in the Hartwell Project. Once again, submarines—not German U-boats, but rather Soviet snorkeling submarines—were posing a threat. The purpose of the Hartwell Project, a Navy program, was to recommend an appropriate anti-submarine response.[200]

Soon afterward, the State Department enlisted Purcell's help in combating the Soviets in the intensifying war of propaganda. Voice of America radio broadcasts were being jammed behind the Iron Curtain, and Purcell was put in charge of the technical section, organized at MIT, whose goal it was either to prevent the jamming or to broadcast through it. They failed to invent an effective remedy.

Also in 1952, Professor Purcell became involved in the Beacon Hill Project. A technical study of the possibilities of photographic reconnaissance, its conclusions became the basis for much of the development of such reconnaissance in the years that followed, both by airplanes and later by satellites, and marked the beginning of extensive work in that area by Purcell.[201]

In 1954, two years after receiving the Nobel Prize in physics, Dr. Purcell became involved in a broad-based assessment of the United States defense posture, headed up by Dr. James Killian. Then president of Massachusetts Institute of Technology, Killian had taken a leave of absence to chair the secret commission at the request of President Eisenhower who, along with other government and military leaders, had become concerned about the danger of a surprise attack. The concern was more than post-Pearl Harbor syndrome. According to author Michael Beschloss, a top-secret report by analysts at the Rand Corporation in California had warned that a preemptive Soviet strike could eliminate up to 85 percent of the Strategic Air Command's bombers. Wrote Beschloss:

> By September 1954, [Killian] had assembled 46 experts and staff in the gray 19th-century splendor of the Executive Office Building next to the White House. The Technological Capabilities Panel (or Killian Commission, as members soon called themselves) worked fast and hard, for the President wanted a report on his desk by

February. Except for field trips to the CIA, Pentagon, SAC and elsewhere, members worked behind locked doors manned by Air Force guards. . . . The most secret unit was the intelligence panel chaired by Edwin Land.[202]

Edward Purcell was assigned to the intelligence panel headed by Land, a role in which he soon had contact with President Eisenhower who, unlike some of his successors, valued the input of the scientific community.

Killian had extremely good relations with Eisenhower [said Purcell]. In fact, a number of the people knew Eisenhower and were trusted by him. We had direct access to the President on any really important matter when decisions had to be made. There was no holding back.[203]

Already during this period, one could see hints, according to Purcell, of the hawk-dove split that would become more obvious a decade later, and perhaps, if one reads between the lines, even the basis for Eisenhower's parting expression of concern about the dangers of the military-industrial complex:

You could see the shadow of things ahead in some controversies at that time. I think particularly of the question of the ANP, nuclear propelled aircraft . . . the military in the nuclear industry were very determined to make an airplane that was nuclear powered, and every scientific study of the thing showed that it was a bad idea. And yet it couldn't be killed. You could never kill the thing because G.E. or somebody would always revive it. So for about 10 years the nuclear-powered aircraft was a project which most of us thought was stupid but couldn't stop. . . . This ridiculous object would have flown at subsonic speed and would have been a sitting duck and was not good for anything.[204]

President Eisenhower in his memoirs, *The White House Years: Waging Peace, 1956-1961,* wrote of the Killian Commission:

In February of 1955 a . . . scientific committee, headed by Dr. James R. Killian, recommended that we develop, along with the ICBM, an intermediate-range ballistic missile (IRBM) with a range of fifteen hundred miles. By the summer of 1955 the Air Force research and development ICBM program had been given the highest priority, and by December we concluded it wise to assign highest priority to programs for two ICBMs, Atlas and Titan, and two IRBMs, Jupiter and Thor. To these programs we devoted all the resources that they could usefully absorb at any given time.[205]

It was out of the Killian Commission that the President's Science Advisory Committee (PSAC) was formed. Although a Science Advisory Committee had existed under the Office of Defense Mobilization for some time, in late 1957 it was the orbiting beep-beep of a Soviet satellite called Sputnik that got the attention of the president.

There were two problems created by the Soviet Sputnik, [wrote Eisenhower]. The first, a short-term one, was to find ways of affording perspective to our people and so relieve the current wave of near-hysteria; the second, to take all feasible measures to accelerate missile and satellite programs. To discuss these matters I asked the members of the Science Advisory Committee of the Office of Defense Mobilization, a group of distinguished scientists, to meet with me. As the group gathered in mid-October, I said that I had invited them in order to learn what ideas and proposals they might like to advance. . . . Dr. Isidor Rabi, of Columbia University, was the first to reply.[206]

As the chairman of the Committee, Rabi told the president that although the United States still enjoyed a number of advantages over the Soviets, it was possible that "unless we take vigorous action, they could pass us swiftly." Rabi's suggestion to Eisenhower was to abolish the Committee as it was currently organized, name a new committee responsible directly to the president, and appoint a full-time scientific advisor to the White House staff. To facilitate his suggestion for a full-time scientific advisor, a role he was unwilling to take, Rabi said he would resign as chairman of the existing committee.[207] In November, Eisenhower followed Rabi's suggestion:

As spurs to action [wrote Eisenhower], I announced a number of specific decisions, among them: I was appointing Dr. James R. Killian, president of the Massachusetts Institute of Technology, as Special Assistant to the President for Science and Technology, a new post. He would be aided by a staff of scientists and by an advisory group—the existing Science Advisory Committee of the Office of Defense Mobilization, now enlarged, reorganized, and elevated to the White House.[208]

Both Rabi and Purcell were appointed as members of the new committee. It was a role that Purcell would fill with clarity and thoughtful insight for two non-consecutive terms under three presidents—Eisenhower, Kennedy and Johnson. As James Killian has written: "[Edward Purcell] did not speak often, but when he did, there would be enormous silence in the room because everybody knew that whatever he said was going to be worth listening to with careful attention."[209]

In the period immediately following Sputnik, it was an open question as to whether the development of space technology should be solely the province of the military or placed under a new or revised government agency. In the end, it was decided to expand the existing National Advisory Committee for Aeronautics, renaming it National Aeronautics and Space Administration (NASA).

One of the influencing factors in opening space up to the broad-based interests of science was a booklet called the *Space Primer*. Written by Edward Purcell of Harvard and Edwin Land of Polaroid along with Frank Bello of *Fortune* magazine, and issued by President Eisenhower, its purpose was to educate as many as possible about the exciting prospects of space exploration, a purpose it fulfilled admirably. "I think our little *Space Primer* really stands up very well," Purcell said. "We talked about eventually going to the moon. Our timetable wasn't too far off, although it was a little more expensive than what we said. We talked about weather satellites and what that might do and a number of things like that, which have all come true."[210]

The education process was not meant just to inform the American public, said Purcell, but people in responsible positions in Washington as well.

Herb York and I had a little talk that we prepared that we gave jointly, equipped with some charts for the easel and so on, and we went around Washington giving this little tutorial lecture on space. We gave it twice in the Cabinet Room, once to the President and the Cabinet and once to the President and the Security Council. Eisenhower is one of the people I've given the same lecture to twice.[211]

How did they respond? "Like good students," said Purcell. "Each was interested in his own way. I recall that the chairman of the Security Council at the time was a fellow named Bobby Cutler,* who kept insisting that we give him a legal definition of outer space. It was clear that we were heading into a time when the notion of what a country had jurisdiction over would be very difficult to deal with."[212]

How difficult was made clear even before the end of the Eisenhower administration with the downing of the U-2 and Francis Gary Powers by the Soviet Union. From as early as the Beacon Hill Project in 1952, Purcell had been involved with the development of photo reconnaissance from aircraft. With the advent of space exploration and satellite reconnaissance, the question of who owned space intensified, although the problem was eventually resolved, "more or less," said Purcell, by "simply going ahead and making the assumption that space was open to all."[213]

The polarization in the physics community that began in 1954 with the Oppenheimer case and which continued with the question of arms limitations throughout the Eisenhower and Kennedy years reached its peak with the Vietnam War under Johnson and Nixon. Although Purcell's second term as a presidential science advisor came to an end in 1965, he continued to serve on a technical panel concerned with reconnaissance—until the bombing of Laos.

> I didn't sever all my connections with PSAC [Purcell said] until the middle of the Vietnam War when I finally wrote a letter just resigning flatly from everything. I'm ashamed to say how late it was. I think it wasn't until maybe the bombing of Laos, and then I just withdrew from all government connections. Anything connected with the White House I resigned from.[214]

Post-Nobel Prize Research

In between his frequent trips to Washington throughout the 1950s and '60s, Purcell continued with his teaching and personal interests in research. Because of these demands as well as his own "style," he "kind of slipped," he said, "into the role of not taking graduate students. I guess

---

* Robert Cutler, an Army general and a Boston trust-company executive, was Eisenhower's Special Assistant for National Security Affairs, the same position held by McGeorge Bundy in the Kennedy administration.

the reason is that after a long period with NMR stuff, I just didn't have any new ideas I wanted to work on . . . so I was dabbling in different things in an opportunistic way."[215]

A cursory scan of Purcell's bibliography after 1951 reveals that "NMR stuff" continued to occupy the research Purcell was able to conduct in the 1950s. Following a one-and-a-half year intermission in the early 1960s at Brookhaven National Laboratory in which he searched in vain for magnetic monopoles, Purcell's research began to be directed into two broad categories: 1) astrophysics of interstellar dust and gas, and 2) biophysics of bacterial motion.

The Search for the Elusive, Perhaps Nonexistent, Monopole—Deep in the heart of a mountain in the Italian Alps, a massive, football-field sized instrument waits in readiness. The sole purpose for its mega-lira existence is to welcome, after mega-light years of non-interrupted travel, a heavenly intruder known as a magnetic monopole. The solid limestone of the mountain is intended to serve as a sort of cosmic filter, to keep out the less energetic rays that bombard the mountain and to allow only the precious monopoles through—if they exist. If they do exist, they must be remnants of the Big Bang and only the Big Bang as nothing else could have created the massive explosion needed to create such entities. The detector is still waiting.

Three decades earlier, Edward Purcell waited for a more than a year at Brookhaven National Laboratory for the same thing. Compared to the Italian detector, the device he and his associates assembled to catch monopoles was very small, an ultra-light fly fishing rod, so to speak, compared to a multi-acre tuna net that requires a massive electric winch to bring aboard. Purcell didn't catch any monopoles, either. Either they weren't biting or they weren't there.

To add to the challenge of monopole fishing, it's difficult enough to imagine a magnetic monopole, much less catch one. From experience, we can only relate to magnetic dipoles, magnets with two poles, a north and a south. Any normal attempt to divide a dipole into a monopole would be futile, as Purcell points out:

If you have a magnet, you can't cut off one pole. It's almost like saying, 'Look, hand me the end of a piece of string. Well, I cut the string, and it makes two ends. If I cut it again, it makes two more ends. So the question is, Can I have a piece of string that has only one end? And the answer is no, at least the answer that theory gives.[216]

To a fisherman, it's fun to spend hours and days lying in wait for the big one that hasn't been enticed by anyone else's bait. To a physicist like Purcell, it's hard to imagine anything more fun than trying to catch something that may or may not exist. So what would you do with a monopole if you ever caught one? Purcell has a ready answer for that question.

Had we found a monopole, then the question would have been immediately, Where was it made? What was it made of? But since we didn't find any, that became in the classic phrase, academic. They still have not been found. At this point, the theoreticians aren't sure whether they ought to be there or not.[217]

It was theoretician, Paul A.M. Dirac, who, in 1948, provided the hypothesis for the existence of monopoles.[218] If they did exist, Dirac suggested, they were probably created in pairs in very energetic processes— hence the Big Bang connection as hypothesized by present-day believers in the monopole.

In the paper in which he published the negative result of his Brookhaven experiment, Purcell agreed that, based on the law of charge conservation, monopoles were probably created in pairs. On the same premise, Purcell believed that—and this is very important if you are the one looking for them—once separated from its partner, "an isolated pole cannot vanish. Given the manifest scarcity, not to say absence, of monopoles in ordinary matter," continued Purcell, "this promises practically unlimited life to any monopole once it has been macroscopically separated from its partner in creation."[219]

Other scientists were also challenged at the time by the possibility of the monopole and searched for them experimentally. One of them, W.V.R. Malkus[220] looked for monopoles as early as 1951 in the earth's atmosphere, but had found nothing.

Later several teams turned to the big guns, the alternating-gradient synchrotrons at CERN and Brookhaven National Laboratory. Purcell went to Brookhaven to conduct his search. Working with four collaborators from that Long Island laboratory, along with others from the BNL staff, and using 30-GeV-accelerated protons, Purcell worked on his experiment between 1960 and 1962, one of a number of high-energy experiments that were taking place at the same time at Brookhaven.

In a long, straight section of the accelerator, an evacuated box with an 8-inch inside dimension was targeted for a high-energy proton-nucleon interaction. If a successful hit resulted in the creation of monopoles, they expected these "sample" monopoles to have a mass, more than 2.4 BeV. (See Figure 2.)

To catch a fraction of these monopoles, they mounted in the top of the box a 3-foot round column, sealed at the bottom and containing pump oil to a depth of about 11 inches. The oil was there for two reasons: 1) They knew that the thin aluminum wall of the trap was "too thin to stop such energetic monopoles," and 2) it was to serve as a target "for possible electromagnetic production of monopole pairs by the energetic photons which traverse the well."[221]

The remainder of the vertical column was an evacuated solenoid that served to attract to the surface of the oil any trapped monopoles (which happened to be of the right sign), to accelerate them upward, and to focus them for detection just beyond the upper end of the column, which was sealed with Mylar. If their calculations were correct, they expected such a monopole to arrive at the detector with a kinetic energy of 1.1 BeV. Two methods of detection were tried: 1) "a xenon scintillator consisting of a quartz tube filled with pure xenon and viewed by two photomultipliers," and 2) nuclear emulsions.

Nothing in the way of magnetic monopoles was picked up by either detector. In the case of the emulsion detector, reported Purcell, "No monopole-like track was found." Although neither the CERN nor the Brookhaven teams found any monopoles, they were able to establish upper limits for future searches, and Purcell was comforted by his confidence that "only under two sets of conditions, both believed to be unlikely, would monopoles created in our experiment have been systematically missed."[222] As Anatole Abragam summarized the attempt:

> [Purcell] thought up some extremely ingenious methods for detecting magnetic monopoles, should they exist and be produced in particle accelerators, and he spent a couple of years lying in wait for them at Brookhaven. Unfortunately the monopoles did not show up: the best hunter comes home with an empty bag if the game is not there.[223]

Interstellar Dust—For the writer of this book, one of its more enjoyable aspects was the opportunity to be personally taught by Professor Edward Purcell on the two areas of research that have occupied most of his attention during the past 30 years: the astrophysics associated with interstellar dust and the biophysics associated with bacterial locomotion. The major paper for the first was jointly published by Professor Purcell of Harvard

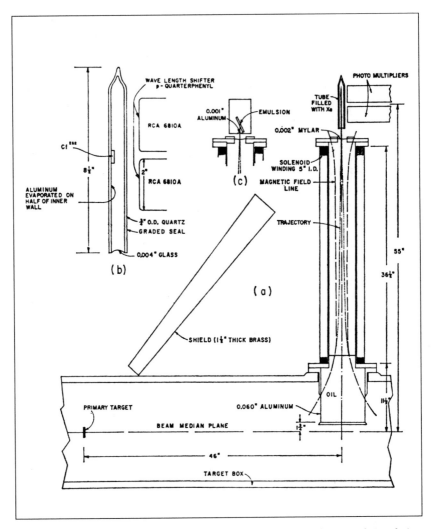

(a) Elevation view of apparatus showing focusing solenoid and oil receptacle in relation to the target and target box of the Alternating Gradient Synchrotron (AGS). (b) Details of counter arrangement. (c) Upper end of focusing solenoid showing the positioning of the emulsions.

Figure 2. Cross-Sectional View of Apparatus Used by
Purcell and Collaborators in Searching for the Dirac
Monopole at Brookhaven National Laboratory (1960-62)

and Professor Lyman Spitzer of Princeton. A widely known paper of Purcell's for the second is entitled 'Life at Low Reynolds Number,' and follows the lead of Harvard biophysicist Howard C. Berg who discovered that a bacterium swims by rotating (rather than waving) its flagellum.

Briefly and off-the-cuff, Professor Purcell described the dusty universe that has captured his attention for so long:

The dust grains and the bacteria that I'm going to talk about are both very small, about the same size, in fact, about one micron in diameter or the size of a particle in cigarette smoke. Here's what we know about the interstellar dust. Interstellar means between the stars in our galaxy. The dust is there, about one grain of dust to two cubic miles of space, and yet its area is enough to eventually stop any starlight that tries to go through it over a galactic distance of 10 light years.

It has the following effects. The first effect it has is to absorb sunlight. The light that comes through the galaxy has been filtered by having to pass this dust. The dust is black and it absorbs some of the light, and that's why we cannot really see the galaxy from our position. If we could see the galaxy, it would be a splendid sight, not dimmed or obscured at all by the dust, but there's enough dust there so that we can't even see to the edge of the galaxy in most places.

We now know what the dust is chemically and how it got condensed, and it's pretty certain what its size is. Lots of people were involved, including myself, in solving that problem.

Now the dust has one other property which is most remarkable, but seldom commented on. The dust makes interstellar chemistry run. The chemical reaction of two atoms coming together in space and forming a molecule is what I would call interstellar chemistry. Upwards of a hundred such different molecules have now been found, usually detected by their resonant absorption, which was the way in which Harold I. Ewin and I first detected the hydrogen emission in space.

The way that the dust works is to catalyze. One important reaction, the simplest reaction there is in space, occurs when two hydrogen atoms meet and form a molecule of hydrogen. That starts the whole chain of chemical reactions leading up eventually to alcohol and anything you want that's an organic molecule in space. The great important point about that is that no other reaction can be catalyzed that way and there's no other way to catalyze the H plus H to get H_2. The dust grain absorbs light and the molecule wants to emit. And when it does emit, it becomes a non-energetic molecule. It's just sitting there until something else comes along and hits it. And there's so little gas in space that if you're a molecule out there waiting to be hit by an atom or if you're an atom waiting to be hit by another atom, you've got to wait about two or three hundred years.

It's mind-boggling from any astrophysical point of view. An atom of interstellar gas travels in a straight line at constant speed just as Newton said it would if you didn't hit it, and it travels for something like 10 light years or more and takes about 50 years to cross the sun's orbit. So that's why astronomers are interested in interstellar dust.

Now it's not a prepossessing object. If you took all of the dust there is in the galaxy and scrunched it down into a ball, what you would have in your hand would be well-described as a dirty snowball. First of all, it's mostly ice and mostly hydrogen, but there's that third item in it which makes it a catalyst. It's like the catalyst in your car's exhaust system. It runs by surface reaction.[224]

Beginning with a 1969 article in *Physica* describing the alignment of interstellar dust and ending with a 1979 article on suprathermal rotation of interstellar grains, Purcell published eight articles shedding extensive light on these light-absorbers. "Somehow, I got hooked on interstellar dust," he said. One of the surprising facts revealed by Purcell's study is that interstellar grains must be rotating at high spead, millions of revolutions per minute.

It's interesting to note that, although interstellar dust is opaque to light, it is transparent to radio waves and thus offered no hindrance to radio astronomy and the 21-cm hydrogen radiation Purcell and Ewen had detected about two-and-a-half decades earlier.

Bacterial Locomotion—In describing his work in the physics of diffusion and bacterial propulsion, it became clear why Professor Purcell is such an effective teacher. In the process of communicating various physical concepts, he constantly uses analogies and common materials to make his point. As a teacher, he places the major responsibility for effective communication on himself, the transmitter, and less on the receiver. When the writer sought to clarify a point, for example, Purcell saw the shortcoming to be his rather than that of the student, although such a conclusion was not necessarily warranted. "I see one or two places from what you said where I could have done better," he said during the phone conversation. "So don't hang up until I try that on you because I think I can make you a low Reynolds number physicist."[225]

The reference to "low Reynolds number" came, of course, from the major paper published by Purcell in which he provided the theoretical physics that enables *Escherichia coli (E. coli)* to get from Point A to Point B, and why. Because the paper is actually an edited transcription of a talk given in 1976 by Purcell in honor of his friend and colleague, Victor Weisskopf,* it retains the warm-hearted camaraderie that accompanied the occasion.

The Reynolds number is a ratio introduced by Osborne Reynolds, an English engineer from the 19th century who correlated the viscosity and density of fluids. In a fluid with a low Reynolds number, viscous forces dominate over inertial forces, and in fluids with very low Reynolds numbers, the effect of inertia becomes largely non-existent. To comprehend such an environment, which is typical for bacteria living within our bodies, Purcell asked the audience to "imagine under what conditions a man would be swimming at, say, the same Reynolds number as his own sperm."

> Well, you put him in a swimming pool that is full of molasses, and then you forbid him to move any part of his body faster than 1 centimeter per minute. Now imagine yourself in that condition: you're in the swimming pool in molasses, and now you can only move like the hands of a clock. If under those ground rules you are able to move a few meters in a couple of weeks, you may qualify as a low Reynolds number swimmer.[226]

(Given the choice, the writer prefers becoming a low Reynolds number physicist to a low Reynolds number swimmer.)

---

*Weisskopf expressed his appreciation in his autobiographical book, *The Joy of Insight*, for the interest that Purcell shared with him of "trying to explain things in the best possible way" to people with no scientific training. "Richard Feynman," wrote Weisskopf, "would have been ready to discuss such problems any time I wanted to, but he lived far away in Pasadena. I was lucky, therefore, to have Edward Purcell nearby at Harvard. Ed was one of the few people who understood and valued such endeavors. He helped me enormously in clearing up vexing points and ambiguities. I always benefited from my talks with him about any kind of problem of that sort. Our approach to physics is very similar, although he is an experimental physicist and I am a theorist, so it was a pleasure to work with him."
—Victor Weisskopf, *The Joy of Insight: Passions of a Physicist*, (New York: Basic Books, 1991), 160-161, 270.

With this basic premise of life at low Reynolds number in mind, Purcell proceeds to analyze methods of propulsion and their relative effectiveness in such an environment. He points out, for example, that swimming in water, which is about as low in viscosity as a liquid gets, will work by reciprocal motion. By changing one's body into a particular shape and then reversing the action, one is propelled forward. Not so at low Reynold's number. In such an environment, he states, "Time . . . makes no difference—only configuration." Which is why Howard Berg's discovery that *E. coli* bacteria move by rotating their corkscrew-shaped flagella rather than waving them is so significant. Reciprocal motion, the type used in waving, is ineffective at low Reynolds number. A helical-shaped twisting motion, such as that provided by the bacteria's flagella is, however, another matter and, in 1973, Berg hypothesized, contrary to accepted belief, that this was indeed the method that the humble *E. coli* uses to get from Point A to Point B. Within a year, it was confirmed experimentally. In "Life at Low Reynolds Number," Purcell provides the physics.

Related to NMR relaxation rates is another topic that Purcell raises in the paper: diffusion. In describing the process, he used ammonia as an example.

> Most people think [said Purcell]—and I've seen biologists make this mistake in textbooks—that smells are some kind of molecule in a gas and smells travel very rapidly. That's their idea. So if I open a bottle of, let's say ammonia, over in a corner of the room and I'm 10 feet away, that smell of ammonia will quickly spread through the room. Not at all. The answer is it will not spread through the room. It will take an extraordinarily long time to spread even a foot.[227]

"If that doesn't seem surprising to you, then I haven't explained it very well," he told the writer, ever mindful as the teacher of how the communication process was coming along. To make sure comprehension was occurring, he gave another example.

> If you take all the cars in the parking lot and turned them on and let them run at 20 miles an hour, they won't go 20 miles the first hour. They'll just reduce themselves to junk. That's the real point. It isn't the speed we're talking about. As soon as we talk about speed and miles per hour or centimeters per second and so on, we've left the real hindrance out of it. That's why we call it diffusion. Diffusion is blind progress by random walking. That's the heart of it.[228]

It also explained why Professor Purcell received the Oersted Medal for excellence in teaching.

Purcell's Contributions to NMR Spectroscopy and Scanning

Long journeys begin with first steps. Standing on the shoulders of others who had accomplished other prerequisite steps, perhaps most notably Professor I.I. Rabi, *et al.* of Columbia, and drawing from his own experience with water absorption in the ill-fated 1.25-centimeter radar program at the Radiation Laboratory, Edward Purcell was the first to induce atomic nuclei within condensed matter to identify themselves by emitting their unique NMR signal to a listening receiver. On the basis of that experiment as well as his subsequent research in NMR, he became a vital contributor to the revolution in chemical analysis that took place in the 1960s.

Relaxation Studies—Significant early on was Purcell's decision to focus on the relaxation times of various substances. As Bloch points out, the initial Purcell and Bloch experiments had "merely confirmed the value of the magnetic moment, known from magnetic resonance in a molecular beam," but until T_1 was found to be about 3 seconds in water, said Bloch, "not even the order of magnitude of the relaxation time had been surmised."[229] Making NMR useful and practical, in other words, required following the path of discovery to its next destination, to determine relaxation times of various substances and to understand what causes them to vary.

Actually, as was pointed out in what is said to be one of the most quoted physics papers ever—known as BPP for Bloembergen, Purcell, and Pound—the study began as a "more or less cursory survey of typical substances and grew, as the theoretical interpretation of the results progressed, into a systematic study of certain types of structures which form the basis for a comprehensive theory of nuclear magnetic relaxation applicable to liquids, some gases, and certain types of solids."[230]

So while Bloch concentrated primarily on determining the magnetic moments of various atomic nuclei, Purcell and his associates studied the details of relaxation, determining the relaxation times of water in its various states, as well as in other liquids, gases and crystals. One finding of particular importance, discovered by Bloembergen, was that as the viscosity of liquids was lowered, T_1 relaxation times increased, with T_1 varying, for example, from 3.5 seconds for low-viscosity petroleum ether to .0013 seconds for highly-viscous heavy machine oil.[231]

The Purcell team attributed these differences and the resultant spectro-scopic line narrowing to the important and "dominant" role that molec-ular motion played in nuclear spin relaxation. "After that was cleared up," said Purcell, "then one understood the physics of spin relaxation and understood why we were getting lines that were really very narrow, which of course eventually became very narrow indeed when the high resolution NMR came in" [spearheaded by Bloch].[232]

"It is because of this motional narrowing [discovered by the Purcell team]," wrote Felix Bloch years later, "that liquid samples offer distinct advantages when high resolution is important."[233]

Chemical Shift Theory—Coincident with the improvements in resolu-tion and playing a vital role in its own right in the NMR spectroscopy revolution was the chemical shift phenomenon. The phenomenon was explained from a theoretical standpoint by Norman Ramsey even before confirmation from condensed matter studies appeared. On the basis of what he had learned from molecular-beam radiofrequency spectroscopy, Ramsey theorized that different chemical bonds cause protons to shift resonance frequencies because of the unique shielding effect produced by a molecule's electrons, or as Edward Purcell explained it in his 1952 Nobel lecture:

> The magnetic field at an atomic nucleus differs slightly from the field externally applied because of the shielding effect of the electron cloud around the nucleus. In different molecules the atom's electron configuration will differ slightly, reflecting differences in the chemi-cal bond. The resulting resonance shifts have been called 'chemical shifts.' They are only a nuisance to the experimenter interested in exact ratios of magnetic moments. But they are interesting to the physical chemist because they reveal something about the electrons that partake in the chemical bond.[234]

The most famous example of this phenomenon, also mentioned by Purcell in his Nobel lecture, was discovered by Arnold, Dharmatti and Packard in 1951[235] from their radiospectral analysis of ethyl alcohol. Although the protons making up the molecule are all chemically equiv-alent and, if isolated, would resonate at the same frequency, instead, because of their unique chemical bonds, each of the three groups of protons making up the molecule resonates at slightly different fre-quencies, producing three spectral lines, each shifted from "normal," thus producing a spectral line combination that serves as ethyl alcohol's "fingerprint."

Other experimental evidence of chemical shifts appeared as early as 1949. In an abstract published that year,[236] Nicolaas Bloembergen noted that in $CuSO_4 \cdot 5H_2O$, the constant magnetic field at the position of each proton was shifted in accordance with the relative positions of the hydrogen and copper atoms and that this shift increased with decreasing temperature. Later the same year, Knight[237] reported that resonance frequencies for certain nuclei shifted by several tenths of a percent in a metallic state compared to their frequencies when in the form of powdered or dissolved salts. Ramsey's theories on chemical shifts, published between 1949 and 1952,[238] would account for several types of these phenomena.

Another paper would be developed regarding chemical shifts in collaboration with Edward Purcell. In 1952, the same year Purcell received his Nobel Prize, Purcell and Ramsey provided the theoretical explanation[239] for a special kind of chemical shift that had been discovered experimentally a year earlier by H. Gutowsky, McCall, C. Slichter and McNeil[240] at the University of Illinois and by Erwin Hahn and D.E. Maxwell[241] at Stanford. Not accounted for by any previously known interaction, the Harvard collaborators attributed the shift to an electron-coupled nuclear spin-spin interaction. The nucleus, they said, was interacting magnetically with the electron spin of its own atom. Subsequent experiments confirmed their hypothesis.

Spin Echo Refinements—Purcell, in collaboration with Herman Y. Carr, would also make an important contribution to the field of NMR spectroscopy by offering in 1954 a variation to the spin echo method first given by Erwin Hahn in 1949.[242]

Hahn and Purcell first met each other in 1947, while Hahn was still a graduate student at the University of Illinois. After working initially on the betatron and becoming disillusioned with spending all his time building power supplies for that large-scale project, Hahn decided he was more interested in "small-table science." Professor Bartlett at Urbana suggested he read what had been published on NMR by Purcell and Bloch and, before long, Hahn had built his own version of the Purcell-Torrey-Pound bridge-circuit apparatus.

It was fortuitous for Hahn that F. Wheeler Loomis was the chairman of the department of physics at Illinois. Formerly at the MIT Radiation Lab, Loomis knew Purcell well from the war-time period and he arranged the financing for Hahn to visit Purcell and Pound at Harvard. (By then,

Bloembergen had returned to Holland to complete his thesis and to work with Cornelis Gorter.)

Hahn was inspired and helped immensely by his visit to Cambridge. "Purcell was very nice to me," he told the author recently:

> I remember Purcell sat down with me and I asked him a few questions, and he made a few sketches for me. He was very kind to me. Here I was a lowly flunkie from graduate school. Pound showed me around. He showed me his permanent-magnet quadrupole work, and so forth. They were both very good to me, partly because Loomis had written to them, and they knew Loomis. Loomis was of course their [personnel] director during the war. Loomis having sponsored me, they treated me very well. So it was very good. It got me catapulted.[243]

After comparing notes with Purcell and Pound, Hahn went back to Illinois and soon had his bridge-circuit tuned and functioning. Less than two years later, he discovered spin echoes, which he quickly told Purcell about by mail. In the months that followed, the two of them would keep up a running conversation by mail on spin echoes and other NMR-related topics. (Both men have copies of their handwritten discourses during that period).

Hahn's spin echoes would have a dramatic impact on both NMR spectroscopy and scanning. The method he used for measuring transverse (T_2) relaxation rates, however, was often severely compromised by molecular diffusion throughout the inhomogeneous external field. In 1954, Purcell and one of his graduate students, Herman Carr (now Professor Carr at Rutgers University) found a way to circumvent the diffusion effect by devising a more convenient variant of Hahn's spin echoes. Employing a combination of 90-degree and 180-degree pulses instead of the equal pulse widths employed by Hahn, Purcell and Carr were able to greatly simplify the process and to interpret the observed data.

The 1954 Purcell-Carr paper[244] was also foundational to the MR imaging idea espoused two decades later by Paul Lauterbur of superimposing a magnetic field gradient onto the main homogeneous magnetic field. Very early in this regard was Robert Gabillard of Paris, France who, in 1951, described the effect of a field gradient on an NMR signal.[245]

As Herman Carr has pointed out, however, also influential in this regard was Erwin Hahn's 1950 paper on spin echoes. As a result of the diffusion effects observed by Hahn in his original spin-echo paper, Purcell and Carr were motivated to superimpose a strong magnetic field gradient onto the main magnetic field. It was this technique, in fact, which enabled them to circumvent the diffusion effects that had troubled Hahn.

> Based on this clue [wrote Carr], Edward M. Purcell and I intentionally superimposed a strong magnetic field gradient onto the main field, giving a linear dependence of the resonant frequency on the spatial position of the diffusing nucleus. The enhanced diffusion effect then enabled us to make accurate quantitative measurements of the self-diffusion coefficient for suitable fluids.[246]

This was not the only NMR imaging precursor that came out of Purcell's Harvard laboratories. Two years before the above paper was published, Carr described a one-dimensional phantom in his PhD thesis under Purcell's tutelage:

> It was constructed [Carr wrote] to produce an NMR response similar to the newly discovered chemical shift in ethyl alcohol. I used the imaging concept, with its superimposed gradient and Fourier transformations, to relate the one-dimensional frequency-encoded spatial structure of the phantom to the NMR response in the time domain. Similar one-dimensional phantoms are currently used in MRI textbooks to introduce the imaging concept.[247]

NMR Scanning and Imaging—By the early 1950s, the prerequisite groundwork was sufficiently complete so that the *raison d'être* upon which MR scanning would be built—tissue differentiation on the basis of T_1 and T_2 values—could follow.

In fact, Purcell, in writing the foreword to a two-volume textbook on MRI, suggested that if two essential ingredients had been present as early as 1950, the transition to MR scanning and imaging could have taken place immediately.

> By 1950, plus or minus a year or two, the basic physics that underlies NMR imaging was for practical purposes completely understood. That includes: the magnetic dipole moments and electric quadrupole moments of relevant nuclei; the relaxation times T_1 and T_2 and their dependence on molecular viscosity; the dynamic behavior of spins of all sorts in oscillating fields, both continuous and pulsed; the chemical shifts that were soon to open up an immense

field of application in organic chemistry. No physicist working with NMR at that time would have been surprised to see a proton resonance with a mouse, or a human finger, in the coil. Its amplitude, as in the case of any other largely aqueous substance, would have been quite predictable. Yet with all this knowledge ready to apply, the realization of medically useful NMR images lay more than 20 years in the future. What essential ingredients were lacking?[248]

Two ingredients were lacking in 1950, he continues, the computer power needed to process the signals and, most important, the idea itself "that a useful interior image was in principle obtainable, and was a goal worth pursuing." For that, he said, Raymond Damadian, Paul Lauterbur and Peter Mansfield deserve "enormous credit."[249]

As alluded to above by Purcell, the idea of looking for a proton signal from biological tissue was not beyond the imagination of NMR physicists as early as 1950. In fact, Purcell, Ramsey, and Bloch all looked for such a signal, as E. Raymond Andrew, an important contributor to the science of NMR who worked as a postdoctoral fellow with Purcell in 1948, has described:

> Soon after the first successful NMR experiments at Stanford, Bloch obtained a strong proton NMR signal when he inserted his finger into the rf coil of his spectrometer. In 1948 Purcell and Ramsey, in turn, inserted their heads into the 2 Tesla field of the Harvard cyclotron; around their heads was a coil connected to a powerful rf generator tuned to the proton NMR frequency. The only sensation recorded was that of the EMFs generated in the metal fillings of their teeth as their heads were moved into and out of the magnet, and detected by their tongues. It is noteworthy that 40 years later [Andrews wrote in the late 1980s] there is no evidence of injury or damage arising from this magnetic adventure by these distinguished physicists.[250]

Idea upon idea, like a photograph awash in a basin of developer, the image in magnetic resonance imaging began to emerge.

First came the idea foundational to magnetic resonance scanning—the understanding that not all tissue emits the same NMR signal. Since tissues vary because of water content, viscosity and interaction with neighboring tissue, each sampled volume, like so many samples of water, emit signals that make it possible to differentiate them from their neighbors. The premise came directly from the T_1 and T_2 data accumulated by Bloembergen, Purcell and Pound. The idea for extending the concept to use it as a method for differentiating between tissue for the purpose of medical diagnosis came from Dr. Raymond Damadian, a medical researcher affiliated with Downstate Medical Center in Brooklyn, New York.

One of the first documents in which Damadian mentioned his idea is a letter he wrote in September 1969 to the scientific director of the Health Research Council of the City of New York in which he requested funds to purchase a high-field spectrometer.[251] In a postscript to his request, he wrote, "I will make every effort myself and through collaborators, to establish that all tumors can be recognized by their potassium relaxation times or H_2O-proton spectra and proceed with the development on instrumentation and probes that can be used to scan the human body externally for early signs of malignancy."[252]

His first publication to that effect came in early 1971 following his successful 1970 experiments proving that cancerous tissue did indeed differ in relaxation rates from non-cancerous tissue and that even normal tissues could be differentiated from one another by their relaxation rates.[253] A patent application for a medical scanner based on these differences soon followed in 1972. (The patent was issued in 1974.[254])

Next came the idea, published in 1973,[255] for displaying this relaxation T_1 and T_2 data in the form of user-friendly pictures. After observing experimental confirmation of Dr. Damadian's T_1 and T_2 research on tissues, a chemist, Dr. Paul Lauterbur, affiliated with the State University of New York at Stony Brook, created what he called "NMR zeugmatography."[256-257]

The innovation of Lauterbur's zeugmatography was that it combined the idea of superimposing a magnetic field gradient onto the main field to obtain spatial localization—an idea published in 1951 by Robert Gabillard of Paris[258] and demonstrated by Edward Purcell and Herman Carr at Harvard in 1954[259]—with the back-projection techniques first introduced by William Oldendorf[260] and then embodied in the first X-ray computed tomography (CT) scanner by Geoffrey Hounsfield at Hammersmith College, London.[261]

Lauterbur initially spelled out his imaging idea in a notebook, suggesting that linear gradients could allow NMR imaging of the body and thereby serve as an application of Damadian's research.[262-263] Lauterbur first published his ideas in 1973.[264] In 1974, Peter Mansfield, an NMR researcher at the University of Nottingham in England published his own ideas for imaging crystals using NMR.[265] Once he realized he could achieve spatial imaging, he looked around for other applications, came across Damadian's findings and he, too, turned his attention to medical imaging.[266]

Even here, however, the rippling effect of Purcell's influence is significant. One of those figuring prominently in the research published in the mid-1970s—and who achieved an early NMR image of a human hand[267]—was E. Raymond Andrew, a colleague of Mansfield's at the University of Nottingham, whose work in NMR can be traced back to postdoctoral research he performed with Purcell at Harvard in 1948.

Although the journey from T_1 and T_2 differentiation of tissues to commercial MR scanning all took place in one short decade—from Damadian's first T_1 and T_2 tissue analysis in 1970,[268] to the first MR image of two tiny tubes of water immersed in a larger tube by Lauterbur,[269] to a cross-sectional chest image of a mouse by Damadian in March 1976,[270] to a cross-sectional chest image of a human by Damadian in July 1977,[271] to the first commercial MR scanner by Damadian in 1980[272]—none of it could have occurred without the foundational work performed by Dr. Edward Purcell and his colleagues at Harvard in the latter part of the 1940s. As Purcell pointed out, all that was needed to take the next step was the computer power and the idea.

When the computer power and the idea came together, Professor Purcell wrote to congratulate the medical researcher who had once audited one of his introductory quantum-mechanics courses and who had now achieved the first human MR image: "Thank you very much for sending me a copy of your historic first picture," he wrote Dr. Damadian. "I congratulate you and shall keep the picture as a perpetual reminder of how little one can foresee the fruitful application of any new physics."[273]

The statement calls to mind another comment Purcell made a quarter-century earlier at the end of his Nobel lecture in Stockholm, Sweden:

> This has been a long story and a complicated one, I'm afraid. We are dealing not merely with a new tool but with a new subject, a subject I have called simply nuclear magnetism. If you will think of the history of ordinary magnetism, the electronic kind, you will remember that it has been rich in difficult and provocative problems and full of surprises. Nuclear magnetism, so far as we have gone, is like that, too.[274] ∎

REFERENCE NOTES:

1. *1989 Keystone Coal Industry Manual*, (Chicago: Maclean Hunter Publishing, 1989), 472-484.

2. Edward M. Purcell, from *The Christian County History, Sesquicentennial Edition, 1880-1968*, published by Christian County Historical Society, 1968.

3. *Breeze-Courier*, Taylorville, Illinois, November 6, 1952.

4. John Lynch in *The Boston Herald*, Nov. 7, 1952. From Harvard University Archives.

5. Ibid.

6. Edward M. Purcell, interview by Katherine Sopka, 8 June 1977, transcript, Center for History of Physics, American Institute of Physics, New York, 2.

7. Ibid., 4.

8. Ibid.

9. Ibid., 2.

10. David C.D. Rogers, "Profile: Edward Purcell" in *The Harvard Crimson*, 8 Dec. 1952.

11. E.M. Purcell, interview by Sopka, 6-7.

12. Ibid., 42.

13. E.M. Purcell, interview by James Mattson, 8 November 1994.

14. E.M. Purcell, notes to James Mattson, January 1994.

15. E.M. Purcell, interview by John Bryant, 14 June 1991, Cambridge, Massachusetts, published in *Rad Lab: Oral Histories Documenting World War II Activities at the MIT Radiation Laboratory*, (Piscataway, NJ: Center for the History of Electrical Engineering, 1993), 241.

16. E.M. Purcell, notes to Mattson, January 1994.

17. R. Kronig and I.I. Rabi, *Physical Review*, February 1927.

18. E.M. Purcell, interview by Sopka, 8.

19. Ibid., 11.

20. Ibid., 12.

21. Ibid., 8-9.

22. Abraham Pais, *Inward Bound: Of Matter and Forces in the Physical World*, (New York: Oxford University Press, 1986), 75.

23. I.I. Rabi, interview by Thomas S. Kuhn, 8 December 1963, transcript, American Institute of Physics, College Park, MD, 1-2.

24. E.M. Purcell, interview by Sopka, 9.

25. "Award E. Purcell, '33, fellowship to Harvard" in *Purdue Alumnus*, Vol. 22, Oct. 1934, Special Collections Library, Purdue University, 5.

26. E.M. Purcell, K. Lark-Horovitz, H.J. Yearian, "Electron diffraction from vacuum-sublimated layers," *Physical Review* **45**, 123 (1934).

27. E.M. Purcell, K. Lark-Horovitz, J.D. Howe, "Method of making extremely thin films," *Rev. Sci. Inst.* **6**, (1935), 401-403.

28. E.M. Purcell, interview by Sopka, 12.

29. Ibid.

30. E.M. Purcell, interview by James Mattson, 11 November 1994.

31. E.M. Purcell, interview by Sopka, 11-12.

32. Ibid., 12.

33. E.M. Purcell, interview by Bryant, 242.

34. Johannes W. van Spronsen, *The Periodic System of Chemical Elements: A History of the First Hundred Years*, (Amsterdam: Elsevier, 1969), 42; quoted by I. Bernard Cohen, *Revolution in Science*, (Cambridge, MA: Belknap Press of Harvard University Press, 1985), 471.

35. Mary Jo Nye, ed., *The Question of the Atom: From the Karlsruhe Congress to the First Solvay Conference, 1860-1911*, (Los Angeles: Tomash Publishers, 1984), 5-11.

36. I. Bernard Cohen, *Revolution in Science*, (Cambridge, MA: Belknap Press of Harvard University Press, 1985), 471.

37. E.M. Purcell, interview by Sopka, 15.

38. Ibid., 14.

39. Alan D. Beyerchen, *Scientists Under Hitler: Politics and the Physics Community in the Third Reich*, (New Haven: Yale University Press, 1977), 27.

40. E.M. Purcell, notes to Mattson, January 1994.

41. Beyerchen, *Scientists Under Hitler: Politics and the Physics Community in the Third Reich*, 173.

42. Ibid., 132.

43. E.M. Purcell, interview by James Mattson, 23 December 1994.

44. E.M. Purcell, interview by Sopka, 15.

45. Enrico Fermi, *Zeitschrift für Physik* **88**, (1934), 161; quoted by Pais in *Inward Bound: Of Matter and Forces in the Physical World*, 418.

46. E.M. Purcell, interview by Sopka, 14-15.

47. E.M. Purcell, interview by Sopka, 15.

48. J.H. Van Vleck, *The Theory of Electric and Magnetic Susceptibilities*, (Oxford: Clarendon, 1932), part of The International Series of Monographs on Physics, edited by R.H. Fowler and P. Kapitza.

49. E.M. Purcell, interview by Sopka, 21.

50. Ibid.

51. Ibid., 22.

52. P. Debye, *Ann. d. Physik* **81**, (1926), 1154.

53. M.H. Hebb and E.M. Purcell, "A theoretical study of magnetic cooling experiments," *J. Chem. Phys.* **5**, (1937), 338.

54. J.H. Van Vleck, *J. Chem. Phys.* **5**, (1937), 338.

55. E.M. Purcell, interview by Sopka, 21-22.

56. I.I. Rabi, "On the principal magnetic susceptibilities of crystals," *Physical Review* **29**, (1927), 174-185.

57. E.M. Purcell, interview by Sopka, 4.

58. R.H. Fowler, *Statistical Mechanics*, second edition, (Cambridge: 1936).

59. E.M. Purcell, interview by Sopka, 19.

60. Ibid.

61. E.M. Purcell, notes to Mattson, January 1994.

62. E.M. Purcell, interview by Mattson, 8 November 1994.

63. E.M. Purcell, interview by Sopka, 19.

64. F.W. Aston, *Phil. Mag.* **38**, (1919), 710.

65. E.M. Purcell, "The focusing of charged particles by a spherical condenser," *Physical Review* **54**, (1938), 819.

66. Ibid.

67. E.M. Purcell, interview by Sopka, 20

68. E.M. Purcell, interview by Mattson, 8 November 1994.

69. E.M. Purcell, "The focusing of charged particles by a spherical condenser," 826.

70. Ibid.

71. Ibid., 824.

72. Ibid.

73. E.M. Purcell, interview by Mattson, 22 November 1994.

74. Ibid.

75. E.M. Purcell, "The focusing of charged particles by a spherical condenser," 826.

76. E.M. Purcell, notes to Mattson, January 1994.

77. E.M. Purcell, interview by James Mattson, 22 November 1994.

78. J.M.B. Kellogg, I.I. Rabi, N.F. Ramsey, and J.R. Zacharias, "Magnetic moments of the proton and the deuteron. Radiofrequency spectrum of H_2 in various magnetic fields," *Physical Review* **56**, (1939), 728.

79. Daniel J. Kevles, *The Physicists* (New York: Alfred A. Knopf, 1978), 320.

80. Ibid., 329.

81. Ibid., 320.

82. E.M. Purcell, interview by Mattson, 22 November 1994.

83. John S. Rigden, Rabi: *Scientist and Citizen*, one of Alfred P. Sloan Foundation Series (Basic Books, New York: 1987), 140.

84. E.M. Purcell, interview by Sopka, 25.

85. Ibid., 25-26.

86. F.H. Hinsley, *British Intelligence in the Second World War*, vol. 3, (London: HMSO, 1981), 517; quoted by Tom Bower in *The Paperclip Conspiracy: The Hunt for the Nazi Scientists*, (Boston: Little, Brown and Co., 1987), 53.

87. S.W. Roskill, *Naval Policy Between the Wars*, (London: HMSO, 1960), 33; quoted by Tom Bower in *The Paperclip Conspiracy: The Hunt for the Nazi Scientists*, (Boston: Little, Brown and Co., 1987), 53.

88. Vannevar Bush, *Pieces of the Action*, (New York: William Morrow, 1970), 88.

89. *Five Years at the Radiation Laboratory*, originally published in 1946 by the Massachusetts Institute of Technology, copyright 1947; republished along with additional material in 1991 as: Five Years, 1991 IEEE MTT-S International Microwave Symposium Edition.

90. I.I. Rabi, quoted by Jeremy Bernstein in "Profiles: Physicist," *New Yorker*, 20 October 1975, 49.

91. John Rigden, "Quantum states and precession: the two discoveries of NMR," *Reviews of Modern Physics* **58**, (1988), 433.

92. Ibid., 440-41.

93. G.E. Pake, interview by Mattson, 27 January 1993.

94. Ibid.

95. E.M. Purcell, interview by Sopka, 31.

96. I.I. Rabi, interview by Barbara Land, 12 November 1962, transcript, Columbia Oral History, Columbia University, New York, 102.

97. E.M. Purcell, interview by Sopka, 31.

98. Ibid.

99. Ibid., 28.

100. David C.D. Rogers in *The Harvard Crimson*, 8 December 1952.

101. *The Who's Who of Nobel Prize Winners* (Phoenix: Oryx Press, 1986), 168.

102. I.I. Rabi, J.R. Zacharias, S. Millman and P. Kusch, "A new method of measuring nuclear magnetic moment," *Physical Review* **53**, (1938), 318; I.I. Rabi, S. Millman, P. Kusch and J.R. Zacharias, "The molecular beam resonance method for measuring nuclear magnetic moments," *Physical Review* **55**, (1939), 526-535.

103. E.M. Purcell, interview by Sopka, 31.

104. Ibid., 29-30.

105. G.E. Pake, interview by Mattson, 27 January 1993.

106. David C.D. Rogers in *The Harvard Crimson*, 8 December 1952.

107. E.M. Purcell, interview by Sopka, 34.

108. G.E. Pake, "Fundamentals of nuclear magnetic resonance absorption, part II," *American Journal of Physics* **18**, (1950), 473.

109. E.M. Purcell, "Nuclear magnetism in relation to problems of the liquid and solid states," *Science* **107**, (1954), 433.

110. I. Waller, Über die magnetisierung von paramagnetischen kristallen in wechselfeldern," *Zeitschrift für Physik* **79**, (1932), 370.

111. E.M. Purcell, interview by Sopka, 34.

112. E.M. Purcell, notes to Mattson, January, 1994.

113. David C.D. Rogers in *The Harvard Crimson*, 8 December 1952.

114. E.M. Purcell, notes to Mattson, January, 1994.

115. E.M. Purcell, interview by Sopka, 34.

116. Leon Lederman, *The God Particle* (Boston: Houghton Mifflin, 1993), 7.

117. E.M. Purcell, H.C. Torrey, and R.V. Pound, "Resonance absorption by nuclear magnetic moments in a solid," *Physical Review* **69,** (1946), 37.

118. Ibid.

119. Ibid.

120. Ibid., 37-38.

121. Ibid., 38.

122. E.M. Purcell, notes to Mattson, January 1994.

123. N. Bloembergen, interview with James Mattson, 1989.

124. F. Bloch, W.W. Hansen, and M. Packard, "Nuclear induction," *Physical Review* **69,** (1946), 127.

125. E.M. Purcell, interview by Sopka, 34.

126. F. Bloch, interview by Charles Weiner, 15 August 1968, Niels Bohr Library, American Institute of Physics, College Park, MD, 43.

127. M. Packard, in private communication to John Rigden, quoted by Rigden in "Quantum states and precession: the two discoveries of NMR," 446.

128. E.M. Purcell, interview by Sopka, 27-28.

129. Profile: Felix Bloch, *Neighborhood News,* Palo Alto, CA, Vol. 2, No. 49, 3 December 1953, Dept. of Special Collections, Stanford University Libraries.

130. E.M. Purcell, interview by Sopka, 27-28.

131. G.E. Pake, interview by Mattson, 27 January 1993.

132. E.M. Purcell, notes to Mattson, January 1994.

133. Anatole Abragam, *Time Reversal, An Autobiography* (Oxford: Clarendon Press, 1989), 160.

134. Felix Bloch, interview by Charles Weiner, 15 August 1968, 43.

135. E.M. Purcell, quoted by Rigden in *Rabi: Scientist and Citizen* , 170.

136. E.M. Purcell, notes to Mattson, January 1994.

137. F. Keesing and R. Lowen, "The Felix Bloch papers," Dept. of Special Collections and University Archives, Stanford, 1989.

138. E.M. Purcell, notes to Mattson, January, 1994.

139. Ibid.

140. Abragam, *Time Reversal, An Autobiography*, 144, 155.

141. Ibid.

142. David C.D. Rogers, "Profile: Edward Purcell" in *The Harvard Crimson,* 8 Dec. 1952.

143. Donald Stokes, author of press release for Stanford University News Service, 4 May 1982, Dept. of Special Collections and University Archives, Stanford.

144. G.E. Pake, interview by Mattson, 27 January 1993.

145. Abragam, *Time Reversal, An Autobiography*, 44.

146. E.M. Purcell, notes to Mattson, January, 1994.

147. Ibid.

148. E.M. Purcell, interview by Sopka, 59.

149. Robert L. Weber, *Pioneers of Science: Nobel Prize Winners in Physics,* Second Edition, (Bristol: Adam Hilger, 1988), 146.

150. E.M. Purcell, interview by Sopka, 58.

151. Raymond V. Damadian, interview with James Mattson, 1993.

152. Sonny Kleinfield, *A Machine Called Indomitable,* (New York: Times Books, 1985), 26.

153. E.M. Purcell, notes to Mattson, January 1994.

154. G.E. Pake and E.M. Purcell, "Line shapes in nuclear paramagnetism," *Physical Review* **74,** (1948), 1184; G.E. Pake, "Nuclear resonance absorption in hydrated crystals," *Journal of Chemical Physics* **16,** (1948), 327; G.E. Pake, "Fundamentals of nuclear magnetic resonance absorption, I, *American Journal of Physics* **18,** (1950), 438; Pake, "Fundamentals of nuclear magnetic resonance absorption, II, 473.

155. R.M. Brown and E.M. Purcell, "Nuclear magnetic resonance in weak fields," *Physical Review* **75,** (1949), 1262.

156. J.H. Gardner and E.M. Purcell, "A precise determination of the proton magnetic moment in Bohr magnetons," *Physical Review* **76**, (1949), 1262-63.

157. H.S. Gutowsky, G.B. Kistiakowsky, G.E. Pake, and E.M. Purcell, "Structural investigations by means of nuclear magnetism, I. rigid crystal lattices," *Journal of Chemical Physics* **17**, (1949), 972-981.

158. H.Y. Carr and E.M. Purcell, "Interaction between nuclear spins in HD gas," *Physical Review* **88**, (1952), 415-416; "Effects of diffusion on free precession in nuclear magnetic resonance experiments," *Physical Review* **94**, (1954), 630-638.

159. F. Reif and E.M. Purcell, "Nuclear magnetic resonance in solid hydrogen," *Physical Review* **91**, (1953), 631-641; G.B. Benedek and E.M. Purcell, "Nuclear magnetic resonance in liquids under high pressure," *Journal of Chemical Physics* **22**, (1954), 2003-2012; G.B. Field and E.M. Purcell, "Influence of collisions upon population of hyperfine states in hydrogen, *Astrophysical Journal* **124**, (1956), 542-549.

160. N.F. Ramsey and E.M. Purcell, "On the possibility of electric dipole moments for elementary particles and nuclei," *Physical Review* **78**, (1950), 807; "Interactions between nuclear spins in molecules," *Physical Review* **85**, (1952), 143-144; N.F. Ramsey, J.H. Smith, and E.M. Purcell, "Experimental limit to the electric dipole moments of the neutron," *Physical Review* **108**, (1957), 120-122.

161. E.M. Purcell, Bibliography of scientific publications, 1992.

162. *Collier's Encyclopedia*, Vol. 19 (New York: P.F. Collier, 1994), 626.

163. Brian J. Robinson, "Hydroxyl radicals in space," Frontiers in Astronomy, Readings from *Scientific American*, (San Francisco, W.H. Freeman: 1970), 184.

164. E.M. Purcell, interview by Sopka, 37.

165. Morton S. Roberts, "Hydrogen in galaxies," *Frontiers in Astronomy*, readings from *Scientific American*, (San Francisco: W.H. Freeman, 1970), 204.

166. Ibid.

167. Ibid.

168. Ibid.

169. E.M. Purcell, interview by Sopka, 37-38.

170. Ibid., 38.

171. E.M. Purcell, notes to Mattson, January 1994.

172. E.M. Purcell, interview by Sopka, 38.

173. Ibid.

174. H.I. Ewen and E.M. Purcell, "Observations of a line in the galactic radio spectrum," *Nature* **168**, (1951), 356.

175. Jan Oort and C.A. Muller, *Nature* **168**, (1951), 356.

176. J.L. Pawsey, *Nature* **168**, (1951), 356.

177. E.M. Purcell, notes to Mattson, January 1994.

178. E.M. Purcell, interview by Sopka, 39.

179. *Collier's Encyclopedia*, Vol. 19 (New York: P.F. Collier, 1994), 626.

180. Roberts, "Hydrogen in Galaxies," 204.

181. E.M. Purcell and N.F. Ramsey, "On the possibility of electric dipole moments for elementary particles and nuclei," 883.

182. N.F. Ramsey, "Earliest criticisms of assumed P and T symmetries," Time Reversal, Arthur Rich Memorial Symposium, *AIP Conference Proceedings* **270**, (1992), 179.

183. E.M. Purcell and R.V. Pound, "A nuclear spin system at negative temperature," *Physical Review* **81**, (1951), 279-280.

184. E.M. Purcell, interview by Sopka, 35-36.

185. N.F. Ramsey and R.V. Pound, "Nuclear audiofrequency spectroscopy by resonant heating of nuclear spin system," *Physical Review* **81**, (1951), 278.

186. Hebb and Purcell, "A theoretical study of magnetic cooling experiments," 338-350.

187. Richard Rhodes, *The Making of the Atomic Bomb,* (New York: Simon and Schuster, 1988), 339-340, 495-496.

188. N.F. Ramsey, "Students, research and publications," unpublished, 14.

189. N.F. Ramsey, "Thermodynamics and statistical mechanics at negative absolute temperatures," *Physical Review* **103,** (1956), 20-28.

190. E.M. Purcell, interview by Sopka, 36.

191. N.F. Ramsey, interview by James Mattson, December 15, 1993.

192. E.M. Purcell, interview by Sopka, 36.

193. E.M. Purcell, interview by James Mattson, 8 November 1994.

194. *Nobel Lectures, Physics: 1942-1962,* (Amsterdam: Elsevier, 1964), 201.

195. Ibid.

196. Ibid., 53.

197. E.M. Purcell, interview by Sopka, 46.

198. Ibid., 26.

199. Ibid., 26-27.

200. Ibid., 45.

201. Ibid., 46.

202. Michael R. Beschloss, *Mayday: Eisenhower, Khrushchev and the U-2 Affair* (New York: Harper & Row, 1986), 74-75.

203. E.M. Purcell, interview by Sopka, 46.

204. Ibid., 47.

205. Dwight D. Eisenhower, *Waging Peace: The White House Years, 1956-1961* (Garden City, NY: Doubleday, 1965), 208.

206. Ibid., 211.

207. Rigden, *Rabi: Scientist and Citizen,* 249-250.

208. Eisenhower, *Waging Peace: The White House Years, 1956-1961,* 224.

209. James R. Killian, Jr., *Sputnik: Scientists and Eisenhower* (Cambridge, MA: MIT Press, 1977), 123.

210. E.M. Purcell, interview by Sopka, 48-49.

211. Ibid., 49.

212. Ibid.

213. Ibid., 51.

214. Ibid., 40-41.

215. Ibid., 54.

216. E.M. Purcell, interview by Mattson, 22 November 1994.

217. E.M. Purcell, interview by Mattson, 23 December 1994.

218. E.M. Purcell, G.B. Collins, T. Fujii, J. Hornbostel, and F. Turkot, "Search for the Dirac monopole with 30-BeV protons," *Physical Review* **129,** (1963), 2326.

219. W.V.R. Malkus, *Physical Review* **83,** (1951), 899.

220. H. Bradner and W.M. Isbell, *Physical Review* **114,** (1959), 603.

221. Ibid., 2336.

222. Abragam, *Time Reversal, An Autobiography,* 160.

223. E.M. Purcell, interview by Sopka, 57.

224. E.M. Purcell, interview by Mattson, 23 December 1994.

225. Ibid.

226. E.M. Purcell, "Life at low Reynolds number," *American Journal of Physics* **45,** (1977), 4.

227. E.M. Purcell, interview by Mattson, 23 December 1994.

228. Ibid.

229. Felix Bloch, "Past, present, and future of nuclear magnetic resonance," *Magnetic Resonance Imaging,* 2nd Edition, Partain, Price, Patton, Kulkarni and James, eds., (Philadelphia, W. B. Saunders: 1988), 5.

230. N. Bloembergen, E.M. Purcell, and R.V. Pound, "Relaxation effects in nuclear magnetic resonance absorption," *Physical Review* **73,** (1948), 679.

231. Ibid., 703.

232. E.M. Purcell, interview by Sopka, 35.

233. Bloch, "Past, present, and future of nuclear magnetic resonance," 5.

234. E.M. Purcell, "Research in nuclear magnetism," Nobel Lecture, 11 December 1952, *Les Prix Nobel 1952*, Nobelstiftelsen, (Stockholm: Imprimerie Royale, 1952), 97-109.

235. J.T. Arnold, S.S. Dharmatti, and M.E. Packard, *Journal of Chemical Physics* **19,** (1951), 507.

236. N. Bloembergen, abstract, *Physical Review* **75,** (1949), 1326.

237. W. Knight, *Physical Review* **76,** (1949), 1260.

238. N.F. Ramsey, *Physical Review* **77,** (1950), 567; **78,** (1950), 699; **83,** (1951), 540; and **86,** (1952), 243.

239. N.F. Ramsey and E.M. Purcell, "Interactions between nuclear spins in molecules," *Physical Review* **85,** (1952), 143.

240. H. Gutowsky, D.W. McCall, C. Slichter, and McNeill, *Physical Review* **82,** (1951), 748; and *Physical Review* **84,** (1951), 589 and 1246.

241. E.L. Hahn and D.E. Maxwell, *Physical Review* **84,** (1951), 1246; and *Physical Review* **88,** (1952), 1070.

242. E.L. Hahn, "Spin echoes," *Physical Review* **80,** (1950), 580.

243. E.L. Hahn, interview by James Mattson, 9 March 1994.

244. Carr and Purcell, "Effects of diffusion on free precession in nuclear magnetic resonance experiments," 630.

245. R. Gabillard, "A steady state transient technique in nuclear resonance," *C.R. Acad. Sci.* (Paris) **232,** (1951), 1551; *Physical Review* **85,** (1952), 694.

246. H.Y. Carr, letter to the editor of *Physics Today*, written August 1992, published January 1993, 94.

247. Ibid.

248. E.M. Purcell, "Foreword," *Magnetic Resonance Imaging*, 2nd Edition, Partain, Price, Patton, Kulkarni and James, eds., (Philadelphia, W. B. Saunders: 1988), xxvi.

249. Ibid.

250. E. R. Andrew, "NMR in medicine: a historical review," *Magnetic Resonance Imaging*, 2nd Edition, Partain, Price, Patton, Kulkarni and James, eds., (Philadelphia: W. B. Saunders, 1988), 12-13.

251. R.V. Damadian, letter as assistant professor in Dept. of Internal Medicine at Downstate Medical Center, State University of New York to George S. Mirick, Scientific Director, The Health Research Council of the City of New York, dated September 17, 1969.

252. Ibid.

253. R.V. Damadian, "Tumor detection by nuclear magnetic resonance," *Science* **171,** (1971), 1151-1153.

254. R.V. Damadian, "Apparatus and method for detecting cancer in tissue," U.S. Patent No. 3,789,832; patent application filed on March 17, 1972, patent issued February 5, 1974.

255. P.C. Lauterbur, "Image formation by induced local interactions: Examples employing nuclear magnetic resonance," *Nature* **243,** (1973), 190.

256. Paul C. Lauterbur, "The first 20 years of MRI and *in vivo* spectroscopy," Magnetic Resonance Imaging: NIH Consensus Development Conference, 26-28 October 1987, National Institutes of Health.

257. P.C. Lauterbur, "Cancer detection by nuclear magnetic resonance zeugmatographic imaging," *Cancer* **57,** (1986), 1899.

258. Gabillard, "A steady state transient technique in nuclear resonance," 1551; 694.

259. Carr and Purcell, "Effects of diffusion on free precession in nuclear magnetic resonance experiments," 630.

260. W.H. Oldendorf, "I.R.E. transactions," *Biomed. Elect.* **8,** 68.

261. G.N. Hounsfield, *Br. J. Radiol.* **46,** (1973), 1016.

262. Ros Herman, "A chemical clue to disease," *New Scientist*, 15 March 1979, 876.

263. P.C. Lauterbur, handwritten laboratory notes written 2 September 1971, countersigned by G.D. Vickers on 3 September 1971.

264. P.C. Lauterbur, "Image formation by induced local interactions: Examples employing nuclear magnetic resonance," *Nature* **243,** (1973), 190.

265. A.N. Garroway, P.K. Grannell, and P. Mansfield, "Image formation in NMR by a selective irradiative process," *J. Phys. C: Solid State Phys.* **7,** (1974), L457.

266. P. Mansfield and A. Maudsley, "Medical imaging by NMR," *Brit JP Radiol* **50,** (1977), 188.

267. E.R. Andrew, P.A. Bottomley, W.S. Hinshaw, G.N. Holland, W.S. Moore, and C. Simaroj, "NMR images by the multiple sensitive point method: application to larger biological specimens," *Phys. Med. Biol.* **22,** (1977), 971.

268. Damadian, "Tumor detection by nuclear magnetic resonance," 1151-1153.

269. Lauterbur, "Image formation by induced local interactions: examples employing nuclear magnetic resonance," 190.

270. R.V. Damadian, L. Minkoff, M. Goldsmith, M. Stanford, and J. Koutcher, "Field focus nuclear magnetic resonance (FONAR): visualization of a tumor in a live animal," *Science* **194,** 24 December 1976, 1430-1432.

271. R.V. Damadian, M. Goldsmith, and L. Minkoff, "NMR in cancer: FONAR image of the live human body," *Physiol. Chem. Phys.* 1977, 97-108.

272. "First clinical trials of diagnostic NMR," *Radiology Nuclear Medicine Magazine,* June 1981, 8-12.

273. E.M. Purcell, letter to Raymond V. Damadian, 26 October 1977.

274. E.M. Purcell, "Research in nuclear magnetism," reprinted from his Nobel lecture, *Science* **118,** (1953), 436.

❖ ❖ ❖

Two American laboratories, one on the East Coast at Harvard, the other on the West Coast at Stanford, working entirely independently, simultaneously detected the NMR response of protons in paraffin and water respectively. . . . For months and even years afterwards, according to whether a physicist spoke of nuclear magnetic absorption or nuclear induction, one could decide whether he came from New England or California, more surely than by his accent.

—Anatole Abragam

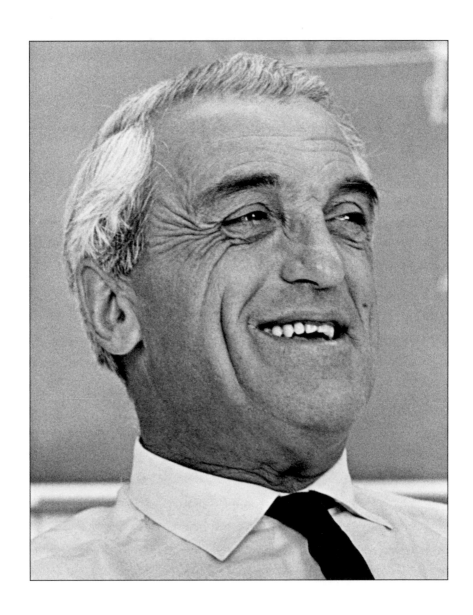

4

FELIX BLOCH

Discoverer of NMR Signal in Condensed Matter Using Nuclear Induction Method

In A MEMORIAL TRIBUTE to Felix Bloch in 1983, physicist Anatole Abragam wrote: "If the Nobel Prize that he shared with Edward Purcell in 1952 was the accolade for the great discovery (in 1946) of nuclear magnetic resonance (NMR for short) or 'nuclear induction' as he liked to call it, at least three other earlier discoveries might have won Bloch the same prestigious award . . . propagation of electrons in crystalline solids; spin waves and Bloch walls; magnetic interactions of slow neutrons with matter, and measurement of the magnetic moment of the neutron." Describing Bloch as "a virtuoso of quantum mechanics," Abragam asserted that "for more than 30 years, nobody used this tool with more originality, elegance and efficiency than Felix Bloch."[1]

As his Stanford colleagues Leonard Schiff and Robert Hofstadter have noted, the "remarkably large" number of formulas or effects that have come to be associated with Bloch's name are evidence of the fundamental nature of his scientific contributions.[2] Included in the list are Bloch wave functions, Bloch spin waves, Bloch walls, the Bethe-Bloch formula, Bloch's theorem, the Bloch-Nordsieck theory and, of particular note with regard to magnetic resonance, the Bloch equations.

In 1928, at the age of 23, Bloch published his PhD thesis on the quantum-mechanical electron theory of metals[3] which established him early in his career as an eminent practitioner of the new quantum mechanics. In addition to providing the basis for modern understanding of electrical conduction, his thesis paved the way for development of the quantum theory of solids that soon followed, and laid the foundation for development of the ubiquitous semiconductor—essential to life as we know it in the late 20th century. These contributions were followed soon afterward by his theory of ferromagnetism at low temperatures, described in terms of "spin waves"[4] and his discovery in 1932 of "Bloch walls,"[5] the transition areas separating the oppositely-magnetized domains of a ferromagnetic crystal.

In 1933, Bloch's academic career in Germany was cut short by Adolf Hitler. Although he was a Swiss citizen and not in immediate danger, he was put on the list of those who were *beurlaubungen*, "forced to leave,"[6] thus opening the door for his emigration to the United States. Bloch once said that Hitler did him "a great deal of favor, but he didn't intend it."[7]

Although he was already recognized as an insightful theoretical physicist and would likely have achieved greatness in almost any environment that allowed him freedom to be creative, Bloch's departure from Germany in 1933 and subsequent emigration to the United States and California's Stanford University in 1934 would result in some of his greatest scientific achievements.

In 1936, intrigued by a nuclear particle called the neutron discovered by James Chadwick just four years earlier at Cambridge University, Bloch suggested an ingenious method[8] for convincing the electrically-neutral particle to reveal its magnetic personality. Unable to draw upon techniques that had been used for making the electrically-charged electron disclose its magnetic moment, Bloch suggested that the job could be done by observing the scattering and polarizing of slow neutrons in iron, confirmed soon afterward by researchers at Cornell and Columbia universities.[9-11]

In 1939, in collaboration with Luis Alvarez, Bloch dramatically improved the accuracy of his own method by incorporating magnetic resonance.[12-13] Bloch's idea for using magnetic resonance to measure neutron magnetic moments actually came to him two years earlier, in 1937.[14-15] Though very similar to I.I. Rabi's 1937 Nobel Prize-winning molecular-beam method which used magnetic resonance to measure magnetic moments of atomic nuclei, the two methods were independently conceived. In fact, Rabi acknowledged Bloch's plan to use the method for another purpose in the letter to the editor of *Physical Review* in which he announced his first magnetic resonance experiment.[16]

Bloch would also meet his future wife in the United States, physicist Lore Misch, with whom he would share 43 years of marriage and a family life which has been described as "happy and stable."[17] A Jewish refugee, Lore left Germany for Switzerland in 1936 and, two years later, emigrated to the United States where she married Felix Bloch in 1940.

Bloch's personal research career was interrupted by the scientific prerogatives of World War II, but five months after the war ended, Bloch and his collaborators, William W. Hansen and Martin Packard, observed their first NMR signals from hydrogen protons in water, using a method Bloch called nuclear induction.[18] Unbeknownst to them, Edward Purcell and his collaborators, Henry C. Torrey and Robert Pound, had discovered just a few weeks earlier the NMR signal from hydrogen protons in paraffin.[19] Seven years later, the Nobel Committee would award them both the Nobel Prize in physics for 1952.

In spite of being at the forefront of the new physics ushered in by the Quantum Revolution , Bloch described his NMR discovery using physics terms that were largely classical, terms such as precession, torque and induction. Bloch's appreciation for the classical perspective came from his close association with Niels Bohr in Copenhagen. "Bohr used to say and kept on saying," said Bloch, "that the dilemma in quantum mechanics is this; that all observations are essentially classical. That is to say, the only way we can make contact with reality is through classical experiments."

Not only was Bloch's NMR experiment classical, as in traditional physics, it was also a classic, as in excellence, and the theory for his NMR discovery was provided in a series of equations which themselves have become classics, the famous "Bloch equations," which in addition to magnetic resonance, have found application in masers, lasers and atomic clocks.

In concluding his tribute to Bloch, Anatole Abragam pointed out that Bloch's works are marked by elegance, conciseness, and "a remarkable sense of experimental realism," and added, "In the age of the computer, when experimental techniques are dominated by the accumulation of data and technical theories by the accumulation of numerical calculations, a whole style of physics based on simplicity and clarity was taken from us with the death of Felix Bloch."[20]

The Early Years

Felix Bloch was born in Zürich, Switzerland on October 23, 1905, the second of two children born to Gustav and Agnes (Mayer) Bloch.

Gustav Bloch was born in German-speaking Bohemia. Then under the jurisdiction of the Austrian monarchy, Bohemia today comprises the western portion of the new Czech Republic. In the late 1890s, Gustav moved to Switzerland where he joined an uncle in his already-established wholesale grain business.*

---

* Bloch is a common surname in Switzerland. Although most of them came from the historic Alsace province of France, theirs was one of the few families, Bloch said, that came from Bohemia.

The "promising young nephew," as Bloch described his father, turned out to be "not terribly successful" as a businessman, despite his fascination with numbers. With his love for books and his interests in geography and languages, his father, Bloch said, "really would have liked best to be a teacher."[21]

Agnes Mayer, who moved to Switzerland somewhat later than Gustav, was from Vienna, Austria, where her brother owned a small textile factory. The two branches of Bloch's family tree were not unacquainted with one another, however, as Gustav and Agnes were first cousins, a fairly common occurrence in close-knit Jewish European communities and which in his family, said Bloch, occurred "rather frequently."[22]

When Felix was nine, he entered an "extremely lonely" period of his life when his 12-year-old sister, to whom he was very attached, died suddenly of blood poisoning. "After my sister died," he said, "I was really not very much interested in the company of other children, because of the grief which I had I felt I couldn't share."[23]

As a further consequence of his sister's death, he became a "doubly only child," he said, when his parents, seeking to avoid the pain of another loss, increased their watchfulness over him. "I was not allowed to do many things that other boys were allowed to do," said Bloch, "because they were afraid that something might happen to me, too, so I became quite a secluded person at that time, I think against my real natural temperament." As a result of his self-imposed seclusion and the over-protectiveness of his parents, he became an avid reader and a very good student.

Early on, Felix decided that he wanted to be an engineer. "I don't really remember how far it goes back, but certain interests in mechanical things I must have had rather early," he said. "I was interested in steam engines and locomotives at that time. I liked bridges and beautiful things like that."[24] Because of his engineering interest and his intention to eventually enroll at Switzerland's Federal Institute of Technology,* considered to be the school to attend for engineering, Bloch decided to take his secondary-school training at the *Realgymnasium,* a school that emphasized mathematics and science.

Although other boys were put off by the engineering profession because of its mathematics requirements, "that didn't scare me at all,"[25]

---

* The Federal Institute of Technology, or Polytechnic, (Albert Einstein's alma mater) is known by a number of names and acronymns, depending on the language used. Based on its German name, it is often referred to as the ETH (*Eidgenössische Technische Hochschule*); in French, EPF (*École Polytechnique Fédérale*); in Italian, SPF (*Svizzera Polytecnica Federale*).

Bloch said. He also received encouragement in that direction from his uncle in Vienna, the one who owned the textile factory, as he had plans for Felix to eventually join him in the business. Something practical like engineering, the uncle thought, might be quite beneficial.

Bloch soon discovered that he had an aptitude for mathematics, although it wasn't initially his primary interest, and that, like his father, he enjoyed studying languages, especially Latin. He also took, like every boy in his class, some music and learned to play the piano. At the time, he was rather ambivalent about the instrument, but later it would become one of his favorite pastimes.

He became very interested in nature and astronomy. "The Swiss mountains meant a great deal to me,"[26] he said. At the age of seven, two years before his sister's death, Felix had gone skiing for the first time in the beautiful Swiss Alps, and it too would be a favorite relaxation of his throughout most of his life. Not until his late 60s, when he broke his leg skiing, would his enthusiasm for the sport finally wane.

Sometime during his first or second year at the *gymnasium,* Bloch came across an old book on astronomy by Simon Newcomb, who had devoted much of his life to the charting of lunar and planetary orbits.

> I thumbed through that [said Bloch] and, although I didn't yet know much trigonometry, I was very much fascinated. Just for myself I solved some problems like, How does the length of the day[light] vary between spring and fall? I developed an approximate formula and checked that it agreed, and it gave me a great deal of satisfaction. So I began to feel, "Well, maybe I am really capable of doing this thing" [referring to engineering].[27]

It wasn't just Bloch's intellect, however, that was stimulated by astronomy; it also appealed to his spirit. Although his family did not practice the Jewish religion, as a young teenager still grieving the untimely loss of his sister, Bloch found in the heavens a constancy and a predictability that gave him comfort.

> My father took me once to an observatory at night and I looked up and saw some stars; I had the feeling that this was very wonderful and apparently people can even understand what goes on up there, although they didn't understand so much at that time. I had quite an early feeling that, "Yes, nature is apparently capable of rational analysis;" and also, because of the great shock of the death of my sis-

ter I very soon got attracted to that because I felt, "Well, life is uncertain, people die; here is something which is certain; this is a sound foundation." And I think that, to some extent, was at that time a narrow but firm basis which made me very fond of mathematics.[28]

The *Realgymnasium* was considered more technical than other schools, but even there Bloch's classmates found mathematics to be "rather sober and dull," as well as difficult, and they turned to Felix for assistance, which was for him a source of "some pride:"

I was very good at mathematics. Our training was excellent, I must say. Our mathematics professor . . . was a man by the name of [Karl] Beck . . . who worked with Pierre Weiss* at that time. [Beck] was actually, although he taught mathematics, a physicist. And he re-did the Einstein-de Haas experiment. [Although de Haas' calculation came out as Einstein had predicted, it was wrong, Bloch reminded his interviewer.] This man did it right.[29] And he was an excellent teacher, so it was really a joy to take mathematics with him.[30]

Calculus was not taught at the school. "Analytic geometry was the last thing we learned, and we learned that very thoroughly," he said. When Felix was 18, however, he obtained a book on calculus, taught himself the elements of derivatives, and realized on his own that this invention of Newton's was "a very simple way of constructing tangents to curves in analytic geometry."[31]

Besides Beck, Bloch also had a "very excellent" teacher in physics, a man by the name of Seiler who had authored a book on the subject. Although he didn't think Seiler was particularly outstanding scientifically, he was nevertheless, Bloch said, an "enthusiastic" and "marvelous teacher" who taught the fundamentals of elementary mechanics, optics, heat and DC electricity very well. Except for electromagnetic theory and quantum theory, which were not included in the course—"I don't remember where I first met the quantum," Bloch said—his *gymnasium* training in physics was, "almost as good a training in basic physics as we teach here now [at Stanford] in introductory courses."[32]

---

* Although Felix Bloch did not realize it when he was at the gymnasium, Pierre Weiss was a well-known physicist who had invented the Weiss magneton. "I knew he was a good teacher," said Bloch, "and I rather liked him, but I didn't know how outstanding he was."
— F. Bloch, interview by Kuhn, 4.

By 1924, Bloch's last year in the *gymnasium*, he began having some misgivings about his choice of engineering as a profession. Ironically, his concern was instigated in part by a visit from the uncle in Vienna who had always encouraged him to take engineering. The uncle visited Zürich shortly before Bloch was scheduled to take the *matura*, the required qualifying examination that determined whether or not a student would be permitted to go on to an institution of higher learning. "That's all very fine [to study engineering]," he told Felix, "but of course you must also be very sure that you get a sound commercial training to be a good businessman."

At that point, said Bloch, "I began to fear that engineering might not be quite what I wanted because my family was interested in engineering from an entirely practical point of view, and this was not what attracted me very much." Nevertheless, after graduation—"I think I got the best grades,"[33] he said—Bloch proceeded with his plan to enter the ETH to study engineering.

He stuck with the program for just one year. He had already become fairly convinced that engineering was not, as he said, "my cup of tea,"[34] but the summer of 1925 cinched his decision. Engineering students were encouraged to use their summer vacations to do practical work that would help prepare them for a career. For Felix, that meant working as a volunteer at a foundry near Zürich, an environment at odds at the time with his leftist views, then in vogue. "It was very clear to me," he said, "that this was not at all what I was looking for." The engineering he found to be very empirical with no scientific interest and he viewed the foundry as "a system of exploitation of the workers, who were very hard driven. I wanted to have no part of it."[35]

He thought momentarily about studying medicine, an interesting consideration in view of the fact that his work with magnetic resonance would lead to one of the greatest breakthroughs in medicine in the 20th century, but he soon abandoned thoughts of being a medical doctor in favor of being a physicist.

He didn't choose physics, however, because of encouragement from physicists. When he asked Professor Seiler what he thought about physics as a career, Seiler told him, "Don't do it. It's a hard job; there is no meat in it. Look at me here; I'm teaching the same thing [for] years." Although he did not know him at the time, Bloch also asked the eminent Hermann Weyl, director of the ETH's *Abteilung für Physik und Mathematik* (School of Physics and Mathematics), what he thought about physics as a vocational choice. Weyl also responded negatively. "No, you shouldn't," he told Felix bluntly.

Based on the situation at the time, Bloch said, "He was quite right. There was absolutely no prospect. If a man was that unsure that he had to ask, I think the sensible advice to him was to say, 'No.' "

"Well, I did it anyhow,"[36] said Bloch.

Bloch's parents were even less enthusiastic about the idea than the physicists, but he was bolstered in his decision with some moral support from a "quite good" physicist at the University of Giessen by the name of Jaffé. When Bloch's parents started asking around, "What is it this boy of ours wants to go into, this futureless occupation of being a physicist?" one of his father's cousins in Zürich, a lawyer, passed the question on to Jaffé, who went to bat for Felix.

> He had seen me or something [said Bloch], and had the good sense to tell my parents that they should be very glad that they had a son who knew what he wanted. . . . My father was rather sad about it, and for years didn't quite understand why I chose such an abstract thing. But he was a very kind man and said, "Well, all right, if that's what you want."[37]

His father, Bloch explained, was not a very wealthy man. From Gustav Bloch's perspective, his son should study something with which he could make a living and even Felix couldn't promise much vocational potential with physics. The only future that he could anticipate was teaching high school, said Bloch, "and even that was uncertain. It was entirely a shot in the dark, and I really have thought, rather proudly now, that I did that simply at that time because I thought I couldn't help it; and never mind what it leads to."[38]

In retrospect, he thought it may have been discussions with fellow students that helped settle the issue for him. "All I know," he said in 1964, "is that when I got into the first contact with real mathematics and real physics, I realized this is a serious and exciting business. Although I was also worried about the material prospects, that I would feel at home in this field I had very little doubt."[39]

It was an advanced laboratory course taught by a *privatdozent** by the name of Bär that gave Bloch his next significant physics experience and a valuable dose of encouragement. Since Bloch was the only one who registered for the course, Bär allowed him to do pretty much whatever he

---

* Title given to a non-salaried university teacher who is paid for his or her services by a small fee paid by the students; not considered a faculty position.

wanted. Bloch had read about Nobel laureate Robert Millikan's oil-drop experiment, reported in 1911, which measured electronic charge by calculating the joint influence of gravity and an electric field on charged drops of oil suspended in air, so Bär suggested that he try duplicating the experiment. After setting up the chamber, Bloch was able to observe with a dark-field microscope the same effect Millikan had observed and to calculate "more or less . . . a number for the electric charge."[40] The primary benefit to Bloch, however, as far as he was concerned, was not the successful duplication of a famous experiment but rather the personal regard and encouragement he received from Bär.

> The main thing was . . . what this man did to me. He was an extremely nice man. I think he has never been quite recognized for the quality of some very fine work—reflection of light rays from sound waves. I think it was he who did it the first time. It was a suggestion of Debye's, but he did it. . . . He gave me extreme encouragement. At that time, this man Bär apparently had quite a high regard for me because of my obvious interest, and I got strong encouragement from that. I also found out at that time that these experiments, although they had been done before, were really interesting.[41]

Bloch also received encouragement from a man by the name of Marcel Grossmann, who taught projective geometry. Grossmann was an early friend of Albert Einstein who, when Einstein was struggling with general relativity, had pointed him to "this so-called Ricci calculus," as Bloch termed it.[42] And now, when Bloch found a proof for a geometry problem that was simpler than the one suggested, Grossmann told the other students, "See, one of your fellows here has better sense." That encouragement reassured Bloch that he was on the right track. "But I was still worried," he said, "because I did not know how much I could do, still."[43]

In 1925, Bloch officially entered Weyl's *Abteilung für Physik und Mathematik* where he was introduced to college physics by the eminent Dutch physicist Peter Debye. It was an introduction for which Bloch would always be grateful. Although he had little contact with Debye during the course—"Debye was a man very remote,"[44] he explained—"without knowing much about his scientific work, I realized from the high quality of his lectures at the Institute that here was a great master of his field."[45]

> Debye had this real fine knack not only of making the basic things very clear to you but indicating, at the right moment, how they were

connected with the more modern things. . . . I knew he was very famous; I began to read some of his papers. I read his paper on the Compton effect . . . collision theory, and I think I knew a little bit already about his theory of specific heat.[46]

There was "a good deal less to be enthusiastic about," said Bloch, "in the other [physics] courses one could take."

Once in a while, a professor would offer a special course on a subject he just happened to be interested in, completely disregarding the tremendous gaps in our knowledge left by this system. Anyway, there was only a handful of us foolish enough to study physics and it was evidently not thought worthwhile to bother much about these 'odd fellows.' The only thing we could do about it was to go to the library and read some books, though nobody would advise us which ones to choose.[47]

Because he "never had a coherent course" in electromagnetic theory, said Bloch, he read Sommerfeld's book on the topic, *Atombau und Spektrallinien* (Atomic Structure and Spectral Lines),* realized that he would need to learn a lot more about electromagnetic waves, and found the information he needed in a book written by Max Abraham. He was then ready to come back and re-read Sommerfeld. Thermodynamics were also never really taught. For that he read the book written by Danke.[48]

Independent reading was also the basis for much of the sophisticated mathematics demonstrated by Bloch in his early papers. Although he had, by this time, taken courses in calculus as well as a seminar on complex functions theory taught by Weyl and Pólya, it was from a book by Richard Courant and David Hilbert† that Bloch "really learned" his mathematics,

---

*In the United States, I.I. Rabi was also reading during the same period Sommerfeld's classic book on spectral lines as well as material published by Bloch's physics professor, Peter Debye.

† Richard Courant, a younger colleague of David Hilbert, was a Jewish professor of mathematics at Germany's Göttingen University, an institution noted for its strong mathematics-physics tradition. When Hitler imposed his Law for the Restoration of the Career Civil Service on April 7, 1933, designed to rid Germany's civil service of those who were "politically unreliable" or of "non-Aryan" descent (read Jews), Göttingen was particularly hard hit as the directors of three of its four institutes for physics and mathematics were Jewish—James Franck, Max Born, and Richard Courant. All three were dismissed, although Born

(Continued on next page)

he said, while in bed with jaundice. Earlier, during another stint with ill-ness during his *gymnasium* years, he had learned applied analytic geome-try by not only reading the text, but by actually doing the calculations. Now, he applied the same discipline to Courant-Hilbert. "This I have done for a long time," Bloch said. "I'm sure that I owe my proficiency [in math-ematics] at a very early stage only to that. I did it as a game, just because I felt this is more entertaining than to solve crossword puzzles."[49]

Because Purcell and Bloch would later share the Nobel Prize for their work with NMR, it is interesting to note a parallel between Purcell's edu-cation and Bloch's during their third year of undergraduate work. For Bloch, it was academic year 1925-26; for Purcell, it was 1931-32. Each of them was given the rather unique opportunity at that point to work, in a self-directed manner, with spectroscopy. As mentioned in Chapter 3, Purcell was shown to the attic of the physics building in his junior year at Purdue University where "there was a Rowland grating and a mount that had not been used for a long, long time," and was instructed to set it up "all on my own" and "examine some spectra." The following year, Purcell would work with electron diffraction and find Debye-Scherrer rings "only five years after electron diffraction had been discovered."[50]

For Bloch, the opportunity to work in spectroscopy came about through Paul Scherrer himself, a faculty member at the ETH who, togeth-er with Debye, had first discovered the rings with which their names became associated. Bloch had read about band spectra, so he asked Scherrer about the possibility of measuring some spectra. Scherrer told him that would be fine and suggested he use the quartz spectrograph they had which measured spectra in the ultraviolet range.

> I didn't quite know how to go about it [said Bloch]. I went to Victor Henry [at the University of Zürich] who was a physical chemist and

---

(Continued from previous page)
and Courant were later notified that they were not affected by the law. By that time, how-ever, Born had already emigrated and Courant had already made arrangements to emigrate to England.

Decimated by Hitler's actions, the Mathematical Institute at Göttingen was left with few to carry on its tradition of excellence. Author Alan Beyerchen noted that "during the 1920s, Hilbert had received a blood transfusion from Courant, so the joke went that [after the dis-missals] there was only one Aryan mathematician in all of Göttingen, and in his veins flowed Jewish blood. By the end of 1933," Beyerchen added, "the joke was no longer amusing."

Sometime afterward, Hilbert was asked by the Nazi minister of education at a banquet, "And how is mathematics in Göttingen now that it has been freed of the Jewish influence?" Hilbert responded, "Mathematics in Göttingen? There is really none any more."
— Alan D. Beyerchen, *Scientists Under Hitler*, (New Haven, CT: Yale University Press, 1977), 6, 33, 36.

had done some spectra, and he gave me some hints, and pointed out to me that to adjust the spectrograph is a major enterprise, not simple. I played around a little bit. We took some spectra with an arc source; we got a discharge, got some ultraviolet light from that and took some spectra, but they were never very good. And I became a little tired of it, and somehow drifted away from the experiment.[51]

The reason for his loss of interest was probably not so much that spectroscopy became boring as that, in 1926, theoretical quantum mechanics suddenly became very exciting, and Bloch was an eyewitness to some of the key events as they unfolded. The opportunity to view history in the making came about, at least in part, because of Bloch's long-standing habit of calculating answers for himself and because he was so presumptuous as to challenge an assumption made by the eminent Peter Debye in the 1923 paper Debye had written on the Compton effect in electron scattering.

Having read a little bit about Sommerfeld, I realized there was an assumption which Debye made in his paper. He takes an electron at rest. Then he says, "Now I come to the collision with a light quantum, and I will calculate its momentum and thereby the momentum and energy of the scattered light quantum." And I said, "Well, there's something wrong here; after all, the electrons are not at rest. I just read in Sommerfeld that they are in motion." And I thought about it, just simply took the Debye formula but started with a moving electron and realized that this had some effect, at least, on the scattered light. I went, rather proud, in to Debye. I screwed up my courage and went to him, and he was rather nice. I said, "I've done that." And Debye said to me, "Yes, well, that may all be quite amusing, but you know, this is not at all any more what people think about the atom. This is all old-fashioned. You should learn about the new mathematics.[52]

The Right Place, The Right Time
Debye's admonition to Bloch to learn about the new mathematics couldn't have come at a more appropriate time—or place. In 1925-26, Zürich was one of several epicenters of the quantum mechanics revolution.

In 1925, a French prince and physicist, Louis Victor de Broglie, had published his doctoral thesis in which he theorized that electrons had both a particulate nature and a wave nature resulting from so-called pilot waves (now called de Broglie waves) that accompanied electrons in their quantized orbits.

At approximately the same time, Bloch began attending physics colloquia that were jointly sponsored and alternately hosted by the ETH and
the University of Zürich. Although the ETH had the larger, more illustrious faculty, said Bloch, physics was also taught at the University of
Zürich where "a certain Austrian" by the name of Erwin Schrödinger
held forth on theoretical physics. At the time, said Bloch, "The news that
the foundations of a new mechanics had already been laid by de Broglie
and Heisenberg had hardly leaked to Zürich yet and certainly had not
penetrated to our lower strata [of undergraduates]."[53]

De Broglie's thesis had not escaped the notice of Peter Debye, however, and it was at one of these colloquia, which attracted as many as a couple dozen physicists "on a good day," said Bloch, that Debye, who ran the
meetings with "firm authority," asked Schrödinger to report on the
recently-published thesis.

Although Bloch wouldn't swear as to the exact words Debye used, he
said he could "vouchsafe" as truth that Debye said something like:
"Schrödinger, you are not working right now on very important problems anyway. Why don't you tell us some time about that thesis of de
Broglie, which seems to have attracted some attention."[54]

Although experiments by C.J. Davisson and L.H. Germer[55] and, independently, by G.P. Thomson,[56] would soon verify the accuracy of de
Broglie's ideas, at the end of 1925 and the beginning of 1926 those ideas
were met with skepticism by most physicists, including Debye.

A few weeks after Debye assigned the de Broglie report to Schrödinger,
Bloch was in attendance at a subsequent colloquium and recalled
Schrödinger giving a "beautifully clear account of how de Broglie associated a wave with a particle and how he could obtain the quantization
rules of Niels Bohr and Sommerfeld by demanding that an integer number of waves should be fitted along a stationary orbit."[57]

Bloch also recalled that Debye, a former student of Sommerfeld who
had been taught that theories must be supported by equations, remarked
during the discussion period that followed that this sounded rather naive
to him. "I don't know whether he used the word 'kindisch' or 'childish' or
something like that—'naive.' . . . But the gist of it," Bloch said, "is that he
felt, quite naturally, that when one talks about wave phenomena, this
should be based on a discussion of the wave equation.[58] *

---

* When Bloch reminded Debye many years later of his remark about the wave equation,
Debye said he had forgotten about it, but then turned to Bloch and said with a smile: "Well,
wasn't I right?"
—F. Bloch, "Heisenberg and the early days of quantum mechanics," *Physics Today*, December 1976, 24.

At any rate, within a few weeks of Debye's skeptical reaction, said Bloch, Schrödinger gave another report at another colloquium which he introduced by saying, "My colleague Debye suggested that one should have a wave equation; well, I have found one!"[59] He then proceeded to spell out the details of his equation which would soon be published under the title "Quantization as Eigenvalue Problem" in *Annalen der Physik*.[60]

Bloch said he was still "too green" to appreciate the significance of Schrödinger's second talk, but he was able to discern from the general reaction of the others in attendance that "something rather important had happened, and I need not tell you what the name of Schrödinger has meant from then on."[61]

It was after the third colloquium, after Schrödinger had announced his equation, that Debye told Bloch not to bother with this "old-fashioned kind of atomic mechanics," but to study instead the new quantum mechanics put forth by Schrödinger.

Well, you would not disobey the authorities [said Bloch], and, of course, he was again quite right. So this is what I did; Schrödinger's next papers on wave mechanics appeared shortly, one after the other. I did not learn about the matrix formulation of quantum mechanics by Heisenberg, Max Born and Pascual Jordan[62-63] * until I read that paper of Schrödinger's[64] in which he showed the two formulations to lead to the same results.[65]

As alluded to in the above statement by Bloch, Schrödinger's wave mechanics was the second major quantum theory to be published in less than a year. In June of 1925, 23-year-old Werner Heisenberg of Göttingen University in Germany had also published a theory of quantum mechanics called matrix mechanics[66] but, because it used a mathematical approach called non-commutative algebra which was foreign to most physicists, it hadn't received an overwhelming response.

Schrödinger's mechanics, on the other hand, which used a traditional approach, was welcomed immediately. Ironically, apart from their mathematical framework, the two theories led to the same results. Of the

---

* Heisenberg's first paper on quantum mechanics did not mention matrix theory directly as he had not yet realized that his mathematical formulations were based on it. The matrix theory connection was made soon afterward in a paper by Heisenberg's colleagues at Göttingen, Max Born and Pascual Jordan and later developed further in a paper by all three authors.

almost unbelievable coincidence, physicist George Gamow wrote, "It was as if America was discovered by Columbus, sailing westward across the Atlantic Ocean, and by some equally daring Japanese, sailing eastward across the Pacific Ocean."[67]

Schrödinger's proof that the two approaches were identical, Gamow commented further, "was just as surprising as the statement that whales and dolphins are not fish like sharks and herring but animals like elephants or horses! But it was a fact, and today one uses wave-and-matrix mechanics intermittently depending on one's taste and convenience."[68]

Before 1927 was gone, Bloch would have an opportunity to work personally with both Schrödinger and Heisenberg. He would also form that year a close friendship with Walter Heitler and Fritz London. They had just finished their PhD's and had come to work at Schrödinger's Institute at the University of Zürich in 1926, where they were working on their theory of covalent bonds. "I must have met them in a seminar," said Bloch, "and it was a great thing for me that they asked me to join them in some of their walks through the forests around Zürich. For us students the professors lived somewhere in the clouds, and that two real theorists at the ripe age of almost 25 should even bother about a greenhorn like me was ample cause for my gratitude to them."[69]

No wonder then that Bloch was distracted from the spectroscopy experiment he had started in the basement of the ETH. After noticing that the apparatus had been left undisturbed for a number of weeks, Paul Scherrer asked Bloch about it, to which he replied, "Yes. Well, I now study quantum mechanics." Scherrer responded, "That's fine, as long as you do anything at all." Said Bloch, "That was the end of my experimental career, at least temporarily."[70]

It was during this same period that Bloch heard, either from Schrödinger or from Heitler and London—he couldn't recall for sure—about a new area of difficulty for physicists that had been brought about by the Schrödinger equation. The problem was one of interpretation. Although Schrödinger had provided a landmark equation for expressing de Broglie's wave theory, Schrödinger's interpretation of the equation's results, notated by the Greek letter psi (ψ), was deficient. What did psi really mean?

Bloch and his physicist friends posed the question in irreverent fashion by composing a verse in German:

Gar Manches rechnet Erwin Schon
Mit seiner Wellenfunktion.

Nur wissen möcht' man gerne wohl
Was man sich dabei vorstell'n soll.

Translated into its approximate English equivalent:

Erwin with his psi can do
Calculations quite a few
But one thing has not been seen—
Just what does psi really mean?

In telling the story, Bloch laughed and said, "The trouble was— Schrödinger didn't know himself! Born's interpretation [of psi] as probability amplitude came later, and of even that interpretation Schrödinger remained skeptical to the end of his life, along with no less company than Max Planck, Albert Einstein and Louis de Broglie."[71]

According to Max Born at the University of Göttingen, psi was not a hard-and-fast number, but rather a probability amplitude for a particular location that, if squared, would indicate your chances of finding an electron home at that spatial address at a particular point in time. This "iffy" development, and its implied abandonment of strict causality, was a dramatic departure from the quantitative certainties that physicists had come to expect.

Bloch recalled attending a seminar much later where someone, he said, "drew certain, quite extended conclusions from the Schrödinger equation." When Schrödinger, who was at the meeting, expressed grave doubts that his equation could be taken that seriously, Gregor Wentzel told him, 'Schrödinger, it is most fortunate that other people believe more in your equation than you do!'"[72]

On the other hand, Schrödinger also claimed more for his wave mechanics than quantum theorists were willing to allow. Whereas Einstein's 1905 paper on the photoelectric effect showed that light sometimes behaves like particles rather than waves, Schrödinger claimed that his wave theory balanced the scales in favor of classical physics with its continuous processes rather than quantum theory with its discontinuous jumps. With that Niels Bohr could not agree.

In a marathon meeting between the two at Copenhagen in the fall of 1926, Bohr sought to convince Schrödinger that his wave mechanics would have to co-exist with quantum mechanics, that both were reflections of reality. Even when Schrödinger became ill, Bohr would not let him rest until he admitted that his interpretation was insufficient to explain Planck's law.

As Heisenberg once told the story, Bohr, sitting by the bed of a miserable Schrödinger, would come back time and time again with: "But you must surely admit that . . ." Finally, Schrödinger responded in desperation, "If one has to go on with these damned quantum jumps, then I'm sorry that I ever started to work on atomic theory," to which Bohr responded consolingly, "But the rest of us are so grateful that you did."[73]

As Schrödinger continued to argue for continuous process and absolute determinism, Werner Heisenberg, also at Copenhagen during the same period, was struggling with some of the same questions but coming to opposite conclusions. Prodded one evening by a paradox that Einstein had once told him in the course of a conversation that "it is the theory which decides what we can observe," Heisenberg conceived what would become known as the Uncertainty Principle. This mathematics-based formulation said that, at the atomic level, one measurement always made a related measurement uncertain and that the product of uncertainties in measurements of position and momentum could not be smaller than Planck's constant h.

According to Heisenberg, the interactive jolt of taking a measurement, challenge enough in the world of classical physics where the impact of a measurement upon a continuum could be minimized, was impossible when applied to the sub-microscopic world of the quantum. In this world, where only discrete steps can be taken, any attempts to experimentally measure, for example, the location of an electron would, in the very act of measuring, alter the experimental data, which are complementary to one another.

Heisenberg's paper establishing his Uncertainty Principle was published in the spring of 1927.[74] The only thing certain, according to the momentous paper, was that "we cannot know, as a matter of principle, the present in all its details." Even if location x of a particle is known exactly, according to the Principle, the experimenter will not be able to exactly determine its velocity or momentum. In other words, know one component, and it becomes impossible to precisely know the other. Because the variables of x, location, and v, velocity, for example, are complementary, they cannot both be measured with precision at the same time. If x is exactly known, v or momentum must be assigned a range of values, with equal probability that v is any one of the values. Conversely, the less accurately you are able to determine location x, the more accurately you can determine the velocity v, all of which makes an environmental impact study of a measurement's effect difficult to determine with certainty.

Correlated with Bohr's Complementarity Principle which recognized a duality between particles and waves, Heisenberg's principle meant the end of determinism in physics and provided a theoretical boost to Born's probability argument with regard to the interpretation of *psi* in Schrödinger's equation.

Related to the "interpretation" problem of psi was the fact that, as Bloch expressed it, "wave packets ran apart, which bothered Schrödinger very much." For a time, said Bloch, Schrödinger thought that a wave packet represented the actual shape of an electron, but it "naturally bothered him that the thing had a tendency to spread out in time as if the electrons would actually get fatter and fatter."

Naively, said Bloch, I went to Schrödinger and told him, "Look, so far people have always spoken about the motion of electrons in an atom, but they haven't taken radiation damping into account. Maybe radiation damping will hold all the waves together."

"Believe it or not," said Bloch, Schrödinger thought it was a good idea and told him to try it, an effort that resulted in Bloch's first published paper, in which he was able to show the effect of radiation damping on a harmonic oscillator. Bloch would later realize that his hypothesis was a "very lousy idea" in regard to wave packets and that he had been "too naive to appreciate the depth of the problem."[75] He would have another chance, however, to explore the problem with Schrödinger's counterpart in the new quantum theory, Werner Karl Heisenberg, in the Weimar Republic of Germany.

Bloch in Germany

In 1927, just as Bloch was ready to begin working on his doctoral thesis, every physicist with whom he would have cared to work left Zürich, succumbing, Bloch said, "to the pull of the large magnet in the North,"[76] Germany's flourishing scientific environment.

Hermann Weyl, strong in relativity theory and mathematics, accepted a position at Göttingen University, a school noted for its strength in mathematics. Although Weyl would not leave until the following year, "it was known that he was going to leave," said Bloch. "Furthermore," he added, "I would not have worked with Weyl because I'm not a mathematician."[77]

Erwin Schrödinger, held in high esteem because of his wave mechanics contributions, went to Berlin, where he had been appointed professor of theoretical physics at Berlin University, succeeding Max Planck, who started the Quantum Revolution in 1900.

Peter Debye, who had derived Planck's law in a few lines in 1910 and had occupied the Einstein chair at the ETH ever since, accepted an appointment as director of the Institute of Physics at Leipzig University.

Had any of them had the prescience to have seen six years into the future, it is likely that none of them would have left neutral Switzerland, a country that had not been involved in a foreign war since 1515 and whose citizens were proud of their personal freedoms. All three—Weyl, Schrödinger and Debye—would be personally affected by Hitler's anti-Semitic Germany.

Weyl was not Jewish, but his wife was. Following Hitler's anti-Semitic civil-service edicts, Weyl resigned his position at Göttingen effective the end of 1933 to accept a position as a colleague of Einstein's at Princeton's Institute for Advanced Study in the United States.[78] Before the trauma of 1933, however, Weyl would publish an important work in Göttingen on group theory[79] and would collaborate with two other renowned mathematicians, Richard Courant and John von Neumann.*

The Austrian-born Schrödinger was not Jewish either, but he joined other petitioners, including Heisenberg, in requesting the reinstatement of Richard Courant,[80] one of three Jewish institute directors who had been dismissed from the University of Göttingen shortly after the enactment of the April 7 Civil Service Law. Later that year, Schrödinger protested the anti-Semitic actions of the Nazis by resigning from Berlin University and leaving for England. Soon afterward, however, he accepted a post at Graz in Austria at a time when Nazism was making its presence felt in that country and, because of his political activities, had to flee with barely enough time to take hand luggage. This time, he emigrated to Dublin, Ireland, where he would later make a seminal contribution to molecular biology with a series of 1943 lectures entitled "What is Life?"[81]

Dutch-born Peter Debye was also not Jewish, but he helped Austrian-born physicist Lise Meitner, who was part Jewish and therefore subject to

---

* John von Neumann, also Jewish, would emigrate to the United States much earlier than other physicists. In 1930, he and Eugene Wigner, who would also publish an important book on group theory in 1931, were hired by Princeton University. Concerning anti-Semitism in Germany in 1930, Wigner, who was Jewish, said, "There was no question in the mind of any person that the days of foreigners [in Germany], particularly with Jewish ancestry, were numbered. . . . It was so obvious that you didn't have to be perceptive. . . . It was like, 'Well, it will be colder in December.' Yes, it will be. We know it well." Von Neumann would later play a vital role at Los Alamos, along with Edward Teller, a Jewish fellow Hungarian, in determining the mathematical feasibility of implosion as a method for detonating an atomic bomb.

—Quote by Wigner from *The Making of the Atomic Bomb*, by Richard Rhodes, (New York: Simon and Schuster, 1988), 187.

Germany's anti-Semitic laws, escape from Berlin to Holland on one-and-a-half hours notice in 1938.[82] * In 1940, Debye would be forced to leave Germany for the United States when he refused to give up his Dutch citizenship and join the Nazi Reich.

In 1927, however, Hitler had not yet been given the opportunity to form, as Bloch would describe it, "a new Germany in his own frightful image."[83] In fact, two years of apparent prosperity still remained before the world economy would collapse in the fall of 1929 and Germany would begin to experience the runaway inflation that would cause them to choose any economic savior, even a diabolical one. To Bloch, the main objective in 1927 was to begin working on his doctoral thesis and get on with his career in physics. With all the professors leaving Zürich that he considered possible mentors, "it was clear to me," said Bloch, "that I had to join the exodus if I did not want my time as a student to drag on much longer."[84]

The question [said Bloch] was only where to go; I was tempted to follow either London's example and go with Schrödinger to Berlin, or Heitler's, and go to Göttingen. Before deciding, however, I went to ask Debye for his opinion, and he advised me to do neither but instead to come to Leipzig. There I would work with Heisenberg whom [Debye], as the new director of the Institute of Physics of the University, had persuaded to accept the professorship for theoretical

---

* Later that year, in exile near Stockholm, Meitner was notified by her long-time chemist collaborator, Otto Hahn, who remained in Berlin (he was not Jewish), that research she had initiated and which Hahn and Fritz Strassmann had continued after her departure from Germany had produced mystifying results. Bombardment of uranium 239 with neutrons had yielded what they thought was barium 138 and masurium 101 (today called technetium). Was that possible? Lise Meitner, together with her nephew, Otto Robert Frisch, also in exile from Germany and working at Bohr's Institute in Copenhagen, performed the calculations that confirmed, yes, it was physically possible for one element to be divided into two other elements lower on the periodic chart, thus validating theoretically the discovery of nuclear fission. [Ref. a]

Although he was not anti-Semitic and was anti-Nazi, Otto Hahn was unwilling to share the credit for the discovery of fission with Meitner who had initiated the experiments that led to it and who, along with Frisch, provided the theory for it when it was found. "Within a month [after the discovery,]" wrote science writer Sharon Bertsch McGrayne, "Hahn was claiming that physics had impeded the discovery and that chemistry alone had solved it." Hahn was awarded the 1944 Nobel Prize in chemistry for his discovery. Strassmann, a gifted experimentalist hired by Meitner, was also not recognized for his important contributions. He was, however, honored posthumously by the Holocaust Memorial in Jerusalem for sheltering a Jew in his apartment during the war. [Ref. b]

— [a] Roger H. Stuewer, "Bringing the news of fission to America," *Physics Today*, October 1985, 50, 53-54; [b] Sharon Bertsch McGrayne, *Nobel Prize Women in Science*, (New York: Carol Publishing, 1993), 51, 60.

physics. Debye's power of persuasion was quite formidable and I could not resist it either, particularly because I had previous evidence of his sound judgment.[85]

On another occasion, Bloch said he may have also chosen Leipzig because he would know at least one professor. At any rate, that October, "before the beginning of the winter semester," said Bloch, "I left my nice home town for the first time, to arrive on a cold gray morning in that rather ugly city of Leipzig."

The little room I found for rent from a family overlooked a railroad yard; the noise and smoke did not help much to cheer me up! As soon as I had completed the simple formality of registering as a student of the University in the center of the city I went to the Physics Institute, which was located near the outskirts.

It was an old building opposite a cemetery on one side and adjoining the garden of a mental institution on the other, but occupied by people who were far from being either dead or crazy.[86]

Because Heisenberg had not yet arrived, Bloch was met at the Institute by physics theorist Gregor Wentzel, who welcomed him into his third-floor apartment. It was quite customary at that time, said Bloch, for professors to have official living quarters in or near their institutes. Young bachelors like Wentzel and Heisenberg were given small but comfortable apartments under the same roof as the Institute. Debye, as the Institute's director, had a villa in a side wing.

Bloch said he was used to "the great distance that separated the students and professors in freedom-loving Switzerland," and therefore, considering "the proverbial discipline of the Germans," expected an "even stricter caste system." Instead, he was welcomed by Wentzel with the "informal cordiality of a colleague" which, said Bloch, "made it almost difficult to address him with the normal 'Herr Professor' but very easy to show him a little paper I had written before I came to Leipzig."[87]

The "little paper" Bloch showed Wentzel was the one he had written on radiation damping of harmonic oscillators. Although he made some kind comments, said Bloch, Wentzel declined to critically analyze the paper, claiming insufficient knowledge of the subject and deferring judgment instead to Heisenberg, who was expected in a few days.

When Heisenberg arrived and met Bloch for the first time, any passer-by seeing the two young men shaking hands would not have suspected that the older was the PhD mentor of the younger. With less than four years difference in age between them—Bloch turned 22 that October and Heisenberg was still two months short of 26—the word "founder" would not have come to mind for describing either of them. Yet Heisenberg was already "very famous," said Bloch, as the founder of quantum mechanics and, within a year or so, Bloch himself would qualify as one of the founders of modern solid-state physics.

With his freckles, red hair and boyish, outdoorsy appearance, Heisenberg may have looked younger than Bloch—even Bloch was taken aback momentarily by Heisenberg's youthful appearance. Five years earlier, Heisenberg had accompanied his mentor, Arnold Sommerfeld, from Munich to Göttingen to hear a visiting lecturer, the eminent Niels Bohr and, during the lecture, had objected to one of Bohr's statements. Rather than being irked by the impetuous youngster, Bohr had sought him out afterward, invited him for a walk over the Hain Mountain, and, even more significantly, invited him to his institute at Copenhagen. As a result, Bohr was congenially "arrested" the next evening at a dinner given in his honor by two uniformed Göttingen "policemen," actually two students, on the charge of "kidnapping young children," referring, of course, to Heisenberg.[88]

One of Heisenberg's friends described him during that period as even "greener" than he was. As a member of the Youth Movement in Germany, he often wore, "even after reaching man's estate," he said, "an open shirt and walking shorts."[89] Richard Rhodes points out that "in the Youth Movement young Germans on hiking tours built campfires, sang folk songs, talked of knighthood and the Holy Grail and of service to the Fatherland," and adds, "many were idealists, but authoritarianism and anti-Semitism already bloomed dangerously among them."[90]

When Heisenberg came to Copenhagen, Bohr, who was Jewish, asked him whether he had personally encountered any anti-Semitism. Acknowledging that he had observed it, Heisenberg attributed it to old officers embittered by World War I, and said, "but we don't take these groups very seriously."[91]

As soon as Bloch and Heisenberg shook hands and Heisenberg started talking in his "simple, natural way," Bloch immediately felt that he was "accepted."[92]

> I had a tremendous impression of Heisenberg, right from the beginning. I mean we struck it off very well; he was extremely kind to me. I was his first student so I had a lot of time [with him]; I participated

immediately in the seminars and established a very close and good connection with Heisenberg and admired him tremendously.[93]

Despite the fact that Heisenberg was only four years Bloch's senior, putting them into the same generation chronologically, to Bloch those four years could have been four decades. "In the time scale of theorists this . . . put him something like two generations ahead of me,"[94] * he said.

Nevertheless, Bloch once described his relationship with Heisenberg as one of "almost friendship,"[95] with the qualifier "almost" paying homage to both the positional gap separating PhD mentor and PhD candidate and the generational gap existing between the leader of a revolution and his disciple. He and Heisenberg would eat lunch together, Bloch said, and on weekends would go skiing on the southern border of Germany, their discussions ranging over a wide variety of topics, including physics but not limited to physics. "Physics and everyday life," explained Bloch, "were not separate in our lives. It was all the same."[96]

They had similar interests. In addition to skiing and mountain climbing, they both played the piano, Heisenberg probably the more proficient of the two—Bloch described him as "excellent,"[97] a description confirmed by George Gamow, who wrote that "in spite of his great fame as a physicist, [Heisenberg] was better known in Leipzig . . . as a first-class piano player."[98]

"It was from Heisenberg, as his first doctorate student," Bloch once told a meeting of The American Physical Society, "that I caught the spirit of research, and that I received the encouragement to make my own contributions."[99]

For Bloch, this spirit of research was more than discovering and accumulating facts about the physical world. It was a mix of experiment and theory, of physics as science and physics as philosophy.

Bloch once recalled coming back to his apartment after dinner and hearing Heisenberg practicing on the piano. Late that evening, Heisenberg came down to Bloch's apartment, confessed that he had been

---

* Physicist Abraham Pais, Detlev W. Bronk Professor of Physics Emeritus at Rockefeller University and a professor at the Institute of Advanced Study in Princeton, New Jersey from 1950 to 1963, has noted the same time warp. "In those times a variance in age of but a few years could amount to a generational difference. To mention but one example, Robert Oppenheimer, who made his mark in quantum field theory, was only four years younger than Pauli. Yet, when in later years I was on occasion together with both, I noted how Oppenheimer understandably treated Pauli as the veteran of battles waged in his childhood."
—Abraham Pais, *Inward Bound*, (New York: Oxford University Press, 1986), 362.

practicing a few bars of a Schumann concerto for three hours, but then told of Franz Liszt who, when he was already a famous pianist, became dissatisfied with his scales of thirds and fifths and canceled all appointments for a full year to devote himself to nothing but those scales before resuming any performances.

Bloch felt that, in telling the story, Heisenberg had told him something important about himself, that just as the audience of Liszt may have felt that his playing of the piano came effortlessly, so Heisenberg's intuitive approach to physics, in which solutions seemed to come to him as if "out of the blue sky," was the result of what Bloch called the "Liszt phenomenon." The dreamy expression on Heisenberg's face even while participating in and enjoying social activities indicated that "in the inner recesses of the brain, [Heisenberg] continued his all-important thoughts on physics," a self-discipline which, in Bloch's estimation, made Heisenberg's accomplishments all the more admirable.[100]

Bloch also credited Heisenberg with the ability to keep divergent concepts of reality in proper perspective, an important trait to Bloch who once said, "the most significant contribution of quantum mechanics . . . has been its influence on our concept of reality."[101] The challenge, said Bloch, is to retain objectivity even as our experiences grow beyond the events of our daily lives. Heisenberg, he said, was able to keep that objectivity. As an example, Bloch told of a conversation they had about space on one of their many walks. Having just read Hermann Weyl's book *Space, Time and Matter,* Bloch proudly informed his mentor that space was simply the field of linear operations, to which Heisenberg responded, "Nonsense. Space is blue and birds fly through it."

"I knew him well enough by that time," said Bloch, "to fully understand the rebuke. What he meant was that it is dangerous for a physicist to describe nature in terms of idealized abstractions too far removed from the evidence of actual observation."[102]

As theoretical physicists, however, neither Heisenberg nor his protégé had much scientific contact with Leipzig's experimental physicists. Although he acknowledged that he was speaking somewhat facetiously, Bloch once said, "There was a certain attitude among the theorists at that time, so to say, we don't really need the experimentalists; we know better. . . . You didn't just go and ask an experimenter for some curve and then you say, 'Aha, now I have to explain this curve.' It was the other way around. You made your theory, and then you came to him, and if his experiments agreed with it, fine. If they didn't, you said he made a mistake."[103]

Because of their rapport, Bloch did not take offense when he showed his paper on radiation damping to Heisenberg and Heisenberg immediately discarded its usefulness with regard to wave packets. As Bloch recalled Heisenberg's reaction, "he only smiled and said that, if anything, it could of course only make them spread even more. Nevertheless he thought my calculations on the harmonic oscillator were a good start, and that I should go on to work them out for the general case."[104]

For Bloch, who was already beginning to doubt the thesis of his paper anyway, Heisenberg's view made him feel, "Well, that settles it. There's no use worrying about that any longer."[105]

"With the help of P.A.M. Dirac's paper on radiation effects," said Bloch, "and a few more tricks, I managed to [make the changes] rather quickly, confirming Heisenberg's prediction, and it became my first published paper. It appeared in the *Physikalische Zeitschrift* as a precursor to the well-known paper of Victor Weisskopf and Eugene Wigner on radiation damping and natural line widths."[106]

Shortly before Christmas break in 1927, Heisenberg suggested to Bloch that it was time to start thinking of a topic to investigate for his doctoral thesis, which Bloch did while skiing in the Swiss Alps. Knowing the importance of Paul Ehrenfest's adiabatic theorem as expressed under the old quantum theory, Bloch thought about reformulating it for quantum mechanics. When he mentioned that to Heisenberg upon returning to Germany, however, Heisenberg told him, "Yes, one might do that, but I think you had better leave such things to the learned gentlemen of Göttingen."[107]

Heisenberg's implication was that the Max Born school in Göttingen was better suited for such a task with its reputation and fondness for, as Bloch expressed it, "elaborate mathematical formalisms." Instead, Heisenberg "sort of in a gentle way," said Bloch, suggested that perhaps he should focus on something "more down to earth" such as either the conductivity of metals or ferromagnetism.[108]

Because Bloch hadn't done much with magnetism at the time, and because Heisenberg seemed to have his own theories about it "already in a nutshell," Bloch took Heisenberg's first suggestion and soon became interested in "this question of metal electrons."[109] As far as he was concerned, there was also a greater challenge in exploring the properties of metals. Heisenberg himself followed up his other suggestion and began studying the question of ferromagnetism, writing a paper that Bloch said laid the groundwork for the modern theory of ferromagnetism. "It wasn't until two years later that I somewhat embellished his treatment," Bloch said modestly, "by the introduction of spin waves."[110]

Electron Theory of Metals

Science historians Lillian H. Hoddeson and G. Baym divide the quantum theory of metals into three periods: 1) Classical, 1900-26; 2) semi-classical, 1926-28; and 3) modern, late 1928 and onward. They associate the classical period with the Paul Drude and H.A. Lorentz model in which a metal was said to contain, as Hoddeson and Baym described it, an "ideal gas of conduction electrons governed by kinetic energy."[111] This model was proven deficient by the end of World War I, and it wasn't until Wolfgang Pauli applied statistics in 1926, which had been independently developed that same year by Enrico Fermi and P.A.M. Dirac, that significant new concepts were added. This foundation was then strengthened by Arnold Sommerfeld and others—primarily his students—who applied the new statistics to the Drude-Lorentz theory.

The resultant hybrid, Sommerfeld's "free electron theory," as it was called, was much more understandable and agreed more completely with experimental data than any previous theory of metals, but because it was a hybrid and did not take full advantage of the quantum-mechanical theories developed by Heisenberg, Schrödinger, and Dirac, it still fell short. It did not always reflect experimental results and it failed to answer certain key questions. Hans Bethe, for example, felt that Sommerfeld should have explained why the electrons in his free electron theory should be considered free. Others felt that Sommerfeld failed to deal with a key question when he neglected to account for interaction between ions and electrons. Yet there was no denying that, at least for the most part, Sommerfeld's theory seemed to work. It just wasn't clear why it should work as well as it did.[112]

That question was answered by a 22-year-old by the name of Felix Bloch. The quantum-mechanical foundation that he provided for Sommerfeld's semi-classical model in his PhD thesis (submitted as an article to *Zeitschrift für Physik* in August 1928[113]) was enough to satisfy the reservations of Hans Bethe who reflected many years later: "I believed the whole [Sommerfeld] theory only when the Bloch paper appeared."[114]

In a 1976 speech to the American Physical Society in which he reflected on the early days of quantum mechanics and his association with Werner Heisenberg, Bloch reviewed the theory of metals as it stood in 1928 and explained how he arrived at his conclusions. Noting the advancements Pauli and Sommerfeld had brought to the field, Bloch pointed out, however, that both men had held on to the Drude-Lorentz idea that conduction electrons were an ideal gas of free electrons, an assumption which, to Bloch, "didn't appear in the least plausible."

> When I started to think about it [said Bloch], I felt that the main problem was to explain how the electrons could sneak by all the ions in a metal so as to avoid a mean free path of the order of atomic distances. Such a distance was much too short to explain the observed resistances, which even demanded that the mean free path become longer and longer with decreasing temperature. But Heitler and London had already shown how electrons could jump between two atoms in a molecule to form a covalent bond, and the main difference between a molecule and a crystal was only that there were many more atoms in a periodic arrangement. To make my life easy, I began by considering wave functions in a one-dimensional periodic potential.* By straight Fourier analysis I found to my delight that the wave differed from the plane wave of free electrons only by a periodic modulation.[115]

In other words, the issue that Sommerfeld had neglected—the interaction of electrons with ions—Bloch had dealt with as the "main problem," and then found it wasn't as big a problem as he had supposed. "This was so simple," he said, "that I didn't think it could be much of a discovery, but when I showed it to Heisenberg, he said right away, 'That's it!' Well, that wasn't quite it yet, and my calculations were only completed in the summer when I wrote my thesis on "The Quantum Mechanics of Electrons in Crystal Lattices."[116]

> I was not the only one who said it was absurd to think that the electrons just run freely through a metal [Bloch once pointed out]. I got so much applause after that, I was quite surprised, but it shows that people had been waiting for that. I was not the only one who thought that [the free electron approach] was crazy.[117]

---

* The key to Bloch's successful physical theory of the periodic electron wave functions, Erwin Hahn has noted, was his use of an important mathematical theorem known as Floquet's theorem.
—Personal communication from Hahn to writer, 22 January 1995.

"It was not until Bloch's paper in August 1928," wrote Hoddeson and Baym, "that the full machinery of quantum mechanics, developed in 1925-26, was brought to bear on solids, thereby spearheading the creation between 1928 and 1933 . . . of the modern quantum theory of solids."[118]

By tracing the wake of this "spearheading" paper, one comes to the clear conclusion, as Anatole Abragam pointed out in a memorial tribute to Bloch, that "with this article he laid the foundations for an electron theory of solids not only applicable to metals but also to crystalline solids in general and in particular to semiconductors, the applications of which are of dominant importance in our present-day industrial civilization."[119]

The far-reaching impact of Bloch's thesis is all the more amazing when you realize that, within a week or two of Heisenberg's suggestion to Bloch that he consider a more "down-to-earth" topic for his thesis such as the conductivity of metals, Bloch had come up with the essential idea "that a periodic arrangement is not really an obstacle for waves, but it's only the thermal vibrations."

> I mean, I didn't know anything [said Bloch]. But anyhow, I did it in an extremely primitive way. All I did was . . . I said, 'Well, I'll make a Fourier analysis; if it is periodic, then I'll make a Fourier analysis of the waves, also.' Then I realized that nothing is happening. By putting the Fourier components together, I realized that it's a wave that's modulated.[120]

H.E. Rorschach, Jr., speaking at a 40th-anniversary symposium commemorating Bloch's 1928 electron theory of metals, stated: "The result of [Bloch's] very beautiful analysis, presented in the opening part of [his 1928] paper, was the discovery of the 'Bloch waves'—plane waves multiplied by a function periodic in the lattice constant, whose character depends on the nature of the interaction." The list of "thoroughly treated topics" covered in the balance of the paper, said Rorschach, is "overwhelmingly impressive," and sufficient alone "to establish Felix Bloch as one of the fathers of solid-state physics."[121]

Although Bloch always readily acknowledged that Heisenberg had suggested the topic of his thesis, he said it was not true that Heisenberg had suggested that he study electrons in the periodic potential, as had been stated in Heisenberg's obituary by Nevill Mott and Rudolf Peierls. What was true, said Bloch, was that Heisenberg said, "Look, there's all that work of Sommerfeld and Pauli on the free electrons, and I think it would be interesting to look into that."[122] Bloch took it from there, coming up himself with his periodic-potential approach, quickly satisfying Heisenberg that he was on the right track.

Had the challenge of formulating a quantum-mechanical theory of metals been presented to Bloch even four years later, it's possible that he may have approached it with more fear and trepidation. Although both he and Heisenberg enjoyed physics as philosophy, neither of them approached that aspect of physics with the same reverence as Niels Bohr. Until late 1931 and early 1932, when Bloch worked with Niels Bohr in Copenhagen, Bloch's approach to physics had been molded by the attitude of the first eminent physicist with whom he had come in contact, Peter Debye.

> My attitude [Bloch said] was, of course, determined through the influence of Debye very much at that time. I mean nobody pushed me into these philosophical problems; I didn't care. I felt, [in regard to some of the 1926 discussions about the interpretation of psi], "Well, there are nice things coming out, and let's see what's coming of it." That there is something profound in it I had a first inkling of, but only an inkling, under Heisenberg, and to the real things my eyes didn't become opened except through Bohr. That was much later. In fact, I had some reluctance at the beginning, a typical Debye attitude. "Why speculate about these things we know how to calculate?"[123]

It's interesting to note the different perspectives of Felix Bloch and I.I. Rabi in regard to the Spirit of Copenhagen. Rabi was in Copenhagen in the fall of 1927 but was transferred to Hamburg two months later. Although he regretted at the time his short tenure in Denmark, he later was thankful that he had escaped the *Kopenhagener Geist,* as he felt it might have changed his approach to experimentation. Felix Bloch would be in Copenhagen four years after Rabi but, in contrast, would be forever grateful that he was affected by the Copenhagen Spirit, which emphasized theoretical discussion over experimentation. A reflection of Bohr himself, who preferred learning by discussion, it was a spirit that could make you shiver.

> Bohr kept on saying [said Bloch], "If somebody doesn't shiver when he learns quantum mechanics, then he hasn't understood it."
> We said, "We are not such cowards. We don't shiver." We realized, of course, what Bohr meant. And this dawned on me only very, very slowly, later, how profound this thing goes, and that one really has to shiver.

Evidently [Bohr] had a rather good opinion of me; he thought it was a shame that this man should run through life and be so blind and not even realize all the dangerous depths. . . . I was more of the aggressive type and felt that solving problems was the interesting thing.[124]

In the fall of 1928, however, the haunts of Bohr's Institute for Theoretical Physics were still three years off in Bloch's career. Instead, now that Bloch had his PhD, Heisenberg thought that Bloch should go to Zürich and work with Wolfgang Pauli, a physicist who could make you shiver with fear because of his caustic tongue. Reflecting on the year he had spent with Heisenberg in Leipzig, Bloch said 36 years later, "It was really a year of tremendous growth . . . at the end of my Leipzig period, when I got my PhD, though there were still very great gaps, I think I was essentially at that time a physicist."[125]

Had Bloch remained in Leipzig a few more months, he would have met Rabi, who had just completed a year at the University of Hamburg working with Wolfgang Pauli and Otto Stern and who was now planning on spending some time working with Werner Heisenberg. Heisenberg, however, didn't know of Rabi's plans—Rabi showed up unannounced—and had already made his own plans to go on a lecture trip to the United States. In the meantime, Pauli moved to Zürich.

Because of Heisenberg's imminent departure for the United States, Rabi's stay in Leipzig lasted only two months and by March of 1929 he, too, was on his way to the University of Zürich to work with Pauli. There, for a period of four or five months, until Rabi's return to the United States to take up a lectureship he had been offered by Columbia University, both he and Bloch would be working with Wolfgang Pauli.

1928-33

It was on Heisenberg's recommendation that Bloch was accepted by Pauli as his assistant, an assignment that Bloch took with some misgivings because of Pauli's reputation for having a sharp, critical tongue. Heisenberg laughed off Bloch's concern, but Bloch had met Pauli before and was afraid of him.

His foreboding was not unfounded. "The transition from Leipzig to Zürich," Bloch recalled later, "was to go from optimism to pessimism."[126] Pauli was often depressed at the time, and felt that things were not going well, a perspective that Bloch attributed to Pauli's personality as well as to the negative view Pauli had in 1928 about the state of physics.

In 1928, when Paul A.M. Dirac published his famous paper in which he generalized Schrödinger's equation by incorporating the demands of the theory of relativity and providing new insights on the electron, most physicists, including Heisenberg, were immediately impressed by it. Bloch, however, was less than impressed by the paper and when he told Heisenberg that he thought its conclusions were "rather obvious," Heisenberg had implied that such a reaction was naive and cocky. When told by an interviewer that he was the first person he had talked to who had ever reacted that way to Dirac's paper on the electron, Bloch replied, "Maybe I'm the first honest person . . . I thought it was trivial."[127] On this, Bloch and Pauli agreed, only Pauli felt that, in addition to the paper being trivial, it was not at all convincing. "He was very critical about Dirac," Bloch said, "he always was. He thought that Dirac was a rather shallow thinker, and of course only a man like Pauli has a right to say that."[128]

At any rate, partly because of Pauli's pessimistic perspectives and partly because Bloch was living at home with his parents again at a time in his life when he had become "too independent and did not want to be the boy any more at home," he too was "rather depressed" during this period and looked for the first opportunity to get away from Zürich. "Indeed," he said in 1964, "I never lived in Zürich again, after that."[129]

As Pauli's assistant, Bloch didn't have very much work to do, beyond correcting the papers of some of Pauli's students. As for research, Pauli thought the theory of electrical conductivity put forth by Bloch in his thesis was fine, but the real interesting problem was superconductivity and that Bloch should now give his attention to that phenomenon.

Bloch did come up with the idea, independently of Lev Davidovich Landau in the Soviet Union, that "the immense stability of superconductive currents could not be just a selection principle, some very highly forbidden transition, because nothing in the world is that highly forbidden," but instead, it must be comparable to spontaneous magnetization, which occurs at the lowest energy state. "For the same reason," said Bloch, "we felt that there must be an energy minimum connected with a current."[130]

Pauli immediately accepted that hypothesis and said, "Yes, of course, that's the explanation." Unfortunately, it wasn't that simple. Although Bloch produced a number of theories, "at the rate of about one every few weeks," he said, it usually took Pauli only about five or 10 minutes to find the flaw and to send him back to the drawing board. In fact, Pauli became rather angry and annoyed by Bloch's repeated failures and would tell him, "This is a simple problem. You're always making these mistakes!" or "Well, that I don't believe. You have neglected this term. . . . I'm not convinced."[131] After correcting all the errors that Pauli pointed out, Bloch would find, once again, that his latest revision also did not account for the phenomenon of persistent currents. Whenever there was an energy minimum, there was also zero current.

One time, when Pauli was either "apparently not awake, or he felt too well," Bloch said, he temporarily convinced Pauli that he had developed the correct theory of superconductivity. "He believed it, so naturally I believed it, too," said Bloch, "and I started already to work on the magnetic field. Otto Stern was visiting Zürich at the time from Hamburg and Pauli told Stern, 'Yes, I think that Bloch knows now the theory of superconductivity. There are some more details about the magnetic field he's worrying about now, but that's not important.' " Before long, however, that attempt too was disproven. "So I got nowhere," said Bloch.[132]

Bloch actually achieved more than he thought. Although he was unsuccessful in formulating a theory of superconductivity, he did clarify the fundamental difficulties in what has come to be known as Bloch's theorem. Jokingly summarized by Bloch as "any theory of superconductivity can be disproven,"[133] it is more accurately stated as "there can be no superconductivity in the absence of external fields."[134]

Bloch made about 10 attempts in all to devise a theory of superconductivity during his time with Pauli in Zürich. "Nowadays," he told Anatole Abragam in 1954, "whenever somebody brings me a theory of superconductivity, I simply say, 'That is my attempt such-and-such.' " Three years later, in 1957, Abragam noted, "Bardeen, Cooper and Schrieffer proposed a theory of superconductivity known as 'BCS,' which Bloch never really liked but had to accept in the end."[135]

After Bloch had been in Zürich about a year, two options became available. One was to go to Göttingen to work as an assistant to Max Born. The other was to go to Holland, to Utrecht, as a Lorentz Fellow to work with Hendrik Kramers. Bloch chose Holland, a decision, he said, that was influenced by both Heisenberg and Pauli, who were somewhat critical of the Göttingen school and its highly formalized mathematics; besides, Bloch felt, he had already been to Germany.

After Bloch's "rather unhappy time"[136] in Zürich, marked both by constant exposure to the perils of Pauli as well as an injury he received while skiing, Bloch had a "very fine time"[137] in Holland. He was immediately accepted by Kramers as a personal friend, and together, they enjoyed music, discussed poetry, talked about Robert Oppenheimer, and, of course, physics.

From a physics perspective, Holland was productive for Bloch in two ways. First, he corrected in a follow-up paper submitted to *Zeitschrift für*

Physik[138] an error he had discovered in his doctoral thesis and, in the process, formulated his famous T^5 law, which proved that his electron theory of metals was also capable of explaining experimental data obtained regarding the resistance of metals at low temperatures. Second, Bloch found that Heisenberg's recently-published theory about ferromagnetism could be improved. "Heisenberg had pulled some rather daring swindles there," he said.[139] Bloch was able to show that, at very low temperatures, almost all the spins are parallel, thus establishing the idea of spin waves. "With the development of the concept of the spin wave," said Rorschach, "Bloch became the founder of all the modern developments based on the idea of quasiparticle excitations."[140]

The first six months of Bloch's time in Holland was spent with Kramers in Utrecht, and the next few months with Adriaan Fokker* in Haarlem. Fokker, then the director of a scientific museum and laboratory called the Teyler Foundation, lived the life of a gentleman there, said Bloch, and basically wanted Bloch to bring him up to date on Pauli matrices and other current developments. "It was just a very nice time," said Bloch, though not particularly productive. Bloch did, however, assist Fokker in his studies of the spinning electron.[141]

Two years after leaving Leipzig, Bloch returned there in the fall of 1930, this time as Heisenberg's assistant. He would be there for one year before departing for Copenhagen and the Niels Bohr Institute as an Oersted Fellow. Notable during that second one-year period in Leipzig was the publication of what Bloch described as "a long and learned paper on ferromagnetism and hysteresis,"[142] thus fulfilling the requirements for his *Habilitationsschrift*, a "second thesis" required for those planning to pursue an academic career at a German university. As with his original thesis, Bloch used the academic requirement as an opportunity to make another significant discovery, the transition areas separating the oppositely-magnetized domains of a ferromagnetic crystal. These areas have since come to be known appropriately as "Bloch walls."

During the time that Bloch had been away from Leipzig, the physics program at the Institute had grown, but there was also a growing feeling among the "younger" people that the revolution was over and, as Bloch said, that "quantum mechanics was getting dull, that one was just doing

---

* Eight years later, Fokker would also be one of those who helped Jewish physicist Lise Meitner escape from Germany through Holland. Others who helped her escape were Peter Debye, Dirk Coster and W.J. de Haas.
— Alan D. Beyerchen, *Scientists Under Hitler*, (New Haven, CT: Yale University Press, 1977), 222n33.

more of the applications, and that the most exciting things were really done."[143] In a way, they were right, as 1930 is seen by many in retrospect as the end of the Quantum Revolution.

> I don't think many of us realized that we had just gone through quite a unique era [said Bloch]; we thought that this was just the way physics was normally to be done and only wondered why clever people had not seen that earlier. Almost any problem that had been tossed around years before could now be reopened and made amenable to a consistent treatment.
>
> To be sure, there were a few minor difficulties left . . . but we were sure that the solutions were just around the corner and that any new ideas that might be called for in the process would be easily supplied in the unlikely event that this should be necessary. Well, the last 50 years have taught us [said Bloch in 1976] at least to be a little more modest in our expectations.[144]

Although he had gotten off the starting blocks quickly with his doctoral thesis and had soon added other significant insights to the theory of metals and magnetism, even Bloch had exhibited what he called "some sleep-walking qualities"[145] that kept him from dealing with the deep, philosophical problems raised by the new quantum mechanics. Neither Debye nor Heisenberg had been greatly concerned with Bloch's somnambulism; Niels Bohr, on the other hand, could not tolerate any avoidance of underlying issues. On Heisenberg's recommendation, Bloch was granted an Oersted Fellowship and in the fall of 1931, he was sent to Copenhagen to be awakened from his slumber by Niels Bohr.

"In those days," Bloch said, "Bohr and especially his brother Harald, noted mathematician, were most widely known for their skill in soccer. Today," he said, "Niels Bohr is clearly part of a team composed, let us say, of Archimedes, Newton, and Einstein, with a fair sprinkling of Socrates and Spinoza."[146]

At the time Bloch worked with him in Copenhagen, Bohr was 46 and Bloch was 25, and when they first met, Bohr asked him if he belonged to "that gang," referring to other young physicists like George Gamow and Mel Delbruck who were becoming known for their practical jokes and frivolous behavior.

When he admitted that he had sometimes played a small part, Bohr smiled, said Bloch, and using the royal 'we' of majesty, responded, "We do not take very seriously their lack of respect!"[147]

The Bohr Institute was a true multi-national environment, with the physicists switching from one language to another, as the need or mood arose. Bloch and Heisenberg, who visited together frequently, usually spoke German, as did Bohr at times. Most of them picked up Danish fairly well, and when they were discussing physics, they would usually speak in English.[148]

If Debye lived by the philosophy, "Why speculate when we can calculate?," Bohr preferred to speculate about the ramifications of quantum physics at length, and he preferred to rehearse his contemplations out loud, in the presence of one or more others. According to Thomas Kuhn, Bohr always dictated his papers, using his "stenographer" as a sounding board. His mother had "done" his thesis, his family his Nobel Prize essay. Even Heisenberg had taken his turn while at the Institute in taking down dictation from Bohr.[149]

> He would walk around the room and dictate, [said Heisenberg] and I would try to put it down on paper. When writing a paper, Bohr would always change the sentence again and again. He could have filled half a page with a few sentences and then everything was crossed out and changed again. And even when the whole paper was almost finished—say, 10 pages or so—the next day everything would be changed again. It was a continuous process of improvement, change and discussions with others. This extreme care in formulating a paper was quite new to me. . . . The final text of Bohr's paper was so subtle. He would think about half an hour whether in a certain case he would use the indicative or the conjunctive and so on. The reader would just read over it and would not realize how much work was put into it.[150]

The same kind of *sorgfalt*, extreme care, said Heisenberg, was taken by Bohr in every activity, whether writing an administrative letter—one simple letter could take hours—or conversing about physics.

Despite Bohr's perfectionism, Heisenberg felt the process had helped him clarify the issues and, in the fall of 1930, it was Bloch's turn for the Bohr treatment. Bloch went to Copenhagen by way of Russia at the invitation of future Nobel laureate L. D. Landau, whom he had met the year before in Utrecht, and with whom he had formed a close friendship. He then traveled on to Denmark by way of Finland and Sweden. Once in Copenhagen, he lived in the same house as Bohr, which gave Bloch an opportunity to take his turn at dictation.

He was always behind in his publications . . . and I promised him that I'd write them up. I would jot a sentence down, which immediately had to be crossed out again. In the meantime, Bohr walked 'round and 'round and 'round. Then he always said, "Let's talk about something else." So in bits and pieces, what I learned from him I got that way.[151]

Rather than becoming exasperated with Bohr's method, Bloch, like Heisenberg, also came to appreciate Bohr's concern for the details, a concern that is probably responsible to some degree for the elegance and clarity for which Bloch's papers are known, as well as his approach to physics itself. "I think from that time on, whatever problem I dealt with, I've always felt more like saying, 'Let's go back to the beginning; let's see what the foundations are,' rather than to produce results. Although I turned away from engineering, I think I was too much of an engineer in regard to physics before I came to Bohr."[152]

It was Bohr's influence, Bloch said, that prompted him to write a paper that he described as "essentially of pedagogical interest" on the stopping power of particles, a paper that Bloch thought he probably would not have written before Copenhagen, but which years later he would look back on with "very great pleasure."[153]

Bohr's skill and dedication to reducing concepts to their simplest terms would have impact on Bloch's skill and dedication in teaching.

Bohr [said Bloch] was a master in classical physics. And once in a while when he was in the mood, he was able to explain to you certain things of classical physics in such an absolutely simple and marvelous way that I've never forgotten.

Once he told me, which I'd never known, in a very simple two lines you can derive, from a classical point of view, the expression for resistance. If you do the right sort of thing with the mean free path you get it in two lines. This is what Bohr was so great at. That is, he could get results within a factor of two or so. In order to understand the basic things you need not much mathematics; that's what I learned from Bohr.[154]

Bloch would devote nearly half a century as a professor at Stanford University with a good share of his teaching directed toward freshman and sophomore students. He once said, "Teaching undergraduates is gratifying—and by no means easy. It means putting complex ideas into their very simplest form. Sometimes this forces one to clarify his own ideas—not a bad thing."[155]

He enjoyed telling a story about Stanford's first president, David Starr Jordan, who listened patiently to a recently-arrived faculty member go on and on about all the great research plans he had and of his intentions to teach only advanced courses.

"That's very good," said Jordan. "You do that. And perhaps after 10 years, you may be qualified to teach the undergraduates."[156] Bloch rejected the idea of academic research divorced from teaching. It is bad, he said, to do nothing but teach, or nothing but research. "You teach while you are doing research, and you learn while you teach. I have always deplored the separation of the two at a university."[157]

Because of the need for clarity in teaching undergraduates, it always took Bloch more time—an average of three to four hours—to prepare the lectures and demonstrations for an undergraduate class than a graduate class. But ever since his course in introductory physics taught by the great Peter Debye, Bloch always felt that the most important courses at a university were the introductory ones. "Fortunately," he said in 1982, "we had the policy at Stanford, then and now, that the introductory courses should be taught by senior physicists. In some other institutions the teaching of the beginners is done by young assistants, but this we have always felt is misguided."[158]

Bloch's close friendship with Bohr, wrote the editors of a *festschrift* honoring Bloch's 75th birthday, "was to last through the trying years of the war and for the rest of Bohr's life." Bloch once remarked that he was in almost continual contact with Bohr through the years, and that the same deep problems never ceased to occupy Bohr's mind.[159]

The editors were referring in the above context to the deep problems of quantum physics, but for the next 13 years, Bohr's mind would also be occupied with another kind of problem, the irrational hatred of anti-Semitism. For one who agonized with such "extreme care"[160] in his search for scientific truth, Bohr must have been pained beyond description by a movement that would seek to deny because of racial prejudice the progress that had been made in his beloved physics. "Aryan" physics, they called it in Germany, and the fact that such a term even existed—as though the discovery of scientific truth was the sole prerogative of blond, blue-eyed scientists—shows the depths to which humans can sink when they attempt to propagate and justify their hate. As Jews, both Bohr and Bloch would feel its impact in a very personal way.

Gathering Storm Clouds

Midway through the "30 years that shook physics,"[161] as George Gamow described the first three decades of the century, a world war, centered in Europe, triggered into political action the hatred already fomenting in the mind of a man called Adolf Hitler. Seeing "the Jew" as a useful tool for gaining political power and a handy scapegoat upon whom he could lay the blame for his nation's ills, he drafted his first party platform in 1919 at a table decorated with a carved caricature of a Jew dangling from a miniature gallows.[162]

Four years later, as Felix Bloch began his studies at Zürich's ETH, Hitler, in Landsberg Prison for his role in Munich's Beer Hall Putsch of November 8, 1923, began dictating his *Mein Kampf*, spilling onto its pages the vile, anti-Semitic poison polluting his own mind and thus corrupting a nation.

In the spring of 1932, when Bloch returned from Copenhagen to Leipzig to resume his position as an assistant to Heisenberg and to take up his new responsibilities as a *privatdozent*, the first rung on the academic ladder, Hitler was running for president against Paul von Hindenburg. Hitler lost, but only by a narrow margin, and nine months later, following further Nazi gains in the Reichstag and compelled by the need to establish political stability, von Hindenburg named his former opponent chancellor of Germany on January 30, 1933.

Aided by a devastating economic depression and by Germany's injured post-war pride, Hitler moved swiftly to enact his agenda and to make his personal prejudices public policy. Less than a month after becoming chancellor, a fire in the Reichstag provided Hitler with the excuse to outlaw the Communist party and to arrest its leaders. Less than one month after the fire, the Reichstag passed the Enabling Act, providing Hitler with four years of dictatorial power. He promptly outlawed all parties except his own, the National Socialist German Workers' Party (NSDAP).

Even though Bloch was quite happy in his new position as *privatdozent* and with his continuing, close relationship with Heisenberg, he nevertheless felt compelled in the fall of 1932 to apply for a fellowship from the International Education Board, funded by the Rockefeller Foundation. The purpose of the Rockefeller Fellowship was to give promising young scientists a sort of sabbatical from their jobs for a year, after which they were expected to return. "It was very clear to me at that time that this might come in very handy in the sense that my staying in Germany would be limited." Even in the fall of 1932, before Hitler was named chancellor, "it didn't take great foresight," Bloch said, "to see that things were coming to an end."[163] Prior to that time, he said, his career course had been "a question which one did not really too seriously consider."

> The hope [Bloch said] was that eventually one would associate oneself with a university. It was by no means clear where that university would be or which it would be. Nor could I say that it really concerned us very much. I think I can truthfully say that we were really so engrossed in our work that the question of where it would lead to materially was, in a certain sense, a secondary question.[164]

When Bloch had let his mind wander in such directions, he saw Germany with its strength in theoretical physics as a likely place to continue his career. "Besides," he said, "it was a large country with many universities, so *a priori* the chances of joining a university were probably greatest in Germany." But there was, of course, also his home country of Switzerland with its strong tradition in physics, and there was America. "I must say that the idea of eventually going to America was by no means a remote or fearful idea at all," he said. "I had discussed that often with my friends, some of whom went to America quite early."[165]

Looking back on 1932 from the perspective of 1968, Bloch said that some of the advantages he and his friends saw in America were increased possibilities for employment and the idea that, with the physics tradition not as highly developed in the United States as it was in Europe, that maybe there would be more chance to "stand on one's own feet." Bloch wasn't so sure, however, but that the latter reason may have been added to his list after the fact, the result of hindsight. "It looks as if I had had prophetic foresight, which I did not have," he said. "I'm sure that the main idea was that, indeed, we were Europeans, and it seemed natural to stay in Europe."[166]

"But it was not," he emphasized, "a matter of prime concern really at that time. We had the confidence somehow or other, rightly or wrongly, that sooner or later we would find a position all right, and we were really in no hurry. We were also very young."[167]

Although they were in no hurry, Hitler felt he had waited long enough. A week after the Reichstag abdicated its powers to Hitler with the Enabling Act of March 23, 1933, Hitler opened his reign of terror by prohibiting Jewish judges and lawyers from practicing in Prussia and Bavaria and by initiating a national boycott of Jewish businesses. To help customers know which businesses to boycott, their addresses were published in newspapers as a public service. Nazi storm troopers were also on hand to provide further aid in directing the violence, both against the businesses and against Jews so misfortunate as to be caught in the streets.[168]

Although dismissals of Jewish academics had begun, according to Bloch, as early as 1932, "they were practically all dismissed,"[169] he said, when Hitler came to power, and to legitimize his actions, the Law for the Restoration of the Career Civil Service was enacted on April 7, 1933. Created ostensibly to restore a "national" career civil service and to streamline administration, its primary purpose was to get rid of unwanted political appointees, those with questionable political activities, and those of "non-Aryan" descent, otherwise known as Jewish.

Although Bloch was a Swiss citizen and had neither been dismissed from his job nor was in immediate physical danger, he knew when it was time to leave, and did. "With my Jewish name . . ."—he didn't finish the sentence, but then continued. "Besides, after all, I despised those guys from the beginning."[170] Bloch left in March of 1933, even before the edict of April 7. "I simply quit," he said. "I went home to my parents in Switzerland."[171]

According to Alan Beyerchen, author of the book *Scientists Under Hitler*, "The students were one of the most vocal forces of National Socialist policy at the universities."[172] and according to Bloch, the students at Leipzig were among Hitler's earliest supporters. Bloch had been observing the rising influence of Nazism for several years. "There was nothing violent about it [initially]," he told science historian Charles Weiner, "but it was quite clear that these ideas were gaining ground. It was quite obvious to me, in any event, that fearful changes were on the horizon."

> I had contact [said Bloch] with students in places where I lived. I rented a room or two in a house with other students together and we talked about these things. There was nothing aggressive in their attitude at that time. But they felt that as an outsider, as a Swiss, as they considered me, I was entitled to some education; and they gave it to me freely. I did not hide the fact that I did not share their opinion, and they accepted that as one of the facts; but it was very clear that they were taken in by this.[173]

Less than a week after the April 7th Civil Service Law went into effect and a few weeks after Bloch left, the German Students Association announced its own initiative "Against the Un-German Spirit," as a prelude to a public book burning that took place a month later. Included in the declaration:

— The Jew can only think Jewish; when he writes German he is lying.

— Students should view Jews as aliens.

— Jewish works should be written in Hebrew and, at the very least, designated as translations if printed in German.

— Students and professors should be selected "according to their guarantee of thinking in the German spirit."[174]

On the 13th of April, the first dismissals under the new law were announced at German universities, and quotas for non-Aryans in German schools soon followed.

In spite of the clear evidence of growing danger, it was possible, like a frog sitting in water that is heated very slowly, to get used to the changing environment degree by subtle degree and to discount what was happening as a temporary phenomenon that would soon pass. After all, not everybody was acting like the radical students. The anti-Semitism that Bloch saw, for example, in Germany in 1932-33 did not yet display itself in open violence. For that reason, it was all the more insidious.

> It was a strange thing in Germany [said Bloch]. You see, anti-Semitism was not a social phenomenon as it is in many other countries. It was almost more of a theoretical attitude. That is to say, I knew many Jews and Jewish families in Leipzig, and I don't hardly recall that they experienced violent anti-Semitism in the sense of beating or things like that, which occurred . . . in Hungary and Austria. That did not exist in Germany. But it was a dogmatic philosophical anti-Semitism, which at that time existed side-by-side with otherwise perfectly normal relations.[175]

You could even call it polite anti-Semitism. Students would say to Bloch: "But *Herr Doktor*, perhaps the Jews are a menace to us. Not all, of course. Not you." But the cloak of friendship could not forever hide the sword of hatred and, until his death, Felix Bloch would never forget the robotic stomp of the Nazi stormtroopers nor the mindless chant of a nation being programmed with prejudice:

> *Wenn's Judenblut vom Messer rinnt,*
> *Erst dann ist Deutschland frei!*

> When Jewish blood runs from the knife,
> Only then will Germany be free![176]

Because he was not a German citizen, Bloch said, he found it easier to take an objective view of the growing dangers. "The liberals, intellectuals and Jews were not as worried as they should have been," he said. "Some got out, but most of them just worried."[177]

To Sup With the Devil

One of the non-Jewish intellectuals who "just worried" was Werner Heisenberg. The one who had once rebuked Bloch for allowing an abstraction to distort the evidence of actual observation would now experience his own denial of reality. In his memoirs, published in 1969, Heisenberg reflected on his inability to recognize the accelerating danger signals of 1933.

The "golden age of atomic physics" now quickly approached its end. The political unrest in Germany grew. Radical groups of the right and left demonstrated in the streets, battled each other in the backyards of the poorer quarter of the city and agitated against one another in public gatherings. *Almost imperceptibly* [italics added] the unrest, and with it anxiety, spread also within university life and faculty meetings. For a time, I tried to push the danger away from myself and ignore the incidents on the streets. But in the end, reality is stronger than our wishes . . .[178]

Sometime in April or May—Bloch couldn't recall exactly—he received a letter from the dean of the University of Leipzig begging him, Bloch said, "to come back and teach my course, which I had announced, and rather ironically promising that I could get guards in my lecture room to prevent any troubles which might arise." The reason it was ironic, said Bloch, was that the only people who would have caused trouble at the time were the guards themselves. Those sitting under his teaching were friends and unlikely, Bloch felt, to initiate any problems. "I didn't even answer that letter," he said.[179]

I'm sorry to say that Heisenberg, rather naively at that time [said Bloch], also felt that I should certainly return. He saw no particular reason why I couldn't go back. And I may say that from the spring until the fall of '33 I had no job. My Rockefeller Fellowship started [in the fall], and so Heisenberg evidently felt: "Well, if he's free anyhow, why can he not at least give us a lecture while he is here?" I mean my very strong feelings about what was going on in Germany, he apparently did not quite understand.[180]

Although Heisenberg had blind spots, such as the example just cited, he was apparently not anti-Semitic. Rather, he saw himself as the protector of the new physics that was being attacked by such Aryan physicists as Philipp Lenard and Johannes Stark and felt that he could have the most positive impact by combating the heresy within Germany.

As a theoretical physicist, a founder of quantum mechanics and a friend of Einstein, Heisenberg was seen—accurately—as an opponent of Aryan physics. A letter to Alfred Rosenberg, the editor of the party newspaper, by a secondary school official in 1934 demanded that, as a supporter of Einstein, Heisenberg should be sent to a concentration camp.[181] Furthermore, as a signer of a petition seeking to have the dismissal of Jewish mathematician Richard Courant from Göttingen University rescinded, Heisenberg was seen as a protector of the enemies within Germany.[182]

Described variously as a "Jew lover" and a "Jewish pawn," it was written of Heisenberg that 1) he was "awarded the [1932] Nobel Prize in 1933 together with the Einstein-disciples Schrödinger and Dirac, a demonstration of the Jewish-influenced Nobel committee against National Socialist Germany," 2) that he "returned his thanks by refusing to sign a proclamation of German Prize recipients for the Führer and Chancellor of the Reich" and 3) that "his fame abroad is an inflated result of his collaboration with foreign Jews and Jew lovers."[183] Because of these and other sins as seen by the Nazis, Heisenberg would be denied the opportunity to inherit the prestigious chair held by Arnold Sommerfeld at the University of Munich, in spite of the fact that Sommerfeld had thrown Heisenberg his personal mantle of support.

Heisenberg was also very visible. In addition to the fact that he was well-known, one of Heisenberg's students was Carl von Weizsäcker, whose father, Ernst von Weizsäcker, was Hitler's secretary of state. The elder von Weizsäcker apparently did help counter some of the attempts to punish Heisenberg for his lack of zeal for the Nazi agenda, however, by pointing out that Germany could not afford to lose a man of his stature.[184]

In 1934, Heisenberg had considered resigning from his position at Leipzig, along with physicist Fritz Hund, mathematician Bartel Leendert van der Waerden, and physical chemist Carl-Friedrich Bonhoeffer (brother of Lutheran theologian Dietrich Bonhoeffer, who was later executed by the Nazis), as an expression of disagreement with the academic dismissals which had occurred, but when he shared his thoughts with Max Planck, the elder statesman of quantum physics advised him: "Hold out until it has passed, form 'islands of stability' and salvage things of value from the catastrophe."[185] The advice resonated with Heisenberg's own inclinations, although a three-part series of articles in *Das Schwarze Korps* (The Black Corps) in July 1937[186] may have caused him to question the wisdom of the advice.

As the official journal of the SS, the terroristic paramilitary organization directed by Heinrich Himmler, *Das Schwarze Korps* was not the kind of publication in which Heisenberg would have chosen to be profiled. After castigating in the first segment "white Jews in scholarship," meant as a disparagement of those who were "Jewish in character" if not Jewish by ancestry, the second article directly attacked Heisenberg "for 'smuggling' a pro-Einstein article into an official party organ in 1936, for taking a vote among physicists on the value of theoretical physics to silence his critics, for becoming a professor in 1928 (when he was too young to have possibly earned such recognition), and for hiring and attracting Jews into his institute in the Weimar period."* Furthermore, the article said that because Heisenberg had refused to sign the 1934 declaration supporting Hitler, he should be made to "disappear" like the Jews.[187]

The declaration Heisenberg and other Nobel laureates had been asked to sign read:

> In Adolf Hitler we German natural researchers perceive and admire the savior and leader of the German people. Under his protection and encouragement, our scientific work will serve the German people and increase German esteem in the world. [188]

Even apart from its inherent demagogic content, it was in conflict with Hitler's attitude toward science as expressed in a conversation he had with Max Planck. "If the dismissal of Jewish scientists means the annihilation of contemporary German science," Hitler is said to have told Planck, "then we shall do without science for a few years!"[189] Hardly "protection and encouragement."

---

* "As a counter-action [to a brochure by Stark on "National Socialism and Science, published in 1934], Heisenberg had delivered an address to the convention of natural scientists in Hannover in September of the same year, clearly formulating the viewpoint of true physics and defending Einstein and his teachings. In addition, this address was published in the Zeitschrift für Naturwissenschaften. Heisenberg's next move, together with Max Wien and [Hans] Geiger, was a public declaration, in which the standpoint of Lenard and Stark was sharply rejected in a carefully prepared text. The declaration was signed by the majority of German physicists. The [Reich Education] Ministry could not tolerate all this, and Heisenberg was rejected [as a candidate for Sommerfeld's chair]."
— Elizabeth Heisenberg, *Inner Exile*, (Boston: Birkhäuser, 1954), 44.

The third segment of the article was a commentary on the first two by Aryan physicist Johannes Stark, discoverer of the Stark effect. Although Heisenberg was not named in the third segment, it wasn't necessary; the association was clear. The immediate objective of the series was to prevent Heisenberg from inheriting Sommerfeld's chair; the longer-range objective to prevent him from continuing his physics career in Germany.

With the handwriting clearly on the wall, Heisenberg, in a bold move, wrote a letter to Heinrich Himmler himself and, to make sure it was delivered, had his mother deliver it in person to Himmler's mother. The Heisenbergs and the Himmlers had been acquaintances of sorts for a number of years, ever since Heisenberg's grandfather and Heinrich Himmler's father had been principals of secondary schools in Munich and part of a circle of colleagues that met periodically to walk together and discuss school matters. As Elisabeth Heisenberg, Werner Heisenberg's wife, told the unusual story:

> My mother-in-law was a religious woman and a bitter enemy of the Nazis. But anxious about the fate of her son and worried for our young, newly-formed family, she called up Mrs. Himmler and asked if she might visit her. Mrs. Himmler still lived in an old, properly middle-class apartment building, a crucifix in a corner of the living room, with fresh flowers arranged in front of it. The old woman listened to everything, took the letter for her son, and kept shaking her head somewhat sadly and with trepidation at what my mother-in-law was relating to her.
>
> Then she said: "If my little Heinrich knew of this, he would certainly put an end to these slanderous accusations. I will talk to him and give him the letter from your son," she resolutely added. Just as my mother-in-law was about to leave, Mrs. Himmler turned to her again and asked, with fear in her eyes: "Or do you think, Mrs. Heisenberg, that my little Heinrich might not be on the right path after all?" My mother-in-law shuddered with fearful horror as she related this macabre scene to us.[190]

By appealing to Himmler, Heisenberg was calling for an investigation in the matters of which he was accused, in order to have the opportunity to directly clarify his position. Although plans were made for a face-to-face meeting between Himmler and Heisenberg, the confrontation never took place. Eventually, world opinion may have influenced Himmler's decision. About one year after the incriminating articles were published, Heisenberg received a letter from Himmler on July 21, 1938 that read:

> Precisely because you were recommended to me by my family, I caused your case to be examined with special care and intensity. I take pleasure in being able to inform you that I do not approve of the attack made against you in the article in the *Schwarze Korps*, and that I have ensured that there will be no further attacks on your person . . .[191]

During this period, Heisenberg was receiving encouragement from a number of sources, including Felix Bloch, to leave Germany while he still had the opportunity. He received a number of offers from foreign universities but, according to his wife, the only offer he seriously considered was the one from Columbia University in the summer of 1937. They repeated the offer in 1938 and 1939. "He had real friends there," wrote Elisabeth Heisenberg, "and that attracted him."[192] One of those friends was I.I. Rabi, with whom Heisenberg had worked for a short time in the early part of 1929 and who had been offered his position at Columbia because of Heisenberg's recommendation.

It wasn't the first time Heisenberg had been given the opportunity to leave Germany. The first time was in 1927, the same year he became professor of theoretical physics at Leipzig. Simultaneously, he had received an offer from the University of Zürich, which he had turned down. Years later, when his wife asked him why he chose Leipzig over the beautiful city of Zürich, he answered with little hesitation, "I preferred to stay in Germany."[193]

In the end, Heisenberg, the formulator of the Uncertainty Principle in physics, would be a victim of his own political uncertainty. As Beyerchen has written:

> To [Heisenberg], the choice of whether to follow the refugees abroad or to stay on and attempt to make the best of things was not unambiguous. . . . The argument in favor of protest, resignation, and emigration, based on moral outrage and the hope that some good would come through a demonstration of opposition to government policies, was unconvincing to Heisenberg. . . . The arguments in favor of remaining were more persuasive. One receives the impression from Heisenberg's account that to a man of Heisenberg's convictions, to emigrate of one's own accord was more akin to desertion of duty than to courageous protest. As he himself stated it, "I almost

envied the friends whose basis for living in Germany had been removed from them by force, so that they knew that they had to leave our land."[194]

Heisenberg took trips to the United States in 1939 and tried to explain to his long-time friends why he was staying in Germany. Pegram at Columbia, the one to whom Heisenberg had recommended Rabi, "was not convinced by his arguments," wrote Heisenberg's wife, "and most of his American friends reacted the same way; it was a painful experience for Heisenberg."[195] Heisenberg apparently did not see Bloch during this trip, which took him to New York and Chicago. At the time, Bloch and his collaborator, Luis Alvarez, were just a few days away from determining the magnetic moment of the neutron using magnetic resonance. Bloch would not see Heisenberg again until after the war. The last time Bloch saw Heisenberg before the war was on a trip he took to Europe in 1937, during which he tried, unsuccessfully, to persuade Heisenberg to emigrate.[196]

It was at the Galvani Conference in Bologna, Italy "long before the war," said Bloch. "It seemed at that time quite possible that he might [emigrate]. He unfortunately decided not to do it."

> He had difficulties with the Nazis at that time [said Bloch], partly because of his former Jewish collaborators, and he was very angry at [the Nazis]. He needed a little push. But I think Debye was really the one who persuaded him that he should not leave, although Debye himself then left.[197]

Caught between the never-comfortable rock and a hard place, Heisenberg decided to stay where he was, his loyalty to his country greater than his opposition to the evil force controlling that country. Had he accepted any of Columbia's offers, it is interesting to contemplate the timing of his emigration and its future ramifications, both for American physics and for Heisenberg personally. If he had emigrated shortly after receiving Columbia's first offer, he would have arrived about the time that I.I. Rabi and his associates were conducting the first successful magnetic resonance experiment. Had he accepted Columbia's 1939 offer, he would have been in the United States shortly after the discovery of fission and who knows where life in the United States might have taken him after that?

A number of Heisenberg's former colleagues, including Felix Bloch, Hans Bethe, Niels Bohr, Enrico Fermi, Rudolf Peierls, Edward Teller and

Victor Weisskopf would end up at Los Alamos working on the Manhattan Project, motivated in large measure by what they saw as the very real possibility that Germany might be working on its own atomic bomb. Having lived in Europe during Hitler's rise to power, they could not bear to envision such a weapon in the hands of such a tyrant. The only hope to keep that from happening, they felt, was to develop the bomb before Germany did.

According to Heisenberg's wife, helping to build an atomic bomb that might be used on Germany was something that he could not bear to envision. "The notion of having to collaborate in the development of an atomic bomb, possibly then to be used on Germany, causing unimaginable death and destruction, was a nightmare to him; he would not do it."[198]

In actuality, at the time the above physicists were at Los Alamos, Germany was working on an atomic bomb—or at least its prerequisite, a sustained nuclear fission chain reaction—and heading up the effort as Germany's counterpart to America's J. Robert Oppenheimer, though on a much smaller scale, was none other than Werner Heisenberg.

As for Heisenberg's concern about contributing to a bomb that might have been used on Germany, he may ironically have contributed more to that effort by staying in Germany and working on their atomic bomb program. Two years after Columbia's 1939 offer, a clandestine meeting in Copenhagen between Niels Bohr and Werner Heisenberg left Bohr, the ever-careful wordsmith, thinking, perhaps mistakenly, that Germany was making great progress toward making atomic weapons and that Heisenberg was a willing collaborator with the Nazis.

According to Robert Oppenheimer, "Bohr had the impression that they [Heisenberg and Carl von Weizäcker, who had come to Denmark with Heisenberg to attend a scientific meeting] came less to tell what they knew than to see if Bohr knew anything that they did not."[199] Heisenberg has claimed to have been distressed by what he saw as a misunderstanding on Bohr's part. At any rate, Heisenberg's words served to alarm Bohr and to spur on Allied efforts in building an atomic bomb that, had events occurred differently, could have been used on Heisenberg's Germany. Regarding Heisenberg's dilemma, Rudolf Peierls wrote, "he had agreed to sup with the devil, and perhaps he found that there was not a long enough spoon."[200]

For Felix Bloch, Heisenberg's first graduate student, it was more pleasant to remember his association with his mentor during the "happier times"[201] before political events placed Heisenberg and Bloch on opposing sides, back when they walked, skied, talked physics, philosophized and enjoyed piano music together. Looking back at that time and the two subsequent periods he spent with Heisenberg in Leipzig, Bloch found that Heisenberg stood "in the center" of his memories from that formative period and said,

> It was not only that he suggested the theme of my thesis, but I owe it to him that I caught the real spirit of research and that I dared to take the first steps in learning how to walk. If I should single out one of his great qualities as a teacher, it would be his immensely positive attitude towards any progress and the encouragement he thereby conferred.
>
> What followed [after 1933, added Bloch], is too well known for me to dwell upon, but I cannot refrain from one sad comment on human nature. Their very devotion to their work and their detachment from the dark irrational passions spreading around them caught most of even the finest German scientists unprepared for the oncoming flood. Those who did not leave were with few exceptions swept along and were left, each in his own way, to struggle with their inner conflicts.[202]

In the deluge of insanity that swept across Germany, Heisenberg found it impossible to follow the advice Max Planck had given him back in 1934. It was too late to form "islands of stability" and there was very little of value to salvage from the catastrophe.

The Summer of '33

As recently as February 28, 1933, the day after the Reichstag fire, Wolfgang Pauli, a native of Vienna, Austria, had been visiting with Edward Teller and others in Göttingen, Germany, and had dismissed the possibility of a dictatorship in Germany as *Quatsch*, as rubbish. "I have seen dictatorship in Russia," he said. "In Germany it just couldn't happen."[203]

Less than two months later, Walter Elsasser, one of the first to leave Germany after the announcement of the April 7 Civil Service Law, went to see Pauli at the physics building of Zürich, Switzerland's ETH. "On entering the main door of this building one faces a broad and straight staircase leading directly to the second floor. Before I could take my first step on it, there appeared at the top of the stairs the moon-face of Wolfgang Pauli, who shouted down: 'Elsasser,' he said, 'you are the first to come up these stairs; I can see how in the months to come there will be many, many more to climb up here.' "[204]

Pauli's second prediction was more accurate than his first. The April 7th law would remove one-fourth of Germany's physicists from their academic positions, including 11 current or future Nobel laureates, and 1600 scholars altogether. With little chance of finding other work, they would have to emigrate to survive. Pauli himself would relocate to Princeton in the United States during World War II. Because he carried an Austrian passport, he was considered a German national once Germany invaded Austria. Pauli was granted citizenship by Switzerland after he was awarded the 1945 Nobel Prize in physics.

Bloch was more fortunate than many. As a Swiss citizen, he could go home, although he didn't have a job lined up in Switzerland. He did, however, have a one-year Rockefeller Fellowship lined up that would start in the fall, the first half of which he planned to spend in Rome with Enrico Fermi, the second half at Cambridge in England. Later he would be invited to lecture that summer for a few weeks at the Henri Poincaré Institute in Paris, but in the meantime, Bloch was one of the many physicists from Germany who showed up at the bottom of Pauli's staircase at the ETH where he worked that spring on quantum mechanics with Pauli and Gregor Wentzel.

Bloch said he had a "very wonderful time"[205] in Paris, where he stayed at the home of physicist Paul Langévin, developer of the theory of paramagnetism in early 1905. A year before Bloch's visit, Langévin had predicted that, with Einstein's emigration, the United States would become "the center of the natural sciences."[206] Already, of course, the United States was enjoying an upsurgence in physics with the return of Rabi and others like him from their sojourns in Europe where they had been learning the new physics, but now, with Hitler in power, the center of gravity began shifting dramatically. One of those who did not emigrate was Langévin's son-in-law, Jacques Solomon, whom Bloch knew quite well from his days in Copenhagen. Solomon would be a casualty of the war, killed by the Nazis.

Bloch also made a return visit to Utrecht, Holland to visit with Hendrik Kramers, where they discussed physics and the events that were taking place in Germany. "It was a very fruitful period," said Bloch. "I knew anyway that I was going to go to Rome in the fall, so the summer went by very interestingly. I cannot say that I was at all unhappy, nor did I lack occupation during that summer."[207]

Bloch didn't know it then—in fact, he wouldn't know it until Charles Weiner informed him of it in an interview 35 years later—but on June 19th of that summer, John von Neumann of Princeton's Institute for

Advanced Study wrote a letter from Budapest to Oswald Veblen, another mathematician at Princeton, informing him of the crisis for Jewish academics. He had just visited Berlin and Göttingen and, on the basis of what he had learned, had made a list of people who had already been dismissed from their positions or soon would be. "He used the term, *beurlaubungen*, 'forced to leave' and your name was on the list," Weiner told Bloch. There were others on the list as well, all prominent theoretical physicists, for whom, wrote von Neumann, "a future in German universities will be impossible."[208] Because of von Neumann's intervention, the name of Felix Bloch was apparently added to a list compiled by the Academic Assistance Council in England and sent to an American group called the Emergency Committee in Aid of Displaced German Scholars. The Committee, in turn, working closely with the Rockefeller Foundation, offered to pay the salary of displaced scholars for two years to universities that showed serious intent to continue their employment if they proved suitable. Emphasizing "preservation of scholarship" rather than "personal relief for scholars," the program specifically excluded aid "to younger German scholars of outstanding promise."[209]

When told of the von Neumann connection, Bloch responded, "That's very interesting. I didn't know that." He knew a list had been circulated, but hadn't known for sure how his name had been included, although he had "sometimes thought,"[210] he said, that he had been nominated by Robert Oppenheimer, who knew Bloch from Zürich and who, as a professor at Berkeley, was in close contact with Stanford University. That, indeed, may have been the case, but the June 19th letter by von Neumann does provide documentary evidence of another possible scenario.

Shortly before going to Rome to begin the first half of his one-year Rockefeller Fellowship, Bloch decided to make another visit to Copenhagen to visit Niels Bohr and other friends at the Institute. Heisenberg also happened to be there at the time. While in Copenhagen, Bloch received a cable from David Webster at Stanford University offering him a position as Acting Associate Professor. How Stanford knew he was in Copenhagen, Bloch couldn't explain. The best he could come up with was that they probably didn't know he had left Copenhagen a year earlier and, "by the sheerest coincidence,"[211] had sent the cable there at the same time he just happened to be at the Institute for a visit.

He also had no idea who David Webster was or where Stanford University was located. The only clue he had that Stanford might be in the United States was that the salary was stated in dollars. Since Heisenberg had been around the world, Bloch showed him the telegram first and asked if he had ever heard of a university by the name of Stanford. Yes, Heisenberg did vaguely recall that it was on the West Coast of the United States and that it was near another university [Berkeley], the name of which he could not remember. Beyond that, the only other information he could offer was that "[the two colleges] steal each other's axes."[212]

Heisenberg's memory of the ax theft problem experienced by Stanford and Berkeley was, of course, based on the schools' long-standing football rivalry and annual efforts by the Berkeley team to spirit away the symbol of the Stanford team, the Native American tomahawk.

When Bloch recited the oft-told story in 1982 to a Stanford University publicist, he still laughed with enjoyment as he recalled his response half-a-century earlier. "Axes! I wondered what sort of place this Stanford was, where people used axes. But then I spoke to Niels Bohr, and he knew immediately. 'It is a very good place,' he said. 'I recommend it. I think you should accept.' "[213]

Bloch did accept Stanford's offer, with the proviso that he start in the spring of 1934 instead of the fall of 1933, as proposed, so that he could proceed with his plans to go to Rome and work with Enrico Fermi. With the approval of the International Education Board, Bloch then relinquished the second half of his fellowship at Cambridge University.

The fact that Bloch's fellowship had not been rescinded is in itself somewhat surprising, based on the experiences of others. Otto Robert Frisch, for example, had also applied for and been awarded a Rockefeller Fellowship to work with Enrico Fermi in Rome prior to the enactment of the April 7 Civil Service Law in Germany. Working with Otto Stern in Hamburg where he was about to lose his position because of the new anti-Semitic laws, Frisch initially thought he could avoid unemployment because of his promised fellowship, but then received word from the foundation that, because he would not have a job to go back to under Hitler's new laws, they would have to withdraw their offer.

Perhaps the difference in treatment can be explained by the fact that Bloch was a Swiss citizen and that the new laws did not affect non-German citizens in the same way they did German citizens. Bloch, for example, had never officially resigned from the University of Leipzig and had never received an official letter of dismissal. Fortunately, Frisch was rescued from his predicament by Niels Bohr, who showed up in Hamburg one day, took him by his waistcoat button, and said: "I hope you will come and work with us sometime; we like people who can carry out 'thought experiments!' " That night Frisch wrote his mother and told her not to worry, "the Good Lord himself had taken me by my waistcoat button and smiled at me. That was exactly how I felt."[214] *

Rome

Enrico Fermi was born about two months before Werner Heisenberg and about four years before Felix Bloch. Like Bloch, he had suffered the loss of an older sibling and, also like Bloch, had found a certain degree of refuge from his grief in books. For Fermi, however, who was 14 at the time he lost his 15-year-old brother, the books were two volumes of physics textbooks published in 1840 and written by a Jesuit physicist. He was so excited by his discovery that he didn't notice until he was finished that they were written in Latin.

Graduating from an Italian *liceo* in 1917 after three years instead of the typical four, Fermi enrolled at the University of Pisa. His assigned entry essay on "characteristics of sound" stunned the examiner, according to physicist and Fermi biographer Emilio Segrè, with its "partial differential equation of a vibrating rod, which Fermi solved by Fourier analysis, finding the eigenvalues and the eigenfrequencies . . . which would have been creditable for a doctoral examination."[215]

When he was 25 years old, Fermi was appointed professor of theoretical physics at the University of Rome, after competing in national competitions. In the latter part of his 20s, financed by the patronage of a Sicilian physicist by the name of Orso Mario Corbino, Fermi began building what would be for a few years another important center of European physics, staffed with Franco Rasetti, Emilio Segrè, and Edoardo Amaldi, all of whom had been seasoned in the centers of European physics. Over them all was Fermi "the Pope," so designated because of his infallibility when it came to quantum physics.[216]

By the time Bloch arrived in Rome in the fall of 1933, Fermi had already made major contributions to the new physics, not the least of which were the Fermi statistics which had contributed so greatly to Sommerfeld's theory of metals and subsequently to Bloch's electron theory of metals.

In Rome, Bloch would play a contributing role in what author Richard Rhodes has called "the major theoretical work of [Fermi's] life, a fundamental paper on beta decay."[217]

---

* In early May 1933, during a visit to the United States, Niels Bohr prevailed upon Max Mason, president of the Rockefeller Foundation, to abolish the foundation's requirement that recipients of Rockefeller Fellowships had to have a position to which they could return.
— Richard Rhodes, *The Making of the Atomic Bomb*, (New York: Simon and Schuster, 1988), 207-208.

That October, about a month or so after Bloch had taken up residence in Rome, Fermi traveled to Brussels, Belgium for the seventh Solvay Conference, which, for the first time, was devoted to nuclear physics. At the conference, discussion was also centered around beta decay, a topic that had surfaced following James Chadwick's 1932 discovery of the neutron, along with various theories of how the new particle fit into the structure of the atomic nucleus.

Nothing conclusive was established at the Solvay Conference, but Abraham Pais has noted that "Fermi must have gone to work right after the Solvay conference"[218] because, in December, he sent a note on beta decay to *Nature*. When it was rejected by the editor for being "too remote from reality,"[219] Fermi resubmitted his theory in more detailed form to *Zeitschrift für Physik*. Included in the all-encompassing package was a previously-unrecognized force, the weak interaction that became known as Fermi's weak force, and a new constant, now known as Fermi's constant. After summarizing these and other essential contributions of Fermi's paper, Pais concluded, "Thus began the modern era in beta-decay theory."[220]

Although Fermi is well known for his development of the theory, less known is the fact that Felix Bloch contributed at least a necessary tool to aid in its construction. *"Fermi,"* wrote Pais, *"was the first to use second quantized spin-1/2 fields in particle physics."* [italics added by Pais].[221] It is noteworthy that Fermi's use of this technique resulted from a suggestion of Bloch's.

Shortly after arriving in Rome, Bloch had begun working, he said, to "understand a little bit better how oscillations—plasma oscillations and oscillations of electron gases—could be explained in terms of the elementary mechanism. I thought at the time that quantized amplitudes might be a good handle to do it, because . . . the quantized amplitudes had wave character. Well, it was sort of a vague idea," said Bloch, and he decided to bounce it off Enrico Fermi.

> I sort of crashed his doors [Bloch said]. That was the only time I ever did, and I started to tell him about the quantized amplitudes. Fermi said to me in Italian, *"Non ci capisco una parola,"* (I don't understand a single word.) It is true. He did not understand quantized amplitudes at that time. He just simply never had studied it. But I think he made a mental note, "Perhaps I ought to look at quantized amplitudes." And he wrote his neutrino paper [on beta decay] a few months later.[222]

Bloch's vagueness in presenting his idea may also have contributed to Fermi's unresponsiveness. As Bloch has observed, "Fermi was not stimulating in the sense of suggesting to you a new problem. But he would always insist on absolute clarity in any discussion."[223]

When questioned further by Charles Weiner about his suggestion to Fermi, Bloch confirmed that it was possible that his discussion with Fermi may have started him on the path to the theory of the neutrino, but Bloch was careful lest anyone misunderstand that he was claiming too large a role in Fermi's theory.

> It was more a technicality. I think the neutrino was almost an exercise for Fermi. Once he understood that, he realized that the theory of the neutrino as he proposed it really essentially required the second quantization. So I don't want to say, by any means, that I suggested to Fermi the theory of the neutrino. It was only that I mentioned to him a certain tool that he was clearly not acquainted with at that time. He felt that it was probably a lot of high-brow nonsense which one didn't need. But then, in typical Fermi fashion, without saying anything, he went home and studied it. Fermi, of course, once he understood something, he really understood it. There was no such thing as half understanding.[224]

For Bloch, working with Fermi was dramatically different than working with either Heisenberg or Bohr. Bohr, for example, enjoyed creating physics by committee, using his collaborators as sounding boards and co-refiners of his concepts. Fermi did not. Said Bloch:

> Interestingly, there was not much contact with Fermi. We had personal contact with him—played tennis and told each other jokes, but very rarely talked physics. Fermi didn't really like very much to discuss physics. He didn't like to solve other people's problems, or to be bothered by other people's problems. He wanted to do his own problems. If people came and tried to push him into a line of thinking in which he was not interested at that time, he didn't like that particularly. I mean he was not impolite, but he made it rather plain that he wasn't too much interested.[225]

Fermi also did not enjoy philosophical physics. "He was simply unable to let things be foggy,"[226] Robert Oppenheimer once said. Even his lecturing style reflected the crisp clarity with which he sought to imbue physics, quite unlike Niels Bohr. Bohr "always dropped his voice at the important words," I.I. Rabi has said, almost as if enunciating such words too clearly might make them too difficult to recall in the likely event he felt it necessary to replace them. Rabi, who was known for speaking his mind, said of Bohr, "In physics, although he did not want to speak more clearly than he knew, which was correct . . . when one speaks this way, one after a time is really lost and finds no sure marker of where one has been or whither one goes."[227]

Fermi on the other hand, who had a deep resonant voice, sent his words out as if on a mission. It has been observed that "to listen to Fermi was a most inspiring experience, not only for the student but also for the hardened worker in physics. He had the knack of all great teachers: he made the student wonder why there had ever been any difficulty in understanding the topic he was presenting."[228]

In spite of Fermi's reticence to discuss physics with his post-doctoral fellows, he did make a suggestion to Bloch that would have a major impact on Bloch's future career. Until then, Bloch had always considered himself a theoretical physicist. Even in Zürich, as an undergraduate, he had dropped the spectroscopy experiment he had been working on in favor of the more esoteric ideas he heard expressed by the theoretical physicists at Debye's colloquia, a bent that had been further encouraged by Heisenberg and Bohr. After working with Fermi in Rome, however, Bloch would begin to think of himself as an experimental physicist, even though he did no experiments while in Rome.

All it was, said Bloch, was "one of these casual remarks that Fermi once in a while made. He said to me in Rome once, 'You know, you should sometimes do some experiments. It's really a lot of fun.' That little remark of Fermi's," said Bloch, "stuck somehow in the back of my mind. When I came to this country [the United States], then I realized that I wanted to do experiments."[229] The magnetic moment of the wily neutron would give him the opportunity to do just that.

Emigration

In the spring of 1934—April, as Bloch recalled—he left Rome, stopped by Zürich to visit his parents, and then sailed for the United States. Disembarking in New York, he was met at the pier by Gregory Breit, physics theorist from New York University and co-developer of the 1931 Breit-Rabi theory.[230]

Because his ship had been shaking for much of his trans-Atlantic voyage, Bloch experienced what he called "this peculiar feeling of land sickness" during the short time he spent in New York. Although he felt depressed, which he attributed to fatigue, he remembered having "especially warm feelings toward Breit," whom he knew from Zürich. "When you arrive at the shores of a foreign country and you meet somebody whom you know and is friendly, this makes a great deal of difference," Bloch remarked.[231]

After spending a day or two in New York City, Bloch boarded a train for California. Coming from Europe, his main recollection of his cross-country trip by rail was the enormity of the country, "these endless plains and endless mountains."[232] Ahead of him in Palo Alto, California was Stanford University, his new academic home where he would spend much of the next half century, but he had no idea what Stanford was like.

I must confess to my shame that I did not know too much what was being done here. I learned, of course, later when I came here that they did very fine work in X-ray physics, but I did not know that at that time. However, I had met Oppenheimer before, and I knew that Oppenheimer was in Berkeley, and so therefore I knew that there would be at least some theoretical physicist with whom I could discuss my work. Although I did realize that I was going rather far away from the [physics] centers, the fact that I was not all by myself, that there was a fellow theorist in the neighborhood, certainly also had its attraction. But otherwise I must confess that if you ask me whether I imagined Stanford the way it was, I must frankly say no; I had no way of knowing what I would find.[233]

Although Bloch didn't know what lay 3,000 miles ahead of him, he did know what lay 5,000 miles behind, and that, with each mile of steel track, he was putting one more mile of distance between himself and the barbarism of Adolf Hitler. Although he would have occasion to return to Europe several times in the next two or three years, Bloch, who had once considered Germany as the most likely place to spend his academic career, now had no plans to ever return to the land of Bach and Beethoven.

It was made so absolutely clear, particularly to the Jews who left Germany, that they were not wanted there anymore, that they could not very well have any serious thoughts of coming back. On the other hand, I knew very well that many of them, to put it very mildly, deeply regretted the fact they had to leave Germany. They felt that there were their roots and that they were torn out of them, and I suppose some of them hoped that they would return. They hoped that this would blow over and that they would return at perhaps not too late a time.

Now, I must say that for me Germany was out and I think I can safely say forever at that time. I would not have considered going back. But, of course, it was a different matter because I was not raised in Germany.[234]

Bloch was met at the train station, as he recalled, by Dr. David Webster, the head of the physics department at Stanford who had first contacted him by telegram in Copenhagen a half-year earlier. Bloch couldn't recall his impressions and activities of his first few days at Stanford, but what did stand out in his mind was the friendly reception he was given. "I had a wonderful feeling of being really wanted," he said, "which, after what had happened in Europe, was not a minor aspect. They were clearly glad to have me here, so that was a very fine start."[235]

Within a few days after Bloch's arrival at Stanford, he and Robert Oppenheimer got together, the first of many such meetings they would have over the next decade. It also wasn't long before they began holding joint seminars between the two schools. Sometimes they would meet at Berkeley, sometimes at Stanford, sometimes in Carmel or San Francisco, approximately once a week as Bloch recalled. Consisting of only half a dozen people or so, with most of them from Berkeley, the meetings were very informal. One of the group would get up and tell about something he had been thinking or reading about, and then there would be discussions which, said Bloch, were at a higher, more technical level than either of the schools' journal clubs which were joint meetings of theoreticians and experimentalists. "It was very stimulating for me," said Bloch. "I did not feel quite as isolated as I would have otherwise."[236]

Eventually, by the time of the war, the group would grow to at least 20 people. Even then, Oppenheimer, who was quite well-to-do, said Bloch, would occasionally take them all out to a favorite fish restaurant in San Francisco and treat them all very generously.

Although the seminar was limited to theory, Bloch quickly realized that the line between theoreticians and experimentalists in the United States was much less defined than it was in Europe. Actually, there were only two theoretical physicists in California at the time, as far as Bloch could recall, he and Oppenheimer. The experimentalists in the United States— "either by need or by desire," said Bloch—knew more theory than their counterparts in Europe. On the other hand, he noted, "the refinements were not known here, particularly in quantum mechanics, which was really a new science at that time. Except in its rudiments," said Bloch, "it was not known here. People knew the principle of it. I was the one who was to preach the gospel."[237]

Part of the good news Bloch would proclaim, and even more significantly, advance through theory and experiment, was that the power of quantum mechanics was also operative within the nucleus of the atom and that its principles could be used to solve some of the mysteries still remaining about a recently-discovered nuclear particle called the neutron.

Enter, the Neutron

In 1932, not long after returning to Leipzig from his months in Copenhagen as an Oersted Fellow, Bloch saw Bohr in Berlin, and it was at that meeting, as he recalled, that Bohr told him about James Chadwick's discovery of the neutron. "He was very excited," said Bloch, "so were we all."[238]

A major reason for their excitement was that the discovery helped resolve some long-standing nuclear accounting problems that physicists were having. The term "atom," which originated in ancient Greece, means "undivided," but with the discovery of the electron in 1897 by J.J. Thomson at Cambridge University's Cavendish Laboratory, the discovery of the nucleus at the same laboratory in 1911 by Ernest Rutherford, and the discovery of the proton soon afterward, it had become clear that the atom was made up of components, that it was not the monolithic entity it was once thought to be. Fitting these subatomic components together in a scheme that complied with other laws of physics, however, was a challenge. The most popular approach up until 1932 when Werner Heisenberg[239] and Ettore Majorana[240] independently postulated a new nuclear model, was to try cramming both positively-charged protons and negatively-charged electrons into the nucleus. The problem was, even if the two entities could be made to fit dimensionally into the atom's tightly-packed core, other considerations which were coming to the fore, including spins, magnetic moments and statistics, were beginning to make the scheme increasingly untenable.

James Chadwick's neutron—also discovered, like the electron and the atomic nucleus, at Cambridge University's Cavendish Laboratory—conveniently took care of many of the objections that had been raised by the early 1930s against the proton-electron model of the nucleus. While Heisenberg was formulating an overall theory of the nucleus, Bloch began focusing more specifically on how such a scheme would affect the magnetic properties of the nuclear components. Shortly afterward, he said, he became somewhat interested in the neutron and nuclear magnetic moments. "Somehow I've always spun the same thread in my whole life," he said, "it was always magnetism. As soon as neutrons and protons were mentioned, I asked what were the magnetic properties. That was something which somehow suited my character."[241]

Bloch remembered one evening in 1932 when Heisenberg had given him a verbal outline of his theory of the nucleus, before it was published, and not long afterward Bloch told Heisenberg that he thought, on the basis of there being equal numbers of protons and neutrons in a nucleus, that the neutron ought to have a negative magnetic moment equal and opposite to that of the proton.

The reason for this hypothesis, Bloch said later, "was completely wrong" even though "the conclusion wasn't so wrong," and Heisenberg liked the idea intuitively.[242] When Otto Stern of the University of Hamburg spoke, however, at one of their joint colloquia in early 1933 about his recent measurements of the magnetic moments of the proton and the deuteron, things suddenly became clearer for Bloch.[243-244] At that colloquium, Stern announced that his molecular-beam experiments had revealed the magnetic moment of the proton to be about 2.5 times larger than the 1 nuclear magneton they had expected and the magnetic moment of the deuteron to be between 0.5 and 1 nuclear magneton. (The nucleus of deuterium consists of one proton and one neutron.) Both of Stern's findings were important in their own right, but taken together, they provided an important clue to the magnetic moment of the neutron. "Then we knew," said Bloch. "[that the neutron] had a negative magnetic moment but not exactly equal [to the proton]."[245]

In recounting the importance of the event in his 1952 Nobel Prize lecture, Bloch said that the figure for the deuteron "indicated from the simplest plausible considerations of the structure of this nucleus that one should ascribe a moment of about 2 nuclear magnetons to the neutron" (if one assumed that the magnetic moment of the deuteron was the sum of the positive moment of the proton and the negative moment of the neutron). The conclusions he derived from Stern's findings represent, said Bloch, "the start from which my own experimental work has followed in an almost continuous line."[246]

Bloch's experimental work did not begin immediately. His discussions with Heisenberg about nuclear structure and Stern's announcement of the proton's and deuteron's magnetic moments all occurred before Bloch left Leipzig. His detective work on the neutron would be further delayed by his Rockefeller Fellowship in Rome and his emigration to the United States.

At Stanford, although Bloch was given free rein to choose an area of research, he did not immediately pursue his interest in neutrons. "In the first place, of course, I immediately became interested because I was in this environment," said Bloch, "in quite different problems than I had worked on before . . . people discussed things and I felt I had the theoretical answer."[247]

"[David] Webster was very interested in X-rays, so I studied X-rays, too. I wrote a number of papers on such aspects as double electron transitions in the X-ray spectra."[248] Two of the professors with whom Bloch worked closely that first year were P.A. Ross (on X-rays) and Norris Bradbury (on gas discharges). Bradbury would eventually succeed Robert Oppenheimer as director of the Los Alamos National Laboratory after the war.

It wasn't until Bloch returned to Europe the following summer (1935) to visit his parents in Switzerland and his friends at the Niels Bohr Institute in Copenhagen, that neutrons went from the back burner to the front burner in Bloch's list of priorities. Here again, Enrico Fermi was probably at least partially influential. For more than a year, Fermi had been using neutrons to systematically bombard the nuclei of a significant number of the elements on the periodic table, and publishing his results in European journals. On his way to Europe in 1935, Bloch attended the Summer School of Theoretical Physics at the University of Michigan in Ann Arbor where Fermi was lecturing. Since his first series of lectures there in 1930, Fermi had become a mainstay at the well-known summer institute, and would return almost every summer until he finally left Italy for the United States permanently in 1938.* "During

---

* The series also served to Americanize Fermi. By 1937, when he taught a four-week summer session at Stanford at Bloch's invitation, he was showing signs of disenchantment with Mussolini and Fascism. Bloch accompanied Fermi back to Europe after the session was completed. While traveling through Italy, Fermi would read aloud the frequent signs reminding Italian citizens that "Mussolini is always right" or admonishing them to "Believe, Obey, Fight," and would add "Burma Shave," picking up on the well-known roadside advertising program he had encountered in the United States. "It was clear that his respect for the regime was gone by that time," said Bloch. "I'm sure this happened to him during the time he spent in America" (from interview of Bloch by Charles Weiner).

A little more than a year later, Fermi and his Jewish wife, Laura, emigrated to the United States, circumventing Italy's anti-Semitic passport restrictions on the pretext that they were just traveling to Stockholm for Professor Fermi to receive the Nobel Prize in physics. Unable to take much of value out of the country, the Fermi's were able to get reestablished in the United States with the cash award that accompanies the Nobel Prize.

this period," it has been noted, "[Fermi] . . . made a summer's stay at the University of Michigan one of the most exciting intellectual adventures in science."[249]

In addition to any influence Fermi may have had on Bloch's interest in the neutron, Bloch was also prodded in that direction by visits he made to the Cavendish Laboratory in Cambridge, England and to the Niels Bohr Institute in Copenhagen.

In 1933, Bloch had been offered the opportunity to spend half a year at the Cavendish as a Rockefeller Fellow, but had given it up when he accepted his position at Stanford. Now, on his European trip of 1935, Bloch was able to make up for some of that loss by visiting the laboratory where, just three years earlier, Chadwick had discovered the neutron. Nearly five decades later, Bloch recalled viewing the apparatus that enabled Chadwick to hunt down and capture on an oscilloscope the evidence of his elusive quarry.

> I remember seeing the [ionization] chamber at Cambridge, England, with which Chadwick discovered the neutron. It was a shabby little instrument, little more than a box which had been painted over with shellac. This was a primitive instrument, but Chadwick knew what to look for. And with it he made his historic discovery.[250]

It was mainly through Bohr's influence, however, that Bloch would be motivated to find out more about the neutron. Bohr was 50 years old that summer, and many of Bohr's old friends gathered at the Institute to wish Bohr well and to talk physics. "I'm sure," said Bloch, "that this idea of neutron work originated on that occasion. It was mainly through Bohr."[251]

Although Bloch had expressed to Heisenberg back in 1933 that he thought the neutron might have a magnetic moment, a hypothesis that had been confirmed indirectly by Stern's proton-deuteron experiments, his first objective in establishing a neutron program at Stanford was not to measure the neutron's magnetic moment. That idea followed soon afterward, but his immediate objective was to start producing neutrons. Only later would he decide what to do with them.

Bloch did not visit Germany on his trip to Europe. He did, however, visit his grandmother in Austria. In 1935, although the situation had clearly not improved, he didn't have the feeling that this would probably be his last trip to Europe before war broke out. That would not be the case on his second trip back to Europe that he made in late 1937 and early

1938. Shortly before the Nazis took over Austria in March 1938, he visited his grandmother in Vienna once more. "I remember," he said, "I left Vienna with great depression, trying to tell my relatives there to take anything they can and leave, and they did not want to. They left eventually," he added.[252]

After that second trip, Bloch would return to the United States and write a letter to physicist Richard Tolman in which he described the persecution of the Jews that was taking place in Europe, and asking for his aid in soliciting the help of Nobel laureate Robert Millikan. It is unclear how much effect Bloch's letter had on Millikan, but, according to historian Charles Weiner, later that year Millikan did join a number of American university presidents in an effort to bring attention to the Jewish plight.

When shown his 1938 letter in 1968, Bloch didn't recall taking that action, but he did remember his concern about what was happening in Europe at the time. "I thought about it. . . . I dreamt about it." By that time, he said, "the impending doom was clear."[253]

In Search of the Neutron's Magnetic Moment, Part I

In Chadwick's neutron, Fermi saw an ideal battering ram that could be used to penetrate an atom's nuclear defenses. As massive as a proton but carrying no electric charge, it could hurtle past electrons, a nucleus' first line of defense, without being affected by their electric force fields. Even the electric energy of the nucleus itself could not act as a deterrent against the powerful neutrality of the neutron. As a nuclear invader, the neutron was unrivaled, as I.I. Rabi described in a published lecture:

> Since the neutron carries no charge, there is no strong electrical repulsion to prevent its entry into nuclei. In fact, the forces of attraction which hold nuclei together may pull the neutron into the nucleus. When a neutron enters a nucleus, the effects are about as catastrophic as if the moon struck the earth. The nucleus is violently shaken up by the blow, especially if the collision results in the capture of the neutron. A large increase in energy occurs and must be dissipated, and this may happen in a variety of ways, all of them interesting.[254]

Because of Bloch's background with ferromagnetics, he was attracted by the magnetic force of the neutron.

> The idea [said Bloch] that a neutral elementary particle should possess an intrinsic magnetic moment had a particular fascination to me,

since it was in such striking contrast to the then only existing theory of an intrinsic moment which had been given by Dirac for the electron. Combining relativistic and quantum effects, he had shown that the magnetic moment of the electron was a direct consequence of its charge, and it was clear the magnetic moment of the neutron would have to have an entirely different origin. It seemed important to furnish a direct experimental proof for the existence of a magnetic moment of the free neutron, and I pointed out in 1936 that such a proof could be obtained by observing the scattering of slow neutrons in iron.[255]

Before he could do anything about providing a "direct experimental proof," Bloch needed a source of neutrons. For that, he suggested to Norris Bradbury, the gas discharge expert at Stanford, that they build such a source by using their 200,000-volt X-ray equipment. Although the voltage would be marginal, Bloch thought it would be sufficient for accelerating deuterons, rather than electrons, to produce the desired neutrons.

The fact that Bloch deemed it important to furnish experimental proof was an important turning point in his career. For the first time in 10 years—the first time since he had "played around with the quartz spectrograph" during his third year at the ETH—Bloch started using the tools of the physics laboratory bench, and just as Fermi had predicted, he found experimental physics to be "fun."

> I had never, except in my early student days when I did some elementary physics lab, had any experimental experience. But it was a great experience then to work with Bradbury and do some of the really "low-brow" work, soldering and whatever is necessary; and so I did acquire at that point—and I must say with great joy—the elements of experimental physics.
>
> And we did build a neutron source. We installed our source, our atom source, which eventually was built in one of the X-ray tubes, and by very primitive means convinced ourselves that we indeed saw some neutrons. Now, of course, that wasn't a great achievement, but nevertheless it was very exhilarating.[256]

Lest he get too far away from the more intangible tools of theoretical physics, Bloch did work during that same period with Arnold Nordsieck, who had been at Leipzig with Heisenberg after Bloch left there in 1933, on what Bloch described as a "rather strange difficulty of [quantum] electrodynamics and solved it. There is a still-famous paper of Nordsieck's and mine, which we wrote at that time,"[257] he said. Always regarded by Werner Heisenberg to be of particular importance,[258] the paper[259] described a phenomenon known as the "infrared catastrophe" and it resulted in another term with which Bloch's name would become permanently associated, the Bloch-Nordsieck theory.

As it turned out, the neutron source that he and Bradbury built never turned out to be worth much, said Bloch. "To me," he said, "it served only as a stimulus to ideas. It was much too weak."[260] As a stimulus for ideas, however, it was very powerful, as it was during that time that Bloch came up with his idea to use polarization for measuring the magnetic moment of the neutron.

Had the apparatus they had been building shown more promise of producing a significant source of neutrons, Bloch may have delayed his July 6, 1936 letter to the editor of *Physical Review* in which he suggested a method for determining the magnetic moment of the neutron.[261] Even as he dropped his letter in the mailbox, he was working to achieve the measurement himself at Stanford. "Experiments are underway here to test the predicted effect and its implications," he wrote.

> We were way behind [said Bloch]. Probably if I had known that we could do the experiment the next week, I might have just done the experiment and then published the paper. But realizing that the experiments were far in the remote future here, I published it anyway. And I wasn't sorry that somebody else did [the experiment]— not at all.[262]

In the opening paragraph of his letter, Bloch stated:

> There are good theoretical reasons to believe that [the neutron] should have a magnetic moment of the same order of magnitude as the measured moment of the proton but having the opposite direction with respect to the angular momentum; these conclusions are partly based on Fermi's theory of beta-decay, partly on the known magnetic moment of the deuteron. Since the Stern-Gerlach method may meet considerable difficulties when applied to neutron beams, we want to propose a different way of obtaining information about the magnetic moment of the neutron which seems considerably simpler and promising in several other respects.[263]

Instead of magnetic deflection of beams of atoms or molecules, the method Stern had used to determine the magnetic moment of protons, Bloch was proposing magnetic scattering of slow neutrons as a method of polarizing neutron beams and for measuring the magnetic moment of neutrons.

A neutron interacting with an atom (or molecule), said Bloch, would be scattered for one of two reasons: 1) Because of an interaction with the atomic nucleus (or nuclei in the case of a molecule), or 2) because of an interaction between the neutron's magnetic moment and the magnetic field of the atom (or molecule). The first interaction would be strong, but short ranged, said Bloch; the second, much weaker, but long ranged. In either case, he predicted, the effect would be of the same order of magnitude.

After establishing the mathematical basis for his theory, Bloch suggested three possible applications: 1) Measuring the magnetic moment of the neutron "by measuring the scattering cross section for very slow neutrons;" 2) producing polarized neutron beams by letting neutrons pass through successive plates of magnetized iron; and 3) studying the distribution of magnetizing electrons in ferromagnets.[264]

Physicists at Columbia, Cornell and Copenhagen[265-268] quickly picked up on Bloch's suggestion, establishing the first direct proof that the magnetic moment of the neutron was approximately -2 nuclear magnetons and proving the method valid for polarizing neutron beams. For Bloch, however, "the most desirable goal to be reached here was that of accurately measuring the magnetic moment of the neutron."[269] For him, -2 nuclear magnetons was not accurate enough. For that, he would use magnetic resonance, an idea he came up with the very next year.

It should be noted that, although John Dunning of Columbia University was one of the first to claim that he had experimentally achieved what Bloch had predicted[270]—that there is a polarization effect upon neutrons by the magnetization of iron, what would come to be known as the "Dunning effect"—Bloch was not convinced Dunning had actually seen the effect. "I was not quite sure," said Bloch, "and I'm not quite sure to this day [in 1968] whether he had seen it. I'm sure he thought he had seen it. It was marginal, and in our case [in 1939 when Bloch and Alvarez looked for it] it was marginal, but it was clear enough that finally we were convinced that there was an effect."[271] *

---

* It wouldn't be until 1941, after Bloch was able to get a cyclotron built at Stanford, that they were able to establish that the mediocre polarization effects that had been obtained—if they had been obtained—were due to magnets that were not fully saturated. With special magnets, they were then able to achieve effects on the order of 20 percent rather than the 1 or 2 percent that had been reported.

Bloch published two papers on magnetic scattering of neutrons, one in 1936,[272] the other in 1937.[273] In spite of the fact that his first method was unable to determine the magnetic moment of the neutron with sufficient accuracy to suit him, he had nevertheless provided a method for directly establishing that the neutron does have a magnetic moment and he had also provided a method for polarizing neutrons, which the editors of Bloch's *festschrift* pointed out has "led to much of our modern understanding of the structure and dynamics of magnetic materials." The editors also noted that "of all his papers, Bloch is proudest of these, since they bring together two widely diverse phenomena: the magnetic properties of materials and those of the neutron."[274] The work he had done with the electron theory of metals and ferromagnetism had paid off richly when he began to explore the properties of the neutron.

An interesting sidenote to Bloch's 1936 paper on neutron scattering is that a future Nobel laureate by the name of Julian Schwinger took note of it and submitted a response to *Physical Review* in which he predicted that, as a result of the nearly eight pages of calculations that followed, "it will appear . . . that the expression for the scattering cross section given by Bloch is in error." The difference between the two results, he wrote, could be attributed to the fact that he, Schwinger, used "the correct Dirac value of the current density and the corresponding magnetic field."[275]

Although Bloch discounted the validity of Schwinger's correction in his follow-up 1937 paper on neutron scattering, he would later acknowledge in a 1968 interview that Schwinger had found an error. "He was very proud of it and rightly so because he was so young. It was his first paper,"[276] Bloch said.

Schwinger *was* young—just 18—but it was not his first paper. His first paper, which dealt with a problem in relativistic quantum mechanics, had been published a year earlier, the same year he was discovered by I.I. Rabi and was about to flunk out of City College in New York because he was doing very poorly in his non-technical courses. Rabi tried to get him a scholarship to Columbia, but the director of admissions would not consider admitting him. With the help of Hans Bethe and George Uhlenbeck, a scholarship for the mediocre student was obtained and Schwinger graduated from Columbia College as a Phi Beta Kappa, with all the work completed for his PhD thesis. He stayed on at Columbia for two more years, working as a theorist in Rabi's laboratory, in order to satisfy the school's two-year graduate-student residence requirement.[277]

In Search of the Neutron's Magnetic Moment, Part II

It was during Fermi's visit to Stanford in the summer of 1937 that Bloch came up with the idea of using magnetic resonance in order to get "an exact measurement of the neutron moment."

> I sort of remember that I mentioned it to [Fermi] orally. That was a much more complicated arrangement that had to do with polarizing and analyzing a neutron beam with a constant magnetic field and a radio-frequency field in between. It is closely related to the technique that Rabi then used for molecular beams.* . . . And I had this same idea independently, but I didn't publish it.[278]

Fermi had come to Stanford at Bloch's invitation to teach a four-week summer session. "That was marvelous," said Bloch. "I think I got more out of Fermi [at Stanford] than I ever got in Rome, because he was here for no other purpose than talking, and we went together to the Sierras and to the coast and so on."[279] Bloch had initiated the summer series in 1936 with George Gamow as the guest lecturer. In 1938, the lecturer was I.I. Rabi; in 1939, Victor Weisskopf; and in 1940, Hans Bethe.

After the summer session, Bloch returned to Europe with Fermi, where Bloch remained until the following spring. After returning from Europe in 1938, Bloch began developing in earnest, in collaboration with Norris Bradbury and Howard Tatel, his first attempt at using magnetic resonance as a tool for measuring the neutron's magnetic moment. Rabi was there for four weeks that summer, and he would check in every morning, said Bloch, to see how it was going. It didn't go well. Bloch said their equipment was more important as a source of inspiration than of neutrons.[280] "We had a radium source [of neutrons]," said Bloch, "and did it with very primitive means. [We] hoped that we could do it and found out that it wasn't possible."[281]

In September of 1938, Hans Staub, a Swiss physicist who was attending the ETH in Zürich when Bloch was working with Wolfgang Pauli, became an instructor of physics at Stanford at Bloch's invitation. "He wanted very strongly to have the position filled with an experimentalist in nuclear physics," remembered Staub, "since together with Norris Bradbury and Howard Tatel he had just started the attempt to measure

---

* Rabi would not actually incorporate the magnetic resonance method mentioned above into his apparatuses at Columbia University until September of that year, after Dutch physicist C.J. Gorter suggested using a radiofrequency oscillator. (See Chapter 1.)

the magnetic moment of the neutron." As Staub recounts the sequence of events:

It was quite clear that the first pathetic experiments using Ra-Be [radium-beryllium] sources for neutrons could not succeed for intensity reasons, although the temporal constancy of intensity was a great advantage. Keeping in mind that even a few hundred dollars were quite hard to pry loose from the department budget, we decided to build a d-d accelerator to be operated on the 170 KV voltage source that had been in existence at Stanford for some time and that was used for the famous X-ray work of Webster, Kirkpatrick, and Hansen [with whom Bloch would later collaborate in his nuclear induction experiment]. The machine, practically all home made, was completed in the summer of 1939, but it was never used for work on the magnetic moment of the neutron. While the machine was still under construction, Felix got quite unexpectedly the opportunity to do the first successful magnetic resonance experiment [with neutrons] with Luis Alvarez[282-283] at the Berkeley Radiation Laboratory's 37-inch cyclotron.[284]

"It may well have been Rabi's advice," said Bloch, which convinced them that the Stanford source of neutrons would never do and that they should try doing it with the Berkeley cyclotron. "So I spoke to [E.O.] Lawrence, and he was very kind and understanding, and also felt this would be an important experiment. I don't know whether he asked Alvarez but Alvarez said he would like to do it with me. So that started my collaboration with Alvarez. I think it started in the fall of '38."[285]

In the fall of 1938, 27-year-old Luis W. Alvarez had been on the faculty of the University of California, Berkeley, for two years. He received his PhD at the University of Chicago in 1936. The cyclotron they would be using for their experiment was the 37-inch machine* (measured across the magnetic poles) that had begun accelerating protons into the

---

* In September 1938, Berkeley's 37-inch cyclotron made history when it was used to radiate cancer with neutrons for the first time in a human patient. The patient was the mother of Ernest Lawrence and his brother, John, a physician. After successfully treating their mothers' cancer with the 37-inch machine, the brothers made plans to use the new 60-inch machine they were building to further their research.
—Richard Rhodes, *The Making of the Atomic Bomb*, (New York: Simon and Schuster, 1988), 240.

million-volt range in January 1932, the same month Chadwick discovered the neutron.

The following is Alvarez's recollection on how his collaboration with Felix Bloch came about:

> One day the telephone rang and it was Felix Bloch whom I had never heard of, and he said he wanted to speak with Ernest Lawrence. Ernest got on the line and later told me that Felix had said, 'I have just thought of how to measure the magnetic moment of the neutron; can I come up and do it?' And Ernest said, 'Fine, how long do you think it will take?' And he said, 'Oh, I don't think it'll take more than a few days.' I think he had the feeling he could probably do it that afternoon.
>
> His idea was that neutrons would be polarized in going through magnetized iron, and he wanted to be able to see the difference in the scattering of neutrons on magnetized and unmagnetized iron. That was the basic idea, that neutrons would be polarized and they would scatter differently. And his original idea was that if you measured the scattering from a piece of iron that was in the magnetic field of the cyclotron and then you took the iron and heated it above the Curie point, then you should see a difference in the number of scattered neutrons. I think this is what Felix thought he could do that afternoon. Maybe it wasn't quite that extreme, but anyway, it seemed like a very, very trivial experiment.[286]

Bloch acknowledged that he probably underestimated the difficulties when they started, and that it gradually became clear that it was not so simple. "This is always true in research," he said. "I think very few people can make a proper forecast of how long it will take, because you never know what difficulties you will run into. But then we had, of course, always our little encouragements and discouragements."[287]

When Bloch told Alvarez that he planned to use the Rabi technique in the experiment, Alvarez said he "immediately thought [Bloch] meant running a beam of neutrons down between shaped magnetic pole pieces, lining them up."

> I told him that there wasn't nearly enough intensity [Alvarez said], that he was doing us a great compliment by saying this, but we couldn't possibly do it. Then he came up to Berkeley and told me that he planned to use big slabs of iron as polarizers and analyzers and he

would use the Rabi technique for flipping [the neutrons] over. And that made sense. I was the only one who had a neutron beam and detecting equipment available, so I was the obvious candidate to implement his idea.[288]

As for who should get the credit for the experiment, Alvarez said:

The magnetic moment of the neutron was done because a theoretical physicist—namely Felix Bloch—50 miles away, suggested the idea, and then he actually came up and worked long hours with me. I was the one who made the equipment run. Felix helped take the data and gave me encouragement and did a lot of hard manual labor, pushing magnets around and lining things up.[289]

Lawrence's cyclotron was "practically the only working cyclotron in the world" at the time, said Bloch, and "it didn't work too well, either."

There were frequent interruptions. In fact, once we had our apparatus built, I remember for weeks and weeks what we did mostly was sit around waiting until the cyclotron beam was on, which sometimes happened once a day. Sometimes it didn't happen for three days. Sometimes it lasted five minutes, and sometimes it lasted three hours. Whenever it was ready, we had to work.[290]

To build the beam-analysis portion of the apparatus and to conduct the experiment, Bloch commuted daily between Stanford and Berkeley, except for an occasional night that he would spend at Emilio Segrè's home in Berkeley, with whom Bloch had worked in Rome five years earlier.

In general, the design of the apparatus was very similar to that suggested by Bloch in his 1936 paper. A beam of neutrons, supplied by the cyclotron, was aimed at two successive magnetized iron plates called the polarizer and the analyzer. The plates took months to develop. Borrowing from techniques others had used, they first tried Armco steel and failed to see the difference in neutron intensity Bloch had predicted in his first paper. They attributed the failure to insufficient magnetic saturation of the iron.

Picking up on a report that Swedish iron would show the magnetic effects at lower fields, they wrapped Swedish iron with flat copper strip and passed current through the copper. Again, there was no difference in neutron transmission.

Finally, they took the Swedish iron, removed the copper strip, and magnetized it between the pole pieces of a Weiss magnet. This time, when they looked for the effect, it showed up.

According to Alvarez, they first found the effect on May 3, 1939. Since they had started looking for it as early as Thanksgiving 1938, they had spent at least six months looking for an effect which, wrote Alvarez, "we should have been able to find at once—at least that is the fundamental rule of experimental physics. If one person can do it, and describes it in the literature, then any other competent person should be able to do it very quickly, if he has all the necessary equipment."[291]

Professor Dunning at Columbia University, for whom the effect was named, had done a "first-class" investigation, noted Alvarez, magnetizing the iron almost to saturation, but the other two groups, one at Niels Bohr's Institute in Copenhagen (Otto Frisch, et al.) and the other at Cornell University (J.G. Hoffman, et al.), had seen an effect that Alvarez and Bloch didn't believe was there.

> These two groups [wrote Alvarez] found that the Bloch-predicted effect appeared when the magnetization of the iron was quite far from saturation, and in fact the Copenhagen group "saw" the effect when the iron was not subjected to an external magnetizing current, but simply existed in its remanent field. . . Felix and I spent six months finding out for ourselves that these two groups had been wrong."[292]

Other than the source of the neutrons, the primary difference between the early experiments and the Bloch-Alvarez experiment was the addition of a strong homogenous magnetic field and an oscillating field in the region between the polarizer and analyzer. This was the equivalent change Rabi and his team had made in 1937 when they made the same additions to the center of their molecular-beam apparatus. As Bloch and Alvarez described it in their paper:

> Its principle consists in the variation of a magnetic field H_0 to the point where the Larmor precession of the neutrons is in resonance with the frequency of an oscillating magnetic field. The ratio of the resonance value of H_0 to the known frequency of the oscillating field gives immediately the value of the magnetic moment.[293]

It was virtually the same technique that Rabi and his associates had used, slowly changing the magnet current while a beam of lithium chloride molecules wended their vacuous way from oven to detector and noting when the bottom dropped out of the beam intensity, an indication that almost all of the lithium nuclei had reoriented at the point of resonance. For Bloch and Alvarez, the *neutron* beam dropped off in intensity at the point of resonance. Plotted on a graph, the magnet strength compared to the beam intensity resulted in the same kind of resonance dip the Rabi team had obtained.

According to Alvarez, on June 1, 1939, Felix wrote in his notebook, "Dip at 0.8, corresponding to 2.2 nuclear magnetons." That was the first entry, said Alvarez in reviewing the notes, in which any mention is made of the existence of a dip. The next page, he said, showed a dip corresponding to 2.3 nuclear magnetons, and a curve a couple of pages later showed a dip at 2.25.

We had, of course [noted Alvarez], hoped that the magnetic moment would not simply be the difference between the deuteron moment and the proton moment, so we were delighted that the apparent measured moment was more than 1.93. But then as we achieved more and more precision, the moment came down to the "expected" value of 1.93.[294]

More precisely, Bloch and Alvarez found the magnetic moment of the neutron to be 1.935 ± 0.02 nuclear magnetons.*

It was during the time that Bloch and Alvarez were working on their neutron experiment that the announcement was made to the world that neutrons had been used to split the uranium atom. Alvarez remembered exactly where he was when he first learned of the historic event.

I was sitting in the barber chair in Stevens Union having my hair cut, reading the *[San Francisco] Chronicle*. I didn't subscribe to the *Chronicle*, I just happened to be reading it, and in the second section, buried away some place, was an announcement that some German

---

* In 1949, just a short time before Erwin Hahn arrived at Stanford to work with Bloch, Hans Staub and his graduate student, Emery Rogers, determined the signs of proton and neutron magnetic moments directly by using a true rotating field instead of an oscillating one. The sign of the neutron magnetic moment was found to be negative. "I remember vividly," wrote Staub, "how pleased Felix and also I.I. Rabi were, that the transition experiment was done for once with a true rotating field."

—E.H. Rogers and H.H. Staub, *Physical Review* 76, (1949), 980; Hans Staub, "Ten years of neutron physics withFelix Bloch at Stanford, 1938-1949," *Felix Bloch and Twentieth-Century Physics*, (Houston: Rice University Press, 1980), 195.

scientists had found that the uranium atom split into two pieces when it was bombarded with neutrons—that's all there was to it.

So I remember telling the barber to stop cutting my hair and I got right out of that barber chair and ran as fast as I could to the Radiation Laboratory where my student Phil Abelson [who was later editor of *Science*] had been working very hard to try and find out what transuranium elements were produced when neutrons hit uranium. He was so close to discovering fission that it was almost pitiful. He would have been there, guaranteed, in another few weeks. . . .

I said, "Phil, I've got something to tell you but I want you to lie down first." So being a good graduate student, he lay down on the table right alongside the control room of the cyclotron. "Phil, what you are looking at are not transuranium elements, they are elements in the middle of the periodic table." I showed him what was in the *Chronicle* and, of course, he was terribly depressed. That afternoon, he got out the critical absorbers and, sure enough, identified what he'd been looking at as the eight-day iodine 129.[295]

In Search of the Neutron's Magnetic Moment, Part III

Bloch's original expectation in 1933 that the neutron would have a magnetic moment of -2 nuclear magnetons, estimated on the basis of the deuteron's magnetic moment, was not that far off from his 1939 experimental results. (Bloch had predicted the -2 magneton figure for the neutron by subtracting the proton's magnetic moment from the deuteron's.) Although magnetic resonance had enabled them to measure the neutron's magnetic moment much more accurately, Bloch still wasn't satisfied with the 1 percent uncertainty contained in the number they submitted to *Physical Review* in October 1939. A less-than-optimum magnetic field was partly to blame for the uncertainty; the dependability of the neutron supply was another factor. Bloch wanted to achieve an accuracy to at least three significant digits. After nearly a year of commuting between Stanford and Berkeley, and endless waiting for time on the cyclotron, Bloch wanted his own machine, a machine that would produce a reliable stream of neutrons.

Hans Staub stated it more emphatically, "Felix's mind was now dead set on getting a cyclotron" that would accelerate deuterons to more than a million electron volts (MeV) and which would have the temporal constancy of a radium-beryllium source but would provide a more intense stream of neutrons. "I too shared his desire, but I was appalled to think of the financial consequences," said Staub.[296]

Important assistance, however, was provided by E.O. Lawrence and I.I. Rabi. From Lawrence came encouragement and advice; from Rabi came both encouragement and the critical funding assistance Bloch needed.

[Rabi] took me to see Dr. Weaver, who later was president of the Rockefeller Foundation [Bloch recalled]. Rabi knew him. I'm sure it was due to Rabi's support that they gave me $4000. At that time, the Rockefeller Foundation almost entirely sponsored medical work [rather than the basic science that Bloch was proposing to do with his experiment], but nevertheless, they gave me that. . . . Rabi was very much interested in this experiment.

So then I went back to Stanford and saw the president and said: "I want to build a cyclotron." He said, "Who will raise the money?" I said, "I've just raised $4000, but I don't think it will do." We made a very close estimate and we thought it would run over $5000. He said, "I'm sorry—I don't have any money." This was Ray Lyman Wilbur. So I said to him, "Do you think I should start anyhow?" And sort of with a twinkle in his eye, he said, "Well, if I were you, I would start anyway." Somehow, we financed it. We didn't get a real gift from the University, but we got a little bit of money here and a little bit there. We scraped together the last thousand dollars. There was no need to convince the University. You could do anything you wanted as long as it didn't cost any money.[297]

The cyclotron that Bloch, Bradbury, Staub and William Stephens built in the basement of the physics building was very similar—"practically a copy," said Bloch—to an earlier cyclotron. "It was the simplest design we could find," he said. "We just wanted, for the money we had, to get the strongest neutron source we could."[298]

"Felix proved himself to be not only an outstanding theoretician of magnetism, but also a very able constructor of a large magnet," noted Staub.

Concurrently with the construction of the cyclotron [Staub continued], we had to build all the clumsy electronic and neutron counters, which also required much room and power, by ourselves. The idea of having a technician or a machinist working full-time on our experiments never even entered our minds. Felix was a marvelous collaborator. Within a short time he became quite an expert in electronics and enjoyed these simple techniques. When a circuit he had built with his own hands worked just the way it was expected to, he was as pleased as a child with a toy.[299]

Bloch also got a great deal of pleasure from an arrangement they were able to make with the Stanford power station manager, a story he obviously enjoyed telling a Stanford newspaper reporter in 1982:

> "Let me tell you how we got our power!" [he told the reporter]. "We found that the power station at Stanford had a standby generator, in case the main one failed. So we went to the manager of the station and said, 'Look, why don't you put the standby generator in the basement of our physics department; then we could use it for our cyclotron. It could have a switch on it so that any time you need it in an emergency, all you would have to do is pull the switch.' "
>
> "The power station people were very nice about it, and generously said they agreed. Then came the problem of mounting the generator. It had to be mounted on concrete. We got a bill for $25 from the contractor who cast the concrete."
>
> Bloch could hardly contain his mirth. "Then! We had the nerve to go to the power station people and say to them, 'Listen, this is your generator.' " Bloch was so happy with the thought that each word became punctuated by a laugh: "Why . . . should . . . we . . . pay . . . for . . . your . . . generator?"
>
> When he recovered he wiped his eyes and went on: "Well, they paid. You see? In those days we had to scrounge. How often we have laughed over what we got up to in those days."[300]

According to Staub, the "immense antiquated double pole-double throw switch" that was installed to do the switchover in the case of an emergency was never used.[301]

When completed in the fall of 1941, the Stanford cyclotron did provide the strong beam intensity they had wanted—about 10 µamp of 2.5 MeV deuterons—but the machine would not be used immediately to measure the magnetic moment of the neutron. In fact, seven more years would pass before Bloch and his associates would measure the neutron's magnetic moment with more accuracy than he and Alvarez had achieved in 1939.

It's possible they could have achieved it in late 1941 or early 1942, but Bloch was approaching his second attempt very painstakingly, according to Staub. Niels Bohr had influenced Bloch to be more philosophical and methodical in his approach to physics and perhaps that mindset now influenced the way in which Bloch approached his latest experiment.

It was typical of Bloch [Staub said] that after the cyclotron was successfully operating, he would not attack the main experiment, the precision determination of the neutron magnetic moment, without thorough preparation. In order to do a thorough experiment, we had to get not only an intense slow neutron beam but even more important, a highly polarized one.[302]

As Bloch described his approach:

When our cyclotron was functioning in '41, the first thing we did was to go back and investigate what it was that caused these rather poor polarization effects [in the 1939 experiment]. And we found, although there was some theoretical guidance on that, that one had to push the saturation of the iron very, very close to completeness. At that point then, we built special magnets for that, and then we achieved effects of the order of 20 percent instead of 1 or 2 percent. That was a systematic investigation we did, so that we knew from then on one could get much higher polarization effects.

But then the Manhattan Project got underway, and I was in this early group with Bethe and Teller and Oppenheimer. Oppenheimer called me up one day and told me I should come and see him in Berkeley. I realized then that things had completely changed, and we were told then the first problems about the atom bomb.[303]

The Stanford cyclotron had been operational for only two or three months when Pearl Harbor was bombed by the Japanese on December 7, 1941. The next day, the United States declared war against Japan and, three days later, against Germany and Italy. Although Bloch's preliminary work on his neutron experiment continued until the summer of 1942, it was brought to an abrupt end when he was one of eight physicists recruited by J. Robert Oppenheimer for a summer study to determine the feasibility of producing an atomic bomb. (The others were Hans Bethe, Edward Teller, John Van Vleck, Robert Serber, Emil Konopinski and two post-doctoral assistants.[304]) Gathering behind the locked doors of Oppenheimer's office at Berkeley, the "luminaries," as Oppenheimer called them, agreed early on that fission bombs were indeed achievable, and then took on the question of whether a fusion bomb, the thermonuclear hydrogen bomb, as proposed by Teller, was feasible. Whether "the Super" could be developed was still an open question by the end of the summer but that the Germans were working on a fission bomb was, at that time, a commonly-held presumption.[305]

That summer, Bloch and the rest of the "luminaries" were asked to join the Manhattan Project and to do "whatever we could," said Bloch.

> It was assigned to us here at Stanford to determine the energy distribution of the neutrons emitted in the fission process, which was a rather important question for the chain reaction. This is what we did. The laboratory—down in a light well—was closed. It was done under strict security regulations.[306]

Staub has written that "any further work on the magnetic properties of the neutron came to an abrupt end in midsummer of 1942, when Felix and I, with the collaboration of M. Hamermesh and D.B. Nicodemus and others, took over a contract with the Manhattan District project prior to the formation of the Los Alamos Laboratory. Our task was the determination of the spectral distribution of the neutrons from fission induced by thermal neutrons in [uranium] 235."[307] As alluded to by Bloch, the new cyclotron was also recruited for the task, which was completed by June of 1943. Shortly afterward, Staub and Bloch relocated along with some of the equipment to Los Alamos.

Love and War

In April 1939, just a month or so before he and Alvarez discovered their own evidence of the "Dunning effect," Felix Bloch discovered Lore Misch. He had traveled east to a meeting of the American Physical Society and, while in New York, had met her at the home of a friend to whom he had been introduced by Franco Rasetti. Rasetti, one of the original Fermi collaborators in Rome, had emigrated to the United States in 1935.

Born in Berlin, Lore Clara Misch, also a Jewish physicist and the daughter of a professor, had obtained her PhD degree in 1935 at the University of Göttingen. Trained in X-ray crystallography under world-renowned geophysicist and mineralogist Viktor Moritz Goldschmidt, also Jewish, both mentor and protégé left Germany to escape Hitler in 1936, Goldschmidt to Norway and Misch to Switzerland by way of Copenhagen. She served as an assistant in physics for two years at the University of Geneva before emigrating to the United States in 1938. In the United States, Misch became a research associate at Massachusetts

Institute of Technology in George Harrison's spectroscopy laboratory, where she was employed when she met Bloch the following April.

In September 1939, not long before he began commuting regularly to Berkeley for his collaboration with Alvarez, Bloch spent five weeks on the East Coast and during that period, Felix and Lore decided to get married. On March 14, 1940—shortly after construction of Stanford's cyclotron was started—they were married in Las Vegas. Ten months later, on January 15, 1941—shortly before construction of the cyclotron was completed—they became the parents of twin boys, George Jacob and Daniel Arthur. (Four years later, a third boy, Frank Samuel, would be born on January 16, 1945. He would be just over one year old when his father would submit the announcement of his successful nuclear induction experiment to *Physical Review*. Four more years and the family would be complete on September 15, 1949 with the birth of a daughter, Ruth Hedy.)

When the Blochs and their two-and-a-half-year-old twin boys moved from Palo Alto, California to Los Alamos, New Mexico, the husband and father of the family was having mixed emotions. "I wasn't sure, first of all," he said, "what I would do there and whether I could really live in this military atmosphere. But nevertheless I felt it was my duty at least to try."[308]

In Los Alamos, Bloch was first assigned to Hans Bethe's group but found that the theoretical work that was going on there just didn't interest him. "I didn't fit in there," he said. "That was Bethe's group, and he had his people compute it. I found that was not what I wanted to do. I got interested in the implosion, in [Seth] Neddermeyer's group."

In Neddermeyer's group, Bloch did both theoretical and experimental work to show that the velocities and pressures predicted by Neddermeyer were, indeed, achievable. "People were not convinced of it," said Bloch. "I must say I had very little doubt about it, but they needed experimental proof, and I did that."

At that point, Bloch decided that his usefulness at Los Alamos was over. "Besides," he said, "I just could not live under this atmosphere."

It was a military atmosphere. Letters were opened and one was under constant surveillance and so forth. Maybe that's a rationalization. The only reason I joined the project, like many of us, was the fear that the Germans might develop [the bomb] first and might be ahead of us. I had no real evidence for that, but I felt that this was not very likely to happen. If it had happened, I probably would have felt very badly, but it did not happen. So I left, somewhat to the annoyance of some of my friends, in particular, Oppenheimer.[309]

Although Lore Bloch didn't mind Los Alamos, she, too, was "perfectly glad to leave,"[310] said Bloch, when he was offered a position at Harvard's Radio Research Laboratory (RRL) back in Cambridge, where she had lived before their marriage. In November 1943, the four of them headed east. When they arrived in Cambridge, they moved into a home on Bates Street, just two blocks away from Rabi's home on Avon Hill Street, where Rabi and his wife Helen had lived since the beginning days of the Radiation Laboratory in late 1940.

By that point in the war, the Germans had begun developing radar and the RRL's task was to find effective counter-measures against it. As a result, the RRL had even higher security than that of the MIT Radiation Laboratory. Physicist John Van Vleck of Harvard, an old friend of Bloch's, was the head of Bloch's group.

At Los Alamos, Bloch had felt that his usefulness was over and was ready to leave. At the RRL, he also didn't know whether his work was of great use or not. Under the direction of Stanford engineer Frederick E. Terman, Bloch found his new job to be "pretty straightforward . . . nothing really terribly profound," but he found his new environment to be "much more congenial," he said. "We lived in the city, and we had a civilian life. . . . It was a good time I had in Cambridge. And actually I didn't realize that what I did there was going to be much more useful for my post-war work than what I had done and learned in Los Alamos."[311]

Although his work was primarily theoretical, Bloch did find opportunity to do some experiments, for which he had acquired a taste since moving to the United States nine years earlier. And the experiments, which involved working with microwaves to test the reflectivity of certain materials, gave him practical work with radio techniques, so that, by the end of the war, he said, "I knew what a receiver and an antenna was, and I knew what noise was. . . . I knew very little about radio techniques before I joined this Harvard laboratory." The new knowledge that he gained would prove to be "all-important"[312] in the task he would later begin working on in the evenings of early 1945.

The Copenhagen Spirit of 1943

A month before the Blochs moved from Los Alamos to Cambridge, Bloch's friend Niels Bohr, his wife Margrethe, and his brother Harald, the mathematician, moved from Denmark to Sweden by fishing boat under cover of night, each carrying one bag.[313]

The summer of 1943 had seen a tightening of the screws by Germany against its northern neighbor, Denmark. Although the Nazis had occupied the country since the early part of 1940, they had allowed the Danes to keep their constitutional monarchy and self-government to avoid triggering resistance from its many small-acreage farmers, suppliers of much-needed food for Germany. For agreeing to cooperate with Germany's less-than-total occupation, Denmark also exacted another condition, one that Hitler eventually could not tolerate, the safety of its 8,000 Jews, most of them in Copenhagen.

With Germany's surrender at Stalingrad and the impending loss of Italy to the cause, Hitler demanded in late August that the Danish government declare a state of national emergency, impose curfews, censor the press, forbid strikes and meetings, and outlaw firearms. When the government refused, Copenhagen was reoccupied, the army disarmed, and the royal palace blockaded. Besides the frustrations caused by military reversals, another major reason for Hitler's crackdown was his unwillingness to exempt Denmark's Jews from participating as victims in his Final Solution, a euphemistic term for his plan to systematically exterminate European Jews, a plan which by 1943 had shifted into high gear.

Although Nobel laureate Niels Bohr was high on the Nazi list for removal, and other notable Jews had been arrested, the Nazis had delayed apprehending the well-known scientist until a more general round-up of Jews was made, to make his arrest less odious to the world. In late September, however, the Swedish ambassador hinted to Bohr that his turn was coming in a few days. This was soon confirmed from another source who had seen the actual orders for arresting and deporting him and his brother, Harald. On September 29, Niels and Margrethe Bohr, and Harald Bohr made their escape but not before Niels heard that the Nazis were planning to gather up all the rest of the Jews the following evening. (Niels Bohr's son, Aage, who would also become a Nobel laureate in 1975, would escape soon afterward.)

When Niels Bohr alerted Swedish authorities in Stockholm to the German plan, he found that the Swedes had already protested to Germany and had offered to intern the Danish Jews, but that the Germans had denied any plans to go after the Jews. Actually, they were trying to carry out their plans even as Bohr was trying to intervene. Fortunately, except for nearly 300 nursing-home residents who were captured, most of the Jews in Denmark had also gotten word and had been concealed by their fellow citizens. At this point, however, it was not still not known to them that Sweden was offering a safe haven.

Requesting a meeting with the king of Sweden, Bohr urged him to make Sweden's private protest to Germany public so as to alert the Jews in Denmark and to bring world attention to their plight. The king, in turn, agreed to talk to the Foreign Minister. On October 2, Swedish radio made the broadcast Bohr had requested, and signaled an escape route. In 1922, Bohr had visited Stockholm to receive the Nobel Prize in physics. Now, nearly 21 years later, he had again found himself in Stockholm and this time, with the help of the Swedish government, had secured the greatest prize of all, the saving of many lives. More than 7,000 Jews fled to Sweden in the next two months, many of them with the help of the Swedish coast guard.

It is quite probable that the latter prize—the saving of so many lives— may not have been achieved had Bohr not been awarded the Nobel Prize. Because of who he was and the high esteem in which he was held, his appeal for help had carried more weight.

Even the Germans had recognized his political clout and had delayed his arrest, hoping to minimize negative world opinion. It is a well-estab- lished principle: Exposing human-rights violations is more effective in their reduction than is silent acquiescence, and the higher the level of the person making the exposure, the greater the impact.

In 1937, Felix Bloch had recognized this principle when he sought to obtain, through Richard Tolman, the help of Nobel laureate Robert Millikan in sponsoring action that would help reduce the persecution of the Jews in Europe.

After Felix Bloch was awarded his own Nobel Prize, he recognized the added responsibility that went with it. In 1982, he said,

> The weight that has been added to my name because of my Nobel Prize makes it a matter of conscience for me to speak up for the caus- es in which I believe. One of them is to help the Jewish scientists of Russia, many of whom are singled out for punishment under false accusations. Many of them want to emigrate, as I did. So I add my voice, together with many others, to appeal for them.[314]

Prelude to Nuclear Induction

"In early '45," said Bloch, "the end of the war was very much in sight. At that time, I began to think about what one could do after the war. I talked with Rabi quite a lot at that time," he said. "The Rabis lived only two blocks from us in Cambridge, so we saw each other quite often."[315] During one of their conversations, Bloch told Rabi that he would like to go back to his neutron work after the war. The problem of polarizing iron had been solved before the duties of war had taken Bloch and his associates away from their experiment, but there was still one problem they needed to deal with, the measurement of the magnetic field.

Because he planned to use the same magnetic resonance method he had used in 1939 with Alvarez, Bloch knew there were really just two parts of the experiment, now that the polarization problem had been solved. The first was to measure the frequency of the oscillating field— that was easy—and the second to measure the strength of the magnetic field—that was not so easy. Rabi, of course, was familiar with the problem because of his own work with molecular beams.

"We had all sorts of ideas," said Bloch. "[including] perhaps we could ship a permanent magnet to Columbia for calibration with molecular beams and then it would be shipped back to us. It sounded extravagant, as one would never know what happened to the magnet in shipment." Somewhere in the process, however, Bloch began shifting his focus somewhat from neutrons to nuclei.

I began to think whether one could not do it in some other way [other than molecular beams]. And then I found out that one doesn't really need molecular beams to study the nuclear magnetic resonances—Rabi did only molecular beams—but that one should be able to do it in condensed matter, not in a vacuum, in liquids in fact. I thought almost exclusively of water from the beginning. So I had this idea then of what I called nuclear magnetic induction.

I invented the phrase "nuclear induction" because I wanted to state that nuclear magnetic resonance was not our invention. That had been done by Rabi and his people before. But the fact that the signal was received by induction in the Faraday sense, induction in a coil, is why I called it nuclear induction. However, the word didn't stick. It is now used in a very special sense.[316]

Bloch did his initial theoretical development of nuclear induction while living in Cambridge. "I did my work mostly in the evening—my calculations—convincing myself that this should at least be possible; that the size of the signals were big enough."[317] He began by calculating the voltage that would be induced by precessing protons in 1 milliliter of water at room temperature, subjected simultaneously to a strong static field superimposed by a radiofrequency field positioned perpendicularly to the main field. He was amazed, he once told Erwin Hahn, how his simple calculation had yielded such large voltage signals, well above amplifier noise. In spite of his theoretical expectations of large signals, shown by calculation, his gut feeling told him that, since the magnetic energy of spins coupled to the applied field was a million times smaller than the energy of random thermal vibrations, the signal would be drowned out by the thermal noise. , although he was concerned about how long it might take to reach thermal equilibrium.[318-319] Even though Bloch was surprised by the large signal his calculations had theoretically uncovered, he was still, according to Hahn, much concerned that, since the magnetic energy of spins coupled to the applied field was a million times smaller than the energy of random thermal vibrations, the signal would be drowned out by thermal noise.

While still in Cambridge, Bloch secured the help of his first collaborator on the project, William Webster Hansen. Hansen knew radios. A colleague of Bloch's from Stanford, he had co-invented, together with Russell and Sigurd Varian, the "klystron" vacuum tube, which had been incorporated as the receiver tube in practically all microwave radar systems. On leave of absence from Stanford from 1940 to 1945, Hansen had divided most of his time during the war between Long Island's Sperry Gyroscope Company in Garden City, New York where he worked on further development of the klystron, and the MIT Radiation Laboratory, where he had served as a consultant. In 1944, he had been awarded the Morris Liebmann Memorial Prize, selected by the National Institute of Radio Engineers, for his outstanding contributions to radio engineering.

Bloch and Hansen knew each other well from Stanford, and with Hansen making almost weekly trips to Cambridge, they got together quite often. On one of Hansen's trips in 1945, Bloch enlisted Hansen's help in the new project he'd been working on in the evenings.

> I remember very well how we walked over the Charles River to a restaurant to have lunch and I told Bill that this was something I wanted to do when I came back to Stanford. We knew [the end of the war] would come pretty soon. He was very much interested and promised his collaboration. Even though I knew something about radio techniques, I needed somebody, and Bill Hansen was a great expert. He immediately thought of ways of how that could be put into practice.[320]

Hansen also told Bloch on the same occasion of his own plans to build what has since come to be known as a linear accelerator. Hansen had started his career at Stanford by seeking to accelerate electrons and in the process had co-invented the klystron. Because of his expertise, he had served as a sort of tutor to the physicists at the Radiation Laboratory who knew a great deal about cyclotrons and X-rays, but little about microwaves. In the process, the Radiation Laboratory had been able to achieve tremendous gains in microwave power and Hansen now realized that, with what they had learned, much larger electron accelerators could be built. "So two really great projects were brewing for Stanford," said Bloch. "When Bill and I went back, we both had our hands full."[321] (W.W. Hansen would not live to see his dream completely fulfilled. He died of emphysema May 23, 1949, four days short of his 40th birthday.)

Bloch moved back to Stanford in the summer of 1945, and immediately began putting his plan into action. He only had $450 with which to construct the apparatus for his experiment. This was before large amounts of money began being released for physics research after the war. Three hundred dollars was needed just for the cathode-ray oscillography equipment, and virtually all the radio equipment would have to be built from scratch. For that, Bloch and Hansen enlisted the help of a 24-year-old graduate student by the name of Martin Everett Packard, who built the radio equipment according to Hansen's design. Bloch worked mainly on the magnet portion of the apparatus.

The team was now complete and the letter they would submit to the editor of *Physical Review* in late January of 1946 would bear the names of Bloch, Hansen and Packard. Had Bloch's collaborator from his pre-war cyclotron days been able to get away from Los Alamos sooner, the experiment would also have been credited to Hans Staub. Writing for Bloch's 1980 *festschrift,* Staub recalled how close he had come to working on the project.

In September 1945, I returned for a few days' visit to Stanford. Felix had already been back for some time and had started peaceful work with great enthusiasm. I remember very well how, on a sunny afternoon in his garden, he told me that he believed he had found the really decisive method for comparing the magnetic moments of the neutron and proton. In his familiar and simple way, using purely classical ideas and models, he explained his experiment, and I heard for the first time about nuclear induction. He urged me to return immediately to Stanford to participate in this work, but much as I regretted it (and I still do), I had to return to Los Alamos until February 1946 for a lot of clean-up work. When I finally returned, Felix, Bill Hansen, and Martin Packard had just completed successfully the first nuclear induction experiments, using the same old 3-inch lecture demonstration magnet we had used for the neutron polarization experiments, whenever it was not needed for lecture demonstrations.[322]

Nuclear Induction

Thus far, three phases of Bloch's search for the magnetic moment of the neutron have been described:

1) His plan to develop a neutron source at Stanford, inspired by his 1935 trip to Europe, soon became directed toward experimentally determining the neutron's magnetic moment. When Bloch's radium-beryllium source of neutrons proved to be inadequate, he published his idea for using magnetized iron to scatter and polarize neutrons and to measure their magnetic moment. Other experimenters soon used his suggestion to confirm that the neutron's magnetic moment was equal to approximately -2 nuclear magnetons.

2) Bloch's collaboration with Luis Alvarez, completed in 1939 and using magnetic resonance, resulted in their detection of the polarization effect Bloch had predicted (claimed earlier by John Dunning and others) and the establishment of the neutron's magnetic moment at -1.935 ± 0.02 nuclear magnetons. It was definite progress as far as accuracy was concerned, but not as accurate as Bloch wanted. He also was not satisfied with the strength of the polarization effect they had detected.

3) Together with Hans Staub and others, Bloch was able to get a cyclotron constructed at Stanford. After its completion in 1941, Bloch, Staub and M. Hamermesh began a careful, methodical approach to measure again the neutron's moment, but first Bloch wanted to understand why the polarization effect had not been more pronounced in his previous attempt. By 1942, they were able to significantly improve the polarization effect, but a more accurate measurement of the magnetic moment was halted by the demands of the Manhattan Project.

The conversation Bloch had with I.I. Rabi in 1945 had focused on continuing his work with neutrons after the war. Only afterward did Bloch begin to think of getting away from beams—either molecular or neutron—and to contemplate the possibility of measuring the magnetic moments of atomic nuclei in condensed matter. But this was more an evolution of method than of purpose. In other words, Bloch had not decided to abandon measurement of the neutron's magnetic moment in favor of the proton's; he had instead found a method that would allow him to measure the magnetic moments of the neutron, proton, deuteron and even the triton.

He was not aware, however, that attempts had already been made to detect magnetic resonance in condensed matter, as Erwin Hahn, a colleague of Bloch's in the early 1950s, points out:

> He [Bloch] was unaware that Gorter had failed in 1936 and in 1942 to carry out such an experiment in a crystal. This is not surprising since Bloch was not a conscientious surveyor of the literature. He preferred to rediscover and work out things for himself—a marked characteristic of his independent personality.[323]

It should also be mentioned that just a few months before the Bloch-Alvarez experiment in 1939, and three thousand miles to the east, I.I. Rabi, Norman Ramsey and their associates had discovered that the deuteron also has an electric quadrupole moment,[324] which Bloch and Alvarez had acknowledged in their 1939 paper. Two years later, in 1941, William Rarita and Julian Schwinger had shown theoretically that, because of the quadrupole moment, it was invalid to assume that the magnetic moment of the neutron was essentially the difference between the proton's magnetic moment and the deuteron's magnetic moment.[325] Experimentation was needed to confirm the theory and to measure those values precisely.

That these developments were considered by Bloch in conceiving nuclear induction is evident in his theoretical paper on the subject, published in October 1946:*

> The exact measurement of the magnetic moments of the neutron, the proton, and the deuteron is at present one of the most interesting

---

* Two comprehensive papers on nuclear induction were published in October 1946. The first, mentioned here, is authored by Bloch only and provides the theoretical foundations for nuclear induction. [Ref. a] The second, published in the same issue right after the first, was authored by Bloch, Hansen and Packard and describes the experimental apparatus in detail. [Ref. b] The original publication on nuclear induction, a letter to the editor of *Physical Review* by Bloch, Hansen and Packard, was submitted in late January 1946 and published soon afterward. [Ref. c]

— [a] F. Bloch, "Nuclear induction," *Physical Review* **70**, (1946), 460; [b] F. Bloch, W.W. Hansen, and M.E. Packard, "The nuclear induction experiment," *Physical Review* **70**, (1946), 474; [c] F. Bloch, W.W. Hansen, and M.E. Packard, "Nuclear induction," *Physical Review* **69**, (1946), 127.

problems, concerning nuclear forces. The main difficulty in this comparison was until now the sufficiently accurate calibration of the resonance field. It can be completely avoided by repeating the experiment of Alvarez and Bloch for neutrons and by observing through nuclear induction simultaneously and in the same field the resonances of protons and deuterons. The problem of comparison of their magnetic moments is thus reduced to that of their respective resonance frequencies and can be solved with high accuracy. It was indeed with this experiment in mind, and while searching for a suitable method of comparison, that the author was led to the thought of nuclear induction, and preparations are now under way at Stanford to carry out the measurement in the near future.[326]

What is nuclear induction? In the introduction to his theoretical paper, Bloch pointed out that magnetic resonance had already been used to measure the magnetic moment of the neutron (by Bloch and Alvarez) and of various nuclei (Rabi and associates) and that the principle feature of the method had been "the observation of transitions, caused by resonance of an applied radiofrequency field with the Larmor precession of the moments around a constant magnetic field."[327]

"The question arose," Bloch continued, "whether nuclear transitions could not be detected by far simpler electromagnetic methods, applied to matter of ordinary density." Citing a 1937 attempt in this direction by Soviet physicists B.G. Laserew and L.W. Schubnikow and the 1942 attempt by C.J. Gorter and L.J.F. Broer, which were unsuccessful, and the 1945 experiment of Purcell, Torrey and Pound, which was successful, Bloch pointed out that both the Gorter attempt and the Purcell achievement had looked for a "relatively small reaction upon the driving circuit."[328] In other words, when Purcell's apparatus achieved resonance, the two-sided bridge circuit used in the experiment had become unbalanced.

In contrast, Bloch pointed out, his experiment used a larger radiofrequency field so that a "considerable change of orientation of the nuclear moments would occur," and secondly, rather than detecting resonance by its "relatively small reaction upon the driving circuit," his experiment allowed him to directly observe an "induced electromotive force in a coil, due to the precession of the nuclear moments around the constant field and in a direction perpendicular both to this field and the applied r-f field. This appearance of a magnetic induction at right angles to the r-f field," he wrote, "is an effect which is of specifically nuclear origin and it is the main characteristic feature of our experiment."[329]

At the heart of the Bloch apparatus, the hydrogen-containing sample, 100 milligrams of water sealed in a glass sphere,* was surrounded at nearest proximity by a receiver coil sensitive to variations in flux in the *yz* plane and, outside of that coil, by a transmitter coil, which produced flux in the *x* direction. This double-coil arrangement was then placed between the three-inch diameter poles of the lecture-demonstration electromagnet mentioned by Staub. Oriented in the *z* direction, this static magnetic field, uniform to within 2 gauss according to their measurements, was capable of easily producing "the necessary fields of a few thousand gauss" required for the experiment. (The strength they used in their experiment was 1826 gauss.)[330]

The idea behind the experiment was that when the sample of water was placed between the poles of the static-field magnet, the nuclear magnetic moments would tend to align themselves with that field—either parallel or anti-parallel. "In matter of normal density," read one of the papers, "thermal equilibrium may be established, in which case there will be a paramagnetic polarization in the *z* direction."[331] The fact that there are slightly more that line up in the parallel direction is what makes magnetic resonance methods work. According to a 1954 paper of Edward Purcell's, if 1,000,000 nuclei are lined up parallel to the field,[332] 999,993 will be lined up in the opposite direction.

The Bloch team, like the Purcell team with its hydrogen-containing paraffin, did not initially know how long it would take for thermal equilibrium to be established. According to John Van Vleck, Bloch asked him "whether there was any relaxation process fast enough to make the experiment work,"[333] and Van Vleck had been unable to help resolve the question. To help the process along, Bloch added a set of auxiliary pole pieces in the fringe field of the main magnet to act as pre-polarizers, just in case the nuclei happened to be polarization-resistant. And there was even an unconfirmed rumor that, while he was waiting for the water sample to relax in its new magnetic environment, Bloch relaxed by going on a skiing trip.[334] As a time filler, the trip was unnecessary. The relaxation time required for water, a mere 2.3 seconds, turned out to be much shorter than the relaxation time taken by Bloch.

Once thermal equilibrium was reached, the researchers could proceed with the rest of the experiment. While the transmitter coil superimposed on the sample a 60 cycle-per-second radiofrequency field (oscillating in

---

* In subsequent experiments, the amount of water was increased to about 1 gram.

the x direction), the strength of the static electromagnetic field was adjusted to coincide with the anticipated point of resonance. The collaborators could have done it another way, leaving the magnetic field at a preset value and adjusting the radiofrequency until resonance was reached. Bloch decided to change the static magnetic field because, he said, it "seemed easier."[335] When resonance was reached, the nuclei flopped from the z-direction to the y-direction, where they continued to precess. As they did so, the receiver coil picked up the radiofrequency flux in the y-direction (at the same frequency as the transmitted frequency, but much smaller in magnitude) and manifested it as an induced voltage across its terminals. It was this voltage, the product of nuclear induction, which was "led off to a receiver to be measured."[336]

According to Erwin Hahn, the team's first attempt to measure nuclear induction which took place in the fall of 1945, was a failure, even though they sought for resonance with the field adjusted to the proper 1826 gauss at 7.76 megacycles (or MHz). Shortly after Christmas, 1945, about two weeks after the Purcell team achieved success, the Bloch team momentarily saw a blip appear on the oscilloscope screen as they dropped the magnetic field through the point of resonance. To improve the signal, they added paramagnetic iron nitrate to the water to shorten the relaxation time further and confirmed that they had indeed achieved nuclear induction.

Hahn said that shortly afterward, the Bloch team tried to show an audience what they had found, but they couldn't detect any signal—"the spins," wrote Hahn, "were still shy about exposing themselves to the public, having been left alone in their incoherent privacy for an eternity."[337]

Bloch once said that they had gone "rather slowly" at the experiment and said that he had gotten the first results early in January 1946. "I heard just about at that time from Professor [Otto] Stern at Berkeley* that Purcell had a similar idea and had developed something. I didn't quite know what it was, but it was clear to me that it was in principle the same idea."[338]

---

* In 1922, experiments on space quantization by Otto Stern and Walther Gerlach had made a deep impression on I.I. Rabi, then a graduate student and, in 1927-28, Rabi worked with Stern on molecular beams at the University of Hamburg. Five years later, Stern's 1933 findings on the magnetic moments of the proton and the deuteron would significantly influence Bloch's early interest in looking for the magnetic moment of the neutron. That same year, Stern emigrated to the United States to escape the Nazis and took a position at Carnegie Institute of Technology in Pittsburgh. Stern relocated to the West Coast and the University of California at Berkeley in 1945.

Bloch's recollection appears to essentially jibe with that of his collaborator, Martin Packard, who informed author John Rigden that "it was quite clear to us that it was the same phenomenon, but we were simply approaching it from a different experimental viewpoint. . . . It is true that prior to Bloch's meeting with Purcell, he could not accept the fact that the results were equivalent."[339]

The first meeting between the two future Nobel laureates took place at the spring meeting of the American Physical Society in Cambridge, held April 22-24, 1946. Although Purcell and Bloch had once attended the same party in celebration of I.I. Rabi's 1944 Nobel Prize, they had never met personally. At the APS meeting in Cambridge, both physicists presented brief papers describing their different but equivalent approaches.

Although the Bloch experiment was successful in measuring the magnetic moment of protons using nuclear induction, which was reported first in a brief letter to the editor of *Physical Review*[340] and then described in much more detail by all three authors in the October 1946 issue of *Physical Review*,[341] it was the theoretical paper on nuclear induction authored solely by Bloch[342] (also published in October 1946) that contained what would become known as the Bloch equations.

These equations described not only the theory for nuclear induction but also the theory for the two types of relaxation time, what Bloch called "thermal" or "longitudinal" relaxation time, or T_1, and "transversal" relaxation time, or T_2. These values would come to be much more useful as far as chemical analysis was concerned than the determination of the proton's magnetic moment, and a quarter century later, when a medical researcher by the name of Raymond V. Damadian would take NMR another giant step, from chemical analysis to medical diagnosis, it would be on the basis of the T_1 and T_2 relaxation times first described by Felix Bloch. Damadian's two-pronged discovery,[343] 1) that diseased tissue has significantly different T_1 and T_2 relaxation times than healthy tissue and 2) that healthy tissues also exhibit different though less pronounced T_1 and T_2 relaxation times, would give the clinical basis for MR scanning and its derivative, MR imaging.

Although the division of labor between Purcell's group and Bloch's group was in a state of flux for some time, eventually it became the Purcell group, and in particular, Nicolaas Bloembergen, who would concentrate more heavily on measuring relaxation times for a wide variety of substances and who would develop the theory for why liquids display substantially shorter relaxation times than non-liquids.[344]

The Harvard group also concentrated more heavily on crystals, while the Bloch group, during the same period, concentrated more heavily on determining the magnetic moments for a wide range of nuclei dissolved in solutions.

> We had several machines going then in the basement [said Bloch]. And that was one line which we followed through, simply the precision measurement of every possible nucleus. Every one posed some problems of its own because we always wanted to have them in liquids. It was a question of solutions in which they could be dissolved and so forth. But once that was done, it was usually very simple to measure the moments with accuracy and determine signs.[345]

In Search of the Neutron's Magnetic Moment, Part IV

During the two-year period immediately following his return to Stanford, Bloch did not set aside his plan to determine with more precision the magnetic moment of the neutron. In fact, as soon as Hans Staub returned from Los Alamos, Staub and D.B. Nicodemus, together with Felix Bloch, resumed the polarization work they had left off before the war.

An important by-product of the Bloch-Hansen-Packard experiments was the development of techniques, using nuclear induction as a tool, for measuring and stabilizing magnetic fields. Early on, said Bloch, they realized that nuclear induction was "the ideal magnetometer."

> If you put a proton sample, water let us say, into a magnetic field, then all you had to do is to measure the resonance frequency and you knew the field to a very great accuracy. But we did even better than that. Packard built a magnet stabilizer. That is to say, you can use the signal which comes out to readjust the field automatically electronically. And since we needed not only a very homogeneous field but also a very constant field for the neutron experiment, we combined [nuclear induction with the magnet stabilizer and] measured the field with great accuracy. . . . Then we did the experiment for the neutron moment once more, and did it with very great accuracy.[346]

In his tribute to Bloch, Hans Staub also mentions the neutron experiment, stating that he, Bloch and Nicodemus were able to achieve an accuracy using nuclear induction that "was not improved by an order of magnitude until more than 25 years later."[347] (When that improvement did come, it was accomplished by Norman Ramsey and his collaborators at a laboratory in Grenoble, France.)

As a result of the improvements that Bloch and his associates were able to make in achieving accurate magnetic fields, they were able to make impressive gains in resolution.

> I think I may claim that as altogether our project [said Bloch]. I mean some people thought: "Oh, well, if you have it to a part in a million, why do you want it to a part in a hundred million?" But to me it was a sort of fascinating question. And, of course, my paper had dealt a great deal with the theory of relaxation time and I really wanted to understand what was going on there. Then, out of this, later in 1960 or so, grew probably the most important application of all this.[348]

Bloch was referring at the time (1968) to the revolution in chemical analysis made possible by high-resolution NMR spectroscopy and not to what others might define as "the most important application," the use of NMR for detection of disease. In fact, two more years would pass before Raymond Damadian would use NMR to provide a clinical basis for disease detection with his proof of prolonged relaxation times for cancer tissue as well as significant variations in relaxation times even between normal tissues. Because of the discovery of various types of chemical shifts* at MIT, Harvard, Stanford, and the University of Illinois in the early

---

* A discussion of chemical shifts occurs several times throughout this book, in this chapter as well as in the Ramsey and Bloembergen chapters. Erwin Hahn, cautioning against an overly generic use of the term, has written: "To get the story strictly correct, what was known as the chemical shift was first discovered experimentally in the MIT laboratory of the late Francis Bitter by a graduate student named William Dickenson way back, even before I found spin echoes. The original chemical shift results from the additional local magnetic field produced by the atomic currents of bonded circulating electrons in molecules, added to the external applied field. This shift is relatively easy to resolve because it is larger than another shift which was discovered experimentally later at Illinois and Stanford, independently by Hahn and by the team of Gutowsky and Slichter. Harvard followed up these experimental discoveries afterwards with seminal theoretical interpretations. This second shift is not the "chemical shift" alluded to above. It is rather another interaction, like a shift but much smaller that involves the contact of the electron clouds with mutually bonded nuclear moments and is called the indirect spin-spin hyperfine interaction, identified by Ramsey and Purcell. Hence, credit is due to Harvard because of the theoretical interpretations made, first by Ramsey on the Dickenson chemical shift, and then by Ramsey and Purcell theory on the hyperfine coupling, now called the "J interaction."
—Erwin Hahn, personal communication to James Mattson, 22 January 1995.

1950s,[349-356] combined with a theoretical explanation for several of them by Norman Ramsey starting in 1949 and later, collaboratively, with Purcell and Liddell, [357-363] NMR spectroscopy was, by 1968, well recognized for its ability to provide "fingerprint" identification of chemicals by their unique combination of spectral lines.

One of the most-cited examples in reference to chemical shifts—ethyl alcohol—took place in Bloch's laboratory at Stanford. Although the protons making up the ethyl alcohol molecule are all chemically equivalent and, if isolated from one another, would resonate at the same frequency, Arnold, Dharmatti and Packard[364] found that because of the chemical's unique bonds, each of the three groups of protons making up the molecule resonated at slightly different frequencies. As a result, instead of one spectral line, there were three, each shifted from "normal," producing a spectral line combination that serves as ethyl alcohol's "fingerprint."

Bloch particularly enjoyed the way Niels Bohr once described the chemical shift phenomenon when used as a tool for chemical analysis:

> I visited Copenhagen frequently after the war [said Bloch]. At one point, I gave a talk in Copenhagen, and then afterwards we met with Bjerrum. Bjerrum was a chemist and a great friend of Niels Bohr. . . . Bohr said to him: "You know, what these people do is really very clever. They put little spies into the molecules and send radio signals to them, and they have to radio back what they are seeing." I thought that was a very nice way of formulating it. That was exactly how they were used. It was not anymore the protons as such. But from the way they reacted, you wanted to know in what kind of environment they are, just like spies that you send out. That was a nice formulation.[365]

During the same period that Arnold, Dharmatti and Packard were working on chemical shifts, Erwin Hahn, who had recently discovered a phenomenon called "spin echoes," came to work with Bloch at Stanford.

> He came from [the University of] Illinois [said Bloch], a very original man; and he had developed . . . spin echoes. That was his own version or really a variation, a very interesting variation, of our game where, instead of applying the radiofrequency at a constant wave form, he put in pulses and observed what came out from that. He developed it very ingeniously. He also, when he came here, started to work on substances other than water and found some peculiar structure which he interpreted as chemical effects [or shifts].[366]

Hahn came to Stanford as a post-doctoral fellow in 1950, and remained for an additional year as an instructor before moving on to IBM, Columbia University and later, to the University of California, Berkeley. Before he came to Stanford, he had already developed an appreciation for the multi-purpose Bloch equations; at Stanford, Hahn developed a deep appreciation for the multi-talented and personable Felix Bloch himself.

Felix was a wonderfully clear teacher. His fundamentalism was evident in his use of the original works of J.W. Gibbs as a text in his course on statistical mechanics. After his retirement, Felix began the writing of a text on statistical mechanics based on his rigour of interpretation, which was unfinished at the time of his death. . . . I learned recently that Felix had a small hobby of doing this sort of thing in another vein. During short visits to Israel he resorted to the original Hebrew in carrying out translations of the Old Testament, which was so stated in his honorary degree *Laudatio* at Oxford University. . . .[367]

It was in his nature to have a profound influence on his students. His love for physics took a high priority in his life, which induced him continually to avoid the impediments of formal rules of bureaucratic restraints that [could have] prevented him from doing things for himself. He always invited others to share in his search for answers, and did not distance himself from anyone who would join him in the search, regardless of his or her status. What many of his students gained from him intellectually was often merged with his advice and counsel. Felix was a devoted family man, and not incidentally, he was also an accomplished pianist.[368] . . . He was an accurate and inspired performer. His style of playing exhibited a perfectionism, in constant awareness of nuances demanded by the composer.[369] . . . With his good wife Lore and the family, the invitations to participate in activities of family life, with musicals, hikes and parties, were all occasions indeed memorable, giving positive incentive and enjoyment in learning physics from Felix.[370]

It was the same awareness of nuances demanded by the physical world if one was to properly interpret it, combined with a superior intellect, that made Felix Bloch such a great physicist. He would credit Heisenberg and especially Bohr with developing much of his philosophical approach to physics, for teaching him to examine the foundations, but the propensity to do so, though perhaps latent for a time, had been there all along, as evidenced by his conclusions after visiting the observatory in Zürich many years earlier with his father. To repeat his recollection of that important event in his young life:

> I looked up and saw some stars; I had the feeling that this was very wonderful and apparently people can even understand what goes on up there, although they didn't understand so much at that time. I had quite an early feeling that, "Yes, nature is apparently capable of rational analysis."[371]

Young Felix had been right, and throughout his adult life, he would be an avid investigator of that physical world and an effective communicator of what he had learned.

The Nobel Prize

The scientific community was well aware of the importance of nuclear magnetic resonance or, as Bloch preferred to call it, nuclear induction, and there were frequent discussions as to when it would be recognized by a Nobel Prize.

> What gets a Nobel Prize and what doesn't [Bloch pointed out], is not so sure to say. I had some inklings a few weeks before I received the prize but not before that. And then, there is always the usual gossip among physicists, to which one better pay no attention. . . . "I'm sure you'll get the Nobel Prize next year," and so on. I think quite largely it was a pleasant surprise [said Bloch, but then added] I must say in all modesty that it didn't come entirely out of the blue sky.[372]

When the call came, it was actually a night sky. "They called me from Associated Press at 4 o'clock in the morning, I think," said Bloch, "and I got up and was so sleepy. When they told me, my reaction was 'Nonsense, I must be dreaming.' But then very soon the telegrams started coming in."

Actually, the day before, Bloch had gotten his first warning. Someone from Stanford's information office had come to him and said that he had been hearing rumors; maybe Bloch should be prepared for something the next day. Before Felix and Lore Bloch went to bed that night, he had said to her, "You know, of course, it may all be a false rumor. But even to think that it is possible is a very nice thought."[373]

It wasn't long after hearing that he and Edward Purcell were sharing the prize that Felix Bloch sent his own telegram to his co-winner:

> I think it's swell that Ed Purcell
> Should share the shock with Felix Bloch.[374]

The ditty was so catchy that Harvard's Norman Ramsey remembers his young daughters going around the house for days singing the congratulatory message as joyful accompaniment to their childplay.[375]

A year or so after he received the Nobel Prize, the editor of a local Palo Alto newspaper asked Professor Bloch just how one goes about receiving a Nobel Prize.

"All you do," he said, "is to start with an idea. Then you get paper and pencil and write down some numbers to see whether the idea might work. Then, if necessary, you build a machine to prove it."[376] That's exactly what Bloch had done, and for his achievement, he received many other accolades in addition to the Nobel Prize in physics.

He was elected to the National Academy of Sciences in 1948 and served as president of the American Physical Society in 1965. In addition to the honorary degree conferred by Oxford University (mentioned previously by Erwin Hahn), Bloch also received degrees from the University of Grenoble, the Hebrew University of Jerusalem, the University of Zürich, Gustavus Adolphus College, Brandeis University, and the University of Pavia.

Bloch was a member of the Board of Governors of the Weizmann Institute in Israel and, in 1958, was elected an honorary fellow of the Weizmann Institute of Science. He was also named an honorary member of the Royal Dutch Academy of Sciences in 1958, a fellow of the Royal Society of Edinburgh in 1966, and an honorary member of the French Physical Society in 1970.

Except for his leave of absence from Stanford during the war and a one-year leave as director of the European Center for Nuclear Research (CERN), he remained on the faculty of Stanford as Max H. Stein Professor of Physics until his retirement in 1971, at which time he was named Professor Emeritus of Physics.

Back to Europe . . . for a Year

I.I. Rabi was influential right after the war in establishing Brookhaven National Laboratory on the east end of Long Island, and soon afterward he proposed its European counterpart, the European Center for Nuclear Research (otherwise known as CERN) in Geneva, Switzerland. It has been called "the most significant international cooperative exchange program in science,"[377] and it was of major concern when it was founded that the right person be selected to direct its activities.

The person chosen for the task was Felix Bloch. Although he was not anxious to leave Stanford and his own research agenda, he felt compelled, especially with the strong urging he received from Niels Bohr and Werner Heisenberg, to accept the responsibility.

> The first idea about [my directing of] CERN [said Bloch] came up in the fall of 1953. I received a letter—I believe it was from Bohr—telling me about the importance of this new laboratory and asking me whether I would consider the directorship. I went through great struggles at that time, first feeling, "This is sheer nonsense. I shouldn't go into this kind of thing. I'm not made for administrative work," then thinking that perhaps it wasn't altogether administrative.
>
> Well, finally, in the spring of '54, upon the insistence of Bohr, I went to Copenhagen and talked it over with him. He urged me very strongly at that time to take the directorship of the laboratory. He felt that it was important that an active physicist should head the laboratory, and he believed and gave me the impression that, as director, still my main function would be scientific. And although many of my friends warned me and said, "Don't believe it—it's not going to be that simple," nevertheless I felt at that point that I should try it. . . . Heisenberg was also very eager. I think it was mainly Heisenberg and Bohr who wanted very much that I should take that job.[378]

"I think I can say psychologically," Bloch reflected in 1968, "[that my decision to accept the CERN position] was due to the feeling that my necessity of staying with nuclear induction was not so great anymore. At least my own heydays were over."[379]

Nevertheless, part of the bargain he struck for taking the job was that he would be able to continue some of his research.

> It is true [Bloch said] that I did take some equipment to Geneva. Arnold packed it before I went to Geneva and actually did go with me, because I didn't want to be entirely separated from nuclear induction work. They set up a laboratory at Geneva at the University. What little my time allowed me then, I still came and was interested in this.[380]

Less than five months after his arrival in Geneva in October of 1954, Bloch announced that he would resign effective the end of August, 1955.

"I must confess I was rather unhappy," Bloch said later. He had found that not only were his scientific interests "practically unused," but equally negative, he found his time almost all taken up with administrative work. "In retrospect," said Bloch, "I must say it was an interesting, enjoyable experience, but I'm certainly glad I did not carry it further."[381]

Physicist Anatole Abragam spent two months working with Bloch during Bloch's short stay in Geneva, a time that Abragam recalled with pleasure in 1989.

> Felix Bloch, the great Felix Bloch, who had been chosen as the first Director General of CERN, invited me to spend a few months with him in Geneva. The choice of the first Director of CERN had been delicate: was not there a danger from the beginning of exhibiting the ascendancy of one of the member states? The member states chose someone who was a European by his Swiss birth, but American by his citizenship, and his residence, and a great physicist as well.
>
> There was one flaw in this choice: Bloch disliked "Big Science" and hated administration. Since in the autumn of 1954 the big machines were at the project stage, or at best at the stage of excavation works, all that was left was administration, which filled him with disgust. He had accepted his position out of good will towards old Europe, to which, after 20 years of exile, he still felt very close, and towards CERN as a common European enterprise; but there is no denying that he was bored in Geneva. He wanted to have someone near him with whom he could talk about his beloved magnetic resonance, to "hold his hand," as he put it, and I was flattered to be chosen for this task, from the whole of Europe. . . .
>
> I was not the only one to have been summoned to Geneva to provide cultural amusement for the Maestro; a heavier type of entertainment was on the programme. Bloch had arranged to ship a large permanent magnet from Stanford to Geneva. It weighed several tons, and was specially designed for high resolution NMR by two of his disciples, Jim Arnold and Weston Anderson. . . . My contact with these two men, especially Arnold, was both pleasant and fruitful for me. As soon as they arrived, they uncrated the magnet, installed the electronics, and went to work. "This way at least we'll get a little physics going in CERN," commented Bloch.[382]

The magnet shipped to Geneva in 1954 wasn't the first magnet Bloch was influential in exporting across the Atlantic that year. As a member of the Board of Governors of Weizmann Institute in Israel, he played a key role in the building of the first NMR magnet in Israel. Prior to Bloch's departure for CERN, Solomon Meiboom and Shlomo Alexander had studied at Stanford with Bloch for the purpose of preparing them for spearheading NMR research in that old, new nation (then only six years old since its new birth in 1948).

At the close of a 1968 interview with Felix Bloch, science historian Charles Weiner asked him, "In summing up the work you've done through the years, what has given you the most personal satisfaction?"

For the immediate satisfaction [said Bloch], one of the greatest joys that a scientist can have is when a good idea hits him. That is, when headaches which have been brewing in his mind for some time come together to a solution. That happened to me a few times. But those are moments almost. Those are moments of elation which might last for a day or a week or two, or something like that.

There was a paper with Nordsieck where we stewed and worried for a long time, and suddenly I realized, "Ah, this is the crux of the matter." That gave me great satisfaction.

I'm sure that when I first realized this idea of the nuclear magnetic resonance—just on paper it came, in checking and rechecking and saying, "Yes, by God, I haven't made a mistake. I'm not fooling myself. It should really be possible." That was also a moment of great joy.

Then, of course, there are also long-range satisfactions—that is to say, the development of a certain line, like this resonance work after the war, which extended over many years. It was not a period of constant happiness. I mean there were ups and downs, but by and large it was a time of great satisfaction.[383]

And which of Bloch's contributions has had the most impact?

I would say probably two [he responded]. The one goes way back to my thesis. That was my work on conduction of metals. That certainly has had a great impact. And the second was, I think, the discovery of induction. The work based on my early work on electron conduction is still going on. It's very important in solid-state physics. And nuclear induction has become a tool which is made use of widely.[384]

That was in 1968. Damadian's research revealing the potential of NMR for medical diagnosis would not be completed until 1970 and would not be published until March of 1971, and the first commercial MR scanner would not be shown to the world until 1980. Fortunately, Felix Bloch lived to see the beginning of the magnetic resonance revolution in medical diagnosis and, before his death in 1983, told physicist Erwin Hahn and others that the extension of magnetic resonance to humanitarian practical use was of great satisfaction to him.[385] ∎

REFERENCE NOTES:

1. Anatole Abragam, "A virtuoso of quantum mechanics," Felix Bloch (1905-1983), European Laboratory for Particle Physics, Geneva, CERN/DOC, August 1984, 6-7.

2. L.I. Schiff and R. Hofstadter, "Felix Bloch: A brief professional biography," *Physics Today* **18**, (December 1965), 42.

3. F. Bloch, "Quantum mechanics of electrons in crystal lattices," *Zeitschrift für Physik* **52**, (1928), 555.

4. F. Bloch, "Temperature variation of electrical resistance at low temperatures," *Zeitschrift für Physik* **59**, (1930), 208.

5. F. Bloch, "Theory of the exchange problem and of residual ferromagnetism," *Zeitschrift für Physik* **74**, (1932), 295.

6. F. Bloch, interview by Charles Weiner, 15 August 1968, transcript, Niels Bohr Library, American Institute of Physics, College Park, MD, 7.

7. F. Bloch, interview by Lillian Hoddeson, 15 December 1981, transcript, Niels Bohr Library, American Institute of Physics, College Park, MD, 77.

8. F. Bloch, "On the scattering of neutrons," *Physical Review* **50**, (1936), 259.

9. J.G. Hoffman, M. Stanley Livingston, and H.A. Bethe, "Some direct evidence on the magnetic moment of the neutron," *Physical Review* **51**, (1937), 214.

10. J.R. Dunning, P.N. Powers, and H.G. Beyer, "Experiments on the magnetic properties of the neutron," *Physical Review* **51**, (1937), 51.

11. P.N. Powers, H.G. Beyer, and J.R. Dunning, "Experiments on the magnetic moment of the neutron," *Physical Review* **51**, (1937), 371.

12. Luis W. Alvarez and F. Bloch, "The magnetic moment of the neutron," *Physical Review* **57**, (1940), 352.

13. Luis W. Alvarez and F. Bloch, "A quantitative determination of the neutron moment in absolute nuclear magnetons," *Physical Review* **57**, (1940), 111.

14. Norman F. Ramsey, conversation with Luis Alvarez mentioned in "Early magnetic resonance experiments: roots and offshoots," *Physics Today*, October 1993, 42.

15. F. Bloch, interview by Weiner, 15 August 1968, 28.

16. I.I. Rabi, J.R. Zacharias, S. Millman, P. Kusch, "A new method of measuring nuclear magnetic moment," *Physical Review* **53**, (1938), 318.

17. M. Chodorow, R. Hofstadter, H. Rorschach, and A. Schawlow, eds., *Felix Bloch and Twentieth-Century Physics*, (Houston: Rice University Press, 1980), ix.

18. F. Bloch, W.W. Hansen, and M. Packard, "Nuclear induction," *Physical Review* **70**, (1946), 460.

19. E.M. Purcell, H.C. Torrey, and R.V. Pound, "Resonance absorption by nuclear magnetic moments in a solid," *Physical Review* **69**, (1946), 37.

20. Abragam, "A virtuoso of quantum mechanics," August 1984, 7.

21. F. Bloch, interview by Thomas Kuhn, 14 May 1964, transcript, Niels Bohr Library, American Institute of Physics, College Park, MD, 1.

22. Ibid.

23. Ibid., 2.

24. Ibid.

25. Ibid., 3.

26. Ibid.

27. Ibid.

28. Ibid., 3-4.

29. E. Beck, *Annalen der Physik* **60**, (1919), 109-48.

30. F. Bloch, interview by Kuhn, 4.

31. Ibid.

32. Ibid., 4-5.

33. Ibid., 5.
34. Ibid., 6.
35. Ibid.
36. Ibid., 7.
37. Ibid.
38. Ibid.
39. Ibid., 8.
40. Ibid., 9.
41. Ibid.
42. Ibid., 8.
43. Ibid.
44. Ibid., 9.
45. F. Bloch, "Heisenberg and the early days of quantum mechanics," *Physics Today*, December 1976, 23.
46. F. Bloch, interview by Kuhn, 8-9.
47. Bloch, "Heisenberg and the early days of quantum mechanics," 23.
48. F. Bloch, interview by Kuhn, 10.
49. Ibid., 11.
50. Edward M. Purcell, interview by Katherine Sopka, 8 June 1977, transcript, Center for History of Physics, American Institute of Physics, New York, 8-9.
51. F. Bloch, interview by Kuhn, 10.
52. Ibid., 11.
53. Bloch, "Heisenberg and the early days of quantum mechanics," 23.
54. Ibid.
55. C.J. Davisson and L.H. Germer, "Diffraction of electrons by a crystal of nickel," *Physical Review* **30**, (1927), 705.
56. G.P. Thomson, "Experiments on the diffraction of cathode rays," *Proceedings of the Royal Society (London)* **117A**, (1928), 600 and "The diffraction of cathode rays by thin films of platinum," *Nature* **120**, (1927), 802.
57. Bloch, "Heisenberg and the early days of quantum mechanics," 23.
58. F. Bloch, interview by Kuhn, 13.
59. Bloch, "Heisenberg and the early days of quantum mechanics," 24.
60. E. Schrödinger, "Quantisierung als eigenwertproblem" ("Quantization as eigenvalue problem"), *Annalen der Physik* **79**, 361, 1926; English translation in *Collected Papers on Wave Mechanics* by E. Schrödinger, transl. J. Shearer and W. Deans, (Glasgow: Blackie, 1928).
61. Bloch, "Heisenberg and the early days of quantum mechanics," 24.
62. M. Born and P. Jordan, "Zur quantenmechanik," *Zeitschrift für Physik* **34**, (1925), 858.
63. M. Born, W. Heisenberg, and P. Jordan, "Zur quantenmechanik ii," *Zeitschrift für Physik* **35**, (1926), 557.
64. E. Schrödinger, "Über das verhältnis der Heisenberg-Born-Jordanschen quantenmechanik zu der meinen," *Annalen der Physik* **79**, (1926), 7634.
65. Bloch, "Heisenberg and the early days of quantum mechanics," 24.
66. W. Heisenberg, "Über quantentheoretische umdeutung kinematischer und mechanischer beziehungen," *Zeitschrift für Physik* **33**, (1925), 879.
67. George Gamow, *Thirty Years That Shook Physics, The Story of Quantum Theory*, (Garden City, NY: Doubleday & Company, Inc., 1966), 3.
68. Ibid., 105.
69. Bloch, "Heisenberg and the early days of quantum mechanics," 24.
70. F. Bloch, interview by Kuhn, 16.
71. Donald Stokes, "Felix Bloch tells how his decision led to a Nobel Prize," *Campus Report*, 28 April 1982, 3.

72. Bloch, "Heisenberg and the early days of quantum mechanics," 24.

73. W. Heisenberg in *Niels Bohr*, edited by Stefan Rozental, 1967, North-Holland, quoted by Richard Rhodes in *The Making of the Atomic Bomb*, (New York: Simon and Schuster, 1988), 128-129; W. Heisenberg, *Physics and Beyond*, Harper, 1971.

74. W. Heisenberg, "Über den anschaulichen inhalt der quantentheoretischen kinematik und mechanik,"*Zeitschrift für Physik* **43,** (1927), 172.

75. F. Bloch, interview by Kuhn, 15-16.

76. Bloch, "Heisenberg and the early days of quantum mechanics," 24.

77. F. Bloch, interview by Hoddeson, 28.

78. Alan D. Beyerchen, *Scientists Under Hitler: Politics and the Physics Community in the Third Reich*, (New Haven, CT: Yale University Press, 1977), 32.

79. H. Weyl, *Gruppentheorie und Quantenmechanik*, Hirzel, Leipzig 1928; in English: *The Theory of Groups and Quantum Mechanics*, transl. H.P. Robertson, Dover, New York.

80. Beyerchen, *Scientists Under Hitler: Politics and the Physics Community in the Third Reich*, 25.

81. Ibid., 46-47, 222 note 31.

82. Ibid., 222 note 33.

83. Bloch, "Heisenberg and the early days of quantum mechanics," 27.

84. Ibid., 24.

85. Ibid., 24-25.

86. Ibid., 25.

87. Ibid.

88. Gamow, *Thirty Years That Shook Physics, The Story of Quantum Theory*, 51.

89. Robert Jungk, *Brighter Than a Thousand Suns*, (Harcourt Brace), 26, quoted by Rhodes in *The Making of the Atomic Bomb*, 116.

90. Rhodes, *The Making of the Atomic Bomb*, 116.

91. Ibid.

92. Bloch, "Heisenberg and the early days of quantum mechanics," 25.

93. F. Bloch, interview by Kuhn, 19.

94. Ibid., 25.

95. F. Bloch, interview by Hoddeson, 6.

96. Ibid., 7.

97. Bloch, "Heisenberg and the early days of quantum mechanics," 27.

98. Gamow, *Thirty Years That Shook Physics, The Story of Quantum Theory*, 117.

99. Bloch, "Heisenberg and the early days of quantum mechanics," 23.

100. Ibid., 27.

101. Donald Stokes, "Bloch looks back on nearly 50 years research, Nobel Prize," *Campus Report*, Stanford University, 5 May 1982, 4.

102. Bloch, "Heisenberg and the early days of quantum mechanics," 27.

103. F. Bloch, interview by Hoddeson, 6.

104. Bloch, "Heisenberg and the early days of quantum mechanics," 25.

105. F. Bloch, interview by Kuhn, 19.

106. Bloch, "Heisenberg and the early days of quantum mechanics," 25.

107. Ibid.

108. Ibid.

109. F. Bloch, interview by Kuhn, 21.

110. Bloch, "Heisenberg and the early days of quantum mechanics," 26.

111. Lillian H. Hoddeson and G. Baym, "The development of the quantum mechanical electron theory of metals: 1900-28," *Proceedings, Royal Society of London* **A 371,** (1980), 8.

112. Ibid., 8-17.

113. F. Bloch, "Über die quantenmechanik der elektronen in kristallgittern," *Zeitschrift für Physik*, **52,** (1928), 555.

114. Interview with Bethe by T.S. Kuhn in Archive for History of Quantum Physics, (A.Q.P.), New York, Copenhagen, Berkeley and Minneapolis, 21, quoted by Hoddeson and Baym in "The development of the quantum mechanical electron theory of metals: 1900-28," 17.

115. Bloch, "Heisenberg and the early days of quantum mechanics," 26.

116. Ibid.

117. F. Bloch, interview by Hoddeson, 23.

118. Hoddeson and Baym, "The development of the quantum mechanical electron theory of metals: 1900-28," 8.

119. Abragam, "A virtuoso of quantum mechanics," August 1984, 7.

120. F. Bloch, interview by Kuhn, 21.

121. H.E. Rorschach, Jr., "The contributions of Felix Bloch and W.V. Houston to the electron theory of metals," *American Journal of Physics* **38,** (1970), 901-902.

122. F. Bloch, interview by Hoddeson, 22.

123. F. Bloch, interview by Kuhn, 17.

124. Ibid., 33.

125. Ibid., 25.

126. Ibid., 28.

127. Ibid., 25.

128. Ibid., 28.

129. Ibid., 29.

130. Ibid., 27.

131. Ibid.

132. Ibid., 28.

133. F. Bloch, interview by Hoddeson, 40.

134. Schiff and Hofstadter, "Felix Bloch: A brief professional biography," 42.

135. Anatole Abragam, *Time Reversal: An Autobiography*, (New York: Oxford University Press, 1989), 180.

136. F. Bloch, interview by Kuhn, 28.

137. Ibid., 30.

138. Bloch, "Temperature variation of electrical resistance at low temperatures," 208.

139. F. Bloch, interview by Kuhn, 30.

140. Rorschach, "The contributions of Felix Bloch and W.V. Houston to the electron theory of metals," 902.

141. Felicia Keesing and Rebecca Lowen, "The Felix Bloch Papers: Guide and Inventory of the Collection," Dept. of Special Collections and University Archives, Stanford University Libraries, 1989, 3.

142. F. Bloch, interview by Kuhn, 31.

143. Ibid., 32.

144. Bloch, "Heisenberg and the early days of quantum mechanics," 26.

145. F. Bloch, interview by Kuhn, 31.

146. Stokes, "Felix Bloch tells how his decision led to a Nobel Prize," 4.

147. Ibid.

148. Ibid.

149. W. Heisenberg, interview by Thomas S. Kuhn and John Heilbron, 30 November 1962 to 12 July 1963, transcript, Niels Bohr Library, American Institute of Physics, College Park, MD, session 6, 8-9.

150. W. Heisenberg, interview by Kuhn and Heilbron, session 6, 8-9.

151. F. Bloch, interview by Kuhn, 34.

152. Ibid.

153. Ibid.

154. Ibid., 35.

155. Schiff and Hofstadter, "Felix Bloch: A brief professional biography," 43.

156. Stokes, "Bloch looks back on nearly 50 years research, Nobel Prize," 4.

157. Ibid.

158. Ibid.

159. Chodorow, Hofstadter, Rorschach, and Schawlow, eds., *Felix Bloch and Twentieth-Century Physics*, vii.

160. W. Heisenberg, interview by Kuhn and Heilbron, session 6, 8-9.

161. Gamow, *Thirty Years That Shook Physics, The Story of Quantum Theory*.

162. Rhodes in *The Making of the Atomic Bomb*, 175.

163. F. Bloch, interview by Weiner, 3.

164. Ibid., 2.

165. Ibid.

166. Ibid., 3.

167. Ibid., 2.

168. Rhodes, *The Making of the Atomic Bomb*, 185.

169. F. Bloch, interview by Weiner, 4.

170. F. Bloch, interview by Hoddeson, 69-70.

171. F. Bloch, interview by Weiner, 5.

172. Beyerchen, *Scientists Under Hitler: Politics and the Physics Community in the Third Reich*, 16.

173. F. Bloch, interview by Weiner, 3.

174. Beyerchen, *Scientists Under Hitler: Politics and the Physics Community in the Third Reich*, 16.

175. F. Bloch, interview by Weiner, 4.

176. Stokes, "Felix Bloch tells how his decision led to a Nobel Prize," 3.

177. Ibid., 4.

178. W. Heisenberg, *Der Teil und das Ganze: Gespräche im Umkreis der Atomphysik*, (Munich: R. Piper, 1969), 174; quoted by Beyerchen, *Scientists Under Hitler: Politics and the Physics Community in the Third Reich*, 58.

179. F. Bloch, interview by Weiner, 5.

180. Ibid.

181. Beyerchen, *Scientists Under Hitler: Politics and the Physics Community in the Third Reich*, 161-162.

182. Ibid., 25.

183. Elisabeth Heisenberg, *Inner Exile: Recollections of a Life with Werner Heisenberg*, (Boston: Birkhäuser, 1954), 48.

184. W. Heisenberg, "Der Kampf um die sogenannte 'Deutsche Physik,' " Heisenberg Papers; Ernst von Weizsäcker to Sommerfeld, 30 September 1937, Sommerfeld Nachlass; as noted by Beyerchen, *Scientists Under Hitler: Politics and the Physics Community in the Third Reich*, 161.

185. Heisenberg, *Inner Exile: Recollections of a Life with Werner Heisenberg*, 40.

186. Stark, et al., " 'Weisse Juden' in der Wissenschaft," *Das Schwarze Korps*, Berlin, 15 July 1937, 6; discussed by Beyerchen., *Scientists Under Hitler: Politics and the Physics Community in the Third Reich*, 158.

187. Beyerchen, *Scientists Under Hitler: Politics and the Physics Community in the Third Reich*158.

188. Ibid., 118.

189. Edward Y. Hartshorne, *The German Universities and National Socialism* (London: Allen & Unwin, 1937), 112; quoted by Beyerchen, *Scientists Under Hitler: Politics and the Physics Community in the Third Reich*, 43.

190. Heisenberg, *Inner Exile: Recollections of a Life with Werner Heisenberg*, 54.

191. Ibid., 57.

192. Ibid., 60-61.

193. Ibid., 34.

194. Beyerchen, *Scientists Under Hitler: Politics and the Physics Community in the Third Reich*, 63.

195. Heisenberg, *Inner Exile: Recollections of a Life with Werner Heisenberg*, 64.

196. F. Bloch, interview by Weiner, 29.

197. Ibid., 29.

198. Heisenberg, *Inner Exile: Recollections of a Life with Werner Heisenberg*, 67.

199. Rhodes in *The Making of the Atomic Bomb*, 385.

200. Ibid., 386.

201. Bloch, "Heisenberg and the early days of quantum mechanics," 26-27.

202. Ibid.

203. Rhodes in *The Making of the Atomic Bomb*, 185.

204. Ibid., 188.

205. F. Bloch, interview by Weiner, 6.

206. Daniel J. Kevles, *The Physicists: The History of a Scientific Community in Modern America*, (New York: Alfred A. Knopf, 1978), 221.

207. F. Bloch, interview by Weiner, 6.

208. Ibid., 7.

209. Finn Aaserud, "Niels Bohr as fund raiser," *Physics Today*, October 1985, 41.

210. F. Bloch, interview by Weiner, 7-8.

211. Ibid., 8.

212. Ibid., 9.

213. Stokes, "Felix Bloch tells how his decision led to a Nobel Prize," 4.

214. Rhodes in *The Making of the Atomic Bomb*, 190.

215. Ibid., 206.

216. Ibid., 207-208.

217. Ibid., 208.

218. Abraham Pais, *Inward Bound: Of Matter and Forces in the Physical World*, (New York: Oxford University Press, 1986), 418.

219. According to Emilio Segrè in *Enrico Fermi, Physicist*, (Chicago: University of Chicago Press, 1970), 72; quoted by Rhodes in *The Making of the Atomic Bomb*, 208-209.

220. Pais, *Inward Bound: Of Matter and Forces in the Physical World*, 422.

221. Ibid., 418.

222. F. Bloch, interview by Kuhn, 38-39.

223. F. Bloch, quoted by Chodorow, Hofstadter, Rorschach, and Schawlow, eds., *Felix Bloch and Twentieth-Century Physics*, viii.

224. F. Bloch, interview by Weiner, 11.

225. F. Bloch, interview by Kuhn, 39.

226. J. Robert Oppenheimer, quoted by Nuel Pharr Davis in *Lawrence and Oppenheimer*, (New York: Simon and Schuster, 1968), 266; requoted by Rhodes in *The Making of the Atomic Bomb*, 206-207.

227. I.I. Rabi, interview by Barbara Land, 12 November 1962, transcript, Columbia Oral History, Columbia University, New York, 82.

228. Henry A. Boorse, Lloyd Motz, and Jefferson Hane Weaver, *The Atomic Scientists: A Biographical History*, (New York: Wiley, 1989), 349.

229. F. Bloch, interview by Weiner, 21.

230. G. Breit and I.I. Rabi, "Measurement of nuclear spin," *Physical Review* **38**, (1931), 2082-2083.

231. F. Bloch, interview by Weiner, 13.

232. Ibid.

233. Ibid., 10.

234. Ibid., 11.

235. Ibid., 14.

236. Ibid., 18.

237. Ibid., 15.

238. F. Bloch, interview by Kuhn, 37.

239. W. Heisenberg, *Zeitschrift für Physik* **77,** (1932), 1; *Zeitschrift für Physik* **78,** (1932), 156; *Zeitschrift für Physik* **80,** (1933), 587.

240. E. Majorana, *Zeitschrift für Physik* **82,** (1933), 137.

241. F. Bloch, interview by Kuhn, 38.

242. Ibid.

243. Robert Frisch and Otto Stern, *Zeitschrift für Physik* **85,** (1933), 4.

244. I. Estermann and Otto Stern, *Zeitschrift für Physik* **85,** (1933), 17; *Physical Review* **46,** (1934), 665.

245. F. Bloch, interview by Kuhn, 38.

246. F. Bloch, "The principle of nuclear induction," Nobel Prize lecture reprinted in *Science* **118,** (16 October 1953), 426.

247. F. Bloch, interview by Weiner, 21.

248. Stokes, "Bloch looks back on nearly 50 years research, Nobel Prize," 3.

249. Boorse, Motz, and Weaver, *The Atomic Scientists: A Biographical History*, 345.

250. Stokes, "Bloch looks back on nearly 50 years research, Nobel Prize," 4.

251. F. Bloch, interview by Weiner, 25.

252. Ibid., 31.

253. Ibid.

254. I.I. Rabi, *Science: The Center of Culture* (World, 1970), 16; quoted by Rhodes in *The Making of the Atomic Bomb*, 190.

255. Bloch, "The principle of nuclear induction," 426.

256. Ibid., 22.

257. Ibid.

258. Chodorow, Hofstadter, Rorschach, and Schawlow, eds., *Felix Bloch and Twentieth-Century Physics*, viii.

259. F. Bloch and A. Nordsieck, "Radiation field of the electron," *Physical Review* **52,** (1937), 54.

260. F. Bloch, interview by Weiner, 26.

261. Bloch, "On the magnetic scattering of neutrons," 260.

262. F. Bloch, interview by Weiner, 27.

263. Bloch, "On the magnetic scattering of neutrons," 259.

264. Ibid., 260.

265. Dunning, Powers, and Beyer, "Experiments on the magnetic properties of the neutron," 51.

266. Hoffman, Livingston, and Bethe, "Some direct evidence on the magnetic moment of the neutron," 214.

267. Powers, Beyer, and Dunning, "Experiments on the magnetic moment of the neutron," 371.

268. Otto Frisch, H. von Halban, and J. Koch, "A method of measuring the magnetic moment of free neutrons," *Nature* (London) **139,** (1937), 756.

269. Bloch, "The principle of nuclear induction," 426.

270. Dunning, Powers, and Beyer, "Experiments on the magnetic properties of the neutron," 51.

271. F. Bloch, interview by Weiner, 33.

272. Bloch, "On the magnetic scattering of neutrons," 259.

273. F. Bloch, "On the magnetic scattering of neutrons, II," *Physical Review* **51,** (1937), 994.

274. Bloch, quoted by Chodorow, Hofstadter, Rorschach, and Schawlow, eds., *Felix Bloch and Twentieth-Century Physics*, ix.

275. J.S. Schwinger, "On the magnetic scattering of neutrons," *Physical Review* **51**, (1937), 544.

276. F. Bloch, interview by Weiner, 27.

277. Jeremy Bernstein, *The Life It Brings: One Physicist's Beginnings*, (New York: Ticknor & Fields, 1987), 61.

278. F. Bloch, interview by Weiner, 28.

279. Ibid., 23.

280. Keesing and Lowen, "The Felix Bloch papers: guide and inventory of the collection," 6.

281. Bloch, interview by Weiner, 29.

282. Alvarez and Bloch, "The magnetic moment of the neutron," 352.

283. Alvarez and Bloch, "A quantitative determination of the neutron moment in absolute nuclear magnetons," 111.

284. H. Staub, "Ten years of neutron physics with Felix Bloch at Stanford, 1938-1949," *Felix Bloch and Twentieth-Century Physics*, (Houston: Rice University Press, 1980), 195.

285. F. Bloch, interview by Weiner, 32.

286. Luis Walter Alvarez, interview by Charles Weiner and Barry Richman, 14 and 15 February 1967, transcript, Niels Bohr Library, American Institute of Physics, College Park, MD, 27.

287. F. Bloch, interview by Weiner, 33.

288. L. Alvarez, interview by Weiner and Richman, 28.

289. Ibid., 29.

290. F. Bloch, interview by Weiner, 32.

291. L. Alvarez, in letter to Charles Weiner, February 2, 1972.

292. Ibid.

293. Alvarez and Bloch, "A quantitative determination of the neutron moment in absolute nuclear magnetons," 113.

294. L. Alvarez, in letter to Charles Weiner, February 2, 1972.

295. L. Alvarez, interview by Weiner and Richman, 41.

296. Staub, "Ten years of neutron physics with Felix Bloch at Stanford, 1938-1949," *Felix Bloch and Twentieth-Century Physics*, 195.

297. F. Bloch, interview by Weiner, 35.

298. Ibid.

299. Staub, "Ten years of neutron physics with Felix Bloch at Stanford, 1938-1949," *Felix Bloch and Twentieth-Century Physics*, 197.

300. Stokes, "Bloch looks back on nearly 50 years research, Nobel Prize," 3.

301. Staub, "Ten years of neutron physics with Felix Bloch at Stanford, 1938-1949," *Felix Bloch and Twentieth-Century Physics*, 197.

302. Ibid.

303. F. Bloch, interview by Weiner, 37.

304. Rhodes, *The Making of the Atomic Bomb*, 416.

305. Ibid., 416-420.

306. F. Bloch, interview by Weiner, 38.

307. Staub, "Ten years of neutron physics with Felix Bloch at Stanford, 1938-1949," *Felix Bloch and Twentieth-Century Physics*, 198.

308. F. Bloch, interview by Weiner, 39.

309. Ibid.

310. Ibid., 40.

311. Ibid.

312. Ibid., 41.

313. Much of the historical information contained in the following account is based on information provided by Rhodes in *The Making of the Atomic Bomb*, 481-484.

314. Stokes, "Felix Bloch tells how his decision led to a Nobel Prize," 4.

315. F. Bloch, interview by Weiner, 40.

316. Ibid.

317. Ibid., 41.

318. Erwin L. Hahn, personal communication to James Mattson, 22 January 1995.

319. Erwin L. Hahn, "Felix Bloch and magnetic resonance," *Bulletin of Magnetic Resonance*, **7**, 85.

320. F. Bloch, interview by Weiner, 41.

321. Ibid., 42.

322. Staub, "Ten years of neutron physics with Felix Bloch at Stanford, 1938-1949," *Felix Bloch and Twentieth-Century Physics*, 199.

323. Hahn, "Felix Bloch and magnetic resonance," 85.

324. J.M.B. Kellogg, I.I. Rabi, N.F. Ramsey and J.R. Zacharias, "An electrical quadrupole moment of the deuteron," *Physical Review* **55**, (1939), 318.

325. William Rarita and Julian Schwinger, "On the neutron-proton interaction," *Physical Review* **59**, (1941), 436.

326. F. Bloch, "Nuclear induction," *Physical Review* **70**, (1946), 460.

327. Ibid.

328. Ibid.

329. Ibid., 460-461.

330. F. Bloch, W.W. Hansen, and M.E. Packard, "The nuclear induction experiment," *Physical Review* **70**, (1946), 478.

331. Ibid., 474.

332. E.M. Purcell, "Nuclear magnetism in relation to problems of the liquid and solid states," *Science* **107**, (1954), 433.

333. John Van Vleck, "A third of a century of paramagnetic relaxation and resonance," Magnetic Resonance: *Proceedings of the International Symposium on Electron and Nuclear Magnetic Resonance*, Melbourne, edited by C.K. Coogan, Norman S. Ham, S.N. Stuart, J.R. Pilbrow, and G.V.H. Wilson (New York: Plenum, 1970), 1; quoted by John Rigden in "Quantum states and precession: The two discoveries of NMR," *Reviews of Modern Physics* **58**, (April 1986), 444.

334. Martin E. Packard in private communication with Rigden, mentioned in "Quantum states and precession: the two discoveries of NMR," 444.

335. F. Bloch, "Nuclear induction," *Physical Review* **70**, (1946), 478.

336. Ibid., 475.

337. Hahn, "Felix Bloch and magnetic resonance," 86.

338. F. Bloch, interview by Weiner, 43.

339. Martin E. Packard in private communication with John Rigden, quoted in Rigden's "Quantum states and precession: The two discoveries of NMR," 446.

340. Bloch, Hansen, and Packard, "Nuclear induction," 127.

341. Bloch, Hansen, and Packard, "The nuclear induction experiment," 474.

342. F. Bloch, "Nuclear induction," *Physical Review* **70**, (1946), 478.

343. R.V. Damadian, "Tumor detection by nuclear magnetic resonance," *Science* **171**, 19 March 1971, 1151-1153.

344. N. Bloembergen, E.M. Purcell, and R.V. Pound, "Relaxation effects in nuclear magnetic resonance absorption," *Physical Review* **73**, (1948), 679.

345. F. Bloch, interview by Weiner, 45.

346. Ibid., 47.

347. Staub, "Ten years of neutron physics with Felix Bloch at Stanford, 1938-1949," *Felix Bloch and Twentieth-Century Physics*, 199.

348. F. Bloch, interview by Weiner, 46.

349. N. Bloembergen, abstract, *Physical Review* **75**, (1949), 1326.

350. W.G. Proctor and F.C. Yu, *Physical Review* **77**, (1950), 717.

351. W.C. Dickinson, *Physical Review* **77**, (1950), 736 and *Physical Review* **78**, (1950), 339.

352. N. Bloembergen and W.C. Dickinson, *Physical Review* **79**, (1950), 179.

353. W.G. Proctor and F.C. Yu, *Physical Review* **81**, (1951), 20.

354. M.E. Packard and J.T. Arnold, *Physical Review* **83,** (1951), 210.

355. H. Gutowsky, D.W. McCall, C. Slichter, and McNeill, *Physical Review* **82,** (1951), 748 and *Physical Review* **84,** (1951), 589 and 1246.

356. E.L. Hahn and D.E. Maxwell, *Physical Review* **84,** (1951), 1246 and *Physical Review* **88,** (1952), 1070.

357. N.F. Ramsey, "The internal diamagnetic field correction in measurements of the proton magnetic moment," *Physical Review* **77,** (1950), 567.

358. N.F. Ramsey, "Magnetic shielding of nuclei in molecules," *Physical Review* **78,** (1950), 699.

359. N.F. Ramsey, "Dependence of magnetic shielding of nuclei upon molecular orientation," *Physical Review* **83,** (1951), 540.

360. N.F. Ramsey, "Chemical effects in nuclear magnetic resonance and in diamagnetic susceptibility," *Physical Review* **86,** (1952), 243.

361. U. Liddel and N.F. Ramsey, "Temperature dependent magnetic shielding in ethyl alcohol," *Journal of Chemical Physics* **19,** (1951), 1608.

362. N.F. Ramsey and E.M. Purcell, "Interactions between nuclear spins in molecules," *Physical Review* **85,** (1952), 143.

363. N.F. Ramsey, "Electron coupled interactions between nuclear spins in molecules," *Physical Review* **91,** (1953), 303.

364. J.T. Arnold, S.S. Dharmatti, and M.E. Packard, "Chemical effects on nuclear induction signals from organic compounds," Letter *in J. Chem. Phys.* **19,** (April 1951), 507.

365. F. Bloch, interview by Weiner, 49.

366. Ibid., 48.

367. E.L. Hahn, "Felix Bloch reminiscences," *International Journal of Modern Physics* **B, 4.6** (1990), 1283-1288.

368. Hahn, "Felix Bloch and magnetic resonance," 89.

369. Hahn, "Felix Bloch reminiscences," 1288.

370. Hahn, "Felix Bloch and magnetic resonance," 89.

371. F. Bloch, interview by Kuhn, 3-4.

372. F. Bloch, interview by Weiner, 51.

373. Ibid

374. E.M. Purcell, interview by James Mattson, 10 February 1994.

375. Norman F. Ramsey, conversation with James Mattson, February 1994.

376. *Neighborhood News*, Vol. 2 No. 49, December 3, 1953, Palo Alto, California, 15.

377. From press release announcing Rabi's death, Office of Public Information, Columbia University, 11 January 1988, 1.

378. F. Bloch, interview by Weiner, 51-52.

379. Ibid., 50.

380. Ibid., 51.

381. Ibid., 53.

382. Abragam, *Time Reversal: An Autobiography*, 179-180.

383. F. Bloch, interview by Weiner, 55.

384. Ibid.

385. Hahn, "Felix Bloch and magnetic resonance," 89.

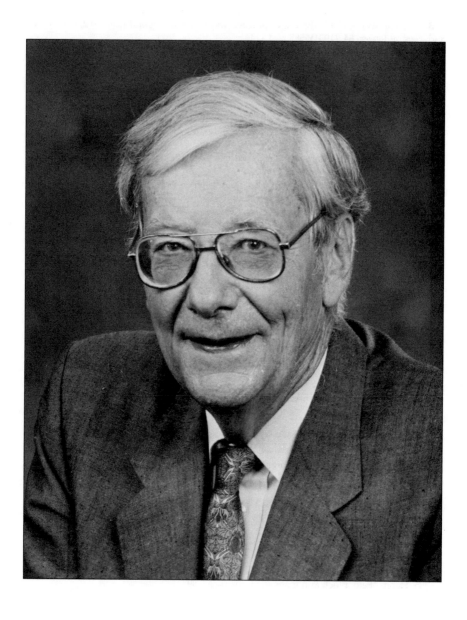

5

NICOLAAS BLOEMBERGEN

Nobel Laureate for Nonlinear Optics and Spectroscopy
Helped Set Stage for Human MR Scanning

DURING PERIODS OF REVOLUTION and upheaval, time often seems compacted by the press of events. Whereas a generation is normally equal to 30 years, the 30-year Quantum Revolution is seen by physicists to encompass many generations of thought and development, often with one generation succeeded by another in as little as two years.

Thus it was that Felix Bloch, who was only four years younger than Werner Heisenberg chronologically, saw him as two generations older when it came to theoretical physics;[1] Robert Oppenheimer, who was four years younger than Wolfgang Pauli, viewed the latter as a veteran of physics battles waged in Oppenheimer's childhood;[2] and Nicolaas Bloembergen would revere Professor I.I. Rabi, who discovered magnetic resonance in molecular beams when Bloembergen was 17, as "the grand old man" when they met nine years later, although Rabi was then a middle-aged 47.[3]

By the time Bloembergen began working on his doctoral dissertation in 1946, Rabi's Nobel Prize-winning discovery was nearly a decade in the distant past—a past that seemed even further removed in time because of a war that had commanded the world's attention from 1939 to 1945. Yet, within a two-year period, Bloembergen would become a major contributor to the science of NMR.

Although he would be awarded the 1981 Nobel Prize in physics for his achievements in nonlinear spectroscopy and optics and not for NMR *per se*, Bloembergen would continue to use the principles of NMR in his contributions to both the maser and the laser. "Many people aren't aware, but I certainly was," he said, "that all of these techniques—the theory of magnetic resonance—could be theoretically translated to what happens at optical frequencies. These frequencies are 10,000 times larger than the microwave frequencies," said Bloembergen, "but they can all be described in the same language developed first to describe magnetic resonance—the Bloch equations and so forth."[4]

Presently Gerhard Gade University Professor Emeritus at Harvard University, Nicolaas Bloembergen got started on his illustrious career by being in the right place at the right time. Accepted as a graduate assistant in early 1946 by Edward M. Purcell of Harvard shortly after his arrival in the United States from war-torn Holland, Bloembergen was assigned the task of following up the findings of Purcell and his associates, Henry C. Torrey and Robert V. Pound, who had detected NMR in paraffin about six weeks earlier.

Bloembergen's research, culminating in his doctoral thesis in 1948, contributed significantly to the body of knowledge available on NMR. He was the first to determine quantitatively the T_1 and T_2 relaxation times for a host of different substances, including pure water, ice, ionic solutions and glycerine. Bloembergen also drew attention in his thesis to the motional narrowing of magnetic resonance, the fact that spectral lines get very sharp due to the molecular motion in the liquid. The practical significance of this for the use of NMR in chemical analysis and later, for MR spectroscopy in medicine, is that without narrow, sharply-peaked spectral lines, there is no high resolution.

His findings did not go unnoticed. Anyone familiar with the physics of nuclear magnetic resonance is also familiar with a paper commonly referred to as "BPP." For the uninitiated, BPP stands for Bloembergen, Purcell and Pound, co-authors of one of the 10 most cited physics papers ever published. Officially entitled "Relaxation Effects in Nuclear Magnetic Resonance Absorption" and published in the April 1, 1948 issue of *Physical Review*,[5] BPP contains essentially the same material as Bloembergen's PhD dissertation, which included some additional theoretical and experimental details. After completing the research for his dissertation, Bloembergen received his PhD degree from the University of Leiden in 1948. Following several non-commercial reproductions of his thesis in the years that followed, including distributions in Japan and the Netherlands, it was republished by popular demand as a monograph[6] in 1961 by W.A. Benjamin in New York.

Although he went on to other areas of study in the years that followed, Bloembergen's direct involvement with the science of NMR in the years 1946-1948 gave him the opportunity to know personally most of the people of NMR during that important period. Now in his mid-70s, Professor Bloembergen was interviewed for this book in his office on the third floor of Harvard University's Pierce Hall. Located adjacent to Lyman Laboratory of Physics, where Edward Purcell's office is located, and near the site of the first successful attempt to detect nuclear magnetic resonance in condensed matter, Pierce Hall has been Bloembergen's academic home for over four decades.

From Many Waters

As Europe's Rhine River exits the broad fertile valley it has carved into the western highlands of Germany and levels off as it approaches the flat lower lands—the *nether* lands, the *hollow* land—it has helped form with ages of alluvial deposits, it abandons its former single-minded rush to the North Sea and, like water poured slowly on a flat table-top, seeks a number of more languid escapes. First, it divides in two, becoming the Lower Rhine River and the Waal River, with both heading west in roughly parallel paths. Before long, however, the Lower Rhine, which is actually the upper of the two routes, divides again, with the new tributary taking a northerly course—the IJssel River—in what appears to be an attempt at a more hasty escape from the flatness of Holland.

It turns out to be the slowest. Flowing into what used to be a large mini-sea off the North Sea called the Zuider Zee, it finds its escape frustrated by the tenacious Dutch who have dammed the sea and made it into a lake, the IJsselmeer, a lake that has grown ever smaller as the Dutch have insisted, even more astoundingly, on converting a significant fraction of it into dike-protected polders, land dry enough for agriculture.

Meanwhile, the westward flow of the Lower Rhine divides again. Its right fork becomes the Curved Rhine and then the Old Rhine, flowing past Utrecht and Leiden. Once a major waterway that made Utrecht accessible to the sea, the Old Rhine, like the IJssel, has been becalmed, its energy dissipated by Dutch-made dikes, dams and canals. The lower course was allowed to flow unobstructed past Rotterdam, but not without a name change. Before it reaches Rotterdam, it becomes the Lek River and after Rotterdam, the Nieuwe Maas. Thus, the Rhine River, at least by that name, never reaches the North Sea. Even with a pseudonym, it doesn't arrive at the sea in one clearly-defined channel, but in a multitude of estuarial veins, well mingled with waters from France and Belgium.

Still further to the south, also flowing westward is the Waal River. Before reaching Dordrecht, it divides in two and after leaving Dordrecht, it divides again. Some of its water takes a northwestward course in the direction of Rotterdam, where it links up with the Nieuwe Maas. The rest heads southwestward, where it mixes with the waters of the Maas and

Schelde, originating in France and Belgium. A large area of brackish water is formed in various sea arms between numerous islands. At low tide, the water is permitted to flow into the North Sea through sluice gates in giant dikes built after the devastating floods of 1953. The Dordrecht-Rotterdam area is famous for water tourism, fisheries, commercial shipping lanes and nature reserves.

Such a lengthy description of Holland's primary waterways is not unrelated to the story of Nicolaas Bloembergen for, even more than the typical Hollander, young Nicolaas was well acquainted with his country's myriad waterways. With his father and older brother, he navigated many of them by kayak, camping on their serene and pristine banks while nearby windmills lazily converted energy from wind to water in scenes straight out of paintings by 17th-century Dutch masters.

But that was before 1940, before the Netherlands was raped, its agricultural and industrial bounty confiscated and its people starved, before more than 120,000 of its 140,000 Jewish inhabitants were herded into tightly-packed railroad cars like so many ill-treated cattle and shipped to slaughter, and before a quarter-million of its non-Jewish inhabitants were deported to Hitler's Reich to work as slaves of the enemy, many never to return.

Because of its flat, no-place-to-hide topography, the Netherlands, a haven for Jews from Germany and Eastern Europe during the early years of Hitler's regime, would become a trap for Jews from 1940 to 1945. Apart from the coastal marshlands, there were few natural hiding places and the sea prevented flight to the west and north. To escape the ruthless hunters, the hunted would have to find refuge with compassionate strangers, many of them Catholic and Protestant Christians.

Nicolaas Bloembergen wasn't Jewish, but he was a student and therefore, as far as the Nazis were concerned, part of the Dutch Resistance, eligible for either deportation or worse. If deported, he would be made, like a quarter-million other Hollanders, a slave laborer for the German state. The Nazis knew where he lived, on the basis of a tip from a Dutch Nazi informer—an "NSB-er" as the Dutch called such traitors, members of the Dutch National Socialist Bond. For a couple of years, Bloembergen too would have to go into hiding.

The Early Years

On March 11, 1920, Nicolaas Bloembergen was born in Dordrecht, a thousand-year-old city on the Waal branch of the Rhine. Here it was 302 years earlier that 180 leaders of the still-young Protestant Reformation met to settle, in the Synod of Dort, the thorny theological question of predestination. It was a question that had come to be sharply debated by two professors at the University of Leiden. Professor Gomar took Reformer John Calvin's position—you were either predestined to damnation or to salvation and your free will was not free. Professor Arminius, on the other hand, taught that God, unwilling that any should perish, gave the choice to man while urging him to make the choice in favor of eternal life. Although the will of the gathered assembly at Dort was in favor of predestination, both Calvinists and Arminians would continue to co-exist in Holland.

Bloembergen remembers virtually nothing, however, from his time in Dordrecht. He was destined to move from there when he was one-and-a-half and, by the time he entered grade school, his family had moved again, the second time to Bilthoven, a residential suburb of Utrecht that would be young Nicolaas's hometown for the remainder of his growing-up years.

They moved to Bilthoven in 1925. Although it was an important year in the history of quantum mechanics with the publication of Werner Heisenberg's paper on the subject, five-year-old Nicolaas wouldn't learn about quantum theory for another 13 years, when he would read about it on his own during his first year at the university. In fact, he would never complete a formal course in quantum mechanics as the course, too, would be terminated by the war.

Nicolaas was the second of six children—four boys and two girls—born to Auke and Sophia Maria (Quint) Bloembergen. A chemical engineer in a fertilizer company started by his father, Auke had learned the business from the ground up. Eventually he had risen through the ranks to the position of executive director only to find that he liked working with the people on the production line better than he did working in the main corporate office with the chief executive officer. As a result, he looked forward to vacation opportunities when he could escape from business by camping with his two oldest sons.

> I think my father was unhappy in his executive work [said Bloembergen]. He didn't like the office work, and he had a CEO who . . . there was some friction there I can see now, many years later. So on his vacations he took his two eldest sons on kayak trips, and we camped all around the country. You couldn't do it anymore, it's so dense the farmers wouldn't let you put a tent up anywhere. But in those days you could, more than half a century ago. We knew all the waterways in Holland, all the rivers, the lakes, the canals, the locks. The water geography of Holland is very familiar to me.[7]

Although these father-and-sons outings took place in idyllic settings, they were not taken leisurely because, for Auke Bloembergen, productivity was just as important in the pursuit of leisure as it was in setting manufacturing goals. "My father liked performance," said Professor Bloembergen. "He encouraged us to do sports, and on those kayak trips we had to do a certain minimum distance each day. I didn't realize it then, but looking back, I think that performance was encouraged—and sometimes imposed."[8]

On holidays when he and his sons weren't kayaking the watery thoroughfares of Holland, the elder Bloembergen would take his family to a cabin he owned on a lake near Utrecht, where they did a lot of sailing. The sailboat, a 20-footer with a movable centerboard for a keel, was actually a gift to Nicolaas from his father during a time when Nicolaas was suffering from osteomyelitis in a heel bone. Bloembergen credits the boat with helping him through a two-year period when he was incapacitated from participating in rougher sports. During those two years, he spent a lot of time sailing on Holland's lakes and canals, learning to use the vectors of the wind to his advantage by tacking back and forth in narrow channels only six times wider than the length of his craft.[9]

The osteomyelitis was eventually taken care of with surgery. "A successful operation," Bloembergen said, "finally cured me completely from this disease which was dreaded in pre-penicillin days."[10]

On two occasions, Auke Bloembergen took his family on trips out of the country, once to Sweden and once to Germany. They could have afforded many more trips than they took, Bloembergen felt. His parents were more austere in their lifestyle than their income demanded.

> The Dutch attitude of frugality reigned supreme in our family, and so we were held short on food and outings. The budget could have afforded a little more freedom, I would say. But that's a typical Dutch trait which is well described in a book by a Harvard colleague, Simon Schama. Called *The Embarrassment of Riches,* it is on the Dutch 17th century.[11] On the one side, the people were very wealthy. But on the other hand, they were very frugal, and there was a sort of conflict. But this was a general attitude of the Dutch well-to-do classes. They were not ostentatious.[12]

The Dutch aversion to the flaunting of wealth can be attributed partly to the strong Protestant work ethic instilled by its Calvinist ministers and partly to the humanist tradition initiated by Desiderius Erasmus, the revered 15th-century Dutch philosopher. As Schama has pointed out,

"The official creeds of both Calvinism and humanism . . . were agreed that lucre was indeed filthy, and that devotion to its cult constituted a kind of polluting idolatry. . . . This strong sense of the reprehensible nature of money-making persisted, even while the Dutch amassed their individual and collective fortunes."[13]

This financial schizophrenia sometimes resulted in hyperfine distinctions between the sacred and the secular. Although it was considered a possibility, Schama wrote, that a Christian merchant was not a contradiction in terms, there was little question about bankers. Because of their usurious occupations, bankers were excluded by a Calvinist ordinance passed in 1581 from receiving communion, as were pawnbrokers, actors, jugglers, acrobats, quacks and brothel keepers. Wives of bankers were permitted to partake provided they renounced their husband's occupations as repugnant. Although the ordinance was repealed in 1658 under pressure from the state, the spiritual stigma likely remained.

Just recently, Bloembergen said,[14] he had acquired a genealogy of his paternal ancestors which traced the direct male line back to 1774 when they were bankers in Friesland, Frisia, in the northern part of Holland. Considering the Calvinist view of banking, it may help explain why Auke Bloembergen was not religious.

Auke's wife, on the other hand, Sophia Maria (Quint) Bloembergen, was religious, a Dutch Mennonite, not to be confused, said Bloembergen, with other Mennonite denominations. All Mennonites trace their spiritual heritage back to Menno Simons, a converted Roman Catholic priest (ca. 1496-1561) who organized Anabaptist congregations in Holland, who preached against any union between church and state, and whose teachings were codified in a confession of faith hammered out, also in Dordrecht, in 1632. Beyond that, many of Simon's spiritual descendants have little in common. Frank Mead's *Handbook of Denominations* lists 13 Mennonite categories in the United States, ranging from conservative, Amish-type Mennonites to those of more liberal persuasion.[15] In Holland, the Quint family were adherents of Mennonism at the liberal end of the movement's spectrum. To emphasize the difference, Bloembergen pointed out that "here [in the United States] Mennonites are pretty strict and rigid. Those are the Mennonites who found Holland too liberal. They moved out and left. But the Mennonites in Holland are very liberal in their religious outlook."[16]

Sophia Maria Bloembergen was not so liberal, however, when it came to overseeing her household. According to Bloembergen, she ran a rather tight ship, instilling in him and his siblings a rather large dose of the

Protestant work ethic. Although she had an advanced degree for teaching French, she devoted herself to her family. "My mother was always very busy running the large household," said Bloembergen, "and taking care of the small children."[17]

With six children, she recognized the benefits of delegating authority. "I was often entrusted to the supervision and authority of my older brother," noted Bloembergen and added, "My parents had the wisdom to send us to different high schools."[18]

"My family was all for intellectual activity and studying," Bloembergen said. "My mother encouraged a lot of reading, literature, the French language, and that sort of thing."[19] Her father, a high school principal in The Hague, had a PhD degree in mathematical physics. His mentor, in fact, was a Nobel laureate, Johannes Diderik van der Waals of the University of Amsterdam who received the Nobel Prize in physics in 1910 for describing the relationship of liquids and gases with regard to pressure, absolute temperature and volume.

In spite of the natural tendency for one to suppose that the grandfather passed on his interest in physics to his grandson, Professor Bloembergen denies any link except the possible genetic one. His grandfather died in 1917 from the Spanish grippe, the epidemic of influenza that devastated much of Europe several years before Nicolaas was born. It is tempting, nevertheless, to note the commonality between Nicolaas Bloembergen's PhD dissertation and his grandfather's. Bloembergen's thesis was on nuclear magnetic relaxation, with special emphasis upon the effect that motion in liquids has upon the narrowing of spectral lines. Grandfather Quint's thesis was a mathematical physics treatment of turbulent motion.

In spite of his environmental and genetic heritage, Professor Bloembergen noted that he was "apparently a rather slow starter," pointing out that he was called "dumb Nick" for awhile by relatives. The unkind moniker didn't stick for long. The "Nick" name was abandoned suddenly when, at the age of four, Nicolaas Bloembergen beat an inattentive uncle in checkers.

In elementary school, he lacked challenge. At age six, out of boredom, he learned the Greek alphabet forward and backward and throughout grade school, often did his homework twice, for lack of something better to do. "The educational philosophy in the school system," Bloembergen said, "was strict and did not encourage initiative. Being obedient, if not meek, I was content with getting high scores."[20]

He doesn't remember experiencing emotional highs or lows during those years. "My childhood was obviously rather comfortable and was probably considered to be a happy one. Nevertheless," he noted, "I cannot recall either being happy or very unhappy during the first decade of my life."[21]

In spite of the fact that intellectual pursuits were definitely encouraged in the Bloembergen home, they were not pushed to the exclusion of other priorities. For example, to keep their second son's tendency toward bookishness from becoming too pronounced, his parents decreed that his brothers and sisters should tear him away from books at certain hours to participate in other activities. In addition to kayaking and sailing, these included swimming, rowing, field hockey and skating—at least when the brief periods of cold weather in Holland permitted it. Contrary to popular belief, the canals of the Netherlands are suitable for skating—at most—two weeks out of the year. "Of course, it is a very popular sport," Bloembergen said, "and when it does freeze over, all the schools and offices are given a holiday."[22] He credits the physical regimen he received during those early years to his lifelong effort to keep fit with tennis, hiking, and skiing.

His parents' efforts to train their children in both mind and body paid off. All six siblings are still alive. The eldest brother obtained a Doctor of Laws degree and culminated a successful and varied business career as CEO of the largest publishing firm in the Netherlands, the VNU. One sister married a medical doctor, a general practitioner, and raised a large family in Roermond, a town on the Maas River. The younger sister has a Master's degree in French and was a high school teacher. One brother obtained a medical degree and had a general practice in Gorinchem, a town on the Waal River. The youngest brother, also with a Doctor of Laws degree, was a professor of civil law at the University of Leiden, until he accepted a nomination as justice on the Dutch Supreme Court.

High School
In 1932, at the age of 12, Nicolaas Bloembergen entered the prestigious *Stedelijk Gymnasium* in Utrecht, daily bicycling the five- or six-mile distance between the school and his suburban home in Bilthoven. Founded as a Latin school in 1474, the curriculum of the *gymnasium* was still heavily weighted toward the humanities, with courses in Latin, Greek, French, German, English and Dutch all required for graduation, along with history and mathematics. The school also offered an excellent program in the sciences, Bloembergen said, particularly in the final three grades, with laboratory opportunities in physics, chemistry and biology. Nearly all of the teachers in the school held PhD degrees.

Although for most students the rigorous curriculum was traumatic, Bloembergen thrived on it. He found that he enjoyed Latin as much as mathematics, that physics and chemistry were his favorite subjects and Dutch literature his least favorite.

It was not a foregone conclusion, however, that he would ultimately concentrate on science; in fact, for a while he considered a career in languages. That was partly because the school's emphasis on the humanistic values of Erasmus did not encourage, in spite of its excellent science curriculum, the pursuit of science as a career and partly because his extracurricular activities in the school's theater club and debating society were nudging him toward the humanities.

The debating society included opportunities for discussing natural philosophy, which ranged from Leibniz and Kant to Einstein's concept of relativity, as well as poetry reading, which ranged from Homer to Rilke. In the process, the society also instilled in its members, said Bloembergen, "an unusual degree of intellectual snobbism." At the time, he considered himself well on his way toward becoming a well-rounded, educated person, but in retrospect, he said, "it is clear that there was a complete void in my understanding of social relations, psychology, government and politics."[23] In a school that prided itself on its classical approach to academics, he had not had any courses in social science, political science or economics, and the history courses he had taken were taught as though history ended with the 18th century and Holland's Golden Age. "Looking back," he said, "that was a very serious gap in my upbringing."[24]

It was increased exposure to the sciences in Bloembergen's later years at the *gymnasium* that began shifting his focus away from the humanities. Both physics and chemistry were well taught. It was a chemistry course that inspired Nicolaas and a friend to set up a small laboratory for themselves in a barn, but it was physics that became his favorite subject, not because it came easily, but because it was hard. In fact, had Bloembergen made his career choice on the basis of which subject was easiest, he would never have been awarded the Nobel Prize in physics. "I liked the challenge," he said. "And I still find it the most difficult field, even now," he stated in 1992.[25]

Probably for the same reason his grandfather decided to become a mathematical physicist, Bloembergen was intrigued by the way mathematics and physical facts correspond to one another. To this day he continues to be ever more fascinated, he said, by the "uncanny adaptability of abstract mathematics to describe physical phenomena."[26]

In retrospect, he realized that he had been attracted to physics for a long time, ever since childhood, although he was a little concerned to read, upon beginning his studies in physics, that the beginning student shouldn't think he could become a good physicist just because he had construct-ed a good radio. The trouble was, that wasn't Bloembergen's assumption. "What worried me about this," he said, "was that all my experience was completely theoretical. I had never even constructed a radio. My educa-tion was in an old-fashioned European kind of Latin school . . . certainly we had nothing in the way of practical applications. . . . As it turned out, it didn't really make any difference."[27]

Bloembergen was not exposed during his *gymnasium* years to quantum mechanics. "It was classical," he said. "You didn't learn about nuclear physics. That wasn't in the textbooks yet. [We were taught] mechanics, electricity, and some atomic physics, a little bit."[28]

Ironically, it would not be an academic environment but the competi-tive sport of field hockey that would give Bloembergen his first brief edu-cation about a social, psychological and political phenomenon called Nazism that was quickly enveloping the country just across Holland's eastern border and which would soon spread across all of Europe.

In the Netherlands, sports were not extracurricular school activities, but were organized by private clubs or on an individual basis. Field hockey was a favorite. All of Bloembergen's brothers and one of his sisters took part in the nearly year-round sport, and sometimes the competition was international within Europe. In 1934, when Bloembergen was 14, the game took him to Germany. Little more than a year had passed since Hitler's rise to power, but the teenagers on his field hockey team, said Bloembergen, "were pretty shocked by what was going on there already."[29] *

"It should have been obvious [what was happening in Germany],"[30] Bloembergen said, in analyzing his own youthful complacency about the madness developing within the powerful nation whose border lay as close as 40 miles from his home in Bilthoven. If it should have been obvi-ous to a 14-year-old, how much more obvious should it have been to the Dutch government? But they were no different than the French and British who, as one writer put it, "each looked to the other for reinforce-

---

* Bloembergen would not return to Germany for over 45 years. Three decades after emi-grating to the United States, he realized that he felt more negatively toward the country that had occupied his homeland during the war than did his relatives who had remained in Europe. "I came to the United States in '46 and my attitude toward the Germans was emo-tionally fixed at that point," he said. In a deliberate attempt to expunge feelings that were no longer justified, he chose to do his 1979-80 sabbatical in Germany. "I went back to Munich twice and we have plenty of friends there now. I am more relaxed now and see that the German situation has changed."
— From interview by James Mattson, 19 July 1994.

ment of its own weakness rather than confirmation of a strong resolve, and both were well satisfied."[31]

Like their neighbors, the Dutch found it easier to live in denial than to risk confrontation, and more pleasant to hope for the best than to be prepared for the worst or, as another writer expressed it in 1944:

> Which of the nations that are now united against the Fascist powers can fairly point a finger at any other? All are guilty of a complacency that was almost criminal and could barely escape a fatal issue. The Kingdom of the Netherlands erred like the rest in deferring to the Axis; it also made the mistake of taking itself too modestly. . . . Most of its people suffered from delusions of the country's smallness and comparative insignificance. The taste for neutrality induced an illusory sense of detachment from world affairs. Germany kept assuring the Netherlands and its other small neighbors that they had nothing to fear . . . and it was incredibly effective.[32]

Dutch citizens were generally aware in 1934 of the changes taking place in Germany, but many of them minimized the dangers they posed for Holland. During World War I, even as neutral Belgium fell victim by reason of its location to a Germany intent on defeating France, Holland's neutrality, less vital to the Kaiser's* strategy, had been honored. Why should it not be honored again was the conventional wisdom.

That's how Bloembergen recalled the general attitude of the country, too, although he was too young, he said, to really describe the political mood from personal observation. "I mean, my life was concentrated on just high school work and sports. I was not politically concerned."[33] Within six years of his visit to Germany, however, Hitler's pro-Aryan, anti-Semitic message would result in the destruction of four out of every five Dutch Jews and Hitler's dreams of empire would result in the nightmare of deportation for tens of thousands of Holland's youth.

In the spring of 1938, Nicolaas Bloembergen graduated from the Utrecht municipal *gymnasium* as the valedictorian of his class, 464 years after the founding of the school. As had been done for the last century, the

---

* The grave of Germany's Kaiser Wilhelm II is in Doorn, a town in the province of Utrecht located about 10 miles from Bloembergen's home city of Utrecht. The Kaiser retired there in 1918 after Germany's defeat in World War I and died peacefully after spending his exile days hewing oak trees.

ceremonies were enacted with great pomp in *Pieterskerk,* a church with Romanesque architecture dating back to the 1100s. Bloembergen was 18 when he graduated and his valedictory address, delivered in white tie and tails, was on the reconciliation of scientific facts with spiritual values in natural phenomena.

Forty-three years later, at the age of 61, Nicolaas Bloembergen, Gerhard Gade University Professor at Harvard, donned the same white tie and tails in Stockholm, Sweden to receive the most prestigious award given a scientist—the Nobel Prize. "I got back in shape," he said. "I don't think I would have fit it in middle life, but I fit it again in '81 with some alterations. I didn't have to rent another suit."[34]

College and the War Years

In the fall of 1938, Bloembergen matriculated at the University of Utrecht as a student of physics. The reason he chose Utrecht, he said, was more for social traditions and for its proximity to his home than for academic considerations. Besides, at the undergraduate level, he pointed out, all of the Dutch state-supported universities held to the same high academic standards. If he had chosen, however, an alma mater from purely scientific considerations, especially from a physics standpoint, he probably should have chosen, he said, the University of Leiden.

As of 1938, three of the four Nobel Prizes awarded to Dutch physicists had gone to Leiden scientists. In 1902, Pieter Zeeman and Hendrik Antoon Lorentz had shared the prize for their contributions to the Zeeman effect; Zeeman for discovering the effect of magnetism on spectral light and Lorentz for explaining it. In 1913, Heike Kamerlingh Onnes had received the Nobel Prize in physics for his experiments with low temperatures and for liquifying helium. As mentioned earlier, the fourth Nobel laureate, Johannes van der Waals, the mentor of Bloembergen's grandfather, was from the University of Amsterdam.

Utrecht also had a strong physics tradition, however. In 1912, Professor Julius, a solar physicist from Utrecht, had enticed Albert Einstein to think seriously of accepting a professorship at the school, but lost out when Einstein's alma mater, the ETH in Zürich, Switzerland, made a counteroffer. Einstein then suggested that Utrecht contact Peter Debye, the eminent Dutch physicist who had replaced him a year earlier at the University of Zürich. Debye accepted Utrecht's offer, although he would not remain long at the school.

From 1926 to 1934, Hendrik Anthony (H.A.) Kramers, who had made a substantial contribution to quantum physics with his derivation of the dispersion formula, had held the theoretical physics chair at Utrecht and in 1929-30, when Felix Bloch spent an academic year as a Lorentz Fellow in Holland, he had chosen to spend most of that year at Utrecht with Kramers.

Coincidentally, Bloch had spent the remainder of that year— Bloembergen was only nine years old at the time—with Adriaan Fokker at Teyler's Foundation, a scientific laboratory and museum in Haarlem. Fokker, the founder of The Netherlands Physical Society, is a distant relative of Bloembergen, an uncle "two or three times removed" on his father's side. Associated with the Fokker-Planck equation and Fokker's action principle, the one-time University of Delft professor had studied with Einstein at Zürich shortly before the First World War.[35] When Bloch visited him in Haarlem, Fokker had given up his professorship at Delft a few years earlier to succeed H.A. Lorentz as the director of Teyler's Foundation.

Between 1936 and 1939, another major contributor to quantum mechanics, George Uhlenbeck, was at the University of Utrecht. More than a decade earlier, in 1925, Uhlenbeck and Samuel Goudsmit, then PhD candidates at Leiden, had discovered that electrons have spin and therefore magnetic properties. Two years later, immediately after receiving their doctorates, the two physicists left for the University of Michigan at Ann Arbor where they had accepted positions as instructors. Uhlenbeck returned to Holland, however, in 1936 to succeed H.A. Kramers at Utrecht, a position Uhlenbeck held until August 1939, when he returned to the United States. Bloembergen would not have the opportunity to take any courses from Uhlenbeck, however. In 1938, when Bloembergen entered college as a freshman, the only physics courses open to undergraduates were classical.

Just because there were no courses in quantum mechanics available to undergraduates didn't keep Bloembergen from learning about the new physics. What really stimulated him in atomic physics and quantum theory was a book he read that year by Max Born,* a series of 10 lectures that the eminent co-founder of quantum mechanics gave to general audiences.

About the same time, Bloembergen also read a book entitled *Physik als Abenteuer der Erkenntnis*, which means *Physics as Adventure of Perception*.

---

* Five years earlier, in 1933, Max Born, one of the founders of quantum mechanics and director of the Institute for Theoretical Physics at Göttingen University in Germany, was placed "on leave" from his position because he was Jewish. Rather than fight the suspension, he resigned from Göttingen and a few months later accepted a post at Cambridge University in England where Norman Ramsey heard him lecture during his time at Cambridge between 1935 and 1937.

Written in 1937 by Albert Einstein in collaboration with Leopold Infeld, it described, Bloembergen said, "the example of two people falling in an elevator and then they don't feel the gravitational force, and that sort of thing. That book stimulated me." Published in 1938, the popular book enjoyed wide acceptance. "I read it in German," Bloembergen commented, "which was easier than English."

Politically in the fall of 1938, Europe was still hoping, in spite of evidence to the contrary, that Hitler could be trusted.

Three years earlier, in 1935, the Saar area between France and Germany, long an area of contention between the two countries and awarded to France following Germany's defeat in World War I, had been reincorporated by Germany as the result of a plebiscite.

In March 1936, Germany moved troops into the Rhineland, that part of Germany west of the Rhine River which had been demilitarized by the Versailles Treaty at the end of World War I.

In March of 1938, Hitler annexed Austria, suddenly turning Austrian Jews, in effect, into German Jews, with all the lack of human rights that were guaranteed by the 1935 Nuremberg Laws.

At 8:45 p.m. on March 11, 1938—the same day Nicolaas Bloembergen turned 18—Adolf Hitler gave the order for his troops to enter Austria at daybreak the next morning.[36] With little opposition, Hitler accompanied his troops into his native country to cheering crowds, declared Austria a province of Germany, and made a pro-Nazi Viennese lawyer by the name of Artur Seyss-Inquart the provincial governor. (The name Seyss-Inquart would come to be despised by Dutch citizens a couple of years later.) Germany's entrance into Austria was sudden, but it hadn't come without warning; bringing Austria under Germany's umbrella was an objective Hitler had clearly stated on page one of *Mein Kampf* 14 years earlier.

Hitler's invasion of Austria was bad news for physicist Lise Meitner. An Austrian citizen then working in Germany at the Kaiser Wilhelm Institute for Chemistry in Berlin-Dahlem, Meitner had been exempt from many of the laws enacted against German Jews between 1933 and 1938. But then came the *Anschluss*—the annexation of Austria to Germany— and suddenly she became a German citizen, which meant she was, in effect, no citizen at all. Although Hitler had suspended a number of basic rights from all German citizens shortly after becoming chancellor in 1933, the 1935 Nuremberg Laws made it clear that whatever rights other German citizens retained did not belong to Jews. In addition to being

denied marriage rights with Aryan Germans, they were denied the protection of the state, access to law and law courts, employment, the opportunity to graduate, and the right to participate in the German economy.

Lise Meitner didn't need the Hebrew prophet Daniel to interpret the
handwriting that was now on the wall, but physicist Max von Laue, a
Prussian Nobel laureate (1914) who had become a symbol worldwide for
refusing to cooperate with the Nazis, sought Meitner out anyway and
told her it was time to leave Germany. He had heard that Heinrich
Himmler, the head of the Nazi SS and chief of German police, had
ordered that no more academics be allowed to emigrate. With the help of
Dutch physicists Peter Debye, Dirk Coster, W.J. de Haas, Adriaan
Fokker*—the distant uncle of Bloembergen—and a sympathetic Dutch
government that promised to admit her into Holland with no visa and an
expired passport, Meitner left Germany by train, a flight to freedom that
she recalled years later:

> I took a train for Holland on the pretext that I wanted to spend a
> week's vacation. At the Dutch border, I got the scare of my life when
> a Nazi military patrol of five men going through the coaches picked
> up my Austrian passport, which had expired long ago. I got so fright-
> ened, my heart almost stopped beating. I knew that the Nazis had
> just declared open season on Jews, that the hunt was on. For 10 min-
> utes I sat there and waited, 10 minutes that seemed like so many
> hours. Then one of the Nazi officials returned and handed me back
> the passport without a word. Two minutes later I descended on
> Dutch territory, where I was met by some of my Holland colleagues.[37]

The Dutch had rescued, and the Nazis had allowed to slip through
their fingers, the physicist who had initiated the experiments that would
result before the end of the year in the discovery of nuclear fission.
Meitner and her nephew, Otto Robert Frisch, exiled in Sweden and
Denmark respectively, would be the first to confirm, from a theoretical
physics standpoint, that their former collaborators, Otto Hahn and Fritz
Strassmann, had indeed derived barium (Ba) and masurium (Ma), today
called technetium (Tc), from uranium 239.

---

* It was also Adriaan Fokker who, four years earlier, had helped von Laue surreptitious-
ly get word to physicists outside of Germany that not all of their German colleagues were
in agreement with the views of the anti-Semitic "Aryan" physicists.
—Beyerchen, *Scientists Under Hitler,* 242.

In late September of 1938, as Bloembergen started college, Neville Chamberlain, the prime minister of Britain, met with Hitler in Munich, Germany and agreed, as did France, to Germany's annexation of Czechoslovakia's German-speaking Sudetenland, without asking the opinion of Czechoslovakia. "I believe it is peace in our time," declared Chamberlain upon returning home. His successor, Winston Churchill, assessed the situation differently. "The British and French cabinets at this time," he wrote later, "presented a front of two overripe melons crushed together; whereas what was needed was a gleam of steel."[38] Eleven months later, on September 1, 1939, Adolf Hitler would attack Poland and two days later, Britain and France would declare war on Germany to start World War II.

Even as his military machine efficiently polished off Poland, Hitler was reassuring the Netherlands and Belgium that they had nothing to fear, but his words, intended to promote continued apathy among the Dutch, would echo mockingly a few months later when he invaded neutral Norway and Denmark. Although they continued to hope that they would be spared from invasion, there was little to do now but anxiously mobilize their resources as best they could. As Riemens wrote in 1944:

> They saw much too late that their long-maintained pacifist attitude and their deathly dread of a budgetary deficit might be perfectly adapted to an ideal world but were wholly inappropriate for a nation that had Hitler's Germany for its close neighbor. As public opinion swung around to a sounder view, not one foreign country could or would sell armaments to the Netherlands in substantial quantities, and there was not time enough to build up an adequate armament industry at home. . . . The Netherlands had to try to stay neutral at least for the time being, not so much because neutrality was its time-honored policy as because there was no alternative in 1939, when the democracies were almost utterly devoid of offensive weapons.[39]

For the first two years of his college career, Nicolaas Bloembergen lived a relatively care-free life at the University of Utrecht, renting a room near the campus on one of the city's old canals. He joined a student social fraternity, complete with hazing and drinking parties. "Looking back on it," he said, "it was a pretty irresponsible way of living."[40] He also went out for the rowing team and made stroke on the varsity 150-pound crew. (Stroke, or stroke oar, is the term for the rower nearest the stern of the long, thin racing shell who sets the pace for the other members of the crew.) Rowing put a stop to the alcohol consumption, said Bloembergen; it wasn't compatible with the rigorous training requirements. The years of kayaking around Holland with his father and brother now paid off in a tangible way. "To the surprise of many, including myself," he said, "our lightweight crew won two regattas in its class." In the spring of 1939, participating in the famous Student Varsity, Bloembergen won two silver medals as he competed on the canals of Holland against teams from six other universities.

When Bloembergen returned for his second year of college in the fall of 1939, Professor George Uhlenbeck had been replaced by Professor Léon Rosenfeld, who was just back from what had been an exciting six-month stay at the Institute for Advanced Study in Princeton, New Jersey.

A graduate of the University of Liège in Belgium, Rosenfeld was a close friend of Niels Bohr and had collaborated with him in the past. When Bohr had begun finalizing plans, therefore, to spend the second semester of the 1938-39 academic year as a visiting professor at the Institute for Advanced Study in Princeton and was thinking about a collaborator with whom he might work during that period, he thought of Léon Rosenfeld. By then a full professor in Liège, Rosenfeld was an expert on the problem of measurement in quantum electrodynamics, the same problem Bohr wished to address during his stay in Princeton.

Shortly before they set sail for the United States, however, Bohr was informed by Otto Robert Frisch of the recent experimental discovery of nuclear fission by Otto Hahn and Fritz Strassmann in Germany and of the theoretical confirmation Frisch and his aunt, Lise Meitner, had provided. Bohr, in turn, told Rosenfeld about the discovery but forgot to tell Rosenfeld that the news was to be kept confidential until Frisch had a chance to send an announcement of the Meitner-Frisch interpretation to *Nature*.

As a result, when Rosenfeld arrived at Princeton just in time for the regular Monday meeting of Princeton's Physics Journal Club and was asked if he had anything to report, he told them about nuclear fission and the extensive discussions he and Bohr had had during the voyage.

By coincidence, I.I. Rabi of Columbia University, who was on sabbatical at the Institute that year, was at the meeting, and Willis Lamb, also of Columbia, was at Princeton for a brief visit. They quickly informed their colleagues back in Columbia's Pupin Hall of the event—Lamb told Enrico Fermi—and because of their early access to the news, physicists at

Columbia University were the first in the United States to duplicate the results achieved in Europe.[41]

As a sophomore, Bloembergen was not yet able to take graduate courses from Rosenfeld. He did take, however, a course from Leonard S. Ornstein, professor of experimental physics at Utrecht, which gave him, as he phrased it, "a contact with real science."[42] Ornstein, who had directed the university's center for optical spectroscopy for a number of years, was a well-respected physicist who had made important contributions to the field. Back in 1927, his spectroscopic analysis of singly ionized molecular nitrogen had contributed to a finding by Ralph de L. Kronig that disputed the proton-electron model of the nucleus.[43] In 1929, Ornstein had been invited as a guest lecturer to Massachusetts Institute of Technology and had also lectured at the University of Minnesota.[44]

Bloembergen's laboratory partner for the course was J.C. Kluyver, Jr., the son of a very famous Dutch professor of microbiology who, together with Ornstein, had secured Rockefeller Foundation funding for a biophysics laboratory at Utrecht. Although young Kluyver and Bloembergen were both sophomores and in the same physics class, Kluyver was the more advanced of the two, partly because of his father's influence in getting him enrolled in an advanced laboratory course and partly because of a year he had already spent studying in Geneva, Switzerland. When Kluyver, Jr. was allowed to bypass some of the more mundane lab routines assigned to other students and assist a graduate student in his PhD research project, the question arose about what to do with his lab partner, Nicolaas Bloembergen. They decided to let Bloembergen have the same privilege, "so I got some acceleration in that way," he said.

As a result of the research assistance they provided graduate student G.A.W. Rutgers, Bloembergen and Kluyver were listed as collaborators with him in a 1940 article in *Physica*. "We were thrilled," Bloembergen wrote later, "to see our first publication, 'On the Straggling of Po-a-particles in solid matter,' in print."[45-46] J.C. Kluyver, Jr. would later become a professor in high-energy physics at the University of Amsterdam.

Before his article appeared in print, however, life as Bloembergen had known it for his first 20 years came to an abrupt end. On the dawn of May 10, 1940, following an interim period known as The Phoney War, Hitler launched his western offensive. Without warning, highly-trained German troops—some of them wearing Dutch uniforms—began invading the skies over Holland with gliders and parachutes. Key to

Germany's strategy was their immediate control of the vital bridges crossing the Nieuwe Maas River south of Rotterdam and estuaries of the Maas at Dordrecht and Moerdijk. Without control of those bridges, Hitler's ground forces moving westward from Germany would be severely hampered in their drive toward Holland's population centers— The Hague, Amsterdam, Utrecht, Rotterdam and Leiden.

The plan went off almost without a hitch. All the bridges were secured the morning of May 10, before Dutch forces could blow them up. Hitler's element of surprise had been effective. "Never in my life will I sign a declaration of war," he said one month after invading Holland. "I will always strike first."[47] Although warning signs had been increasing in the months prior to the invasion, Hitler's long string of comforting reassurances to Holland had finally been revealed for what they really were—lies.

Dutch forces resisted the invasion bravely, but they were no match for Germany's air superiority. William Shirer in *The Rise and Fall of the Third Reich* wrote, "To the bewildered Dutch was reserved the experience of being subjected to the first large-scale airborne attack in the history of warfare. Considering their unpreparedness for such an ordeal and the complete surprise by which they were taken they did better than was realized at the time."[48] By May 13, only 10 of the 248 Netherlands planes available on the first day of the invasion were still flying, and then they too were shot down.[49]

Despite the lack of air cover, the Dutch destroyer *Jan van Galen* tried to assist the Dutch marines still holding the Germans off at Rotterdam by approaching the city through narrow, mine-infested waters. Although she was able to shoot down some enemy planes near The Hague as it headed toward Rotterdam, the complete air supremacy enjoyed by the Germans made the task impossible. With her guns still firing, the ship finally sank while her crew escaped to continue their fight on land.[50] By May 14, it was clear there was no alternative but for the Dutch army to surrender. Then came the most stunning blow of all.

Although German forces had secured the bridges south of Rotterdam, its tanks were unable to cross them immediately. In the meantime, the Dutch sealed off the northern ends of the bridges. Hitler then issued a directive in which he stated: "The power of resistance of the Dutch army has proved to be stronger than was anticipated. Political as well as military considerations require that this resistance be broken speedily."[51]

Even as negotiations for Holland's surrender proceeded—a Dutch officer had just come to German field headquarters to discuss the terms—the order was given for the bombing of Rotterdam. With no opposition from the Dutch air force, German planes knocked out what remained of the anti-aircraft guns surrounding Rotterdam, opening the way for bombers to rain 94 tons of bombs on the city's center. According to one source, "thousands met their death within a few hours, other thousands were crippled, and the entire heart of the city became one huge pile of wreckage."[52] The center of Rotterdam is only 25 miles from the center of Utrecht, as a bomber flies, and Bloembergen remembers seeing from Utrecht the huge cloud of black smoke rising in the south-western sky.

The initial reports stating that between 25,000 and 30,000 Dutch were killed were in error—the actual number claimed by the Dutch at the post-war Nuremberg Trials was 814—but reality was shocking enough. In addition to the deaths, several thousand were wounded and 78,000 made homeless.[53]

The Germans declared that the same fate awaited Amsterdam, Utrecht and The Hague, the most populous cities in the nation, if there was any more resistance. As the Dutch royal family and governmental ministers escaped to England to establish a government in exile, the Dutch military, under the command of General Winkelmann, surrendered on May 14.

Militarily, the attack had been swift and complete, a *blitzkrieg* (lightning war) that had accomplished its strategic objectives before Holland could mount an effective defense, but Germany could not eliminate Dutch resistance against its occupation.

> The Kingdom of the Netherlands was invaded but not conquered in 1940 or in the years following [wrote Hendrik Riemens in 1944][54]. . . . That the German military machine could easily conquer a small country was plain from the outset. The German successes never bewildered the Netherlanders as they did the French. But no merely material power could command the people's souls. The more brutal the conqueror, the more he is scorned. Firing squads cannot compel friendship; quite the other way![55]

As Nicolaas Bloembergen has pointed out in another context, the Dutch love stubbornness, and indeed, its people continued to resist in whatever ways a nation can which is held hostage by a vastly superior military power. One of the many ways the Dutch—both Catholic and Protestant—sought to subvert the intentions of the enemy was in protecting its Jewish population, a population that had swelled by the thousands after 1933 when Hitler first began systematically persecuting Jews in Germany.*

For years, long before 1933, Holland had been a refuge for Jews, an island of relative safety in a sea of racial hatred.† During the 17th century, fleeing unjust persecution, many Jewish people had viewed old Amsterdam like a city of refuge described in the Torah and had declared it to be the new Jerusalem. By 1940, about 10 percent of that city was Jewish.[56]

With the German invasion of Holland, the security which Jews had found in that country evaporated and those living in Amsterdam found their "new Jerusalem" as dangerous as ancient Judea's old Jerusalem when it was overwhelmed by the legions of Rome. Of the estimated 140,000 to 150,000 Dutch Jews in the country at the time of the invasion, between 104,000 and 120,000—as many as 85 percent—would be destroyed with the systematic regularity of trains departing stations.[57] According to one source, 110,000 were deported by the trainload to the concentration camps of Germany and Poland. Of these, only 6,000 survived.[58]

> Eminent scholars have been thrown into concentration camps [wrote one author] and even killed in cold blood. Nothing can ever restore to the Netherlands a great part of its Jewish population, such a necessary leaven in its otherwise somewhat dull and all too placid makeup. Wholesale deportations and killings such as modern man did not think was possible any more are bound to have deep and ineradicable effects. How such crimes can ever be expiated by the many guilty amongst the Germans who will survive this war it is all but impossible to conceive.[59]

---

* Although anti-Semitism had been present in Europe for hundreds of years, periodically erupting like a chronic putrefying ulcer, Jews in Western Europe during the latter part of the 1800s had experienced increasing emancipation which gave them the civic rights normally given to other citizens, including the right to vote, run for office, enter the professions, and join the military. For many Jews in 19th-century Germany, civic emancipation and cultural assimilation went hand in hand. Seduced by the culture of Germany, many Jews had chosen to overlook its sickness, a fast-growing cancer that would soon metastasize throughout all of Europe.

† The same spirit of tolerance had also extended to the Dutch colonies. In the early 1600s, when Holland established a colony in America known as New Netherlands—and a city called New Amsterdam, known today as New York City—it was the first place in the New World that permitted Jews, although its colonial governor, Peter Stuyvesant, had, on one occasion, thrown every Jew in New Amsterdam into jail. Many of their descendants would eventually settle in a borough of New York City called Brooklyn, the Anglicized name of a village near Utrecht called Breukelen.

Because Professor Ornstein of the University of Utrecht was Jewish, he was one of those who was dismissed and, before 1941 was history, he would also be one of the dead, "not through violence," said Bloembergen, "but from enormous stress and undernourishment." Soon after Ornstein's dismissal, all Jewish students were expelled. "These were only the forerunners," Bloembergen said, "of the much harsher measures of persecution and deportation that were to follow soon."[60]

By the early part of 1941, the harsher measures began in earnest. In February, disturbances in Amsterdam between Jewish workers and German and Dutch Nazis resulted in a retaliatory raid by the Nazis in which 425 Jewish men between the ages of 20 and 35 were picked up at random and sent east to death camps. At the time their fate was unknown, but none of the Jews arrested that day would survive.

A few days later, a series of strikes by production workers in the provinces of North Holland and Utrecht brought martial law and the imposition of heavy fines on the inhabitants of three cities: Amsterdam, Hilversum, and Zaandam.

In July of 1941, it was ordered that the letter "J" be added to the identification cards of all Jews; restrictions on their travel were made in September and October; and Jewish ghettos were established in Amsterdam as corrals to aid in their eventual round-up. After May 1942, Jews had to wear the yellow Star of David. Other restrictions soon followed, including: 1) a curfew to keep Jews off the streets between 8 p.m. and 6 a.m.; 2) shopping was allowed only between 3 p.m. and 5 p.m.; 3) use of public transportation was prohibited except with special permission; and 4) Jews were prohibited from entering the homes of non-Jews.

With the nation's Jewish population now largely immobile, Adolf Eichmann began scheduling their evacuation by rail to Auschwitz in June of 1942. An initial quota of 100,000 Jews from Western Europe called for 40,000 from Holland. Before the genocide was halted, 115,000 would be sent to Auschwitz, Sobibor, Theressienstadt, Bergen-Belsen, and other killing centers in the east. Other reductions in the Jewish population would result from emigration and flight (4,000), aggravated deaths and suicides (2,000), and an abnormal increase in deaths compared to births not attributed to the causes already mentioned. By the end of the war, fewer than 20,000 of the original 140,000 Jews in Holland remained.

One of those who committed suicide was a friend of Nicolaas Bloembergen. "He was in Amsterdam," Bloembergen explained. "They had to wear the yellow stars and that sort of thing and he would have been caught, but he threw himself in front of a streetcar."[61]

It wasn't only Jews who were at risk. Students in general were viewed with suspicion as likely sources of resistance. If the Nazis determined that a student was politically active, it meant either shipment to a concentration camp or on-the-spot execution.

Political activity wasn't required, however, to place one in danger. "One student," said Bloembergen, "was a mild young man, not politically active, but he was taken hostage when a German was killed and shot along with 10 others in a reprisal."[62]

Asked if he had seen the movie, *Schindler's List*, Bloembergen responded that he had and then added, "It's all true. It wasn't overdramatized; it was *under*dramatized. The pictures—also those at the Holocaust Museum in Washington, DC—were very familiar to me, just the way I saw it and remember it."[63]

In addition to violence and killing, hunger became an ever-present reality for many Dutch citizens soon after the German occupation began. With much of its agricultural bounty confiscated by the Nazis for use in Germany, Holland had to make do with the leftovers. At the University of Utrecht, Bloembergen became a member of a student committee that ran a central kitchen for the students. With the help of Dutch government officials, the committee was able to distribute hot vegetable and potato soup without requiring ration coupons.

"There were agonizing discussions [by the students] about what forms of protest to mount," said Bloembergen. "The University of Leiden adopted a strong stand in 1941 and was closed by the German authorities.* Most of the Leiden students transferred, however, to the other universities. These, including Utrecht, remained open and functioned until the spring of 1943."

In spite of the less-than-optimum academic environment that existed under the German occupation, Bloembergen completed the Dutch equivalent of a bachelor's degree, the Candidate in Philosophy (Phil. Cand.) in

---

* According to Cornelis Gorter, who was a professor at the University of Amsterdam at the time, the first Jewish professor at Leiden to be dismissed was Meyers, the president of the Dutch academy of sciences. When another professor (Cleveringa) protested the action in a speech on November 26, 1940, he and a number of others were arrested. Later, when a second Jewish professor, Kranenburg, was dismissed, many of the Leiden professors agreed to resign *en masse* the next time a dismissal occurred. As Gorter recalled in an interview nearly 20 years later, about 40 Leiden professors did resign as a block in 1941, resulting in the closing of the university.

— C.J. Gorter, interview by John L. Heilbron, part of the Archives for the History of Quantum Physics project, 13 November 1962, American Institute of Physics, Center for History of Physics, College Park, MD, 26.

1941, just two-and-a-half years after entering the university. "I made good use of the continental academic system," he said, "which leaned heavily on self-study with a minimum of formal courses."[64]

He immediately began working toward the Dutch equivalent of the Master's degree, the *Doctorandus* in Philosophy (Phil. Drs.) which signifies that all doctoral requirements are completed except the thesis. He also began working part-time as a research assistant, obtaining laboratory experience which would stand him in good stead a few years later when he applied to Harvard University. In addition to becoming exposed to vacuum-tube electronics which, at the time, was the state of the art and learning to deal with the problems of fluctuations and noise in photoelectric detectors, Bloembergen also wrote the lecture notes for a seminar on Brownian motion given by Professor J.M.W. Milatz. The Brownian motion work would pay off handsomely a few years later for Bloembergen when he wrote his doctoral thesis which focused, in part, on the effect which molecular motion of liquids has on the width of NMR spectral lines.

As a graduate student, Bloembergen was now eligible to take courses from Professor Rosenfeld, the professor of theoretical physics, who gave one course each year. The first course Bloembergen took from Rosenfeld was statistical mechanics which, he said, was "very exciting. I really learned that well."[65]

In the fall of 1942, Bloembergen finally had his first formal introduction to quantum mechanics when Rosenfeld gave a course on the topic. Unfortunately, Rosenfeld spent the first half of the year setting the stage.

> He did it the old-fashioned way [said Bloembergen], that is, he first prepared you in the Hamiltonian formulation of classical mechanics using Poisson brackets, and so forth, and then, halfway through the whole year course, about February, he started quantizing things. And that is just when the Germans interrupted the university's academic life. So I never finished a formal course in quantum mechanics.[66]

Most of the other courses Bloembergen took as a graduate student were essentially self-directed. "I taught myself some applied mathematics, mechanics and electromagnetic theory," he said, "from standard German textbooks."[67]

About three months before the Germans closed down the University of Utrecht, they started tightening the screws on any students who still remained enrolled by requiring them to sign a declaration of loyalty pledging they would do nothing against the occupational forces of the Third Reich. The penalty for refusing to sign? Deportation to Germany as a forced laborer.

Fewer than half of the students signed it and, consequently, many of them disappeared.

Ten percent of the students I knew [said Bloembergen] didn't return, didn't survive. They picked up any student off the list they had. Lots of them. Some were politically active in the Resistance. They were just executed or sent to a concentration camp. Because the country is so densely populated and there are no mountains or uninhabited regions to hide in, Dutch resistance work was very difficult and treacherous.[68]

Those deported for slave labor would experience extreme suffering and hardship. Often, they were required to produce munitions and other products that would be used against their own nation.

By the end of September 1944 [wrote historian William Shirer], some seven and a half million civilian foreigners were toiling for the Third Reich. Nearly all of them had been rounded up by force, deported to Germany in boxcars, usually without food or water or any sanitary facilities, and there put to work in the factories, fields and mines. They were not only put to work but degraded, beaten and starved and often left to die for lack of food, clothing and shelter. . . .

In the massive deportations of slave labor to the Reich, wives were torn away from their husbands, and children from their parents, and assigned to widely separated parts of Germany. Even top generals of the Army cooperated in the kidnapping of children, who were carted off to the homeland to perform slave labor.

Increasing terrorization was used to round up the victims. At first, comparatively mild methods were used. Persons coming out of church or the movies were nabbed. In the West especially, SS units merely blocked off a section of a town and seized all able-bodied men and women."[69]

The country was also robbed of its material assets with approximately two-thirds of its national income extracted by the Germans to cover their "occupation costs" and that didn't include the nation's natural resources or its agricultural and manufactured goods which were confiscated without so much as the formality of payment.[70] Soon after the invasion, for example, Auke Bloembergen's fertilizer plant was closed down, its chemical-making machinery dismantled and sent to Germany. "The Nazis just robbed the country of everything," said Bloembergen. "Half the railroad tracks were broken up."[71]

Overseeing these and other atrocities was the Austrian lawyer Artur Seyss-Inquart, the occupational administrator called upon by Hitler to whip a country into subservience following its military conquest. After an initial stint as provincial governor of Austria, Seyss-Inquart's skills were called upon in the fall of 1939 to help bring Poland under control. After less than nine months as Deputy Governor in Poland, he was appointed *Reichskommissar* of Holland, responsible directly to Adolf Hitler. A member of the *Schutzstaffel*, the Blackshirts, he could not be characterized as a benevolent administrator. Indeed, William Shirer described him as the butcher governor of Holland.

Because of increasing evidence that the university would likely be shut down before long, as well as the constant risk of apprehension and deportation to Germany, Bloembergen tried very hard, he said, to get his *Doctorandus* degree completed in the spring of 1943, between February and May. In order to achieve his goal, he had to pass tests in statistical mechanics, electricity, magnetism, quantum mechanics and mathematics under less-than-ideal circumstances.

> I passed tests—nearly all individual oral examinations—in these subjects as quickly as I could, because the threat of the closing of the university was very real. The next to last test was conducted at the home of a lecturer in mathematics, 40 miles from Utrecht. It was unsafe for young men, especially students, to be in or near the city. The police tried to pick me up one night at home, but I had been warned of the raid and was hiding with an old aunt in the countryside.[72]

The reason the police tried apprehending Bloembergen was on the basis of a traitorous tip from a fellow member of his field hockey club. An official in the Dutch National Socialist Bond—a Nazi—he knew which members of the hockey club were students and he had their addresses. Once alerted to the treachery of his former team member, Bloembergen stayed with his elderly aunt for two months.

When the Nazis knocked on his parents' door, they asked first for Nicolaas Bloembergen's older brother, but his parents told them he was married, was already independent, and lived elsewhere. Then they asked for Nicolaas, to which his parents replied, "Well, he's a student. We don't know where he is." Nicolaas Bloembergen also had two younger brothers, but both of them, at age 16, were too young for the deportations then taking place. Throughout that stressful two-month period, Bloembergen continued working to finish his examinations. Because of the ever-present danger, arrangements were made for him to take his tests in other venues, to which he traveled clandestinely by train.

In April 1943, just a few weeks before the Nazis closed down the university, Bloembergen was granted his doctoral candidate degree, even though he had not yet taken his exam in quantum mechanics. Professor Rosenfeld had told him they would forgive him that shortcoming for the time being and Bloembergen had responded, "Well, I'll take that exam later. I promise I will."[73] Not long afterward, the university was formally closed.

In the summer of 1943, when Bloembergen told Professor Rosenfeld that he had learned quantum mechanics and was prepared to take the examination, Rosenfeld set a date and invited Bloembergen to his home for the exam. The oral exam consisted of one question. After discussing it for quite a while, Rosenfeld said, "Well, you've passed," and started writing out a slip of paper to that effect. When Bloembergen reminded the professor that he didn't require the certification as he already had his degree, Rosenfeld responded good-naturedly, "Oh, you should have told me that at the beginning; then we could have dispensed with the whole thing."[74]

Getting his *Doctorandus* degree before the university closed turned out to be an "enormous advantage," said Bloembergen,

> because that meant I was not legally a student anymore. I didn't have to sign a declaration [of loyalty]. In fact, I became an assistant in the university and I got a stamp on my identity card—everybody had an identity card with a picture that entitled you to food coupons and if you didn't have that it was terrible. They put a little seal on the card that said I belonged to the fire brigade of the university. If there was a fire in the lab, I had to help put it out. So that meant I could still travel for a year-and-a-half rather freely and didn't have to worry.[75]

Scientific work had come to a virtual standstill, however. "The laboratory was unheated and there were no new supplies," said Bloembergen. "We fiddled with some obsolete equipment and a clandestine radio."[76] Actually, he did more than fiddle. When he wasn't in the laboratory,

Bloembergen was spending "a fraction of the time just keeping alive," he said, "growing some vegetables, and so on."[77]

Having a radio was, in itself, a dangerous proposition as they had been confiscated by the Nazis in an attempt to keep the Dutch people uninformed and isolated. Many Dutch citizens held on to their radios, however, in order to maintain their link with the outside world, sometimes concealing them in such disguises as thick, hollowed-out books.[78]

The following summer, those radios would finally tell them that the Allies had invaded the mainland of Europe on D-Day—June 6, 1944—and had begun their eastward push to wrest Europe from the death grip with which it was held by Hitler. The deliverance would not come easy.

For much of the one-year period between D-Day and the liberation of the Netherlands, Bloembergen was hiding out. "I survived at home," he said, "or rather its substitute, because my parents' house had been requisitioned by the military occupation forces." Assigned a little house in Bilthoven, the Bloembergens' own, much larger, home was confiscated by the Nazis to provide "recreation" for troops on leave from the front lines. "These troops were relieved every few weeks behind the lines in a safer place," Bloembergen explained, "and they just camped in [our house]."[79]

In September of 1944, a railroad strike was ordered by the Dutch government-in-exile to make it more difficult for the Germans to slow down the advance of Allied troops. Dutch citizens complied by completely paralyzing the country and the Germans, in turn, cut off what little remained of the nation's food supplies. In addition, for the next nine months, until its liberation in May of 1945, much of Holland would be without gas, electricity or coal.

As the Germans fought Allied troops, they continued to punish the citizenry of Holland. "The whole country was mutilated," said Bloembergen. "Then any man between 16 and 50 could be picked up from the street and sent to forced labor by the Germans, so you had to be very, very careful. In one street, you were safe. In the next street, they shot people or picked them up."[80]

While Bloembergen was hiding out at home, many other Hollanders were also concealing themselves from the Nazis. *Onderduiken*, they called it, or its literal translation, diving under water.

Going into hiding was practiced not only by Jews but also by men who had been called up for labor service in Germany, and by resistance workers. Vast numbers of people lived through the war in cupboards and attics, spending hours every night with little crystal radio sets that brought news via the BBC in London. Hiding was far from easy in a country as flat and open as Holland, and luck played a major part in survival. Those who hid the *onderduikers* also risked their own lives, of course. Some were eminently brave, while others demanded large sums of money from their guests.[81]

By the summer of 1944, there were almost as many *onderduikers* submerged in the hiding places of Amsterdam alone as had disappeared to the Reich as forced laborers. All over Holland, people were "diving under water" and holding their breath, as it were, for months on end.

At war's end, 7,000 Jews were still in hiding throughout Holland. One of them was Lèon Rosenfeld's former assistant, Abraham Pais, presently Detlev W. Bronk Professor of Physics Emeritus at Rockefeller University in New York City. Soon after the dismissals of Jewish academics and students, Pais left Utrecht in 1941 for Amsterdam, where he hid out for the duration of the war in one room of an attic. Bloembergen knew Pais and knew he was in hiding, but the only physicist who knew *where* Pais was hiding was the esteemed physicist H.A. Kramers. He would visit Pais in his hideaway from time to time and together they would discuss their current work in physics theory.[82]

During the latter part of the war, Bloembergen was also hiding out with Kramers—not the man but the book. "I read through the book *Quantum Theorie des Elektrons und der Strahlung* by H.A. Kramers, with the light of an oil lamp." The storm lamp Bloembergen used was designed to burn kerosene, however, not the leftover No. 2 heating oil that he had to use. "That was awful," he said, "because the heating oil carbonizes the wick. So every 20 minutes I had to clean out everything, clean the soot from the glass and cut the wick."[83]

With the increased reprisals against the Dutch, finding food was becoming increasingly difficult. Bloembergen's parents did "an amazing job of securing the safety and survival of the family,"[84] he said. "My mother," said Bloembergen, "tended an ailing brother and other sick members of the family. . . . My father did a fantastic job of foraging . . . on far-away farms."[85] The man who had once preferred working with the production people at his fertilizer plant now found himself trying to keep his former employees and his family alive by exchanging fertilizer for food. "My father made trips on the bicycle for 50 miles and hauled back some potatoes and whatever he could get,"[86] Bloembergen recalled.

The "whatever" also included tulip bulbs. Like many Hollanders, Bloembergen remembers eating many of the bitter bulbs just to fill his stomach. "They have no caloric value," he said, "and you have to boil them for six hours."[87] Even then, he pointed out, they were tough "like raw potatoes"[88] and indigestible. "At that point," he said, "I left Utrecht and was in hiding with my parents. The [Utrecht] suburb of Bilthoven was pretty quiet for awhile."[89]

By the time Allied soldiers were able to stave off Hitler's last-ditch offensive in December 1944 in the Battle of the Bulge, Dutch citizens were fighting an intense battle to stave off hunger. They called it the "hunger winter." By that winter, virtually everyone was hungry. Cats and dogs would mysteriously disappear only to reappear in meat markets as "roof rabbit." The official per capita ration was 400 calories a day, far less than the 1200 to 1600 calories needed for subsistence, and Eisenhower's food drops to the Dutch, made even before the Germans relinquished control of the country, would not begin until April of 1945. In the meantime, twenty thousand Hollanders would die.

"If you look at the death rate," said Professor Bloembergen, "it increased exponentially in the spring of '45. Terrible, terrible. So many people died. Everyone over age 60 was dying, and infants were dying."[90]

During that "winter of starvation," Dutch citizens, deprived of access to normal heating fuels, found themselves scavenging everywhere for any combustible alternatives. For many, the only available source was the vacant homes of missing Jews. In Amsterdam, where 80,000 Jews had lived prior to the invasion, 70,000 would disappear by the end of the war. In The Hague, where the prewar Jewish population was 17,000, only 1,700 would be left. Desperate for fuel, respectable citizens decimated the beautiful Hague Woods and even found themselves gutting the vacant homes of their former Jewish neighbors for anything that would burn.

In The Hague, one of those gutted-out homes belonged to the parents of Jewish physicist Samuel A. Goudsmit. Near the end of the war, Goudsmit, co-discoverer with George Uhlenbeck of the electron's spin, was back in Europe on the heels of the Allied invasion forces to search, as scientific head of the Allies' Alsos team, for Werner Heisenberg and the rest of the German atomic physicists. In The Hague, he stopped by his former home—just recently liberated from the Germans—where he had lived with his parents during high school and college.

Five years earlier, just four days before the Germans invaded the Netherlands, Goudsmit's parents had received their final papers to emigrate to the United States. Tragically, they were unable to get out of the country fast enough. The last their son heard from them was in a letter he received from them in 1943 from a Nazi concentration camp. Later, because of the Nazi propensity at times to document their evil deeds, he would find that both of his parents were put to death in a gas chamber on his father's 70th birthday. Although the full story of the Holocaust was not yet known the day he stood in the wreckage of his former home, the emotional toll was beyond measure.

> The house was still standing [wrote Goudsmit] but as I drew near to it I noticed that all the windows were gone. Parking my jeep around the corner so as to avoid attention, I climbed through one of the empty windows. The place was a shambles. Everything that could possibly be burned had been taken away by the Hollanders themselves to use as fuel that last cold winter of the occupation. The stairways had been torn down, doors ripped out, parts of the ceiling, the walls—anything and everything that was combustible. But the framework still stood. . . .
>
> As I stood there in that wreck that had once been my home I was gripped with that shattering emotion all of us have felt who have lost family and relatives and friends at the hands of the murderous Nazis—a terrible feeling of guilt. . . . If I had hurried a little more, if I had not put off one visit to the Immigration Office for one week, if I had written those necessary letters a little faster, surely I could have rescued them from the Nazis in time. Now I wept for the heavy feeling of guilt in me. I have learned since that mine was an emotion shared by many who lost their nearest and dearest to the Nazis. Alas! My parents were only two among the four million victims taken in filthy, jam-packed cattle trains to the concentration camps from which it was never intended they were to return.[91]

The nightmare finally ended in May of 1945. When the southern part of the country was liberated in the latter part of 1944, the Dutch government-in-exile moved quickly to restore its civil authority and on May 6, 1945, one of Queen Wilhelmina's councilors was finally able to announce that Germany had surrendered and that its destructive occupation of the Netherlands was over.

Hurry Up and Wait

As soon as the war was over, 25-year-old Nicolaas Bloembergen with a *Doctorandus* in physics was ready to get on with the research needed to get a PhD. "I had made up my mind that I wanted to get out of the badly ravaged country and do some 'real physics.' "[92] Although he had completed the qualifying examinations for his doctorate at the University of Utrecht and had already done some research on the photoelectric effect* (for which a paper was published in 1945), he had been unable to complete his doctoral thesis. As Bloembergen saw it, although he "knew what research was all about," he had nothing in the works that would evolve into a PhD thesis.

Before the war, he had planned to broaden his perspective by doing his thesis research in England, France or Germany. After the war, with those options clearly impractical, he turned his attention to the United States, an idea that came from his older brother.

> I was pretty depressed [said Bloembergen] about what to do. I still wanted to get my PhD and I had always had the idea of doing my thesis research somewhere else. I didn't want to stay in Utrecht anyway, even if times had been normal. But with the ravages of the war, there was really no place to go. I had no contacts in Sweden. That might have been a possibility, otherwise. So my older brother suggested, "Why don't you try to do your work in the United States?" And so I wrote to three [U.S.] universities in June or July, 1945. They were the University of Chicago, the University of California in Berkeley, and Harvard University.[93]

The reason he chose those three schools was based entirely on impressions he had gathered in reading *Physical Review*. "I didn't know much about the United States," he explained. "I had seen just a few copies of the *Physical Review*, and I knew they were places that had a fairly impressive record of papers I usually couldn't understand. I knew some names," he said, "but I wasn't familiar with anybody. I had heard of [Enrico] Fermi [then at the University of Chicago], and I had heard of some names at Berkeley like [E. O.] Lawrence."[94] Bloembergen spent days, he said, writing letters to the schools in longhand. Since he knew no one, he addressed his correspondence to the chairman of each school's physics department.

What he didn't know was that both the University of Chicago and the University of California at Berkeley were heavily involved in the

---

* Albert Einstein's hypothesis that light is composed of individual quanta called photons which are not only wave-like but also have the properties of particles earned him the 1921 Nobel Prize for physics. Einstein's theory helped explain the photoelectric effect, why some solids emit electrons when struck by light.

Manhattan Project at the time and not likely, for security reasons, to accept a foreign physics student. Although he was on an official Dutch government list of 20 or so promising students who should receive priority from any available scholarship funds, it was up to him to make the necessary contacts. Students of the humanities on the list majoring in Chinese literature, U.S. history and the like were sponsored quickly by the Rockefeller Foundation, but in May of 1945 it was considered questionable to even *accept* foreign physics students on U.S. campuses, much less finance their presence.*

The University of Chicago didn't even bother answering Bloembergen's letter of inquiry. Berkeley was courteous in their rejection, but what they told Bloembergen took him completely by surprise.

They said they would love to consider my application at a later time [said Bloembergen] but they couldn't have alien students as long as the war lasted. Now for me in Europe, the war was finished. Nobody in Europe was really realizing that the war with Japan was still raging. That was before the atom bomb. So I was quite surprised by that letter.[95]

At Harvard, the department chairman in 1945 was Professor Otto Oldenberg, a native of Germany and one of the first Jewish physicists to emigrate to the United States in the 1930s.† Oldenberg wrote back to Bloembergen and asked that he send some more documentation, copies of his degrees, letters of reference and so on, and they would be happy to consider his application. Soon after Harvard received the requisite materials from Bloembergen, they wrote back, welcoming him to Harvard's Graduate School of Arts and Sciences for the 1945-46 academic year. (Years later, the other two universities would write letters to Bloembergen

---

* Abraham Pais who, like Bloembergen, would eventually become a member of the U.S. National Academy of Sciences, was the other physicist on the list of recommended scholarship recipients. Also shut out from U.S. scholarships in physics and lacking adequate Dutch resources of his own, Pais would have to wait another year before getting his chance to go to the United States.

† Oldenberg had come initially for study at California Institute of Technology (Cal Tech) in Pasadena and ended up at Harvard when he settled permanently in the United States in 1930, the same year Eugene Wigner and John von Neumann emigrated. Another NMR pioneer, Edward Purcell, had taken a graduate-level laboratory course from Oldenberg in the mid-1930s.

offering him faculty positions which he would turn down, preferring to stay at Harvard.)

To be accepted by Harvard was one thing; getting there was another. With no U.S. scholarship money, Bloembergen would have to accept his father's offer to finance his time in Cambridge with Dutch guilders, but Dutch guilders could not be freely changed into U.S. dollars in 1945. Permits to do so were almost impossible to obtain.

> I went to the Department of Education in The Hague [said Bloembergen] and I said, "Look, I'm on your official list to go to the United States for a fellowship. Now I don't have the fellowship, but I have been admitted by a first-rate university. My father is willing to put up the Dutch money, so the least you can do now is get me a permit to change it into dollars."[96]

In a nation where men insist on turning the sea into dry ground, stubbornness is valued highly and Bloembergen's logical tenacity impressed the officials at the Dutch Department of Education. "I must say, they accepted that argument," said Bloembergen. "So I got a *valuta* permit to change my five thousand guilders at the official pre-war rate to $1800 which was enough at that time, because the Harvard tuition was $400 a year and the remaining $1400 was just enough to live for one year."[97]

At the time, however, there was only one bank, the official Netherlands Bank in Amsterdam, that could exchange guilders into dollars. Although it's only a 20-minute ride today and trains leave Utrecht for Amsterdam every 10 or 15 minutes, in the period right after the war only one or two trains a day were operating between those cities, and they were freight trains that took two hours to make the trip.

At the bank, even with the rare permit in hand, Bloembergen still had to justify his request to an incredulous bureaucrat who said the permit was for the largest amount he had ever seen.

"Well, who normally gets these permits?" Bloembergen asked, and the man responded that there were two categories: 1) professors renewing their international contacts, and 2) tulip bulb dealers seeking orders for delivery in the spring. Because tulips were about the only thing Holland was capable of exporting in those early days after the war, bulb dealers were given special treatment by the government because of the hard currency they brought back into the country. "Well," Bloembergen explained to the official, "they only go for three to six weeks, but as a student I have to go for a whole year. That's why I get more."[98]

From the time Bloembergen began responding to Oldenberg's request for additional admission documentation until the time he set sail for the United States, about eight months would pass. In the interim, he would apply for a Dutch passport and a U.S. student visa, obtain the permit to exchange Dutch guilders to U.S. dollars, and schedule passage out of Rotterdam, a port that had been destroyed by the war. There were delays at almost every step.

As he waited for bureaucratic wheels to turn in a country where the normal administrative functions of the government had been usurped for five years, Bloembergen could only watch and fret as the date he had been scheduled to start at Harvard approached and then receded into the distant past. In the fall of 1945, there were no regularly-scheduled ocean liners and there were no airlines. His best option was to try and book passage on a Liberty ship, one of the many hastily-built freighters built by the United States in a crash program to replace the hundreds of freighters torpedoed by German U-boats in the Atlantic.

Manufactured under the leadership of California contractor Henry J. Kaiser, the 441-foot-long Liberties were not impressive to look at. Powered by old-fashioned steam, they were also not very fast, but they could hold 10,800 tons of cargo, and could be built quickly and inexpensively using prefabricated components that could be shipped to the shipyard by rail. By the end of 1942, 597 Liberties had been launched and, for the first time since the beginning of the war, were coming out of shipyards faster than ships were being sunk in the Atlantic. By 1943, 140 Liberty ships were being completed every month and, at the peak of production, shipyard workers were able to assemble one of them in just 80 hours and 30 minutes.

For the Dutch, the Liberty ships became lifesavers toward the end of the war when General Eisenhower told the Germans he was commencing food drops behind enemy lines to alleviate severe food shortages. After the war, 8,000 tons of food bound for Holland aboard a Liberty would be replaced by 2,000 tons of sea water in the ship's ballast tanks to keep the empty freighter from riding too high in the water. About a dozen passengers could also be accommodated on the return trip.

Bloembergen was finally able to book passage on a Liberty ship scheduled to leave from Rotterdam in mid-January 1946. By that time, it seemed, at least four precious months had been lost. Unbeknownst to Bloembergen, however, he would be arriving in Cambridge, Massachusetts at just the right time.

The Discovery

If anyone happened to notice the three young men—the oldest was 33, the other two still in their 20s—who entered the small, wood-frame building attached to Harvard's Lyman Laboratory of Physics on the afternoon of December 15, 1945, it is unlikely the observer would have viewed the occasion as momentous. They might have wondered, of course, what was so interesting so as to command anyone's attention for so many hours in a structure not much larger than a garden shed. Maybe there was another entrance to the main building through the shed? Or maybe they were meteorologists taking weather measurements? They would have wondered even more if they had noticed that one of the men, the tall, thin one who wore glasses, had stayed overnight in the shed the night before.

That afternoon, however, as Christmas shoppers watching for bargains filled Boston and Cambridge stores, the three men in the shed were intently watching for the slightest deflection of a needle on a microammeter as they methodically adjusted the current for a large electromagnet powered by a noisy motor-generator.

It wasn't the first time the three men—Edward Purcell, Henry Torrey and Robert Pound—had tried the experiment. On Thursday, the 13th, they had methodically adjusted the magnet current through a pre-selected range of values, but had seen nothing. Perhaps thermal equilibrium hadn't yet been achieved, they thought. Maybe if they "pre-soaked" the paraffin for at least 10 hours in the strong magnetic field, they would see what they were looking for. That's why Purcell had been there all night on Friday night; you couldn't leave the generator running unattended. But now it was late Saturday afternoon and it still wasn't working.

They were about to give up for the day and go home when they saw it, a brief, but definite, deflection. That was it! That was the signal they were looking for and to the three researchers the moving needle spoke volumes. In order for it to have deflected as it did, all of the following actions had to have transpired.

1) The hydrogen protons in the two pounds of paraffin they had bought at a nearby grocery store had to have come into thermal equilibrium with their molecular environment. Before being positioned between the poles of Professor Street's powerful electromagnet, these atomic nuclei or spins had been randomly oriented in the weak magnetic field of the earth. Once positioned in the powerful magnet, however, they had, because of their spin-induced nuclear magnetism, responded to their new environment by aligning themselves both with and against the strong magnetic field. Slightly more than half—the lower-energy spins—

had become *aligned with*, or *parallel* to, the external field. The minority group—the higher-energy spins—had become *aligned against*, or *antiparallel* to, the field. For hydrogen nuclei, those were their only two options.

2) With an oscillator tuned to 30-megacycles creating a radiofrequency field at right angles to the main field, the current for the main field was adjusted with a rheostat until the resulting frequency had matched—or come into resonance with— the Larmor frequency, unique to hydrogen nuclei, with which the spins were precessing around the main magnetic field. On the basis of the "new physics" of quantum mechanics, the three experimenters knew that, at the point of resonance, more transitions from the lower spin state to the higher spin state would occur than vice versa.

3) As this resonance occurred, the team's two-sided "bridge circuit," which had been carefully balanced like an electronic teeter-totter, had suddenly become unbalanced and had registered the imbalance as a needle deflection on the microammeter.

Because the strength of the main magnetic field and the frequency of the radiomagnetic field were both roughly known at the point of resonance, the Purcell team was able to approximate the magnetic moment of the spinning protons to be 2.75 nuclear magnetons. The proximity of their calculated value to the more precise value determined by Rabi's molecular-beam method—2.7896 nuclear magnetons—further assured Purcell, Torrey and Pound that their experiment had been a success. On Christmas Eve, the first time in six years that Saint Nicolaas had been able to make his annual visit to Hollanders without the presence of German soldiers in the streets, the Purcell team mailed the announcement of their discovery of NMR in condensed matter to the editor of *Physical Review*. It was a Christmas present that Nicolaas Bloembergen would not find out about for another six weeks.

The Right Place, The Right Time

In mid-January 1946, the Liberty ship Bloembergen had boarded at Rotterdam steamed past the Hook of Holland into the North Sea and headed southwest toward the Straits of Dover and the English Channel which was still mine-infested following the recent war. Both the British and Germans had sown the coasts they controlled with thousands of the deadly devices and, although international agreement permitted the use of contact mines only—mines that detonated when struck by a ship's hull—Germany had disregarded the agreements and had used magnetic mines. Planted in the seabed under shallow coastal waters by submarines, ships and airplanes, they would explode if a ship's hull even came near them.

Since Liberty ships lacked modern mine-detection systems, it was necessary for a seaman to stand at the prow of the ship and search for them visually. If he saw something suspicious, he would get the attention of the ship's navigator on the bridge by shouting and pointing. "It was an unbelievably primitive operation," said Bloembergen.[99]

Because of stormy conditions in the North Atlantic that could break a nearly-empty, high-riding Liberty ship in two, the captain decided to take a long detour by way of the Azores, which are due west of Portugal. His prudence was well founded. Enroute, they heard radio distress signals from two other vessels that had broken apart near Iceland. The trip across the Atlantic took 18 days as they were unable to avoid one storm that slowed their progress to only two miles in 24 hours. When the ship finally arrived in the United States, it was not permitted to dock in the port of New York because of a longshoremen's strike, so they proceeded down the New Jersey coast and then up the Delaware River to Philadelphia, where they disembarked in early February 1946.

From Philadelphia, Bloembergen took a train to Boston, but stopped enroute for two days in New York City for sightseeing and to visit the physics department of Columbia University. Although both I.I. Rabi and Norman Ramsey had returned to Columbia by that time from their wartime venues in Cambridge and Los Alamos, Bloembergen did not meet them at that time, but he did meet Professor George Pegram, the chairman of the department.

Seventeen years earlier, when Bloembergen was only nine years old, Pegram, on the recommendation of Werner Heisenberg, had hired Isidor I. Rabi as a lecturer. As a result of that decision, magnetic resonance had been discovered at Columbia University by Rabi and his associates in 1937. A few months later, Norman Ramsey, one of those associates, had been the first to detect multi-spectral lines using radiofrequency spectroscopy. It had been the first instance of multiple-line spectroscopy using coherent electromagnetic radiation, a characteristic not only of radiofrequency spectroscopy, but also of the microwave and laser spectroscopy that would follow years later.

Bloembergen also met Professor John Dunning on his visit to Columbia. Nearly a decade earlier, Dunning had experimentally determined the magnetic moment of the neutron—without using magnetic resonance—on the basis of Felix Bloch's famous 1936 paper in which he suggested using magnetized iron as a way to measure the magnetic properties of these nuclear particles. Three years later, Bloch had modified his own method and had used magnetic resonance to obtain significantly more accurate results. Much of this information was still unknown, however, to Bloembergen when he visited with Professors Pegram and Dunning that day, but he was treated as though he was a visiting professor.

"They thought I was an important man," said Bloembergen. "I was nothing. I was not quite finished as a student, but they had so few foreign visitors that I was taken to lunch by George Pegram in the Columbia Faculty Club."[100]

When Bloembergen arrived at Harvard in Cambridge, Massachusetts, Professor Oldenberg also took him out for lunch to welcome him to the school and to discuss Bloembergen's research program. Because Bloembergen had passed the examinations for his doctorate before the University of Utrecht was closed in 1943 and had already done some research, he was one of the few students at Harvard who could start his thesis research immediately.

"It was all a matter of very fortunate coincidences," said Bloembergen. Although the spring semester of 1946 had brought a great influx of bright, well-motivated graduate students who were returning to the academic world for the first time after serving in the military, "practically nobody," said Bloembergen, "was ready for research. They all had to take courses." He was also better off at Harvard than if he had remained at the University of Utrecht to do his PhD research. When his alma mater in Holland reopened in 1945 after being shut down for more than two years, the graduate students who returned essentially had to start over from scratch, he said.

As for how Bloembergen should get started in research, Oldenberg suggested a straightforward approach. "Just look around and see who you can do research with," he told Bloembergen.[101]

"The contrast between the anemic state of academic affairs in the wartorn Netherlands and the exhilarating pulse of scientific research in Cambridge, Massachusetts was bewildering at first," Bloembergen said, "but members of the Harvard physics faculty were most helpful and sympathetic."[102] One of those with whom Bloembergen spoke was Professor J. Curry Street, who was interested in resuming the cosmic-ray research he had postponed because of the war.

In the 1930s, Street had constructed a large electromagnet, the yoke of which came from a generator discarded by the Boston Street Railways, and in 1937, he and Assistant Professor E.C. Stevenson had used the magnet, together with a cloud chamber, to photograph a previously-unknown particle called the muon.[103]

In late 1940, Street's academic career, like that of many other U.S. physicists, had been interrupted by the desperate situation in which Britain found itself following the collapse of Holland, Belgium and France. With Hitler unleashing his nightly bombers against England in the Battle of Britain, it appeared to be just a matter of time before it too would be overwhelmed. Propitiously, however, just the year before, British science had developed the resonant cavity magnetron, a device that dramatically increased the power and viability of radar. They needed the help of their American allies, however, to integrate that power into a militarily-useful system. The Americans had responded heroically. In response to Britain's dire crisis and the increasing possibility that the United States would also be drawn into the conflict, the Radiation Laboratory had been established on the campus of Massachusetts Institute of Technology in Cambridge and physicists had been quickly recruited from around the nation.

The Rad Lab, as it came to be called, had fulfilled its purpose beyond the most optimistic imaginations of those who founded it and, by midway through the war, its primary product—radar—had become an indispensable "eye" for the Allies that was used both defensively and offensively. Defensively, in combination with other strategic methods, it had done an outstanding job in reversing the substantial threat posed by German U-boats.

Street, an invaluable contributor to that effort, was on the Steering Committee of the Radiation Laboratory and, by war's end, had been put in charge of Division 10 radar developments, known as Ground and Ship. By early 1946, with the war behind, Street was ready to resume the cosmic ray research he had set aside five years earlier and discussed with Bloembergen the directions his research might take.

Had he gone with Street, Bloembergen might well have ended up in the "big science" of high-energy physics tracking atomic particles for the rest of his career instead of the "little science" of microwave, radio, and non-linear spectroscopy. The move would have likely been a mistake as three years later, when Bloembergen did make a brief, two-year switch toward high-energy physics, he came to the conclusion that such large-group, large-machine research was incompatible both with his personality and his intellectual approach to science. At any rate, after "shopping around" for a suitable thesis topic for about 10 days in early February of 1946, he had "the good fortune," Bloembergen said, "to talk with Purcell," another alumnus of the Radiation Laboratory who had just made his Nobel

Prize-worthy discovery of NMR in a solid.[104] In fact, Purcell had made his discovery using Street's cosmic-ray magnet.

Bloembergen's timing couldn't have been better. Purcell was very interested in getting a graduate student to assist in the follow-up experimentation he needed done. In early 1946, Purcell, Torrey and Pound were all busy writing the tomes they had been assigned in the 28-volume Radiation Laboratory Series and Purcell, recently promoted to associate professor at Harvard, was also busy preparing to resume his teaching career.

The writing for the Radiation Laboratory Series was particularly time consuming. Conceived by I.I. Rabi in late 1944 as a way to share the wealth of knowledge about microwave and radar technology gained during the war, Rabi also recognized that such a massive record—he described it as "the biggest thing since the Septuagint"[105]—might also come in handy should Congress investigate what had happened to all the money it had invested in the Rad Lab. Rabi's concern for preserving the information they had accumulated and making it available to everyone proved to be farsighted, although at first some thought it was a waste of time, considering that the war was still being fought. "All this microwave and radio stuff," Bloembergen pointed out, "was very important in doing research after the war. Suddenly, the field of radio and microwave spectroscopy came into bloom. There was an awful lot of science to be done right after the war with these new radio techniques."[106]

For Bloembergen, who wanted to be on the cutting edge of physics, the choice was fairly clear.

> [NMR research with Purcell] appealed to me more [than cosmic-ray research, said Bloembergen], because it was a new experimental technique and it was somewhat related to Dutch work on magnetic relaxation. More important was the fact that Professor Purcell needed a pair of hands for a follow-up on the pioneering experiment.
>
> Fortunately, I had brought with me a preprint of pre-doctoral research work carried out at the University of Utrecht. It involved the development of a low-noise photoelectric amplifier coupled to a phase-sensitive AC galvanometer. On this basis, Purcell accepted me tentatively as his first graduate student and as a quarter-time laboratory assistant.[107]

Actually the "preprint" was nothing more than a typewritten manuscript of an article that would appear later in 1946,[108] but it was enough to convince Purcell that Bloembergen was familiar with some electronic techniques and was qualified to handle the research. "He liked that paper," said Bloembergen, even though Bloembergen's galvanometer-based, lock-in phase-sensitive detection scheme was old-fashioned compared to the Dicke amplifier Purcell planned to use on his next generation of apparatus. "That's what we are going to use," he told Bloembergen, "the lock-in scheme."[109]

Despite Purcell's readiness to accept Bloembergen as a protégé and part-time assistant, he also recognized Bloembergen's need for outside counsel on the matter before locking himself into a particular program and he personally knew two men who could provide such a perspective—two well-respected former countrymen of Bloembergen's:

> Purcell arranged for me to discuss my decision with [Samuel] Goudsmit and [George] Uhlenbeck, who were both still associated with the Rad Lab at that time. Goudsmit suggested that I send my preprint with an application to the University of Michigan, "because there my limited dollar funds would last twice as long." The Cambridge cost of living was twice that in Ann Arbor. Uhlenbeck told me that I could not go wrong in casting my lot with Ed Purcell.[110]

Although Bloembergen had completed the course requirements for his PhD, Purcell did advise him to take two graduate courses at Harvard, one on electromagnetism by Julian Schwinger and the other on statistical mechanics by E.C. Kemble.

Schwinger was the 17-year-old genius I.I. Rabi had discovered in 1936 at Columbia University about one year before Rabi discovered magnetic resonance in molecular beams. At the time, Schwinger was about to flunk out of City College in New York because of poor performance in his non-technical courses. With the help of Rabi, Hans Bethe and George Uhlenbeck, Schwinger had been rescued from his academic demise and given a scholarship to Columbia, where he graduated as a Phi Beta Kappa.

By the time 26-year-old Bloembergen took a class from 28-year-old Schwinger in 1946, the latter was a seasoned veteran, having worked as a theorist in Rabi's laboratory at Columbia before the war and having made major contributions to waveguide theory during the war at the Radiation Laboratory. In the commemorative publication entitled *Five Years at the Radiation Laboratory*,[111] published in 1946, a photo of Schwinger studying an equation-filled blackboard is accompanied by the following caption: "Example of men who seldom stirred out of the Laboratory but whose work exerted profound influence was Julian Schwinger, whose method of solving electromagnetic field forms will probably outlive most radar design." Two decades later, Schwinger would share the 1965 Nobel Prize in physics with Richard Feynman (U.S.) and Sin-itiro Tomonaga (Japan) for his basic work in quantum electrodynamics, or QED.

In 1946, the 57-year-old Edwin (E.C.) Kemble, a member of Harvard's physics faculty since 1919, was twice Schwinger's age. Born in 1889, only 10 years after the death of classical physicist James Clerk Maxwell and six years before the discovery of X rays, Kemble would still be associated with Harvard when he died in 1984 at the age of 95. In 1915, as a student caught between classical physics and the new quantum physics, Kemble had written:

> I presume that all of us would agree that the quantum theory is quite distasteful. In working with the theory we have no definite mechanical picture to guide us nor have we any definite clear-cut principle as a basis of operations—physicists everywhere have been making strenuous efforts to find a method of escape from the theory. If such a method could be found I presume that we should all breathe a sigh of relief and sleep better thereafter.[112]

By 1946, of course, many of the frustrations associated with the old quantum theory had been resolved in the new quantum mechanics developed in the mid-1920s by Werner Heisenberg, Erwin Schrödinger, Pascual Jordan, Max Born and Paul Dirac, and Kemble had become a devoted disciple committed to spreading the gospel of quantum mechanics to a generation of American physicists.

Because of his February arrival at Harvard, Bloembergen had to start both the Schwinger class and the Kemble class several weeks late, but found that he was not greatly handicapped. "Since I had taken both subjects before with Lèon Rosenfeld in Utrecht, I had no trouble with either course and spent most of my time in the laboratory," he noted.[113] He also attended lectures by John H. Van Vleck, the renowned authority on the quantum theory of magnetism who would receive the Nobel Prize for his contributions to the field in 1977. Bloembergen enjoyed both the courses and the lectures and profited quickly from all of them because of the solid foundations he had been provided by the Dutch educational system and from his own independent study while hiding out in Holland.

My plodding study during the grim war years in Holland started to pay off [said Bloembergen]. The traditional Dutch system had given me a very solid background in the fundamentals of physics. I was well prepared to catch up quickly with the advances made in the free countries during the war. So I plunged into a room in the basement of Lyman Laboratory, never noticing the lack of daylight.[114]

It wasn't just Bloembergen's educational background, however, that was paying dividends; it was also his hard work at Harvard. Not only did he not see daylight in the laboratory, he also didn't see it when he emerged at the end of each workday. "I devoted all my time in that lab until midnight most days," he said. "It was exciting."[115]

Getting Started in NMR

The first task assigned Bloembergen was to make a "mud pie" from a recipe that called for calcium fluoride powder and mineral oil. After thoroughly mixing the transparent fluorite crystals with mineral oil, purchased from a local druggist, he began stuffing the concoction into a small coupling hole of the resonant cavity, the same cavity used in the original NMR experiment about two months earlier. By the time the cavity was filled, in a manner not unlike stuffing toothpaste into a tube, he had wormed about a liter of the mud through the small hole. He was rewarded for his patience a few days later when he witnessed his first NMR signals. As Pound monitored the electronic equipment and Purcell adjusted the magnet current, Bloembergen was able to see the proton resonance signal followed by the resonance signal for fluorine.

Since Purcell and Pound were still occupied full time at the Radiation Laboratory, Bloembergen had plenty of time to catch up, he said, with the NMR state-of-the-art as it existed in early 1946, a process that was further aided by the team's decision to construct a second-generation apparatus. As Purcell had told Bloembergen in his initial interview, he wanted to incorporate a Dicke lock-in amplifier in his new NMR apparatus and he now put his new assistant to work in building the device.

Princeton physicist Robert Dicke had been a member of Purcell's Fundamental Development Group at the Radiation Laboratory and, as part of his work there, had invented a microwave radiometer, a tool which had proved very helpful toward the end of the war when Purcell's group encountered a problem with their new 1.25-cm radar program (see Chapter 3). Dicke had used his radiometer to measure the water vapor absorption line in the atmosphere and had confirmed that, coincidentally, it was almost identical to the Rad Lab's new, shorter-wavelength radar. As a result, transmitted radar energy was not being reflected back to its source. Dicke had also used also his invention while at the Radiation Laboratory to measure oxygen absorption at six millimeters, to observe a partial solar eclipse, and to make a measurement of the sky temperature, setting an upper limit on the density of what is now known as the isotropic microwave background radiation. Eventually the Dicke radiometer would come to be a basic tool of radio astronomers and microwave spectroscopists.[116]

Incorporated in the Dicke radiometer was a lock-in amplifier/detector and in 1946, years before it was commercially available, Bloembergen made his own copy, based on an article by Robert Dicke published in an early 1946 issue of *Review of Scientific Instruments*. After familiarizing himself with RCA vacuum tubes, electronic components and chassis punches, Bloembergen set to work. With little money available for the project, he had to make do with what little he had. There was a machine shop on the premises and a machinist, but no money with which to pay the machinist, so he did the shop work himself. "My craftsmanship was marginal," he said. "The lock-in performed reasonably during my 18 months at Harvard, but was relegated to the scrap heap soon after my departure."[117]

"The Grand Old Man" and the Gorter Connection

In April 1946, several months after Bloembergen arrived at Harvard, Professor I.I. Rabi came by to visit Purcell and to view the NMR apparatus for the first time. To 25-year-old Bloembergen, the 47-year-old Columbia University professor was "the grand old man," not so much for his age as for his scientific contributions. Already considered by many as the dean of American physicists for his work with molecular beams before the war, Rabi had risen even further in their esteem when he was awarded the Nobel Prize in 1944 for his 1937 discovery of magnetic resonance.

In pointing out the fundamental nature of Rabi's contributions, Bloembergen noted that "people still talk about the famous Rabi precession which also occurs in the laser field. That is universal. People still talk about the Rabi Frequency just as people talk about the Bloch Equations. They are very basic and they are used not only in magnetic resonance but also in lasers."[118]

Purcell, of course, was very anxious to show Rabi an NMR proton signal. Unfortunately, balancing the radiofrequency bridge circuit was still "a tricky art," said Bloembergen, and when he tried to show the "grand old man" the well-known resonance signal using water, he was unable to coax the signal out of hiding.*

Naturally, Purcell was quite disappointed, so after Rabi and Purcell left the laboratory, Bloembergen continued to tinker with the apparatus. By retuning the controls from scratch, he was able to get the signal back within an hour or so. "I rushed upstairs to Purcell's office," he recalled. "Fortunately, Rabi was still there and they were both happy to see the NMR signal."[119]

Although Rabi was the first to detect magnetic resonance, he was not the first to search for the phenomenon. In fact, in his thesis Bloembergen credits Professor C.J. Gorter, who by then had become his PhD mentor in Holland, with being "the first to point out how the phenomenon [of magnetic resonance] could be used to detect nuclear magnetism."[120] In fact, Gorter had tried unsuccessfully to detect magnetic resonance in 1936, and the oscillator technique that Rabi used in his successful attempt one year later was suggested to him by Gorter.

When Bloembergen arrived at Harvard and heard for the first time about magnetic resonance, Purcell had explained to him that it was related to studies on magnetic relaxation in Holland done by Cornelis Gorter. "Well, that's a connection," Bloembergen had said.

Although Bloembergen had never met Gorter, he was aware of Gorter's work on paramagnetic relaxation. In fact, said Bloembergen, "Gorter had published a little booklet on the subject, which we read very carefully. But those were non-resonance studies," Bloembergen explained.

The Gorter connection would turn out to be much more significant than Bloembergen could possibly have anticipated at the time he was talking with Purcell. Eighteen months later, he would return to Holland as an associate of Professor Gorter and, under Gorter's mentorship, would receive his PhD degree in 1948 from the University of Leiden, just one more example of how the four-month delay in Bloembergen's arrival at Harvard was turning out to be positive rather than negative.

C.J. Gorter

In 1907, 13 years before Bloembergen was born, Cornelis J. Gorter was born in Utrecht, the same metropolitan area in which Bloembergen

---

* Martin Packard of the Felix Bloch team had a similar disappointing experience. Not long after they observed the NMR signal using the nuclear induction method, Bloch was speaking on the topic at a seminar and Packard, wanting to back up the discussion with demonstration, transported the apparatus to the lecture room only to find, to his embarrassment, that he was unable to produce the signal.
—J.R. Rigden, *Reviews of Modern Physics* **58**, (1988), 445.

would live for most of his youth. Raised in a family of "third-generation intellectuals," as he described them, Gorter grew up in The Hague, the seat of the Dutch government and monarchy, where he attended what he said was "the best [secondary] school of the country."[121] The rector of the school was Rommert Casimir, a progressive educator and university professor, and the father of Hendrik Casimir who, along with Gorter, would become another well-known Dutch physicist.

The two of them, in fact, would later collaborate in the development of the two-fluid model of superconductivity, but during their teens didn't know each other well, even though they attended the same *gymnasium*. Casimir was two years younger, a difference that almost qualifies as a generation gap at the *gymnasium* level. Both Gorter and Casimir excelled academically in secondary school, however, and passed their final examinations at the ages of 16 and 15 respectively, well ahead of the average age of 19.

At the *gymnasium*, it was a physics teacher by the name of Korfer who instilled in Gorter the desire to become a physicist. "This teacher just convinced me," he said. "Every year the people started studying physics because he was such a marvelous teacher. He was a student of Lorentz, and he told us much about it. Lorentz and Kamerlingh Onnes and Zeeman and van der Waals [the Nobel laureate mentor of Bloembergen's grandfather] were very central personalities when we were young," he said.[122]

In 1924, at the age of 17, Gorter enrolled as a student at the University of Leiden with majors in mathematics and physics and a minor in chemistry. A little over two years later, not yet 20, he graduated with a bachelor's degree. During that period, like the other physics majors at Leiden, he didn't bother attending the general courses in physics that included students from other disciplines. "These courses were of no importance," he said. "We passed the examinations, but we didn't follow the courses because we learned it from books. . . . We developed ourselves, more or less," he said. As far as he was concerned, real development in physics came from the specialized courses taught on thermodynamics and radiation, from personal reading, from four to five hours of weekly interaction in a student-organized society called The Leiden Flask, headed up the George Uhlenbeck,* and from a weekly colloquium led by Leiden's theoretical physicist, Paul Ehrenfest.

It was through Ehrenfest's colloquium that 22-year-old Gorter became "very good friends" with 24-year-old Felix Bloch. The connection is note-

---

* Uhlenbeck and Goudsmit would make their discovery of electron spin the year after Gorter matriculated at Leiden and two years later, in 1927, would receive their doctorates.

worthy since both Gorter and Bloch would be pioneers in magnetic resonance. In Bloch's October 1946 article in *Physical Review* in which he provided the Bloch equations and the theoretical foundation for nuclear induction, Bloch would acknowledge the 1942 attempt by C.J. Gorter and L.J.F. Broer to detect NMR in a solid.

During the year that Bloch spent in Holland (1929-30) as a Lorentz Fellow, working with H.A. Kramers and Adriaan Fokker, he attended whenever possible the Wednesday evening by-invitation-only Ehrenfest colloquia held in Leiden. These meetings often featured rather aggressive give-and-take discussions with Ehrenfest frequently the primary aggressor. Gorter remembered one of the meetings in particular that Bloch attended:

> I remember Felix Bloch . . . telling about his electron theory of metals. Well, Ehrenfest attacked him so much, he couldn't move forward nor backward, and Bloch is not a man who is easy to stop. But he couldn't move; he was just completely pinned down on certain weak points of this single-electron model, which was too simple according to Ehrenfest. He just proved this to Bloch during the colloquium; we enjoyed it.[123]

In spite of, or maybe because of, Ehrenfest's sometimes prickly exterior and unconventional ways—he cut his hair once a year, in April—he instilled enthusiasm for physics in his young students. In fact, he gave more time and attention to his younger students than his senior students, said Gorter. It was Ehrenfest to whom Gorter credited the direction for much of his early scientific work.

> To Ehrenfest I owe two suggestions [said Gorter] which guided the choice of the first scientific work I did after completing my thesis on low-temperature paramagnetism in 1932 under the supervision of W.J. de Haas. [1] W. Lenz and Ehrenfest had pointed out in 1920 that interaction with thermal motion is essential to obtain the Curie-Langevin magnetization in a paramagnetic substance. This meant that relaxation phenomena should occur, which Gregory Breit tried in vain to detect with the insufficient means at his disposal in 1926 during his Leiden time. [2] After a visit to an industrial laboratory, Ehrenfest once exclaimed to me that, although he understood hardly anything of the wonderful techniques being developed in the radio industry, he felt that such techniques might become of great benefit to pure scientific research.[124]

Probably as a result of his earlier conversation with Ehrenfest, Gorter included a proposition in his thesis in which he advocated the use of short radio waves in conducting spectroscopic research with hydrogen in a magnetic field. To that extent at least, he anticipated the radiofrequency spectroscopy that Norman Ramsey would pioneer at Columbia University six years later with I.I. Rabi, Jerome Kellogg and Jerrold Zacharias.

Even before receiving his PhD degree, Gorter was appointed conservator of the prestigious Teyler's Foundation in Haarlem by Adriaan Fokker, Bloembergen's distant uncle. He would remain at the foundation until 1936, making fundamental contributions to the thermodynamics of superconductivity, including the paper mentioned earlier in which he collaborated with Hendrik B.G. Casimir. It was also during his association with Fokker at Teyler's Foundation that Gorter began learning about radio techniques and made his first attempt at detecting paramagnetic relaxation.

The search for the frequency dependence of the magnetic susceptibility in paramagnetic substances began in the 1920s. According to Norman Ramsey, the earliest reported search was in 1922 by M.H. Belz who looked for the dependence unsuccessfully in various solutions of paramagnetic salts. Four years later, Gregory Breit, acting on the Lenz-Ehrenfest suggestion, also searched in vain for such a frequency dependence. "Perhaps this disappointment," speculated Ramsey, "contributed to Breit's decision to concentrate in theory, where he had a highly productive career."[125] In 1931, Breit would collaborate with I.I. Rabi in developing the Breit-Rabi formula. This theory of hyperfine structure permits the determination of nuclear spin magnitudes and magnetic moments.

In 1936, 10 years after Breit's failed attempt to detect paramagnetic relaxation, Gorter succeeded by using a calorimetric method. In his first attempt, he tried to detect relaxation by observing, he said, "the mechanical couple acting on a paramagnetic substance in a low-frequency rotating magnetic field."[126] The result was not conclusive.

For his next attempt, which was performed at nearby Leiden at the invitation of his mentor, W.J. de Haas, Gorter was able to detect with a gas thermometer an increase in the temperature of the sample when radiating it with a strong, radiofrequency field. Since, according to the Curie law, the paramagnetic susceptibility of a substance is inversely proportional to absolute temperature, an increase in temperature indicated a drop in paramagnetic susceptibility and a dependence of paramagnetic susceptibility on frequency. Gorter was able to show this dependent relationship of susceptibility to frequency with a number of alums.

The establishment of paramagnetic relaxation is actually the first step in the detection of nuclear magnetic resonance, and Gorter tried to use the same radiofrequency-heat measurement technique in 1936 to observe nuclear magnetic resonance for lithium (^{7}Li) in lithium chloride and for hydrogen (^{1}H) in aluminum potassium alum. For this experiment, he used what he called "a primitive but sensitive foil manometer"[127] in his attempt to detect a sudden rise in the temperature of the sample as it passed through resonance. By very slowly changing a transverse magnetic field, he searched for a temperature rise within the range of radiofrequencies in which NMR of lithium-7 and hydrogen could be expected but the effect did not show up.

In 1936, Gorter left Teyler's Foundation and was appointed a reader at the University of Groningen in the northern part of Holland. As he continued investigating paramagnetic relaxation as well as paramagnetic dispersion, he determined to continue his search for the detection of magnetic resonance. With that in mind, he made plans to spend the summer of 1937 in the United States. According to Gorter, he had two options: 1) Columbia University where I.I. Rabi was working with molecular beams, a method that Gorter thought might have benefits in getting around the spin-temperature problems associated with his first attempt, and 2) the University of Michigan at Ann Arbor, where C.E. Cleeton and N.H. Williams had observed the absorption of ammonia gas, a first step in the field of microwave spectroscopy that would later mushroom after World War II.

Although he was welcome at both universities, Gorter chose Ann Arbor, in part, he said, because he thought Professor Williams' work in microwaves might be useful as a starting point for detecting electron spin resonance and also because of the school's well-known summer symposium for theoretical physics.

Unfortunately, a secretary had failed to inform Williams of Gorter's plans, and he was about to leave on vacation just as Gorter arrived. That left the summer symposium where, said Gorter, "I spent a very interesting time . . . and particularly enjoyed lectures by Enrico Fermi, George E. Uhlenbeck and Luis Alvarez but learnt hardly nothing about microwaves."[128]

After the symposium was over, Gorter departed by Greyhound bus for the East Coast and the ship waiting to return him to Holland. Upon his arrival in New York, however, he stopped off at Columbia University to visit I.I. Rabi, where "one of Rabi's collaborators," said Gorter, "showed me the details of the various atomic beam apparatuses." (The collaborator was Norman Ramsey, who had just recently arrived at Columbia to work with Rabi on molecular beams after spending two years at Cambridge University.) The following is Gorter's recollection of the event.

> Seeing the set-up in which the beam passed through a magnetic field, the direction of which rotated in space so that the sign and approximate magnitude of the magnetic moments of the nuclei could be evaluated, I realized that replacing this magnetic field by a constant plus a transverse radiofrequency field would make the apparatus immediately suitable for the observation of nuclear magnetic resonance.
>
> I then asked to see Rabi, whom I had earlier shown around the Leiden laboratory, and suggested to him the introduction of a radiofrequency magnetic field into his apparatus, showing by a simple calculation that a small oscillator would be sufficient to obtain a strong depolarization of his beam. I did not succeed in convincing him of the advantages of my proposal over his constant field rotating in space, but he promised to consider the matter at his ease. I understood that he intended to visit us soon in Holland and would then continue the conversation. But a few months later I could congratulate him and his collaborators on the discovery of nuclear magnetic resonance announced in a Letter to the Editor of the *Physical Review*.
>
> I cannot deny that I felt some pride, mixed with the feeling that my contribution had been somewhat undervalued though my advice was acknowledged in the Letter. I realized quite well, however, that it would have cost us years to set up the adequate equipment in our small group at Groningen. Some time afterward in California, Alvarez and Felix Bloch who apparently had arrived at the same ideas independently, measured the magnetic spins of neutrons by passing a beam of them through a similar transverse radiofrequency magnetic field.[129]

"Rabi immediately recognized," said Bloembergen, "[the potential of the resonance technique suggested by Gorter] and really pushed experimental techniques to combine molecular beams with his magnetic resonance equipment. And that gave very famous results on the nuclear magnetic moments and quadrupoles, and really opened up the field of radiofrequency spectroscopy."[130]

It also gave Rabi the 1944 Nobel Prize, recognition Gorter would never receive. Gorter's collaborator Hendrik Casimir has said of Gorter that he is the man who "almost discovered nuclear spin resonance, who almost was the first to orient nuclear spins. . . . Certainly, he has been close to results that would probably have earned him a Nobel Prize."[131]

There is, of course, another side to the story. Out of fairness, it needs to be pointed out that Rabi had already published a paper in *Physical Review*—it was submitted in February 1937 and published in April of that year—entitled "Space Quantization in a Gyrating Magnetic Field."[132] In that paper, Rabi set the stage for magnetic resonance but he expressed it in terms of a gyrating or rotating field rather than an oscillating field. As Ramsey has pointed out, the resonance equation provided by Rabi in the paper would become the basis for all subsequent magnetic and electric resonance experiments. The form of the equation, however, "obscured the resonant nature of the result," noted Ramsey, "and Rabi failed to see it immediately."[133]

Although Gorter felt his comment had been tabled for further thought and future discussion, it had not fallen on deaf ears, a fact which Rabi has acknowledged. "Gorter's visit was a stimulus," Rabi told his biographer, John Rigden. "I knew about his work; in fact, he didn't tell us anything we didn't know. But he asked me, 'Why aren't you doing it this way?' Well, I liked what we were doing [with the T-field method], but I saw that he might go after it [magnetic resonance] and we might get some competition. So I said, 'Let's do it.' Gorter's visit stimulated me into saying, 'It's time to do it the other way.' "[134]

According to Norman Ramsey, Rabi and another collaborator, Jerrold Zacharias, had once briefly discussed, in fact, the benefits of using an oscillator to produce a magnetic field that rotated with time but, because of other pressing duties, had given the idea little further thought until September 1937 when Gorter came to Pupin Hall. On that day, the word "oscillator" took on new significance with regard to their molecular beam apparatus. After Gorter left, no time was lost in making the shift to the magnetic resonance method. Gorter's visit was on Saturday. Two days later, on Monday morning, Rabi's research team began modifying their molecular-beam apparatuses to incorporate a transverse oscillating field as Gorter had suggested.

When Rabi and his collaborators announced their discovery in an early 1938 issue of *Physical Review*, a footnote to the letter to the editor cited the earlier attempt by Gorter and then continued: "We are very much indebted to Dr. Gorter who, when visiting our laboratory in September 1937, drew our attention to his stimulating experiments in which he attempted to measure nuclear moments by observing the rise in temperature of solids placed in a constant magnetic field on which an oscillating field was superimposed."[135]

Rabi did not, however, detect nuclear magnetic resonance in condensed matter, and in 1942, Gorter, in collaboration with L.J.F. Broer, made another attempt. By that time, Gorter had been appointed the successor to Pieter Zeeman, Nobel laureate and discoverer of the famous Zeeman effect, at the University of Amsterdam where he was able to build, he said, "a small but able research team . . . in spite of the war and German occupation which did not make my Amsterdam years a particularly agreeable period."[136] (Certainly, that qualifies as an understatement. During this period, Gorter was living in the Jewish quarter of Amsterdam, an area experiencing a rapid drop in population as Hitler continued his efforts to rid Europe of all Jews.)

Although Gorter was a professor at Amsterdam in 1942, he was permitted to do his NMR research at the University of Leiden where there were better low-temperature facilities. This time, he tried to detect energy dispersion.

> The idea [said Gorter] was to observe the frequency shift of an LC oscillator as it slowly approached the nuclear-magnetic-resonance line so that no energy absorption would equalize the occupations of the higher and lower energy levels. The results of a few days' observations were again negative for lithium-seven in lithium chloride and fluorine-19 in potassium fluoride, although we sometimes saw apparently irreproducible irregularities in our frequency.[137]

As they stepped the strength of the applied magnetic field through the anticipated point of resonance, Gorter and Broer were hoping they would see the NMR effect as an inductive pulling or shifting of the self-excited radiofrequency oscillator. They were again disappointed.

"Several years later," said Gorter, "we understood that we had used too pure chemicals and therefore had still too long relaxation times. Nicolaas Bloembergen then measured the relaxation time of the lithium-seven spins in our sample and, in fact, found several minutes at liquid-helium temperatures."[138]

The two sentences seem to contradict one another. If the chemicals had been too pure, it seems unlikely that Bloembergen would have been able to detect NMR using the same crystals a few years later. The reason for the second failed attempt continues to remain somewhat of a mystery. Citing Bloembergen's successful detection of NMR using one of Gorter's original samples, Professor Norman Ramsey has stated that the reasons for failure were "probably due to detection inefficiencies."[139] Professor John Van Vleck has stated:

[Gorter's apparatus] was primitive but the real difficulty arose from the fact that he used too much power and too pure materials, things that are advantages in most physical experiments. He tried to detect the resonance in LiCl, where the nuclear resonance times are inordinately long, sometimes minutes or so, although this was not known at the time. In consequence, the line saturates exceedingly easily. In other words, the populations of the upper and lower states become substantially equal.[140]

In recounting his retest of the lithium chloride sample used by Gorter and Broer, Bloembergen noted:

I measured [the T_1 relaxation time of lithium-7] to be 10 minutes at 2.1° K., caused by some undetermined paramagnetic impurity. It is likely that they saturated this resonance on their first scan and consequently no reproducible signal could be found in subsequent transversals. They would have had a better chance if they had used a less pure crystal, or had observed the influence of dispersion on the resonant frequency with a marginal oscillator.[141]

There is no question, however, that Gorter was an important contributor to the science of NMR, as evidenced by the early Rabi, Purcell and Bloch papers in which they all acknowledged Gorter's attempts to make the same discoveries they had made.

As for Bloembergen's assessment of Gorter's contributions and his place in the history of NMR, he has noted that "the possibility of resonance transitions between nuclear spin Zeeman levels was conceived by Gorter, who reported two unsuccessful attempts at detecting such transitions."[142]

[Gorter] was early on concerned with nuclear magnetism [said Bloembergen] and he deserves a lot of credit. But he wasn't a good enough experimenter. I always felt that if he really had seen the significance of his suggestion, what he should have done was to stay at Columbia University with Professor Rabi and be a participant. Now there are many reasons why he probably couldn't—because he had a job (he was a professor in Holland), he probably had to go back to teach—but he missed out on the big prize. He was a very perceptive scientist.[143]

Gorter wasn't the only one who missed out on the "big prize." As Bloembergen has also noted, E. Zavoisky, working in Kazan in the war-ravaged Soviet Union, would actually be the first to obtain a positive indication of magnetic resonance in condensed matter, not nuclear magnetic resonance at the nuclear spin level, but electron paramagnetic resonance at the much-higher-frequency electron spin level.

[Zavoisky] investigated paramagnetic relaxation phenomena at frequencies that were higher than those described by Gorter. He observed a maximum in the radiofrequency magnetic susceptibility, as the function of a direct current magnetic field applied at right angles to the RF field. Frenkel gave a brief theoretical description of this phenomenon. [Frenkel's] equations may be considered precursors of the Bloch equations.[144]

Announcement of Zavoisky's experimental achievement and Frenkel's theoretical explanation of it would appear in three articles published in the *Journal of Physics USSR* in 1945.

East Meets West

In addition to Rabi, two other visitors who came by to visit at Lyman Laboratory in early 1946 were William W. Hansen and Felix Bloch. Hansen, one of Bloch's collaborators on the nuclear-induction discovery of NMR, came in February, not long after Bloembergen's arrival. Hansen had been the "real experimental wheel"[145] on the Bloch team, said Bloembergen. Whereas Bloch had supplied the theory and the idea for the experiment and had worked on the magnet, it was Hansen who had designed the radio system and, when the experiment failed to work, had invented the "paddle system" which controlled the magnetic flux from the transmitter coil. Martin Packard, the third member of the team, had assembled the radio equipment according to Hansen's design.

In spite of the fact that both the Purcell and Bloch teams had discovered the NMR signal in condensed matter, it was not immediately apparent to either of them that they had achieved the same result. "When Bill Hansen came east," Purcell said, "we talked with each other for over half an hour before either of us understood exactly what the other was doing."[146]

In April 1946, Bloch traveled east for a meeting of the American Physical Society held in Cambridge, a meeting at which both the Harvard and Stanford groups presented papers describing their experiments. It was evident, according to Bloembergen, that "Bloch clearly had a much bigger reputation than Purcell, deservedly so."[147] In 1946, Bloch was the better known of the two physicists, having established a solid reputation in theoretical physics even before emigrating to the United States in 1934 at the age of 28. His theory for measuring the magnetic moment of the neutron, published in 1936, and his 1939 experiment in which he and Luis Alvarez expanded on his 1936 proposal by incorporating magnetic resonance, had only served to make that reputation more solid. As a result, Bloch was invited to give a 40-minute paper at the Cambridge gathering. When he needed more time, Rabi convinced the chair of the session to give Bloch an additional 10 minutes. Purcell had to settle for presenting two 10-minute papers. His reputation would grow rapidly, however, in the following years.[148]

Bloch met with Purcell during that trip and had a chance to compare notes. According to Packard, it was the first time Bloch was able to accept that the results were really equivalent. For one thing, the communication process had been hindered by the fact that the Stanford group had used very strong radiofrequency fields and the Harvard experimenters had used a very weak RF field. Bloch also acknowledged that, for a time, "we were speaking an entirely different language."[149]

That same communication problem would continue to plague physicists for some time, often with geographic overtones, as physicist Anatole Abragam has described:

> For months and even years afterwards, according to whether a physicist spoke of nuclear magnetic absorption [Purcell's method] or nuclear induction [Bloch's method], one could decide whether he came from New England or California, more surely than by his accent. The situation was reminiscent of that following the birth of the quantum theory when the devotees of the de Broglie and Schrödinger wave mechanics appeared to be speaking a different language from those who followed the matrix algebra of Born and Heisenberg. And just as the adherents of these two theories came finally to the realization that they were really two different formulations of the same more general theory, quantum mechanics, the champions of nuclear induction and nuclear absorption came to appreciate that these were merely two different aspects of the same

phenomenon, now generally if not universally known as nuclear magnetism.[150]

For Felix Bloch especially, the realization that his nuclear induction approach and Purcell's nuclear absorption approach were equivalent must have seemed at times like scientific *déjà vu* as Werner Heisenberg had become Bloch's PhD mentor only a year or so after the equivalency of the Heisenberg-Schrödinger approaches was established.

NMR on a Shoestring

After using Curry's monstrous cosmic-ray magnet for the early NMR experiments, Purcell, Pound and Bloembergen came to realize that it also had monstrous inhomogeneities, so they obtained another magnet made by the Societé Genevoise. Built in 1905, the "new" magnet was older than any of the scientists using it and, according to Bloembergen, "it turned out to be a beast."

> I had to build a regulating supply for it [he said], because it had a curious oscillation. It was fed by rectified 60 cycles, but there was a big ripple on the supply at about 1 cycle, and we had to build a new electronic feedback and so on, but it was impossible to get that out. At first, of course, they wouldn't believe me. Then Pound, who was the electronics expert—at 12 years he was already making radios—he looked at it, and he finally agreed. I wasted two months on that.[151]

It turned out that the "curious oscillation" was caused by a "curious fault in the winding" and that the time constants were not very constant at all. "So what we did," said Bloembergen, "we bought a set of surplus heavy-truck batteries to run that magnet DC."[152]

That brought up another problem. Since they didn't have a rheostat suitable for changing the magnet current, they had to improvise again. "I remember taking manganin resistance wire*," said Bloembergen, "stretching that thing to the ceiling, and then, with a hand-held clip sliding along the wire, I got the magnetic resonance. It was very, very primitive equipment—no money. Purcell had so little money that he couldn't offer me even a research assistantship." When it later became apparent

---

* Manganin, which consists mainly of copper along with some manganese and nickel, is commonly used to provide variable resistance in electrical heating elements and rheostats.

that Bloembergen needed more than the 12 months originally planned to finish his project, Purcell would scrounge up enough money, Bloembergen said, to pay him for a month, and then take him off the payroll again. "I just extended my stay to a year-and-a-half that way," said Bloembergen. "But, by that time, we had all the major results of our BPP [paper]."[153]

The large electromagnetic cavity resonator was also replaced with an old-fashioned lumped parameter LC radiofrequency circuit. Now, instead of the sample surrounding a center post in the cavity about which a radiofrequency-induced magnetic field circulated, the sample was surrounded by a coil. And instead of samples that measured a whopping 850 cubic centimeters, they could now use samples that measured approximately 1 centimeter by 0.5 centimeter, an improvement of about three orders of magnitude.

With the new coil system, instead of trying to force the contents of a "mud pie" through a small hole into a large cavity, Bloembergen now cut his own crystals of calcium fluoride in the shape of a cylinder, customized to fit the coil.

Even the bridge circuit itself Bloembergen rebuilt. "It was very primitive," he said, "because I didn't know that much about electronic theory—couldn't buy those things—so I built my own RF bridge."[154] The new bridge was more symmetrical with orthogonal adjustments of amplitude and phase, so that the in-phase and out-of-phase part of the nuclear magnetic susceptibility could be measured independently. By turning up the RF power and increasing the balance of the bridge while keeping the input to the RF amplifier constant, the team was now able to observe saturation of the NMR resonance.

For the first seven months or so of Bloembergen's time at Harvard, Purcell and Pound continued to work full time at the Radiation Laboratory at MIT, a situation which, from Bloembergen's perspective, worked out "very well. It gave me a breather," he said, "to really catch up with them. Sometimes I knew more than they did, because I was spending all my time on it. . . . Since they were still so busy with the Rad Lab, I had a lot of ideas on my own to do."[155]

On the other hand, both Purcell and Pound would come by from time to time to see how things were going in the basement of Lyman Laboratory and these occasions were also very beneficial for Bloembergen, with discussions that were, he said, "most stimulating."[156]

By the time Purcell returned to Harvard that fall to resume teaching—the first time in nearly six years—Bloembergen had made most of the changes needed in the group's NMR apparatus and was ready to begin the experimental and theoretical activity that would provide the primary substance of his thesis, most of which would be accomplished by the end of the year. Both Purcell and Pound, finally free of their responsibilities at the Radiation Laboratory and able to devote more time to the field they had introduced nearly one year earlier, were now showing up frequently in the basement of Lyman Hall, and everyone profited from the stimulating synergism that developed. In the process, Bloembergen noted, he evolved in the last three months of 1946 "from a lab assistant to a full-fledged research partner."[157]

That fall, nearly 6,000 miles east of Cambridge, Massachusetts, Artur Seyss-Inquart, the Austrian who had betrayed his own country to the Nazis and had then served Hitler as administrative butcher in Poland and Holland, was on trial for his war crimes, along with 20 other leaders of the Third Reich. The day before Hitler committed suicide, the Führer had dictated his last will and testament, calling Seyss-Inquart "honorable" and naming him Foreign Minister in the government Hitler was appointing to carry on after his death. As for the millions of deaths that had occurred on the battlefields and for Hitler's massacre of the Jews, Hitler blamed the Jews, giving them "sole responsibility."

The Nuremberg trials were an attempt by the International Military Tribunal to mete out justice, but like the "honor" bestowed by Hitler, "justice" had little meaning when it came to prosecuting the accused. "An eye for an eye" equivalence between crime and punishment was impossible to achieve considering the millions who had died at their hands. About an hour-and-a-half after midnight on October 16, 1946, Artur Seyss-Inquart was one of 10 who took his turn at mounting the gallows in Nuremberg prison. The butcher of Holland was dead.

Before "E Mail"
George E. Pake had arrived in Cambridge to begin working on his PhD in physics at about the same time that Bloembergen's Liberty ship docked in Philadelphia. Although Bloembergen and Pake arrived on the campus of Harvard only two or three days apart, they would be unaware of each other for a number of months. They would soon share, however, the distinction of being Edward Purcell's first two graduate students and of being, both figuratively and literally, on the ground floor of NMR.

The younger of the two by four years, Pake had spent the previous three-and-a-half years in much different settings than Bloembergen. When the Germans invaded Holland in May of 1940, Pake was finishing his sophomore year in high school; Bloembergen was finishing his sophomore year at the University of Utrecht. For Pake, the war would not come "home" until the middle of his senior year in high school when the Japanese bombed far-away Pearl Harbor.

In the fall of 1942, Pake entered Carnegie Institute of Technology in Pittsburgh (now called Carnegie-Mellon University) where he majored in physics, although he later withdrew to enlist in the Air Force. When he was rejected by the Air Force because of a congenital back defect, his draft board told him that if he returned to Carnegie, obtained his degree and then joined the war effort they would declare him ineligible for military service. "So that's in effect," he said, "what I did."

> I went back to Carnegie and, by that time, with the war on, the idea of taking summers off was done away with and we went to school around the calendar. Each calendar year contained three semesters, three-halves of an academic year. If you figure it out, from the fall of 1942 until the end of the spring semester in 1945 was eight semesters. And in that time I got my Bachelors degree in physics and also a Masters degree. Very intensive. Two years and eight months from high school to a Masters degree.[158]

After graduating in late April of 1945, Pake was hired at Westinghouse's research laboratories where he worked for the duration of the war on a component for an airborne radar system.

As soon as the Pacific war ended for the United States in August 1945, Pake was ready to get back to graduate school to work on his PhD. Although he was, as he recalled, "pretty broke" at the time, with the help of a fellowship from the National Research Council in Washington, DC, he was able to join the large post-war class of graduate students that showed up at Harvard in the spring of 1946.

Unlike Bloembergen, who was already credited with a couple of scientific papers when he came to Harvard, Pake was unable to get immediately involved in direct research. Within weeks of his arrival on campus, however, he did have the opportunity to hear both Edward Purcell and W.W. Hansen describe the Harvard and Stanford versions of the 1945-46 NMR experiments and was fascinated by the two discoveries.

During the summer of 1946, while taking a required laboratory course which taught techniques for conducting experiments in modern atomic physics from Professor Otto Oldenberg, Pake was asked by the chairman of the Harvard physics department if he had given any thought to the research he would do for his PhD thesis. Well, he had thought about it, but hadn't made a decision yet, although "I was very interested," he recalled, "in these hot new experiments done by Purcell."[159] He told Oldenberg that he would like to work with Purcell's research group, but was concerned that it might be such a glamourous topic that Purcell might be oversubscribed with students. Oldenberg didn't think that was the case, he told Pake, but if he was interested in working with Purcell, Pake could write to him in York, Pennsylvania, where he was visiting his in-laws.

So I did that [said Pake] and I got a letter back in a couple weeks. Purcell said he would be back soon at Harvard, that he thought this looked like a good match and that we ought to meet to discuss whether I should become his research student. We did and I did. So in the fall of '46, he assigned me to a laboratory downstairs, next to Bloembergen, and that's where I got to know Bloembergen.[160]

Through a hole in the wall was *how* Pake got to know Bloembergen. Sometime before either Bloembergen or Pake inherited their small, adjacent rooms in the basement of Lyman Hall, another researcher with a project too large for one room had found it necessary to invade the adjacent one by cutting a rectangular aperture in the wall between them. Measuring somewhere between a foot-and-a-half to two feet high by three or four feet wide, this small opening now served as Pake's window of opportunity.

Bloembergen was almost like a second professor for me [Pake said], although he was a graduate student. He was older and had a lot more experience. When I was starting out, I knew nothing about magnetic resonance and I would shout through the hole in the wall to Bloembergen who would give me tips as to how to get out of my particular dilemmas. And I really liked that, because his experimental operation was way ahead of mine.[161]

Relaxation T_1 and T_2

In early 1946, there was little time to give much thought to future applications of NMR. "We were so busy with the basic physical phenomena," said Bloembergen, "that, rightly or wrongly, we didn't worry about applications. When I arrived here, they had seen the effect and then the next question was, 'What can we do with it?' "[162]

In publishing the results of their original NMR experiment in *Physical Review*, Purcell, Torrey and Pound had identified four areas that could be further investigated using their magnetic resonance method: 1) measurement of magnetic moments for other atomic nuclei; 2) analysis of spin-lattice coupling; 3) standardization of magnetic fields; and 4) determination of the sign of magnetic moments.

Although the phrase "relaxation time" was not mentioned as an area for potential investigation, "longitudinal" spin-lattice relaxation, also known as T_1 relaxation time, was subsumed under the second area suggested—"analysis of spin-lattice coupling." In fact, it was this very question of how long it would take for nuclear spins to release energy to their environment and thereby achieve thermal equilibrium that had concerned both the Purcell and Bloch teams and which may also have been a significant shortcoming in the ill-fated 1942 attempt by Cornelis Gorter to observe nuclear magnetic resonance in a solid.

Operating on the same principles as the electron paramagnetism described by Paul Langevin in 1905, nuclear paramagnetism is influenced by the temperature of the nuclear spins. The higher the absolute temperature of a magnetic moment, the greater the thermal agitation that opposes parallel alignment with the external field. Lower the temperature, in other words, and increase the paramagnetic polarization of the sample. Raise the temperature, and decrease the polarization. Just as electron paramagnetism varies in inverse proportion to the absolute temperature of a substance (the Curie Law), so does nuclear paramagnetism, but in 1945 it wasn't known how long it would take for such nuclear paramagnetic polarization—or thermal equilibrium—to develop.

What was available in 1932 was a theoretical study by Swedish physicist Ivar Waller which predicted relaxation times for electron spins on the order of several hours. To allow for the possibility that the spin-lattice relaxation time of hydrogen nuclei might also be a matter of hours, both the Harvard and Stanford groups had gone to extra lengths in their original experiments to make sure that thermal equilibrium had been achieved prior to looking for the NMR signal. (Spin-lattice relaxation will begin to occur in a sample placed in a steady magnetic field whether a transverse radiofrequency field is present or not. Its detection, on the other hand, requires an oscillating or rotating magnetic field.) Fortunately, both the Purcell and Bloch experiments were set up in such a way that they were able to detect the NMR signal in spite of spin-lattice relaxation times that were much shorter than expected, a matter of just seconds.

Did Purcell have a specific objective that he wanted Bloembergen to work toward in early 1946? "Purcell was very noncommittal," said Bloembergen. "He had the effect. I took part in the early discussion of what to do. I said I'd rather do a study of the relaxation phenomena than measure nuclear moments and he agreed with that."

[At the time] few magnetic moments were known [said Bloembergen]. . . . We could try to search for other nuclei and that's what Bloch first did. He looked for helium-3. It was an important nucleus to know the magnetic moment of. He did find it at Los Alamos but we decided from the beginning that we were going to study the relaxation times. . . . How do these nuclear spins achieve a magnetization in a material—the so-called nuclear paramagnetism? We knew it goes inversely proportional to the temperature and that is why at low temperatures you get bigger signals in general. So that we understood. But we wanted to know the details. How long does it take for such an equilibrium to be established? That's what relaxation is all about. How long does it take for nuclear paramagnetic polarization to develop?[163]

"In the first half of 1946," wrote Bloembergen, "there was no explanation for the reasonably short values of T_1 in the samples used, and the spin-spin relaxation time T_2 was thought to correspond to a linewidth equal to the root-mean-square value of internal local field produced by neighboring nuclear spins. It was therefore natural," he stated, "for the NMR research team at Harvard to concentrate its experimental efforts on measuring these quantities."[164]

As part of the paper Bloch presented in April 1946 at the Cambridge meeting of the American Physical Society, he reported, he told science historian Charles Weiner, "about something called the relaxation time— that is, the time which it takes for these nuclei in water, for example, to realign themselves and establish equilibrium. We measured that and found it to be about two seconds. I think later measurements gave it somewhat more accurately at something like three seconds." The later measurements referred to by Bloch were done by Nicolaas Bloembergen, who determined that T_1 for water was 2.3 seconds. "I measured it right," Bloembergen said. "I shouldn't brag, but it's still 2.3 seconds."[165]

Was there competition between the Purcell team at Harvard and the Bloch team at Stanford? "Oh, there was friendly competition," said Bloembergen.

Purcell had the discussions with Bloch. I didn't. I was just a graduate student and I did my job and a lot of experiments and also a lot of theory at the same time. It was fascinating. It's quite clear that there was competition, but it was always friendly. Bloch might suggest we study this and he would study that and then Purcell wouldn't commit himself. He said, "You go your way. We'll go our way." And I think neither party begrudged the other in that.[166]

In July of 1946, Bloch submitted the theoretical explanation for his nuclear induction experiment to *Physical Review*. Published in October, the paper included what would come to be known as "the Bloch equations," a masterful set of formulations that included equations for both T_1 (spin-lattice relaxation time) and T_2 (spin-spin relaxation time).

T_1 is the measure of how fast the spins within a population *achieve* a net magnetization by aligning themselves, both with and against (or parallel to and anti-parallel to) a strong, static magnetic field. The net magnetization results from the fact that slightly more than half of the spins line up with the external static field. T_1 may be thought of therefore in two ways: 1) how long it takes for a spin population to line up with the main field and achieve thermal equilibrium after its initial placement in the field, and 2) how long it takes for a spin population to return to that equilibrium following the absorption of RF energy. The first was the concern of both the Harvard and Stanford groups when setting up their original experiments, as the experiments could not proceed until that equilibrium was reached. The second is what is most commonly meant by the term T_1.

T_2, on the other hand, is the measure of how fast a spin population *loses* its net magnetization after being stimulated by a radiofrequency field oscillating at the Larmor frequency of the spins. When that stimulation occurs, the spins not only flop from one orientation to another, they also begin precessing in synchronized formation, creating a net magnetization that is not there when they are precessing out-of-phase with one another. It is as though they were under the influence of a performer spinning tops at a carnival who not only keeps all the tops spinning simultaneously, but is able to make them gyrate or precess in perfect unison. An imperfect analogue of T_2 is the time it would take for the gyrating tops to get out of phase with one another if the performer were to stop paying attention to his perfectly synchronized set of gyrating tops and walk away. In the case of nuclear spins, this decay in synchronism and the resultant loss in net magnetism stems from the fact that each spin is a magnet and eventually their multiple magnetic interactions overcome the synchronized unity of the spins. Other components are also opposing the in-phase unity of the spins, including inhomogeneities within the static field and zero-frequency components lying along the axis of the static field.

Both signal measurements—the T_1 recovery of net magnetization and the T_2 loss of net magnetization—are important contributors to the science of NMR and, because of the understanding that he would provide about these relaxation mechanisms, Nicolaas Bloembergen would likewise contribute greatly to the science of NMR.

Motional Narrowing

Not long after Purcell and Pound returned to Harvard on a full-time basis, Bloembergen mentioned to Pound one day that the NMR signal appeared to change in magnitude after the probe was reinserted into the magnet gap. As Pound began to systematically move the probe around in the gap, they discovered that the narrowest resonance with the largest peak signal was not at the center of the gap where one might assume it to be, but rather near the edge of a pole piece. The reason? Inhomogeneities in the magnet material of the pole caps. At the so-called "sweet spot" of minimum inhomogeneity in the main field, the minimum line width in water and other fluid samples was about 0.14 gauss while the resonance in their calium fluoride (CaF_2) sample remained broad. As a result of this finding, Purcell, Bloembergen and Pound decided that they would find the true resonance width of calcium fluoride, also called fluorite.

> We realized [noted Bloembergen] that this width would be a minimum when the magnetic field was pointed along the body diagonal of the cubic lattice. In this orientation, the nearest neighbors would not contribute a static local field component parallel to the external field. It is the magic angle δ between the body diagonal and the cubic axis. I spent a few days cutting a cylinder with its axis along a face diagonal out of a natural CaF_2 crystal. This cylindrical sample could be rotated inside the RF coil. Our observed line widths were in agreement with a formula for the second moment of internal dipolar fields derived by [Professor John H.] Van Vleck. Purcell spent hours on a Marchant mechanical calculator to evaluate the dipolar lattice sums for a cubic lattice. This resulted in a joint publication[167] with Purcell and Pound.[168]

In sharp contrast to the broad resonance lines of crystals like CaF_2 were the narrow resonance lines of fluids. Because of the magnetic field inhomogeneity with which the Harvard team was saddled, they knew it was impossible to measure the true line widths associated with these fluids but that they could measure their T_1 relaxation times.

They quickly recognized, however, that fluidic motion tended to "average out" variations in the local magnetic fields associated with neighboring nuclei and very soon the term "motional narrowing" was coined. Had someone poked their head in the door as Bloembergen, Purcell and Pound discussed the concept, they may have felt they had cause for concern. Standing in close proximity to one another, the three scientists would have appeared to be performing some kind of finger puppetry without puppets. Actually, said Bloembergen, they were moving their index fingers through space relative to one another in order to better visualize the time dependence of dipolar interactions. It was all serious scientific work. "The variations of the local field with time," Bloembergen pointed out, "were the important clue to magnetic relaxation problems."[169]

Another experiment performed that fall, conceived by Purcell and Pound but conducted in collaboration with Bloembergen,[170] used hydrogen gas to observe the effect of increased pressure. At room temperature, with the RF coil contained inside a small brass cylinder filled with tank hydrogen, the pressure of the gas was varied between 10 atmospheres and 30 atmospheres. Whereas the width of the line appeared unaffected by pressure—a factor difficult to measure because of the field inhomogeneity—the T_1 relaxation time, they found, was directly proportional to the gas pressure.

Referring to the 1939 molecular-beam experiment performed with H_2 by Norman Ramsey in which six proton resonance peaks were observed over a 90-gauss-wide region, Purcell, Pound and Bloembergen noted that their single-peak observation of tank hydrogen resulted from molecular collisions, to which the hydrogen molecules observed by Ramsey et al. in 1939 were largely immune because of the isolating effects of the evacuated molecular-beam chamber. Colliding with one another with greater frequency than the radiofrequency used in the experiment, the local nuclear fields in the Purcell experiment were fluctuating rapidly and very nearly averaging out.

Although the inhomogeneity prohibited direct observation of the true line width, the term "pressure narrowing" was introduced as a result of the experiment, a phenomenon that contrasts sharply, said Bloembergen, with the "pressure broadening" that occurs in optical spectroscopy.

"The process described," the team concluded in their letter to the editor of *Physical Review*, "is a potent one for thermal relaxation. It should lead to a relaxation time proportional to the pressure. We have measured the relaxation time by observing the onset of saturation as the r-f voltage is increased and find that the relaxation time [T_1] does in fact increase with increasing pressure, and in a proportional manner within the accuracy of our measurement, which is not great. . . . We suggest that a related process may be important in liquids."[171]

By now, Bloembergen was thoroughly immersed in collecting the data he would later report and explain in his PhD thesis and he was concentrating his attention on the time-dependent local field in liquids. "Fortunately," he stated, "I had followed a seminar on Brownian motion and noise given by J.M.W. Milatz in 1942 at Utrecht. I had written the lecture notes for it which had been distributed in mimeographed form. I was therefore familiar with the concept of power spectral densities of random variables."[172] A book by Peter Debye, *Polar Molecules,* recommended to Bloembergen by Purcell, also proved to be of great help with its explanation of random rotation of electric dipole moments which causes dielectric relaxation in polar liquids.

That fall, Bloembergen worked out the spectral density of the various terms in the dipole-dipole interaction between two proton spins caused by the random rotation of a water molecule. He also calculated, for spins in various molecules, the contributions of translational Brownian motion to local field spectral density. Realizing that the Fourier components in the local field at the Larmor frequency and at twice the Larmor frequency were responsible for the longitudinal relaxation process, Bloembergen determined T_1 theoretically. In particular, he recalled developing explicit equations for T_1 in water between Christmas 1946 and New Year's Day 1947. Prevented from going to the laboratory by a bad cold, he came up with the equations in the eerie quietness of his dormitory room while other students spent the holidays with their families.

Bloembergen also determined that the transverse relaxation process, T_2, also had a contribution from Fourier components near zero frequency, and that the motional narrowing phenomenon associated with liquids commences when the spectral density of the local field has a correlation time shorter than T_2.

All of these insights were theoretical. Their validity could only be tested by actually measuring the relaxation rates of fluid samples which varied in viscosity. "I prepared scores of samples," Bloembergen noted, "with hydrocarbons from light to heavy oils, water-glycerin mixtures, and measured their viscosities." His experimental measurement of T_1 in the samples agreed "nicely," he said, with the theories he had developed.[173]

In 1947, the annual meeting of the American Physical Society was slated to be held in January at New York City's Columbia University and Edward Purcell decided that the presentation of his team's work on NMR relaxation in liquids should be given by Nicolaas Bloembergen.

> My mandate was to get the essential ideas of T_1 in fluids across in only 10 minutes. Thanks to a rehearsal at Harvard before a critical audience consisting solely of Purcell and Pound, I was able to finish the presentation in accented English before a packed audience at Columbia University a few seconds before the chairman's bell rang.[174]

An abstract of the presentation was published soon afterward in *Physical Review*.

Bloembergen spent the spring of that year in rounding out the experimental data for his thesis. To confirm, for example, the dependence of T_1 on what he termed the correlation time of fluid motion, he compared the relaxation findings for glycerin over a wide temperature range. To maintain the sample at the required low temperature long enough to take his readings, he designed his own mini-refrigeration system.

> I soldered some copper tubing around the brass pipe containing the RF coil. I put a can filled with acetone and dry ice above the magnet gap. I started siphoning action by sucking some cold acetone which then dripped into another can below the magnet gap. The temperature of the sample was monitored with a thermocouple. Thus the smell of acetone was added to the acrid smell from the overnight battery recharging process in the basement room of Lyman Laboratory. Environmental regulations did not impede the pace of progress in NMR research in early 1947.[175]

Bloembergen also made further modifications to the team's NMR apparatus, including a way to display on an oscilloscope the inhomogeneous broadening of the line width in water.

> I turned off the current in the modulation coils. The RF field would then saturate the protons in that part of the sample where the resonance condition was satisfied. I next turned up the modulation cur-

rent to a large value so as to sweep through the whole resonance broadened by the field inhomogeneity. This resonance showed the saturation dip. I called it "eating a hole out of the inhomogeneous distribution." The dip filled up in a time of a few seconds. I was so excited by this observation, made during Thanksgiving weekend 1946, that I immediately called Purcell at his home. A few days later, we filmed the disappearance of the "hole" with an 8 mm movie camera and determined that T_1 equals 2.3 seconds in water. Of course, we also checked that the resonance in CaF_2 was homogeneously saturated and showed no dip.[176]

From the beginning, the Purcell team had been less-than-satisfied with the reliability of their bridge circuits. "Purcell had been very active in trying to design various ways to make that bridge," George Pake recalled. "Then Bloembergen took over a particular form of what was designed," he said, "and improved upon it. And I built something that was based on Bloembergen's concept."[177]

To extend his T_1 measurements to a lower frequency, Bloembergen built in the spring of 1947 an RF bridge circuit operating at 4.8 MHz which enabled him to verify the dependence of T_1 with regard to both frequency and the correlation time of fluid motion.

The lower frequency also permitted the detection of magnetic resonance in deuterium's deuteron. In the process of observing magnetic resonance in the deuteron, Bloembergen detected for the first time in condensed matter what Rabi, Ramsey, Kellogg and Zacharias had detected for the first time in molecular beams—the nuclear quadrupole of the deuteron.

> In a 50-50 mixture of light and heavy water, I found the relaxation time of D [the deuteron] to be much shorter than that of H [the proton]. I realized that the explanation should be found in terms of a time-dependent quadrupolar interaction, and I subsequently calculated the spectral density of the electric field gradient explicitly. This observation of the relaxation time in heavy water is an early manifestation of a nuclear quadrupole interaction in condensed matter.[178]

With the arrival of 1947, the visits of Purcell and Pound to the basement laboratories of Bloembergen and Pake became less and less frequent. Pound had shifted his attention to the study of nuclear quadrupole interactions in crystals and Purcell was busy not only with teaching, but also with mentoring other graduate students who had arrived in the spring of 1946 and who were now ready to start their research projects.

Before moving on to those other projects, however, Purcell had designed a new magnet—a permanent magnet with a field of about 6000 oersted and a gap of approximately 2 centimeters which would be used by George Pake to study the line shape of NMR in a gypsum crystal. In April of 1947, Bloembergen and Pake temporarily moved the permanent magnet to the Physics Lecture Hall to give a public demonstration of NMR at the Harvard Physics Colloquium where Bloembergen had been invited to speak. "By this time," said Bloembergen, "the experimental work for my thesis was essentially complete."[179]

With his research completed and most of his thesis completed, Bloembergen could have finished the PhD process at Harvard. To do so, however, would have required the time and money associated with passing Harvard's qualifying examinations, a waste as far as Bloembergen was concerned since he had already completed the equivalent exams at Utrecht four years earlier. It was thus very timely that Professor C.J. Gorter of the University of Leiden was scheduled as a guest lecturer at Harvard for the summer of 1947.

Gorter taught paramagnetic relaxation that summer, based largely on the book he had written during the last years of the war. Bloembergen had never met Gorter before, but when Bloembergen explained his degree status and told him that he wanted to submit his PhD thesis with Gorter back in Holland, "Gorter was enthusiastic," said Bloembergen, "and immediately offered me a research position at the Kamerlingh Onnes Laboratorium in Leiden."[180] He would start in September.

> Purcell was quite understanding [said Bloembergen] and agreed to this arrangement. He and Van Vleck, who was then chairman of the Physics Department, were however interested in my eventual return to Harvard. They arranged for me to be interviewed by the Senior Fellows of the Society of Fellows before my departure. I was to hear in 1948 in the Netherlands about the outcome of this interview.[181]

In the months that remained before his return to Holland, Bloembergen completed the rough draft of his thesis, which he discussed with both Gorter and Purcell. Purcell then retained a copy of Bloembergen's handwritten notes to serve as the basis for a comprehensive paper the three of them—Bloembergen, Purcell and Pound—were planning to submit to

Physical Review. The paper would become the oft-cited BPP. Because so many physicists have referred to it so frequently over the years, the paper is a Citation Classic, ranking among the top 10 physics papers in the Science Citation Index during the period 1945-1988.

When a report on related work by B.V. Rollin and others at Oxford University appeared in *Nature* closely paralleling that of Bloembergen, the three Harvard researchers decided to also submit a condensed version of their research on nuclear magnetic relaxation to the same journal. It was published as a note in *Nature*[182] in 1947.

Back to Holland

Although Oxford University's Clarendon Laboratory in England had now become involved in nuclear magnetic resonance, study of the phenomenon had not yet crossed the English Channel to the European continent. "Gorter and I were both keen," said Bloembergen, "on introducing NMR techniques to the Continent and extend the relaxation investigation to liquid helium temperatures. We decided that we could make a quick start by duplicating the Harvard setup."[183]

Before boarding the ocean liner, therefore, Professor Gorter and his new associate visited the local Radio Shack outlet in Boston and bought all the electronic equipment and components they would need. They didn't need to worry about constructing magnets as the Kamerlingh Onnes Laboratory was well equipped with good electromagnets and cryostats. At Leiden, Bloembergen would also not need to concern himself with playing the dual role of physicist and machinist.

> The machine shops there were supervised by highly professional master technicians and instrument makers. It was not appreciated, or even permitted, for scientists to do an amateurish job, as I had done at Harvard. If one went through the established channels, however, beautiful gadgets were delivered on a surprisingly fast schedule. The liquefaction of hydrogen and helium was entirely in the hands of the technicians and no mortal scientist was allowed to touch a helium dewar. Liquid helium was only available on Thursdays and my low-temperature experiments had to be scheduled well in advance.[184]

Within one month of Bloembergen's return to Holland, he had his NMR apparatus set up and operating. "Gorter left me an awful lot of freedom," he said. "He was director of the whole lab and didn't have so much time for all of these details."[185]

After concentrating on liquids with their "motional narrowing" for his thesis, Bloembergen was ready to learn about the relaxation details of solids that didn't exhibit large-scale atomic motion. He knew about Swedish physicist Ivar Waller's work published in 1932 which predicted extremely long relaxation times with regard to the interaction of nuclear spins with phonons. It was the same paper, in fact, which had been used as the basis for the Purcell team's 1945 expectation that it might take several hours to achieve thermal equilibrium in their sample, even though they recognized that Waller's investigation of the interaction between electron spins and lattice vibrations was somewhat of an 'apples and oranges' situation when compared with nuclear interactions. By calculating the change in local fields produced by the classical motion of vibrating atoms, Bloembergen found that his results agreed with Waller's.

Clearly [Bloembergen noted], paramagnetic impurities might play a role. They would have to produce local fields at the nuclear Larmor precession frequency and it occurred to me that the z-component of the electron spin might produce such Fourier components as it executed random transitions through the interaction with lattice vibrations in the paramagnetic relaxation process.[186]

To quantitatively test his hypothesis about paramagnetic impurities, Bloembergen grew a series of potassium aluminum crystallites which he doped with varying concentrations of iron ions [Fe+++] ranging from a few parts per million to a few percent. By measuring the relaxation time of these samples at temperatures ranging from that of liquid helium to room temperature, Bloembergen was able to confirm the influence of paramagnetic impurities on nuclear spin relaxation time, even at concentrations as low as a few parts per million. At such low concentrations, of course, Bloembergen knew that the relative distance from most spins to an impurity were great, seemingly too great to account for the rapid relaxation the impurity induced. This difficulty was resolved with the introduction of a concept called "spin diffusion."[187]

The relaxation pathway [Bloembergen explained] is as follows: The z component of the electron spin of the impurity, undergoing random flips by an electron spin-lattice relaxation mechanism causes flips of nuclear spins in its vicinity. Nuclear spins farther away from the paramagnetic impurity can relax by means of a process called spin diffusion, which consists of mutual nuclear spin flip-flops that can transport Zeeman energy to the vicinity of the impurity.[188]

A 1936 theory by Walter Heitler and Edward Teller regarding the effect of conduction electrons on nuclear spin relaxation in metals predicted reasonably short T_1 relaxation times. Bloembergen tested this by measuring the relaxation times of copper powder particles embedded in paraffin. His experimental results agreed with the Heitler-Teller model.[189]

In 1948, Bloembergen obtained what may well have been the first experimental evidence of a chemical shift. To test his hypothesis that fast electron spin exchange, in a way similar to fast electron spin-lattice relaxation, would prevent excessive broadening of a nuclear spin resonance curve, Bloembergen performed a radiofrequency spectroscopy analysis of a $CuSO_4 \cdot 5H_2O$ crystal he had grown. At room temperature, the proton resonance of the crystal was readily observable, its width primarily determined by the local fields of other protons. When the crystal was cooled down to 20° K, however, the line broadened and assumed a complicated pattern. Cooled still further, down to liquid helium temperatures, the pattern split into 10 well-defined lines which extended over a 400-gauss range and corresponded to a variation of over seven percent.

The 10 resonance curves each corresponded to one of 10 distinctive proton positions in the unit cell, each with a different time-averaged local field produced by the average magnetizations of the copper ions. "These paramagnetic shifts are large," noted Bloembergen, "but they attracted much less attention than the Knight shift in metals [noted in 1949], caused by the temperature-independent paramagnetism of conduction electrons."[190] The following year, Norman Ramsey of Harvard published the first in a series of articles that would provide the theoretical explanation of chemical shifts.

Ramsey wasn't aware of Bloembergen's priority in chemical shift experiments until 1993. "I had to tell him just in the last year," said Bloembergen. "I said, 'Norman, you have all these shifts, but I really had a very big chemical shift independently, just before the other ones, which people aren't aware of.' I was a little earlier [than Knight],"[191] Bloembergen explained.

Later, before returning to the United States in 1949, Bloembergen submitted a 10-minute paper on his chemical-shift findings which he planned to present at the January 1949 meeting of the American Physical Society. "I was anxious to publish this work and get it known," said Bloembergen, "but I couldn't deliver the paper because I was delayed in

Isidor I. Rabi (1898 - 1988)

"The tradition of science teaches us that no vested interests in institutions or systems of thought should escape continual reexamination merely because they have existed and have been successful. On the other hand, it also teaches us to conserve what is operative and useful. Science teaches us self-discipline. One must continually look for the mote in one's own eye. The history of science shows that it is always there. The help of others in this search is not to be despised."

—I.I. RABI

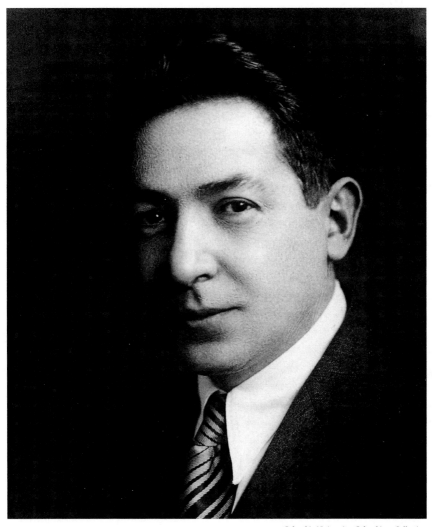

—*Columbia University, Columbiana Collection*

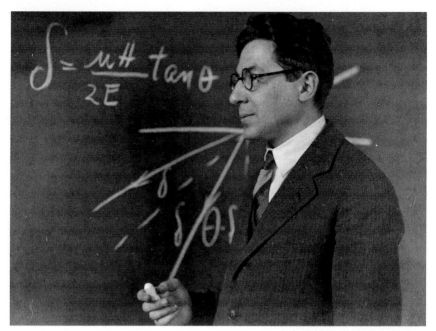

I.I. Rabi began his career as a lecturer in Columbia University's physics department in the fall of 1929 at the age of 31. His association with Columbia would span nearly 60 years.

—*AIP Emilio Segrè Visual Archives*

UPPER RIGHT:
Rabi's molecular-beam apparatus, 1938.
—*Research Corp. photo,
AIP Emilio Segrè Visual Archives*

LOWER RIGHT:
Magnet for Rabi's molecular-beam apparatus, 1937. Typewritten caption provided with photo reads: "This magnet is 20 inches long and is wound with four turns of heavy copper (water cooling). With the orthodox design, a magnet equally effective would weigh several tons. The entire magnet is inside the vacuum system."
—*Research Corp. photo,
AIP Emilio Segrè Visual Archives*

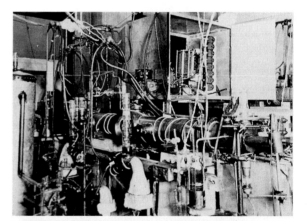

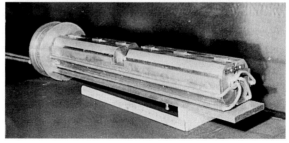

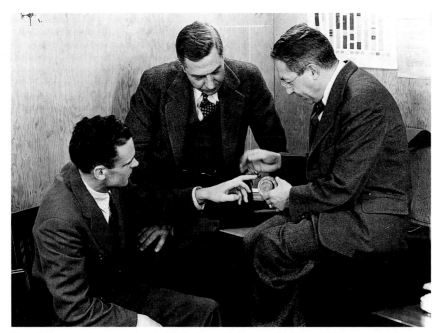

Examining a cavity magnetron in 1943, similar to the one first brought from England to the United States by the Tizard Mission in 1940, are: E.G. "Taffy" Bowen, British liaison to the MIT Radiation Laboratory; Lee DuBridge, director of the "Rad Lab;" and I.I. Rabi, who became associate director of the World War II radar research and development facility.

—*The MIT Museum*

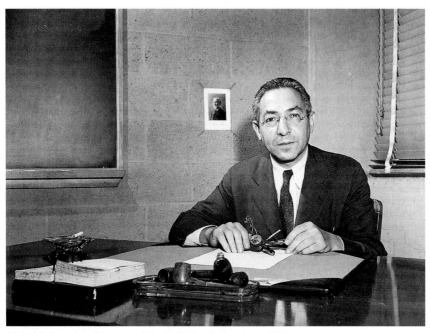

I.I. Rabi, Associate Director of the Radiation Laboratory, 1945. —*The MIT Museum*

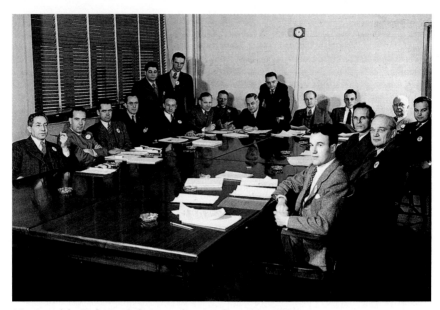

Meeting of the Radiation Laboratory Steering Committee, 1944.
Seated from left to right: I.I. Rabi, E.C. Pollard, T.W. Bonner, J.W. Hinckley, R.G. Herb, L.C. Marshall, L.N. Ridenour, L.A. DuBridge, J. Trump, D. Ewing, C. Turner, I. Getting, J. Lawson, F. Loomis, B. Chance. *Standing:* J. Zacharias, L. Haworth, D. White in attendance for H. Gaither. *Absent:* J.R. Killian, Jr., J. Street, L. Turner, and M. White.

—*The MIT Museum*

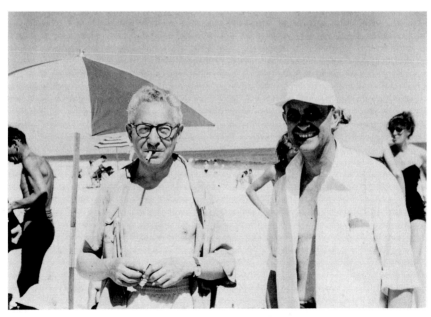

I.I. Rabi and Enrico Fermi around 1950. Fermi, 1938 Nobel laureate in physics and the first to demonstrate a self-sustaining nuclear chain reaction, died of cancer in 1954.

—*AIP Emilio Segrè Visual Archives, Bainbridge Collection*

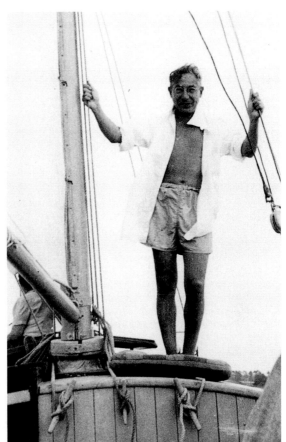

RIGHT: Photo of I.I. Rabi
taken about 1947.
—*AIP Emilio Segrè Visual Archives,*
Bainbridge Collection

BELOW: Niels Bohr, James
Franck, Albert Einstein and
I.I. Rabi around 1952.
—*AIP Emilio Segrè Visual Archives,*
Margrethe Bohr Collection

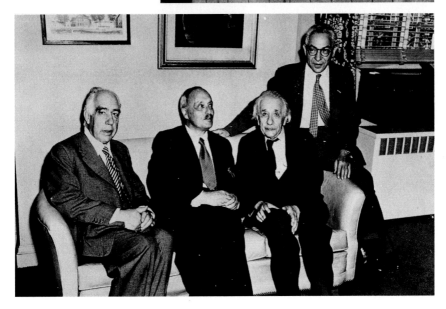

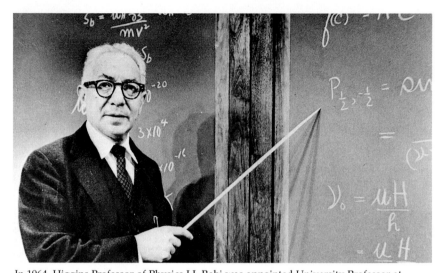

In 1964, Higgins Professor of Physics I.I. Rabi was appointed University Professor at Columbia, the first to be given that title in the University's 210-year history. Upon his retirement in 1967, he was named University Professor Emeritus. In 1979, a Rabi Visiting Professorship was established, funded by the Sloan Foundation. In 1985, the Isidor Isaac Rabi Chair in Physics was established. Funded by David and Rosalie Rose, the chair is presently held by Nobel laureate Melvin Schwartz. *—Columbia University, Columbiana Collection*

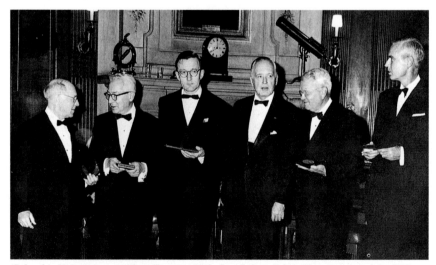

Columbia University president Grayson Kirk, fourth from left, with recipients of the 1961 Alexander Hamilton Award given by Columbia's Alumni Association for distinguished service in any field of human endeavor. *From left to right:* **Edward C. Kendall,** one of three recipients of the 1950 Nobel Prize in physiology/medicine for discoveries of cortisone and ACTH; **I.I. Rabi,** 1944 Nobel laureate in physics for discovery of magnetic resonance in molecular beams; **Polykarp Kusch,** 1955 Nobel laureate in physics for determining the magnetic moment of the electron; **Grayson Kirk,** president of Columbia University from 1953 to 1968; **Harold C. Urey,** recipient of the 1934 Nobel Prize in chemistry for his discovery of deuterium (heavy hydrogen); and **Willis Lamb,** 1955 Nobel laureate in physics for discoveries on the structure of the hydrogen spectrum.*—Columbia University, Columbiana Collection*

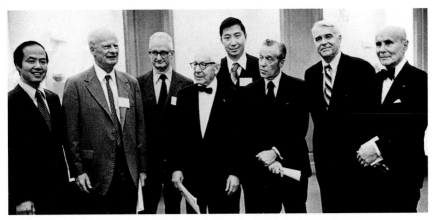

Columbia University president William J. McGill, second from right, with seven Nobel laureates present at the 50th anniversary of Columbia University's Pupin Physics Laboratories on November 4, 1977. *From left to right:* **Tsung Dao Lee,** co-winner with Chen Ning Yang of the 1957 Nobel Prize in physics for disproving the law of conservation of parity; **Hans Bethe,** recipient of the 1967 physics prize for his contributions to the theory of nuclear reactions, especially his discoveries on the energy production in stars; **James Rainwater,** co-recipient of the 1975 Nobel in physics with Aage Bohr and Ben Mottelson of Denmark for their work on the structure of the atomic nucleus; **I.I. Rabi,** 1944 Nobel physics laureate for recording the magnetic properties of atomic nuclei; **Samuel Chao Chung Ting,** co-recipient with Burton Richter of the 1976 Nobel physics prize for their discovery of an elementary nuclear particle called the *psi,* or *J,* particle; **Julian Schwinger,** co-recipient with Sin-itiro Tomonaga (Japan) and Richard Feynman (U.S.) of the 1965 Nobel Prize in physics for basic work in quantum electrodynamics; **President McGill; André Cournand,** co-recipient with Dickenson Richards, also of Columbia, and Werner Forssmann (Germany) of the 1956 Nobel Prize for physiology and medicine for using a catheter to chart the interior of the heart. *—Columbia University, Columbiana Collection*

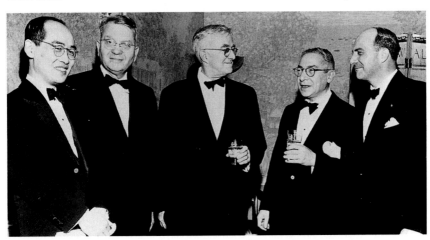

I.I. Rabi, fourth from left, with **Hideki Yukawa** of Japan, recipient of 1949 Nobel Prize in physics for his discovery of the meson; **Harold C. Urey,** 1934 Nobel laureate in chemistry for discovery of deuterium; **Irving Langmuir,** 1932 Nobel laureate in chemistry for discoveries in surface chemistry; and **John Dunning,** dean of Columbia University's School of Engineering and Applied Science from 1950 to 1969. *—Columbia University, Columbiana Collection*

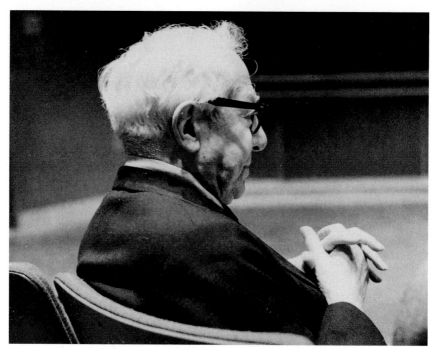

I.I. Rabi, elder statesman of physics and articulate advocate for control of nuclear energy, at Harvard University in 1976 at the age of 78. Rabi once said that "science is a great game. It is inspiring and refreshing. The playing field is the universe itself." Science, he said, should be taught in relation to the great personalities who have affected it and it bothered him, it was reported in the *New York Times*, that, while political history is recorded "blow by blow," there are "no really great historians" of science who present its history in jargonless prose. Even minor literary figures, he pointed out, are the subjects of volumes of biography while the scientist remains "an invisible man."

—*John H. Martin photo, AIP Emilio Segrè Visual Archives*

Norman F. Ramsey (1915 -   )

"A large part of my life has been spent doing research, mostly in collaboration with graduate students. My association with the students has been close and friendly. At any one period of time, if I were asked to name my 20 closest and best friends, about 10 of them would have been my then current graduate students. Our relations were much more those of joint collaborators than of professor and student."

—NORMAN F. RAMSEY

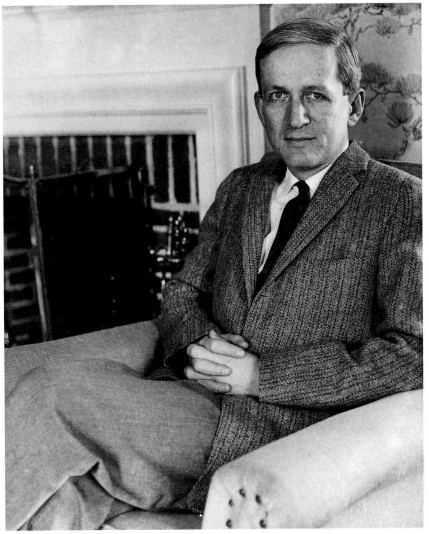

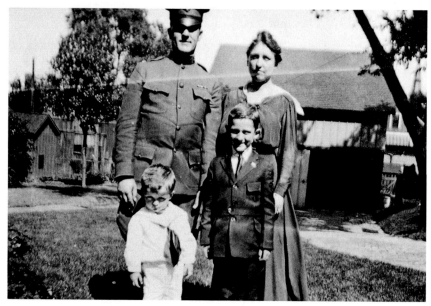

A West Point graduate and a general in the Army Ordnance Corps, Norman Ramsey, Sr. frequently changed assignments. Norman Ramsey, Jr. was born in Washington, DC. By the time he began college, Army duties had taken the Ramseys to Topeka, Kansas, to Paris, France, to Picatinny Arsenal near Dover, New Jersey, to Fort Leavenworth, Kansas, and to Governor's Island in New York City harbor. Mrs. Ramsey, the former Minna Bauer, was once a mathematics instructor at the University of Kansas. In the above photo, taken in Topeka, Kansas, Norman Ramsey, Jr. is on the left next to his older brother, John.

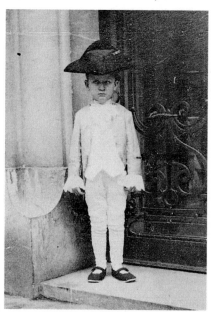

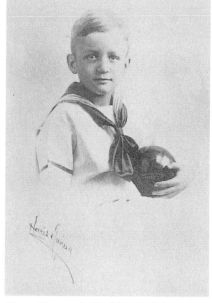

Norman Ramsey, Jr. at a 1920 Washington birthday party at the U.S. Embassy in Paris.

Young Norman in Washington, DC in 1921.

RIGHT: Norman and Elinor Ramsey in New Hampshire in 1941. A year earlier, shortly after Ramsey and Elinor Jameson of Brooklyn, New York were married, the couple had moved to Urbana, Illinois where Ramsey had been hired as a member of the physics faculty at the University of Illinois. They moved back East to Cambridge, Massachusetts only weeks later, however, after Dr. Ramsey was recruited to help in radar development at the MIT Radiation Laboratory.

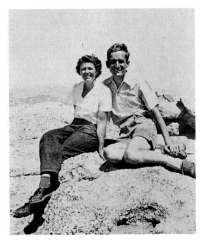

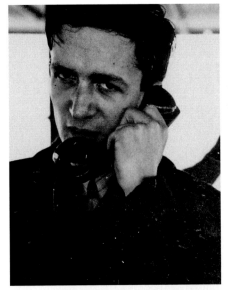

LEFT: Ramsey supervising ballistics testing of various atomic bomb designs at Muroc Dry Lake, California. After playing a key role in the development of 3-centimeter radar at the Rad Lab, followed by a one-and-a-half year stint as Expert Consultant to Secretary of War Henry Stimson, Ramsey was recruited for the Manhattan Project by J. Robert Oppenheimer. At Los Alamos, Ramsey was head of the Delivery Group, the group responsible for delivery of the Project's atom bombs to their targets.

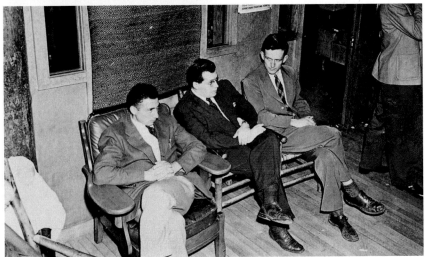

Physicists Bernard Feld, Julian Schwinger and Norman Ramsey at Los Alamos in 1944.

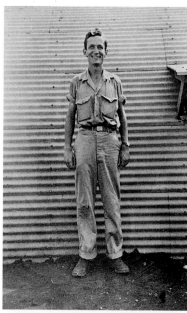

LEFT: The day after the world's first atomic bomb explosion at the Trinity test site near Alamogordo, New Mexico, Ramsey left for Tinian Island in the Pacific where, as chief scientist of the Delivery Group, he oversaw final assembly of the two atomic bombs that would suddenly end the war in the Pacific.

BELOW: Ramsey with a molecular beam apparatus at Harvard in 1952. After the war, Ramsey returned to the East Coast where he was on the physics faculty of Columbia University. During this period, as head of the Ramsey Panel, he played a key role in the founding of Brookhaven National Laboratory on Long Island, serving as the head of its physics department while on the faculty at Columbia. In 1947, he accepted an invitation to join the physics faculty at Harvard University where he took charge of developing that school's first molecular beam laboratory.

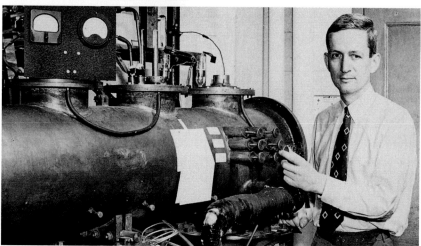

RIGHT: Luis Alvarez, a collaborator with Felix Bloch in measuring the magnetic moment of the neutron and a Nobel laureate in physics (1968) for his contributions to the knowledge of subatomic particles, confers with Norman Ramsey during a meeting at Oxford University in 1954.

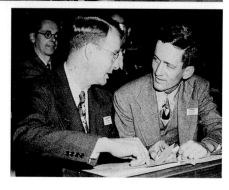

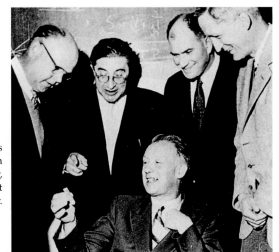

At Heidelberg in 1958, Hans Kopfermann (seated) with, from left to right, Ralph H. Fowler, George Placzek, Otto Robert Frisch and Norman Ramsey.

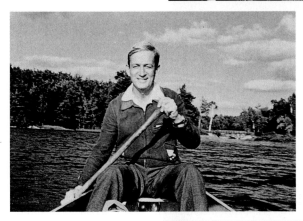

Norman Ramsey on Mystic Lake near Winchester, Massachusetts in 1957.

S. Cramton, Norman Ramsey and Daniel Kleppner examine an atomic hydrogen maser at Harvard in 1966.

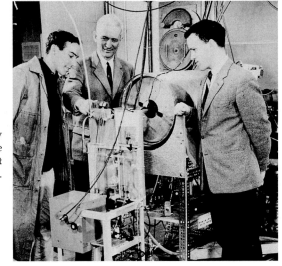

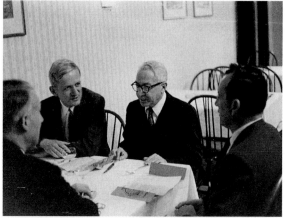

LEFT: Hans Kopfermann,
Norman Ramsey, I.I. Rabi
and William Nierenberg.
*—AIP Emilio Segrè Visual Archives,
V.W. Cohen Collection*

BELOW: Ramsey with
students at Harvard, 1971.

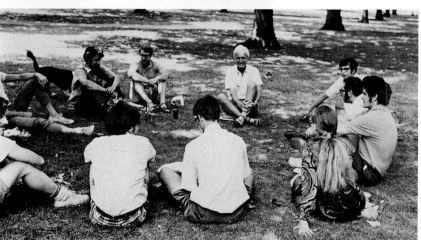

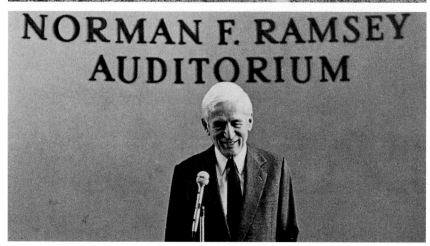

Norman F. Ramsey at the 1984 dedication of the auditorium named in his honor at Fermi
National Accelerator Laboratory, otherwise known as Fermilab, in Batavia, Illinois.

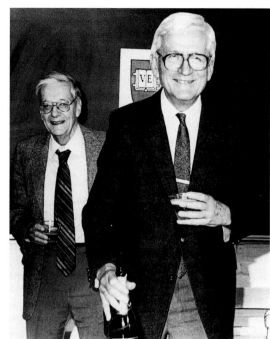

Nicolaas Bloembergen, 1981 Nobel laureate in physics, helping Ramsey celebrate his selection as a 1989 recipient of the Prize.

—Harvard University photo, AIP Emilio Segrè Visual Archives

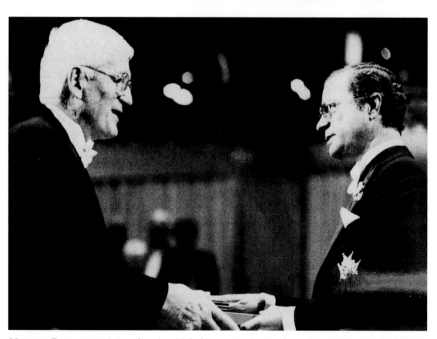

Norman Ramsey receiving the 1989 Nobel Prize in physics from Sweden's King Carl XVI Gustaf for work that led to the atomic clock. Also receiving the Nobel Prize in physics in 1989 were Hans G. Dehmelt (U.S.) and Wolfgang Paul (Germany) for isolating and measuring single atoms.

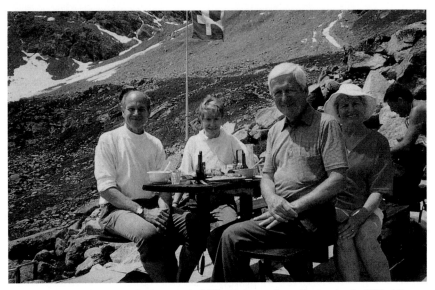

Jim and Annette Cronin with Norman and Ellie Ramsey above Pontresina in 1991. After Ramsey's first wife died in 1983, he married Ellie Welch of Brookline, Massachusetts. James Cronin and Val Fitch (U.S.) shared the 1980 Nobel Prize in physics for their research on subatomic particles revealing that a fundamental law of symmetry in nature (time reversal) could be violated.

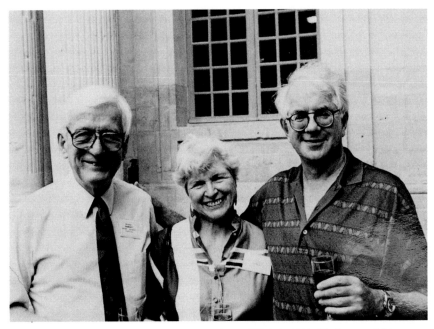

Norman and Ellie Ramsey with Sheldon Glashow at Blois in 1992. Glashow and Steven Weinberg (U.S.) together with Abdus Salam (Pakistan) were awarded the 1979 Nobel Prize in physics for developing a principle that unifies the weak nuclear force and the force of electromagnetism.

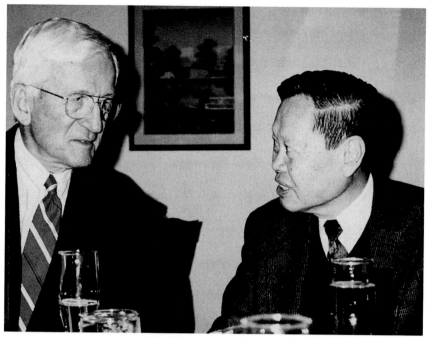

Norman Ramsey and Chen Ning Yang at the State University of New York at Stony Brook in 1993. Yang and Tsung Dao Lee, in photo below, were awarded the 1957 Nobel Prize in physics for disproving the law of conservation of parity.

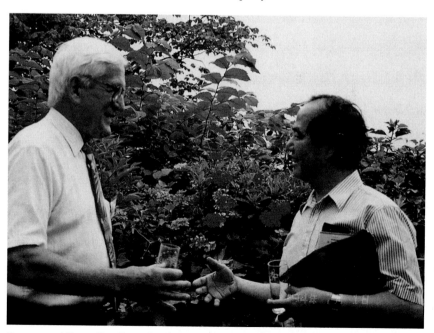

Ramsey and Tsung Dao Lee at Lindau in 1994. (See caption above.)

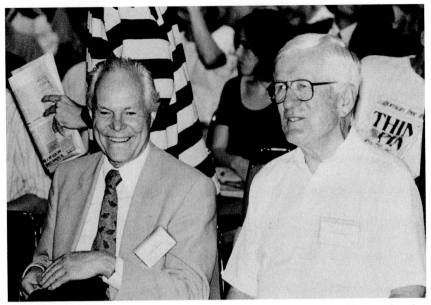

Rudolph Mössbauer and Norman Ramsey at Lindau in 1994. Mössbauer (Germany) and Robert Hofstadter (U.S.) shared the 1961 Nobel Prize in physics, Mössbauer for his research on gamma rays, Hofstadter for his studies of nucleons.

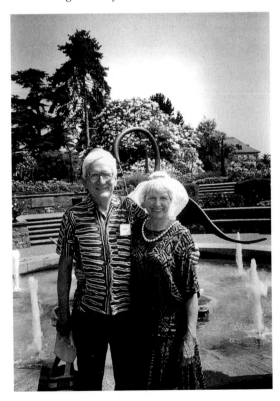

Norman and Ellie Ramsey at Minau Island, Germany in 1995. The Ramseys have a combined family of seven children and a growing group of grandchildren.

Edward M. Purcell (1912 -   )

"To tackle the problem of delineating a space program, as requested by the president, I appointed a panel of PSAC members consisting of General Doolittle, Edwin Land, Herbert York, and Edward Purcell, with Purcell, the gifted Harvard physicist and Nobel laureate, serving as chairman. In this role Purcell made a lasting contribution to the U.S. space program, and he won the confidence and admiration of the president. . . . Robert Kreidler . . . spoke almost with awe of [Purcell's] impact on PSAC. 'Ed Purcell did not speak often,' he said, 'but when he did, there would be enormous silence in the room because everybody knew that whatever he said was going to be worth listening to with careful attention.' "

—JAMES R. KILLIAN, JR.
Chairman, President's Science Advisory Committee
under President Dwight D. Eisenhower

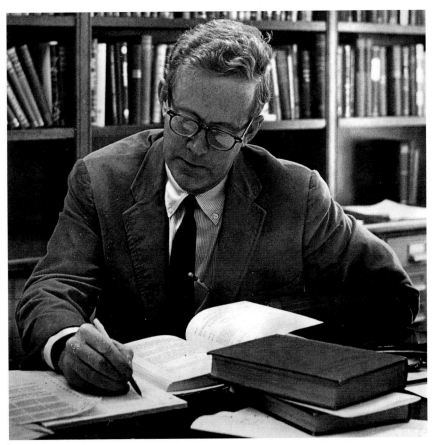

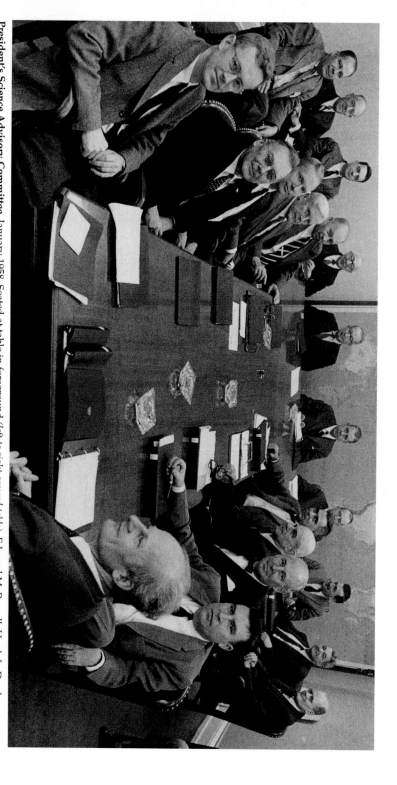

President's Science Advisory Committee, January 1958. Seated at table in foreground (*left to right around table*): Edward M. Purcell, Hugh L. Dryden, William O. Baker, Alan T. Waterman, George B. Kistiakowsky, Emanuel R. Piore, Gen. James H. Doolittle, Lloyd V. Berkner, Herbert F. York and Hans A. Bethe. Seated at table at the rear of the room (*left to right*): Albert G. Hill, Detlev W. Bronk, Edwin H. Land, I.I. Rabi, Robert F. Bacher, J.R. Killian, Jr., James B. Fisk, Jerome B. Wiesner, Jerrold R. Zacharias and Caryl P. Haskins.

—*Life Photo by Paul Schutzer*

RIGHT: In late 1940, at the age of 28, Purcell, then a physics instructor at Harvard University, was recruited by the MIT Radiation Laboratory to help in the development of radar. After Norman Ramsey, the first leader of the Fundamental Development Group, left for Washington, DC in 1942, Purcell became the head of that group, which was part of Division 4, Rabi's Research Division. Twice a week, Julian Schwinger, who was in the Theory Group, would come in and lecture on his latest findings, after which, said I.I. Rabi, people like Edward Purcell and Robert Dicke, who was also in Purcell's group, "would invent things like mad."

—*Photo, AIP Meggers Gallery of Nobel Laureates*

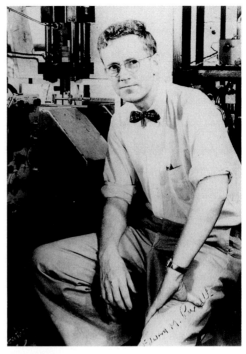

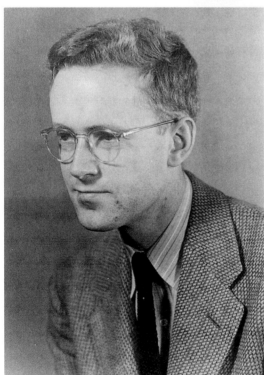

LEFT: Edward Purcell at the time he was the leader of Group 41 at the MIT Rad Lab.

—*The MIT Museum*

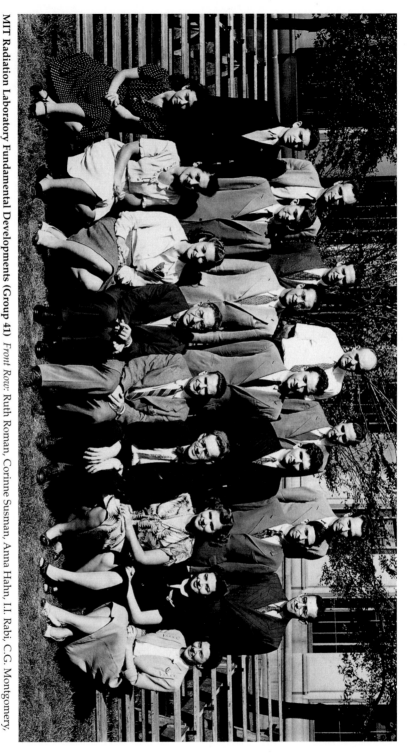

MIT Radiation Laboratory Fundamental Developments (Group 41) *Front Row:* Ruth Roman, Corinne Susman, Anna Hahn, I.I. Rabi, C.G. Montgomery, E.M. Purcell, Miriam Newhall, Rosemarie Saponaro and Dorothy Montgomery. *Middle Row:* C.W. Zabel, E.R. Beringer, N. Marcuvitz, H.R. Worthington, Jr., R.H. Dicke, E.L. Younker and R.S. Bender. *Back Row:* H.E. Kallmann, J.E. Coyle, E.C. Ingraham, F. Maxwell and W.F. Millett.

—*The MIT Museum*

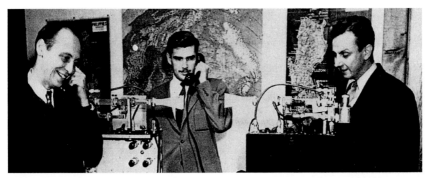

Robert Pound (center) and **Henry Torrey** (right), two of Purcell's collaborators in the historic experiment that detected nuclear magnetic resonance absorption, are shown together in this photo from the commemorative publication, *Five Years at the Radiation Laboratory*. Both men were members of Group 53, the Radiofrequency Group, which developed and engineered RF components, experience which would prove useful in the December 1945 NMR experiment. The third person in the photo is **J.B.H. Kuper,** also a member of Group 53. It was noted in the same publication that the Kupers and the Rabis gave the "nicest and finest parties."   —*The MIT Museum*

BELOW: Robert Pound, described by Bloembergen and Pake respectively as an "electronics whiz kid" and an "electronics wizard." A native of Canada, Pound said he never really considered being anything other than a physicist. His father, also a physicist, held the fourth PhD awarded in physics from the University of Toronto. Involved in amateur radio at the age of 12, Pound had built many electronics devices by the time he began attending college in Buffalo, New York. "I never learned much about electronics in college," he said. "I knew more than I ever learned in college before I came." He began

working at the Radiation Laboratory when he was just 23 and soon became section chief of microwave mixers and converters. In addition to the work Pound did as a participant in Purcell's 1945 NMR experiment, he also played an important advisory role in the design of the receiver used by Edward Purcell and Harold Ewen in detecting the 21-centimeter hydrogen line in space. In his own right, he has made important contributions in the area of Mössbauer and gamma ray spectroscopy.

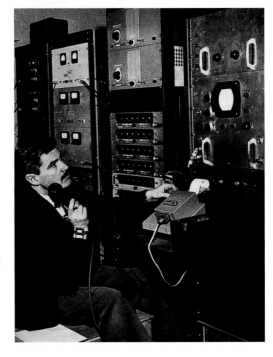

—*Pound quotes from* Rad Lab: Oral Histories Documenting World War II Activities at the MIT Radiation Laboratory, *produced by the IEEE Center for the History of Electrical Engineering; Harvard University photo, AIP Emilio Segrè Visual Archives.*

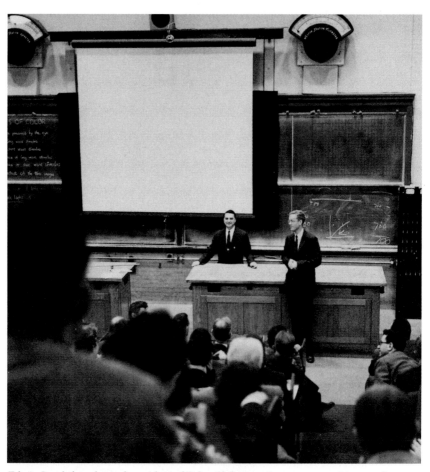

Edwin Land, founder and president of Polaroid Corporation, was a guest in one of Edward Purcell's classes at Harvard on November 18, 1958. About nine months earlier, President Eisenhower had announced the selection of a panel, drawn from his Science Advisory Committee, whose purpose was to recommend, as James Killian described it, "the outlines of a space program and the organization to manage it." Chaired by Purcell and known as the Purcell Panel, the group played a key role in educating both public officials and members of the public on the new frontier of space at a time when the orbiting *Sputnik*, launched only a few months earlier, was fueling many misconceptions and fears.

Rather than compiling a technical report that would reach a limited audience, the Purcell Panel decided to publish what Purcell has referred to as a "space primer." Drafted in Cambridge by Purcell and Land together with Francis Bello, then an editor of *Scientific American*, the result, Killian stated, "was an authoritative, literate essay under the title 'Introduction to Outer Space.' " Endorsed with enthusiasm by President Eisenhower, the publication was disseminated widely and proved to be quite accurate in predicting the future of the U.S. space program, although it had not counted on the accelerated push by President Kennedy to get a man on the moon by the end of the 1960s.

Political powers would ultimately determine the shape of the agency which would come to be known as the National Aeronautics and Space Administration, or NASA. Nevertheless, the Purcell Panel played an important role in helping to determine the course of space exploration. —*Quotes by James R. Killian from* Sputnik, Scientists and Eisenhower, *(Cambridge, MA: The MIT Press, 1977); photo by Paul H. Donaldson of Harvard University, AIP Emilio Segrè Visual Archives.*

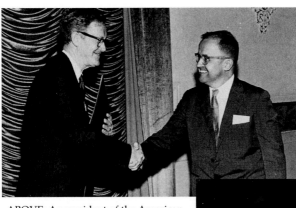

ABOVE: As president of the American
Physical Society in 1970, Edward
Purcell gave the High Polymer Award
to William Spence Slichter.

—AIP Emilio Segrè Visual Archives,
Physics Today Collection

RIGHT: APS President Purcell with
Dr. Yoichir Nambu.

—AIP Emilio Segrè Visual Archives,
Physics Today Collection

BELOW: Purcell with Nicolaas
Bloembergen in October 1981 when
Bloembergen was named a Nobel Prize
winner in physics. Bloembergen ws
Purcell's first graduate student.

—Photo by A.J. Dionne, Harvard:
AIP Emilio Segrè Visual Archives.

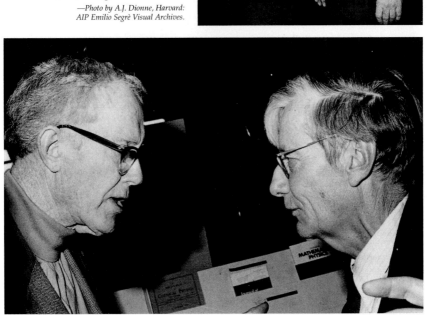

Felix Bloch (1905 - 1983)

"Bloch had a ready sense of humor. On his way to Stockholm to pick up his Nobel Prize by ship, he related that an old lady asked him in the moonlight on the deck what he did for a living. He said he 'dealt with magnetic moments' without further explanation, and she replied, 'Oh, how nice! Then you must be in the perfume business.' "

—ERWIN L. HAHN

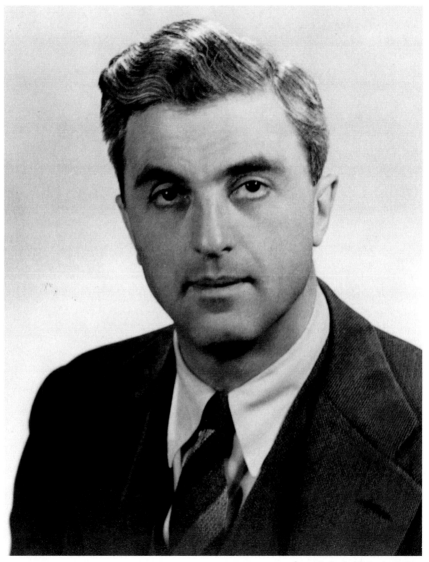

—*The Stanford University Archives*

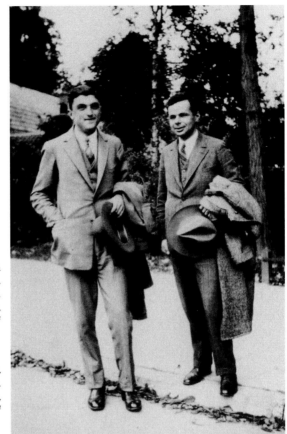

RIGHT: Felix Bloch with
Lothar Wolfgang Nordheim,
photo taken about 1929.
*—AIP Emilio Segrè Visual Archives,
Uhlenbeck Collection*

BELOW: George Uhlenbeck,
Enrico Fermi and Felix Bloch.
*—AIP Emilio Segrè Visual Archives,
Uhlenbeck Collection*

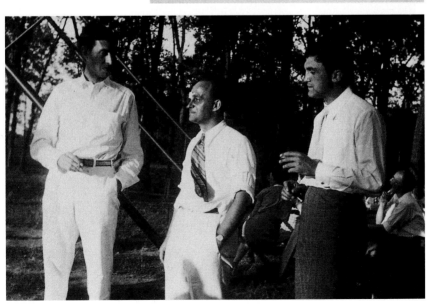

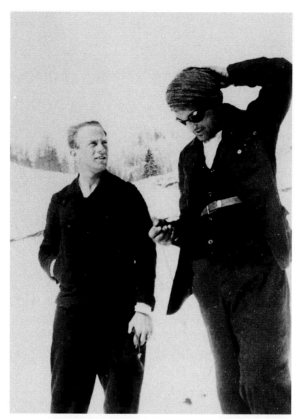

LEFT: Werner Heisenberg and Felix Bloch, photo taken about 1931. Heisenberg was Bloch's PhD mentor. At the time of Bloch's departure from Leipzig in response to Hitler's expulsion of Jewish professors, Bloch was an assistant to Heisenberg as well as a *privatdozent*.

—*Max Planck Institute, AIP Emilio Segrè Visual Archives*

BELOW: At Leipzig in 1931: *(In front)* Rudolf Peierls and Werner Heisenberg; *(in back)* G. Gentile, G. Placzek, G. Wick, Felix Bloch, Victor Weisskopf and F. Sauter.

—*AIP Emilio Segrè Visual Archives, Peierls Collection*

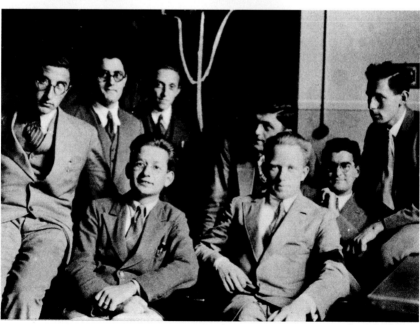

RIGHT: Felix Bloch with magnet used to perform 1946 nuclear induction experiment.
—*Stanford University News and Publication Service*

BELOW: Felix Bloch and William Hansen. Co-developer of the klystron tube with Russell Varian, Hansen was one of Bloch's collaborators in his nuclear induction discovery of NMR.
—*Stanford University News and Publication Service*

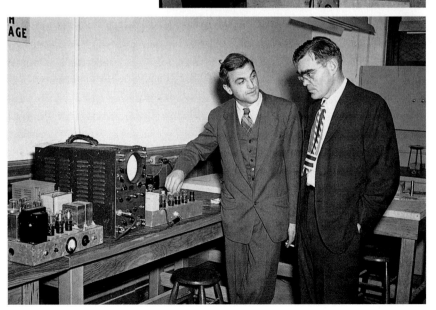

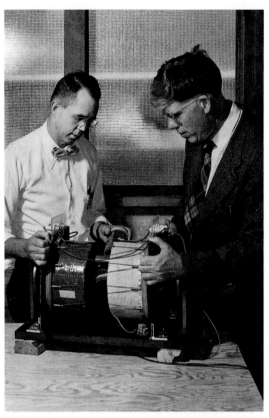

LEFT: Martin Packard and Russell Varian examine the first proton free-precession magnetometer, 1953. (See Ernst chapter for further discussion.) Another of Bloch's collaborators, Packard later joined Varian Associates where he was involved in the development of NMR spectrometers.

—Varian Associates photo,
AIP Emilio Segrè Visual Archives

BELOW: Felix Bloch in his Stanford University laboratory. In a 1953 speech, Bloch said: "One sometimes gets the impression that a science department is essentially a more or less well-oiled machine for conversion of new discoveries into dollars or vice versa . . . this is both false and dangerous . . . my little boat has been sailing here [at Stanford] far more under the famous winds of freedom than from steam generated by the burning of dollars."

—Quoted by Donald Stokes, Campus Report,
5 May 1982, page 4; Stanford University photo,
AIP Emilio Segrè Visual Archives

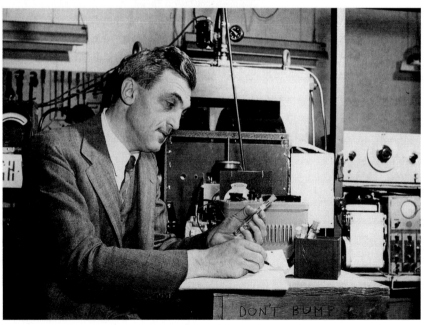

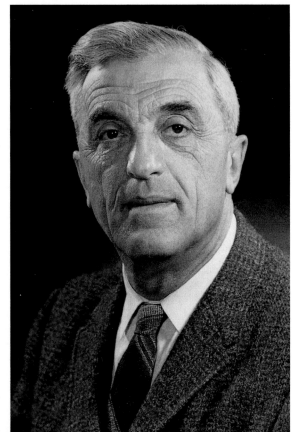

RIGHT: Felix Bloch.
—*The Stanford University Archives*

BELOW:
Felix Bloch, Robert Bacher,
Owen Chamberlain and
Karl K. Darrow.
—*AIP Emilio Segrè Visual Archives,*
Physics Today *Collection*

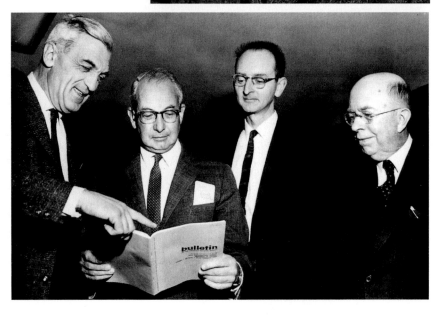

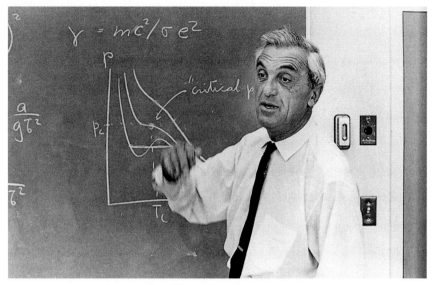

Bloch teaching at Stanford. "It is an obligation when teaching young people," said Bloch, "to try to think in the way they do. You must adjust yourself. In that sense, it is a very good thing to teach the young. I have always been indebted to my young students. Always they forced me to explain things in a way that would be clear to them."

—*Quoted by Donald Stokes,* Campus Report, *5 May 1982.*
Photo provided by Stanford University News and Publications Service

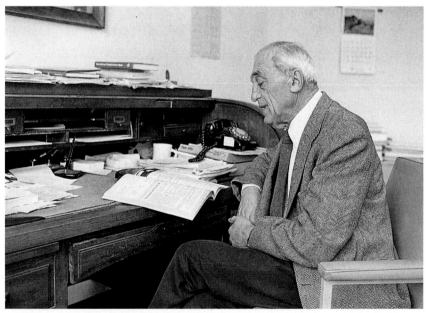

Felix Bloch at his desk. During a 1982 interview with a Stanford publicist, Bloch patted the very large rolltop desk at which he sat and said, "This used to belong to Bill Hansen, who had the office next to mine. This has great sentimental value to me." It was during Bloch's tenure at the Radio Research Laboratory at Harvard that he first told Hansen his plans for a nuclear induction experiment following the war.

—*Quoted by Donald Stokes,* Campus Report, *28 April 1982.*
Photo provided by Stanford University News and Publications Service

Nicolaas Bloembergen (1920 -   )

"I think what attracts me most about this field is the eternal fascination of discovering in my laboratory or seated here behind my desk something that no one else before me has found."

—NICOLAAS BLOEMBERGEN

from 1961 interview by Evarts Erickson of *The Microwave Journal*

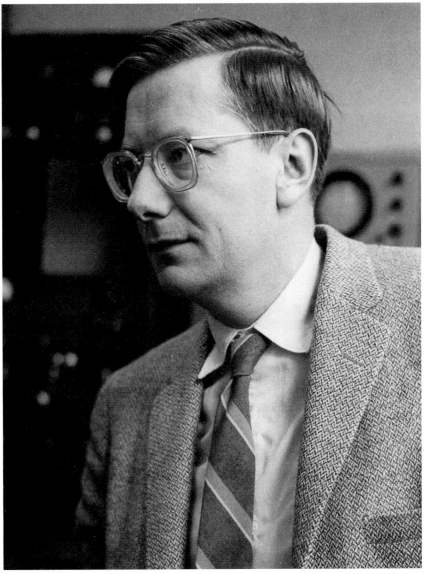

—*Harvard University*

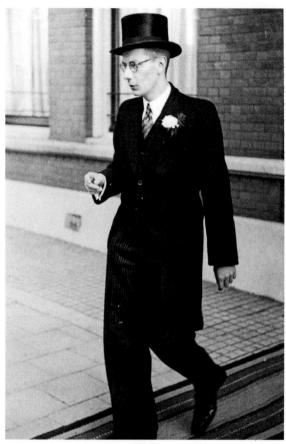

LEFT: Nicolaas Bloembergen attending family wedding in 1942.

—AIP Emilio Segrè Visual Archives, Bloembergen Collection

BELOW: In 1946, when this photo was taken, Nicolaas Bloembergen had been in the United States for just a few months. It was during this period, as a graduate assistant of Edward Purcell, that Bloembergen did much of his research on the relaxation mechanism of NMR. The person on the left is Harvard professor Philippe Le Corbeiller.

—Harvard University

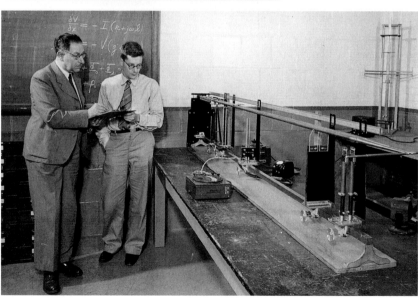

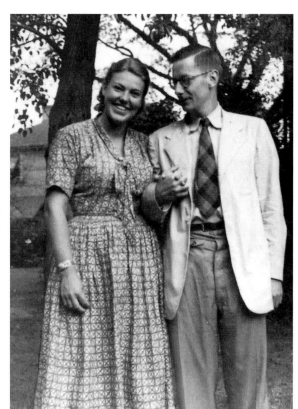

RIGHT: A 1949 photo of Nicolaas Bloembergen with his fiancée, Huberta Deliana ("Deli") Brink, in Cambridge, Massachusetts.
—*AIP Emilio Segrè Visual Archives, Bloembergen Collection*

BELOW: Bloembergen with Cornelis J. Gorter on Lake Chuzenji near Nikko, Japan in 1955.
—*AIP Emilio Segrè Visual Archives, Bloembergen Collection*

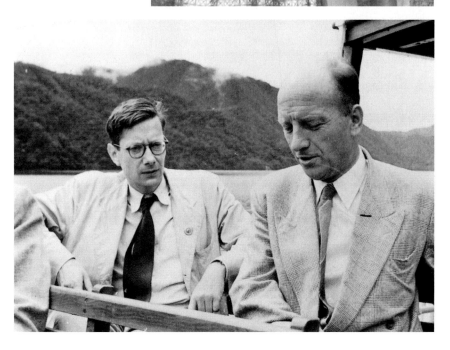

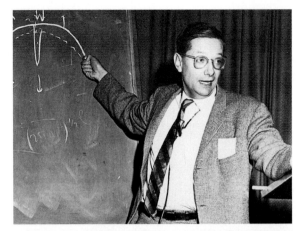

Bloembergen lecturing, 1957.

—Photo by Bill Gamble,
AIP Emilio Segrè Visual Archives

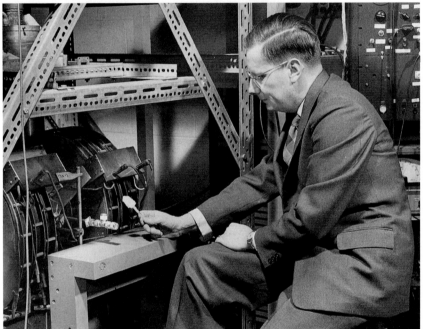

This 1958 photo, taken the year he became a U.S. citizen, shows Professor Bloembergen with a crystal of potassium cobalticyanide, grown in his Harvard laboratory for his development of the three-level solid-state maser. In the background is some of the equipment used in his earlier magnetic resonance experiments. Dr. Bloembergen likes to tell the story of when he and Professor Charles Townes, 1964 co-recipient of the Nobel Prize in physics for his development of masers and lasers, were co-recipients of the Oliver Buckley Prize at an annual meeting of the Institute of Radio Engineers (IRE) in New York City. The prizewinners' wives were also in attendance. "The two ladies started chatting," Bloembergen told the writer. "Mrs. Townes had a beautiful ruby pendant made by her husband in commemoration of the ruby maser he had developed. After dinner, back in the hotel room," said Bloembergen, "my wife asked me—but not this crudely—'So when are you going to get me a ruby?' So I said, 'Well, my dear, my maser works with cyanide.' "

—Harvard University

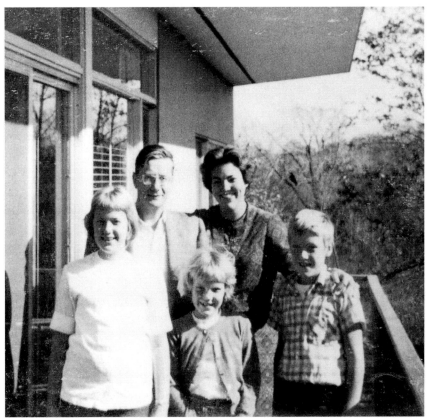

Nicolaas and Deli Bloembergen with their three children, from left to right, Antonia, born in 1951, Juliana, born in 1955, and Brink, born in 1953. "In retrospect," Bloembergen has noted, "it is difficult to overrate the accomplishment of my wife who raised the family in a country of adoption on a modest budget of a young faculty member, and supported me while I was devoting nearly all my efforts to establish a reputation in the world of physics."

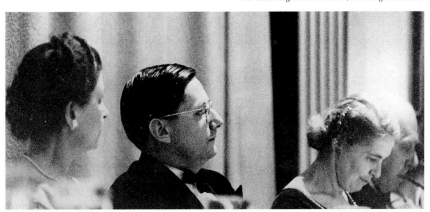

Mrs. E. Hutchisson, Nicolaas Bloembergen, Mrs. Karl Darrow and Niels Bohr.

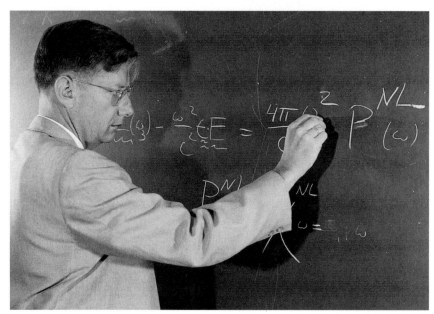

The above photo, taken in 1964, shows the future Nobel laureate writing an equation for nonlinear optics. If he were to be recognized as the "father" of anything, said Professor Bloembergen, he would like to be recognized as the father of nonlinear optics, a significant subfield of physics that opened up with the advent of lasers with high peak powers. As he pointed out in his lecture before the Swedish Royal Academy of Sciences when he received the 1981 Nobel Prize in physics, there are numerous applications for this technology in chemistry, biology, medicine, materials technology and especially in the field of communications and information processing. "Alfred Nobel would have enjoyed this interaction of physics and technology," said Bloembergen. —*Harvard University*

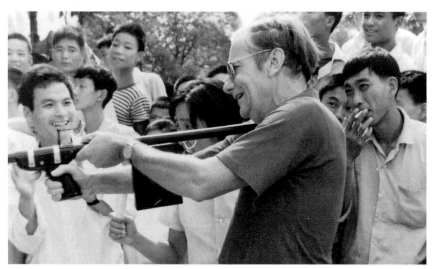

While visiting Shanghai in 1975, Bloembergen lined up the sights of a laser gun, just one of the innumerable technological applications made possible by the science he helped pioneer.
—*AIP Emilio Segrè Visual Archives, Bloembergen Collection*

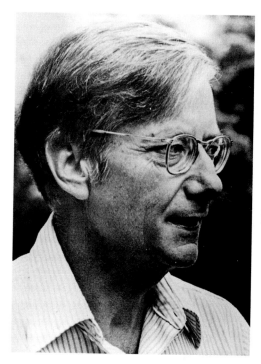

LEFT: Nicolaas Bloembergen. Bloembergen and Arthur Schawlow shared one-half of the 1981 Nobel Prize in physics for their work in laser spectroscopy. The other half of the Prize was awarded to Kai Siegbahn for electron spectroscopy. "I made it clear in my Nobel lecture that my significant contributions were really in the pumping scheme [used in masers and lasers] and in nonlinear spectroscopy," said Bloembergen.

—*AIP Meggers Gallery of Nobel Laureates*

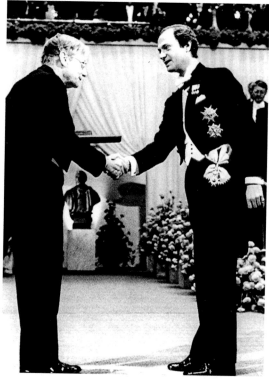

RIGHT: On December 10, 1981, wearing the same white-tie-and-tails that he wore as an 18-year-old when giving his valedictory address at the *gymnasium* he attended in Holland, 61-year-old Professor Bloembergen received the coveted Nobel Prize in physics from King Carl XVI Gustaf.

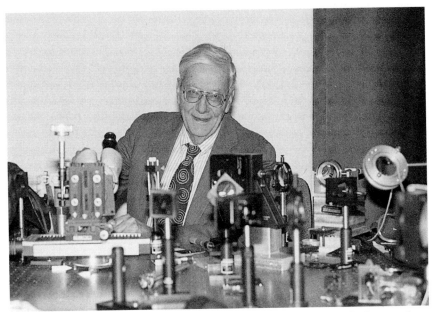

Surrounded by laboratory laser apparatus, Nicolaas Bloembergen can look back on nearly five decades of scientific breakthroughs in the fields of nuclear magnetic resonance, masers, lasers and nonlinear optics, all of which have been significantly advanced by his research.

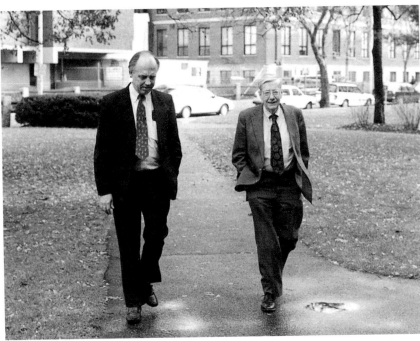

Nicolaas Bloembergen and author James Mattson outside Pierce Hall on the campus of Harvard University. Most of Professor Bloembergen's historic contributions have taken place in Pierce Hall, where his office is located, and the adjacent Lyman Laboratory of Physics.

Erwin L. Hahn (1921 -   )

"I decided one day—this was during the summer of 1949—to increase the intensity of the pulses and shorten them to squeeze in more points. After seeing the usual signals on top of the pedestals in sequence, a strange symmetric signal appeared on the screen with no pedestal under it. I discounted the latter as a false signal from the multivibrator, kicked the apparatus, let go with a few obscenities, and was happy to see that the signal finally disappeared. In retrospect, I tremble at the thought that by this particular 'ignoration' I could have missed completely the discovery of free precession and spin echoes."

—ERWIN L. HAHN

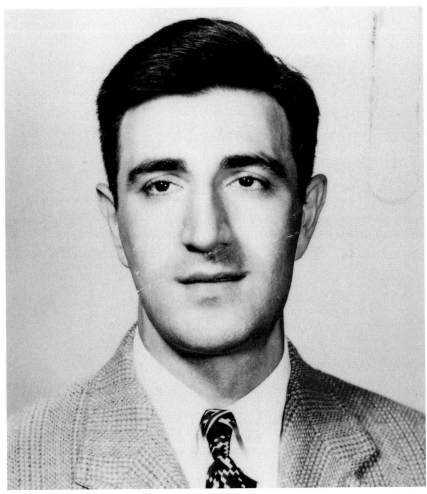

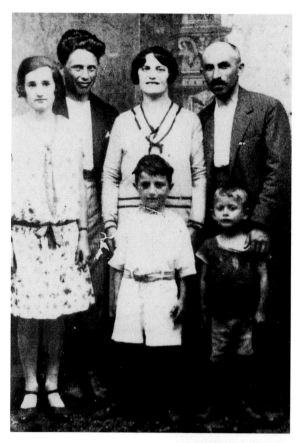

LEFT: Photo taken during Mary (Weiss) Hahn's 1926 trip back to her childhood home in Boni Had, Hungary accompanied by her youngest son, Erwin, then age 5.

From left to right, Michael Weiss, Mary's brother; Michael Weiss' wife, Katerina; Mary Hahn with her son Erwin in front of her. To the right of Erwin is Joseph, a cousin of Erwin's on Katerina's side, together with his father. Both son and father would perish in a Nazi death camp during World War II. Katerina and Michael Weiss would both escape to Israel.

RIGHT: In 1943, after he began graduate studies at Purdue University, Erwin Hahn met Marian Failing, an undergraduate at Purdue from Terre Haute, Indiana who was learning electronics for the purpose of editing Air Force technical manuals. The couple married on April 8, 1944, prompting Los Alamos to drop its offer of employment to Hahn. As a result, Hahn ended up in the Navy teaching radar, work which would eventually lead him into pulsed NMR.

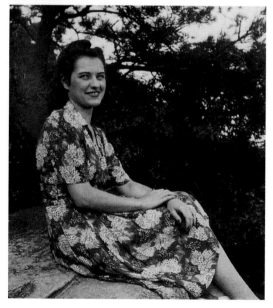

RIGHT: Erwin Hahn and Marian Failing on their wedding day with, from left to right, Erwin's mother and Marian's mother. Because Erwin was Jewish and Marian Catholic, their wedding took place at a teachers' college in Terre Haute, Indiana, a change from their original plans for a church ceremony made in deference to the wishes of Mary Hahn. Erwin's mother appreciated the minister's reference in the ceremony, however, to the Old Testament book of Ruth where Ruth told her mother-in-law that she would accompany her back to the land of Judah after the death of their husbands, telling her that "your people will be my people."

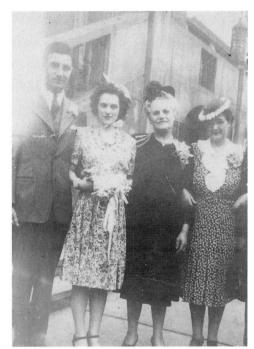

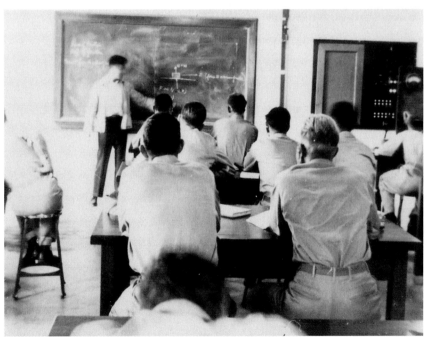

At Purdue, Hahn was deferred from military duty because he was teaching physics to GIs under the Army Special Training Program (ASTP). The class shown above, an introductory physics class, stood out especially in his mind. "All of a sudden," he said, "most of them disappeared. Army orders sent them to Anzio Beach [in Italy] and they were all killed."

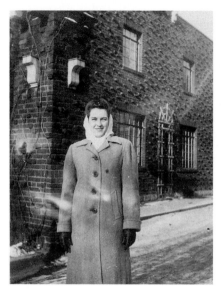
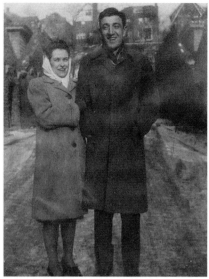

From October 1945 through March 1946, Erwin Hahn taught radar and sonar to shipboard Navy combat personnel, assigned to the Educational Department at Navy Pier on Lake Michigan near the Chicago Loop. At the time the above photos were taken of Erwin and Marian Hahn on January 23, 1946, he was unaware of the successful attempts at Harvard and Stanford to detect nuclear magnetic resonance in condensed matter, experiments that would directly affect the course of his future career.

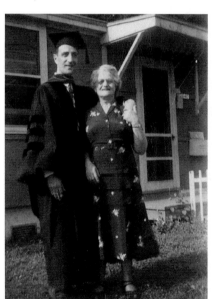
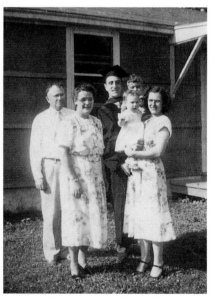

A couple months before he discovered spin echoes, Erwin Hahn graduated from the University of Illinois at Urbana with a PhD in physics. LEFT: Erwin with his mother, Mary Hahn. RIGHT: Hahn with Marian's parents, Mr. and Mrs. Failing, his wife Marian, and their first two children, David and Deborah. The couple would have one more child, Katherine. After 34 years of marriage, Marian died of cancer in 1978.

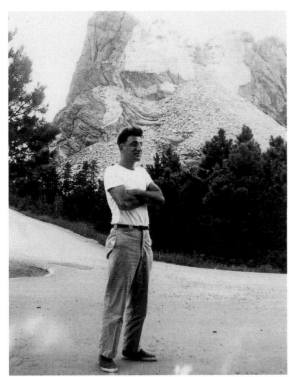

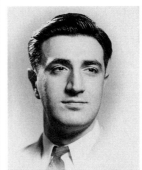

LEFT: "Competing profiles," Professor Hahn wrote regarding this photo of himself taken against the backdrop of Mount Rushmore's presidential likenesses.

BELOW: Another more formal portrait of the physicist.

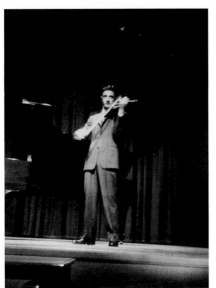

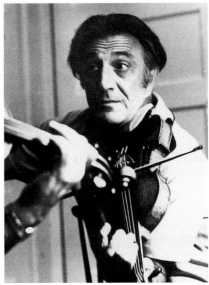

Since childhood, music has been an important part of Erwin Hahn's life, both avocationally, as violinist, and professionally, as a physicist teaching the physics of music. LEFT: Hahn as an undergraduate at Juniata College, performing a Mendelssohn concerto on the violin with piano accompaniment. RIGHT: A few years later, Hahn, self-described in this photo as a "mad violinist," compares notes with another of similar persuasion.

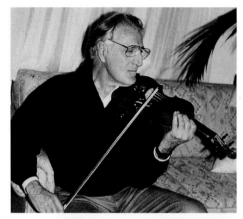

Throughout his career, Hahn has played music with colleagues who share his passion for music, including Karl Lark-Horovitz, Sidney Drell, Leonard Schiff, Felix Bloch, Edward Teller and Otto Robert Frisch. Science is like music, Hahn has said. "When you accomplish a revelation in a physics experiment and you work out its theory, no matter how minor it is, and you confirm something or you predict something, there's a sense of beauty in it, an exultation. It's a private experience."

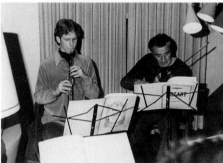

Hahn playing a duet with William Bennett, the principle oboeist of the San Francisco Symphony.

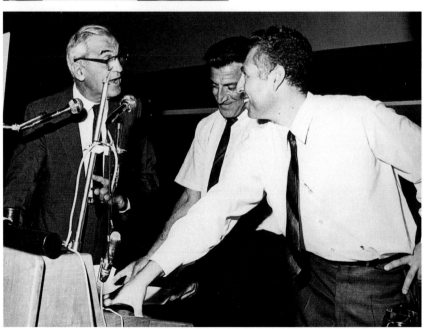

In a ceremony held in Israel, Felix Bloch (left) and Daniel Fiat (right) present Professor Hahn (center) with first International Society of Magnetic Resonance Prize, awarded in 1971.

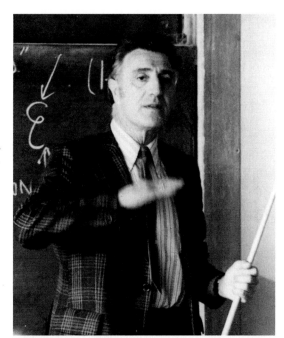

Hahn in his role as classroom teacher.

Erwin Hahn with his good friend, Anatole Abragam of Saclay, France, noted author of *The Principles of Nuclear Magnetism* and, like Hahn, a periodic visitor to Oxford University.

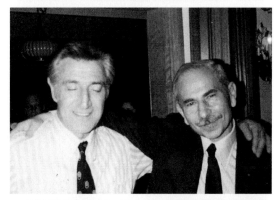

Abragam (left) with Nicholas Kurti, eminent thermodynamicist of Oxford University, and Alexander Pines of the University of California at Berkeley. Officially retired, Hahn continues his research under a National Science Foundation grant in the chemistry department at Berkeley, where he has been working in collaboration with Alexander Pines. Both Hahn and Pines are Wolf Prize laureates, Hahn in physics and Pines in chemistry.

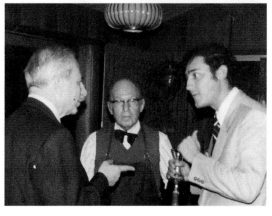

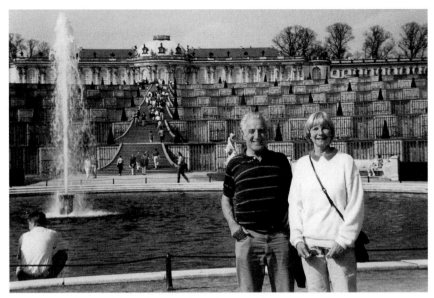

Erwin Hahn and Natalie Woodson Hodgson were married on April 12, 1980. These days, they enjoy frequent travel together, much of it international. This May 1994 photo shows them at the palace of Frederick the Great at Potsdam in northeast Germany. One of their favorite destinations is Oxford University, where Professor Hahn has twice done research as a Guggenheim Fellow and where Natalie has been a much-appreciated volunteer researcher at the historic Bodleian Library.

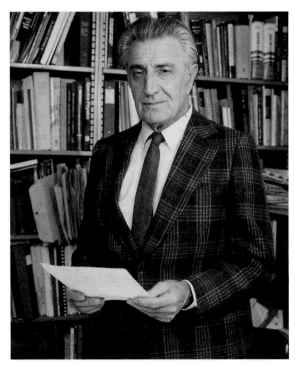

A 1985 photo of
Professor Erwin Hahn.
—Univ. of California, Berkeley
Public Information Office

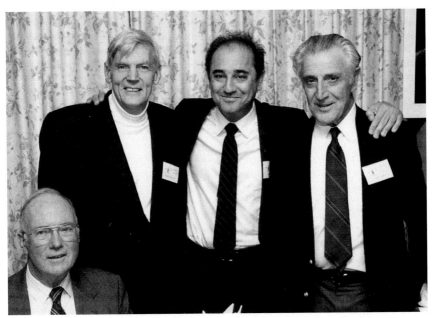

At Hahn's 70th birthday retirement party, from left to right: **Charles H. Townes,** pioneer of the maser (seated); **Sven Hartmann,** first to observe photon echoes and collaborator with Hahn in what is known as Hartmann-Hahn cross-relaxation; **Alexander Pines,** co-recipient with Richard Ernst of the 1991 Wolf Prize in chemistry for multiple-quantum and high-spin NMR; and **Erwin Hahn**.

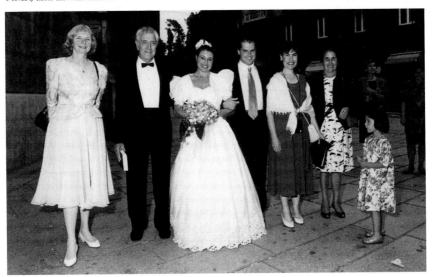

LEFT TO RIGHT: **Natalie and Erwin Hahn** in Genoa, Italy, at the wedding of Professor Hahn's youngest daughter, **Katherine,** to **Carlo Caruso**. Katherine lives in Zürich, Switzerland and is employed by the ETH. The fifth person from the left is Hahn's older daughter, **Debbie,** who lives in Marin County near San Francisco and is employed by a pharmaceutical company. Professor Hahn's son, David (not pictured), is a medical doctor. Specializing in epidemiology, he has made important contributions to the study of asthma.

Richard R. Ernst (1933 -   )

"In the early '60s we were looking for ways to improve the NMR spectrometers which were becoming more widely used for molecular structure determinations. In 1963 we heard through Warren Proctor, who was at the Varian applications laboratory in Switzerland, that a bright, young PhD student at the Swiss Federal Institute of Technology (ETH) in Zürich might be interested in coming to the United States. . . . After working with Ernst, it became apparent that he was not only bright and productive, but also had a marvelous sense of humor. He made the laboratory a happier place."
—WESTON A. ANDERSON

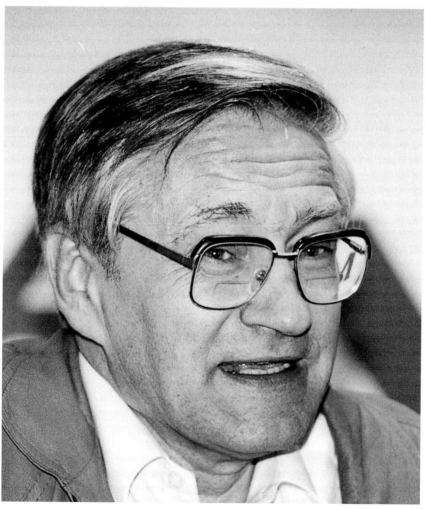

AP/Wide World Photos

RIGHT: Richard Ernst responds with a broad smile after receiving congratulatory flowers upon his arrival at New York's John F. Kennedy International Airport on October 16, 1991. He was en route from Moscow to the United States where he was to receive the Louisa Gross Horowitz Prize at Columbia University when the pilot informed him that he had been selected as the 1991 Nobel Prize winner in chemistry for his contributions to Fourier transform NMR and multidimensional NMR spectroscopy.

—*AP/Wide World Photos*

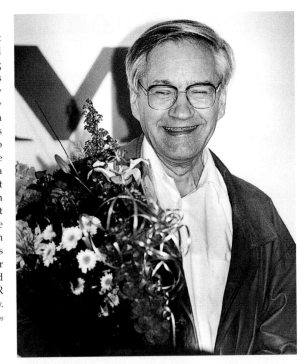

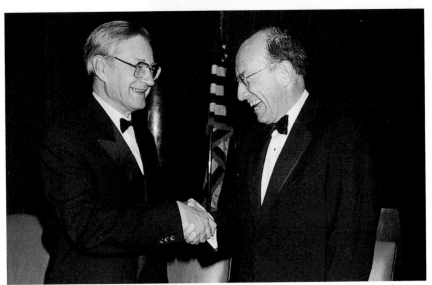

Professor Ernst, newly-named Nobel Prize winner, is congratulated by Michael Sovern, president of Columbia University, at the October 17, 1991 awards ceremony during which Ernst received the Louisa Gross Horowitz Prize. The Horowitz prize is given for outstanding basic research in the field of biology or biochemistry. Also awarded the Horowitz prize on the same occasion was Kurt Wüthrich of the ETH, with whom Ernst collaborated for a period of 10 years in the development of two-dimensional spectroscopy in molecular biology.

—*AP/Wide World Photos*

Raymond V. Damadian (1936 -   )

"When I first began developing the MR scanner in 1970, I would meet new people and they would ask, 'What is it that you do?' After explaining that I was working on a new invention that would someday scan the entire body non-invasively, hunt down cancer deposits and provide scans of all the body's organs using radio signals and magnets, they would commonly respond by saying, 'Yeah, sure.'

"Well, it's 22 years later, there are approximately 4,000 MR scanners installed worldwide and it has become a multibillion-dollar industry and a world-famous technology. I still meet new people and they still ask me what it is that I do. Now I tell them that I invented the MR scanner. They still say, 'Yeah, sure'—and one chap added, 'And my uncle's President of the United States.' "

—RAYMOND V. DAMADIAN
addressing the Washington Patent Lawyers Club in 1992

BELOW: Dr. Damadian with "Indomitable," the first whole-body MR scanner, on permanent exhibit in the Hall of Medical Sciences at the Smithsonian Institution.

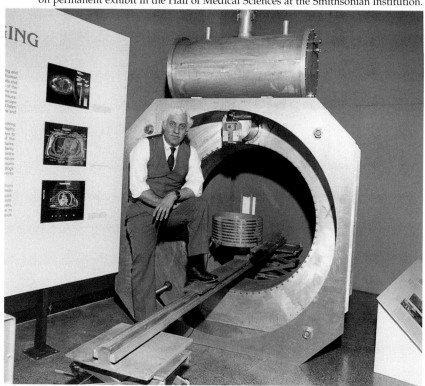

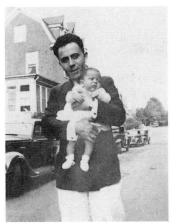
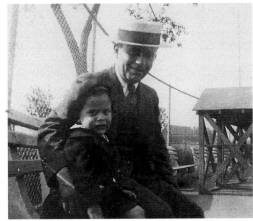

Young Raymond Damadian as an infant of 3-1/2 weeks and as a toddler with his father, Vahan Damadian, who worked as a photoengraver at the *New York World,* which later became the *World-Telegram.* An Armenian, Vahan Damadian was born in 1903 in Turkey. At the age of 12, Vahan together with his sister and his mother miraculously escaped death during the 1915 Armenian genocide. Following World War I, the Damadians were reunited in the United States with two of Vahan's brothers who had emigrated earlier.

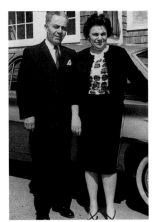
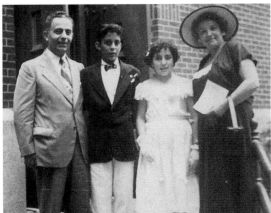

ABOVE LEFT: Vahan and Odette Damadian. Vahan married Odette Yazedjian, the daughter of a French mother and an Armenian father, in 1932. The couple was living in Manhattan when Raymond was born on March 16, 1936. Shortly after his birth, they relocated to Queens where Raymond's sister, Claudette, was born.

ABOVE RIGHT: Raymond Damadian with his parents and sister, Claudette, at his graduation in 1949 from Public School 101, located in the Forest Hills Gardens section of Queens. At age 15, while attending Forest Hills High School, Damadian received a Ford Foundation Pre-Induction Scholarship (university admission without completion of high school) and subsequently attended the University of Wisconsin in Madison where he received his Bachelor of Science degree in 1956.

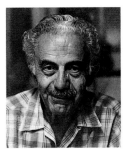

RIGHT: Raymond Damadian's father, Vahan.

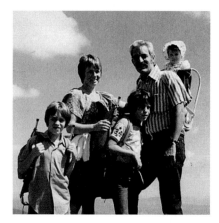

LEFT: Dr. Raymond Damadian and his wife, Donna, and their children, left to right, Timothy, Jevan and Keira. Damadian first met the former Donna Terry in Westhampton on Eastern Long Island where he worked in the summers as a tennis pro at the Dune Deck Hotel to help earn money for medical school.

RIGHT: Raymond Damadian with his sister Claudette (lower right), their parents Vahan and Odette Damadian, and the grandchildren, Calton Chan and Keira Damadian (held by Odette), Jevan Damadian (in front of Dr. Damadian), and Timothy (behind Claudette).

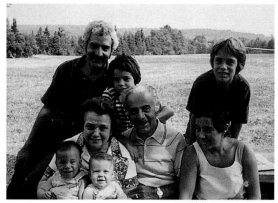

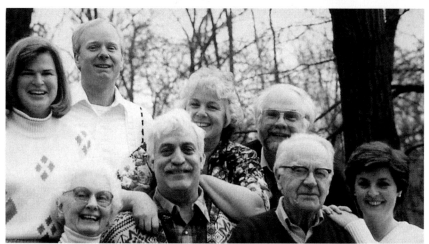

Raymond and Donna Damadian (center) with Donna's parents, Amy and Donald Terry (front); Donna's brother Thomas and his wife Sherry (left); and Donna's brother David and his wife Constance (right). David Terry has played an active role in Damadian's MR scanner project from the beginning, from raising funds to help finance the building of the scanner to his present role as head of stockholder relations for FONAR Corporation.

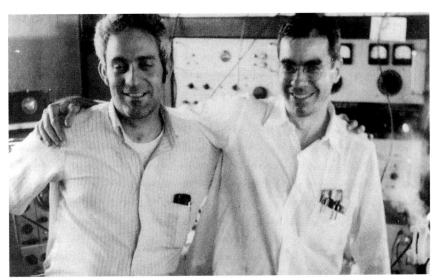

Dr. Raymond Damadian with scientist-physician Dr. Freeman Cope. It was a 1969 collaborative effort by Damadian and Cope in which they were the first to detect potassium in living tissue using NMR that led Damadian, about nine months later, to determine whether or not cancer tissue exhibited different relaxation times than normal tissue. Not only did he find that malignant tumors exhibited dramatically different relaxation times; he also discovered and reported that there were significant differences in relaxation times between normal tissues. Damadian's findings were made public in an article entitled "Tumor Detection by Nuclear Magnetic Resonance," published in the March 19, 1971 issue of the journal *Science*.

RIGHT: Professor Damadian analyzing tissue samples with NMR at Downstate Medical Center. Recalling the first time he compared relaxation times of tumors to normal tissue, Damadian said, "After a few more days of measurements to be confident I was measuring T_1 in the different normal rat tissues reliably, I decided to attempt the cancer measurement. [The date was June 18, 1970.] To my mind, this was the measurement that would make or break my NMR body scanner idea. I needed that abnormal cancer signal if there was to be any hope of a human scanner that could hunt down cancer deposits in the body. I held my breath and made the first measurement. It was different—dramatically different!"

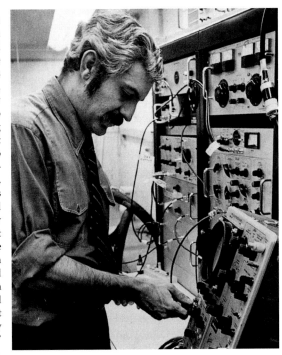

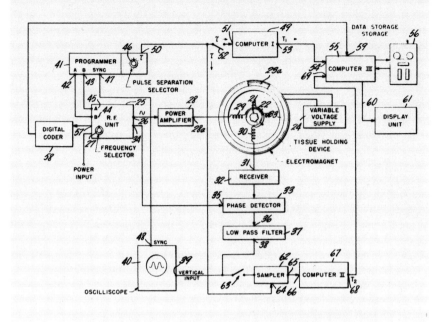

3,789,832

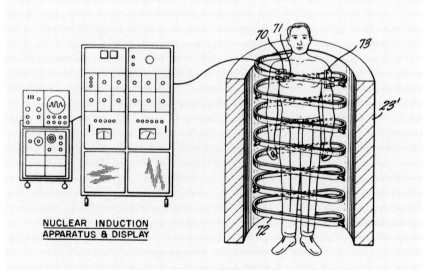

NUCLEAR INDUCTION APPARATUS & DISPLAY

The "Pioneer Patent" of NMR scanning, U.S. Patent 3,789,832 describing an "Apparatus and Method for Detecting Cancer in Tissue," was the first description ever of a device for scanning the human body by NMR. The patent application was filed by Damadian on March 17, 1972, two days less than one year after *Science* published his article entitled, "Tumor Detection by Nuclear Magnetic Resonance."

Building "Indomitable" . . .

"The 53-inch bore superconducting magnet and associated dewar was constructed by Damadian and his colleagues who had no previous experience in superconducting technology—a truly remarkable feat. . . . The ultimate goal of whole-body imaging was first achieved by Damadian using his f.o.n.a.r. technique in 1977. . . . He was followed shortly afterward by [Peter] Mansfield and colleagues using a line-scanning method, and by many other academic and commercial concerns since."
—PETER G. MORRIS
Department of Biochemistry, University of Cambridge
Nuclear Magnetic Resonance Imaging in Medicine and Biology

Although he had never built a magnet before, Damadian set about to build a 5,000-gauss superconducting magnet, the ninth largest in the world. For an electromagnet to be superconductive, it has to be kept immersed in liquid helium below minus 269 degrees Celsius, nearly absolute zero. That required a Thermos-like device called a dewar to drastically slow down the three main types of heat transfer—conduction, convection and radiation. Damadian's magnet design called for the construction of three huge, hollow metal rings to isolate the heart of his magnet—the windings—from the heat of the outside world (see following page).

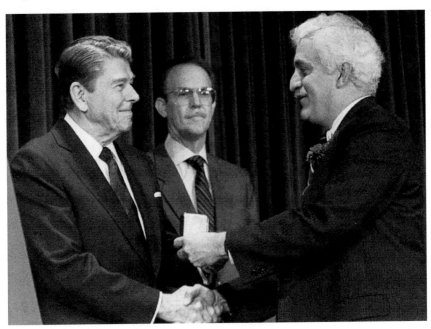

Dr. Damadian receiving the National Medal of Technology, the nation's highest honor in technology, from President Ronald Reagan at the Executive Offices of the White House on July 15, 1988. In giving the award, President Reagan cited Damadian for his "independent contributions in conceiving and developing the application of magnetic resonance technology to medical uses, including whole-body scanning and diagnostic imaging."

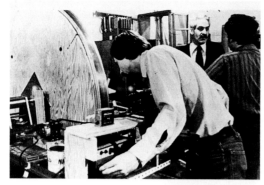

LEFT: Niobium-titanium wire, obtained at the "miraculous" price of 10 cents on the dollar from Westinghouse Corporation, was tightly and precisely wound off a wooden spool onto two large hoops, each containing 30 miles of wire, an almost trance-producing process that went on for weeks at six days a week, 16 hours a day.

RIGHT: The smallest, inner-most doughnut, made of polished stainless steel, contained the wire hoops comprising the magnet and the liquid helium in which the magnet was immersed. To reduce heat conduction, the magnet was prevented from touching its container with the use of special supports made of a material that was a poor conductor of heat.

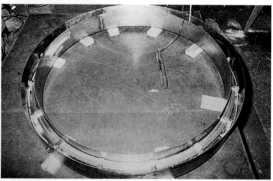

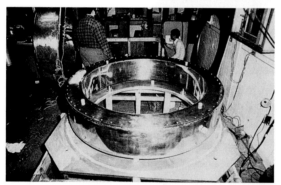

LEFT: Finally, the third and largest doughnut, an aluminum "can" with half-inch-thick walls, helped prevent heat transfer by surrounding its two inner containers with a convection-reducing vacuum atmosphere of 10^{-9} TORR.

RIGHT: Though surrounded by liquid nitrogen and encased in a vacuum atmos-phere, the liquid helium had to be replenished daily. To store extra helium, Damadian and Minkoff built a reservoir that sat astride the huge magnet. Unfortunately, it leaked intolerably and required weeks of valuable time for the team to find and fix the leaks.

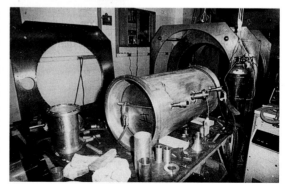

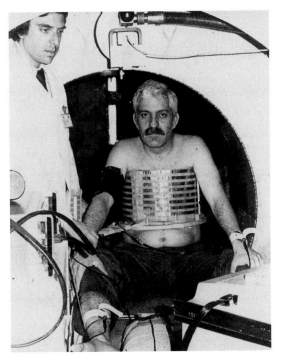

LEFT: The first attempt at a whole-body human scan was made with Dr. Damadian sitting in the scanner. A blood-pressure cuff was affixed to his right arm, an EKG was wired to his chest, and oxygen was kept handy. The cardiologist (standing at left in photo) was there just in case the magnetic field produced any strange cardiac effect on Damadian. However, no signal was received from the scanner. The team decided that the professor was oversized for the cardboard vest housing the antenna and that the antenna must have been detuned. A thinner "guinea pig" was needed.

RIGHT: Although Minkoff was smaller and fit the antenna vest better, he wasn't anxious to risk his health for an experiment that had never been done before. But finally, on July 2, 1977, Minkoff told Damadian that he would go into the machine. That very evening, shortly before midnight, Minkoff took his shirt off and put on the cardboard vest. As soon as the machine was turned on, there was a signal. Four hours and 45 minutes later, after Minkoff had been incrementally moved via the adjustable seat into different positions, the first whole-body human scan showing a cross-section of Minkoff's chest was complete. An ecstatic Damadian noted his jubilant reaction in Goldsmith's notebook (NEXT PAGE).

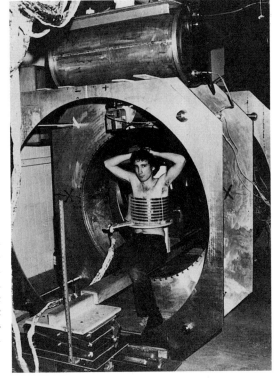

LEFT: The data from Michael Goldsmith's notebook where he and Damadian recorded signals received from Larry Minkoff's chest on the night of the first whole-body MR scan. Each of the 106 numeric values was given a corresponding color which, when drawn on a sheet of grid paper, indicated a rough, but otherwise accurate, representation of Minkoff's chest.

BELOW: Damadian's jubilant hand-written notation, "Fantastic Success!" marked the historic event in Goldsmith's notebook.

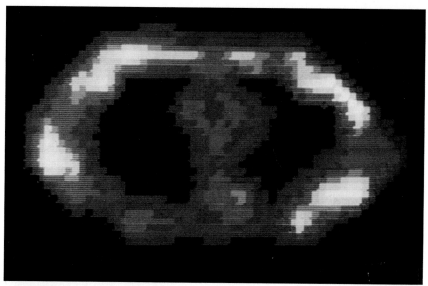

ABOVE: Later, the data was fed into a computer and interpolated to produce the first image of the live human body, known as "MINK 5."

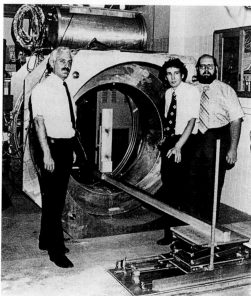

LEFT: Professor Damadian, Lawrence Minkoff and Michael Goldsmith stand next to the completed "Indomitable."

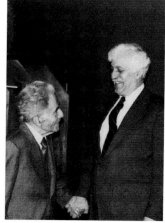

RIGHT: Vahan Damadian and his son, Dr. Damadian, share a light-hearted moment during the ceremony in which Indomitable was inducted into the Smithsonian Institution in Washington, DC.

Paul C. Lauterbur (1929 -   )

"How does one associate a particular NMR signal with a small localized region in the human body? Paul Lauterbur took one of the first steps toward this goal in 1973 when he proposed developing spatial maps of elements of nuclear magnetization by NMR zeugmatography."

—GEORGE E. PAKE
from an October 1993 article in *Physics Today*

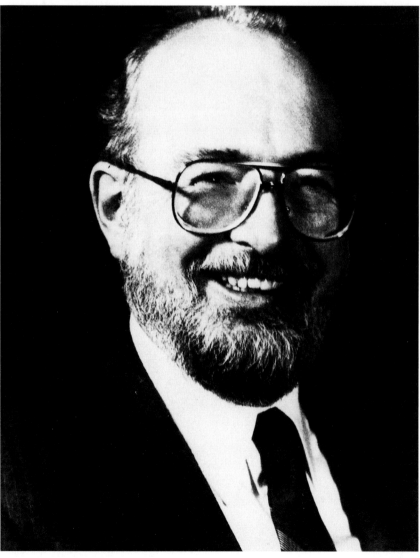

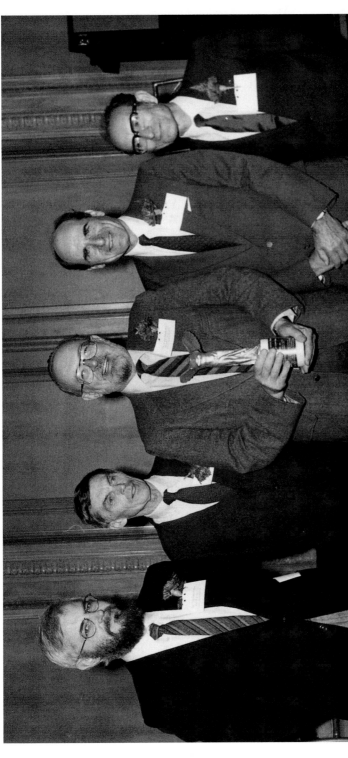

Paul Lauterbur receives the $15,000 Albert Lasker Clinical Research Award on November 14, 1984 in New York City. From left to right: **Dr. Michael Potter,** chief of the Laboratory of Genetics at the National Cancer Institute and National Institutes of Health; **Dr. Georges J.F. Kohler,** member of the Basel Institute of Immunology; **Dr. Paul C. Lauterbur,** professor of chemistry and research professor of radiology at the State University of New York at Stony Brook; **Dr. Cesar Milstein,** head of the Protein Chemistry Subdivision of the Laboratory of Molecular Biology, Medical Research Council, Cambridge, England; and **Dr. Henry J. Heimlich,** professor of advanced clinical science at Xavier University, Cincinnati, Ohio.

—*AP/Wide World Photos*

my passage by visa and still another freighter problem. So I came too late for the January meeting. So that was never presented, but the record is there." The information he planned to present to the American Physical Society was published in a paper in *Physica*[192] a year later but "because it wasn't *Physical Review*, it didn't get the attention it deserved. I did the work in 1948 in Leiden and it's completely written up in this paper in *Physica*."[193]

In May 1948, 28-year-old Nicolaas Bloembergen defended his PhD thesis, "Nuclear Magnetic Relaxation," in a grand public ceremony in the centuries-old aula of the University of Leiden, where he arrived, said Bloembergen, "in white tie and tails in a horse-drawn carriage according to an ancient ritual which has since succumbed to modern efficiency."[194]

Present at his thesis defense, in addition to 300 others that included faculty, relatives, and student friends was Professor Adriaan Fokker, Bloembergen's distant uncle. "I had to answer questions of the faculty," explained Bloembergen, "and one of those was Fokker."

I remember Fokker saying a very nice thing. I've translated it, of course, because he said it in Dutch. "Well, it's a very interesting and nice work," he said, "but even the sun has spots." He had discovered that there was an inconsistency of signs in the beginning of the thesis. On one page I had a plus, and on another page, in a corresponding place, I had a minus sign. So I said, "Well, obviously one of these is incorrect. I will check it and I will let you know which sign is wrong," which I did. But [his remark] meant that he had read the thing with some care.[195]

The first printing of Bloembergen's thesis totaled 500 copies, half of which he distributed among faculty, colleagues, family and friends. The other half were quickly sold out through the offices of the Nyhoff publishing house located in The Hague. During the following decade, Bloembergen's thesis would be reproduced in various formats in Japan, the Netherlands, and "possibly elsewhere," said Bloembergen. In 1961, because of continuing popular demand, New York publisher W.A. Benjamin reprinted it again as part of its Frontiers in Physics series, with the addition of comments and corrections in an appendix to relate it to subsequent developments and improvements.[196]

By the summer of 1948, Bloembergen felt that the basic nuclear spin relaxation mechanisms in solids, liquids and gases were understood and he was invited to speak on the topic at an international conference in

Zürich, devoted to postwar advances in high energy and nuclear physics. Although the international renown of Bloch and Purcell was already high, considerations of time and expense prevented them from attending the conference. In 1948, transatlantic travel was still predominantly by ocean liner.

> I was honored [said Bloembergen] to introduce the emerging field of NMR to a critical audience, which included among others [Walter] Heitler, [Wolfgang] Pauli and [Victor] Weisskopf. In the hallway I heard afterwards the comment that 'the experimenters had gotten ahead of the theoreticians.' This reinforced my view that a combination of these two aspects of physics is more than the sum of the separate parts.[197]

Bloembergen also attended a low-temperature conference at Oxford University with Professor Gorter where he met B. Bleaney and M.H.L. Pryce, who had been working on electron spin resonance at microwave frequencies, as well as B.V. Rollin and J. Hatton, whose work more closely paralleled his own. There was a significant difference, however, Bloembergen felt, between his approach to NMR and theirs. "I had the impression that they considered NMR as an amateur sport. For me it was not only fun, but also a serious professional pursuit. Therefore, our experimental and theoretical results were more systematic and quantitative and received subsequently much wider attention."[198]

Perhaps Bloembergen's approach to NMR was a carryover from his early days when he and his brother kayaked around the rivers and canals of Holland with their father who, even while enjoying the sport of kayaking, set minimum distance goals, encouraged performance, and sometimes imposed it.

Physicist Anatole Abragam has written of Professor Nicolaas Bloembergen: "Endowed with an ingenious and fertile mind, and an indefatigable worker, Bloembergen is moved, more than anyone else perhaps, by a spirit of competition which is apt to generate a certain amount of tension around him, and which took him all the way to the Nobel Prize."[199] Backhanded compliment or not, Auke Bloembergen would have been proud.

Deli

If vigorous kayaking in his youth paid off handsomely in Bloembergen's professional achievements, sailing, another sport he had enjoyed as a teenager, came to have romantic benefits when he was 28. In the summer of 1948, not long after receiving his PhD, Bloembergen joined a sailing camp organized by Leiden's Christiaan Huyghens Physics Club—Huyghens was a famous Dutch astronomer—and it was there that he met Huberta Deliana Brink, "Deli," who, two years later, would become his wife.

Eight years younger than Nicolaas, Deli was a citizen of Holland who had been born in the Dutch colony of Indonesia in 1928 and had grown up in East Java where her father, who held a PhD degree in biology, was involved with tropical agriculture, including the production of sugar, coffee and rubber. In 1942, however, the Japanese in their island-hopping conquest of the Pacific had also taken over Java and Deli had spent the rest of the war years restricted to a Japanese concentration camp.

The end of World War II, however, had not brought an end to fighting in Indonesia. Nationalist forces, led by Sukarno and Hatta, proclaimed a republic, which would eventually be recognized by the Dutch in 1949 after four years of armed conflict. Deli, however, was repatriated to Holland where she was about to begin pre-medical studies at the University of Amsterdam when she met Nicolaas Bloembergen.

If romance was to blossom for the couple, however, it appeared that it would have to be cultivated from a distance, as Bloembergen was making plans to return to Cambridge, Massachusetts in January 1949. He had been offered and had accepted a Junior Fellowship by Harvard's Society of Fellows, a position Robert Pound had once held. Deli Brink soon revealed her own resourcefulness.

> When I returned to Harvard in 1949 to join the Society of Fellows [Bloembergen wrote], she managed to get on a student hospitality exchange program and traveled after me to the United States on an immigrant ship. I proposed to her the day she arrived and we got married in Amsterdam in 1950. Ever since, she has been a source of light in my life. Her enduring encouragement has contributed immensely to the successes in my further career.[200]

She would also bring music into Bloembergen's life. Along with the educational void he had experienced at the *gymnasium* in social relations, psychology, government and politics, he had never been exposed to music. A naturally talented pianist and artist, Deli Bloembergen has worked to develop her gifts and has passed on her love for music to her children.

The same resourcefulness she showed in getting to the United States has also been a source of strength for her family. Although she liked life in the United States much better than the more confined social structures of Holland, said Bloembergen, and found it similar to the freedom she experienced growing up in Indonesia, nevertheless the absence of relatives "implied," he said, "an absence of emotional support for our young immigrant family."

> My wife showed enormous strength and the capability to firmly establish our family in a new environment. . . . In retrospect, it is difficult to overrate the accomplishment of my wife who raised the family in a country of adoption on a modest budget of a young faculty member, and supported me while I was devoting nearly all my efforts to establish a reputation in the world of physics. . . . Fortunately, my tenure appointment in 1951 [as an associate professor at Harvard] helped to provide a sense of financial security and facilitated our taking root.[201]

The Bloembergens have three children, all born in Cambridge, Massachusetts: a daughter, Antonia, in 1951; a son, Brink Auke, in 1953; and a daughter, Juliana, in 1955. Soon after the birth of Juliana, the Bloembergen family moved to a new home they had built in Lexington, Massachusetts and it was there that they became integrated into a community and where the children attended public schools. Deli Bloembergen taught the children music; Nicolaas Bloembergen took them hiking, swimming and skiing. In April 1958, Nicolaas and Deli Bloembergen joined their children as citizens of the United States.

Today, the children are grown and pursuing their own successful careers. In comparing himself to his father's expectations of performance, Professor Bloembergen smiled and said:

> I think I may have been too lax. All my three children, they looked at their father. They said, "That's a lot of hard work." And then they grew up with [their father receiving] rather little pay as a junior faculty member, so they all decided to get MBA's and they are doing financially very well.
>
> But I didn't pay perhaps enough attention, you know, stimulate them in their scholastic performance. I did take them on trips and so forth. I never pushed them, but maybe I never encouraged them, either. I think they looked at their father and said, "That is too much work for too little compensation."[202]

Other Physics and More NMR

After Bloembergen's return to the United States in 1949, he took leave of NMR for awhile, using his two-and-a-half years in the Society of Fellows to broaden his exposure to other subfields of physics.

> For starters, I wanted to acquire some first-hand experience with microwave techniques. I studied the electron spin resonance at the transition from ferromagnetic to paramagnetic resonance near the Curie point of nickel. [The Curie point is the temperature above which ferromagnetic substances lose their remanent magnetism.]

Next, I joined the Harvard cyclotron group to learn some nuclear physics. At the end of my term in the Society of Fellows I obtained a tenured faculty position [Associate Professor of Applied Physics] in the Division of Engineering and Applied Physics in July 1951. [The division had just been established, with Professor Van Vleck serving as its first dean.] There was no vacancy in the Physics Department, where R.V. Pound, E.M. Purcell and N.F. Ramsey already directed experimental research programs in magnetic resonance.

Research in solid state physics was to be carried out in the Division. I was glad to return to NMR and apply its techniques to the study of solids. Although the NMR enterprise had grown tremendously during the intervening years 1949 to 1951, I found that many nuggets remained to be unearthed.[203]

The mental picture of a lone prospector finding nuggets is also suggestive of the way Bloembergen liked to work. "I preferred," he said, "the smaller scale experiments of spectroscopy, where an individual, or a few researchers at most, can master all aspects of the problem."

> I welcomed this opportunity [Bloembergen noted] to turn away from the questions of nuclear physics . . . I much preferred the smaller scale experiments. Significant results could be obtained without working with a large team, without the need of large central facilities or huge budgets. There was an immediate connection with the electromagnetic and mechanical properties of matter. The research also had many points of contact with electronics, solid state devices and other aspects of applied physics, which in turn produced many connections with individuals working in industrial and governmental research organizations. The questions of physics which occupied me were not as fundamental and fashionable as those of weak and strong interactions in elementary particle physics or gravitational interactions in astrophysics, but they were

both intellectually stimulating and relevant to the needs of a technological society.[204]

Bloembergen now acquired graduate students and post-doctoral research fellows and his role changed from carrying out experiments with his own hands to the conception and design of new lines of investigation. Concentrating on nuclear spins as a probe for the structure of solids, Bloembergen and his NMR group found that nuclear quadrupole interactions play an important role in alloys and imperfect ionic crystals. The anisotropy of the Knight shift was discovered in non-cubic metals. Indirect electron-coupled nuclear spin interactions were demonstrated in metals and insulators. Bloembergen and his collaborators also determined that different relaxation and energy exchange processes occur in more complex magnetic systems, including ferromagnetics, and that cross-relaxation between lithium and fluorine spin systems is described by cross-relaxation times, intermediate between T_1 and T_2. The influence of an externally applied electric field on nuclear spin resonances was also discovered and explained.

Bloembergen's life as a professor was, of course, rather different from his life as a student, although his hard work in interesting science continued. He participated regularly in national and international meetings. His contacts with the rapidly growing number of NMR scientists quickly multiplied and he became a consultant to government and industrial research organizations. He was elected as a correspondent of the Royal Dutch Academy of Arts and Sciences in 1956 and was elected a member of the National Academy of Sciences in Washington, DC in 1959. It falls outside the scope of this book to analyze all of Bloembergen's NMR activities in detail, but the bibliography listed in the appendix reveals his further contributions to the field.

From NMR to Masers, Lasers and Nonlinear Optics

The biggest nugget Bloembergen unearthed in his work on relaxation phenomena in NMR and electron paramagnetic resonance (EPR) was the pumping scheme to achieve continuous wave maser action in crystals.

It is fitting that a Dutchman would develop such a pump. "God made the world," goes the saying, "with the exception of Holland, which was made by the Dutch." Without taking anything away from the Creator, it is true that in the 1930s, the Dutch, seeing that the Almighty hadn't chosen to deliver them overnight from the invasive Zuider Zee as He had the children of Israel from Pharaoh's army at the Red Sea, decided to pump thousands of acres of their sea dry, lowering it one centimeter per day over a period of 12 years until it became arable cropland. In fact, H.A. Lorentz, who is remembered by physicists, among other notable achievements, for his interpretation of the Zeeman effect, is revered in Holland for his leadership in reclaiming the land under the Zuider Zee.

Although pumping out the Zuider Zee may be viewed as a bigger project than pumping some atoms from one level to another, it may well be argued that the impact of the second pump is far greater than that of the first. This claim becomes even more persuasive if one considers the example cited by Bloembergen in his Nobel lecture on December 8, 1981.

Lasers are sources of coherent light, characterized by a high degree of monochromaticity, high directionality, and high intensity or brightness. To illustrate this last property, consider a small ruby laser with an active volume of 1 cubic centimeter. In the Q-switched mode it can emit about 10^{18} photons at 694-nanometer wavelength in about 10^{-8} second. Because the beam is diffraction limited, it can readily be focused onto an area of 10^{-6} square centimeter, about 10 optical wavelengths in diameter. The resulting peak flux density is 10^{13} watts per square centimeter. Whereas 0.1 joule is a small amount of energy, equal to that consumed by a 100-watt light bulb, or to the heat produced by a human body, each one-thousandth of a second, the power flux density of 10 terawatts per square centimeter is awesome. It can be grasped by noting that the total power produced by all electrical generating stations on the earth is about 1 terawatt.[205]

A pumping scheme that contributes to such awesome power cannot, when viewed in these terms, be considered small scale.

Every maser (an acronym for *M*icrowave *A*mplification by *S*timulated *E*mission of *R*adiation) and laser (an acronym for *L*ight *A*mplification by *S*timulated *E*mission of *R*adiation) uses a pumping mechanism to stimulate emission of either microwave or visible-light radiation in amplified, coherent form. The seed for both types of amplifiers was planted by Albert Einstein in 1916 when he published a proof of Planck's law and, in the process, provided new insights into the emission and absorption of light from atoms and molecules.

Although additional contributions had been made in the intervening years, Edward Purcell and Robert Pound had helped push open the door to masers and lasers in 1951 when they demonstrated that they could invert spin populations, making the system an emitter of radiation rather than an absorber, and introducing the idea, then considered heretical, of negative absolute temperatures.[206] A few years later, in 1956, their Harvard colleague, Norman Ramsey, would provide the theoretical foundations for such a system.[207] Two years earlier, however, maser action had already been demonstrated experimentally in a molecular beam apparatus utilizing ammonium molecules by Charles Townes and co-workers at Columbia University in New York, and by N.G. Basov and A.N. Prokhorov in Moscow.

The ammonia maser was a great amplifier in that it vastly increased the sensitivity of microwave receivers over conventional receivers, but its shortcoming was that it could amplify only a very narrow bandwidth of frequencies and it provided very limited tunability. Researchers experimented with other media, but, as two-level systems, they also had other shortcomings. First, since they were stimulated by intermittent pulses, they could not run continuously, and second, they were restricted to solids with very long relaxation times.

In her history of the development of the laser,[208] Joan Lisa Bromberg notes that in May 1956, Nicolaas Bloembergen was stimulated to provide an answer for these shortcomings by a colloquium he attended at Massachusetts Institute of Technology in which MIT physicist Woodrow Strandberg was urging his hearers to develop solid-state masers for the purpose of providing ultra-low-noise microwave amplification. At the time, in addition to his work at Harvard, Bloembergen was a consultant for Lincoln Laboratory, which was working to provide the Department of Defense with radar, communications and computer systems, and for him, the benefits of such an amplifier were clear.

For several weeks, Bloembergen considered ways to overcome the disadvantages associated with two-level masers and then on June 12 and 13, the breakthrough came. His June 12 entry in his notebook reads in part: "Got an idea. Overhauser effect may be used to obtain negative temperatures under certain conditions." That statement is followed by three horizontal lines separated by two equal spaces and another note: "Equal splitting won't do."[209]

Early on, Bloembergen had seen the merits of a prediction by Allan Overhauser, a postdoctoral student at the University of Illinois, who had promoted the idea of spin resonance saturation to dramatically increase nuclear polarization in metals. Just as there were those who had felt that the Purcell-Pound paper on negative absolute temperatures violated the Second Law of Thermodynamics, now there were those who felt Overhauser was doing the same. Bloembergen, however, was not among them, and he drew from the Overhauser effect to develop a three-level continuous action maser.

Bloembergen's notebook entry on June 13 shows three more horizontal lines, this time unevenly spaced, and the triumphant statements, "This will do it! I am bound to get stimulated emission either at frequency v_{32} or v_{21}."[210]

With his unequally-spaced, three-level approach, Bloembergen proposed pumping from the lowest level to the highest level, to equalize the population in Level 1 and the population in Level 3, but giving both of them larger populations than Level 2. He could then get stimulated emission by radiation from Level 3 to Level 2 or, when Level 2 had a larger population than Level 1, by radiation from 2 to 1. By separating the pumping action from the masing action, continuous masing could be achieved.

The next hurdle was to find a suitable material that would allow such transitions, and this Bloembergen overcame by positioning the internal axis of the crystals he was considering at an angle to the direction of the external magnetic field, an idea that harked back to his experiments with the magic angle δ during his pre-PhD days at Harvard.

Not long after Bloembergen came up with his three-level approach, H.E. Derrick Scovil of Bell Laboratories independently came up with a similar approach, which he prepared to announce in *Physical Review.* When Bloembergen, who was hoping to patent his idea, heard about Scovil's work, and when Bell Laboratories, who had their own plans to profit from the device, heard about Bloembergen's work, they agreed to meet to head off a possible confrontation. As a result of their meeting, at which Bloembergen presented his results, Bell Laboratories agreed to apply for the patent for Bloembergen and both parties agreed they would work independently and in competition with one another to produce the first three-level working maser. Scovil, who recognized the priority of Bloembergen's work, did not send his paper to *Physical Review.*

The concept of the three-level solid-state maser developed by Bloembergen was published in *Physical Review* in 1956.[211] The device was soon reduced to practice by many different groups, but in December 1956, Scovill and his associates at Bell Laboratories became the first to operate a three-level maser. It has been used as an ultra-low-noise receiver in radar systems and radiotelescopes.

Incidentally, it is interesting to note another connection between Edward Purcell and Nicolaas Bloembergen. It was Purcell and Harold Ewen who discovered the 21-centimeter hydrogen line in outer space and it was Bloembergen who developed the maser that was used in a Harvard radiotelescope to study that line in the years that followed. Solid-state masers are still operative in the deep-space satellite tracking stations of NASA and in transatlantic microwave communications systems. Today, solid-state masers are still used to amplify the faint radio signals received from outer space, but they never attained widespread application. Microwave parametric devices, which do not require cooling to liquid helium temperature, are the most widely-used microwave receivers.

Bloembergen's principle of population inversion by pumping in multilevel systems, however, was soon afterward used in lasers. It was incorporated by Arthur Schawlow and Charles Townes in the design of their laser and the first operating laser, a ruby laser designed by Theodore Maiman, was also directly based on Bloembergen's pumping scheme.

> Rightly or wrongly [said Bloembergen], I had held the opinion that it would be impossible for an academic laboratory without previous specialization in optics to compete successfully in the invention and realization of lasers. As a matter of fact, nearly all laser types were first developed in industrial laboratories. When the laser art was developing rapidly in the years between 1960 and 1962, I recognized that my laboratory should also exploit the new research opportunities that presented themselves. It was decided to study the properties of matter at very high light intensities. This choice proved very fruitful and led the development of the new subfield of physics, now commonly called "nonlinear optics."[212]

In the 19th century, James Clerk Maxwell had explained to most everyone's satisfaction the nature and behavior of electromagnetic radiation. Those same formulations, however, did not always apply to the electric and magnetic intensities ushered in by the laser, and a new field of study, nonlinear optics, was created.

"With the development of various types of lasers," Nicolaas Bloembergen stated in his Nobel lecture, "the stage was set for a rapid evolution of the study of nonlinear optical phenomena."[213] No one has been more at the forefront of this area of study than Bloembergen, as a simple comparison of the development of scientific laws for linear and nonlinear optics quickly reveals.

From the time Hero of Alexandria formulated the law of reflection for linear optics in the first century until Snell formulated the law of refraction in 1621, more than one-and-a-half millenia had passed. Nearly 200 more years would pass before Fresnel formulated the theory for comparing the intensity of reflected and refracted light. Only 10 years went by, however, before Hamilton and Lloyd provided the theory and experimental proof for conical refraction in linear optics.

For nonlinear optics, however, the corresponding formulations have occurred much more quickly, and Bloembergen has participated in every one of them. Three of them, the law of reflection, the law of refraction, and the intensity comparison of reflected and refracted light were all provided by Bloembergen and his associate, P.S. Pershan,[214] in 1962. The fourth, the theory for conical refraction, was provided by Bloembergen and H. Shih[215] in 1969, and the fifth, the experimental proof for conical refraction, by Bloembergen and A.J. Schell[216] in 1977. From the beginning of these formulations until their completion in 1977, only 15 years had passed compared to 1.8 millennia for linear optics.

When Bloembergen was asked how he made such quick strides forward in nonlinear optics, he responded with a smile:

> How did it happen [that Onnes discovered superconductivity]? He just took a high-school textbook and, after every paragraph, he asked, "What happens at low temperature?" So he measured the resistance of metals at low temperature and, of course, lead became superconductive. And he did the same with vibrations. "What happens to sound at low temperature?"
>
> I had a colleague here at Harvard who was almost three times my age when I arrived, [Percy] Bridgeman. He was the expert on high pressure and he measured everything under the sun at high pressures. And he got a Nobel Prize in '46.
>
> So when the lasers came along, I said I've got to measure any optical property at high intensity and that gives rise to the birth of nonlinear optics. And it was a very fertile field. So I took a textbook and, after every paragraph, I said, "What happens at high intensity?"[217]

In 1962, Bloembergen and his associates, J.A. Armstrong, J. Ducuing and P.S. Pershan, published a comprehensive paper[218] which contains the general framework for the description of many nonlinear optical phenomena. These ideas were extended into a monograph by Bloembergen in 1965.[219]

Although it was Bloembergen's idea for the pumping mechanism that dramatically improved the maser and which, when lasers came along, made them much more practical, he is quick to discount those who would take credit for the theory of the laser away from Charles Townes and his brother-in-law, Arthur Schawlow (Schawlow later shared the 1981 Nobel Prize with Bloembergen for his work with laser spectroscopy). Nevertheless, Bloembergen's pumping scheme was, to use Bloembergen's word, "absolutely" basic to both the maser and the laser. Although the Nobel Committee did not explicitly recognize this important contribution, Bloembergen's lecture before the Swedish Academy of Science gave him the opportunity to make the connection for them and he is philosophical about not receiving the Nobel Prize for his continuous-action pump:

The Nobel Committee has a rule that, at most, three people can share [a Nobel prize]. In '64, the prize went to Charlie Townes who was obviously No. 1 in the maser field and to two Russians, Nikolai Basov and Alexander Prokhorov, who independently conceived the first maser.

But then there was Townes' close collaborator and colleague in Schawlow, and there was me. So after another 17 years, in '81, they decided to have us share the prize.

Clearly, the Nobel Committee had to compromise in 1981. Schawlow and I shared one-half of the prize for laser spectroscopy, the other half was awarded to Kai Siegbahn for electron spectroscopy, a rather unrelated field. I made it clear in my Nobel lecture that my significant contributions were really in the pumping scheme and in nonlinear spectroscopy.

I'm sure that Schawlow had been on the nomination for years and I was, too. That's the way the cookie crumbles. The main requirement is to get old enough, to live long. Norman Ramsey got it at an even older age. I was only 61 [said Bloembergen]. But Purcell got it when he was under 40. And that is not all that nice, because you're too young and you peak too soon.

Some people who want to detract can say that the proposal for a laser by Schawlow and Townes put the idea of parallel mirrors [the Fabry-Pérot resonator] and the pumping mechanism together, but I think that is not fair to them. They fully deserved all the honors they got. They proposed the laser and then the first laser was built by Dr. [Theodore H.] Maiman in 1960. And then there was Mr. [Gordon] Gould, who owns an important patent which was much discussed in the newspapers. Gould was more aware of the applications than some others.

I think it's the combination. I think my contribution of suggesting the pumping mechanism for condensed matter is very important. I think a detailed history shows that the whole field really exploded after the pumping mechanism had been proposed and worked.[220]

Bloembergen is very happy and fascinated by the fact that his work in both NMR and nonlinear optics have led to important technological applications, not foreseen by him. His study of relaxation times in water, to name one, became a cornerstone for magnetic resonance scanning of the human body for the detection and diagnosis of disease.

He was the first to determine quantitatively the T_1 and T_2 relaxation times for a host of different substances, including pure water, ice, ionized water and glycerine. Bloembergen's findings became the take-off point for the efforts in the early 1970s by a medical researcher, Dr. Raymond V. Damadian at Downstate Medical Center in Brooklyn, to determine if the water of cancerous tissue was quantitatively different from the water of normal tissue.

The seminal event that initiated magnetic resonance scanning was the discovery by Dr. Damadian that the NMR signal from cancerous tissue was recognizably different, based on T_1 and T_2 values, from the NMR signal from normal tissue. Prior to this discovery, no one had considered nuclear magnetic resonance as the basis for a medical scanner that would detect disease.

The NMR scanning signal is the starting point for all NMR images. NMR images are simple constructs of scanning signals obtained from cross-sectional slices of the human body. Today's MRI scanners make extensive use of differences in T_1 and T_2 in various tissues to detect tumors in the brain and other parts of the human body.

Damadian published his idea under the title, "Tumor Detection by Nuclear Magnetic Resonance" in the March 1971 issue of *Science* magazine. "In principle," he wrote, "nuclear magnetic resonance (NMR) techniques combine many of the desirable features of an external probe for the detection of internal cancer."[221]

"T_1 and T_2, everybody uses those quantities," said Professor Bloembergen. "Dr. Damadian's contribution was to apply it to living tissues. That's the big step and that's not so easy."

I knew that Damadian was talking about it and working on it in the early '70s. And, you know, we sort of wished him luck and waited to see what would come out. I was very fascinated to see that cancerous tissue would have different relaxation times [from non-cancerous tissue].

Dr. Damadian deserves credit for calling attention to the fact that differences in NMR relaxation times T_1 and T_2 in human cells existed and he used this to determine whether the cell was normal or diseased (cancerous). He further demonstrated that such measurements can be made on a living human body. He produced the first body scans.

A second important step was that of Dr. Paul Lauterbur who combined Damadian's results and faster data acquisition with CAT scanning techniques. The latter had been developed by Professors Hounsfeld and Cormack, who received the Nobel Prize for its application in X-ray diagnostics.

In my opinion, Dr. Raymond Damadian's contribution is as important and as significant as the second step made by Lauterbur.[222]

Unwittingly, Bloembergen would also participate in another significant, but little known way, to the evolution of MR imaging. Shortly after Lauterbur came up with the imaging method which he called "zeugmatography," he was explaining his imaging approach at a conference in Bombay, India in December 1972, a meeting at which Bloembergen was also in attendance. The projection-reconstruction method Lauterbur was suggesting, however, seemed unnecessarily slow to Bloembergen and he raised the question to Lauterbur, "Why not use pulsing?"

Coincidentally, there were three others in attendance at the conference who would come to be major contributors to the science of MR imaging: E. Raymond Andrews, the chairman of the physics department at the University of Nottingham, along with Waldo Hinshaw and Paul Darbyshire, also from the University of Nottingham. On the way back to London, Hinshaw, prompted by Bloembergen's inquiry of Lauterbur, began discussing ways that Bloembergen's idea could be used. As a result, Hinshaw developed the pulse-driven sensitive line or multiple sensitive point method and soon afterward, another colleague of his at Nottingham, Peter Mansfield, developed the faster, pulse-driven line scan technique.

Giving Credit Where Credit Is Due

Although Bloembergen made major experimental and theoretical contributions to the understanding of NMR relaxation, he was not recognized for his NMR contributions with a Nobel Prize.

The record is clear [said Bloembergen] that Purcell got the Nobel Prize for it and he deserves it. I was his student. I did a lot of good work, but then I had my students who did a lot of the work in nonlinear optics, so I don't feel too bad about it.

It was quite clear to me that if I really wanted to be a father of something, I couldn't be the father of magnetic resonance, so I had to do something else. If you're going to call me the father of anything, I wouldn't mind being called the father of nonlinear optics. That's what I got the Nobel Prize for.[223]

Was this a conscious decision, to choose an area where his contributions would have a greater chance of leading to a Nobel Prize?

Well, as an ambitious young scientist, you always think about it some [he said]. The main thing is that the most excitement [occurs] while you do it, finding things that nobody has ever seen before. Having it recognized is nice. It depends on what age you get it. I got it late enough so that it didn't change my personal life that much. It's nice to get that recognition.[224]

The recognition began arriving early in Bloembergen's illustrious career. In 1957, he was named Gordon McKay Professor of Applied Physics, a chair he held until 1980. For six years of that period, he was also Rumford Professor of Physics. In 1980, he was named Gerhard Gade University Professor.

In his four-and-a-half decades as a faculty member of Harvard University, Bloembergen has also had the opportunity to live in many parts of the world. In 1957, he was a Guggenheim Fellow and visiting lecturer at the École Normale Supérieure in Paris; from 1964 to 1965, visiting professor at the University of California in Berkeley; in 1973, Lorentz guest professor at the University of Leiden and visiting scientist at the Philips Research Laboratories in the Netherlands; in the fall of 1979, Raman Visiting Professor at Bangalore, India; in the first semester of 1980, Von Humboldt Senior Scientist in the *Institut für Quantum Optik* in Garching, near Munich, Germany, as well as visiting professor at the *Collège de France* in Paris. He has also had two exchange visits to what was then the Soviet Union and three visits to the People's Republic of China.

In addition to the 1981 Nobel Prize in physics, he has been awarded the following: 1) the Oliver Buckley Prize, awarded by the American Physical Society in 1958; 2) the Morris E. Liebman Award, awarded by the Institute of Radio Engineers in 1959; 3) the Stuart Ballantine Medal, awarded by the Franklin Institute, Philadelphia in 1961; 4) the National Medal of Science, awarded by the President of the United States in 1974; 5) the Lorentz Medal, awarded by the *Koninklijke Akademie van Wetenschappen*,

Amsterdam in 1979; 6) the Frederic Ives Medal, awarded by the Optical Society of America, in 1979; and 7) the Medal of Honor, awarded by the Institute of Electrical and Electronics Engineers (IEEE) in 1983.

He has also been a correspondent of the *Koninklijke Akademie van Wetenschappen* in Amsterdam since 1956, a fellow in the American Academy of Arts and Sciences since 1956; a member of the National Academy of Sciences in Washington, DC since 1959; a foreign honorary member of the Indian Academy of Sciences in Bangalore since 1978; and *Associé Étranger* of the *Académie des Sciences* in Paris since 1980.

In 1975, when Bloembergen summarized his career in an unpublished autobiography, he stated that his academic career at Harvard University had afforded him "not only the stimulation of interaction with many distinguished colleagues but also with the younger generations of students and postdoctoral fellows." (He has worked with 57 PhD candidates and a similar number of postdoctoral research fellows.)

> Such contacts [Bloembergen stated] help in keeping the aging mind alert. I enjoy the teaching in the moderate amounts required. It forces one to obtain a deeper understanding of the fundamentals by exposing them to successive bright new generations of students. I have taught courses in solid state physics, electron physics, magnetism, electromagnetic theory, statistical mechanics, quantum mechanics, quantum electronics and nonlinear optics. The freedom to participate in summer schools and conferences, and in consulting activities with governmental and industrial organizations also enhances the professional life. So do, of course, the membership and meetings of professional societies. The sabbatical leaves afford the opportunity to travel farther and live in a different geographic environment for a longer period of time.[225]

The combination of activities Bloembergen mentioned in 1975 have obviously worked in keeping his mind alert. Twenty years later, although he is now retired and is now Gerhard Gade Professor Emeritus, there is little evidence of tapering off in his schedule. When he isn't traveling internationally—which is still frequent—there's a good chance that he is in his office on the third floor of Pierce Hall, where he continues to keep in touch with and participate in what is happening in the world of physics. ∎

REFERENCE NOTES:

1. F. Bloch, "Heisenberg and the early days of quantum mechanics," *Physics Today*, December 1976, 25.

2. Abraham Pais, *Inward Bound: Of Matter and Forces in the Physical World*, (New York: Oxford University Press, 1986), 362.

3. Nicolaas Bloembergen, interview by James Mattson, September 1988.

4. Ibid.

5. N. Bloembergen, E.M. Purcell, and R.V. Pound, "Relaxation effects in nuclear magnetic absorption," *Physical Review* **73,** (1948), 679-712.

6. N. Bloembergen, *Nuclear Magnetic Relaxation*, (New York: W.A. Benjamin, 1961).

7. N. Bloembergen, interview by James Mattson, 19 July 1994.

8. Ibid.

9. Evarts Erickson, "Microwave people: Nicolaas Bloembergen," *Microwave Journal*, November 1961, 26.

10. N. Bloembergen, unpublished autobiography prepared for National Academy of Sciences, March 1975, 4.

11. Simon Schama, *The Embarrassment of Riches*, (New York: Alfred A. Knopf, 1987).

12. N. Bloembergen, interview by Mattson, 19 July 1994.

13. Schama, *The Embarrassment of Riches*, 334.

14. N. Bloembergen, interview by Mattson, 19 July 1994.

15. Frank S. Mead, *Handbook of Denominations in the United States*, (Nashville: Abingdon, 1980), 167-173.

16. N. Bloembergen, interview by Mattson, 19 July 1994.

17. Bloembergen, autobiography, 2.

18. Ibid., 2.

19. N. Bloembergen, interview by Mattson, 19 July 1994.

20. Bloembergen, autobiography, 2.

21. Bloembergen, autobiography, 2.

22. Erickson, "Microwave people: Nicolaas Bloembergen," 26.

23. Bloembergen, autobiography, 4.

24. N. Bloembergen, interview by Mattson, 19 July 1994.

25. N. Bloembergen, interview by Mattson, November 1992.

26. Bloembergen, autobiography, 3.

27. Erickson, "Microwave people: Nicolaas Bloembergen," 26.

28. N. Bloembergen, interview by Mattson, 19 July 1994.

29. Ibid.

30. Ibid.

31. Gerhard L. Weinberg, *The Foreign Policy of Hitler's Germany: Diplomatic Revolution in Europe, 1933-36* (Chicago: 1970), 245; quoted by Alan Bullock in *Hitler and Stalin: Parallel Lives*, (New York: Alfred A. Knopf, 1992), 530.

32. Hendrik Riemens, *The Netherlands: Story of a Free People*, (New York: Eagle Books, 1944), 286-287.

33. N. Bloembergen, interview by Mattson, 19 July 1994.

34. Ibid.

35. Pais, *Inward Bound: Of Matter and Forces in the Physical World*, 209.

36. Alan Bullock, *Hitler and Stalin: Parallel Lives*, (New York: Alfred A. Knopf, 1992), 566.

37. Rhodes, *The Making of the Atomic Bomb*, (New York: Simon and Schuster, 1988), 236.

38. Rhodes, *The Making of the Atomic Bomb*, 245; quoted from Winston Churchill, *The Gathering Storm*, (Houghton Mifflin, 1948), 301.

39. Riemens, *The Netherlands: Story of a Free People*, 291-292.

40. N. Bloembergen, interview by Mattson, 19 July 1994.

41. Roger H. Stuewer, "Bringing the news of fission to America," *Physics Today*, October 1985, 49-56.

42. Bloembergen, autobiography, 6.

43. L.S. Ornstein and W.R. van Wyk, *Zeitschrift für Physik* **49**, (1928), 315; R. de L. Kronig, *Naturw.* **16**, (1928), 335; also *Naturw.* **18**, (1930), 205.

44. Katherine Russell Sopka, *Quantum Physics in America*, (Tomash Publishers, 1988), 325.

45. G.A.W. Rutgers, J.C. Kluyver, and N. Bloembergen, "On the straggling of Po-a-particles in solid matter," *Physica* **7**, (1940) 669-672.

46. N. Bloembergen, autobiographical sketch, *Les Prix Nobel 1981*, (Stockholm: Nobel Foundation, 1982), 59.

47. Bullock, *Hitler and Stalin*, 671.

48. William L. Shirer, *The Rise and Fall of the Third Reich*, (New York: Simon and Schuster, 1960), 721.

49. Riemens, *The Netherlands: Story of a Free People*, 295.

50. Ibid.

51. Shirer, *The Rise and Fall of the Third Reich*, 722.

52. Riemens, *The Netherlands: Story of a Free People*, 296.

53. Shirer, *The Rise and Fall of the Third Reich*, 722.

54. Riemens, *The Netherlands: Story of a Free People*, 3.

55. Ibid., 316.

56. Ibid., 109.

57. Bullock, *Hitler and Stalin*, Appendix, 989.

58.. Bullock, *Hitler and Stalin*, 810.

59. Riemens, *The Netherlands: Story of a Free People*, 317.

60. N. Bloembergen, interview by Mattson, 19 July 1994.

61. Ibid.

62. Ibid.

63. Ibid.

64. Bloembergen, autobiography, 6.

65. N. Bloembergen, interview by Mattson, 19 July 1994

66. Ibid.

67. Ibid.

68. Ibid.

69. Shirer, *The Rise and Fall of the Third Reich*, 946-947.

70. Ibid., 943.

71. N. Bloembergen, interview by Mattson, 19 July 1994.

72. Bloembergen, autobiography, 6.

73. N. Bloembergen, interview by Mattson, 19 July 1994.

74. Ibid.

75. Ibid.

76. Bloembergen, autobiography, 7.

77. N. Bloembergen, interview by Mattson, 19 July 1994.

78. Hans Koning, *Amsterdam*, (Amsterdam: Time-Life International, 1977), 139.

79. N. Bloembergen, interview by Mattson, 19 July 1994.

80. Ibid.

81. Koning, *Amsterdam*, 128.

82. Pais, *Inward Bound*, 448-449.

83. N. Bloembergen, interview by Mattson, 19 July 1994.

84. Bloembergen, autobiographical sketch, 60.

85. Bloembergen, autobiography, 7.

86. N. Bloembergen, interview by Mattson, 19 July 1994.

87. Ibid.

88. Erickson, "Microwave people: Nicolaas Bloembergen," 95.

89. N. Bloembergen, interview by James Mattson, 1989.

90. Ibid.

91. Samuel A. Goudsmit, *Alsos*, first published in 1947, republished by Tomash Publishers and the American Institute of Physics, 1983, 46-49.

92. Bloembergen, autobiography, 6.

93. N. Bloembergen, interview by Mattson, 19 July 1994.

94. Ibid.

95. Ibid.

96. Ibid.

97. Ibid.

98. Ibid.

99. Ibid.

100. Ibid.

101. N. Bloembergen, interview by Joan Bromberg and Paul L. Kelley for Laser History Project, American Institute of Physics, College Park, MD, 2.

102. N. Bloembergen, "My early years in NMR, 1946 to 1948," unpublished, 1993, 2.

103. J.C. Street and E.C. Stevenson, "New evidence for the existence of a particle of mass intermediate between the proton and electron," *Physical Review* **52**, (1937) 1003; mentioned by John S. Rigden in "Quantum states and precession: the two discoveries of NMR," *Reviews of Modern Physics* **58**, (1986), 442.

104. N. Bloembergen, interview by James Mattson, November 1988.

105. John S. Rigden, *Rabi: Scientist and Citizen*, (New York: Basic Books, 1987), 164.

106. N. Bloembergen, interview by Mattson, November 1988.

107. Bloembergen, "My early years in NMR, 1946 to 1948," 2.

108. N. Bloembergen and J.M.W. Milatz, "The development of an a.c. fotoelectric amplifier with a.c. galvanometer," *Physica* **11**, (1946), 449-64.

109. Bloembergen, interview by Bromberg and Kelley for Laser History Project, 3.

110. N. Bloembergen, personal communication to James Mattson, 16 November 1994.

111. *Five Years at the Radiation Laboratory*, originally published in 1946 by the Massachusetts Institute of Technology, copyright 1947, and reprinted in 1991 for the 1991 IEEE International Microwave Theory and Techniques Society Symposium, 34.

112. Sopka, *Quantum Physics in America*, 35.

113. Bloembergen, "My early years in NMR, 1946 to 1948," 2.

114. Bloembergen, autobiography, 10.

115. N. Bloembergen, interview by Mattson, 19 July 1994.

116. E.M. Purcell, interview by Katherine R. Sopka, American Institute of Physics, College Park, MD, 29.

117. Bloembergen, "My early years in NMR, 1946 to 1948," 3.

118. N. Bloembergen, interview by Mattson, November 1988.

119. Bloembergen, "My early years in NMR, 1946 to 1948," 3.

120. N. Bloembergen, *Nuclear Magnetic Resonance*, (Utrecht: Drukkerij Fa. Schotanus & Jens, 1948), 18.

121. Cornelis J. Gorter, interview by John L. Heilbron, American Institute of Physics, Center for History of Physics, College Park, MD, 1.

122. Ibid., 2.

123. Ibid.,12.

124. C.J. Gorter, "Bad luck in attempts to make scientific discoveries," *Physics Today*, January 1967, 76.

125. Bloembergen, "My early years in NMR, 1946 to 1948," 2.

126. Gorter, "Bad luck in attempts to make scientific discoveries," 76.

127. Ibid.

128. Ibid., 78.

129. Ibid.

130. N. Bloembergen, interview by Mattson, November 1988.

131. Hendrik B.G. Casimir, *Haphazard Reality: Half a Century of Science,* (New York: Harper and Row, 1983), 175; quoted by Rigden in "Quantum states and precession: the two discoveries of NMR," 442.

132. I.I. Rabi, "Space quantization in a gyrating magnetic field," *Physical Review* **51,** (1937), 652-654.

133. N.F. Ramsey, "Early magnetic resonance experiments: roots and offshoots," *Physics Today,* October 1993, 40.

134. Rigden, *Rabi: Scientist and Citizen,* 96.

135. I.I. Rabi, J.R. Zacharias, S. Millman, and P. Kusch, "A new method of measuring nuclear magnetic moment," *Physical Review* **53,** (1938), 318.

136. Gorter, "Bad luck in attempts to make scientific discoveries," 79.

137. Ibid.

138. Ibid.

139. N.F. Ramsey, "Origins of magnetic resonance," (1993), unpublished, 4.

140. Rigden, "Quantum states and precession: the two discoveries of NMR," 442.

141. Bloembergen, "My early years in NMR, 1946 to 1948," 11.

142. N. Bloembergen, "Retrospective comments on magnetic resonance and relaxation," *Concepts in Magnetic Resonance* **6,** (1994), 185.

143. N. Bloembergen, interview by Mattson, November 1988.

144. Bloembergen, "Retrospective comments on magnetic resonance and relaxation," 186.

145. N. Bloembergen, interview by Bromberg and Kelley for Laser History Project, 6.

146. Rigden, "Quantum states and precession: the two discoveries of NMR," 445.

147. N. Bloembergen, interview by Bromberg and Kelley for Laser History Project, 7.

148. N. Bloembergen, personal communication to Mattson, 16 November 1994.

149. F. Bloch, interview by Charles Weiner, August 15, 1968, American Institute of Physics, Center for the History of Physics, College Park, MD, 43.

150. Anatole Abragam, *Reflections of a Physicist,* (Oxford: Clarendon Press, 1986), 9-10.

151. N. Bloembergen, interview by Bromberg and Kelley for Laser History Project, 4.

152. Ibid.

153. Ibid.

154. Ibid., 5.

155. Ibid., 5, 3.

156. Ibid., 3.

157. Ibid., 6.

158. George E. Pake, interview by James Mattson, 27 January 1993.

159. Ibid.

160. Ibid.

161. Ibid.

162. N. Bloembergen, interview by Mattson, November 1988.

163. Ibid.

164. Bloembergen, "Retrospective comments on magnetic resonance and relaxation," 186.

165. N. Bloembergen, interview by Mattson, November 1988.

166. Ibid.

167. E.M. Purcell, N. Bloembergen, and R.V. Pound, "Resonance absorption by nuclear magnetic moments in a single crystal of CaF_2," *Physical Review* **70,** (1946), 988.

168. N. Bloembergen, interview by Bromberg and Kelley for Laser History Project, 4.

169. Ibid., 5.

170. Purcell, Pound, and Bloembergen, "Nuclear magnetic resonance absorption in hydrogen gas," *Physical Review* **70,** (1946), 986-987.

171. Purcell, Pound and Bloembergen, "Nuclear magnetic resonance absorption in hydrogen gas," 988.

172. Bloembergen, "My early years in NMR, 1946 to 1948," 1993, 5.

173. Ibid., 6.

174. Ibid.

175. Ibid., 7.

176. Ibid.

177. George E. Pake, interview by Mattson, 27 January 1993.

178. Bloembergen, "My early years in NMR, 1946 to 1948," 7-8.

179. Ibid., 8.

180. Ibid.

181. Ibid., 8-9.

182. N. Bloembergen, E.M. Purcell, and R.V. Pound, "Nuclear magnetic relaxation," *Nature* **160**, (1947), 475-476.

183. Bloembergen, "My early years in NMR, 1946 to 1948," 9.

184. Ibid., 10.

185. N. Bloembergen, interview by Mattson, November 1988.

186. Bloembergen, "My early years in NMR, 1946 to 1948," 10.

187. Ibid.

188. Bloembergen, "Retrospective comments on magnetic resonance and relaxation," 187.

189. N. Bloembergen, "Nuclear magnetic relaxation in metallic copper," *Physica* **15**, (1949), 588-592.

190. Bloembergen, "My early years in NMR, 1946 to 1948," 11.

191. N. Bloembergen, interview by Mattson, 19 July 1994.

192. N. Bloembergen, "Fine structure of the magnetic resonance line of protons in $CuSO_4 \cdot 5H_2O$," *Physica* **16**, (1950), 95-112; abstract published, *Physical Review* **75**, (1949), 1326.

193. N. Bloembergen, interview by Mattson, 19 July 1994.

194. Ibid.

195. Ibid.

196. Bloembergen, *Nuclear Magnetic Relaxation*.

197. Bloembergen, "My early years in NMR, 1946 to 1948," 12.

198. Ibid.

199. Anatole Abragam, *Time Reversal: An Autobiography*, (Oxford: Clarendon Press, 1989), 44.

200. Bloembergen, autobiographical sketch, 60.

201. Bloembergen, autobiography, 17.

202. N. Bloembergen, interview by Mattson, 19 July 1994.

203. Bloembergen, "My early years in NMR, 1946 to 1948," 13.

204. Bloembergen, autobiography, 13.

205. N. Bloembergen, "Nonlinear optics and spectroscopy," *Science* **216**, (1982), 1057.

206. E.M. Purcell and R.V. Pound, "A nuclear spin system at negative temperature," *Physical Review* **81**, (1951), 279-280.

207. N.F. Ramsey, "Thermodynamics and statistical mechanics at negative absolute temperatures," *Physical Review* **103**, (1956), 20-28.

208. Joan Lisa Bromberg, *The Laser in America, 1950-1970*, (Cambridge, MA: The MIT Press, 1991), 31-41.

209. Ibid., 36.

210. Ibid.

211. N. Bloembergen, "Proposal for a new type solid state maser," *Physical Review* **104**, (1956), 324-327.

212. Bloembergen, autobiography, 14.

213. Bloembergen, "Nonlinear optics and spectroscopy," 1059.

214. N. Bloembergen and P.S. Pershan, "Light waves at the boundary of nonlinear media," *Physical Review* **128,** (1962), 606-622.

215. N. Bloembergen and H. Shih, "Conical refraction in nonlinear optics," *Optics Communications* **1,** (1969), 70-73.

216. N. Bloembergen and A.J. Schell, "Laser studies of internal conical diffraction: I. Quantitative comparison of experimental and theoretical conical intensity distributions in argonite," *J. Opt. Soc. Am.* **68,** (1978), 1093-1098; N. Bloembergen and A.J. Schell, "Laser studies of internal conical diffraction: II. Intensity patterns in an optically active crystal, α-iodic acid," *J. Opt. Soc. Am.* **68,** (1978), 1098-1106; N. Bloembergen and A.J. Schell, "Laser studies of internal conical diffraction: III. Second harmonic conical refraction in α-iodic acid," *Physical Review* **A18,** (1978), 2592-2602.

217. N. Bloembergen, interview by Mattson, November 1992.

218. N. Bloembergen with J.A. Armstrong, J. Ducuing and P.S. Pershan, "Interactions between light waves in a nonlinear dielectric," *Physical Review* **127,** (1962), 1918-1939.

219. N. Bloembergen, *Nonlinear Optics,* (New York: W.A. Benjamin, 1965). Republished as Advanced Book Classic, Addison-Wesley, 1992.

220. N. Bloembergen, interview by Mattson, November 1992.

221. R.V. Damadian, "Tumor detection by nuclear magnetic resonance," *Science* **171,** (1971), 1151-1153.

222. N. Bloembergen, interview by Merrill Simon, April 1988.

223. N. Bloembergen, interview by Mattson, November 1992.

224. N. Bloembergen, interview by Mattson, November 1988.

225. Bloembergen, autobiography, 15.

Purely accidental discoveries of a basic nature are exceedingly rare in physics. In a sense, every unexpected result could be considered accidental, but a careful experimenter recognizes the unusual, provided it falls within his range of imagination.

—Morris H. Shamos

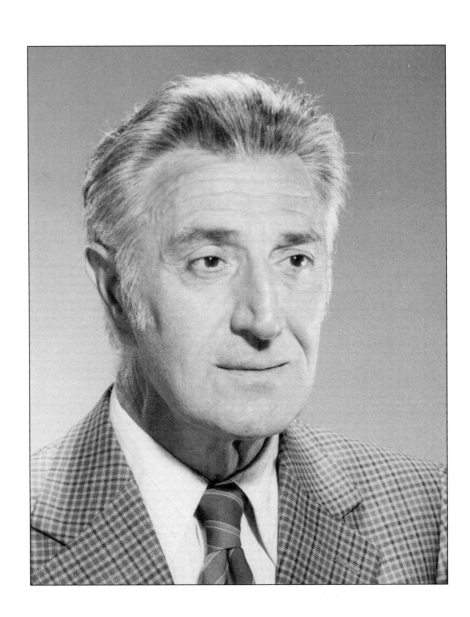

6

ERWIN L. HAHN

Discoverer of Spin Echoes and Free Induction Decay

LIKE "The Three Princes of Serendip"[1] whose amazing discoveries were unexpected by-products of their quest for a dragon-destroying secret formula, Professor Erwin Hahn has had the pleasure of making significant scientific discoveries that turned out to be more significant than the original object of his search. Perhaps most notable of these and of particular interest in the context of this book was his 1949 detection of spin echoes. First regarded by Hahn as an "annoying glitch"[2] on the screen of his oscilloscope, the silent echoes he had discovered would come to be recognized as a key contribution to the science of NMR, important both to the revolution that took place in chemical analysis in the 1960s and the on-going revolution in medical diagnosis whose foundations were laid in the 1970s.

To attribute the success of Hahn's subsequent career to a single serendipitous event would be, however, grossly unjust; his scientific contributions have been too many and their significance too great to be relegated to mere good fortune, as noted by physicist D.M.S. Bagguley of Oxford University's Clarendon Laboratory:

Hahn's contribution . . . has not been limited to the spin echo, despite his thorough and wide ranging work to establish the consequential phenomena which derive from this effect (chemical shifts, J-coupling, quadrupole resonance, population transfer techniques: the list is very long). The first demonstration of free induction decay may not excite the same surprise for students aware of the impulse response . . . methods of time domain electric circuit theory, but the whole field of modern Fourier transform spectroscopy stems from that observation. Again, the later contributions to coherent optics together with the discovery of self-induced transparency reveal a quite unique continuing ability to discover unexpected and significant experimental results.[3]

Hahn's original discovery of spin echoes should also not be described as a "fluke" or "happenstance." To do so would be to negate the creative process involved in scientific research. He would not have sighted his first nuclear echo had he not been experimenting with pulses in the first place nor would he have known what he had found had the "glitch" that he initially cursed not aroused his scientific curiosity. In the process of pursuing its source and nature, he joined the likes of Wilhelm Roentgen, who "accidentally" discovered X-rays, Alexander Fleming, who "accidentally" discovered penicillin, and a host of other curious scientific investigators who, because of their investigative persistence, have "accidentally" made our lives better.

Marriage and Misdiagnosis Led to Spin Echoes

The direction a person's life takes is influenced by factors too numerous to count, but at least two events in Hahn's early adult years can be seen to have had a direct influence on his discovery of spin echoes. The first was his marriage in 1944 and the second was a misdiagnosis by Hahn's dentist.

Deferred from the military draft for a year while a graduate student at Purdue because he was teaching GIs, Hahn had applied to work on the Manhattan Project at Los Alamos and had been accepted. In between his acceptance by Los Alamos and his move west, however, he married Marian Failing, an undergraduate student at Purdue from Terre Haute, Indiana who was learning electronics for the purpose of editing Air Force technical manuals. When he contacted Los Alamos to inquire on available housing for married couples, they withdrew their employment offer. "They had no living quarters for married, young guys like me," he said. "Therefore, I was drafted in the Navy. If I wasn't married, I would probably have gone to Los Alamos and my career would have been entirely different."[4]

The apparent setback in his scientific career was soon followed by a setback in his military career. If he was going to be in the military, Hahn figured he might as well be an officer. "In those days," he explained, "you felt you didn't make it if you weren't an officer."[5] But that was also not to be. Prior to enlisting in the Navy, Hahn had suffered for a time with a jaw infection, which a dentist had treated using a surgical procedure to drain the infected area, but had misdiagnosed as chronic osteomyelitis. At his induction physical, when asked to list on the medical history form any preexisting medical conditions, Hahn indicated he had 'chronic osteomyelitis.' Even with penicillin, which had been introduced just a few years earlier, osteomyelitis was still considered quite serious and the examining doctors told him he was physically unqualified to enter officer training. Thus, instead of graduating a few months later as a second lieutenant, junior grade, Hahn was shunted off to technical school to learn electronics.

In retrospect, his career was very much on course. "If I had become an officer," he said, "I would have just been one of these 90-day wonders and would have been shunted someplace where I wouldn't have learned anything" except "superficially, to direct other guys." Fortunately for physics, chemistry, medicine, and Hahn—"it's the best thing that could ever have happened to me,"[6] he said—he was sent to radar school where he learned about echoes and pulsing.

Five years later, he would submit an article to *Physical Review* entitled simply, "Spin Echoes."[7] It was an article that would forever change the young field of NMR. As Anatole Abragam expressed it in 1992:

> To me, during the first forty-five years of the existence of NMR, there have been in this field three (well, perhaps four) great articles (as distinct from short notes). Not important, or brilliant, or seminal, or most frequently quoted, but great. Some will say five or more, and I will not argue, but in my selection of three (or four), you will find Erwin Hahn, *Phys. Rev.,* Nov. 15, 1950. There was NMR before it, there is NMR after. It is not the same NMR.[8]

Land of Promise

In a moving 133-page autobiography completed in 1979 when she was nearly 94, Mary Weiss Hahn Guggenheim, the mother of Erwin Hahn, recalled for her family the joy and the pathos of her long life. Because an account of her life sheds light on the influences that molded Erwin Hahn, portions of that account are included as part of his story. In transmitting the unpublished document to the writer, Erwin Hahn wrote: "My mother lived to be 96. She was a strong, compassionate and intelligent woman."[9]

Just as surely as Erwin Hahn's original spin-echo paper would one day separate the world of continuous-wave NMR from that of pulsed NMR, so June 18, 1907 separated the Old World of 22-year-old Mariska [pronounced Ma-rish-ka] Weiss, daughter of Rabbi Weiss, from the New World of Mary Hahn, wife of Israel Hahn and future mother of Erwin Hahn. That was the day she boarded the steamship *Hamburg* of the Hamburg America Line in Bremerhaven, Germany and allowed it to transport her thousands of miles away from her home and parents in Vrbas, Vojvodina, Hungary to marry the man to whom she was engaged, but had never met.

Like most of the passengers onboard the *Hamburg*, Mariska had her own dreams and aspirations, but it was the past more than the future that influenced her emigration to America. It was tradition, specifically the tradition of the assigned bride, that placed Mary's name on the ship's manifest of passengers, a tradition as old as that observed by her ancient ancestor Abraham when he sent his servant to find a wife for his son Isaac and as contemporary as the one celebrated by Tevye in the musical, *Fiddler on the Roof*. For Abraham's son Isaac, it was Rebekah, the great-niece of Abraham. For Israel Hahn, it was Mariska Weiss, the great-niece of a distant relative of Israel Hahn's mother.

From the start, Mariska had not been enthusiastic about the match, but she knew her rabbi father couldn't afford the kind of dowry that was normally expected in her native Hungary. Even though self-appointed matchmakers would bring potential suitors around in hopes of facilitating the culture's expectations of marriage at a young age for women, unfortunately for Mariska they all wanted money. "I was not hard to look at," she wrote, "and I was liked, even with my shyness . . . but the money was always the main object. . . . They all wanted at least 1000 gulden, some agreed on 800 gulden or so."[10] I felt like a cow on the bargaining block, she said. Although her father, whom she dearly loved, had always said that the congregation would help him with the money, Mariska was firmly opposed to that idea.

While she was opposed to her father's solicitation of dowry money from his congregation, her father was against her aspirations for singing and acting. Early on, she had shown an aptitude for music and, upon graduation from a four-year girl's *gymnasium* in Vrbas, the school principal recommended to Rabbi Weiss that he send Mariska to a college or university in Budapest.

He said I have great talents and should be developed [wrote Mary many years later], but my father who was very much against women's emancipation told the principal that I know enough to be a wife, mother and housekeeper. The principal tried hard to change my father's mind about this, but with no result. And he said in German, *"Schade für das Mädchen."* It means, "It's a pity for the girl, a wasted talent." So I learned all the things to be a mother, a cook, a wife.[11]

In spite of her disappointment, Mariska didn't stop her singing.

> I loved to sing. I sang even when I scrubbed the floor. I sang when I cooked, baked or did whatever. . . . I had a very good singing voice and I could act. . . . We had a very nice park, and there were occasional holiday celebrations on national holidays. My parents befriended a schoolteacher and his wife, who also was a teacher. They both belonged to a club which organized the plays in the park, and through them I was asked to be in the play. . . . One day, a music and singing teacher attended one of our park affairs and saw me acting and heard me singing. He was from Budapest. He came to my parents and told them that I have a fortune in [my] throat, told them to send me to the Conservatory in Budapest, to learn music and to educate my voice. He said that I could become a great actress or singer or both. I think my mother would have let me go, but not my father. He didn't want his daughter to become an actress or anything like it. He said they are all immoral. And there and then I lost another chance. But maybe it was better this way. Who knows?[12]

As a young adolescent, Mariska had dreamed of the prince who would come and rescue her and make everything rosy and beautiful, but in real life the only one she really cared for, the brother of one of her friends, had never told her that he cared. At the time, she was about 15 or 16 and living in a society in which, as she noted, "a girl . . . was an old maid at the age of 20."

> I remember, how unhappy it made me [wrote Mary]. He was polite and the perfect gentleman, but that was all. But one day, he asked me whether I loved him. I was terribly embarrassed. I thought, if he loved me, he should tell me so, and I didn't answer him. I went on, my heart aching, but nothing changed. One day my father came home and told us that he—the one I cared for—went to Szolnok, where he had a married sister living, to see a girl she wanted to match him up with. He came home, and after about six weeks, he married that girl and brought her to Vrbas. And with her he received a dowry of 4000 gulden. That was a lot of money; and he needed it. He opened a mon-

ument establishment. Of course, he couldn't marry me. I had no dowry, period. I cried much, after that, but I got over it. I learned early in life, that whatever is impossible, just to forget about it.[13]

Four or five years after losing her chance to marry the man she loved, negotiations began for Mariska's marriage to Israel Hahn. Israel's mother, a distant relative of Mary's great aunt in Bonyhád, then located in Hungary, had emigrated to the city of Pittsburgh in the United States after the birth of 16 children and the death of her husband only to find that Israel, who had emigrated about five years earlier, was single and unable to find the girl he wanted to marry. The girls in America are very demanding, he told his mother. "I suppose they are, and good for them," Mary wrote in an editorial aside in her autobiography, and then continued telling the rest of the story:

> So Mother Hahn said to him, "I know a nice girl in Europe, I will try to get her for you; and that girl was I. And she wrote to my aunt to approach the idea to us. When the letter came I was sort of depressed. I told you about the love I felt for the brother of my girl friend so I decided that it doesn't make any difference whom I marry, because a match by a matchmaker would be an unknown, just the same. . . . I think it was an attractive idea to [my parents], not to have to worry where the money would come from for a dowry so we wrote to my aunt that we would negotiate. So the correspondence began between us and the Hahns, Mother Hahn and Israel Hahn, my father and me. Israel wrote in German, sort of very short notes. I answered [with] elaborate letters about myself and my hopes, but in his answers there were no responding ideas. Israel had no imagination. I was idealistic and romantic. Nevertheless, I tried to believe that it is well and I accepted the situation, because I knew that I had to marry somebody.[14]

After a going-away visit from the one she loved in which he told her, "I hear you go to America to get married. I am sorry that I didn't marry you; maybe I would be better off,"[15] and after a tearful goodbye from her mother—"I still can see poor mother standing by the gate crying and saying, 'Will I ever see you again,' "[16]—Mary left home. She was accompanied as far as Budapest by her father. There they met Mrs. Fischel, her chaperone for the rest of the journey. A friend of Mrs. Hahn, Mrs. Fischel had returned to Hungary for a visit. She and a friend, a Mrs. Berg who, along with her two sons, was also emigrating to America, would accompany Mary Weiss from Budapest to New York.

Compared to the steerage passengers confined to the hot, throbbing bowels of the ship for the two-week journey to America, Mary Weiss, age 22 years and one week on the day of her departure, had quite comfortable accommodations. Assigned a second-class compartment across the hall from the others in her group, Mary reported that the ship was "nice, clean and the service quite all right. The weather was nice, we spent a lot of time on the deck, we got acquainted with some Hungarians, one a Catholic priest. He was young, he wore priestly clothes, but sometimes I doubted his priestliness. Anyway, he was good company. Most of us were Jews."

The other Hungarians on the ship [Mary wrote], traveled steerage, mostly people to come to work in mills and make money. Most of them returned back home, after they made enough money, to pay off the mortgage on the farms or buy some horses or cows; some of them, because of circumstances, remained here in America. I guess they [the ones who remained in America] were the lucky ones.[17]

Tragically, the numbers would confirm her comment about "the lucky ones." Three decades after their Atlantic crossing to the United States, many of those who returned to their homes in Europe would be among the approximately 200,000 Hungarian Jews annihilated by Hitler (out of a previous Jewish population of 403,000). Some of those who returned to Hungary ended up in Yugoslavia when maps were redrawn after World War I. In Yugoslavia, between 55,000 and 65,000 Jews would be killed out of a total Jewish population of 75,000.

Mary ate her first non-kosher meal while on board ship. Although her father had requested that Mrs. Fischel arrange kosher meals for her, Mrs. Fischel informed Mary after they were underway that, to do so, would require that she eat at a different table and a different time. "So I ate the first 'trife' meal on the ship," Mary wrote. "I sort of felt guilty in a way, but I got over that feeling. I figured, I can keep my kosher diet again."[18]

Because Mary was traveling second class and not in steerage, she did not have to suffer the indignities that were often associated with immigration processing on Ellis Island. Typically, first- and second-class passengers were processed and inspected by immigration officers and medical inspectors aboard ship while anchored at the entrance to the Lower Bay of New York Harbor. After this inspection, which was more courteous than the ones given at Ellis Island, the ships were allowed to proceed to a Manhattan pier, where those who had been inspected were free to disembark and those who had languished in steerage for the duration of the journey were sent by barge to Ellis Island for processing. Mary and her fellow travelers were ferried to a railroad terminal in Hoboken, New Jersey where they were met by Mrs. Fischel's husband and Israel Hahn for the trip west to Pittsburgh.

Mary's impression of Israel in person was even less positive than the one she had from his short letters and, if anything, was an ominous sign for the future. "He stood there," she wrote, "looking me over, but didn't do anything, just stood there. So Mr. Fischel said to him, 'Kiss her, you *shlemiel*,' so Israel kissed me very awkwardly, mechanically. As far as I was concerned, it didn't make any difference. His appearance did not excite me at all."

> He was not really bad looking [Mary wrote]. In fact, he was handsome, but overweight. His face was full of pimples, his teeth yellowed by nicotine. He was dressed very stylish, according to those days. His pants was a baggy style, green in color, his coat was light brown, almost yellow, his shoes lemon color. Well, I really don't know what his first impression was about me, he never told me.[19]

He did tell her, however, that she had beautiful hair. "I had thick, long tresses wound all around my head," she said, "and I was a blond, not very light, my eyes were bluish grey." The topic of her hair would bring one of Mary's first confrontations with her mother-in-law. She told Mary she was to cut it and wear a wig in the Orthodox Jewish tradition for married women. Before leaving for America, Mary had asked her father what she should do about her hair and he had told her to cut it only if your husband requests it. When she asked Israel, he told her he didn't want to sleep with a bald woman. "Mother Hahn was a domineering woman," said Mary, "but in this case, she lost."[20]

About two weeks after Mary's arrival in the United States, she and Israel were married, but they were not to live happily ever after. Mother Hahn's loss on the hair issue would turn out to be one of the few disagreements with Mary that she would lose.

Mary and Israel began their married life in Sewickley, Pennsylvania, then a small town about five miles up the Ohio River from Pittsburgh, where Israel operated a cleaning and dyeing store. Unfortunately for Mary, however, it was well within easy train-ride distance from Mother Hahn, who lived in the city.

Mother Hahn went by some 2,000- to 3,000-year-old law [wrote Mary], when a man married a slave; and, in fact, I became one. . . . I soon found out that I didn't marry Israel alone. I married the whole family, and they lived my life. There was nothing that they didn't interfere with. Israel told his mother everything he was planning . . . but I was not considered. . . . It was a tough beginning. I was very unhappy and, of course, homesick. I was altogether dependent on the Hahn clan.[21]

After a one-night honeymoon in a cheap, third-rate hotel in Pittsburgh—"it was noisy, dirty, drunks roaming around and questionable women squealing in some of the rooms"—Israel introduced his new bride to her new home. It was midnight when they arrived and what Mary saw made her heart sick.

Everything was very dirty, the stove a black iron one, burned milk, eggs. etc. smeared all over, dirty dishes on the floor, on the table, the floor so dirty you couldn't see the boards. . . . The wallpaper [was] dirty and in places torn where the plaster was broken and the lathes underneath showed. And the bathroom, so filthy and dirty, beyond description. It was late when we got to the place, so we went to bed. The bedclothes were dirty and smelly, but there was nothing I could do about it right then.[22]

Mary wasn't able to sleep very well that first night. For one thing, the bed fell apart and they were temporarily trapped under its headboard until Morris, Israel's brother who also lived in the apartment, came and rescued them. But she still had difficulty sleeping. Her body itched all night long and she didn't know why. The next day, she found that the whole place was infested with bedbugs, something she had not experienced in Europe.

The bedclothes, even the pillows were full of [bedbugs]. I took out all the feathers, put them in the bathtub, and washed them with soap powder. I spread a sheet on the attic floor and spread the feathers on it to dry. I washed the tickings and when the feathers dried, I filled them. . . . But when it was all cleaned, Mother Hahn came and took them, saying that the bedclothes belonged to her.[23]

Every month following their marriage, Mother Hahn would inquire if Mary was pregnant. After three months had gone by and there was no sign of a grandchild on the way, Mother Hahn "lamented," wrote Mary, "that I was a barren woman and she blamed herself [for getting] such a woman for her son. I began to think of myself as a failure as a wife, but then it happened, and I was pregnant."[24] Simon was born the following July.

Although for many, the year 1907 would always be associated with a severe recession known as the Panic of 1907, business was thriving for Israel Hahn. "All businesses were bad," Mary recalled, "only the cleaning business flourished, especially in Sewickley. All those rich people had their old garments renovated and cleaned, so Israel made money."[25] After Mary became pregnant, they moved to a different apartment—"a palace compared with that dump I was in before," said Mary and soon afterward, when the landlord raised the rent from 20 dollars to 22 dollars, Israel decided to build a 10-room house on an acre of land he had purchased. "It was a nice house," said Mary, "well built, real walls, beautiful wood work, not like these cardboard houses of today."[26]

In the dozen years between 1907 and 1919, six children were born to Israel and Mary Hahn. "The babies came regularly, 16-18 month intervals,"[27] Mary wrote. After Simon came two more sons, Harry and Milton, then a daughter Debora, followed by two more sons, Jack and Philip. Debora, named after Mary's paternal grandmother, filled a special spot in the home for both Israel and Mary, so that even the pronouns Mary used in her autobiography changed from "I" to "we."

> We were so happy with her [Mary wrote]. Israel gave the district nurse an extra bonus on her pay. She was pretty, my little Debora. She had reddish blond hair—curly—and dark brown eyes. She had a very fair skin. We idolized her. I made her dresses, I dressed her in a different dress every day.[28]

Debora even seemed to improve Mary's relationship with Mother Hahn. For some time, it had been going from bad to worse—for months Mary was barred from accompanying Israel to Pittsburgh for his weekly visits with his mother—but after telling how much Debora meant to them, Mary added, almost parenthetically, "Meanwhile, I made up with Mother Hahn."[29]

Tragically, the light Debora brought to the Hahn home would shine for just a short time. In what Mary described as "the most important and sad episode of my life," Debora died March 3, 1919, a casualty of the 1918-19 influenza epidemic. Everyone except Israel had become sick from the flu and all Mary could remember in her feverish state was when they brought a casket to her bed and told her that Debora had died. "I did not comprehend fully at that time the real tragedy. I looked and I saw a little face, black from the burning fever, the hair tousled and almost gray. She looked terrible."[30] Numb from the shock, and weakened by the flu, it wasn't until Mary took Debora's clothes to a charitable organization that she realized that her little girl was really gone.

Mother Hahn was also gone, having died shortly before the flu epidemic struck, and was thus, wrote Mary, "spared the agony of losing her little granddaughter Debora."[31]

Gone also was the prosperity, followed soon afterward by the house they had built. Mortgaged to finance a second store, a tailor trimming shop that Israel opened in Pittsburgh, the house had to be sold to make ends meet after the Pittsburgh store failed. The Hahn cleaning business in Sewickley also went into a tailspin, a casualty of a decision to fire the tailor hired to operate the business when he was caught stealing. When Israel brought charges against the tailor, apparently with strong evidence, and the judge asked the defendant why he stole the item in question, he replied that he thought it was proper to steal from a Jew because the Jews have stolen enough from us. "As unbelievable as it seems," wrote Mary, "Israel lost the case."[32] He also lost much of his business. The tailor opened up his own cleaning shop in Sewickley and convinced most of Hahn's customers to switch.

As the end of World War I drew near, Mary also learned of other losses she had suffered. During the conflict, she knew nothing about the status of her parents and other relatives in Europe because mail from Europe had virtually stopped. "I didn't hear anything from them," said Mary. "Finally, the Blue Cross announced that if we want some news from overseas relatives, they can and will try to help locate them. So I went and told them about where my folks lived, telling them that I have brothers who, I am sure, had to go into the army. So one day, the Blue Cross ladies informed me that I have a brother, a prisoner in a Russian camp, and gave me the address to write to him. It was my brother Mike."[33] She wrote to him, and he answered once, but then didn't hear from him again.

Finally, after the war ended, the tailor who would later defeat Israel in court, informed her about her family. Besides the brother she knew had been taken prisoner by the Russians, her youngest brother, age 14, had died, a victim of scarlet fever and diphtheria. Another brother had fallen in battle in Trieste. After the war, when the region of Hungary where Mary had lived for most of her youth was given to Yugoslavia as national boundaries were redrawn, Mary's two sisters had left home and smuggled themselves over the border so they could remain in Hungary.

All along, come to find out, letters from Mary's family had been getting through, but they had not been given to her. When Mary confronted Israel as to why she had been ignorant about her folks for so long, he responded that we Jews are not for spreading bad news. "I thought it silly," said Mary many years later, and then added in Israel's defense, "Well, perhaps he meant well."[34]

Following the death of their daughter Debora and the demise of their Sewickley dry cleaning establishment, the Hahns moved to the east end of Pittsburgh and opened another cleaning store. It failed. Israel went into the scrap iron business. That failed. Now all they had was an old house on Hays Street in Pittsburgh which Israel had purchased after selling their nice home in Sewickley. "It was like a barn," said Mary. "The children had no decent clothes. I had no fineries. We ate, but not too much, and very plain. I never had any money."[35] When Israel learned of a jewelry store and pawnshop for sale in Farrell, Pennsylvania, about 50 miles away, that he could purchase for about $200 down, he sold the house, netting about $800, and the family moved north.

Farrell

On January 16, 1919, a constitutional amendment prohibiting the manufacture, sale and transportation of intoxicating liquors in the United States was ratified, thus starting a one-year countdown until "Prohibition," as it was called, became law. Fourteen years later, Prohibition would be repealed, but the years in between would become synonymous with lawlessness as ordinary citizens and notorious gangsters alike sought to circumvent the attempt to legislate temperance with regard to alcohol.

Farrell, Pennsylvania was one of many U.S. communities whose social structure was adversely affected by the well-intentioned amendment. Located in the Shenango River Valley immediately adjacent to the somewhat-larger Sharon, Pennsylvania and only a dozen miles or so from the rough-and-tough steel-making city of Youngstown, Ohio, Farrell had a population in 1920 of 15,586, nearly three times its present-day population. Included in that number were crooked law enforcement officials, bootleggers, prostitutes, and a large contingent of gamblers, a combination that made the big-little town a less than desirable place to raise a family but a good location for a pawnshop.

For a time, the Hahn pawnshop flourished, especially on weekends when gambling was at its peak. Unfortunately for the business, Israel became acquainted with a junk dealer, a "fanatic about religion," according to Mary, who convinced Israel to close the pawnshop on Saturdays. Business immediately dropped off when Israel's customers decided to take their business to the other pawnshop in town. When Mary pointed to the sharp drop in income and demanded that Israel keep the store open on Saturdays, he became angry and called her a *meshumed*, an unbeliever, so she decided to open the store herself on Saturdays.

That didn't work, either. Mary Hahn always offered significantly less for pawned items than their cross-town competitor, a strategy that might have helped profits if customers had gone along with it. They didn't. She got out of the pawnshop business though when a gambler tried to redeem a diamond ring for less than the amount owed on it. She didn't give in and the man finally paid the full amount, but he was apprehended by the police for "cheating, robbery and assault" soon after leaving the store. That was it for Mary. The shop would again be closed on the Sabbath.

The apartment Israel rented in Farrell, just three rooms tucked in behind a grocery store and butcher shop, was in the worst section of town, "a very rough neighborhood," according to Mary. The bootlegger landlord who had once lived there, she noted, had made enough money to move to the good section of town. One night, the Hahns were awakened about 1 or 2 a.m. by three men, apparently clients of the former occupant, demanding whiskey. When they were told that there was no whiskey on the premises, they demanded money. That, too, Israel told them, was unavailable. Fortunately, after conferring together about their available options, the three decided to leave without inflicting physical harm. After that episode, the Hahns also decided to leave for a better section of town, this time a house on Wallis Avenue near Idaho Street, the main street of Farrell. It was while they were living there that their last child was born June 9, 1921. They named him Erwin Louis. "So my baby," wrote Mary Hahn, "which I hoped would be a girl, was a boy, Erwin. He was not a handsome baby, like [his brother] Philip was, but he was a healthy baby." Their business, however, was not so healthy.

Business was bad [Mary wrote]. I had a farmer, who delivered milk for us. Finally, I told him I was unable to pay for it, but he said he will wait [for payment]. I shouldn't worry about it, and he kept on bringing us milk. I still couldn't pay and I told the farmer so. Then he told me that he was glad to let me have the milk, he had to spill some even at that, he even fed it to the pigs, and he was happy to know that my children could have it. He didn't expect to get paid for it.[36]

Although Mary was embarrassed to accept charity, she was secretly glad the farmer wasn't put off by her protestations. Israel's junk-dealer friend, a Mr. Stahl, wasn't so accommodating, however. With Erwin growing and becoming more difficult to carry, Mary needed a baby buggy. Unfortunately, the only one she could afford was high up on a pile in Stahl's junk shop.

> It didn't look too bad [said Mary]. So I told him, I [would] like to buy the buggy and I asked him to get it down for me. He told me to get it myself. He did not respect women; a woman was only a vassal to him. Israel [who happened to be there at the time] just sat there, didn't make a move to help me get the buggy down from the pile, so I did it myself. Stahl laughed, a very insulting way. But I had a baby buggy. I cleaned it and it was quite all right.[36]

It was during their time in Farrell that Harry, Israel and Mary's second son, then 12 years old, developed behavioral problems. When he was born, the district nurse assisting in the delivery had broken the placenta prematurely in an effort to slow down what she thought was a too-fast delivery, but the delivery had not taken place for many hours and when the doctor came he had to use a forceps to delivery Harry in what he termed a "dry birth." Whether his problems were birth-related or not, Mary recognized that from the beginning, Harry was not like her other children. He didn't cry much or move much, and as he grew older, she noticed that he was very quiet and never laughed. When he began developing behavioral problems, Mary at first discounted it as just that, misbehavior, until a teacher informed her that Harry was mentally incapable of attending classes. When she brought him to a medical doctor for a series of examinations, he confirmed that Harry's intelligence had plateaued at the level of a five- or six-year-old and that he could not tolerate the stress of the mental performance expected in a school classroom. Eventually, when he became more violent, Mary realized he would have to be placed in an institution.

With the aid of a senator in Sharon, Mary was able to get him placed in a large group home in Polk, Pennsylvania about 30 miles away that Mary thought was a nice enough place considering it was an institution, but it was heart-rending every time Harry came home for a visit and then had to return. "No one knows how bad I felt about it, but there was no other way out,"[37] she wrote. "Israel never lifted a finger to help," she said. Although the administrator recommended keeping Harry at the institution for several years before bringing him home to visit, Israel would go and pick him up and leave the unpleasant task of returning him to the institution to Mary. "Poor Harry already recognized the country, when we neared Polk, on the train, and he cried, he didn't want to go back. I just couldn't do anything but cry with him."[38]

Meanwhile, the Hahn pawn business continued to deteriorate. This time, Israel went to his brother Sig, who owned the Hahn Furniture Store in Pittsburgh, for financial assistance. With Sig's help, Israel was able to buy a jewelry store and a house in Aliquippa, Pennsylvania, about 20 miles upstream from downtown Pittsburgh on the Ohio River. "The house wasn't bad and the neighborhood was nice," said Mary. "We hardly had any furniture; only the most necessary things like a stove, table, chairs and beds. No carpets nor any nice things like lamps and knick-knacks, not even curtains on my windows."[39]

When the jewelry store proved insufficient to provide enough income to support the family, Israel started in the cleaning business again, putting a pressing machine in the living room. "I didn't like it," said Mary. "The house was full of steam and odor from the cleaning fluid and the floor wet from the machine. . . . We had many fights and arguments. Israel tried to run both places, jewelry and cleaning, expecting me to do the work in the cleaning."[40]

In the end, neither business was successful. "So it wasn't very long," she said, "before we were all finished in Aliquippa. I believe we were there only about a year. So what to do? Israel sold the house, and had a few hundred dollars out of it, and we moved back to Sewickley."[41] By that time, 1923, Mary's youngest, Erwin, was about two years old.

A Trip to Europe

As for the time he and his family lived in Farrell and Aliquippa, Erwin Hahn would remember virtually nothing. "I remember I entered kindergarten in the town of Sewickley at the age of five," he said. "That's where my memory kind of starts."[42] That was also the year—1926—that Mary Hahn went back to Europe for the first time after her emigration, and she took Erwin along.

"Erwin was a very lively boy," she wrote. "He ran all over the ship, sometimes I didn't know where he was. One time we found him in one of the lifeboats."[43] When they disembarked from their ship in Hamburg, young Erwin, noting that everybody was speaking German, decided that would be his *lingua franca* for the balance of his stay in Europe. He wouldn't talk one word of English while in Europe, his mother recalled.

In the ensuing 19 years since her departure for America, many things had changed, including, as mentioned earlier, the name of the country. Mary's father had died, his health and spirit broken by the deaths of two of his sons during the war. Many other things, however, had not changed as much as Mary had expected.

I didn't like what I saw, nothing changed in 20 years. The same old dusty roads; . . . whenever I came or left any place, I had to register in the City Hall, and on the trains I always had to show my passport, at every border, and they always opened my baggage and messed it up. I met my old friends I knew, but they were strangers to me then. I also met [the man] who I loved, but never admitted [that I loved him], and when I saw him, I wondered, why did I love him?[44]

Relatives and neighbors in Vrbas were less than impressed with five-year-old Erwin. His grandmother, for one, wasn't pleased when he chased the landlady's chickens around the backyard and the neighbors weren't pleased when he played roughly with their son. "People said it was a disgrace," Mary said, "to bring a bad boy like that."[44]

Their opinion was not without merit. "I was something of a menace," said Professor Hahn recently.

When my mother took me to visit Hungary, we went through Berlin via the port of Altona. In Berlin, we were walking in the area of *unter den Linden,* a famous stretch in the business district in 1926. My mother always reminded me that I was something of a five-year-old brazen kid who wore an American Indian costume. Dressed in that costume, I came up to a Berliner policeman and kicked him in the shins, complaining *"du bist zu dich,"* meaning he was too fat. My mother was almost incarcerated because of my behavior.[45]

Mother and son stayed in Europe for almost six weeks. In addition to visiting her mother in Vrbas, Mary visited her brother in Budapest and her sisters in Bonyhád and Novi Sad.* After nearly two decades of sepa-

---

* Novi Sad is the largest city in the area and the city where both Mary's brother Philip and Albert Einstein's first wife, Mileva Maric, attended *gymnasium.* Mileva Maric's home town, Titel, and Mary's home town, Vrbas, are both about 25 miles from Novi Sad.

ration, she was surprised to find that absence had not made her heart grow fonder, that her feelings and compassion for her mother had become dormant. Not until they had talked about old times, refreshed faded memories and discussed the passing of Mary's father and brothers did she find herself identifying more closely with her mother. Even then, however, Mary found herself bored in what had once been the center of her world and she would have returned to America sooner had she not wanted to avoid hurting her mother's feelings.

Looking back on how her perspectives had changed in the intervening years, Mary decided that time and distance had made the difference. "As years go by, we change," she wrote. "We are never always the same— time makes some of us better people, and some of us worse. You form your own character, for this is the power God gave you."[46]

As they set sail for America and Mary watched Europe disappear into the misty horizon for the second time in her life, it was a much different Mary than the one who had left Europe 19 years earlier. For her, Europe had truly become the Old World. Although the world awaiting her on the other side of the Atlantic had not always shown itself to be a land flowing with milk and honey, it was clear that it had become her world. In addition to the son who was with her, she had five other sons depending on her. And then there was her husband Israel. Although he had not proven to be the prince she had once imagined in her adolescent daydreams, she did care about his welfare and was still able to find excuses for his shortcomings.

As young Erwin Hahn left Europe for America, he didn't realize, nor would he have cared, that it had been a momentous summer for the new physics of quantum mechanics. He didn't know, for example, that another Erwin, an Austrian by the name of Schrödinger, had just published a paper proving that the new wave mechanics he had formulated earlier that year was equivalent to a very different formulation of matrix mechanics published in 1925 by Germany's Werner Heisenberg. He didn't know that Felix Bloch, who would one day be his personal friend and a fellow musician as well as a colleague at Stanford University in California, was just then preparing for his illustrious career in physics at the Swiss Federal Institute of Technology in Zürich. As tugboats maneuvered the ship away from the Hamburg pier and into the main channel of the Elbe River, young Erwin was unaware that an American by the name of Isidor I. Rabi, who would one day be a colleague of Erwin Hahn's at Columbia University and whose work in molecular beams would be a precursor to Erwin Hahn's work with spin echoes, would be arriving at the same port the following year to begin his work in molecular beams with Otto Stern. For young Erwin, exploring the fascinating world of an ocean liner was more important just then than exploring the unseen but very real world of the atomic nucleus.

Israel and Mary's marriage would last for seven more years, for a total of more than 25 years, but they would be years of increasing conflict, abuse, and lack of communication.

For awhile, business continued to thrive and Israel opened additional stores in other communities by obtaining loans with promissory notes. Eventually, however, the interest load alone on the debts became more and more burdensome and, one by one, the stores had to be closed. Mary and three of their sons, Simon, Milton and Jack, operated the Sewickley store, managing somehow to make money in spite of a sharp increase in competition from Pittsburgh-based dry cleaning chains, but any money they made was quickly siphoned off by Israel on bad business investments. He even took the money she gave him to purchase a steamship ticket for her mother to emigrate to the United States—money she had borrowed—and used it elsewhere; he invested it in the business, he finally told her, after refusing, for a long time, to even discuss the matter.

Finally, after Israel went to visit his sister in Detroit and didn't return or write for almost a full year, Mary knew it was time to begin divorce proceedings. "I told him," she wrote, "that I can't go on with his ways. I want my boys to have a chance and I am tired of worrying whether there will be enough to eat tomorrow."[47]

In 1933, Israel and Mary Hahn were divorced, in spite of her hopes for reconciliation. She paid all the court and lawyer costs, did not sue for alimony, and assumed on her own the responsibility for all of Israel's outstanding promissory notes. "I didn't have to pay them, if I didn't want to, but Sewickley being a small community I decided to pay them, in order to keep up the good relationship." The house they were living in was sold, its profits given to Israel, and Mary retained ownership of the Sewickley dry cleaning store.

Israel Hahn moved to Pittsburgh. Mary, age 48, and her six boys, ranging in age between 13 and 25, moved into a second-floor apartment on Beaver Street in Sewickley.

> I told the boys to visit their father in Pittsburgh [Mary wrote]. He had a furnished room on Walnut Street in Shadyside. I had no control over the older boys. I insisted [that] Erwin regularly visit his father, but eventually he refused. Israel never supported them. I

don't think he ever gave a nickel to Erwin for an ice cream cone. I
kept working as usual. . . . Milton opened the store. I got up early,
cleaned the house. By 9-10 o'clock, I went to the store. I cooked my
dinners always the night before. I did my laundry on Sundays, and
took the ironing to the store on Monday. When the boys grew up, I
had as many as 30-40 shirts to iron, but it didn't hurt me. I was
young, and healthy.[48]

The Great Depression, the Great Divide

Mary Weiss Hahn's emigration to America had been the fateful water-
shed in her life that forever separated the relatively care-free world of her
childhood from the world of an unhappy marriage, a new culture and a
new language. For her sons, the trauma of the Great Depression would
have a significant effect on their future careers, their ability to take risks
stifled by a pragmatism that squelched youthful dreams of adventure
and replaced them with an overriding concern for security. The severity
of the Depression's impact on their psyche would vary in proportion
with age. Fortunately for his own aspirations and for science, Erwin
Hahn was the youngest in the family.

The normal vagaries of a retail service business like dry cleaning with
its constantly changing competitive pressures are sufficient to test anyone's mettle. For the Hahn dry cleaning establishment in Sewickley, the
Great Depression made a chronic problem acute. When a dry cleaning
chain called Peter Pan opened up in Sewickley and charged just 19 cents
for cleaning a garment, the pressure became intense. "But I held on,"
wrote Mary Hahn, "just getting by."[49]

> It was a hard life [said Erwin Hahn]. I remember when I was a kid
> my mother used to say, "I'm not sure we have enough money to eat
> next week." It was always hand to mouth, particularly through the
> '30s—from '28 through the '30s. [The Depression] was really psycho-
> logically scarring. Particularly I noticed that in my older brothers. A
> job to them was as essential as education is today. Getting a job was
> more essential than going to school. The first step today, relatively
> speaking, is to seek an education rather than a job, although I get the
> impression these days that the education process is abused by many,
> adopted as a delay in a kind of purgatory before confronting the
> notion of getting a job.[50]
>
> I and my brother next to me [Philip] had the opportunity of going
> to college whereas the others had to work [said Professor Hahn], and

then my third brother [Milton] went to college after the war. The Depression inhibited [the older ones] from getting a complete education. So I was lucky in being the youngest in that sense, also my brother next to me.[51]

When Simon graduated from high school, Mary wanted him to go to the University of Pittsburgh, but Israel said no, he needed him to help make deliveries. Later, after serving during the war as a warrant officer in New Delhi, India, Simon got a job working for his uncle Sig who owned a chain of furniture stores in the Pittsburgh area. Simon was very intelligent, said his brother Erwin, but "he made the mistake of working for [his uncle] all his life, which was bad because of nepotism. He couldn't make any headway."[52] Simon Hahn died in 1991 at the age of 83.

Harry, Israel and Mary's second son, remained institutionalized at Polk until shortly before his parents' divorce. When Israel brought him home for a visit, Mary refused for the first time to return him. When she finally relented and tried to return him, the administrator at Polk refused to accept him back because they had exceeded the allotted release time. For a time, Harry remained at home, but eventually Mary was able to find another facility for him in Woodville, where he remained until his death.

Milton Hahn, their third son, wanted to be an actor. After performing frequently at the Pittsburgh Playhouse, he followed his dream to New York City, but then was drafted into the Army Air Corps. After the war, his mother encouraged him to get a college education under the GI bill, but Milton, who was then in his mid-30s, felt he was too old to start college at that point. Eventually, he went into real estate and today lives in Miami, Florida.

Jack was also drafted and saw extensive action with the infantry in Sicily, at Normandy and in Africa. Since he was younger than Milton, Mary Hahn insisted that he take advantage of the GI Bill of Rights, passed in 1944, which provided educational and housing benefits to military veterans. In 1949 Jack graduated with an electrical engineering degree from the University of Pittsburgh and obtained employment with the Department of the Navy in Philadelphia. A few years later, however, he was diagnosed as having brain tumors. Although the growth of the tumors was successfully halted with surgery, his health never returned fully and he had to take early retirement. Today, Jack still lives in Philadelphia.

Philip Hahn, the next to the youngest and the first in the family to graduate from college, was the only son other than Harry who did not serve in the military during World War II. Although Philip tried to enlist, he was turned down because of a heart murmur which really was not serious and, in fact, like Erwin's osteomyelitis, was a misdiagnosis. He has never been troubled by heart problems since. After going into the second-hand furniture business for a time, he returned to school to obtain a graduate degree in business administration. Upon graduation from Northwestern University, he joined the faculty of Youngstown State University in Youngstown, Ohio. Philip also has an MBA from Harvard Business School. Now retired, he lives in California.

Growing Up in Sewickley

Situated about 10 miles downriver from the city center of Pittsburgh, where the confluence of the Monogahela and Allegheny Rivers form the Ohio, Sewickley, Pennsylvania is today one of a series of communities north of Pittsburgh that attract white-collar workers who want the best of both worlds—easy access to and nightly escape from a large city, with the added benefit of close proximity to Pittsburgh International Airport.

White collars have been replacing blue collars in Pittsburgh ever since economic forces wiped out the city's steel industry in the 1970s and it has been easier to keep those collars white because of drastic measures the city has taken to reduce dirt and air pollution. When civic leaders in Pittsburgh became increasingly concerned in the late 1940s about their city's pollution problems and turned to architect Frank Lloyd Wright for a solution, he told them bluntly, "Abandon it." In the end, however, the solution was a combination of strict air-quality regulation and unplanned market forces that removed the polluters.* For those who were still thinking of Pittsburgh stereotypically in 1985 as an environmental disaster, its No. 1 ranking that year as the best place to live in America came as somewhat of a shock.[53]

Although Sewickley has not been untouched by crime and other negative sociological forces, it has also handled the aging process with a certain degree of dignity. "It's more of a boutique town now," said Hahn, "and not particularly rancid like some places have become, like parts of

---

* Pittsburgh's turnaround did not come without pain, however. Two of those who were personally affected were Sig Hahn, Israel Hahn's brother, who owned the Hahn Furniture Company, and Simon Hahn, Erwin Hahn's brother, who worked for Sig. Because the company's sales were primarily to blue-collar workers, the loss of Pittsburgh's steel industry also wiped out Sig's furniture business.

Berkeley and Oakland have become. [Sewickley] maintained the amenity of gracious living more than most areas."[54]

In the early '30s, however, when Erwin Hahn was in elementary school, Sewickley was rural and more isolated, separated from the vices, dirt and smoke of the Steel City by family farms and contemplative cows.

> In those days, Pittsburgh was really mucked up with a lot of dirt and soot, but we lived outside of it [said Hahn]. Sewickley was a nice town to grow up in. I went through high school and developed a sense of accomplishment through the community activities which were very nice, I think, in retrospect. I went up to the YMCA a lot and there were a lot of directed activities—football, basketball, exercises in the gym. In those days, when a person did something you sort of reaped appreciation for it in the community and I find today it's not that way anymore. There wasn't this sinister, gang stuff that goes on today among the kids. It was all very healthy, I think partly because the community was semi-isolated from other communities. Crime was relatively low.[55]

In spite of his parents' less-than-ideal relationship and in spite of an economic depression that reduced the hopes and aspirations of his elder brothers, Hahn views his formative years positively with regard to their impact on his career.

> I believe my earliest years set the stage for my career development. Loneliness in just the right amount as a child and boy led me to develop a curiosity about things around me. My small town environment was pleasantly insular, and my family respected achievement. I was not over-programmed by family or school, nor was I witness or victim of the kinds of tensions we see today. Yet I saw the Depression leave its scars on my elders, which provided some needed humility for the later appreciation of educational opportunities.[56]

Although the combined forces of Israel Hahn and the Depression kept Simon Hahn from attending college, he did contribute to his brother Erwin's interest in chemistry and thus, at least indirectly, to the chemical revolution that his youngest brother would help propagate.

> I was sort of a loner [said Erwin Hahn]. I used to frequent the library a lot, reading books that I didn't understand as a kid around

sixth or seventh grade. My brother sensed my interest in science and he got me this chemistry set. He just gave it to me for a present. That really set me off. I started fiddling around and became an amateur chemist, burning up the carpets and all that stuff. I learned chemistry on my own, as a kid would, and then went to college and majored in chemistry. I got enthused with it and that's the way it began.[57]

He credits his mother with providing the glue that held his family together. "My mother was a strong woman, and she kept us in line," he said. "I didn't get into any serious trouble."[58] Another stabilizing force in young Erwin's life was the discipline imposed by music. His love for music was probably inherited from his mother, whose early desire for stage performance finally found expression in the late 1940s in amateur shows put on to raise money for the Sisterhood of the Poale Zedeck Temple in Pittsburgh. "I was always the star, the singer,"[59] she wrote in her autobiography. Her son Erwin's appreciation for music, however, was not always appreciated by other boys his age.

I was a nerd in the sense that I didn't conventionally do what all the other kids did, was sort of shy and didn't screw around. I did a little bit, but not like the other guys did. And I played the violin. All my colleague kids used to call me a sissy. In those days, if you were a football hero, you made it. You know, the macho stuff labeled you as a successful person. If you did all this cultural stuff, you know, you were just decadent. You didn't have the guts to do he-man things. Well, I felt that all my youth to some extent, but I didn't give a damn. I just figured, well, I'll go ahead on my own. That's the way you buck the tide.[60]

Although Erwin Hahn's decision to choose the violin over sports was viewed with disdain in the blue-collar, steel-making culture of Western Pennsylvania, his musical skills would later be appreciated by the viola-playing Karl Lark-Horovitz, with whom Hahn would play in a string quartet while in graduate school at Purdue. "He always wanted to play too fast—and too loud," Hahn recalled, laughing at the memory. "We always had to calm him down."[61] Later, at Stanford and Berkeley, Hahn would play sonatas together with piano-playing physicists such as Felix Bloch and Edward Teller. (Bloch was at Stanford; Teller was at Berkeley.)

When Erwin Hahn was at Stanford, Otto Robert Frisch, the nephew of Lise Meitner who collaborated with her in the physical interpretation of nuclear fission,* was there for a summer and Hahn played sonatas with him, Frisch playing the piano. Later, when Hahn went to Oxford University, Frisch invited him over to Cambridge University where they played more sonatas while Lise Meitner was listening. "That's name dropping now," Hahn said, chuckling. "Frisch was also a good sketcher," added Hahn. "I remember at parties at the Blochs that Frisch would stand in a corner and sketch people."[62]

In 1978, when Hahn was named a Faculty Research Lecturer by the University of California in Berkeley, a summary of his career by the University's Academic Senate noted, "An accomplished amateur violinist, Hahn has amiably sawed his way through much of the string quartet literature in company with friends of long standing in Berkeley."[63]

"Teller and I played a number of times here at Berkeley. He was pretty good. All of those theoretical physicists seemed to be pianists. I also used to play in violin quartets quite a bit with Sidney Drell, both at Illinois and at Stanford."[64] [Drell would later become well-known as an arms expert who took an active role in arms reduction.]

"A lot of physicists play instruments as a sideline," Hahn pointed out. "Victor Weisskopf played the piano. At Stanford, Sidney Drell played the violin and Leonard Schiff the clarinet. There is a connection."[65]

For a generation of students who signed up for his course at Berkeley on the physics of music, Hahn would seek to make that connection clear.

Science is a beautiful thing [he said]. It reveals beauty in symmetry and harmony when you get into it. It's fascinating. It's like playing a Mozart symphony or quartet. You get a sensation out of it. When you accomplish a revelation in a physics experiment and you work out its theory, no matter how minor it is, and you confirm something or you

---

* While in Germany recently as a Humboldt Foundation Visiting Fellow, Professor Erwin Hahn, speaking at a colloquium at the Free University of Berlin, mentioned that he is sometimes confused with Professor Otto Hahn, the German chemist who received the 1944 Nobel Prize in chemistry for the discovery of nuclear fission: "After a good friend of my wife read the newspaper a few months ago about the new element Hahnium, not naming Otto Hahn himself, . . . this friend wrote a note to my wife congratulating her on the great honor bestowed upon her husband. And there was another incident on the occasion of a formal dinner at an Oxford college, where my wife was seated somewhere else at the banquet table. The man sitting next to wife thought she was Mrs. Otto Hahn, and expressed surprise to her that I was alive after my wife pointed me out sitting at the other end of the table."

Professor Otto Hahn was born in 1888, making him six years older than Professor Erwin Hahn's mother.

predict something, there's a sense of beauty in it, an exultation. It's a private experience. You can't transfer it literally to somebody else.[66]

As for the scientific benefits of being a nerd, Hahn saw a direct relationship. "In order to be a scientist, you have to be crazy. You have to be somewhat eccentric and a loner. Otherwise, if you do the conventional things, you don't take the time to burrow into the details of something that's different. You have to be a nerd."[67]

The benefits of such a role, of course, are more obvious to your peers once you become a physicist and discover a phenomenon like spin echoes. They are less apparent when your brother, who is also strong academically, is a football and basketball star.

When Philip Hahn was about to graduate from Sewickley High School with high honors, the principal of the school, an alumnus of Juniata College in Huntingdon, Pennsylvania, talked with Mary Hahn about sending him to college. She told him she couldn't afford it, but he assured her that Philip could get a scholarship and the remainder probably wouldn't cost her more than about five dollars a week. "Even that seemed too much for me under the circumstances,"[68] wrote Mary, but she consented and Philip was given a scholarship to Juniata College where he excelled in both sports and academics for the next four years.

When Philip's younger brother, Erwin, graduated from high school in 1939, the principal also urged him to consider Juniata. After taking an examination, he was granted a scholarship and matriculated at the school in September 1939.

Juniata College, situated on a rural campus 80 miles due east of Pittsburgh in south-central Pennsylvania, was founded in 1876 by members of the Church of the Brethren and is today home to approximately 1100 undergraduates. In 1939, the enrollment was about 600 students. A Christian denomination, the Church of the Brethren was first established in the United States in 1719 when William Penn granted the persecuted sect land in Pennsylvania after they had been driven from Central Germany into Holland and Northern Germany.

Although the group follows the mainstream of Protestant theology within Christendom, some of its distinctives include pacifism, abstinence from alcohol, a dedication to a simple life that shuns unwholesome amusements and luxuries, opposition to class distinctions, and faithful adherence to the teachings of Christ rather than rigid following of ecclesiastical forms. Because of their opposition to war and hence their opposition to the American Revolution, they were sometimes regarded with suspicion earlier in American history. Their outstanding relief efforts following World War II, however, made them "one of the most honored bodies in American Protestantism."[69]

As a Jew attending a Church of the Brethren college, however, Hahn would have to do some more bucking of the tide.

> In those days it was very fundamentalist [said Hahn]. I had to go to chapel every day and was an object of proselytization by preministerial students. In a way, I enjoyed the experience and learned a lot from them. In fact, I was a roommate with two preministerial students the last couple years. As requirements for all students, we had to take courses in ethics and Bible. I really don't regret the experience. I was a convenient target as a rare Jewish student, and they worked on me. For example, the fundamentalist female students would tell you when they would pray for you. I wasn't the only one they prayed for. They had a roster of people—Christians as well—and they included me. The day before, they would say they were going to stay awake all night in the church tower and pray for us. So I said, "Fine, good." Then after they'd pray for me, I'd say, "Thank you very much," and that was it. They were well meaning and nice people. I was virtually a course that could have been called Proselytization 1 and Proselytization 2, but I never succumbed.[70]

Hahn was careful to point out that he did not experience the distaste of anti-Semitism at Juniata. "I didn't feel abused," he said. Given the anti-Semitism displayed throughout the centuries by those who have angrily labeled Jews as Christ killers, however, it's understandable that the arguments put forth by Hahn's fellow collegians as to why they thought Jesus was the prophesied Jewish Messiah would encounter a major hurdle. With Erwin Hahn, they encountered two hurdles: first, the traditional resistance of Jews to Christian claims about Christ; second, the fact that Hahn was already turned off on religion by what he saw as inconsistency in his father's practice of Judaism.

> My father only practiced religious ceremonies when he was in trouble. He would put on all the accouterments of the praying at the wall, like they do in Israel, if there were problems. But when there were no problems, he didn't pray. It was all phony to me. I saw it even when I was a kid and that turned me off. What turned me off, I remember, as a kid was when he hired a rabbi to teach us to read

Hebrew and we were taught to read the words without understanding them. I said to myself, "This is stupid." And I said that to myself when I was 13 years old, 14. So I'm not really a practicing Orthodox Jew. I'm sort of a rebellious one.[71]

Hahn's live-and-let-live tolerance of the Christians at Juniata College who tried to convince him to accept their beliefs was probably due in part to his mother's upbringing by her rabbi father. In her autobiography, she remembered one childhood episode in particular when two Jewish girls whom she considered "fanatics" came over for a visit:

It was a nice summer day, so we went for a walk, and we passed the Catholic church on our way. There in front was the crucified Jesus Christ monument and, to my horror, the girls spit on it. I got mad and told them that I thought that this was sacrilege. They got mad at me and said I was a *mashumeh*, a disbeliever, [and] that [they] wouldn't want to be my friends anymore. I left and told my father about this. My father said, you are right, we must respect anybody's religion and told me that I didn't lose much by losing the friendship of such people.[72]

A year after graduation from college, Erwin Hahn would be the first in the family to marry. When he told his mother that his fiancé was a gentile, Mary Hahn* had to admit, she said, that she was a bit shaken because of the difference in religion, and then added:

Marian was and is a very nice girl and a very lovely daughter-in-law to me. But when I was notified that they intended [to have] a church wedding, I objected. So there was a compromise. The wedding was held in the teachers' college in Terre Haute [Indiana, Marian Failing's home town]. It was a nice reception and I liked the minister's speech about Ruth who went with her mother-in-law telling her that "your people will be my people" according to the Bible story.[73]

---

* Ten years later, in 1954, Mary Weiss Hahn was married to Jonas Guggenheim. "Jonas always liked to talk about the fact," said Erwin Hahn, "that as a child growing up in Ulm, Germany, he was a schoolmate of the young boy Albert Einstein, who was also born in Ulm."
—Erwin Hahn, personal communication to James Mattson, 24 March 1995.

Hahn graduated summa cum laude from Juniata College with a major in chemistry, although, in his own mind, he had already made the switch to physics. "I became weary," he said, "of the pure memorization of chemical formulas. I was impressed by the fundamental concepts of physics, and so I began to major more in physics in my senior year, although I graduated as a chemistry major."[74] Officially, he minored in mathematics, but he took enough music courses to qualify for at least an unofficial secondary minor.

Hahn's switch in focus from chemistry to physics is also evident from the adjunct work he performed as a student at Juniata. From September 1940 to June 1943, he worked as a laboratory assistant and unofficial teaching assistant to chemistry professor Dr. Donald Rockwell. From September 1942 until his graduation in 1943, his work with Dr. Rockwell was overlapped by laboratory and classroom work he performed for physics professor Paul Yoder.[75]

Although Yoder only had a Master's Degree, Hahn identified him as one of two key influences from his undergraduate years. The other key influence was chemistry professor N.J. Brumbaugh. Brumbaugh, said Hahn, "was inspiring in the sense that he worshiped science more than he knew it."

> He put me in awe a little bit about science. He was rich and he financed the chemistry department at Juniata. He wasn't a very profound scientist himself, but he knew the history of chemistry particularly very well and he knew enough fundamentals to get undergraduates educated to a certain level and that was it."[76]

Part of Brumbaugh's worship of science was the recognition and encouragement of those students at Juniata who were showing great potential for its practice. He saw that potential in Erwin Hahn and thus Hahn was awarded the A.B. Brumbaugh Chemistry Prize, named in honor of Brumbaugh's father.

In addition to the personal attention Yoder gave him as a professor, said Hahn, he played an even more significant role in getting him into graduate school. At a time when anti-Semitism was still flagrant among American colleges and universities, Yoder's advice to his Jewish research assistant was to go west rather than east. "In those days," said Hahn, "there was a quota on Jewish students and anti-Semitism at Harvard and Princeton. Yale was quite open and up front [about their anti-Jewish attitude]."[77] Yoder was well aware, however, that the chairman of the physics department at Purdue, Karl Lark-Horovitz, was Jewish.

Educated in Vienna, Lark-Horovitz had held research fellowships in the United States and Canada before becoming a professor of physics at Purdue in 1928, one year before Edward Purcell entered the school as a freshman. "The Lark," as he was known, had made his mark on the school very quickly and by 1930 had been named director of the physical laboratory and head of the physics department. By 1943, his reputation in physics extended well beyond Purdue, and his solid-state laboratory at Purdue was under contract with the government through the Radiation Laboratory at Massachusetts Institute of Technology. (The latter, of course, was not well known at the time because of the need for security during World War II.)

In response to Hahn's application to enter the graduate physics program at Purdue, Lark-Horovitz arranged for Hahn to take an entrance examination at Juniata and when he passed, he was offered a teaching assistantship. For the next year, from June 1943 to June 1944, Hahn would assist with recitation in the introductory college physics course and for part of that time, from January 1944 to May 1944, would also assist in research conducted on Purdue' s cyclotron.

It wasn't easy working for Lark-Horovitz. In some ways, he may have reminded Hahn of his own father as he used similar terminology in describing the two men. Of his father, Hahn said he had the "European style of domineering the situation."[78] Of Lark-Horovitz, Hahn said:

> He was a martinet; good physicist, but a European domineering type of guy. He was intolerant in many ways, but nevertheless an inspiring scientist. Lark-Horovitz was something like a worshiper of science like Brumbaugh was. He gave you an awesome appreciation of the fact that you should learn physics. I mean he really worshipped and devoted his life to physics. He gave an image and a meaning of what science is and wanted you to work hard. But "the Lark" was a hard man to get along with. I wouldn't want to live with him.[79]

With so many physicists culled from the academic ranks for government service in World War II, the teaching staff at Purdue was somewhat decimated, said Hahn. "There were a few staff people there and the graduate courses were rather slim, but Lark-Horovitz was there and taught, as well as a few other people of some excellence."[80] Three physicists from Purdue listed as references by Hahn on a University of Illinois form in December 1945 were Dr. R.B. Withrow, Dr. Edward Akeley, and Dr. K.W. Meissner.

Another reference listed on the same form with a Santa Fe, New Mexico post office box was Mr. Robert E. Carter. Carter was a fellow graduate student of Hahn's at Purdue who, together with Purdue graduate student Harry Daghlian, was hired in 1944 to work at Los Alamos. Erwin Hahn, in fact, had also been accepted for employment at Los Alamos but shortly after receiving his notification had gotten married on April 8, 1944. When he wrote to Los Alamos informing them of his new status and inquiring about housing arrangements, Los Alamos withdrew its offer of employment.

At Juniata, Hahn had been deferred from the draft because of his undergraduate status. At Purdue, as a graduate student, he was deferred because he was teaching physics to GIs under the Army Special Training Program (ASTP). One of the beginning physics classes he taught under that program stood out especially in his mind. "All of a sudden," he said, "most of them disappeared. Army orders sent them to Anzio Beach and they were all killed. That really disturbed me. That was very upsetting."[81] * When the ASTP program expired, Hahn's deferment expired and without the Los Alamos position in hand, he was obliged to go into the military. He chose the Navy.

Although Hahn and Carter each went their separate ways for the duration of the war, they kept in contact and Carter was later very helpful in Hahn's obtaining an assistantship at the University of Illinois. Harry Daghlian, the first victim of a nuclear radiation accident at Los Alamos,

---

* Anzio is a town in west-central Italy on the Tyrrhenian Sea about 35 miles south of Rome where an Allied invasion took place on January 22, 1944. Because another movement by the Allies from the south was occupying the attention of the Germans holding the area, the landing itself was met with only slight opposition. Because of restraint by General Mark Clark, however, in issuing orders to quickly advance inland and corresponding conservatism by the field commander, General John Lucas, nine days passed before a two-pronged drive was sent inland toward the Alban Hills, giving the Germans time to regroup and prepare a counterattack. In one of the Allied prongs sent out on January 30, a U.S. attack led by Army Rangers met disaster. Thinking they had surprised the enemy, the Rangers were instead ambushed. Of the 767 Rangers who began the drive, only six returned. In another battalion from the U.S. 3rd Division, approximately 650 out of 800 were killed. After failing to make progress inland, all of the troops were ordered back to the small beachhead they had gained at Anzio where they would remain under heavy pressure from the Germans. Finally, on May 23, 1944, the troops were able to break out of their tiny beachhead at Anzio called Hell's Half Acre and advance toward Rome.
—Robert Wallace, *The Italian Campaign*, (Alexandria, VA: Time-Life Books, 1978), 130-151.

would never return from the New Mexican mesa alive. "Carter was there," said Hahn, "and gave me the details of how he died."

It happened during the war [said Hahn]. There was a party going on on Saturday night and [Daghlian] was in the lab tinkering with a block of plutonium. They didn't have the safeguards then. Somehow or other, by accident, Daghlian placed a slab of cadmium too close to the plutonium block and the cadmium reflected the neutrons [from the plutonium] back into the block. That built up a chain reaction—a minor one—and in a split second he was fatally irradiated, without feeling anything at first. He died about two weeks later. His flesh just rolled off his body. There was a second physicist named Sloton who died of the same [kind of] accident. Somehow or other at Los Alamos, the precautions against such an accident were not implemented until after Sloton died—Sloton was more famous while Daghlian was just a flunky graduate student.[82]

Prevented from becoming a Navy officer because of an incorrect medical diagnosis that said he had osteomyelitis, Hahn was assigned to the Radio Technicians program, RT, to become what was known as a technician's mate. His assignment lacked both the mystique of working on a top-secret program in the mountains of New Mexico and the action of naval combat in World War II, but the experience couldn't have been better for his future career. After reporting initially to Great Lakes U.S. Naval Training Center in North Chicago (about 30 miles north of Chicago's downtown Loop), Hahn was sent west for three months to the Naval Training School on Monterey Peninsula south of San Francisco. He was then selected to be an instructor and was assigned to the Educational Department at Navy Pier. Located near the Loop, Navy Pier is about two miles north of Meigs Field and present-day McCormick Place.

For the next year-and-a-half, from the early part of October 1945 through March 1946, Hahn taught radar and sonar to shipboard Navy combat personnel, experience that gave him exposure to pulsing and an interest in transient phenomena. Although the material he was teaching was directly related to the work that had been going on for five years at the Radiation Laboratory at MIT, Hahn knew very little at the time about the Rad Lab's contribution to what he was teaching.

I knew more [said Hahn] about what was going on at Los Alamos because people at Purdue were bombarding targets of materials and looking at cross-sections. I got a hint that there was some bomb-making going on, but didn't say anything. You know, the security on that really wasn't as tight as people pretended. I had a vague idea of what was going on just by osmosis when the researchers were going in and out of the cyclotron at Purdue, but I was busy being a student.

But as far as radar and sonar were concerned, I didn't know much about that until after I got out of the Navy. That was more secret to me than the activity at Los Alamos, in a way, because I met more people who went to Los Alamos than who went to MIT.[83]

After serving nearly two years as an enlisted man on active duty in the U.S. Naval Reserve, Hahn was discharged as an Electronics Technicians Mate, Second Class. Soon afterward, he paid a visit to Karl Lark-Horovitz at Purdue to inquire about readmission. "He didn't have any money for graduate student research assistants or teaching assistants—at least in my case,"[84] said Hahn. In fact, he recommended that Hahn go to the president of Purdue and ask for money. "I thought that was kind of naive; you know, a guy with no clout at all to go to the president of the university. I felt like saying, 'Why don't you go to the president?' So I went to Illinois instead and continued my graduate work there and got my MS and PhD."[85]

It was Bob Carter, Hahn's friend from Purdue who had gone to Los Alamos, who told him about the assistantship that was then open at Urbana-Champaign. At Los Alamos, Carter had worked with Donald W. Kerst, the University of Illinois professor who had invented the magnetic induction particle accelerator known as the betatron and who was then preparing to build his latest and largest version. (A 20 MeV and a 50 MeV betatron were already in operation.) When Kerst returned to Illinois from Los Alamos, Carter went with Kerst as a graduate assistant rather than returning to Purdue and he recommended to Kerst that he also select Erwin Hahn as a graduate assistant.

It fell to Hahn's lot to develop a power supply for the accelerator. Initially, it was a useful experience, but after a couple of years Hahn began to feel he was stuck in the role of a technician. He was also disillusioned with the large-scale nature of the project and the limitations it placed on his imagination. "Around the latter part of 1948, I rebelled,"[86] he said. "Kerst kept me on as a flunky technician pounding drills into walls and building power supplies. You know there's only so much you're going to learn there and you have to go on to something else. . . . I preferred small-table science."[87]

It was a perspective that reflected Hahn's own growing-up years when as "a lonesome kid" he regularly visited the local public library and sought out information on his own.

With the betatron [said Hahn] I sensed I was locked into a group, and felt I was not free to imagine, or at least, [not free] to implement my imagination. . . . I had great respect for Kerst's pioneering betatron research, but felt I was not temperamentally suited to the style of collective integration among many people doing research in high-energy physics.[88]

When Kerst finally gave Hahn a chance to do something else, that project also ended in frustration.

I began a two-week experiment with a guy named William Koch, who later became head of the American Institute of Physics in New York. Koch was working for Kerst. I became a colleague of his working on a cloud chamber. We took data day and night for two weeks on what was called triplet production. That involves the use of the gamma ray from the betatron. You plow it into a gas and statistically, every now and then, the gamma ray will produce an electron and a positron together with a recoil electron—in other words, two electrons and one positron. That's called triplet production. A cloud chamber was used to detect these. Sometime during the run—we don't know when—the cloud chamber partially shorted and we really didn't know exactly what the magnetic field was. After two weeks of hard labor, the data was useless. I wasn't enamored with the betatron anyway and this was really my first experiment with it and I said, Oh, to hell. So I looked around for something else to do, and that's how I got into NMR.[89]

In his frustration, Hahn talked his problem over with Professor J.H. Bartlett, a theoretical physicist. "I said to him, 'Look, I'm unhappy. I'm not learning anything.' "[90] In response, Bartlett showed Hahn the 1946 *Physical Review* articles by Harvard's Purcell, Torrey and Pound and by Stanford's Bloch, Hansen and Packard in which they explained how they had come to observe the NMR signal in condensed matter.[91-94] Also available by then, in addition to the 1946 articles, was the April 1948 *Physical Review* paper that would come to be known as BPP. Entitled "Relaxation Effects in Nuclear Magnetic Resonance Absorption" and authored by

Bloembergen, Purcell and Pound, the paper provided helpful information about circuit refinements that had taken place at Harvard following the original experiment as well as information about the extensive experimental and theoretical progress that had been made at Harvard on NMR relaxation, especially liquids. After reading the material, Hahn agreed that he would be interested in doing NMR research, that it appealed to his desire for 'small science' of table-top dimensions where he could work on his own and take him as far as his own capabilities would permit. As a result of his defection to NMR, said Hahn, "Kerst was really mad at me. He thought I was a traitor. I wasn't loyal to his project."[95]

Although Bartlett was willing to support Hahn in his rebellion against the 'big science' of Kerst and the betatron, eventually acquiring Hahn as his thesis student and giving him space in the laboratory connected to Bartlett's office, he wasn't able to provide a great deal of help. For one thing, he hadn't worked personally with NMR and for another, he would depart for a year's sabbatical before Hahn would complete his thesis. With no other NMR expert on the physics staff at the University of Illinois, Hahn would be on his own. "However, with the umbrella support of an Office of Naval Research (ONR) Physics Department block grant, I was able to forge ahead on my own and build a copy of the Harvard CW [continuous-wave] NMR rig."[96] It was essentially the same bridge circuit described by Bloembergen, Purcell and Pound in BPP.

I pack-ratted all kinds of equipment to build up my lab, particularly an old electromagnet nobody seemed to want. Whether to this day I indulged in thievery I am not quite certain. Anyway, maybe it was thievery because I am now punished with a bad back—the surgeons say it is congenital—originating in part from my stupid, zealous, impetuous youth in lifting the magnet myself with my bare hands in order to appropriate it.[97]

The reason Hahn went with Purcell's resonance-absorption apparatus rather than Bloch's nuclear induction version was, he said, "partly psychological."

I chose it because I thought it was easier than Bloch's. I had looked at both papers and thought that I understood the circuitry of two circuits better than the Bloch method where you had to use a little paddle cross-coil. I thought that was a bit complicated. I could understand the circuitry of balanced bridges—tuned circuits—better than I could the coupling with the cross-coil, although both of them are equally good. It was the choice of one versus the other. Either way would have worked.[98]

The connection between Purcell and F.W. Loomis, who had returned as chairman of the University of Illinois physics department after spending the war years as associate director of the MIT Radiation Laboratory, may also have helped tip the scales in favor of the Cambridge-based version. Certainly Loomis' offer to Hahn of an expense-paid trip to Harvard to meet with Purcell, just a few months after Hahn became involved in NMR, helped favor the continued development of the Harvard approach.

I had built their apparatus as a start [based on their papers]. Then they showed me their apparatus and I learned a lot more from them. And I went back and kept working on it, got it to work. They inspired me by my visit there. Purcell was very nice to me. He sat down with me and I asked him a few questions, and he made a few sketches for me. He was very kind to me. Here I was a lowly flunky from graduate school. Pound remembers that visit. Pound showed me around, showed me his permanent magnet quadrupole work, and so forth. They were both very good to me, partly because Loomis had written to them, and they knew Loomis. Loomis having sponsored me, they treated me very well. So it was very good. It got me catapulted.[99]

Around the same time that Hahn visited Harvard, H.S. (Herb) Gutowsky of Harvard joined the faculty of the chemistry department at the University of Illinois. Gutowsky had used NMR at Harvard to investigate the structure of crystals in collaboration with Purcell, Pake and George Kistiakowsky and was planning to investigate its utility in chemical analysis at Illinois. (Chemical shifts were just beginning to be discovered experimentally at the time.) Gutowsky, who was by that time very familiar with NMR apparatuses, was naturally curious about the direction Hahn planned to take with the NMR apparatus he was building, and Hahn, who was just getting into NMR, wasn't at all sure what he was going to do with it. According to Hahn:

At the time, I had no idea about what I wanted to measure with my newly constructed apparatus. I was happy just to see a signal from protons. . . . I felt I was an ignorant peasant graduate student, preoccupied with learning the rudiments of NMR. Herb asked me what I was going to do with the rig I built for my physics thesis. By the time of his query I had cooked up a vague idea that perhaps I could follow the progress of a chemical reaction, maybe by looking at the changes in relaxation times in liquid systems. I decided I needed experience first by measuring relaxation times in the time domain using a pulse saturation method. Why did I choose of all things the heretical subject of measuring the "progress of a chemical reaction" for a graduate physics thesis? The reason: My undergraduate degree was in chemistry, so that was about the only original thing I could think of at the time.[100]

Nicolaas Bloembergen had been back in Holland for about a year and a half at the time Erwin Hahn visited Harvard. In May 1948, a month after BPP was published in *Physical Review* and a few months before Hahn became interested in NMR, Bloembergen's doctoral thesis was published and he received his PhD from the University of Leiden.

Both BPP and Bloembergen's thesis described a transient phenomenon called the "wiggles." According to the authors of BPP, the effect had been observed "rather early" in the course of their research and the decision to mention it briefly in their paper on relaxation effects was justified, they wrote, "if only because it can complicate the interpretation of nuclear absorption experiments in some cases."[101] Later that same year, B.A. Jacobsohn and R.K. Wangness would provide a theoretical analysis of "the wiggles,"* but unbeknownst to both the Harvard team and to Jacobsohn-Wangness, this so-called complication was actually evidence of free precession, the fundamental mechanism behind spin echoes. Although free precession was timidly calling attention to itself through "the wiggles," its presence wasn't being noticed because of the overwhelming noise being generated by the ever-present CW. Had Bloembergen, Purcell, and Pound been pulsing the applied radiofrequency field rather than using a continuous-wave (CW), slow-passage sweep through resonance, the source of "the wiggles"—free precession—would have been more apparent.

---

* Hahn has described the phenomenon of "the wiggles" as follows: "This is a beat phenomenon seen often in [continuous-wave] NMR, after a small sweep magnetic field passes through the resonance condition, and the nuclear spins are tipped slightly to produce a transverse precessing magnetization. The Larmor frequency of this magnetization tracks with the externally swept DC field, and beats with the fixed driving RF field after the resonance condition is traversed."
—E.L. Hahn, "Fifty years of NMR: What happened in the beginning?" speech transcript, 9.

In addition to the "wiggles," which were caused, it could be said, by too-fast slow passage through resonance, Bloembergen's thesis also referred to another transient phenomenon known as the 'nutation effect,' the response of a polarized spin population to a rotating or oscillating magnetic field that was suddenly activated at the point of resonance. According to theory, the sudden perturbation would induce a repetitive flopping of the spins—from the ground state to the excited state and back to the ground state—resulting in an oscillatory motion somewhat analogous to the periodic wobble induced in a spinning gyroscope after it is tipped away from its spin axis. The theory for this nutation had been provided by Julian Schwinger[102] and I.I. Rabi[103] in two adjacent articles in the April 15, 1937 issue of *Physical Review*. Since the effect had not yet been observed experimentally in condensed matter, Hahn decided to look for it and examine its characteristics for his PhD dissertation.

After reading the published thesis of Nico Bloembergen, which contained an analysis by J. Schwinger of the nutation effect (often referred to as the "Rabi flop"), I dropped the fuzzy idea of measuring a chemical reaction and decided to measure instead the nutation dynamics of protons in the rotating frame. The experiment appealed to me as a former radar technician and instructor in the U.S. Navy. These pulses would also be useful for carrying out saturation in order to measure spin-lattice relaxation times.[104]

Hahn didn't know it at the time, but Henry C. Torrey, a member of Purcell's original NMR team who was conducting NMR research at Rutgers University in New Brunswick, New Jersey, had already begun using radiofrequency pulses to search for the same nutations. Although Hahn was the first to announce, via an abstract published in *Physical Review*, that he had experimentally discovered these nutations in condensed matter, Torrey's article, which appeared a few months later, made up in content what it lacked in priority of publication. Torrey's paper, said Hahn, "scooped me completely."

I only went as far as publishing an abstract and continued instead to do more nutation measurements with increased rf pulse power, thinking that the larger-amplitude and higher-frequency nutation signals might be a useful way of achieving better NMR sensitivity. That was a naive idea of no value, but the experimental setup provided conditions for the accident by which I discovered spin echoes.[105]

Unfortunately for Torrey, the pulses he had been using were too long and periodic for either free precession or spin echoes to get a word in edgewise. Instead, it would be Erwin Hahn, the 'new kid' on the NMR block, who would give free precession and spin echoes the opportunity to be "heard."

Erwin Hahn, Doctor of Spins

Since Professor James Bartlett was on a sabbatical when Hahn was completing his thesis, Arnold Nordsieck took over as his nominal advisor. In 1937, Nordsieck had co-authored a paper with Felix Bloch on the infrared catastrophe[106] which Werner Heisenberg "always considered to be of particular importance,"[107] but Nordsieck's interest was not, said Hahn, in magnetic resonance. "He guided me, you might say, by signing my research request chits. His interest wasn't in magnetic resonance at all, and he didn't really steep himself in that discipline. In truth, I more or less was on my own."[108]

In June 1949, upon completion of his thesis on spin nutations, the University of Illinois conferred the PhD degree, Doctor of Philosophy, upon Erwin Louis Hahn. Had the institution known the direction his research would take a month later and the impact of that research, they might have considered awarding him at the same time an honorary DS degree, Doctor of Spins, for the outstanding achievements Hahn would make in manipulating atomic nuclei, achievements that eventually would contribute to the development of magnetic resonance imaging. As Anatole Abragam has noted, "One of the reasons, which in my view will in the future bring NMR imaging far ahead of X-ray imaging is its tremendous flexibility. My old friend Erwin Hahn, the discoverer of spin echoes, a man who probably had more bright ideas in our field than anyone else, used to say: 'There is nothing that nuclear spins will not do for you, as long as you treat them as human beings.' "[109] The University did not grant a degree for doctors who treated spins, of course, and the slang term "spin doctor" would be coined a few decades later to describe public-relations agents seeking to put the desired "spin" on the words and actions of politicians.

After graduation, Hahn stayed on at Illinois as a post-doctoral research associate, his work supported in part by the Office of Naval Research. In the latter part of the summer of 1949, he discovered spin echoes.

"Many people have asked," Professor Hahn said recently, "how I came upon the spin echo effect, particularly because I operated under conditions where I had no real research advisor in NMR, and began my investigations with an ignorance coefficient of 1.00. The answer is, 'By happy accident,' or, as they say, 'Via serendipity.' "[110]

The other question that naturally comes to mind and one that Hahn himself has asked Torrey is, Why didn't Torrey discover free precession during his work with nutations? "Mysteriously, Torrey stated in his paper that no one had yet observed free precession signals," Hahn points out, "and yet he himself did not go ahead and look for an FID simply by turning on a very short pulse after a very short 90-degree pulse 'nutation,' allowing the transverse magnetization to produce a signal with no driving RF present."[111] Torrey's *mea culpa* response to Hahn's question was, "Because I was stupid," to which Hahn responded in an effort to comfort:

> In that case, one could argue that Bloch and Purcell were even more stupid. Purcell and his cohorts were at the forefront of radar pulse technology at the MIT Radiation Laboratory, and yet they did not exploit transient pulse response for NMR. In his pioneering paper, Bloch mentioned that free precession would result after the sudden reorientation of spins by a non-adiabatic field pulse,* but did not emphasize that experimentally one could use an RF pulse extending over many periods.[112]

In Hahn's earnest attempt to console Torrey, he may have forgotten that Torrey also spent the war years at the Radiation Laboratory as a vital member of the Radio Frequency Group and one of Purcell's "cohorts."

The following is a first-hand account by Hahn of his "happy accident," his discovery of spin echoes and free precession (a term often used interchangeably with free induction decay, or FID):

> Lucky for me [wrote Hahn] I was destined to discover free induction and spin echoes by accident because I turned on RF pulse power

---

* "Not only a weak r-f field, acting at resonance over very many Larmor periods, can produce an appreciable nuclear change of orientation, but also a strong field pulse, acting over only a few periods. Once the nuclear moments have been turned into an angle with the constant field, they will continue to precess around it and likewise cause a nuclear induction to occur at an instant when the driving pulse has already disappeared. . . . The main difference between this proposed experiment and the one which we have actually carried out lies in the fact that it would observe by induction the free nuclear precession while we have studied the forced precession impressed upon the nuclei by the applied r-f field." Nobel laureate Richard Ernst has noted that "without experimental confirmation," this paragraph from Bloch's paper on the theory of nuclear induction, "may be considered as the moment of birth of time domain magnetic resonance."
  —F. Bloch, "Nuclear induction," *Physical Review* **70**, (1946), 461; R.R. Ernst, "The multidimensional importance of time domain magnetic resonance," *Pulsed Magnetic Resonance: NMR, ESR, and Optics: A Recognition of E.L. Hahn*, (Oxford: Clarendon Press, 1992), 96.

over shorter periods of times, using pulse sequences in pairs in order to measure relaxation times. . . . My use of pulses permitted measurement of short spin-lattice relaxation times in the millisecond domain. The scheme was as follows: When an RF pulse was turned on, it lasted long enough for a 60-cycle, one-half sine wave of magnetic sweep field to pass through nuclear resonance at the middle of the pulse. The pulse voltage was balanced to a sufficient null by a bridge circuit so that the receiver was not saturated and could detect the absorption "v mode" signals which appeared on top of a pedestal, a small leakage of the pulse itself due to a slight bridge imbalance.

Starting at thermal equilibrium with a first pulse, the signal at the top of the pedestal due to that pulse was compared, after a known time delay of no RF excitation, to a small "v mode" signal on top of a second delayed pedestal caused by an applied second pulse. The second signal amplitude relative to the first one indicated spin-lattice relaxation recovery of magnetization following the saturation caused by the first pulse. By varying known times between first and second pulses, spin-relaxation times were determined in proton samples such as glycerine and water. All signals were synchronized with 60 cycles. In a sweep time of one period of 60 cycles, the oscilloscope face displayed a single "v mode" signal on top of each pedestal, and zero signal during sweeps with time delay and no RF pulse excitation.

Finally one day the weird signal appeared. For no good reason, except maybe to measure as many points as possible, I increased the pulse power and narrowed the pulse widths considerably, to a time of the order of a millisecond or less. The result: A "v mode" type of signal, which looked strangely symmetric, appeared on the oscilloscope in the absence of a pulse and its corresponding pedestal. But I did not admit to that observation at the time as a genuine signal, and cursed it as an annoying glitch. I twiddled the pulse width knob back to a wider pulse and the glitch went away. Offhandedly, on the day of that observation in the late summer of 1949, I blamed the glitch on an erratic misfiring of a multivibrator gate.

A week went by and luckily I fooled with the pulse width knob again. Up popped the signal with no pulse to account for it. This signal, of course, was the spin echo, and this time I nursed and cajoled the then-mysterious blip with various maneuvers. I realized that the 60-cycle modulation was an annoyance and removed it. The symmetric signal had a definite amplitude dependence on pulse intensity and pulse width. After displaying the two-pulse sequence in one

slow single sweep (from protons in glycerine), all the standard characteristics of echo behavior fell out in front of my astonished eyes like
a cornucopia from Mother Nature.

I stuck a screwdriver in the magnet and the echo narrowed because
of the increase in field inhomogeneity. Later, I looked at the echo
decay envelope of protons in water and the envelope decay behavior
was startlingly different. Compared to glycerine, the water decay
envelope no longer looked exponential, but was rather Gaussian in
character. This was the signature of self-diffusion, a deduction which
took me a while to realize only after I noticed that the Gaussian decay
depended on the strength of the field gradient. In short order, all of
the characteristics of damping and various echoes with their delays
showed up with more than two pulses. At the same time, the
inevitable FID signals showed up after each pulse. The FID told me
immediately that I had free precession, but to figure out the various
echoes from three pulses, including the very interesting stimulated
echo, I had to sit down with Bloch's equations and figure out first
why two equal pulses produced an echo.

This effort would have been simplified considerably if I had conceived of the vector model directly and started out with the 90-180
degree pulse echo model demonstrated later by Carr and Purcell. I
devised my own two-dimensional vector models for primary and
stimulated echoes following the application of two and then three
identical pulses. After I announced the discovery of the echo, I was
honored by a letter of congratulations from Ed Purcell in which he
sketched his three-dimensional 'eight ball' picture of the 90-90 degree
spin echo. To say the least, so many new effects came out in such a
short time that I was bewildered and shaky with excitement. It was
only a few days after I confirmed the signal as genuine that I happened to look at the echoes from protons in alcohol and saw the beat
modulation of the echo envelope. That was too much! I had a lot of
explaining to do![113]

"In retrospect," Hahn has said, "I tremble at the thought that [by ignor-
ing the 'glitch'] I could have missed completely the discovery of free precession and spin echoes. The dangerous situation was that I was completely alone with no one to advise me; and then on the other hand it was
a good thing for me to go it alone. A week later, fortunately, the signal
came back, and this time my wheels turned."[114] D.M.S. Bagguley saw
Hahn's response, however, as more than luck.

Modulated signals which occur following an initial impulse excitation of a periodic system are, of course, familiar in the form of
beat phenomena derived from a linear superposition of the individual responses for a set of oscillators having either slightly different frequencies, or the same frequency but loosely coupled
together. It was the genius of Hahn to appreciate that he should not
force his observations to conform with such models and to realize
that he had discovered a pulse sequence which provided a
response at time intervals controlled by the investigator, in contrast to the usual beat signals which are controlled by frequency
differences specific to the sample (and so do not give rise to a variable parameter).[115]

Purcell wrote his letter of congratulations to Hahn in the late fall of
1949. When Hahn responded in a letter written on December 8, he said:

Your 3-dimensional spin echo model takes the prize for simplicity
and purposes of explanation. . . . Thanks for your interest, and if you
care to pass on any other ideas I will be very much interested. As you
say, this stuff is intriguing—when I first found the echoes, you can't
imagine what a daze I was in and still am![116]

In 1994, the emotions Hahn had felt nearly 45 years earlier were still
fresh in his mind:

The private experience I had in discovering the spin echo was just
unbelievable. Here I was, an ignorant peasant—here I stumbled on
something and nobody else knew about it and here I was, the first
guy in the world who's ever seen it and I had no training to get it. I
felt I had found something in the jungle that nobody else found and
was confronted with the task of explaining it. That was really a very
giddy experience. You have this possessive idea. Boy, you don't want
to give it away. You want to figure it out first, and I didn't have the
full artillery of theoretical training to do it. I had just finished graduate school and didn't know a damn thing, I mean in retrospect. Still I
worked out the empirical ideas pretty well with equations that I
could work with.

It's like you're an explorer. It doesn't have the appeal to the public
eye like discovering the source of the Nile. Everybody understands
what it means by finding the source of a river. They don't understand

what it means when you find the source of a phenomenon. But it's the same sensation, but in a different, non-macroscopic sense.[117]

In September 1949, just after Hahn discovered spin echoes, Charles Slichter moved to Urbana to become a physics instructor at the University of Illinois. A graduate student of Purcell's, Slichter had done his thesis on electron spin resonance in paramagnetic salts and had received his PhD in June 1949, the same month Hahn received his PhD. In Slichter, Hahn finally had a person on the Illinois physics staff who appreciated the potency of Hahn's findings and to whom Hahn could turn for assistance when it came to NMR. With the discovery of so many new effects in such a short time, said Hahn,

> I was absolutely bewildered in trying to explain everything, which I could not. I worked out the prediction of the echoes and FID from Bloch's equations; and when Charley Slichter arrived from Harvard to become an instructor, he became the first person in the Illinois physics department who understood the significance of my discoveries. Finally, here was someone with whom I could talk and get some helpful suggestions, particularly about the spatial spin diffusion effect in the magnetic field gradient.[118]

In a 1986 interview, Hahn said, "Charlie Slichter . . . is one who, to this day, I believe is one of the most profound intuitive NMR scientists in the world."[119] The respect is mutual. For a substantial *festschrift* published by Oxford University's Clarendon Press on the occasion of Hahn's 70th birthday, Slichter wrote:

> Erwin Hahn's contributions of pulsed NMR and spin echoes launched the two main branches of present day NMR, high resolution pulsed NMR of liquids and pulsed NMR of solids. The techniques he introduced totally dominate physical, chemical, and biological applications of NMR. . . . Our year together was a total delight. . . . The year of working with Erwin launched me, together with the students I inherited (and those I subsequently acquired) on pulsed NMR.[120]

Slichter's first graduate research student at Illinois was Richard Norberg whose 1951 PhD thesis would constitute the first pulsed NMR study of a solid. "Dick Norberg . . . shared lab space with me," said Hahn, "in the so-called 'Physics Penthouse Loft' on the top floor of the old physics building. Dick was a beneficial stimulus in bringing up all sorts of interesting questions, and encouraging me not to further delay the writing of a major paper because I was trying to solve all the mysteries at once before doing so."[121]

Aboard the Rotating Frame

Earlier in this chapter, Hahn was quoted as saying that it was after reading Bloembergen's thesis that he "dropped the fuzzy idea of measuring a chemical reaction and decided to measure instead the nutation dynamics of protons in the rotating frame."[122] Compared to the laboratory frame of reference whose x, y and z axes remain stationary, the rotating frame concept requires somewhat of a mental exercise in the riding of whirligigs. Spectroscopists working in high-resolution NMR would be able to sit out the wild rides ushered in by Hahn's spin echoes for two more decades, until approximately 1970 when the use of computers for data manipulation in the NMR laboratories became more common. Although the major impact of Hahn's spin echoes with regard to computerized spectroscopy would thus be delayed, awaiting the development and availability of computers, researchers who wanted to learn more about the magnetic world of atomic nuclei were compelled to climb aboard right away.

Since the laboratory frame of reference is stationary, spins precessing about the static field (which is oriented in the z-direction) or even flopping from the z-axis to the y-axis and back again are fairly easy to follow when standing outside that frame of reference. With the advent of pulsed NMR and the rotating frame of reference, however, the person who was unwilling to mentally climb aboard the rotating frame was at a distinct disadvantage. To contemplate the path of precessing magnetic vectors in the laboratory frame and not in the rotating frame was, as Peter Morris of the University of Cambridge put it, "rather akin to a parent wishing to communicate with a son or daughter on a fairground roundabout."

His best solution is to get onto the roundabout himself. Likewise, our best means of investigating the motion of the nuclear magnetization vectors is from the standpoint of a reference frame revolving around the static field direction at the Larmor frequency. This is known as the rotating frame, whose coordinates are designated by the primed quantities x', y', z': the corresponding laboratory frame coordinates being x, y, z.[123]

For a parent standing on the platform of a carousel as the carved mount on which their son or daughter is riding oscillates just within the circumference of the machine in large-amplitude sine waves, it seems fairly straightforward to trace the leaps of the stallion through the music-filled air, simple in fact if only the vertical movement of the horse is considered and not the rotation of the entire merry-go-round assembly. The same principle applies to the rotating frame of atomic nuclei, though the mechanics are different. In the 1950 paper in which Hahn provided the theory for his spin echoes, he referred to this rotating frame concept as the "moving coordinate representation."[124] It's a ride Hahn would take many times over the course of his career, as was noted in 1978 when he was named Faculty Research Lecturer at the University of California, Berkeley by Berkeley's Academic Senate, the highest award the faculty can award its members.

Hahn thinks very well in a rotating frame of reference; that is, he transfers his consciousness to a set of mathematical coordinates rotating at very high frequency and in so doing simplifies the analysis of coherent phenomena. The exercise that leads to discovery for Hahn makes most people simply dizzy.[125]

The Basis for the Echo
The following is a step-by-step description of what was happening within the rotating-frame world of the hydrogen protons in Hahn's original sample of glycerine: At the beginning of the experiment, the spins in Hahn's sample were at thermal equilibrium with slightly more of them precessing with the static field (the z direction) than against it (the $-z$ direction). At this point, in other words, the net magnetization of the spins was in the z direction with regard to the laboratory frame of reference. (See Figure 1.)

Upon introduction of Hahn's first radiofrequency pulse along the x axis, at a frequency which coincided with the sample's Larmor frequency, the net magnetization vector began to tip away from the z direction into the x-y plane and began to precess slowly about the RF field (the x' axis) while continuing to precess rapidly about the z axis. From the laboratory frame of reference with x, y, and z coordinates set within a sphere for clarity of demonstration, a downward, circumnavigating spiral would have been traced on the wall of the sphere by the net magnetization vector as the spins continued to precess around the primary z axis. At the end of this first "90-degree pulse," the net magnetization vector was tracing a line around the equator of the sphere, as seen from the lab-

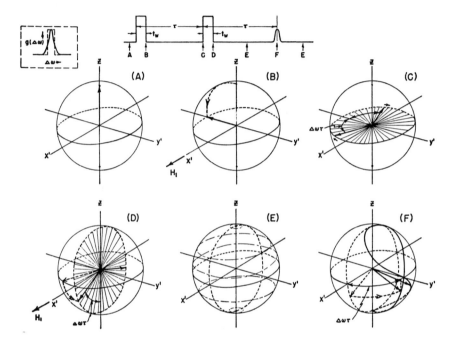

For the pulse condition $\omega_1 t_w = \pi/2$, the formation of the eight-ball echo pattern is shown in the coordinate system rotating at angular frequency ω. The moment vector monochromats are allowed to ravel completely in a time $\tau \gg 1/(\Delta\omega)_{1/2}$ before the second pulse is applied. The echo gives maximum available amplitude at $\omega_1 t_w = 2\pi/3$.

—From "Spin echoes," by E.L. Hahn, *Physical Review* **80**, (1950), 583.

Figure 1. The Formation of a Hahn
90-Degree-Plus-90-Degree Spin Echo

oratory frame, although the line would have appeared somewhat skewed as a result of the nutation or periodic gyration introduced into the system by the secondary precession of the spins around the smaller RF field.

If Hahn could have climbed aboard the rotating frame at that point and observed the process from inside the sphere, he would have seen the same actions but they would have appeared differently to him. Instead of seeing a spiral traced on the wall of the sphere by the net magnetization vector as it descended, he would have seen a straightforward 90-degree tipping of the vector and since the RF field was directed perpendicular to the main field along the x-axis, he would have observed the net magnetization vector precessing only around the x'-axis, even though in 'reality' the x'-axis was itself spinning around the z-axis of the laboratory frame at a much quicker rate than the net magnetization vector was precessing around the x'-axis. Focusing on the precession pattern of the net magnetization vector from within the "carousel," the background outside of the carousel would have appeared as just a blur, although the blur would actually have been evidence of the vector's continuing primary precession around the z-axis of the laboratory frame.

Even after the oscillations driving the secondary field were turned off after one millisecond of pulse time had elapsed, the net magnetization vector continued to process perpendicularly to the z-axis, evidence of free precession. Compared to the one millisecond pulse time, this period of quietness was relatively long. For a time, the net magnetization vector, consisting really of a bundle of individual magnetization vectors, continued precessing in phase in the x'-y' plane, creating an electromotive force that could be picked up as an induction signal by a coil perpendicular to that plane. This signal, called a free induction decay signal, or FID, began to decrease in strength, however, as inhomogeneities within the main field began to affect the precession rates of the spins contributing to it. The spins in the higher-strength portions of the main field began precessing faster than the spins in the lower-strength portions of the main field and, from a somewhat larger perspective, the individual magnetization vectors or "isochromats" contributing to the net magnetization vector began fanning out along the circumference of this "pancake" of precession until all 360 degrees of the pancake were equally filled with isochromats. The time from the end of the pulse until the FID signal was lost due to inhomogeneities was equal to the T_2 relaxation time of Hahn's sample.

Hahn's decision to pulse the "ride" button again before the sample's T_2-relaxation time was completed converted what could be visualized as a relatively sedate ride on a carousel of spins into a heart-stopping escapade that dipped and flipped unlike any ride at an amusement park. The second RF pulse applied by Hahn suddenly "flipped" his "pancake" 90 degrees, however, so that it was now occupying the x'-z' plane of the rotating frame, with the isochromats precessing around the y'-axis. The radio pulse was again turned off after one millisecond, the same time period as the first pulse, and another relatively long quiet period began. These quiet periods are a major benefit of the spin-echo method. With the system free of the radio noise driving the oscillating field, there is less interference in picking up signals.

The last part of the ride before the echo was formed was probably the most hair-raising of all, if one has a good imagination. If you were sitting astride one of the magnetic moment vectors, the path traced by the center of the moment's cone of precession would have made an elongated "figure 8" pattern before finally returning to the relative calm of thermal equilibrium. At the point the isochromats formed the "figure 8," they were also regrouping to form an echo.

The three-dimensional, six-sphere series of drawings ending with the figure-8 was Edward Purcell's contribution to Hahn's task of explaining the echo. A year later, in 1950, Purcell and Herman Carr, then a doctoral candidate working with Purcell at Harvard, would provide a variation on Hahn's original echo that consisted of one 90-degree pulse and one 180-degree pulse* instead of two 90-degree pulses. (The variation was published in 1954.[126]) Although the same effect causes the echo in both methods, for simplicity's sake the second version will be used to further illustrate the basis for the echo's formation.

Up until the second pulse, everything is identical with the Carr-Purcell sequence. Prior to the second pulse, the isochromats have begun fanning out as in the earlier explanation. (See Figure 2.) When the second pulse

---

* Hahn was aware of the 90° - 180° pulse in the early part of 1950, as evidenced by a footnote included with his theoretical explanation of spin echoes submitted to *Physical Review* on approximately May 20, 1950 in which he states, "It is interesting to note that the configuration at $t=t_w$, namely, $M_{xy}=M_0$, can in principle be exactly repeated at $t=2\tau$ by doubling the second r-f pulse width with respect to the first one which is at the pulse condition $\omega_1 t_w=\pi/2$. ... Actual experiment indicates that the inhomogeneity in H_1 throughout the sample prevents this from exactly taking place. ..." The 1954 paper by Carr and Purcell would explain how to eliminate the effect of diffusion, a primary contributor to echo reduction.

In a letter from Hahn to Carr dated November 14, 1950, Hahn noted that the 90°-180° pulse sequence was the one he always used in explaining the echo.

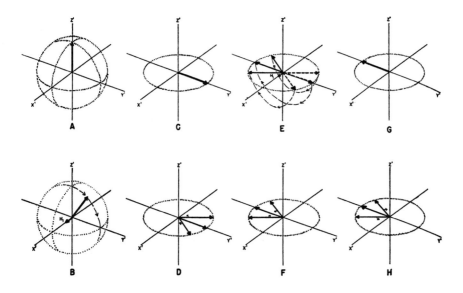

The formation of an echo. Initially the net magnetic moment vector is in its equilibrium position (*A*) parallel to the direction of the strong external field. The rf field H_1 is then applied. As viewed from the rotating frame of reference the net magnetic moment appears (*B*) to rotate quickly about H_1. At the end of a 90° pulse the net magnetic moment is in the equatorial plane (*C*). During the relatively long period of time following the removal of H_1, the incremental moment vectors begin to fan out slowly (*D*). This is caused by the variations in H_z over the sample. At time $t = \tau$, the rf field H_1 is again applied. Again the moments (*E*) begin to rotate quickly about the direction of H_1. This time H_1 is applied just long enough to satisfy the 180° pulse condition. This implies that at the end of the pulse all the incremental vectors are again in the equatorial plane. In the relatively long period of time following the removal of the rf field, the incremental vectors begin to recluster slowly (*F*). Because of the inverted relative positions following the 180° pulse and because each incremental vector continues to precess with its former frequency, the incremental vectors will be perfectly reclustered (*G*) at $t = 2\tau$. Thus maximum signal is induced in the pickup coil at $t = 2\tau$. This maximum signal, or echo, then begins to decay as the incremental vectors again fan out (*H*).

—From "Effects of diffusion on free precession in nuclear magnetic resonance experiments," by H.Y. Carr and E.M. Purcell, *Physical Review* **94**, (1954), 632.

Figure 2. The Formation of a Carr-Purcell
90-Degree-Plus-180-Degree Spin Echo

is activated and held on for twice as long as the first pulse, the "pancake" flips 180 degrees instead of 90, initiating a reverse process that serves as the basis for the echo. Previously, as inhomogeneities took effect, the isochromats fanned out. Flipped 180 degrees, the isochromats begin to regroup and after the second waiting period has elapsed, which is equal in length to the first waiting period, the isochromats have become as one with the same signal strength originally displayed by the net magnetization vector precessing in the $x'-y'$ plane. The coil perpendicular to that plane picks up the induction signal, free of radio interference from the oscillator.

To explain his discovery, Hahn began using a variety of illustrations, including a number of examples from other mechanical systems. One impressive example used by Hahn (contributed by C.A. Hutchison) involves the use of a dye streak in a clear viscous fluid. After first dispersing the dye in the fluid, Hahn reverses the mechanical action and the dye streak is reformed in its original arrangement.

A hypothetical analogy used by Hahn to illustrate the concept, also mentioned by Bagguley, involves a group of runners. Prior to the starting gun, as the runners warm up, randomness is displayed, analogous to the period before the first pulse. As the pulse is initiated, the runners line up at the starting blocks and, at the end of the pulse, take off simultaneously. This race is not to see who comes in first, however. This is a race meant to end in a tie, although the runners will "compete" at different speeds. The faster runners soon outpace the slower runners and, for a time, it appears that there are going to be winners and losers. But these runners are playing by different rules. At some point in time, analogous to the end of the first waiting period used in Hahn's spin echo, the starting gun is fired again. The runners know that this means they are to return to the starting point of the race at the same speed at which they ran the first part of the race. Since the faster runners have farther to return and the slower runners have less distance to travel, maintaining the same velocities for the second half of the race will ensure that all runners arrive at the starting blocks simultaneously. (Incidentally, should the racers all run past the starting blocks and repeat the race in the opposite direction with a third gunshot telling them to turn around again and return to the starting blocks, the same runner dispersal and reformation process would be repeated.)

The racing analogy was used fairly soon after the discovery of spin echoes, as indicated in a letter from Hahn to Herman Carr at Harvard dated November 14, 1950:

By the way, Prof. Bloch tells me he was with Purcell on the boat to Europe (the Amsterdam conference) and Bloch mentioned Purcell's analogy about the rabbits. I took a cue from this in one of the colloquiums I gave, and compared echoes to a bunch of race track contestants who run with different speeds. You know the rest, except you prefer rabbits. One thing though, spins don't multiply like rabbits![127]

The Benefits of the Echo

Understanding the way spin echoes are obtained and how they form also helps one understand their benefits.

One major benefit of spin echoes which has already been mentioned, for example, is the fact that interference from the oscillator driving the RF field is absent during collection of the echo signal, resulting in dramatically improved signal-to-noise ratios. At the end of the first pulse, the net magnetization vector is precessing around the main field in the x'-y' plane just as strongly as it will be later when the echo is formed, but the signal cannot be harvested cleanly at that instant. Two waiting periods later, however, when the echo forms in silence without noise from the high-powered excitation pulse, the collection apparatus is ready and waiting "all ears," so to speak, for the all-important signal.

The idea of a radio pulse followed by silence was, in fact, an idea taken directly from the radar systems developed at the Radiation Laboratory. In radar, the total pulse repetition period might be 1 millisecond (one-thousandth of a second) in length, for example, while the pulse itself might be only 1 microsecond (one millionth of a second) in duration. Much of the "silent" time between pulses is thus available for echo listening free of the noise interference associated with radio transmission. As a radar instructor during the war, Hahn was very familiar with this "duplex" alternation of transmission and reception. That's why he still continues to be amazed by the fact that "those guys at Harvard" who had worked at the Radiation Laboratory didn't figure it out first.

> That I don't understand. . . . They should have been inclined to do it because they had been living with radar longer than me. . . . What inspired me was the fact that I wanted to look at nutations, and nutations required a step function. You turn a pulse on and you turn it off. Knowing that I could saturate in a short time with a pulse and knowing that I wanted to measure relaxation, I wanted to turn on two pulses, the first pulse to saturate, the second one to monitor how much recovered, and then start over again. Well, by virtue of this

application of two pulses and then waiting and then starting over, that set the stage for seeing an echo without my predicting it. It's as simple as that. Now why those guys at Harvard didn't do it is beyond my comprehension because all the time dependence of that approach is inherent in the Bloch equations. And they had the Bloch equations, but they didn't exploit it. It isn't that I was a genius, it just happened I did it first. I mean, it would eventually have been done by somebody else.[128]

(Incidentally, although spin echoes, like radar, use radio pulses, the term "spin echoes" is not meant to imply that a reflection process similar to radar is utilized to obtain NMR signals. Any "reflections" associated with spin echoes have more to do with the "mirror images" of reversed action than they do with "bounced-back" radio waves.)

The fact that echoes form cleanly even after the net magnetization vector has fanned out to all points of the x'-y' compass because of field inhomogeneities is strong evidence of their usefulness in separating useful chemical data from misleading data supplied by the apparatus.

In many cases the dominant factor controlling R_2^* [equal to $1/T_2^*$], the rate constant for decay of the FID, is the magnetic field inhomogeneity rather than the spin dynamics that contain useful chemical information. There is an important experiment that allows us to examine the rate at which the magnetization would decay in the absence of field inhomogeneity, i.e. the true R_2. This two-pulse experiment, which produces a 'spin echo,' was initially developed in 1950 [publication date] by Hahn to study transverse relaxation, but it has become one of the key components embedded in modern pulse sequences.[129]

In addition to improving signal-to-noise and minimizing the effect of inhomogeneous fields, Hahn's spin echo also provided a direct method for measuring spin-spin relaxation times (T_2), a more efficient approach for finding unknown resonances, and a way to avoid the tedious tuning and balancing procedures associated with both bridge- and crossed-coil NMR systems.

Some of the inherent advantages of spin echoes such as improved signal-to-noise data collection would also not be fully utilized until the advent of vastly improved digital measuring devices and more affordable computer systems, many of which did not become available until at least two decades after the discovery of spin echoes. Because of the capability of computers to control all aspects of an NMR experiment, including radiofrequencies and pulse timing, it became possible to accurately reproduce the data collection process over and over again. By taking multiple "shots" and superimposing them with signal averaging techniques, signal-to-noise ratios could be improved even more.

R. Freeman of Cambridge University has called attention to another capability made possible for the first time with spin echoes—spin choreography—which would become a vital tool in the hands of chemists.

> Very soon after the initial discovery of nuclear magnetic resonance, E.L. Hahn performed an experiment that, in conceptual originality and elegance, transcended all that had preceded it—the spin echo experiment. Here was an idea to inspire the young scientists reading about NMR for the first time. Not only could one work with these strange new entities called spins, but also *manipulate* them like a conjurer with a pack of cards. . . . Once Hahn had shown the way, the idea that nuclear spins could be manipulated in quite complicated ways gradually gained acceptance.[130]

Although spin choreographers began teaching atomic nuclei some new steps right away, introduction of the more complicated dance routines for spins would wait until the computer became a common laboratory tool in the 1970s. About the same time "disco" was becoming a common household word, a whole new set of acronyms for spin dances were becoming common among spectroscopists, as physicist Anatole Abragam pointed out in 1992.

> No one benefited more from Hahn's discovery of spin echoes than the chemists and biochemists. They have reached a degree of sophistication and refinement which often baffles me and sometimes even Erwin.
>
> I remember my last Gordon Conference in 1985. I was sitting next to Erwin while young brilliant chemists described, one after the other, the beauties of MLEV, WALTZ, COSY, DEPT, FOCSY, SECSY, INEPT, BLEW, etc. After a while Erwin leaned toward me and asked, "Anatole, remember the time when we explained things to chemists?"[131]

Abragam was first introduced to Hahn, the physicist, at the famous radiofrequency spectroscopy conference in Amsterdam in 1950. Hahn wasn't there. "I met him by proxy," Abragam explained.

Ed Purcell told me there about the spin echoes, in his luminously intuitive way as usual. I was lucky to have that introduction. My interests at the time were in ESR, not NMR, and when a few months later the famous *Physical Review* article, which was to change the face of NMR for the next forty years, arrived in Saclay [France], I might have missed it then if Ed had not warned me about spin echoes. I have been following Erwin the physicist ever since.[132]

Abragam, who would meet Hahn a few years later during a visit to the University of California at Berkeley, has also introduced his readers to Erwin, the person.

Elsewhere,[133] I have described Erwin as "an extrovert genius with an extensive collection of funny stories of all kinds: some, whose gentle wit would enchant a country vicar, others, whose robust gaiety would cause a mule skinner to blush." I remember riding with Erwin in a streetcar in Ljubljana. We were going to the Institute of Physics where our conference was taking place. To relieve the tedium of the ride Erwin was telling me some delightful stories (of the second type, I am afraid). I cautioned him against the possibility of being overheard by our fellow travelers. "Nonsense, what do they understand, peasants, peasants all of them." "Is not the Institute the next stop?" I asked Erwin. "No sir," said one of the peasants, "the Institute is three stops ahead."

What finally transformed my liking of Erwin into brotherly love was the discovery that Erwin's father bore the same Christian name (perhaps I had better say the same *first* name) as my own father— Israel. [Editor's note: Both Hahn and Abragam are Jewish.][134]

Spin Diffusion and Stimulated Echoes

Since the discovery of spin echoes resulted from Hahn's decision to use pulses to measure spin-*lattice* relaxation times, it is ironic that one of the first benefits he found for his echoes was the direct measurement of T_2, spin-*spin* relaxation times. At the time of Hahn's 1949 experiments with nutations, the standard method for measuring T_2 relaxation time was by the line-width method, measuring the width of the spectral line at half its maximum height. When Hahn compared the T_2 plots obtained with his direct spin-echo method, however, for protons in a water solution with a high concentration of ferric ions versus the T_2 plots obtained for the same solution with the line-width method used by Bloembergen, et al. in

BPP,[135] he found remarkable agreement, with all of the plots having a clear linear relationship.[136]

Although T_2 could be measured directly using spin echoes, Hahn discovered and reported in his 1950 spin echoes article that spin diffusion, especially within lower-viscosity liquids, had the potential for diminishing the strength of the echo. Essentially, diffusion is the transport of nuclei within a substance and in liquids. This transport could occur rapidly enough to increase the dephasing rate between the second pulse and the echo. Hahn's paper provided an analysis of the effect so that its impact on T_2 measurements could be minimized. Although Hahn's analysis of the effect of diffusion was correct for the first part of the spin-echo sequence, it contained an error in its analysis of later pulses. This shortcoming was corrected by Carr and Purcell in their 1954 paper on 90°-180° pulse sequences and they provided a method for eliminating the effect of diffusion.[137] For those interested in measuring diffusion rates within liquids, however, Hahn's discovery provided a convenient method of measurement.

Within a week of discovering his first spin echo and measuring T_2, Hahn devised a three-pulse spin-echo variation called a "stimulated echo" (see Figure 3) with which he could measure self diffusion and the effect of T_1. It was the first time multiple echoes were sighted. Although it would be expected that discovery of an echo after two pulses would have prompted Hahn to find out what happened after a third, conjuring up stimulated echoes was more complicated than merely pulsing the sample at equal time intervals *ad infinitum*,* as the source of stimulated echoes was different than that of standard echoes. Whereas standard echoes with their "time reversal" were a manifestation of "phase memory" in the $x'-y'$ plane, stimulated echoes manifested the history of spins along the z axis. Hahn found that this z-axis, T_1-related history could be recalled if the interval between the second and third pulse was different than that of the interval between the first and second pulses and if the third pulse was initiated before the T_1 period following the first two pulses had elapsed. Because stimulated echoes were formed on the basis of z-axis history and not the more short-term memory of the $x'-y'$ axis, the effect of diffusion on stimulated echoes was negligible.

---

* Carr and Purcell would later show that one may build a train of echoes by adding more 180-degree pulses onto their basic 90-degree-plus-180-degree sequence.

—H.Y. Carr and E.M. Purcell, "Effects of diffusion on free precession in nuclear magnetic resonance experiments," *Physical Review* **94**, (1954), 630.

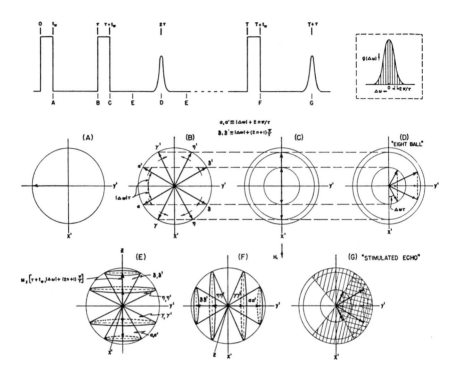

A vector representation which accounts for the stimulated echo at $t = T+\tau$ is shown under conditions of the special case for the primary echo model in Fig. 1 [of original paper]. For a given $|\Delta\omega|$, the symbols α, α' and δ, δ' denote those moments which have Larmor frequencies such that they precess angles $|\Delta\omega|\tau + 2n\pi$ and $|\Delta\omega|\tau + (2n+1)\pi$ respectively in time $t = \tau$. n is any integer which applies to frequencies within the spectrum which will lie in a pair of cones corresponding to a specific $|\Delta\omega|$. These cones provide M_z components (after the pulse at τ) which are available for stimulated echo formation after the pulse at T. The shaded area in G indicates the density of moment vectors. The absence of vectors on the $-y'$ side leaves a dimple on the unit sphere.

—From "Spin echoes," by E.L. Hahn, *Physical Review* **80**, (1950), 588.

Figure 3. Formation of a Hahn Stimulated Echo

The Mystery of the Echo Envelope Beats

Within a few months of his discovery of spin echoes, Erwin Hahn discovered another phenomenon in his experiments which he would later call the "echo envelope modulation effect" in his 1950 spin-echo paper. By that time, he was aware of chemical shifts that had been observed in other laboratories* and he recognized that what he was observing on his oscilloscope screen at the University of Illinois was also evidence of a chemical shift, or what he referred to at one point in his paper as the "chemical Larmor shift effect."

At Illinois, I was aware of chemical shifts. I didn't discover them but they showed up in the echo signal as beats between different species. In other words, I would hit two nuclei of the same species but shifted and they would beat with one another.[138]

In his paper, Hahn showed echo patterns obtained with his pulse sequence from fluorine (F^{19}) nuclei in three different organic compounds. In each case, the free induction decay signals and spin echoes revealed heterodyne beat patterns of differing frequencies indicating, wrote Hahn, that "two or more spin groups [were] contained in the same molecule and [had] non-equivalent molecular environments in the same sample." Spin echoes, he observed, offered simultaneous detection of shifts and faster search times, while providing resolution "at least as good"[139] as previous resonance methods.

It was less clear, however, as to what was causing another echo phenomenon mentioned by Hahn in his 1950 article on spin echoes, an oscilloscope trace that he referred to as the "echo envelope modulation effect." Although he observed the effect with a number of organic compounds,

---

* In 1949, Nicolaas Bloembergen and Walter Knight had published in *Physical Review* the first reports of fairly-large shifts that had occurred in their laboratories under somewhat special circumstances and in early 1950, W.C. Dickinson at MIT and W.G. Proctor and F.C. Yu at Stanford had announced their observation of smaller resonant-frequency shifts that occurred when identical nuclei occupied different chemical environments. At Illinois, Herb Gutowsky and Charles Slichter were also beginning to delve into the phenomenon. Hahn was also aware of two theoretical treatments on the subject of chemical shifts by Norman Ramsey, the second of which, not yet published, Hahn references in a footnote in his 1950 paper.
    —N. Bloembergen, *Physical Review* **75**, (1949), 1326; W. Knight, *Physical Review* **76**, (1949), 1260; W.C. Dickinson, "Dependence of the F^{19} Nuclear Resonance Position on Chemical Compound," *Physical Review* **77**, (1950), 736; and W.G. Proctor and F.C. Yu, "The dependence of a nuclear magnetic resonance frequency upon chemical compound," *Physical Review* **77**, (1950), 717.

the echo envelope modulation effect he showed in his 1950 paper was the one he obtained from protons in C_2H_5OH.

In general, the oscilloscope signal dropped off with time, reminiscent of a normal free induction decay pattern, but the drop-off was not steady. Instead of the normal continuous downward slope typical of a FID, the slope on this oscilloscope trace consisted of a sharply undulating beat pattern which was in violation, according to Hahn, of the normal decay caused by self-diffusion and T_2 relaxation. The period of the modulation, observed Hahn, was generally greater than the echo lifetime and inversely proportional to the applied radiofrequency field. Ruling out the possibility that the effect was that of a normal chemical shift, Hahn observed that "this modulation effect cannot be attributed to an interference between several spin groups" and speculated that perhaps it was due to an interaction between a nuclear spin and its molecule that interfered with the normal echo-forming process. He promised to treat the subject in greater detail in a later paper. The puzzle would occupy much of his time during his next two years at Stanford.

From Illinois to Stanford

When Hahn's one-year stint as a postdoctoral research associate was completed at Illinois, his spin echoes provided him entrée to a research fellowship at Stanford.

> Spin echoes . . . gave me a mark of distinction, if I may put it that way. I learned through the grapevine that my application for a National Research Council Fellowship (to work where, I wasn't certain) was at the bottom of the pile until one of the judges, J.W. Beams of the University of Virginia, put it near the top because he noted my discovery of spin echoes. So with the Fellowship in hand, Professor Nordsieck who was at Illinois and who previously did some theoretical work with Felix Bloch at Stanford, suggested that further studies on NMR at Stanford would be most appropriate with my Fellowship.[140]

Although Nordsieck had been Hahn's advisor in name only and had neither followed his research nor taken interest in the spin echoes he discovered, he did provide valuable assistance when it came time for Hahn to move on. "He was so preoccupied," said Hahn, "with the design and construction of an analog computer that he absolutely avoided all distractions. Nevertheless, I owe my thanks to Nordsieck. As a theoretician who at one time had worked with Felix Bloch, Nordsieck convinced Bloch to take me on as a postdoc fellow at Stanford when it came time for me to leave Illinois."[141]

Hahn looked forward to Stanford for two reasons. First, he was attracted to the climate of Northern California, having spent a few months on Monterey Peninsula during the war. Located in Palo Alto, about 60 miles north of Monterey near the south end of San Francisco Bay, Stanford University offered mild, springlike weather for 10 months out of the year. Second, Hahn looked forward to working with the formulator of the equations which had been so helpful in explaining his echoes.

> Among the versatile contributions of Felix Bloch to physics [said Hahn], the Bloch equations of nuclear induction have played a major role in guiding researchers and students in the interpretation of resonance experiments. From personal experience, the direction of my research in physics would have been quite different without recourse to the Bloch equations. As a graduate and one-year postdoctoral student at the University of Illinois, my start in NMR research was based on these equations. Since I did not know how to use quantum mechanics, the classical pictures allowed by Bloch's equations saved my neck because they afforded a reasonable macroscopic interpretation of spin echo experiments. [142]

By the time Hahn arrived at Stanford in the fall of 1950, nearly five years had elapsed since Bloch's discovery of NMR in condensed matter, or as Bloch preferred to call the phenomenon, nuclear induction. Following that discovery, Bloch had embarked on a systematic program to "apply" the power of nuclear induction to the measurement of nuclear magnetic moments. He did not forget, however, his reason for inventing nuclear induction in the first place, to improve the accuracy with which he could measure a magnetic field and thereby increase the accuracy with which he could measure the magnetic moment of the neutron. Although Bloch's 1940 measurement of the neutron's magnetic moment in collaboration with Luis Alvarez had been a model of elegance, Bloch was not satisfied with the 1 percent uncertainty in accuracy imposed on his experiment by a flip-coil field measurement with a minimum uncertainty of 0.4 percent. Instead of getting results that were accurate to one part in a hundred, Bloch wanted results that were accurate to at least one part in a thousand.

In fact, while still in Cambridge where he worked at the Radio Research Laboratory for the last two years of the war, Bloch had even talked with I.I. Rabi about the possibility of shipping a permanent magnet from Stanford to Columbia for calibration with molecular beams and then having it shipped it back to Stanford. "It sounded extravagant," Bloch acknowledged to science historian Charles Weiner in 1968, "as one would never know what happened to the magnet in shipment."[143]

Although Bloch hadn't followed through with that idea,* his commitment to achieving a reliable, highly-calibrated magnetic field was unswerving and by 1948 he and his colleagues, Hans Staub and D. B. Nicodemus, were able to achieve, using Bloch's nuclear induction method, a highly stabilized magnetic field which contributed greatly to their improved accuracy in measuring the neutron's magnetic moment. (Another 25 years would pass before their 1948 results would be improved by another order of magnitude.)

Concomitant with the increased resolution in the neutron experiment came improved resolution in the measurement of nuclear magnetic moments. After measuring the moments of the proton, the deuteron and the triton in the latter part of the 1940s as well as the moments of a host of other atomic nuclei, both known and unknown, the Stanford laboratory had begun making dramatic contributions in 1950 to NMR spectroscopy, most notably in the area of chemical shifts.

The first of these chemical-shift discoveries had been made, as noted earlier, by Warren Proctor and Fu Chung Yu, and others had followed

---

* Although he didn't mention it in his interview with Weiner, Bloch actually did have a permanent magnet shipped from Columbia to Stanford after the war, but for a different purpose. According to Willis Lamb, who visited Bloch at Stanford in the latter part of 1945, Bloch requested on that occasion that Lamb send him a permanent magnet of the type used in radar magnetrons, a rather small horseshoe magnet. "On return to New York," Lamb said, "I hastened to get a spare magnet and to magnetize it as strongly as I could. I then sent this to Bloch by parcel post. Even after the wonderful discovery of nuclear induction in 1946 I had no idea why he had wanted the magnet."

Some years later, Bloch told him the reason. Since it was not known at the time how long it would take for the protons in his sample of water to reach thermal equilibrium, he thought he would use the magnet Lamb sent him to "pre-soak" the sample in an effort to ensure a net nuclear magnetism. In the end, however, the magnet was not used for that purpose. "As the work proceeded," Lamb explained, "Bloch realized that doping a liquid sample by paramagnetic impurities would work much better. Hence the sample of protons soaking for many months in my magnet was never used. . . . Bloch never offered to return the magnet. He did, however, say that he did not think it was as strongly magnetized as I had measured it to be. I suppose the postal authorities may have opened the package and partially demagnetized the strange steel object.

—Willis Lamb, "Five encounters with Felix Bloch," *Felix Bloch and Twentieth-Century Physics*, (Houston: Rice University Press, 1980), 140.

soon afterward. One of the most famous was the proton resonance signature of ethyl alcohol (CH_3CH_2OH) found by Arnold, Dharmatti and Packard.[144] Obtained in a highly homogeneous field without pulses, the Larmor frequencies of the three "types" of hydrogen protons in the compound were clearly shifted from one another by their local chemical environment and the amplitude of the three proton lines varied in direct ratio to their individual concentrations within the molecule. In 1952, Edward Purcell, noting in his Nobel lecture that "it is an old story in physics that higher resolving power leads to new effects," would point to the ethyl alcohol spectrum obtained at Stanford and declare, "No laboratory has more assiduously pursued high resolution than Professor Bloch's."[145] (A later field-independent spectrum of alcohol revealing fine-structure splitting would turn out to be, said Hahn, "the steady-state counterpart of the mysterious echo envelope beats I first saw in alcohol."[146])

It was thus a propitious time for Hahn's arrival. With NMR activity booming, "the entire NMR clan," said Hahn, "worked in a big basement full of several rigs."[147] At one time or another during the two years that Hahn would remain at Stanford, the "clan" would include, in addition to Hahn, James Arnold, S.S. Dharmatti, Carson Jeffries, Eliott Levinthal, Martin Packard, Warren Proctor, Emery Rogers, Kenneth Trigger, Harry Weaver, Fu Chung Yu and of course Felix Bloch, the "father" of the clan.

> When I first arrived as a postdoc at Stanford in 1950 [wrote Hahn], I remember vividly my first contact with Felix Bloch. He was sitting on a lab stool in the basement of the old "Physics Corner" hunched over a chart recorder, inspecting NMR signals newly obtained by his students, huddled around him. That image of Felix epitomized his relationship toward experimentalists. He did theory for experimentalists, and liked to fancy himself also as an experimentalist. It was marvelous the way Felix could apply quantum mechanics with ingenuity and elegance directly to experiments. The clean lines of his physics reminds me of the music of Mozart—easy to read but demanding in its playing and interpretation.[148]

"In retrospect," said Hahn, "my first days with Felix Bloch were a precious and privileged experience. Soon after my arrival, Bloch took off several afternoons and grilled me about my spin echo results. I outlined the mystery of the echo envelope beats, and Bloch agreed that I should build an echo rig and track down the cause of the beats."

Those first afternoons would turn out to be the first of many exchanges between Hahn and Bloch, an association, said Hahn, that would have "a profound effect on the way I have done physics ever since."[149]

> At the beginning of my two years at Stanford [said Hahn], I remember distinctly how my propensity for arm-waving vector models somewhat overwhelmed Felix. Nevertheless, with discussions seasoned every now and then with dubious jokes, we soon developed a rapport. Eventually, I learned how to use quantum mechanics from Felix after numerous priceless sessions at the blackboard. His effectiveness as a teacher was evident from his broad ability to shift back and forth between the thinking of phenomenological models and fancy formalism.[150]

For Bloch, "afternoon" began approximately four hours after noon.

> Felix was in the habit [said Hahn] of taking afternoon naps, and then would show up in the lab around four o'clock in the afternoon, ready and eager for activity, while the rest of us developed some fatigue toward the end of the day. I became aware of a tradition in force that adjusted to this habit of Felix. Every day, one or two of the NMR lab group, at least, were commissioned to remain in the lab to interact with Felix—something like guard duty in the military, not that it was unpleasant, but just to make sure that by coincidence, not everybody might have gone home at the end of the day. Warren Proctor told me that this was a long practice at various times among Dharmatti, Packard, Rogers, Jeffries, West, Weaver, Anderson, Levinthal, Arnold, etc.
>
> Felix would, of course, make inquiries as to how the research was going, and in turn, the group had the policy of preparing a question first in order to distract Felix from that fact that the group had nothing new to report for the day. In making up questions, they tried to steer clear of anything not in his expertise, but once they thought they fumbled completely and asked Felix about an electronic bug they couldn't eliminate. To their amazement, Felix went to the blackboard and wrote down seemingly irrelevant, impractical, formal Maxwell's equations. Finally, he homed in on the final answer, pointing out the particular hardware that had caused the trouble.[151]

The same ability to get quickly up to speed was evidenced by Bloch at Stanford Physics Colloquia.

The speaker would introduce a subject most people knew about [said Hahn], at least from the current literature, which Felix didn't read. For about the first half of the colloquium, Felix would ask apparently dumb questions to bring himself up to date. Then, for the rest of the colloquium, he would chime in and transcend the speaker by telling him where he might have gone wrong and what he or she should do to improve his or her results.[152]

Bloch's avoidance of keeping up with the literature also accounts for his lack of awareness in 1945 of C.J. Gorter's failures to detect magnetic resonance in 1936 and 1942. "He preferred to rediscover and work things out for himself, a marked characteristic," said Hahn, "of his independent personality."[153]

The quantum mechanics that Hahn picked up in his one-on-one, give-and-take sessions with Bloch would stand him in good stead almost immediately. Although Bloch's classical equations had served Hahn well in explaining his original spin echoes, Hahn's armamentarium for explaining what he was observing with the echo envelope modulation beats was incomplete without further understanding of quantum mechanics, and no one was better equipped than Bloch to teach it. Not only had Bloch had his own "priceless sessions" discussing quantum mechanics in Europe with the likes of Heisenberg, Schrödinger, Bohr, and Pauli, he had also early on proven his ability to use the tools of quantum mechanics effectively in his treatments of electrical conduction and ferromagnetics.

In late 1952, after Hahn had already left Stanford, Bloch would be awarded, along with Edward Purcell, the Nobel Prize in physics, timing for which Hahn was personally grateful.

His first interest was in physics and not in wheeling and dealing. That's what I admired about him. I had the grand privilege of spending afternoons—countless afternoons—with him, just talking at the blackboard about various things, and speculating about what this would do and what that would do, and doing calculations. I learned quantum mechanics from him just casually by these tutorial sessions which were unconsciously given to me without any planning. He was a great man, to me and to everybody else. He received his Nobel Prize after I left. I'm sort of glad he didn't get it while I was there because then he would have been distracted.[154]

In mid-November, about two months after his arrival at Stanford, Hahn wrote to Herman Carr at Harvard. After telling Carr he was gratified to hear that they now had echoes at Harvard, Hahn quickly launched into a detailed discussion about spin-echo questions discussed in a previous letter from Carr, some of which were answered he said in the enclosed "mimeo" of his spin echo paper about to be published in *Physical Review*. "About a week ago," he continued, "I completed a preliminary rig for obtaining echoes. However, I am eventually going to have my own magnet, and I'm going to do quite a bit of dirty work in getting the magnet running. The magnet just arrived a few days ago."

Although he was busy preparing for his upcoming research, he wasn't missing out on the other reason he chose Stanford. "The California weather is certainly beautiful," he told Carr. "I don't work on weekends like I did at Illinois, but now go on pleasure auto trips."

Eventually, Hahn got down to a discussion of the mystery that was continuing to challenge him: "Now about the echo envelope modulation effect, for which I have, I think, the best explanation so far out of the many that haven't worked."[155]

Negative Temperatures and Other "Violations"

It is interesting to observe that Hahn, in discussing with Carr in his letter of November 14, 1950 his then-current hypothesis on the mysterious modulation, brought up the possibility of negative temperature states. A controversial concept at the time, negative absolute temperatures were thought by many to be thermodynamically impossible. The topic would soon be aired publicly for the first time by Edward Purcell and Robert Pound in a letter to the editor of *Physical Review*[156] and would prove to be an important antecedent to the stimulated emission concept crucial to the development of masers and lasers. Although the following is taken out of its technical context, it does indicate that Hahn was also contemplating the possibility of negative temperatures and cross-relaxation, the latter an area to which he would return some years later and, together with Sven Hartmann, would make an important contribution known as Hartmann-Hahn cross-relaxation.

By virtue of the BPP-defined noise spectrum in liquid samples [wrote Hahn], the spins, having frequency ω can flip spins of frequency ω' and vice versa. Due to the nature of relative phases determined by τ and $\theta = \omega_1 t_w$, the spin flip angle, it is possible, for instance, to throw the ω spin system into the negative temperature state and simultaneously leave the ω' spin system in the positive temperature state. This occurs in a given homogeneous (local geometric) region of the sample (in H_0 external). The process of course is reversed in other parts of the sample. Due to the fact that the Boltzmann distribution of the ω and ω' spins have been made <u>artificially different,</u> the thermal relaxation for both the ω and ω' systems will no longer obey the simple exponential law. . . . Then something peculiar happens. While, say, spin system ω relaxes to thermal equilibrium, it can become more populated momentarily due to a net flux of spin energy from the ω' system. . . . [underlining included in original][157]

After further discussion, Hahn continued:

The structure seen in the Sb' resonance in SbF⁻ ions in solution form here at Stanford due to the fluorine fields makes one believe something like this can happen. I am still in the middle of many brainstorms on this . . . so I can't make any claims now. Anyway, this is the best lead so far. Of course, I may abandon this idea like I have many others but so far it seems to account best for the experimental facts.[158]

Hahn has pointed out that these initial speculations were "quite vague, in error, and more or less stumbling in the dark," but found it interesting in reviewing his letter to Carr that what he had written did indeed have overtones of the basic idea concerning the Overhauser effect and somewhat of the Hartmann-Hahn cross-relaxation. "I had forgotten what I wrote to Carr," he noted, "but the muse of the idea stayed with me and did blossom forth later. It startles me now to read what I wrote to Carr."[159]

It was not the first time Hahn had flirted with what appeared to be a violation of the Second Law of Thermodynamics. According to J.S. Waugh of MIT, spin echoes themselves were a violation of the Second Law:

The spin echo is still striking to those who see it for the first time, as it probably was to Hahn. A nuclear magnetization, having disappeared in a free induction decay (FID), spontaneously reappears as a giant fluctuation. While the phenomenon is easily understood from a mechanical point of view, it seems to verge on a violation of the Second Law of Thermodynamics. . . . Our point of view will be that echoes *do* violate the Second Law.[160]

Waugh's point was that the Second Law does not adequately establish a time allowance for reaching a state of equilibrium. An intelligent observer could predict, for example, in the case of spin echoes, said Waugh, that equilibrium had been achieved in a sample's spin population after the second pulse had been applied, but a few moments later would be proven incorrect when an echo appeared seemingly out of nowhere. As M. Weger, who is associated with the Racah Institute of Physics of Hebrew University in Jerusalem, has written:

> Erwin Hahn's discovery of spin echoes surprised the scientific community because it seemed to . . . indicate a violation of time reversal. Violating causality is one of the strictest taboos of theoretical physics, the formation of spin echoes seemed to break this taboo.[161]

The solution to the dilemma suggested by Waugh in 1992 was similar to the one proposed by Norman Ramsey in his 1956 theoretical treatment of negative absolute temperatures; continue to uphold the Law itself as valid but add a proviso to make it reflect the reality of spin echoes. Waugh's suggestion: "When a system is in such a state that after any slight temporary disturbance of external conditions it returns rapidly or slowly to the initial state, this state is said to be one of equilibrium."[162] With such a stipulation, spin echoes could continue to appear legally.

Incidentally, years after Hahn's letter to Carr in which he discussed negative temperature possibilities, Theodore Maiman, the first to achieve a working laser, would credit Hahn with a less technical but nevertheless significant contribution to the development of the laser. At the time, in the late 1950s, Hahn was on the faculty at Berkeley and doing consultation work with Harold Lyons of the Hughes Aircraft group on solid-state masers because of Hahn's knowledge of spins, echoes and coherence.

> I remember while I was first there as a consultant that Ted Maiman was not there. I got to know Ted Maiman while he was a graduate student at Stanford under Willis Lamb. Much later I met Maiman at a meeting somewhere and Maiman said, "You know, I'm looking for a job." I said, "You know, I can tell you where to get a job. Just call up Harold Lyons at Hughes. They need guys like you." So that's where he got his start. And every time I've seen Maiman since, he's said, "Hahn, if it weren't for you, I wouldn't have gotten the laser to work." Well, I don't believe that because his ingenuity would have prevailed anywhere else he would have gone.[163]

In 1984, Hahn and Maiman would meet in Jerusalem at Israel's parliament, the Knesset, to receive the prestigious Wolf Prize in physics from the then-president of Israel, Chaim Herzog. Hahn was awarded the prize for his spin echoes and his later discovery of self-induced transparency in laser optics and Maiman for his achievement of the first operating laser, the pulsed three-level ruby laser. The third recipient of the physics prize that year, Peter Hirsch of Oxford University, was recognized for his development and utilization of the scanning electron microscope.

Delving into the Mysterious Modulation

In his Nobel lecture, just before showing the striking chemical shift achieved by Arnold, Dharmatti, and Packard, Purcell observed that to the experimenter interested in exact ratios of magnetic moments, chemical shifts were "only a nuisance, but to the physical chemist they are interesting . . . because they reveal something about the electrons that partake in the chemical bond."[164] It was an accurate observation of the dichotomy that existed in the Stanford laboratory.

Initially, all of the spectroscopy researchers at Stanford had been frustrated when chemical shifts and other interactions began showing up. As specialists in hunting down new spins and measuring magnetic moments, the deviations seemed to be frustrating their attempts to achieve unambiguous results. For that matter, Bloch may have been initially more receptive than the others to their appearance on the basis, said Hahn, that the spectral splittings may have been evidence of "stable nuclear isomers that had slightly different properties." When it became clear that the phenomenon was actually evidence of the other dreaded possibility, "a nasty diamagnetic chemical shift,"[165] Bloch's interest plummeted while the interest of the others increased.

"Later on," said Hahn, "when NMR proved to be extremely important for chemical analysis and MRI, Bloch changed his views and indeed he then became highly interested."[166] Initially, however, Bloch was not interested in these chemical effects and has been quoted as saying, "When chemists get into a field, it's time to get out."[167]

Bloch's ambivalence toward these many-body interactions that could not be understood without an involved series of empirical measurements was shared, said Hahn, by I.I. Rabi.

> I overheard more than once [said Hahn] comments by Rabi and Bloch that they were happy to avoid as much as possible many-body problems. . . . Bloch remained attached in his research interests more

to the physics of simple systems than to systems involving complicated many-body problems of the solid state. Parameters of fundamental particles were the most important to him. . . . Bloch, of course, was famous for his theories of periodic electron functions in solids and Bloch walls in ferromagnetism, and yet he shied away from attempts to analyze the mysterious splittings (first found in antimony coupled to fluorine in the SbF_6^- ion) found in his laboratory in the course of their searches for the resonances of new nuclear magnetic moments.[168]

"I remember distinctly the time," said Hahn, "when Dick Norberg [who was visiting Stanford] and I were in Felix's office, pouring out our resonance research results to him, Norberg on metals, and I with chemical echo modulation effects. Bloch said, 'Norberg, you should be a metallurgist, and Hahn, you should be a chemist!' "[169]

In Hahn's initial discussions with Bloch about the direction his research would take, Hahn had described a model that involved first-order interactions between two groups of spins, coupled to one another, but distinguished by different chemical shifts. That model turned out to be deficient, however, in its ability to predict the modulation beats of the echo envelope, the unknown ingredient which interrupted the envelope's otherwise monotonic decline. In spite of Bloch's lack of enthusiasm for the phenomenon, he was very helpful in providing Hahn with the theoretical tools for conducting his research.

I really did not know how to manipulate the quantum mechanics of spins in a genuine facile manner when I began my research at Stanford [said Hahn]. I learned from Bloch how to calculate echo pulse sequences quantum mechanically, beginning with a pertinent Hamiltonian, rather than just rely on [Bloch's] macroscopic equations. There was no way to predict the envelope beats from modified Bloch equations.[170]

In 1951, Don Maxwell became Hahn's first graduate thesis student and they now began investigating the echo envelope modulation together. Hahn had thought initially that the source of the phenomenon he was detecting with spin echoes could only be elicited with time-domain pulse methods, but independently, back at the University of Illinois, his former colleagues Herb Gutowsky in the chemistry department and Charles Slichter in the physics department had joined their NMR research forces and they were detecting steady-state manifestations of a similar phenomenon. Gutowsky and Slichter, in fact, were observing proton splittings due to local fields of coupled foreign species not at resonance, a condition, explained Hahn, that forbids the occurrence of echo envelope beats.

Eventually, rather than a first-order interaction as originally outlined by Hahn to Bloch, both groups independently came to the conclusion that they were dealing with a second-order spin effect, an indirect nuclear coupling, also referred to when using pulse spectroscopy methods as J-modulation. Although neither group could account for the fundamental mechanism causing the effect, they were able to provide predictions based on the data they observed.

After completing a quantum-mechanical echo calculation that drew upon Heisenberg's model for ferromagnetism, Hahn arrived at what to him was a reasonable justification for why at least two chemically-non-equivalent spin species such as the CH_3 and CH_2 groups in alcohol had to be excited simultaneously by his two-pulse sequence if he was to observe envelope beats and a satisfactory explanation as to why observation of echo envelope "J-coupling" beats would not occur in the absence of chemical shifts.

Hahn's first publication on the subject, a letter to the editor of *Physical Review* co-authored with Maxwell, was published in 1951 alongside a letter by Gutowsky, McCall, Slichter and McNeill from Illinois. Shortly after these two groups published their findings, Norman Ramsey and Edward Purcell published an article in *Physical Review* in which they identified the fundamental mechanism of the "J" coefficient as the effect of indirect exchange, caused by nuclear hyperfine interactions. "At the news of this explanation," recalled Hahn, "Bloch called me into his office and literally apologized to me. He said he should have thought of this idea himself because he was well aware of the nuclear hyperfine interaction."[171] "Oddly enough," said Hahn, "I had speculated that overlap of nuclear wave functions of neighboring atoms would account for our observations," but had discounted its effect because the mechanism seemed so "negligibly and infinitesimally weak."[172]

In 1952, Hahn and Maxwell published a major paper in which they summarized the various types of interactions that had been observed up to that point, including a description of the indirect nuclear spin-spin coupling they had observed in the form of echo envelope modulations and the theoretical basis Ramsey and Purcell had provided for the phenomenon. At the end of their article, they wrote: "The authors are grateful to Professor F. Bloch for many discussions and valuable suggestions during the course of this research."[173] When Bloch read the acknowledgment, he laughed and told Hahn and Maxwell, "You should have acknowledged me for my constant discouragement!"[174]

The indirect spin-spin research conducted independently by Hahn and Maxwell and by Gutowsky and Slichter has had far-reaching impact. Of Hahn's research, in particular, it has been written:

> Of great import in chemical analysis by pulsed nuclear resonance is Hahn's pioneering work, parallel with that of H.S. Gutowsky and C.P. Slichter, in formulating an experimental and empirical basis for a universal exchange interaction which appears in nearly all chemical compounds, particularly in liquids. Hahn showed that transient effects due to the precession of nuclei in chemically inequivalent parts of a molecule are due to a rotationally invariant indirect spin-spin–exchange type of interaction, which he justified rigorously, both analytically and experimentally. Independent work on this effect, from steady-state spectra data, was carried out by Gutowsky and Slichter. . . . Associated with this work, Hahn measured various effects of the liquid chemical environment on the indirect spin-exchange interaction. He was one of the first to show that the fast hydrogen bond chemical exchange contributed to the annulment of discrete spin-spin interactions (in CH_3OH), and he first formulated equations for a proper description of the exchange effects."[175]

Of Hahn in general, and of the major paper by Hahn and Maxwell, Richard Ernst has stated:

> The influence of Erwin L. Hahn on the development of time domain magnetic resonance during the past 40 years has been very significant. Even some of the roots of two-dimensional spectroscopy may be found in his early work together with Maxwell. Although he never mentions the possibility of 2D Fourier transformation, the J-coupling envelope modulation of the spin echo amplitude is much related to the function of the evolution period in 2D experiments (especially in the 2D J-resolved experiment). . . . The author would like to thank Prof. Erwin L. Hahn for his seminal contributions over a period of more than 40 years to the exciting and important field of time domain magnetic resonance, without which the present account [on the multidimensional importance of time domain magnetic resonance] would not have been possible. Whatever is said about time domain experiments reflects in some way Hahn's early work.[176]

Bloch, too, would come to appreciate the chemical effects uncovered and analyzed by Hahn and his associates. Eventually, said Hahn,

Bloch realized that NMR and the many-body effects and statistics of condensed matter could not be avoided and had to be understood. . . . It was an interesting and extremely profitable experience for me to have interacted with Felix Bloch. I learned how to use quantum mechanics from him. He was a fiercely independent thinker.[168]

"When I first came to Stanford," said Hahn, "Bloch in a way had that European style of being the *Herr Professor*, but he kind of mellowed. Bloch was a strong character, just like Horovitz [at Purdue], but in a more informal sense." Bloch's European background, however, also contributed to the personal, tutorial approach he took with Hahn. "Everything was personal, personally exchanged, in ideas and insights and so forth."[177] One of the reasons they got along so well, said Hahn, was Bloch's ready sense of humor. "He responded to me and I responded to him."[178] On one occasion, said Hahn,

Felix was trying to understand a paper by Al Redfield which dealt with the subject of spin-temperature. At first Felix was convinced that the paper was nonsense. Then after he read it again carefully, he finally understood it, was impressed by the paper, and asked me, "Tell me, Erwin, this guy Redfield, he must be Jewish?!" Then, after I read the paper, Felix asked me if I understood it. I said, "Yes, about half of it, so I think Redfield must be half Jewish!" Actually, Al Redfield [explained Hahn in 1984] "is a blue-blooded thoroughbred New Englander Goy, who apropos to this story is now a professor at Brandeis University."[179]

When Hahn was named as a recipient of the Wolf Prize in January 1984, he told a newspaper reporter, "I'm sorry Professor Bloch wasn't alive to see this and the credit that is due to him. It was his particular work that made possible my work." Felix Bloch had died just four months earlier.

IBM and Columbia

Hahn's first year at Stanford as a postdoctoral fellow had been sponsored by the National Research Council. When that year was completed, he became an instructor at Stanford with his research sponsored by the Office of Naval Research. He would have been willing to have made

Stanford his academic home had it not been for a tenureship policy at the top that precluded the hiring of young people and an offer from IBM's Watson Laboratories in New York City.

The policy was—and it was considered a mistake much later, in fact—that they would build their staff from the top down, not from the bottom up with young people. So they told me I couldn't aspire toward tenure there. Bloch and [Leonard] Schiff tried to talk me into staying a third year, but I preferred a position at IBM as a research physicist, considering that Stanford wouldn't keep me. In fact, as I remember, Bloch said that Rabi had suggested to IBM Watson Laboratories that they should hire me, and Bloch complained, "I wish that Rabi hadn't done this," so that I wouldn't have been seduced from Stanford so soon. In those days, if one had the choice of industrial versus academic work, you were considered to be pros-tituting yourself not to stay in academia.[180]

Even apart from Rabi's influence, IBM had its own interest in Hahn's echoes.

When I came to Stanford [said Hahn], Russell Varian [co-developer of the klystron with W.W. Hansen] approached me and said, "You know, you have this spin echo technique which is very suitable for chemical analysis. We'll help you patent it and we'll pay for the patent litigation if you write it up." So I did that and they had free license rights to the patent. They adopted the patent for a period of time and built one or two pulsed apparatuses, but then dropped it about a year later, and the patent reverted to me.[181]

Contributing to Varian's decision, Hahn explained, was the fact that computers weren't sufficiently developed to process transient signals for Fourier analysis, thus diminishing the commercial potential of pulse techniques at the time for chemical analysis. IBM wasn't interested in Hahn's echoes for chemical analysis, however. With their predilection for storing pulses, spin echoes were viewed by "Big Blue" as having poten-tial for digital memory in computers and not wanting to miss any bets, they expressed an interest in hiring the man who had discovered and patented them. Although Hahn wasn't interested in developing a digital memory for IBM as a major career pursuit—he wanted to focus on physics—he was willing to act as an advisor on the project.

During the three years that Hahn was at IBM, a number of patents were issued using the echo technique as a storage method. Although they were "curious and interesting activities," said Hahn, "[they] didn't go anywhere commercially. These patents did secure, for a couple of people, internal company awards, which was about the best thing that came out of them at the time."[182] In addition to the patents they secured for IBM, Hahn and his IBM associates published a paper on spin echo serial storage,[183] although Hahn was also careful to continue development of his "non-commercial" interests.

Technically, our study had some good physics in it, and has been used and reviewed by others later for certain procedures in physics. At IBM, I worked more assiduously on quadrupole echoes and double resonance experiments rather than echo storage, and published a few other papers on quadrupole effects.[184]

Concurrent with his IBM employment, Hahn was also serving as an adjunct associate professor at nearby Columbia University where, in addition to the two courses he gave, Hahn was also assigned a graduate student, Bernard Herzog, with whom he co-authored a number of papers.

At IBM Watson Laboratory [Hahn recalled] I was given the status of an Associate in the Columbia Physics Department and taught a course in atomic physics. I took on Bernard Herzog as a beginning graduate thesis student and we worked on the problem of detecting zero-field chlorine-35 nuclear quadrupole spin echoes using the "workhorse" crystal of sodium chlorate. Zero-field CW NQR [nuclear quadrupole resonance] was first discovered by Dehmelt and Kruger, and it was natural to look for spin echoes in this interesting nuclear quadrupole coupled regime.[185]

Unbeknownst to Hahn, Myer Bloom, a graduate student of Charles Slichter's at Illinois, was doing the same experiment for his thesis. After some "fumbling and bumbling," said Hahn, "we finally got a signal." Apparently, shortly before Hahn and Herzog detected the signal they were looking for at IBM, Bloom detected it at Illinois, but agreed to report on his research in a paper co-published with Hahn and Herzog in *Physical Review*.[186] This and related work would later be covered more comprehensively in a book co-authored by Hahn and T.P. Das entitled *Nuclear Quadrupole Resonance Spectroscopy*, published in 1958.[187] The subject of nuclear quadrupole resonance would also continue to receive further attention by Hahn and his graduate students at Berkeley after Hahn's 1955 move back to California.

Hahn and Herzog also conducted spin-echo double-resonance (SEDOR) experiments with sodium chlorate in which they were able to detect resonance in an unobserved nucleus by observing the effect of its local dipolar field on a signal from a neighboring nuclear ensemble, a deductive approach not unlike telling whether a certain person is at home by how someone else in the household answers the phone.[188-189]

"Those were booming days" at Columbia, said Hahn. "I overlapped with Townes. He was there a year or two, formulating at that time the maser principle. . . . There were good ideas floating around. Others there were Rabi, Foley, Kusch and Brillouin. Lamb was not there then. I overlapped earlier with Lamb at Stanford."[190]

Although Watson Laboratories were "reasonably liberal," considering the traditional commercial concerns for secrecy, and allowed relatively open access between Columbia graduate students and the staff at IBM, Hahn was, he said, "somewhat of a maverick:"

> I led a rebellion against punching the time clock. . . . I always felt, much as I liked IBM, that I was being preened to be a group leader of some sort for later work in applications for the company. I just felt that I wanted to get into the academic world. There were other people there who were very good people who stayed on. Some of them left. I am grateful to IBM for the freedom that they instituted at that time, which was rather novel for the company. . . . But I felt I wanted to get into the university, and I did. I still maintained connections with IBM and consulted with them for a long time afterwards. It was a very amicable relationship and I'm very grateful to the company.[191]

University of California, Berkeley

In 1955, Hahn returned to the West Coast, this time to Berkeley, about an hour's drive north of Stanford. "Actually, I was solicited by two places," said Hahn. "I was solicited by the University of Minnesota, I remember. They offered me a job, and then Bill Nierenberg came from Berkeley. He was on a recruiting binge, and he said, 'We're interested in hiring you. Do you want to come to Berkeley?' and I said, 'Yes,' and that was it."[192]

Berkeley had an advantage with which Minnesota couldn't compete, Northern California weather. "A professor named Nier—Alfred O.

Nier—offered me the job," said Hahn, "but somebody told me it was too cold there," Hahn told the writer, a native Minnesotan. With an average daily low in January of 3.2 degrees Fahrenheit in Minneapolis versus 45.8 for the San Francisco-Oakland area, the numbers were not in Minnesota's favor. Hahn figured that his visit from Nierenberg came about as a result of grapevine discussions between Emilio Segrè at Berkeley and Leon Brillouin at Columbia.

I think the gist of it was that Segrè learned from Brillouin about my merits, and then Segrè must have passed it on to the staff here [at Berkeley]. The staff then was pretty small. . . . It grew like wildfire in the '50s and '60s. Jeffries and Knight were already here. There was an NMR group here, and I added my own two cents to it.[193]

His "own two cents"—hyperbole, of course, but typical as well of Hahn's characteristic tendency to ensure that others are given appropriate credit. Russell Walstedt, one of Hahn's students from that period and presently with AT&T's Bell Laboratories, sees Hahn's contributions for what they are—truly fundamental in nature and foundational for all that has followed.

In the years immediately following Erwin Hahn's discovery of the nuclear spin echo, pulsed NMR was regarded by many condensed matter physicists as an exotic curiosity. . . . As many of us who were graduate students during that formative era realized, however, the pulse techniques that were being fostered almost exclusively in Hahn's laboratory at the University of California at Berkeley possessed great flexibility and potential for future development. With the advent of digital data manipulation and storage technologies, the expansion of pulsed NMR into the fields of chemistry, biology (Fourier transform spectroscopy, multidimensional spectroscopy), and medicine (NMR imaging) has extended far beyond our earlier imaginings. The seminal contributions Erwin Hahn made to this vast development of phenomenology and technique place him in a truly rarefied category of the scientists of our time.[194]

With regard to magnetic resonance imaging, Hahn's spin echoes are a major weapon in the radiologist's armamentarium, as attested by L.E. Crooks and P. Rothschild:

MR imaging has become an accepted clinical technique in many areas. Spin echo imaging is the most versatile approach to general disease detection. Combined with multi-slice imaging, spin echoes made MRI clinically viable.[195]

As the quote by D.M.S. Bagguley pointed out at the beginning of this chapter, Hahn's spin echo discovery and the follow-on studies he conducted with chemical shifts and J-coupling are just a small fraction of Hahn's list of impressive scientific contributions during his career, most of which would be made during his Berkeley years. (Even though officially retired and endowed with the title Professor Emeritus, Hahn's Berkeley years are still continuing in that he can still be found doing research in a Berkeley laboratory.)

After arriving at Berkeley, Hahn continued his research on spin-echo double-resonance spectroscopy and relaxation, some of which was contained in the graduate theses of E.M. Emshwiller and D. Kaplan, while, at the same time, contemplating ways to increase the sensitivity of double resonance. Increasing the scrambling-phase time was the most obvious approach, but was discarded as impractical because the echo memory relaxation time of T_2 for echoes in solids was not long enough, on the order of a few milliseconds at best. Maybe there was some way to achieve the objective by using the longer spin-lattice relaxation time, T_1, instead. Hahn's association with graduate student Sven Hartmann, aided by hints of "rotary saturation" and spin temperature in the rotating frame, contained in a paper by Al Redfield would lead to another powerful NMR weapon known as the Hartmann-Hahn method.

Before that association came about, however, it was time for Hahn's first sabbatical at Berkeley, which he took at Oxford University's Clarendon Laboratory. There Hahn had the opportunity to work with Professor Nicholas Kurti, an eminent thermodynamicist and low temperature physicist. Inspired by the nuclear cooling ideas of Kurti and working with graduate student Russell Walstedt, Hahn succeeded in developing a pulsed nuclear resonance thermometer that could be used to measure spin temperatures below 1 degree Kelvin and in demonstrating the basis for such a thermometer. That first visit to Oxford with its history and traditions succeeded in winning the permanent allegiance of Erwin Hahn. Anatole Abragam, who shares Hahn's sentiment, observed in his autobiography that Hahn "adores Oxford and goes there as often as he can."[196] "As often as he can" turns out to be about once a year.

Upon his return to Berkeley, Hahn resumed his work in spin-echo double resonance and, together with Sven Hartmann, introduced a highly improved method which was much more sensitive, so that measurements of low concentrations of nuclei (on the order of 10^{14} to 10^{16} per cubic centimeters) were possible. The two were able to demonstrate that two species of nuclei with mismatched Larmor frequencies can be made to interact strongly when strong radiofrequency fields were applied simultaneously at the two nuclear Larmor frequencies. By transferring the polarization of one nuclear spin species to another, the Hartmann-Hahn method, it has been observed, "has proven to be of enormous importance for high resolution NMR in physics, chemistry, and more recently biophysics and biochemistry, where it allows the observation of rare spin species with a small nuclear moment."[197] One of the areas in which the method will continue to impact medicine is in the study of enzymes:

The enormous contributions that Erwin Hahn has made to the field of NMR have impacted the study of enzymes in two major ways. The first is the introduction of a whole family of spin echo techniques, which . . . have opened the door to structural studies of mobile domains of very large proteins, as well as forming the basis for many 2D and 3D pulse sequences. The second is the discovery of the Hartmann-Hahn condition, which, apart from enabling the technique of cross-polarization in solids (including biological solids), currently is enabling the development of cross polarization in liquids, and in particular biological solutions.[198]

Following his work with Hartmann, a series of investigations with variations on the theme of double resonance spectroscopy were conducted by Hahn together with Richard Slusher,[199] Russell Walstedt and David McArthur.[200]

For a time, Hahn would take leave of the intensive NMR research pace he had set for himself throughout the '50s and '60s and turn his attention to lasers. Not long after his arrival at Berkeley, he began consulting with Hughes Corporation in Los Angeles in their development of masers. After Nicolaas Bloembergen published his paper proposing the three-level, inverted pumping system, the field expanded rapidly and Hahn's experience with spins, echoes and coherence placed him in much demand. Eventually, although he continued to do research in NMR, he also began branching into the field of lasers which, because of its use of many of the same principles used in NMR, looked like a natural direction to take.

Indeed, he would make substantial contributions to lasers as well, perhaps most notably the discovery of self-induced transparency, a phenomenon whereby a pulse of laser light of a certain intensity and shape can make an otherwise opaque medium transparent. As energy from a strong laser pulse enters a crystal, it is stored briefly before continuing in the original direction of the pulse. The finding is considered the first atomic demonstration of a phenomenon known as the soliton, which is an interchange or sharing of energy involving cooperation of many particles. It was specifically for his discovery of self-induced transparency, together with his discovery of spin echoes, that Hahn was awarded the Wolf Prize in physics for 1983-84.

At the time of his switch to lasers, Hahn was beginning to feel, he said, that "NMR was turning out to be a routine technique and graduate students looked upon it more as a tool where there wasn't much physics left to do. It was for chemists, and the chemistry department here [at Berkeley] was taking up NMR, and meanwhile, the ideas of NMR were spilling over into the laser, as far as I was concerned."[201] NMR's forecasted demise as a field for physicists, of course, turned out to be premature, as noted by D. Stehlik (a former postdoc in Hahn's lab) and H.M. Vieth, physicists now working in Berlin:

> Magnetic resonance still seems great fun, even though Erwin warned us as young postdocs way back in the '60s that 'NMR is dead.' Fortunately, he keeps disproving himself with his continued leading presence in the active research community.[202]

Hahn is quick to clarify, however, that he "never left NMR."

> When I went into lasers, it didn't mean I quit NMR. What I did was add to the laboratory laser capability which turned out to be much more expensive and much slower and I wasn't able to put out experiments as quickly as I did with NMR because a lot of the ideas had been mined and people were doing other things that were more difficult. When I went into lasers, I did NMR in conjunction with the laser experiments. I pushed the idea of doing NMR-analogue experiments using, however, the optical two-level system rather than the NMR two-level system because the equations of motion are very much the same, except for various things that light does that radio waves don't do.[203]

One reason for the explosive growth of NMR in the 1960s, and one which was especially important to his own involvement in the science, Hahn has observed, was its relatively low cost.

The apparatus and technology necessary for NMR in those early years was relatively inexpensive. Here was a field of research that contained the ingredients of a variety of disciplines—from electronics, through chemistry, to frontier's of nuclear structure. The pursuit of magnetic resonance was a 'small science' endeavor and, at the same time, a broad education experience for graduate students that spread rapidly. My Russian colleagues told me, for example, that there were at least as many spin echo research apparatuses in Kazan [where Zavoisky was the first to detect electron spin resonance] as there were branch offices of the KGB.

The record shows that new and significant discoveries in NMR could then be made by young researchers who could forge out on their own, build the apparatus by themselves, and therefore try all sorts of novel experiments without the constraints of a more elaborate installation for doing physics. NMR proved for many to be preferable to particle accelerator research that could be controlled by some *prima donna* boss professor or clique of high-energy physicists, allowing only limited styles of research problems. For this reason I found it a supreme blessing to be doing NMR in the physics department at Berkeley because excellent graduate students came into my laboratory as refugees from LBL accelerator research groups, where the lack of independence did not appeal to them. Each one of them, most of the time, had their own apparatus in my laboratory.[204]

Erwin Hahn Today

Although Erwin Hahn, at the age of 74, has been officially retired for four years from the physics department at the University of California, Berkeley, he continues to work as an active physicist, traveling, speaking, and doing research in NMR. "I'm still doing NMR because I have an NSF (National Science Foundation) grant and I'm doing optical pumping in gallium arsenide where I'm polarizing and detecting the nuclei in collaboration with the chemistry department."

In that department, Hahn is now working with Professor Alexander Pines, co-recipient of the 1991 Wolf Prize in chemistry with Richard Ernst. "Pines is a brilliant young NMR researcher," said Hahn, "who has done many novel and progressive things. He's virtually more of a physicist actually than a standard chemist. Pines has been my working confidant. I can hardly keep up with him. He's Jewish, with roots in Israel, a PhD product of John Waugh at MIT. He has a brilliant reputation as a lecturer and he has quick conceptual and profound mathematical ideas about things that most physical chemists don't even touch."[205]

Hahn and his first wife, Marian, who died of cancer in 1978, had three children, David, Deborah and Katherine. David is a family doctor and epidemiologist who has done important research in identifying the bacterial cause of one form of asthma, which was published in the *New England Journal of Medicine*. Deborah lives in Marin County near San Francisco and is employed by a pharmaceutical company. The Hahn's youngest, Katherine, after obtaining a degree in history from the University of York, taught English as a second language for a while in England and then moved to the Continent where she did the same. She now lives in Zürich, Switzerland and is an academic secretary for the Swiss Federal Institute of Technology, the ETH, where Felix Bloch did his undergraduate work and where Richard Ernst is a professor.

Erwin Hahn's present wife, the former Natalie Woodford Hodgson, is a professional librarian with an undergraduate degree in English literature from Stanford and a masters degree library science from the University of California at Berkeley. During a sabbatical that Hahn spent at Oxford University's Balliol College, she volunteered at the Bodleian Library, researching and cataloguing playbills printed in the 18th and 19th century. "She is known at Oxford for her skills and is always welcomed back," said Hahn. "That is one of the reasons why we like to return to Oxford."[205]

Twice named a Guggenheim Fellow (both times at Oxford University, 1961-62 and 1969-70) and twice a research professor in Berkeley's Miller Institute for Basic Research in Science, Hahn has been the recipient of numerous awards and recognitions, including: Honorary D.Sc. degree from his alma mater, Juniata College; NSF Fellow (concurrent with first Guggenheim Fellowship in 1961-62); Buckley Prize in Solid-State Physics from the American Physical Society (1971); Prize of the International Society of Magnetic Resonance (1971); Honorary D.Sc. degree from his graduate-school alma mater, Purdue University (1975); Alexander von Humboldt Award from the German Federal Government (1976); co-recipient of the Wolf Foundation Prize in Physics (1983); inducted into the California Inventors Hall of Fame (1984); co-recipient of Dept. of Energy Award for Sustained Research in DC Squid NMR (1986); Alumni Achievement Award, Juniata College (1986); Eastman Professor, Balliol

College, Oxford, England (1988-89); Berkeley Citation, University of California, Berkeley (1991), and co-recipient of the 1993 Comstock Prize, awarded by National Academy of Sciences for discoveries in electricity, magnetism or radiation.

In addition, Hahn has also been a member of the following societies since the year indicated: Fellow, American Physical Society (1952); Fellow, American Academy of Arts and Sciences (1971); Foreign Member, Royal Institution of Great Britain (1971); Member, U.S. National Academy of Sciences (1972); Foreign Associate Member of the Slovenian Academy of Sciences (1981); Honorary Fellow, Brasenose College, Oxford (1982); and Foreign Associate Member of the French Academy of Sciences (1992).

When Hahn was awarded the Berkeley Citation in 1991, just a few weeks before his retirement to Professor Emeritus status, he was reminded: "You were one of those rare individuals who, just after obtaining your PhD, achieved immortality by making a great discovery. It might now be called the Hahn Effect if you had not thought of a more catchy name— the spin echo effect."[206]

The discovery of the spin echo effect was, indeed, an accident, but it was observed by an alert witness who painstakingly sought out what caused the "accident." He has firmly held opinions, therefore, about the dangers of conducting research either on the basis of preconceived opinions or for others who might be waiting for an "accident" to happen.

From my own experience, I would like to make a comment, especially for graduate students, about the dangerous tendency to look only for events in research which you expect in advance, like looking for a lost item only under a street light at night. Most of the time, of course, artifacts are artifacts and false glitches are false glitches, but one must be careful to confirm that what is false is false. On the other hand, sometimes false glitches that are persistent can look like real phenomena, so one has to be super careful. . . . As a thesis advisor, I discovered a common psychological problem: a student gets his equipment in a state that displays the phenomenon he wants to work on, and then a kind of quasi-infantile anal-retentiveness sets in where he is not willing to change anything from then on. He derives security from the predictability and certainty of his equipment, like a child's favorite blanket or teddy bear.[207]

"On the whole," Hahn pointed out, "I have been blessed with an array of superb graduate students who made it possible for the productivity of research in my career."[208] He also believes that if ever there was an argument for the benefits of basic research, it is nuclear magnetic resonance.

The advent of MRI is a lesson to those pragmatists who feel that basic research should be severely limited, and that applied research should reign supreme as the sure and only way of making science useful. Both, of course, should have their place, but it is the short-sighted impatience of the quick-reward pragmatists who impose immeasurable damage on future developments by suppressing fundamental research. . . . When I first discovered the spin echo, and Russell Varian sponsored and supported my effort to write up a patent to apply it for relaxation measurements for chemical analysis, the University of Illinois released the patent rights to me, stating that it was a useless natural phenomenon. In fact, it was "useful" and it was a "unnatural" phenomenon. It happens in the history of science over and over again, as in the case of Rutherford who said, "Anyone who says that radioactivity will be of any use is talking moonshine!" When Michael Faraday was confronted by a skeptic who questioned the use of his discoveries, he retorted, "What use is a baby?"[209] ∎

REFERENCE NOTES:

1. Numerous versions of "The Three Princes of Serendip" have been published. One of the more recent was authored by Elizabeth Jamison Hodges, (New York: Athenum, 1964) who pointed out that Serendip was the ancient name for Ceylon (known today as Sri Lanka) and that the story of its three princes "may be as ancient." According to *Webster's New Twentieth Century Dictionary*, 2nd Ed. (New York: Simon & Schuster, 1979), the word "serendipity" was coined by Horace Walpole around 1754.

2. E.L. Hahn, "Pulsed NMR: a personal history," unpublished, 2.

3. D.M.S. Bagguley, "The echo phenomenon," *Pulsed Magnetic Resonance: NMR, ESR, and Optics: A Recognition of E.L. Hahn,* edited by D.M.S. Bagguley (Oxford: Clarendon, 1992), 49.

4. E.L. Hahn, interview by James Mattson, 9 March 1994.

5. E.L. Hahn, interview by Mattson, 9 March 1994.

6. Ibid.

7. E.L. Hahn, "Spin echoes," *Physical Review* **80,** (1950), 580-594.

8. Anatole Abragam, "The physicist Erwin Hahn," *Pulsed Magnetic Resonance: NMR, ESR, and Optics,* (Oxford: Clarendon, 1992), 2.

9. E.L. Hahn, personal communication to James Mattson, 9 November 1994.

10. Mary Weiss Hahn Guggenheim, *The Memoirs of Mary Weiss Hahn Guggenheim,* unpublished autobiography written between 1972 and 1979, 33.

11. M. Weiss Hahn Guggenheim, 29.

12. Ibid., 35.

13. Ibid.

14. Ibid., 39.

15. Ibid., 40.

16. Ibid.

17. Ibid., 44.

18. Ibid., 44-45.

19. Ibid., 46.

20. Ibid., 47-48.

21. Ibid., 50, 53.

22. Ibid., 51-52.

23. Ibid., 53.

24. Ibid., 53-54.

25. Ibid., 59.

26. Ibid., 54, 59.

27. Ibid., 62.

28. Ibid.

29. Ibid.

30. Ibid., 71.

31. Ibid., 72.

32. Ibid., 68-69.

33. Ibid., 66.

34. Ibid. 67.

35. Ibid., 70.

36. Ibid., 77.

37. Ibid., 79.

38. Ibid., 94.

39. Ibid. 80.

40. Ibid.

41. Ibid.

42. E.L. Hahn, interview by Mattson, 9 March 1994.

43. M. Weiss Hahn Guggenheim, 83.

44. Ibid., 80.

45. E.L. Hahn, personal communication to James Mattson, 24 March 1995.

46. M. Weiss Hahn Guggenheim, 85.

47. Ibid., 93.

48. Ibid., 95-96.

49. Ibid., 96.

50. E.L. Hahn, interview by Mattson, 9 March 1994.

51. Ibid.

52. Ibid.

53. Richard Boyer and David Savageau, *Places Rated Almanac*, (Chicago: Rand McNally, 1985), 4.

54. E.L. Hahn, interview by Mattson, 9 March 1994.

55. Ibid.

56. E.L. Hahn, "Thoughts on my life," provided to *Who's Who in America*, Thirty-eighth Biennial Edition, 1974-75 (New Providence, NJ: Marquis' Who's Who, 1974).

57. E.L. Hahn, interview by Mattson, 9 March 1994.

58. Ibid.

59. M. Weiss Hahn Guggenheim, 105.

60. E.L. Hahn, interview by Mattson, 9 March 1994.

61. Ibid., 2 March 1995.

62. Ibid.

63. Career summary of E.L. Hahn released by the Academic Senate of the University of California in Berkeley, 1978.

64. E.L. Hahn, interview by Mattson, 2 March 1995.

65. Ibid., 9 March 1994.

66. Ibid.

67. Ibid.

68. M. Weiss Hahn Guggenheim, 96.

69. Frank S. Mead, *Handbook of Denominations in the United States,* Seventh Edition, (Nashville, TN: Abingdon, 1980), 62-63.

70. E.L. Hahn, interview by Mattson, 9 March 1994.

71. Ibid.

72. M. Weiss Hahn Guggenheim, 27.

73. Ibid., 101.

74. E.L. Hahn, interview by Joan Bromberg at the University of California, Berkeley conducted as part of the Laser History Project, 21 August 1986, transcript provided by Professor Hahn, 1.

75. E.L. Hahn, University of Illinois form entitled "Request for Information Concerning Training and Professional Experience," completed December 10, 1945, provided by University Archives of University of Illinois at Urbana-Champaign.

76. E.L. Hahn, interview by Mattson, 9 March 1994.

77. Ibid.

78. Ibid.

79. Ibid.

80. E.L. Hahn, interview by Bromberg, 2.

81. E.L. Hahn, interview by Mattson, 8 February 1995.

82. Ibid., 9 March 1994.

83. Ibid.

84. E.L. Hahn, interview by Bromberg, 3.

85. E.L. Hahn, interview by Mattson, 8 February 1995.

86. Ibid.

87. Ibid., 9 March 1994.

88. E.L. Hahn, interview by Bromberg, 5.

89. E.L. Hahn, interview by Mattson, 8 February 1995.

90. Ibid.

91. E.M. Purcell, H.C. Torrey, and R.V. Pound, "Resonance absorption by nuclear magnetic moments in a solid," *Physical Review* **69,** (1946), 37.

92. F. Bloch, W.W. Hansen, and M.E. Packard, "Nuclear induction," *Physical Review* **69,** (1946), 127.

93. F. Bloch, "Nuclear induction," *Physical Review* **70,** (1946), 460.

94. F. Bloch, W.W. Hansen, and M.E. Packard, "The nuclear induction experiment," *Physical Review* **70,** (1946), 474.

95. E.L. Hahn, interview by Mattson, 8 February 1995.

96. Hahn, "Pulsed NMR: A personal history," 1.

97. E.L. Hahn, "Fifty years of NMR: What happened in the beginning?" speech presented on several occasions during a 1994 visit to Germany, 5.

98. E.L. Hahn, interview by Mattson, 9 March 1994.

99. Ibid.

100. Hahn, "Pulsed NMR: A personal history," 1.

101. N. Bloembergen, E.M. Purcell, and R.V. Pound, "Relaxation effects in nuclear magnetic resonance absorption," *Physical Review* **73,** (1948), 692.

102. J. Schwinger, *Physical Review* **51,** (1937), 648.

103. I.I. Rabi, "Space quantization in a gyrating magnetic field," *Physical Review* **51,** (1937), 652.

104. Hahn, "Pulsed NMR: A personal history," 2.

105. Ibid.

106. F. Bloch and A. Nordsieck, "Radiation field of the electron," *Physical Review* **52,** (1937), 54.

107. M. Chodorow, R. Hofstadter, H.E. Rorschach, and A.L. Schawlow, editorial introduction to *Felix Bloch and Twentieth-Century Physics,* (Houston: William Marsh Rice University, 1980), viii.

108. E.L. Hahn, interview by Bromberg, 6.

109. Anatole Abragam, *Reflections of a Physicist,* (Oxford: Clarendon Press, 1986), 127.

110. Hahn, "Fifty years of NMR," 8.

111. Ibid.

112. Ibid., 9.

113. Hahn, "Pulsed NMR: A personal history," 2-3.

114. Hahn, "Fifty years of NMR," 8.

115. D.M.S. Bagguley, "The echo phenomenon," *Pulsed Magnetic Resonance: NMR, ESR, and Optics,* (Oxford: Clarendon Press, 1992), 5-6.

116. E.L. Hahn, letter written to E.M. Purcell, 8 December 1949.

117. E.L. Hahn, interview by Mattson, 9 March 1994.

118. Hahn, "Fifty years of NMR," 8.

119. E.L. Hahn, interview by Bromberg, 6.

120. C. Slichter, "Pulsed NMR in solids—then and now," *Pulsed Magnetic Resonance: NMR, ESR, and Optics,* (Oxford: Clarendon Press, 1992), 54, 56.

121. Hahn, "Pulsed NMR: A personal history," 3.

122. Ibid., 2.

123. Peter G. Morris, *Nuclear Magnetic Resonance Imaging in Medicine and Biology,* (Oxford: Clarendon Press, 1986), 30.

124. Hahn, "Spin echoes," *Physical Review* **80,** (1950), 582.

125. Overview of Hahn's life and career printed by the Academic Senate of the University of California, Berkeley on the occasion of his being named one of two Faculty Research Lecturers for academic year 1978-79.

126. H.Y. Carr and E.M. Purcell, "Effects of diffusion on free precession in nuclear magnetic resonance experiments," *Physical Review* **94,** (1954), 630.

127. E.L. Hahn, private communication to Herman Carr, 14 November 1950.

128. E.L. Hahn, interview by Mattson, 9 March 1994.

129. Jeremy K.M. Sanders and Brian K. Hunter, *Modern NMR Spectroscopy: A Guide for Chemists,* (New York: Oxford University Press, 1987), 65.

130. R. Freeman, "Spin choreography," *Pulsed Magnetic Resonance: NMR, ESR, and Optics,* (Oxford: Clarendon Press, 1992), 219-220.

131. Abragam, "The physicist Erwin Hahn," 2-3.

132. Ibid., 1-2.

133. Anatole Abragam, *Time Reversal: An Autobiography,* (Oxford: Clarendon Press, 1989), 167.

134. Abragam, "The physicist Erwin Hahn," 2.

135. Bloembergen, Purcell, and Pound, "Relaxation effects in nuclear magnetic resonance absorption," *Physical Review* **73,** (1948), 708.

136. Hahn, "Spin echoes," *Physical Review* **80,** (1950), 586.

137. H.Y. Carr and E.M. Purcell, "Effects of diffusion on free precession in nuclear magnetic resonance experiments," *Physical Review* **94,** (1954), 630-638.

138. E.L. Hahn, interview by Mattson, 9 March 1994.

139. Hahn, "Spin echoes," 590.

140. E.L. Hahn, interview by Bromberg, 8.

141. Hahn, "Pulsed NMR: A personal history," 3.

142. E.L. Hahn, "Heritage of the Bloch equations in quantum optics," *Felix Bloch and Twentieth-Century Physics,* (Houston: William Marsh Rice University, 1980), 19.

143. F. Bloch, interview by Charles Weiner, 15 August 1968, transcript, Niels Bohr Library, American Institute of Physics, College Park, MD, 40.

144. J.T. Arnold, S.S. Dharmatti, and M.E. Packard, *Journal of Chemical Physics* **19,** (1951), 507.

145. E.M. Purcell, "Research in nuclear magnetism," Nobel lecture reprinted in *Science* **118,** (1953), 435.

146. Hahn, "Pulsed NMR: A personal history," 4.

147. E.L. Hahn, interview by Bromberg, 9.

148. E.L. Hahn, "Felix Bloch reminiscences," *International Journal of Modern Physics B,* **4,** (1990), 1283.

149. E.L. Hahn, "Heritage of the Bloch Equations in quantum optics," 19-20.

150. Ibid.

151. Hahn, "Felix Bloch reminiscences," 1284.

152. Ibid.

153. E.L. Hahn, "Felix Bloch and magnetic resonance," speech given at Felix Bloch Memorial Symposium sponsored by American Physical Society, Washington, DC, April 25, 1984, printed in *Bulletin of Magnetic Resonance* **7,** (1984), 85.

154. E.L. Hahn, interview by Bromberg, 11.

155. Ibid.

156. E.M. Purcell and R.V. Pound, "A nuclear spin system at negative temperature," *Physical Review* **81,** (1951), 279-280.

157. E.L. Hahn, letter to Herman Carr, 14 November 1950.

158. Ibid.

159. E.L. Hahn, personal communication to James Mattson, 29 March 1995.

160. J.S. Waugh, "Spin echoes and thermodynamics," *Pulsed Magnetic Resonance: NMR, ESR, and Optics,* (Oxford: Clarendon Press, 1992), 174.

161. M. Weger, "High-temperature superconductivity and an apparent breakdown of causality," *Pulsed Magnetic Resonance: NMR, ESR, and Optics,* (Oxford: Clarendon Press, 1992), 210.

162. J.S. Waugh, "Spin echoes and thermodynamics," 174.

163. E.L. Hahn, interview by Bromberg, 22.

164. E.M. Purcell, "Research in nuclear magnetism," 435.

165. Hahn, "Felix Bloch and magnetic resonance," 86.

166. Hahn, "Pulsed NMR: A personal history," 7.

167. Abragam, *Time Reversal: An Autobiography*, 215.

168. Hahn, "Fifty years of NMR," 6.

169. Hahn, "Felix Bloch and magnetic resonance," 87.

170. Hahn, "Pulsed NMR: A personal history," 4.

171. Ibid., 5.

172. E.L. Hahn, interview by Bromberg, 10.

173. E.L. Hahn and D.E. Maxwell, "Spin echo measurements of nuclear spin coupling in molecules," *Physical Review* **88**, (1952), 1083.

174. Hahn, "Pulsed NMR: A personal history," 5.

175. "A profile of Erwin Louis Hahn," *Modern Scientists and Engineers*, (New York: McGraw-Hill Book, 1980).

176. R.R. Ernst, "The multidimensional importance of time domain magnetic resonance," *Pulsed Magnetic Resonance: NMR, ESR, and Optics, A Recognition of E.L. Hahn*, (Oxford: Clarendon Press, 1992), 117-118.

177. E.L. Hahn, interview by Bromberg, 12.

178. E.L. Hahn, interview by Mattson, 9 March 1994.

179. Hahn, "Felix Bloch reminiscences," 1286.

180. E.L. Hahn, interview by Bromberg, 12-13.

181. Ibid., 13.

182. Ibid., 13-14.

183. A.G. Anderson, R.L. Garwin, E.L. Hahn, J.W. Horton, G.L. Tucker, and R.M. Walker, "Spin echo serial memory," *Journal of Applied Physics* **26**, (1955), 1324.

184. E.L. Hahn, interview by Bromberg, 14.

185. Hahn, "Pulsed NMR: A personal history," 6.

186. M. Bloom, E.L. Hahn, and B. Herzog, "Free magnetic induction in nuclear quadrupole resonance," *Physical Review* **97**, (1955), 1966.

187. T.P. Das and E.L. Hahn, *Nuclear Quadrupole Resonance Spectroscopy*, Solid State Physics Series, Suppl. 1, (New York: Academic Press, 1958).

188. B. Herzog and E.L. Hahn, "Relaxation time modification by double nuclear resonance," *Physical Review* **98**, (1955), 226.

189. B. Herzog and E.L. Hahn, "Transient nuclear induction and double nuclear resonance in solids," *Physical Review* **103**, (1956), 148.

190. E.L. Hahn, interview by Bromberg, 15.

191. Ibid., 17.

192. Ibid., 20.

193. Ibid.

194. R.E. Walstedt, "The two-pulse spin echo revisited," *Pulsed Magnetic Resonance: NMR, ESR, and Optics*, (Oxford: Clarendon Press, 1992), 242-243.

195. L.E. Crooks and R. Rothschild, "Clinical imaging," *Pulsed Magnetic Resonance: NMR, ESR, and Optics*, (Oxford: Clarendon Press, 1992), 359.

196. Abragam, *Time Reversal*, 297.

197. A. Henstra and W.T. Wenckebach, "Nuclear orientation via electron spin locking in Si:B," *Pulsed Magnetic Resonance: NMR, ESR, and Optics*, (Oxford: Clarendon Press, 1992), 411.

198. J.N.S. Evans, "NMR and enzymes," *Pulsed Magnetic Resonance: NMR, ESR, and Optics* (Oxford: Clarendon Press, 1992), 123.

199. R.E. Slusher and E.L. Hahn, "Sensitive detection of pure quadrupole spectra of nuclei (10^{15} to 10^{18} cm^{-3}) near impurities in NaCl," *Physical Review Letters* **12**, (1964), 246.

200. R.E. Walstedt, D.A. McArthur, and E.L. Hahn, "Nuclear double resonance of Ca^{43} in CaF$_2$," *Physical Review Letters* **15**, (1965), 7.

201. E.L. Hahn, interview by Bromberg, 27.

202. D. Stehlik and H.M. Vieth, "Time evolution of electron-nuclear cross-polarization in RF-ONP," *Pulsed Magnetic Resonance: NMR, ESR, and Optics,* (Oxford: Clarendon Press, 1992), 476.

203. E.L. Hahn, interview by Mattson, 8 February 1995.

204. Hahn, "Fifty years of NMR," 5.

205. E.L. Hahn, interview by Mattson, 2 March 1995.

206. Excerpt from presentation speech when Erwin Hahn was awarded Berkeley Citation, 20 April 1991.

207. Hahn, "Fifty years of NMR," 10.

208. Hahn, personal communication to James Mattson, 24 March 1995.

209. Hahn, "Fifty years of NMR," 10-11.

The joy of insight is a sense of involvement and awe, the elated state of mind that you achieve when you have grasped some essential point; it is akin to what you feel on top of a mountain after a hard climb or when you hear a great work of music.
—Victor Weiskopf

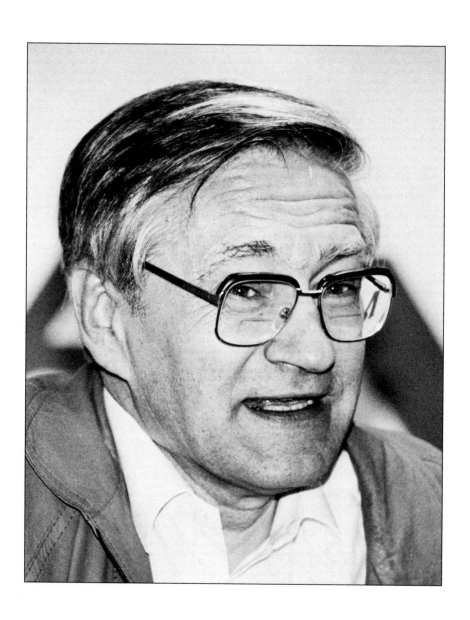

CHAPTER

7

RICHARD R. ERNST

Pioneer of Fourier-Transform NMR and
Two-Dimensional NMR Spectroscopy and Imaging

FIFTY-EIGHT YEARS after his birth in Winterthur, Switzerland, Richard R. Ernst was circling the globe to pick up one more accolade for his scientific achievements when he received word that he had been selected to receive the most prestigious one of all, the Nobel Prize. Notified of the honor by Archie Lindsay, captain of the Pan Am flight from Moscow to New York on which Ernst was a passenger, the Swiss chemist is said to have responded with, "That's great. I'm very pleased,"[1] and "Who are the other two?"[2] Knowing that a Nobel Prize can be split three ways, Ernst said he could imagine several scenarios in which he might be one of two or one of three recipients. There were no others. The honor and the $1 million would be Ernst's alone when he stepped forward to receive the prize from King Carl XVI Gustaf of Sweden in Stockholm on December 10, 1991. Radioed congratulations to the cockpit from the Royal Swedish Academy of Sciences, from the president of his native Switzerland, and from the attendees of a party organized in his honor back in Zürich completed the seven-mile-high event.

According to *New Scientist* magazine, Ernst was called to the cockpit when the flight was somewhere west of Ireland. It was a fitting location because the career that led to the 1991 Nobel Prize in chemistry had also spanned the Atlantic. Swiss in citizenship, allegiance, and training, it was in the United States that Ernst made one of his greatest contributions to science. Perhaps that is the reason he is listed in *American Men & Women of Science*.[3] Or perhaps it's just wishful thinking. Everyone loves a winner.

In the Steps of Bloch

Richard Ernst won the Nobel Prize in chemistry for his achievements in NMR 39 years after another native of Switzerland, Felix Bloch, won the

Nobel Prize in physics for his discovery of NMR in condensed matter. Though there are many differences between the careers of the two men, there are also a number of places where their paths have crossed.

In March 1933, Felix Bloch, presciently aware that the end had come for Jews in Germany, walked out on his job as *privatdozent* and assistant to Werner Heisenberg at the University of Leipzig, and returned to his home in Zürich, Switzerland. He spent the spring and summer of 1933 working at the ETH with Wolfgang Pauli and Gregor Wentzel and visiting his fellow physicists Paul Langévin, Hendrik Kramers and Niels Bohr in Paris, Utrecht and Copenhagen, respectively. It was while visiting Bohr that Bloch received a telegram offering him a faculty position in the physics department at Stanford University in Palo Alto, California, resulting in Bloch's emigration to the United States in the spring of 1934.

On August 14, 1933, about the time Bloch was making preparation to leave Zürich for Rome to commence a half-year of Rockefeller Fellowship-funded research with Enrico Fermi, Richard Robert Ernst was born in Winterthur, Switzerland, about 15 miles from Zürich.

In the summer of 1933, the idea that Ernst, an infant, and Bloch, a 27-year-old physicist already famous amongst his peers for his electron theory of metals, would someday receive, 39 years apart, Nobel Prizes for their contributions to nuclear magnetic resonance would have been so remote as to be incomprehensible.* Although it was known that atomic nuclei had spin and therefore magnetic moments in 1933, the term "nuclear magnetic resonance" had not yet been coined, the first attempt by Dutch physicist Cornelis Gorter to detect the phenomenon was still three years away, Rabi's successful detection of the NMR signal in molecular beams was still four years distant, and Bloch's discovery of NMR in condensed matter more than a dozen years off.

With the passing of years, Bloch and Ernst would also come to have other things in common. In 1956, Ernst would graduate from the Swiss Federal Institute of Technology—the ETH. Bloch graduated from the same institution 29 years earlier. In 1962, Ernst would move to Palo Alto, California, 28 years after Bloch. Ernst's time in Palo Alto would be spent as an employee of Varian Associates, a company with strong Stanford links and for whom Felix Bloch had been a consultant.

---

* In the 39 years separating the 1952 Nobel Prize and the 1991 Nobel Prize, the monetary value of a Nobel Prize would also change dramatically, at least in face value. Bloch and Purcell would split $66,000 between them. Ernst would receive $1 million.

There was also a major difference between the two men, however. Bloch was a physicist and Ernst is a chemist, a division of labor almost as distinct in Bloch's mind as the Bloch walls he had found separating ferromagnetic domains. "When chemists get into a field it's time to get out,"[4] Bloch is said to have stated on at least one occasion. Ironically, despite Bloch's ambivalence toward chemistry, his 1946 nuclear induction discovery and the subsequent contributions by him and his laboratory to high-resolution NMR spectroscopy would result in what has probably been the greatest boon ever for chemists.

A Varian publication on the early history of that company refers to NMR as "the physics experiment that revolutionized chemistry" and quotes Martin Packard, one of Bloch's collaborators in his 1946 experiment. Responding to the question, "What does NMR mean to chemistry?" Packard had replied facetiously, "Without it, they'd be out of business," and then responding more seriously, said:

> Prior to the use of NMR and other less powerful analytical techniques, you could spend literally months and years trying to determine the structure of a molecule. With NMR, infrared, mass spectroscopy, and other such tools, the same problems can often be solved in hours, and the whole field of chemistry has been able to undergo a much more rapid advance and expansion.[5]

One of the chemists who would take NMR, or nuclear induction, as Bloch preferred to call it, and advance its development greatly, first in the field of chemistry and later in magnetic resonance imaging is Richard Robert Ernst.

Growing Up in Winterthur

The Ernst family history goes back a long way in Winterthur, at least to the 15th century, according to Ernst, possibly as far back as 1415 when the city became a free imperial city within the Holy Roman Empire. By European standards, however, Richard grew up in a relatively new house that his grandfather, a merchant, built in 1898. Richard's father, Johannes Robert Walter Ernst, became an architect and, as a professor of architecture, taught at a local secondary-level institution known as Winterthur Technical School. His mother was the former Irma Brunner. In addition to their son, Richard, the couple also had two daughters.

With a present-day population of 90,000, Winterthur is the second largest city in the canton of Zürich. About one-fourth the size of Zürich, it flanks the Töss River, which drains the area north of the Zürichsee and supplies water to the Rhine River separating Switzerland from its northern neighbor, Germany. Strategically located on the populous plateau between the Jura mountains to the north and the mighty Swiss Alps to the south, the city of Winterthur and its larger urban siblings—Zürich, Basel, Luzern, Lausanne and Bern—are connected by a series of fast intercity electric trains. As a terminus for this northern Switzerland railroad network, Winterthur is a city of heavy machinery production that includes the manufacture of railway locomotives and diesel engines.

Winterthur is also a city that appreciates cultural and artistic expression, providing a home for priceless art collections and a well-known symphony orchestra. As a teenager, Ernst was an amateur musician and self-directed chemistry experimenter with dual interests in art and industry that have continued to the present day.

Playing the violoncello [the full name for what is more commonly called the cello in the United States] brought me into numerous chamber and church music ensembles, and stimulated my interest in musical composition that I tried extensively while in high school. At the age of 13, I found in the attic a case filled with chemicals, remainders of an uncle who died in 1923 and was, as a metallurgical engineer, interested in chemistry and photography. I became almost immediately fascinated by the possibilities of trying out all conceivable reactions with them, some leading to explosions, others to unbearable poisoning of the air in our house, frightening my parents.[6]

Fortunately, Ernst and his family survived his early trial-and-error methods. Soon he was reading all the chemistry books he could find, starting initially with some 19th-century books he found in his family's home library and then exhausting the rather extensive collection housed in the city library. By the age of 14, long before exhausting the city's holdings of chemistry resources, he knew what he wanted to be when he grew up; that is, if he could survive his own experiments and escape death by explosion or asphyxiation. He would be a chemist rather than a composer. Instead of seeking to arrange the perfect musical masterpiece, with its points and counterpoints, he would seek to understand nature's rhythms, movements, and harmonic relationships. "I wanted to understand the secrets behind my chemical experiments and behind the processes in nature,"[7] he has stated. Eventually, his search for understanding chemical composition would find expression in NMR spectroscopy, a developing field which he would revolutionize with Fourier-transform NMR in the 1960s and which he would further expand in the 1970s with two-dimensional Fourier-transform NMR.

In some ways, NMR spectroscopy may be seen as a type of music, with spectral signatures providing a sort of musical score of the subtle and majestic interactions taking place within complex molecules. The *crescendoes*, the *fortes*, and the *pianissimos* of spectroscopy all contribute significantly to a chemist's understanding of a molecule's composition. In that sense, NMR spectroscopists are reverse composers, decipherers of a musical score as it is performed, perfectly and precisely, by the tiny "musicians" making up the spectroscopist's sample. By adding the power of the Fourier transform to NMR spectroscopy, Ernst would find a way to detect these patterns much more quickly and with much more sensitivity.

Professor Sture Forsén of the Royal Swedish Academy of Sciences expressed the significance of Professor Ernst's accomplishments eloquently just before calling him forward to receive his Nobel Prize. A significant portion of Forsén's comments are included here to help the reader understand the significance of Ernst's contributions and the historical milieu in which those contributions took place.

One particular methodological development in which this year's Laureate was a leading figure early in his scientific career [said Professor Forsén] was the introduction of Fourier transformation and pulse techniques in NMR spectroscopy, thereby improving the sensitivity of the technique tenfold or even hundredfold. Now I am sure that most of you will shake your head, Fourier transformation and pulse techniques, what is that? Let me try to illustrate it through an analogy. Remember first that spectroscopy is very much concerned with the detection of signals from a sample containing some compound. Assume that you are interested in finding out how well tuned a piano is.

The traditional, "old-fashioned" way of doing this would of course be to hit each key in succession and record the frequencies—the signals from our sample if you wish. Now a modern piano usually has 88 keys and it would take some time to go through them one by one, let us say 10 minutes, i.e. 600 seconds. Now there is a much faster way of getting the same results: stretch out both your arms and hit all keys at once, like this [sound effect]. You have now performed a pulse experiment. The result sounds awkward, but remember that all the tones are there in the response. But how could you possibly extract the individual tones from this cacophony? That you can do by a mathematical analysis called—well, you may have guessed it—Fourier transformation.

A fast modern computer would perform this analysis in less than a second and the output from your computer would be the individual notes [new sound effect—a scale]. So the new way—the FT way—of checking the tuning of a piano would perhaps take six seconds instead of 600 seconds, a substantial improvement in time. This may sound senseless, why this hurry, even if this new method would allow you to tune 100 pianos in the time it took to tune one in the "old-fashioned" way? But, savings in time can be used in another way, to increase sensitivity. To continue our analogy, assume that you had encountered a piano with "signals" from the strings barely audible above the background noise in the room. Now you could improve the detection of these weak signals by hitting the keys of this same piano 100 times every sixth second and *adding* the result. This would improve the signal-to-noise ratio tenfold, in the jargon of scientists.

When Fourier transform NMR was introduced around 1970 it had a tremendous impact on the applicability of the NMR technique to chemistry. It now became feasible to study very weak signals from small amounts of material or from important elements with magnetic nuclei that are rare in nature, for example carbon-13 and nitrogen-15. The Achilles heel of the NMR technique had hitherto been its poor sensitivity, but now *this* obstacle was largely removed.

A later revolutionary development in NMR, in which this year's Chemistry Laureate played a leading role, was the introduction of more than one frequency dimension, 2, 3 or higher. In 2D NMR, the chemical "piano" is hit with pulses of varying lengths and intervals. This allows chemists to extract many parameters of interest from the NMR spectra with great ease. Hopelessly muddled and hard-to-interpret spectra can be spread out and thereby simplify the analysis—much as a two-dimensional map of a landscape would be superior to a mere silhouette. 2D NMR makes it possible to find out which specific atoms in a molecule are closely linked by chemical bonds or which atoms are near each other in space, or which atoms take part in chemical exchange reactions, and much more. A whole new range of experiments have become possible and multidimensional NMR has substantially increased the range of applications to chemistry.

The new method has been a prerequisite for the very important applications of NMR in structural biology that have taken place during the past decade.

Professor Ernst: You have played a leading role in several of the most significant methodological developments that have taken place in the field of NMR spectroscopy over the past two decades; developments that have had a lasting impact on the way modern chemistry is conducted. You have, in an admirable way, combined excellent experimental know-how with extraordinary theoretical insight. In recognition of your services to chemistry, and to natural science as a whole, the Royal Swedish Academy of Sciences has decided to confer upon you this year's Nobel Prize for Chemistry.

Professor Ernst, I have been granted the privilege of conveying to you the warmest congratulations of the Academy, and I now invite you to receive your Prize from the hands of His Majesty the King.[8]

The ETH, Zürich

Upon graduation from the Winterthur public high school in 1952, Ernst matriculated at the famous Swiss Federal Institute of Technology in Zürich, the ETH-Z, with "high expectations and enthusiasm to study chemistry."[9] He was "rapidly disappointed," however, to find that the chemistry he had hoped would help him understand the processes of nature had degenerated in academic practice to a rigid sequence of innumerable facts that were to be memorized more than comprehended. "We students had to memorize incountable facts that even the professors did not understand," stated Ernst. "A good memory, not impeccable logic, was on demand."[10]

The physical chemistry lectures that Ernst attended at the ETH weren't much better than the other chemistry courses. "[They] did not reveal much insight either, they were limited just to classical thermodynamics,"[11] Ernst commented. If he was going to satisfy his curiosity and make a significant contribution, he would have to dig the information out for himself.

Thus, I had to continue, similar as in high school [noted Ernst], to gain some decent chemical knowledge by reading. A book from which I learned a lot at that time was *Theoretical Chemistry* by S. Glasstone. It revealed to me the fundamentals of quantum mechanics, spectroscopy, statistical mechanics, and statistical thermodynamics, subjects that were never even mentioned in lectures, except in a voluntary and very excellent lecture course given by the young enthusiastic Professor Hans H. Günthard who had studied chemistry and physics in parallel.[12]

In a way, the ETH's shortcomings may have worked in Ernst's favor, though less motivated students were doubtless deprived in the process. Forced to find for himself the understanding he was seeking, Ernst sharpened his research skills. Felix Bloch had had somewhat the same experience at the ETH a quarter-century earlier when he changed his major from electrical engineering to physics, an area of study that was viewed by many at the time as having no future. Stuck with an incomplete curriculum but blessed with a great curiosity, "the only thing we could do about it," said Bloch, "was to go to the library and read some books, though nobody would advise us which ones to choose."[13]

For Ernst, one of the benefits of digging out information for himself was a cross-fertilized exposure to both physics and chemistry. When Ernst later moved to California to work at Varian Associates, Weston Anderson, with whom Ernst collaborated on Fourier-transform work, found that Ernst was not your "typical" chemist:

> I call him almost a physicist first [said Anderson], but he did graduate as a chemist. He certainly knows his physics, he knows his chemistry, he knows his electronics and he uses all of these. He's kind of an all-around guy in that sense.[14]

Like Ernst, a number of the NMR pioneers featured in this book have expressed a dissatisfaction with learning facts for facts' sake. Rabi chose electrical engineering by default, knowing he wanted to study the fundamental structure of matter, but not knowing as an undergraduate that the name of the science that would provide those insights was physics. Ramsey planned initially to study engineering, but switched to mathematics with a heavy minor in physics when he became unhappy with engineering's heavy dependence on handbooks and tables. Purcell graduated with a degree in electrical engineering, but by the time he finished his undergraduate years had made the decision to switch over to physics. Bloch started out in electrical engineering, but switched to physics after one year.

It's noteworthy, however, that of the nine scientists in this book, Ernst and Damadian probably used more of an interdisciplinary approach to their research than any of the others. Ernst, a chemist, took large excursions into the field of physics and after gleaning bounty that he found useful to chemists, made important contributions to the field of analytic chemistry. Damadian, trained early on in mathematics and chemistry, earned a medical degree, and then picked up on the physics and chemistry of NMR to propose and achieve a medical breakthrough, a completely new, X-ray-free method for the *in vivo* detection of cancer and other diseases. Ernst would also turn his attention to MRI where he would make significant contributions to image acquisition methods that were then in a state of flux. Ernst's approach would be further refined by scientists at the University of Aberdeen and elsewhere and is now the MRI technique most widely used in clinical applications.

After receiving his *Diplomierter Ingenieur-Chemiker* in 1956, Ernst fulfilled the military service required of all male Swiss citizens who have attained the age of 20, thus delaying the start of his graduate studies until 1957 and age 24.

For researching and writing his PhD thesis, Ernst felt fortunate to be accepted by Hans Günthard, the professor whose elective lecture course had stood out to Ernst as an undergraduate like a sharp, high-amplitude peak in a spectrum of short and insignificant spikes. Günthard, in turn, paired Ernst with Hans Primas, "a young most brilliant scientist," said Ernst. Though lacking in formal studies, Primas had quickly acquired the skills needed for conducting high-resolution NMR spectroscopy, a field still in its infancy. Like the proverbial "iron sharpening iron," Günthard, with his dual focus on chemistry and physics, and Primas, with his emphasis on spectroscopy, would prove to be beneficial associations that would sharpen Ernst's own self-described focus as an "NMR toolmaker."[15]

Both Primas and Ernst would spend much of their time in the design and construction of electronic equipment that would enhance the performance of NMR spectrometers. In the process of doing the hands-on work on the equipment itself, they also developed the theory for the experiments they intended to perform on the improved devices. Because, as Ernst noted, "NMR suffers from a disappointingly low sensitivity that severely limits its applications,"[16] efforts to optimize signal-to-noise ratios became a significant part of his daily routine. These efforts would also serve to heighten his interest in finding methods for circumventing this shortcoming of NMR.

While the statement that the "disappointingly low sensitivity [of NMR] severely limits its applications" would appear to be at odds with the facts from our present-day perspective, it should be emphasized that the NMR signal, while detectable, is indeed feeble. When a suitable sample is placed in a strong magnetic field, a very slim majority of nuclear spins "align" with the magnetic field. The rest are oppositely oriented. The strength of the signal is proportional to the excess of spins aligned with the field, which is limited by the strength of the field and the volume and temperature of the sample. The problem of NMR's low sensitivity would occupy Ernst's attention for much of his early career and NMR's eventual widespread application as a practical analytical tool in chemistry would result, in large measure, from the development of Fourier transform NMR, a methodological development in which Ernst would play an important role. In addition to the improvement Ernst and his collaborators would eventually obtain in signal-to-noise ratios, the Fourier transform technique would also reduce the time needed for collecting NMR data, as Weston Anderson has pointed out, by a factor between 100 and 1000.[17]

While a graduate student, Ernst worked on the construction of high-sensitivity radio frequency preamplifiers and probe assemblies, first for a 25 MHz and later for a 75 MHz proton resonance spectrometer. On the theoretical side, he was concerned with stochastic resonance, that is, excitation of magnetic resonance by random or pseudorandom noise irradiation. In one autobiographical sketch, he summarized his thesis work as follows:

> The goal set by Hans Primas was the usage of random noise for the excitation of nuclear magnetic resonance, following the famous concepts of Norbert Wiener for the stochastic testing of non-linear systems. The theoretical treatment was based on a Volterra functional expansion using orthogonal stochastic polynomials. I tried in particular to design a scheme of homonuclear broadband decoupling to simplify proton resonance spectra. By applying a stochastic sequence with a shaped power spectral density that has a hole at the observation frequency, all extraneous protons should be decoupled without perturbing the observed proton spin. The theoretical difficulties were mainly concerned with the computation of the response to non-white noise. Experiments were not attempted at that time, we did not believe in the usefulness of the concept anyway, and I finished my thesis in 1962 with a feeling like an artist balancing on a high rope without any interested spectators.[18]

If no one else was taking note of Ernst's acrobatics, at least the ETH was. He was awarded the Silver Medal of the ETH-Zürich for his PhD thesis, and, in the end, the exercise which seemed merely academic did turn out to be useful. In the late 1960s, Ernst would return to the subject of stochastic resonance, but this time in the context of sensitivity or signal-to-noise ratio optimization, particularly in relation to pulse-Fourier spectroscopy. In 1962, however, Ernst's perception that his thesis was answering questions that weren't being asked probably played a role in his decision to enter the "real world" of industry a year later. "I thus decided to leave the university forever," wrote Ernst, "and tried to find an industrial job in the United States."[19] He would find that job at Varian Associates.

Varian Associates

Varian has been connected with nuclear induction virtually since its inception, with the possessive "its" referring to both Varian and nuclear induction. The two have been inextricably linked. How Varian Associates came to hold the patent rights for NMR is an interesting story which begins, really, in the 1930s with the invention of a high-power radiofrequency amplifier called the klystron.

In fact, the story begins even earlier with the dream of two brothers, Russell and Sigurd Varian, that they would someday come up with a product that Russell would design and Sigurd would build that would put them on the road to financial security. Despite learning disabilities that made reading a challenge, Russell, the inventor, eventually obtained a degree in physics from Stanford while Sigurd became a barnstorming pilot and eventually a senior captain with Pan American World Airways.

Over the years, they considered many ideas that might fulfill the dream, a number of which were patented, but it was the klystron that became their first big opportunity. As a pilot, Sigurd was keenly aware of the need for devices that would make flying safer, devices that could detect mountains where maps said there were swamps, instruments that could detect approaching planes at night or in poor visibility, or guide a plane to a safe landing. Russell recognized that cloud-penetrating radio waves were the secret to many of these challenges and began working in 1936 on ideas for a device that could generate the high-frequency, short-wavelength radio energy such detection systems would need.

He found the basic component for his "klystron" tube in a "rhumbatron" that his close friend and assistant professor in the Stanford physics department, William W. Hansen, had invented. A cavity resonator which could be tuned to resonate at different frequencies by physically changing its size, much as a glass tumbler can be made to vibrate at different frequencies by changing the amount of water it contains, the rhumbatron had originally been developed by Hansen to generate through resonance the high voltages Stanford was seeking for bombarding atomic nuclei with accelerated particles. Russell Varian saw in Hansen's rhumbatron the potential for obtaining the short-wavelength, high-frequency energy he needed.

To develop the idea further, the Varian brothers felt they needed access to the sophisticated equipment available in the Stanford physics laboratory and the right to consult with Bill Hansen. Russell Varian was hesitant, however, to approach the university. For one thing, although he had completed his masters degree at Stanford and had been urged when he graduated in 1927 to return for a PhD, he had been denied the opportunity to do so when he applied in 1934. Although Russell was a research associate at Stanford at the time he applied, the reasons given by department chairman David Webster were vague as to why he was denied further academic progress, but they implied that he was not of PhD caliber because he knew little German and no French, his mathematics was inadequate, he read too slowly, and he was a poor speller.

Russell Varian's wife Dorothy, who worked closely with him in the founding and early management of Varian Associates, speculated in her book, *The Inventor and the Pilot*, that the rejection of his application may have been due to his image as a technician rather than a scholar.

His most obvious handicap, other than his mathematics, may have been that he had worked around the physics department for so many years as a low-paid technician that the chairman may have continued to look upon him in that capacity rather than as a scholar. It may have been a departmental decision, as the chairman claimed; Russell had been in Philadelphia for two years [where he had made important contributions to the development of television] and few of the newer members of the faculty knew him very well. . . . Bill Hansen was away on a National Research Fellowship.[20]

Felix Bloch was a newer member of the faculty in 1934, but had shown no indication of unwillingness to recognize Varian's scientific aptitude. In fact, he had liked an article Varian had written on photoconduction and the voltaic effect and, after suggesting some mathematical improvements, had sent a letter of recommendation to *Physical Review*, recommending that it be published. Varian was already a prolific inventor and had already demonstrated a strong aptitude for physics. At the time of his PhD application, he had published two articles, a third was accepted, and about a dozen patents were either granted or pending

Sigurd Varian was not so hesitant to ask a favor of the physics department. Although he knew his suggestion would be a departure from usual university policy, he told Webster, they had enough money saved up to support themselves for a year and they would use their own tools whenever possible. All he asked was that they be able to use the physics department equipment when necessary, that they be able to consult with Bill Hansen and others in the department, and that Stanford provide them $100 for the purchase of materials and supplies. In return for these benefits, Stanford University would receive half of any financial returns generated by the klystron. It was a good deal for Stanford. By 1964, Stanford's share of the rewards from their $100 investment would reach nearly $2 million.

It took a while to work the bugs out of their design. Bill Hansen is said to have reported that the device contained "too much haywire." On August 19, 1937, their "Model A" klystron oscillated for the first time, though its performance was unstable. Two days later, after Sigurd virtually rebuilt the device, they were able to pick up RF energy "all over the room." In their excitement, they measured the wavelength of the oscillations to be 6.5 centimeters and were later embarrassed to admit they had measured only half a wavelength. The correct wavelength was 13 centimeters.

Although it was anticipated that the armed services would be the first to be interested in the klystron, nothing came of two visits by the U.S. Navy. However, Sperry Gyroscope Company on Long Island, which had already developed a design for a blind-landing navigation system but which lacked an adequate source of power, was impressed. In exchange for providing annual grants of at least $5,000 and no more than $25,000, Sperry agreed to underwrite the additional research and development needed to bring the device to market. In turn, Sperry would be given exclusive rights to the original klystron patents and any subsequent patents that might result from work funded by the grants.

It was the beginning of an often rocky relationship between the principals involved. With their foot in the door, Sperry demanded to take over one-half of the space allocated to the physics department. As it was, they had already taken over the space previously allocated to Bill Hansen's rhumbatron and Felix Bloch's neutron research, forcing the physics department to roof over a light well in order to find space for Hansen and Bloch to conduct their research. Sperry's subsequent demand for half the physics department was too much for Webster and he informed them, in so many words, that they could hang onto that dream.

Webster and Hansen had less success in getting around a stipulation in the contract that, for the first two years of the project, all of their personal research time had to be spent on the klystron. Although both men initially refused, claiming their right to academic freedom, Sperry refused to compromise.

At one point, Sperry refused to continue Sigurd's $208 per month salary when he became ill with a bout of tuberculosis. They finally backed down when it was agreed Sig's salary would be paid as an advance against future royalties. Although Sperry wanted to continue its relationship with Stanford, they wanted to buy out Russell and Sigurd's interest. Sig was talented, they admitted, but sick and replaceable. Russell, they said, was no longer of value to their organization since his patent work on the klystron was completed. They would be willing to buy out their interests in the patent for what they estimated to be a fair price—$5,000. Only a sharp comeback by Stanford physics chairman David Webster that the whole deal was in jeopardy if Sperry persisted in the action brought such talk to a halt. Despite these struggles, the relationship continued, eventually resulting in moves by Russell and Sigurd Varian as well as Hansen and others to Long Island.

Although the United States' military had shown little interest in the klystron, the British had shown immediate interest and used the klystron to good advantage in equipping their fighters for night bombing during the Battle of Britain. As Edward Ginzton, who was also closely associated with the Varians and the klystron project, later recalled:

The klystron was invented during the summer of 1937 and announced formally to a world on the brink of war by the Varians in the February 1939 issue of *The Journal of Applied Physics*.

The somewhat diffident announcement was apparently overlooked in Germany—but not in England. Already deeply involved in the development of radar, scientists at Bristol University recognized that this ingenious new development would help make airborne radar possible by providing a lightweight source of microwaves for radar receivers. By late 1940—just as the Luftwaffe was switching to deadly night bombing—the RAF succeeded in equipping its night fighters with the klystron radar receivers that would help them win the Battle of Britain.[21]

The joint scientific effort that began in late 1940 between the British and the Americans, resulting in the establishment of the Radiation Laboratory at MIT, further expanded applications for the Varian klystron. The cavity magnetron brought over by the Tizard mission in 1940 became the high-power pulse transmitter for most World War II radar and the klystron tube the lower power, local oscillator for the receiver.

Varian Associates, however, was not founded until 1948, after the war, and from the beginning strong links were forged between Varian and NMR. The company began with about $22,000 in capital, but an even greater storehouse of intellectual capital, in the persons of the Varian brothers, Russell and Sig, and their Stanford physics department colleagues. The company also had an important piece of intellectual property, the patent rights for chemical analysis using nuclear induction.

Although Russell Varian had invented the klystron, Varian Associates was not founded for the sake of capitalizing on that particular invention. A major motivation was to establish a company where scientists and engineers would play a more significant decision-making role. As Russell Varian recounted in 1958:

As time passed, a group of us began to make plans for what we would do after the war was over. We decided that we would return to California [from Sperry in Garden City, New York] and establish a laboratory of our own. There engineers would have a chance to try out their own ideas about how an engineering business should be run.

Shortly before the end of the war, Dr. Hansen returned to Stanford University, largely for health reasons, and Dr. Ginzton accepted an appointment in the Physics Department. I returned to California very shortly after V-J Day and began to actively look around for a location for our new laboratory, and for possible items for development and production. Since the laboratory would be quite small and have limited capital, I more or less eliminated klystrons from the proposed field of our activity. This was because I thought that in order to compete, any company would have to have a considerable number of klystrons, and since I knew that they were quite expensive to develop I did not see any possibility at that time of entering the klystron business.

I was very favorably disposed, however, to select some new development in research that we could continue to develop, and that would preferably grow rather slowly so that we could grow with it. As something meeting these requirements, I took a very deep interest in nuclear magnetic resonance which had been developed by Bloch and Hansen at Stanford, and independently by Dr. E. M. Purcell and Professor Robert Pound at Harvard.[22]

After everyone returned home from their war-time venues, Russell Varian returned to the physics department at Stanford, once again as a research associate, where he observed Felix Bloch and Bill Hansen conducting the research and planning of an experiment that would result in their detection of nuclear induction in early 1946. Recognizing that the phenomenon had commercial application in chemical analysis, Varian urged Bloch and Hansen to patent their ideas. Since neither was inclined to do so, Varian offered to prepare the patent application in their names and handle the filing process, in return for which he would be granted an exclusive license for himself and Sig Varian when the company that they were planning to start began operation.

Bloch and Hansen agreed, and on December 23, 1946, a patent application was filed at the U.S. Patent Office in the names of Felix Bloch and William W. Hansen for a "Method and Means for Chemical Analysis by Nuclear Induction." According to Weston Anderson, who would later get his PhD under Bloch, "chemical analysis" was about the "farthest thing" from Bloch's mind at the time. "He thought it might be useful to a few physicists," said Anderson, "who wanted to measure magnetic moments or measure magnetic fields but he wasn't thinking of chemistry or chemical analysis at all."[23] Bloch and Hansen both would serve, however, as consultants to the fledgling company and Hansen would also serve as a member of the company's first board of directors.

As a result of the Bloch-Hansen patent, the Varian Instrument Division was formed. At the core of the division were Elliot Levinthal and Emery Rogers, both of whom secured their doctorates under Bloch. Not long afterward, Martin Packard, the third collaborator with Bloch and Hansen in the 1946 nuclear induction discovery, joined the company and eventually became head of the Instrument Division.

The first NMR product was a magnetometer designed to very precisely measure and control magnetic fields. In 1950, the company followed up the magnetometer with the first variable, high-resolution NMR spectrometer.

While Russ Varian had envisioned NMR as possibly the first project for the fledgling company, as it turned out, it would be his klystron would that would get the company off the ground:

We had one stroke of very good luck in getting the R-1 klystron contract almost at the start of our operations. This was a contract proposal that had not met with any enthusiasm from the manufacturers because it had an arbitrary allowance for overhead which was unrealistically low. However, this did not, at that time, bother Varian Associates because Dorothy Varian was our entire labor overhead; the rest of us were engineers.[24]

Eventually, Varian Associates would become, in terms of dollar volume, the world's largest manufacturer of klystron tubes as well as the largest supplier of NMR and EPR spectrometers and electromagnets.

As the company quickly grew, the pool of trained engineers and technicians available in Northern California was insufficient to meet its needs, so Sigurd Varian gave many of them on-the-job training until they had the required skills. Many graduate students in physics and engineering were also employed part-time by the company until they were able to complete their degrees. Many eventually became full-time employees.

Weston Anderson Joins Varian

One such employee was Weston Anderson. Anderson had joined Varian in September 1955 about a year after receiving his PhD at Stanford under Professor Felix Bloch. In the intervening period, Anderson, together with James Arnold, another of Bloch's recent PhD graduates, followed their mentor to Geneva, Switzerland when he began his appointment as the first Director General of the European Center for Nuclear Research (CERN). Although Bloch had been assured that his primary role in the position would be scientific and not altogether administrative, he had hedged his bets by making arrangements for Anderson and Arnold to set up a nuclear induction laboratory at the University of Geneva. As Anatole Abragam has pointed out, "Bloch had arranged to ship a large permanent magnet from Stanford to Geneva. It weighed several tons, and was specially designed for high resolution NMR by two of his disciples, Jim Arnold and Weston Anderson. . . . 'This way at least we'll get a little physics going in CERN,' commented Bloch."[25]

Of course, we jumped at the chance [to go to Switzerland, Weston Anderson said]. And so in 1954, the fall of '54, we went to Geneva to CERN and spent a year there. We actually brought along the magnet that we'd been using at Stanford and we set up the lab there and did some experiments. I wouldn't say we accomplished a heck of a lot.

We did some original things on measuring relaxation times in water and heavy water, which was of interest at that time, and we also enjoyed the atmosphere of another country. At the end of the first year, Bloch was sort of tired of administration. He was, of course, Director General and had gotten into more administration than he really liked so he decided he would go back to Stanford instead of staying the second year, which was in the original plan. That left Jim and me with the question, "What do we do now?" I searched around for job offers. I got three different job offers. One of them was from Varian where I had actually worked one summer while I was going to Stanford. Another was from Westinghouse research labs where I'd also worked one summer. The third was from Saclay [France], Professor Abragam's lab there. I chose Varian. So I started here at Varian in the fall of '55.[26]

Russell Varian's Magnetometer: Prelude to the Fourier Transform

Weston Anderson views the proton magnetometer, a device Russell Varian invented and patented to accurately measure the Earth's magnetic field, as one of the first steps on the road to Fourier-transform NMR, a foreshadow of the FT spectrometer that Weston Anderson and Richard Ernst would develop nearly two decades later. Improving its performance was the first task Anderson was assigned when he arrived at Varian. He described the device as follows:

This was a fairly simple concept, at least looking back on it. The idea was that you polarize nuclei in a bottle of water by putting a coil around them and putting current through the coil. You polarize them in a direction that's perpendicular to the magnetic field you want to measure and then you quickly remove the polarization and they start to precess about the magnetic field. They then induce a voltage into the same coil. You amplify that signal and record its frequency and you have a measure of the strength of the Earth's magnetic field. That was Russ Varian's invention. You see, it's very similar to a Fourier transform spectrometer in many respects.[27]

Russell Varian's patent was filed on October 21, 1948 and was entitled "Method and Means for Correlating Nuclear Properties of Atoms and Magnetic Fields."[28] So far as Anderson is aware, it was the first apparatus proposed that made use of free precession. Assigned to the task of improving its performance in 1955, Anderson found that the challenge was to remove the polarizing field without disrupting the magnetization of the water.

You had to be very careful [said Anderson] about how you switch the current off just before you look at the free induction signal. If you switch it off without quickly removing the energy, then you'll get oscillations set up in the coil and that disrupts the magnetization. If you let it decay too slowly, that is, if you pull the energy out of the coil slowly, then the nuclei follow the effective magnetic field and they end up pointing along the direction of the Earth's field. Then you don't have any free precession. So the trick of it was just to quickly remove the energy and switch it to the receive circuit without disrupting the spins.[29]

Asked if he had solved that problem, Anderson replied with satisfaction:

Oh yeah, sure. In fact, the magnetometer was used [in a variety of applications]. One interesting application that really didn't go very far but which caught a lot of interest in people was to find skiers that might be buried under an avalanche. We made this portable little magnetometer. You could just hold it in your hand, and it had a little coil on it that was out in front. The idea was that a skier, before he went up in the ski lift, would fasten a little magnet to his boot. If he happened to get under an avalanche, then a search party would be sent out with a magnetometer to find out where he was, and then they'd dig down and pull him out. They could do that much faster than the classical way, which is to get a bunch of people to just jab poles down through the snow trying to find the skier that way. I don't think Varian made any money off of that, but as I say, it generated a lot of excitement at the time.[30]

Smelling the Cork

In order to appreciate the enormous practical advantages that Fourier transform NMR would bring to chemical analysis, consider that NMR spectroscopy for its first 25 years (1946-1970) was performed using a slow frequency sweep in order to obtain a spectrum. This is a time-consuming process as very slow sweep rates, an extremely stable magnetic field, and a weak radiofrequency irradiation are required to obtain an undistorted spectrum.[31]

It is, of course, the frequency spectrum that spectroscopists are seeking. When the frequency of the transmitted electromagnetic field passes through the Larmor precession frequency of the nucleus under study, which is determined by the strength of the magnetic field in which the sample is placed and the gyromagnetic ratio of the nucleus, a resonance is detected. For multinuclear systems, the resulting spectrum can be quite complex. In any case, the signal amplitude plotted as a function of excitation frequency displays in a most direct way the resonant properties of the system under study and provides clues to the underlying quantum mechanical structure.

This point-by-point measurement of the signal amplitude in response to a single-frequency or monochromatic perturbation is the most intuitively obvious way to determine the spectrum. Of course, while the RF frequency is slowly being swept across the spectrum, the magnetic field must remain very stable, or the spectrum will be smeared. An alternative method for obtaining the so-called continuous wave, or CW, spectrum is to fix the frequency of the applied radiofrequency field and slowly sweep the applied magnetic field. Either way, most of the time is spent collecting off-resonance noise.

Although chemical shifts were discovered experimentally soon after the birth of Varian Associates,[32-33] the most famous being the spectral signature of the ethanol molecule (CH_3CH_2OH) in which the protons in each of the three groups exhibit NMR signals at slightly different frequencies, the initial research intended to unleash NMR's potential for identifying chemical structure was less dramatic and often disappointing.

Indeed, "early work on practical applications was so disappointing," wrote Anderson, "that researcher Martin Packard quipped, 'You could smell the cork on the bottle and almost make the same analysis as those early systems.' "[34] Even with time-averaging techniques that came along later to improve sensitivity, the spectrum still had to be created hundreds or even thousands of times to be considered reliable.[35]

By the time Weston Anderson arrived at Varian Associates, progress in instrumentation had been made and the company had sold one or two NMR machines for chemical analysis. Given his physics background and skills with instrumentation, his role was to try to find ways to improve the device.

There were a number of ways that we were thinking about in those days to make improvements. One of the most obvious, of course, was to operate at higher magnetic field strengths. We were originally operating at 30 MHz which is about 7000 gauss or 0.7 tesla. We moved up to 40 [MHz] not too long after that and then we had a big push. It was called SMOFF, which meant "Sixty Megacycles Or Fifty-Five" if we couldn't hit sixty. We did that one all right.

Continuing that push, we ended up with this magnet series about 100 Mhz. That's around 23 kilogauss or 2.3 tesla. Iron is really starting to saturate at that field and that was close to the end of the line as far as iron magnets went. After that, we started on the superconducting magnet. Harry Weaver [from Stanford] . . . joined Varian and he built the first cryogenic magnet. I think it used niobium titanium as the working material. That first magnet was 200 MHz. Then we quickly went to 220 and the thing has gone up ever since.[36]

Recalling other work that he did at Varian in the 1950s, Anderson said:

I was involved in some of the double-resonance studies. That was another area of particular interest to chemists because you get more chemical information if you irradiate one nucleus and look at the effect on another. You can find out which ones are coupled to each other and so on. The pushers in the field were higher magnetic fields, greater sensitivity, better resolution, better field-frequency stability and double resonance. Those were the areas where we realized improvements could be made, so those were the areas that we generally worked on. And, of course, it was the question of greater sensitivity that led me off into some of the directions that led ultimately to Fourier transform spectroscopy.[37]

With regard to the need for improving sensitivity or signal-to-noise ratios, Anderson pointed out:

I think the thing to remember is that it was the Varian group that really was pushing the sensitivity part. Hahn was very interested in doing spin echoes and using pulse techniques in order to get relaxation times and the like. I guess Lowe and other people talked about the Fourier transform relationship. It was Varian, Russell Varian, who first proposed that you use Fourier transforms to increase the sensitivity of a spectrometer. He actually filed a patent on that in 1956, and that was shortly after I came to Varian.[38]

Russell Varian's Gyromagnetic Resonance Apparatus

This invention was, in retrospect, years ahead of its time. The patent, entitled "Gyromagnetic Resonance Methods and Apparatus," was filed on August 29, 1956.[39] The principal object of the invention was to provide a novel means whereby the time stability of the apparatus could be greatly improved. Varian pointed out, for example, that it would take about 35 minutes to sweep through the entire hydrogen proton spectrum of ethyl alcohol (CH_3CH_2OH) in a polarizing field of 7,500 gauss. This, in turn, meant that, to adequately resolve the spectrum, a time stability of one part in 10^8 was required, a level of stability that is not easily or cheaply attained. As explained in the patent, Varian's invention circumvented this problem by exciting the sample simultaneously at a multitude of frequencies using a broadband frequency source: "The wide band frequency source may comprise, for example, a pulse generator wherein the pulses are regulated to give Fourier components over the desired frequency range or a white noise source having the required bandwidth."[40]

A second salient feature of the invention was the use of a Fourier analyzer to unfold the frequency spectrum of the recorded response. Therein lay the practical problem, how to do the Fourier analysis. Varian proposed two different methods in the patent, which Anderson described as follows:

His idea was that you could irradiate the spectrum continuously using a white noise source and receive the signals or the response from the nuclei and record this response. The way he proposed to do that was, first of all, to beat it down from radio frequencies to some audio frequency so it's easier to handle. Then you record this audio signal on a magnetic tape or wire or some other magnetic recording means for as long as you care to. Of course, the longer you do it, the more sensitivity you're going to get ultimately.

After you've recorded it on this long piece of tape, you take the tape and fasten the two ends together and then put it in a tape player—put the output of the player, say, through a narrow-band filter and rectifier—and then you essentially integrate the output. You play it through once and integrate the output.

Then you either change the speed of the player or you change an offset frequency somewhere so that when you play it through again, say at a higher speed, you will pick out another Fourier component. You send it through the system once for each frequency that you want. At the end, you display the responses at all of these frequencies and that's essentially your Fourier transform. It's a true Fourier transform operation, it's just not very convenient to use. It takes a long time and people judged it to be impractical, but the concept, the idea, is certainly there.

The other technique was that you would record the signal response on film, instead of on magnetic tape, and then use the film as a diffraction grating, and do the Fourier transform that way, which would be an optical Fourier transform.[41]

Even though Varian understood and spelled out in his patent the multiple advantages of this broadband excitation technique coupled with Fourier analysis of the NMR response, namely improved time stability and spectral resolution, shorter data acquisition time, and increased sensitivity, the invention lay dormant for almost a decade. Tragically, Russell Varian did not live to see the realization of his invention in the hands of Anderson and Ernst. Three years after applying for the patent, he died of a heart attack on July 28, 1959 while struggling to moor a charter boat on a stormy night on Alaska's Glacier Bay.[42] The patent for Varian's Fourier analyzer idea would not be issued until November 22, 1966.

Ernst Arrives at Varian Associates

Weston Anderson at Varian Associates first heard of Richard Ernst in February 1963.

In the early '60s, we were looking for ways to improve the NMR spectrometers which were becoming more widely used for molecular structure determinations. In February 1963 we heard through Warren Proctor, who was at the Varian applications laboratory in Switzerland, that a bright young PhD student at the Swiss Federal Institute of Technology (ETH) in Zürich might be interested in coming to the United States. He had done some very good theoretical work on NMR, in particular on instrument optimization. Because of prior commitments that included Swiss military service and getting married, Richard Ernst did not arrive in Palo Alto until November.[43]

"[Proctor] came across this student," said Anderson, "and found that he was interested in a job. Warren wrote to me. I was head of the research group at that time. At first it was called Special Products, but by then we became the Instrument Division. We were interested in hiring him, so we made an offer."[44]

Richard Ernst married Magdalena Kielholz, a teacher, on October 9, 1963. A month later, Richard and Magdalena moved to the United States.

"This was sort of his honeymoon,"[45] said Anderson. The Ernsts would remain in the United States for nearly four-and-a-half years, until their return to Switzerland in February 1968.

Among numerous offers [wrote Ernst], I decided for Varian Associates in Palo Alto where famous scientists like Weston A. Anderson, Ray Freeman, Jim Hyde, Martin Packard and Harry Weaver were working along similar lines as we in Zürich but with a clear commercial goal in mind. This attracted my interest, hoping to find some motivation for my own work. And indeed, I was extremely lucky. Weston Anderson was on his way to invent Fourier transform spectroscopy in order to improve the sensitivity of NMR by parallel data acquisition.[46]

The Prayer Wheel

Ernst has noted that Wes Anderson was "on his way to invent Fourier transform spectroscopy" when he arrived at Varian. In fact, as has already been pointed out, the seeds had been sown by Russell Varian. In a brief historical review article entitled "NMR, The Physics Experiment that Revolutionized Chemistry," Anderson stated:

In the early '60s, I was exploring possible ways to implement Russell Varian's idea of broadband excitation. Rather than use noise to excite the nuclei, I proposed generating a number of coherent [radio] frequencies and using a number of synchronous detectors to detect the response at each frequency.[47]

If one could excite the system simultaneously with multiple frequencies and disentangle the response of the system, Anderson knew, then the time required to gather data, to produce a spectrum, could be shortened considerably. This was exactly the purpose of a mechanical multiple-frequency generator, the "Wheel of Fortune," that Wes Anderson was experimenting with in the early 1960s. Why the long lapse between Russell Varian's proposal and Wes Anderson's attempt at implementation?

I worked on a number of projects [explained Anderson]. Probably more of my effort in the early days was directed towards making magnetic current shims and field-frequency locks and addressing other problems. But the sensitivity question was also in the back of our minds. The technique that I first came up with was essentially a multichannel spectrometer where you irradiate the sample with n discrete frequencies rather than the noise spectrum and you detect it at those n frequencies. You do this all simultaneously.

First I thought of generating them by n separate oscillators—not at radiofrequency levels, but at some lower frequency—and then beating them up and mixing, irradiating the nuclei and beating them down, again with heterodyne techniques. One of the techniques was this wheel idea, which is sometimes called the "Wheel of Fortune." My technician had another name for it. He called it the "Prayer Wheel." Maybe he was praying for good fortune, I don't know. Anyway, the idea was that you generate all your frequencies simultaneously with a light chopper. You have this plastic wheel which is maybe eight inches tall and which rotates at a slow rate, maybe a few revolutions per minute. It's not critical, you can go through the numbers. It depends upon what frequency band you want to work at.

Anyway, you have a number of rulings which are just black and white grating lines around the outside of this wheel and each section has a different number, say it differs by one in the circumference. And that's easy to achieve because you just machine the plastic so it has a slight taper to it. Then you pass light through it from a single source so the light is chopped, and then detected by n photodetectors.

On the detection, you use almost the same technique. You beat it back down to the same frequency. Then you modulate another light on the other side of the wheel. It passes through the same sets of light and dark bands. It demodulates the signal. You integrate the output of those photodetectors and that gives you the n different signals that correspond to the n Fourier components. We never really got that in operation.[48]

The Realization of Fourier Transform NMR

Anderson figured there had to be a better way to achieve the goal than with the mechanical approach used in the "prayer wheel."

Eventually, this chopper wheel landed in the Smithsonian Institution as an example of one step in the evolution of an idea.[49-50] However, before the wheel experiment was finished, I had shifted gears and proposed we use a series of short RF pulses to generate the band of coherent frequencies, and then use Russell Varian's idea of the Fourier transformation to obtain the spectrum. Ernst built the instrumentation to test this new technique and we hit gold.[51]

As Ernst recalled the sequence of events:

After [Anderson's] involvement in the development of a cute mechanical device, the "wheel of fortune," to generate and detect several frequencies in parallel, he proposed to me in 1964 to try a pulse excitation experiment that indeed led to Fourier transform (FT) NMR as we know it today. The first successful experiments were done in summer 1964 while Weston Anderson was abroad on an extensive business trip. In this work, I could take advantage in an optimum way of my knowledge in system theory gained during my studies with Primas and Günthard.[52]

According to Wes Anderson's notebook, he came up with the idea on June 3, 1964. As is the custom in industrial laboratories where patents are at least as important as published papers, Richard Ernst acknowledged that he witnessed and understood Anderson's notes by signing his name and dating it.[53]

The essence of Anderson's suggestion was that a radiofrequency pulse could be used as a broadband frequency source to simultaneously irradiate the entire spectrum. A pulse of short duration Δt corresponds to a wide frequency band $1/\Delta t$; the shorter the pulse, the wider the frequency bandwidth. The representation of a simple square-wave as the sum of an infinite series of sine waves of increasing frequency is a familiar example of the Fourier expansion of a function $f(t)$ in sines and cosines. One can imagine that if a radiofrequency oscillator operating at a fixed frequency ν were switched on and then rapidly switched off, the envelope of the RF power reaching the sample would resemble the top half of the square wave and the sample would be exposed to a range of frequencies centered about ν.

Pulsed NMR experiments were not new in 1964. Indeed, they were described in Bloch's landmark paper[54] and carried out from the early days of NMR, mainly in the context of measurements of the empirical relaxation times T_1 and T_2, for which pulsed NMR experiments are ideally suited. To be sure, the relaxation times characterizing a system could, in principle, be obtained from CW techniques, in particular T_2 from the linewidth of the resonance, but the difficulties of extracting the true linewidth in the face of line-broadening due to magnetic field inhomogeneity and other physical and instrumental effects made the use of CW techniques for such measurements impractical. In any case, chemists were not, in general, much interested in relaxation times.[55]

Hence, the predominance of the CW technique for high-resolution NMR spectroscopy.

The increase in data collection efficiency that Anderson envisioned not only required a broadband frequency source but a means of converting the impulse response into a spectrum. The solution to that problem was obvious: the conversion of the NMR signal, measured as a function of time subsequent to the brief excitation pulse, into a frequency spectrum was to be accomplished by Fourier transformation. Just as a prism decomposes white light into its component colors, the Fourier transform permits the decomposition of a time-varying signal into its component frequencies and their amplitudes.

As it happens, one of the essential features of the experiment, that is, the derivation of the steady-state resonance line shape from the Fourier transformation of the free induction decay following a 90-degree RF pulse, was contained in a paper published in 1957 entitled "Free-Induction Decays in Solids" by Irving J. Lowe and Richard E. Norberg of the Department of Physics at Washington University, in St. Louis, Missouri.[56]

In addition to the paper's importance as an antecedent, it's also of interest for tracing the influence of Erwin Hahn and his spin echoes. In 1949, PhD candidate Norberg had begun working with Professor James Bartlett shortly before Hahn, then a postdoctoral fellow, discovered spin echoes in the fall of that year. About the same time, Norberg took a course in solid-state physics from Professor Frederick Seitz, who had just joined the faculty at Illinois for the purpose of launching a program in solid-state physics. According to Charles Slichter, who joined the physics faculty at Illinois in the fall of 1949, Norberg, after "hearing Seitz's lectures about how absorption of hydrogen affected the properties of Pd [palladium] . . . proposed that for his thesis he use proton NMR to study the H-Pd system. Armed with the knowledge of how spin echoes made possible easy measurements of T_1 and natural T_2s . . . Norberg took much of this data by pulse methods. His thesis," stated Slichter, "constitutes the first pulsed NMR study of a solid. It demonstrated dramatically the rich insight into real solid state physics problems which magnetic resonance could provide."[57]

Eventually, Norberg joined the physics faculty at Washington University in St. Louis where George E. Pake, a former graduate-student colleague of Nicolaas Bloembergen, had become head of the department (Pake left for Stanford in 1956). In 1957, Norberg and his student, Irving Lowe, published the article mentioned above. Regarding the significance of that article, Slichter has stated:

Another important advance . . . was the discovery and demonstration by Norberg . . . and his student Irving Lowe that the free induction decay following a 90-degree pulse applied to the nuclei of a solid is the Fourier transform of the steady state absorption spectrum. Their work pre-dated phase-sensitive detection. If one employs phase-sensitive detection, by proper adjustment of the phase of the detection reference one could pick out signals whose Fourier transform gave either the absorption or the dispersion. The discovery by Lowe and Norberg was of enormous importance. It subsequently revolutionized magnetic resonance technique, but exploitation of its significance was not yet feasible in 1957 because of the numerical difficulty at that time of carrying out Fourier transforms. Indeed, one did not have either the fast Fourier transform algorithms or readily available computers. . . .

Nine years later in 1966, Ernst and Anderson recognized that use of the Fourier transform of the free induction decay could greatly enhance the speed of search for NMR lines in a high-resolution spectrum. Since a single strong radiofrequency pulse could excite all the nuclei, one could avoid wasting time looking for resonances at the empty frequencies between actual resonances.[58]

In the lengthy Norberg-Lowe paper, a general quantum-mechanical description of free-induction decays is developed and it is shown rigorously that, except at very low temperatures, a free-induction decay is the Fourier transform of the corresponding steady-state resonance line shape. Lowe and Norberg then proceed to demonstrate excellent agreement between their experimental induction decay data obtained using a single crystal of calcium fluoride (CaF_2) in a "standard spin-echo apparatus" and the Fourier transforms of the CW line-shape data obtained by C. R. Bruce, published in the publication's preceding paper.[59] Note that Lowe and Norberg used the CW line-shape data to obtain the time-domain signal by Fourier transformation; Ernst and Anderson proposed to go the other way.

From Ernst's system-theory perspective, Lowe and Norberg's derivation and demonstration could not have been too surprising. As he later explained in his Nobel lecture:[60]

It has been known since a long time that the frequency response function (spectrum) of a linear system is the Fourier transform of the impulse response (free induction decay). This was already implicitly evident in the work of Jean Baptiste Joseph Fourier who investigated in 1822 the heat conduction in solid bodies.[61] Lowe and Norberg have proved in 1957 this relation also to hold for spin systems despite their strongly nonlinear response characteristics.[62]

In the brief historical survey of NMR spectroscopy provided in the introductory chapter to his text *Principles of Nuclear Magnetic Resonance in One and Two Dimensions*,[63] Ernst put two and two together as follows:

The fact that a short delta-function-like pulse can be considered as a multifrequency source which allows simultaneous excitation of all resonance frequencies is quite well established.[64-67] According to the superposition principle, which is valid in linear systems, the response to a delta function pulse, known as impulse response, is a linear superposition of the responses of all frequency components. The transfer function can be obtained from the impulse response simply by frequency analysis, i.e. by a Fourier transformation.

It had also been known for many years[68] that the free induction decay, which is equivalent to the impulse response in linear system theory, and the complex spectrum (equivalent to the transfer function) form a Fourier transform pair. Knowledge of these facts leads almost naturally to the recognition that a dramatic sensitivity improvement can be realized by recording the response to a short r.f. pulse in the form of a free induction decay and subsequently computing the desired spectrum by means of a numerical Fourier transformation.[69-70]

Described with textbook hindsight, the development of Fourier transform NMR seems straightforward. The course of science, however, is anything but straight. Lowe and Norberg's work was not about trying to improve the sensitivity nor even the practicality of NMR as an analytical tool. They were bent on understanding the beat structure observed in the free induction or Bloch decays observed in pulsed NMR experiments on various nuclei in solids. To a piano tuner, a beat pattern indicates that two strings are vibrating at slightly different frequencies. To a physicist, induction decay beats suggest the presence of nuclei with slightly different Larmor precession frequencies. In both cases, the exponentially decaying "ringing" is modulated by the interference of the two frequencies.

Lowe and Norberg took their quantum mechanical theory for the shapes of induction decays, applied it to the special case of a rigid lattice of fluorine nuclei (F^{19}), and obtained quite good agreement with the experimentally observed induction decay when a purely dipolar magnetic interaction between neighboring nuclei (2.725×10^{-8} cm apart) was assumed. Lowe earned his PhD based on this work, and new insights into the quantum mechanics of solids resulted.

The power of the proof that the spectrum and the free induction decay after a 90-degree pulse are Fourier transforms of each other was not realized, however, until Ernst and Anderson applied it some seven years later. As Anderson recalled:

When Ernst started working, we weren't even sure [the Fourier transform experiment] was going to work. That's why we did the experiment. Ernst was asked to see if he could do it—build it—and he did. That was his role. He gathered up all of the equipment to do it. He did the laboratory work. I was in charge of the group, so I can't claim very much of the credit for the actual assembling of the hardware. I'm sure he incorporated a lot of his ideas in that, too. In hindsight, the idea might seem pretty obvious in view of all the things that had gone on before, but it sure wasn't obvious at the time.[71]

Despite successfully applying the Fourier transform technique in the summer of 1964, Ernst has written:[72]

The response to our invention was, however, meager. The paper that described our achievements was rejected twice by the *Journal of Chemical Physics* to be finally accepted and published in the *Review of Scientific Instruments*. Varian also resisted to build a spectrometer that incorporated the novel Fourier transform concept. It took many years before, in the competitive company Bruker Analytische Messtechnik, Tony Keller and his coworkers demonstrated in 1969 for the first time a commercial FT NMR spectrometer to the great amazement of Varian that had the patent rights* on the invention.

About six months prior to submitting their paper entitled "Application of Fourier Transform Spectroscopy to Magnetic Resonance"[73] to *Review of Scientific Instruments* in early July of 1965, Ernst and Anderson had con-

---

* Weston A. Anderson and Richard Ernst, "Impulse resonance spectrometer including a time averaging computer and Fourier analyzer," U.S. Patent 3,475,680, filed 26 May 1965, issued 28 October 1969.

tributed two other papers to *Review of Scientific Instruments*. They were published together. The first one was entitled "Sensitivity Enhancement in Magnetic Resonance. I. Analysis of the Method of Time Averaging"[74] and written by Ernst alone. The second in the series was entitled "Sensitivity Enhancement in Magnetic Resonance. II. Investigation of Intermediate Passage Conditions"[75] and written by Ernst and Anderson.

Time averaging is a method of increasing the signal-to-noise ratio of an experiment by making successive, identical measurements of the signal, the idea being that the signals will add coherently while the noise tends to average out because of its incoherence. The introductory paragraph of the paper on time averaging sets the stage so nicely for Fourier transform NMR that it is worth reproducing in its entirety:

> Instrumentation in magnetic resonance spectroscopy has made significant progress in the last few years. But a major demand remains— the demand for the higher sensitivity necessary for many applications in biochemistry and in other fields. There are numerous approaches to increasing the sensitivity. For instance, increasing the magnetization of the sample leads to stronger signals (this can be achieved by using higher magnetic fields, lower temperature, Overhauser experiments, or simply by using a larger sample). The signal can be increased under certain conditions quite effectively by using intermediate passage conditions, as is discussed in the second paper of this series. Often it is possible to reduce the noise by optimizing the input circuitry (probe assembly, preamplifier) and by the use of an optimum filter at the output of the spectrometer. A new approach is the application of Fourier transform techniques to magnetic resonance. It will be treated at another place and shall not be discussed here.[76]

The purpose of Ernst's paper on time averaging was "to give a mathematical basis for a critical evaluation of the time averaging method, especially in comparison with single scan measurements which take up the same total performance time." When time averaging is used, the signal-to-noise ratio is expected to increase as the square root of the number of successive measurements or "scans." Ernst set about to show under what conditions this square-root law holds exactly.

The reason that the time-averaging technique was important to Ernst was simply that it is the basis for the improvement in sensitivity of Fourier transform spectroscopy. Ernst and Anderson did not just take the Fourier transform of the free induction decay following a single 90-

degree RF pulse. Their experiments employed a series of identical RF pulses applied at regular intervals in time. In their 1966 *Review of Scientific Instruments* paper, they pointed directly to potential applications, made indirect reference to Anderson's "prayer wheel/wheel of fortune" precursor and stated quite clearly the origins of the sensitivity improvement:

> The main stimulus to investigate this pulse method was the expected increase in sensitivity, which makes the method of interest to chemists and biologists.
>
> To make the possible enhancement of the sensitivity intuitively clear, it is helpful to consider the problem from another viewpoint. The conventional spectral methods in magnetic resonance use a field or frequency sweep to record a spectrum. At any particular time, the transmitter frequency corresponds to one single point in the spectrum and the rest of the spectrum is for the most part disregarded. . . . It is obvious that the information rate of such an experiment could be greatly increased by investigating the entire spectrum during the total available time. This could be done, at least in principle, by using several transmitters and receivers with different frequencies which correspond to different points in the spectrum. This kind of spectrometer could be called a multichannel spectrometer. The sensitivity improvement which is achievable depends on the total number of channels.
>
> Applying a sequence of equally spaced short rf pulses corresponds to a multichannel experiment. . . .
>
> To obtain an improvement in sensitivity it is essential that the responses after each pulse are added together coherently. This can conveniently be done by using a time averaging computer. The final step is then the Fourier transformation of the time averaged free induction decay. The Fourier analysis is equivalent to using a multichannel receiver. [77]

In their experimental arrangement, Ernst and Anderson used a modified Varian Associates DP60 spectrometer (operating at 60 MHz transmitter frequency) as well as a Varian Associates C1024 time averaging computer, which digitized the free induction decay signal in 1024 sample points, equidistant in time, and added them to the values already stored. That was about all the "on-line" computer did. After a sufficient number of scans (500), a Technical Measurement Corporation Model 220 C data output unit converted the accumulated binary data in the C1024 memory into BCD numbers which were then punched on paper tape using a

Tally Corporation Model 420 perforator. Ernst then had to carry the paper tape over to the nearest IBM 7090 digital computer[78] which calculated the Fourier transform and plotted the spectrum automatically by means of an incremental curve plotter. Of course, the IBM computer used punch cards for input, so the paper tape had to first go through a machine to read the tape and punch IBM cards.[79]

Fortunately for Ernst, at about the same time, Cooley and Tukey at Princeton devised a very clever algorithm for the computation of the discrete Fourier transform. Known as the fast Fourier transform (FFT), it dramatically reduced the time required to carry out the Fourier transform on a digital computer.[80]

Nevertheless, the whole process still took days because it wasn't just the speed of the computer that was important; it was also a question of getting time on the computer. As Anderson pointed out, "It wasn't so easy to do in those days because the only computer we had available was the one that was used for accounting, and it wasn't right handy, anyway."[81] After waiting several days for payroll and factory inventory processing to be completed,[82] said Anderson, "you got the Fourier transform and actually the plotting as well. Of course, if it wasn't phased right, you had to replot it and fix it up."[83]

With characteristic understatement, Ernst recalled the computer aspect of his task at Varian: "The practical realization of pulse Fourier spectroscopy was made possible by the introduction of inexpensive computers in the late-1960s and by the development of the fast Fourier transform (FFT) algorithm."[84] Amplifying that a bit, Anderson noted:

We were all delighted when, within seconds, these first experiments gave us good data that would normally have taken several minutes. . . . In 1965 we continued to await the advances in computer technology that would make the process truly practical—after all, what good was a 10-second data collection if you couldn't see the spectra for several days? The plodding scanning method still generated meaningful spectra faster than FT NMR.

As soon as possible, we ordered a [Digital Equipment Corp.] PDP-8 minicomputer. By today's standards, it was slow, and the 4,000 bytes of memory trivially small. However, it enabled us to transform the data and plot it out in a few minutes.[85]

What kind of sensitivity improvement could one expect from Fourier transform NMR compared to conventional slow-passage frequency- or field-sweep methods? Ernst and Anderson showed that for equivalent signal-to-noise, the savings in time was given approximately by the spectral range divided by the width of a typical line in the spectrum. "A factor of 100 in time can be gained easily,"[86] they claimed in 1966. Once the prerequisite high level of field stability together with the availability of a time-averaging computer are taken care of, they pointed out, the Fourier transform method presents many advantages over direct spectral techniques, even beyond the possibility of obtaining spectra in a much shorter time and with greater sensitivity. (Incidentally, it is much easier to maintain a high level of field stability when using a shorter pulse.) One additional advantage, they pointed out, was the absence of line shape distortions. Pulse experiments, by their very nature, are ideally suited for measuring the transient properties of spin systems, such as the relaxation times. Ernst and Anderson anticipated that the pulse Fourier technique would also permit the study of time-dependent systems such as chemical reactions.

One other point deserves mention here. From Ernst's point of view, the application of a sequence of regularly spaced, identical RF pulses is but "a special case of a wide band frequency source with an arbitrary, discrete or continuous power spectrum."[87] The application of a "white" power spectrum, that is, random noise, had been previously treated by Ernst and his ETH collaborator, Hans Primas, and published in 1963 in the leading Swiss physics journal *Helvetica Physica Acta.*[88] While at Varian, Ernst extended his earlier work on stochastic resonance with the introduction of heteronuclear broadband decoupling by noise irradiation, the "noise decoupling" that led to a rapid development of carbon-13 spectroscopy.[89] In a certain sense, then, Ernst continued mining at Varian the same vein he had begun at the ETH where, at the time, he was ignorant of similar work being done by Russell Varian. Of other work in which Richard Ernst was engaged while at Varian, Anderson has written:[90]

Ernst continued to make important contributions to a number of areas including sensitivity optimization,[91] double resonance line profiles,[92] and the measurement and control of magnetic field homogeneity.[93] He expanded some of the concepts proposed in his thesis and demonstrated NMR spin decoupling using random noise.[94]

Of working with Richard Ernst, Anderson said, "We were very happy with him. He's a very bright guy, very productive, expert at theoretical as well as experimental work. He also has a wonderful sense of humor and is easy to work with.[95]

While it may be true that Weston Anderson handed Richard Ernst the ball, there is no doubt that Ernst took it and ran with it. Along the way, Ernst took NMR spectroscopy into more than one dimension, a development that took place after he left Varian and returned to the ETH in Zürich.

Home Sweet Home

In 1968, after an extensive trip through Asia, Ernst returned with his family to Switzerland. According to Anderson, Ernst wanted to get back into academic life. He would, however, remain a consultant to Varian for a number of years afterwards, and he would assign numerous patents to Varian Associates,[96-99] including patents on two-dimensional Fourier transform NMR and Fourier transform NMR image reconstruction, two very significant developments in modern NMR spectroscopy and imaging brought to light by Ernst.

On his trip through Asia, a brief visit to Nepal sparked what became an "insatiable love"[100] of Asian art. His main interest is in Tibetan scroll paintings, the so-called *thangkas*, which he describes as "a unique and most exciting form of religious art with its own strict rules and nevertheless incorporating an incredible exuberance of creativity."[101]

Back at the ETH-Zürich, Ernst assumed the leadership of the NMR research group in the Laboratory for Physical Chemistry after Professor Hans Primas turned his attention more toward theoretical chemistry.[102] From 1968 through 1970, Ernst was a *privatdozent* or lecturer in physical chemistry. In 1970, he was made an assistant professor and in 1972 he was promoted to associate professor.[103]

Ernst continued to work on methodological improvements of time-domain NMR and further developed stochastic magnetic resonance as an alternative to pulsed Fourier transform NMR. He showed that the maximum signal-to-noise ratio attainable with stochastic excitation is the same as with pulsed Fourier spectroscopy, and that the stochastic method even has some advantages over the pulsed technique.[104] Nevertheless, the "instrumental simplicity and ease of interpretation"[105] of the pulsed FT NMR technique appear to account for its far wider acceptance and application.

More Than One Dimension

In his Nobel autobiography, Ernst recounts the origin of the next significant methodological development in which he played a leading role.

The next fortunate event occurred in 1971 when my first graduate student, Thomas Baumann, visited the Ampère Summer School in

Basko Polje, Yugoslavia, where Professor Jean Jeener [of the Free University in Brussels] proposed a simple two-pulse sequence that produces, after two-dimensional Fourier transformation, a two-dimensional (2D) spectrum. In the course of time, we recognized the importance and universality of his proposal. In my group, Enrico Bartholdi performed at first some analytical calculations to explore the features of 2D experiments. Finally in the summer of 1974, we tried our first experiments in desperate need of results to be presented at the VIth International Conference on Magnetic Resonance in Biological Systems, Kandersteg, 1974 [which he was organizing together with Kurt Wüthrich].[106]

By the early 1970s, time-domain NMR studies were just beginning to be appreciated by chemists. The vast majority of those using continuous wave techniques to obtain high resolution spectra were only dimly aware of the possibilities of pulse methods. Writing in a slender 1971 monograph entitled *Pulse and Fourier Transform NMR*, Thomas C. Farrar and Edwin D. Decker addressed chemists and others familiar with high resolution NMR but with no background in pulse techniques:

Although pulse methods were introduced almost as early as CW methods and have been improved in sophistication and versatility, they have until recently attracted only limited attention from chemists. Within the last few years, however, technical innovations have begun to permit the study by pulse methods of the complex molecules of interest to most chemists; in fact . . . it is possible to obtain the same spectral information from a pulse experiment and subsequent mathematical analysis (principally Fourier transformation) as can be obtained by an ordinary slow passage experiment. However, pulse methods are often much more efficient, thus producing a very significant saving in time or improvement in signal/noise.[107]

Just as chemists were beginning to take advantage of the enormous gain in sensitivity provided by pulsed Fourier spectroscopy, Ernst was about to extend the technique even further, into more than one frequency dimension, thanks to the inspiration provided by his student's careful note-taking during Professor Jeener's summer school lecture. The development of two-dimensional Fourier transform NMR, and subsequently three- and multidimensional techniques, opened up for analysis increasingly complex compounds.

Chemists, it seems, have a fondness for complex spectra. Presented with a complex spectrum, that is, one with more than one resonance or line corresponding to a particular Larmor frequency, chemists want to know what accounts for the multiplicity of lines as well as their shapes and relative amplitudes. As far back as 1949, an atom's chemical environment was known to affect its NMR frequencies. Two well-identified effects are the chemical shift, caused by shielding of the applied magnetic field by the electron "shells" surrounding the nucleus, and the "scalar" or "J coupling" between nearby nuclear spins, mediated by the electron pairs in chemical bonds. A third, the magnetic dipolar interaction, is a pair-wise interaction between nuclear spins that is sensitive to the distance between the nuclei (recall Lowe and Norberg's work in solids). One of the fruits of Ernst's pioneering work in two-dimensional Fourier transform NMR is its ability to, as he puts it, "shed light on the spectral chaos."

One-dimensional spectra that are rendered inscrutable because of severe overlap may be unraveled by separating interactions of different physical origin, e.g. chemical shifts and couplings, thus making it possible to spread the signals in a second frequency dimension much like opening a Venetian blind. In many circumstances, resonances that overlap in conventional one-dimensional spectra can be unraveled in this manner.[108]

As one might infer, two-dimensional spectroscopy results in a two-dimensional frequency spectrum. Imagine a silhouette of the Rocky Mountains at dusk as seen from the Great Plains and then view the same range from an altitude of 30,000 feet. Just as the relationships of the individual mountains become clearer when viewed in two dimensions, so, too, do the relationships of the spectral peaks and valleys.

Just as one-dimensional pulsed Fourier transform NMR largely supplanted conventional CW techniques in elucidating NMR spectra, two-dimensional FT NMR proved superior to methods that had been developed to sort out the pair interactions in nuclear spin systems using one-dimensional spectra, such as the double- and triple-resonance experiments that were pioneered by, among others, Wes Anderson and Ray Freeman at Varian.[109] The double- and triple-resonance experiments, in which two or three RF fields were applied simultaneously, can be considered forerunners of multidimensional spectroscopy in the sense that the signal amplitude can be represented as a complex function of two or three frequencies. However, these are usually parameters rather than continuous variables and as such are not fully appreciated as second- or third-frequency dimensions.[110]

The essence of Jeener's proposal was a simple two-pulse experiment that introduced a true second-frequency dimension. He suggested using two 90-degree RF pulses with a variable time t_1 between them. The usual time variable, call it t_2, was then the time elapsed after the second pulse until detection of the signal. The idea was to repeat the experiment many times, varying the time t_1 between repetitions. Fourier transformation of the signal amplitude, measured as a function of two time variables, would then result in a two-dimensional frequency spectrum.

In the more general case, elaborated by Ernst and others, the initial 90-degree pulse is replaced by a sequence of RF pulses and the second 90-degree pulse is likewise replaced by a pulse sequence. Thus four periods can be identified. The first, called the "preparation" period, consists of a single RF pulse or a sequence of pulses to excite the nuclear spin system. During the second or "evolution" period, "nothing" happens, other than the precession of the macroscopic magnetizations. This period has duration t_1. During the third, or "mixing" period, the system is perturbed by a new RF pulse or pulse sequence. The fourth period is the usual "detection period" during which the signal is measured while the system is in free precession. The second time variable, call it t_2, is the time between the final pulsed excitation of the spin system and the detection of the response, just as in one-dimensional Fourier transform NMR.

This sequence of four periods is repeated with a different duration of the evolution period each run. Thus, the parameters of the digitized data are dictated by as many values of t_1 as there are repetitions of the sequence with different evolution periods and by as many values of t_2 as are needed to adequately sample the signal during the detection period.[111]

The real power of this technique lies in the control it provides over the nuclear spin Hamiltonian. The Hamiltonian is the quantum-mechanical energy operator that incorporates all the known physical interactions that determine the energy levels of the nucleus. By clever manipulation of the pulse sequences, the terms in the Hamiltonian that describe the interaction of the nucleus with external fields can be modified, thus altering the spectrum seen. This kind of manipulation through the pulse sequence is not, of course, peculiar to multidimensional NMR, but rather a feature of pulsed experiments generally. However, the ability to "edit" the spectrum proves particularly advantageous in more than one dimension. As John S. Waugh of the Massachusetts Institute of Technology explains,

"You have a sort of alchemist's power over the nature of the system. You can use that power to get a spectrum that is more easily interpreted than it otherwise would have been."[112]

Of the period following the first successful experimental demonstration of two-dimensional FT NMR by Ernst's group in 1974, he has written:

> From then on, the development of multidimensional spectroscopy went very fast, inside and outside of our research group. Prof. John S. Waugh extended it for applications to solid state resonance, and the research group of Prof. Ray Freeman, particularly Geoffrey Bodenhausen, contributed some of the first heteronuclear experiments. We started [in] 1976 an intense collaboration, lasting for 10 years, with Professor Kurt Wüthrich of ETH-Z to develop applications of 2D spectroscopy in molecular biology. He and his research group have been responsible for most essential innovations that enabled the determination of the three-dimensional structure of biomolecules in solution.[113]

Waugh told *Physics Today* following the announcement of Ernst's Nobel Prize in chemistry, "Two- and multidimensional NMR has had an enormous impact, especially in biological chemistry. It has made possible the relatively routine determination of the geometric structure of complicated molecules."[114]

Fourier Transform in NMR Imaging

In the mid 1970s, at about the same time he was working on two-dimensional NMR, Ernst realized that the 2D spectroscopy principle could be applied to NMR imaging.[115] A couple of years earlier, Professor Paul Lauterbur of the State University of New York at Stony Brook had proposed an NMR imaging method that uses an applied magnetic field gradient to make the resonant frequency vary linearly with position in the object to be imaged.[116] The motivation for this came from the realization and demonstration by Dr. Raymond V. Damadian of the State University of New York Downstate Medical Center that NMR could be used to detect cancer in tissue *in vivo*.[117] The practical implications for medicine and the study of biological processes were staggering.

Ernst realized that the same multichannel advantage of Fourier transform NMR could be applied to NMR imaging. Inefficient point-scan techniques, such as Damadian's field-focused method[118] and line-scan imaging methods, such as those developed by Hinshaw and others, could benefit from the inherently greater sensitivity that the Fourier transform method allowed. First experiments were carried out by Anil Kumar and Dieter Welti in Ernst's laboratory[119] and the method, together with modifications by Peter Mansfield in England, quickly became the method of choice for most commercial NMR imaging devices.

Nobel Prize 1991

Following the formal presentation of the 1991 Nobel Prizes, the Nobel Banquet was held in the Blue Hall of the Stockholm City Hall. In attendance were the king and queen of Sweden, Prince Bertil and Princess Lillian, the Duke and Duchess of Halland, the 1991 prize winners and 128 Nobel laureates from years past. After the prerequisite toasts, including a silent toast to Alfred Nobel, Richard Ernst graciously expressed the emotions he felt on the auspicious occasion:

> It is indeed a great moment for me to stand where I am standing to express my deep gratitude to the Nobel Foundation for this extraordinary honor. Obviously, most of the glory should fall on those standing behind me, my teachers, my colleagues, my coworkers, my school, my 700-years-old country, those whom I represent here as their scientific spokesman. The presence of all the former Nobel laureates gives me a feeling of being carried by a swarm of wild geese, some real high fliers, like in Nils Holgersson, and I am afraid of falling down.

> Science prizes have a tendency to distort science history. Individuals are singled out and glorified that should rather be seen embedded in the context of the historical development. Much luck and coincidence is needed to be successful and be selected. Prizes can hardly do justice to those brave men and women who devote, in an unselfish way, all their efforts and energy towards a goal that is finally reached by others. . . .

> I am one of the very fortunate scientists who have achieved what many claim to be the ultimate form of recognition or even the ultimate form of happiness in this exuberant, splendid, almost unearthly setting. However, I think more important is the responsibility that is being loaded on the shoulders of the laureates who are supposed to suddenly behave like unfailing sages although they might have been just work addicts in the past. The disproportionate importance that is attributed to the Nobel Prize is reflected also in disproportionate expectations from the public. Recently, I got a set of letters,

written by school children from Bedford, Massachusetts, one of them begging me to work hard towards an artificial ozone layer to protect life on earth. I hope that I can live up to a few of these very high expectations . . .[120]

Four years earlier, in the preface to his text on NMR in one and two dimensions, Ernst had singled out three individuals who had had, perhaps, the most profound impact on the course of his own work.

We [the co-authors of the text] would like to express our deep gratitude to those who were instrumental in guiding our interests towards time domain spectroscopy. Professor Hans Primas has contributed much in terms of mathematical tools and basic concepts. Dr. Weston A. Anderson inspired the search for more sensitive NMR methods which led to Fourier spectroscopy and Professor Jean Jeener first expressed the idea of performing spectroscopy in two dimensions.[121]

He went on to give special thanks in that volume to over 50 colleagues and co-workers, a foreshadowing of the acknowledgements he would make in his Nobel Prize lecture when he acknowledged more than 60 co-workers, a dozen or so members of his technical staff and several research groups with whom he had had the pleasure of collaborating over the years.

Ray Freeman, on the other hand, once a fellow employee at Varian with Ernst and now a professor at Cambridge University, placed Ernst's accomplishments in perspective when asked for his reaction to the selection of Ernst for the Nobel Prize. Freeman responded: "He's got it for sustained effort. He created a field that was not there before."[122]

In his Nobel lecture, Ernst also acknowledged the important contributions of Erwin L. Hahn when he said that Hahn "may be regarded as the true father of pulse spectroscopy. He invented the spin echo experiment and devised extremely important and conceptually beautiful solid state experiments."[123] Upon hearing of Ernst's Nobel Prize, Hahn returned the compliment, saying, "He plays lots of music with the pulse techniques. His contributions are beautiful elaborations of fundamental ideas."[124] In a subsequent publication co-authored by Hahn, it was stated:

The Nobel Prize in Chemistry for 1991 was conferred upon Richard Ernst for his development of elegant NMR techniques and fundamental theory applicable to various types of physical and chemical analysis. These include in particular specific innovations and extensions of pulse Fourier transform methods for NMR high resolution spectroscopy and MRI. We of the NMR community especially salute and congratulate Ernst because the Prize brings honor as well upon all of us who have had so much fun in a field that has yielded many innovations over a time period much longer than many of us expected. The field of NMR in its development reached a stage where one could hardly distinguish whether chemists or physicists were doing NMR. Now the chemists, or rather the physical chemists and biologists, have taken over the field of NMR, and they are doing most of the "physics" nowadays. As a consequence, because chemical technology is more "up front" in the public and commercial eye, people know more about NMR than ever before. Also MRI, has had an impact upon the public in the medical and health world, and in scientific research the analytic techniques made possible by NMR have been applied in one form or another to investigations in many disciplines.[125]

Ernst has said that, at the time he did his experiments, he had no idea that NMR spectroscopy and NMR imaging, now known as magnetic resonance imaging or MRI, would become the big industries they are today.[126] He told *Physics Today*, "I never believed in any idea that we were working on. I just had the feeling we were playing with these tools, and it was fun, but I did not expect that it would become as useful and practical as it has."[127] Reflecting on his illustrious career through 1991, Ernst observed:

Looking back, I realize that I have been favored extraordinarily by external circumstances, the proper place at the proper time in terms of my PhD thesis, my first employment in the USA, hearing about Jean Jeener's idea, and in particular having had incredibly brilliant coworkers. At last, I am extremely grateful for the encouragement and for the occasional readjustment of my standards of value by my wife Magdalena who stayed with me so far for more than 28 years despite all the problems of being married to a selfish work-addict with an unpredictable temper. Magdalena has, without much input from my side, educated our three children: Anna Magdalena (kindergarten teacher), Katharina Elisabeth (elementary school teacher), and Hans-Martin Walter (still in high school). I am not surprised that they show no intention to follow in my footsteps, although if I had a second chance myself, I would certainly try to repeat my present career.[128]

For his pioneering contributions, Richard Ernst has received numerous awards, including, in addition to the Nobel Prize in chemistry: 1) the Ruzika Prize (1969), 2) the Gold Medal awarded by the Society of Magnetic Resonance in Medicine (1983), 3) the Benoist Prize, Switzerland (1986), 4) the Ampère Prize (1990), 5) the Wolf Prize in chemistry, Israel (1991), 6) the Louisa Gross Horwitz Prize, Columbia University (1991). In addition, he has been recognized with honorary degrees, fellowships, memberships in academies of sciences, and lectureships. He holds 15 patents related to NMR technology and serves on the editorial board of several scientific journals. ∎

REFERENCE NOTES:

1. Malcolm W. Browne, "European scientists win physics and chemistry Nobel Prizes," *The New York Times*, 17 October 1991, A16.

2. Graham P. Collins, "Nobel chemistry prize recognizes the importance of Ernst's NMR work," *Physics Today* **44**:12, (December 1991), 19.

3. *American Men & Women of Science*, 19th edition, 1995-96, (New York: R.R. Bowker, 1995), 1139.

4. Anatole Abragam, *Time Reversal: An Autobiography*, (Oxford: Clarendon Press, 1989), 215.

5. *Varian Associates: An Early History*, a Varian Associates brochure, courtesy of Weston A. Anderson, 9.

6. R.R. Ernst, autobiographical sketch, *Les Prix Nobel*, 1991, (Stockholm: Almqvist & Wiksell, 1992), 65.

7. Ernst, autobiographical sketch, 65.

8. Sture Forsén, presentation speech for Nobel Prize in chemistry, 1991, *Les Prix Nobel*, 1991, (Stockholm: Almqvist & Wiksell, 1992), 21.

9. Ernst, autobiographical sketch, 65.

10. Ibid.

11. Ibid.

12. Ibid.

13. F. Bloch, "Heisenberg and the early days of quantum mechanics," *Physics Today*, December 1976, 23.

14. W.A. Anderson, telephone interview, 24 May 1995.

15. R.R. Ernst, "Nuclear magnetic resonance Fourier transform spectroscopy," Nobel lecture, 9 December 1991, *Les Prix Nobel*, 1991, (Stockholm: Almqvist & Wiksell, 1992), 70.

16. Ernst, autobiographical sketch, 66.

17. Weston A. Anderson, "NMR, the physics experiment that revolutionized chemistry," *Radiology Today* **9**, (1992).

18. Ernst, autobiographical sketch, 66.

19. Ibid.

20. Dorothy Varian, *The Inventor and the Pilot*, (Palo Alto, CA: Pacific Books, 1983), 153.

21. E.L. Ginzton, "Invention of the klystron" in *Varian Associates: An Early History*, a Varian Associates brochure, courtesy of Weston A. Anderson, 4.

22. R.H. Varian, "The founding of Varian Associates" in *Varian Associates: An Early History*, a Varian Associates brochure, courtesy of Weston A. Anderson, 6.

23. W.A. Anderson, telephone interview, 24 May 1995.

24. Varian, "The founding of Varian Associates," 6.

25. Abragam, *Time Reversal: An Autobiography*, 179-180.

26. W.A. Anderson, telephone interview, 24 May 1995.

27. W.A. Anderson, telephone interview, 24 May 1995..

28. R.H. Varian, "Method and means for correlating nuclear properties of atoms and magnetic fields," filed 21 October 1948, U.S. Patent No. 2,561,490 (issued 24 July 1951); U.S. Patent Re. 23,769 (12 January 1954).

29. W.A. Anderson, telephone interview, 24 May 1995..

30. Ibid.

31. Richard R. Ernst, Geoffrey Bodenhausen, and Alexander Wokaun, *Principles of Nuclear Magnetic Resonance in One and Two Dimensions*, (Oxford: Clarendon Press, 1987), 2.

32. W.C. Dickinson, *Physical Review 77*, (1950), 736.

33. W.G. Proctor and F.C. Yu, *Physical Review 77*, (1950), 717.

34. Anderson, "NMR, the physics experiment that revolutionized chemistry."

35. Ibid.

36. W.A. Anderson, telephone interview, 24 May 1995..

37. Ibid.

38. Ibid.
39. R.H. Varian, "Gyromagnetic resonance methods and apparatus," U.S. Patent 3,287,629, filed 29 August 1956, issued 22 November 1966.
40. Ibid., column 4, line 51.
41. W.A. Anderson, telephone interview, 24 May 1995..
42. Varian, *The Inventor and the Pilot*, 301.
43. Anderson, "NMR, the physics experiment that revolutionized chemistry."
44. W.A. Anderson, telephone interview, 24 May 1995..
45. Ibid.
46. Ernst, autobiographical sketch, 67.
47. Anderson, "NMR, the physics experiment that revolutionized chemistry."
48. W.A. Anderson, telephone interview, 24 May 1995..
49. Smithsonian Institution News, Office of Public Affairs, Smithsonian Institution, Washington, DC 20560, 26 November 1990.
50. IEEE Center for the History of Electrical Engineering, Newsletter No. 24, Summer 1990.
51. Anderson, "NMR, the physics experiment that revolutionized chemistry."
52. Ernst, autobiographical sketch, 67.
53. W.A. Anderson, telephone interview, 24 May 1995..
54. Felix Bloch, "Nuclear induction," *Physical Review* **70**, (1946), 460.
55. Thomas C. Farrar and Edwin D. Becker, *Pulse and Fourier Transform NMR, Introduction to Theory and Methods*, (New York: Academic Press, 1971), 2.
56. I.J. Lowe and R.E. Norberg, "Free-induction decays in solids," *Physical Review* **107**, (1957), 46.
57. C.P. Slichter contributing to the article "Pulsed NMR in solids—then and now," *Pulsed Magnetic Resonance: NMR, ESR, and Optics, A Recognition of E.L. Hahn,* (Oxford: Clarendon, 1992), 56-57.
58. Slichter, "Pulsed NMR in solids—then and now," 62, 64.
59. C.R. Bruce, *Physical Review* **107**, (1957), 43.
60. Ernst, "Nuclear magnetic resonance Fourier transform spectroscopy," Nobel lecture, 73.
61. J.B.J. Fourier, *Theorie analytique de la chaleur,* (Paris: Firmin Didot, Père et fils, 1822).
62. Lowe and Norberg, "Free-induction decays in solids," 46.
63. Ernst, Bodenhausen, and Wokaun, *Principles of Nuclear Magnetic Resonance in One and Two Dimensions,* 4.
64. L.A. Zadeh and C.A. Desoer, *Linear system theory, the state space approach,* (New York: McGraw-Hill, 1963).
65. E.A. Guillemin, *Theory of linear physical systems,* (New York: Wiley, 1963).
66. B.M. Brown, *The mathematical theory of linear systems,* Science Paperbacks (London: Chapman and Hall, 1965).
67. T.F. Bogart, *Basic concepts in linear systems: theory and experiments,* (New York: J. Wiley, 1984).
68. Lowe and Norberg, "Free-induction decays in solids," 46.
69. R.R. Ernst, *Advances in Magnetic Resonance* **2**, (1966), 1.
70. R.R. Ernst and W.A. Anderson, "Application of Fourier transform spectroscopy to magnetic resonance," *Review of Scientific Instruments* **37**, (1966), 93.
71. W.A. Anderson, telephone interview, 24 May 1995..
72. Ernst, autobiographical sketch, 67.
73. Ernst and Anderson, "Application of Fourier transform spectroscopy to magnetic resonance," 93.
74. R.R. Ernst, "Sensitivity enhancement in magnetic resonance. I. Analysis of the method of time averaging," *Review of Scientific Instruments* **36**, (1965), 1689.
75. R.R. Ernst and W.A. Anderson, "Sensitivity enhancement in magnetic resonance. II. Investigation of intermediate passage conditions," *Review of Scientific Instruments* **36**, (1965), 1696.
76. Ernst, "Sensitivity enhancement in magnetic resonance. I. Analysis of the method of time averaging," 1689.

77. Ernst and Anderson, "Application of Fourier transform spectroscopy to magnetic resonance," 96-97.

78. Erwin Hahn, interview by Merrill Simon.

79. W.A. Anderson, telephone interview, 24 May 1995..

80. J.W. Cooley and J.W. Tukey, *Math. Comput.* **19,** (1965), 297.

81. W.A. Anderson, telephone interview, 24 May 1995..

82. Anderson, "NMR, the physics experiment that revolutionized chemistry."

83. W.A. Anderson, telephone interview, 24 May 1995..

84. Ernst, Bodenhausen, and Wokaun, *Principles of Nuclear Magnetic Resonance in One and Two Dimensions,* 4.

85. Anderson, "NMR, the physics experiment that revolutionized chemistry."

86. Ernst and Anderson, "Application of Fourier transform spectroscopy to magnetic resonance," 93.

87. Ibid.

88. R.R. Ernst and H. Primas, *Helv. Phys. Acta* **36,** (1963), 583.

89. Ernst, autobiographical sketch, 67.

90. Anderson, "NMR, the physics experiment that revolutionized chemistry."

91. Richard R. Ernst, "Sensitivity enhancement in magnetic resonance," *Advances in Magnetic Resonance* **2,** (1966), 1.

92. R. Freeman, R.R. Ernst and W.A. Anderson, "Line profiles in nuclear magnetic double resonance," *J. Chem. Phys.* **46,** (1967), 1125.

93. Richard R. Ernst, "Measurement and control of magnetic field homogeneity," *Review of Scientific Instruments* **39,** (1968), 998.

94. R.R. Ernst, "Nuclear magnetic double resonance with an incoherent RF field," *J. Chem. Phys.* **45,** (1966), 3845.

95. W.A. Anderson, telephone interview, 24 May 1995..

96. Weston A. Anderson and Richard R. Ernst, "Magnetic resonance spectrometer employing stochastic resonance by a pseudorandom binary sequence and time-share modulation," U.S. Patent 3,786,341, filed 26 October 1972, issued 15 January 1974.

97. Richard R. Ernst, "Two-dimensional gyromagnetic resonance spectroscopy," U.S. Patent 4,045,723, filed 15 December 1975, issued 30 August 1977.

98. Richard R. Ernst, "Gyromagnetic resonance Fourier transform zeugmatography," U.S. Patent 4,070,611, filed 13 April 1977, issued 24 January 1978.

99. Richard R. Ernst, "Selective detection of multiple quantum transitions in nuclear magnetic resonance," U.S. Patent 4,134,058, filed 28 November 1977, issued 9 January 1979.

100. Ernst, autobiographical sketch, 67.

101. Ibid.

102. Ibid.

103. *Who's Who 1995,* (London: A&C Black Limited, 1995), 598.

104. Richard R. Ernst, "Magnetic resonance with stochastic excitation," *Journal of Magnetic Resonance* **3,** (1970), 10.

105. Ernst and Anderson, "Application of Fourier transform spectroscopy to magnetic resonance," 93.

106. Ernst, autobiographical sketch, 68.

107. T.C. Farrar and E.D. Becker, *Pulse and Fourier Transform NMR, Introduction to Theory and Methods,* (New York: Academic Press, 1971), 1-2.

108. Ernst, Bodenhausen, and Wokaun, *Principles of Nuclear Magnetic Resonance in One and Two Dimensions,* 7.

109. Ernst, "Nuclear magnetic resonance Fourier transform spectroscopy," 77-78.

110. Ernst, Bodenhausen, and Wokaun, *Principles of Nuclear Magnetic Resonance in One and Two Dimensions,* 6.

110. Ernst, Bodenhausen, and Wokaun, *Principles of Nuclear Magnetic Resonance in One and Two Dimensions*, 6.

111. Collins, "Nobel chemistry prize recognizes the importance of Ernst's NMR work," 20.

112. Ibid., 21.

113. Ernst, autobiographical sketch, 68.

114. Collins, "Nobel chemistry prize recognizes the importance of Ernst's NMR work," 21.

115. Ernst, autobiographical sketch, 68.

116. P.C. Lauterbur, "Image formation by induced local interactions: examples employing nuclear magnetic resonance," *Nature* **242**, (1973), 190-191.

117. R.V. Damadian, "Tumor detection by nuclear magnetic resonance," *Science* **171**, (1971), 1151-1153.

118. R. Damadian, M. Goldsmith, and L. Minkoff, *Physiological Chemistry and Physics* **9**, (1977), 97.

119. A. Kumar, D. Welti, and R. Ernst, *Journal of Magnetic Resonance* **18**, (1975), 69.

120. Richard R. Ernst, speech at Nobel Banquet in Stockholm, reprinted in *Les Prix Nobel*, 1991, (Stockholm: Almqvist & Wiksell, 1992), 28.

121. Ernst, Bodenhausen, and Wokaun, *Principles of Nuclear Magnetic Resonance in One and Two Dimensions*, vi.

122. Andy Coghlan, "High-flier wins chemistry Nobel," *New Scientist*, 26 October 1991, 14.

123. Ernst, "Nuclear magnetic resonance Fourier transform spectroscopy," Nobel lecture, 76.

124. Collins, "Nobel chemistry prize recognizes the importance of Ernst's NMR work," 21.

125. David C. Newitt and Erwin L. Hahn, "Detection of two-quantum nuclear coherence by nuclear quadrupole induced electric polarization," *Bulletin of Magnetic Resonance* **16**, (February 1994), 127.

126. Collins, "Nobel chemistry prize recognizes the importance of Ernst's NMR work," 21.

127. Ibid.

128. Ernst, autobiographical sketch, 69.

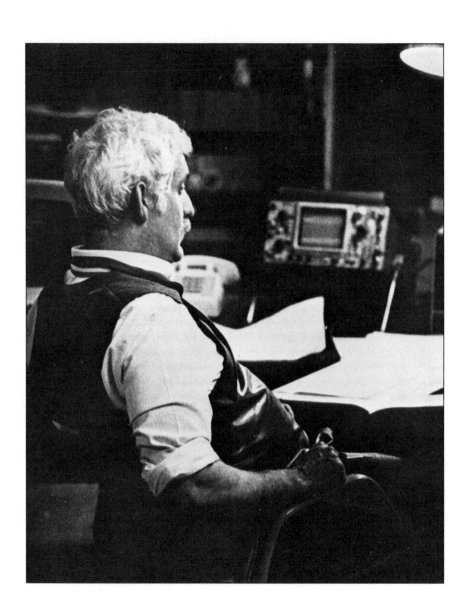

RAYMOND V. DAMADIAN

Originator of the Concept of Whole-Body NMR
Scanning (MRI) and Discoverer of the NMR Tissue
Relaxation Differences That Made It Possible

W HEN A WELL-KNOWN company advertises "We bring good
things to life" and shows a patient being scanned with MRI, television viewers might think that magnetic resonance scanning was
invented and brought to market through the efforts of a large team of
corporate scientists wearing white jackets and working in well-
equipped laboratories funded by one of the giants of industry. View
other advertising and one might conclude this breakthrough technology was developed in Germany, Holland or Japan. None of the above
is true.

In reality, MR scanning was invented, patented and brought to market largely through the efforts of one man, a medical doctor,
Raymond V. Damadian, who was assisted along the way by others
who believed in him and his dream. Instead of a deep-pocketed corporate R&D budget, he had only his salary as a professor and just
enough funding scrounged up from here and there to pay the salaries
of his two graduate assistants and to buy the second-hand components and the liquid helium used for constructing and cooling his
first scanner.

As for white jackets, there weren't any. The academic laboratory in
Brooklyn in which the machine was built, personally gerrymandered
with jackhammer and sledgehammer by Damadian and his associates
from quarters once relegated to laboratory rats, possessed the qualities of a machine shop more than a university medical lab.

In fact, this chapter is unique among all others in this volume.
Unlike the stories of the other pioneers in this book, who are physicists and chemists, this is the story of a medical doctor and scientist,

in the tradition of Robert Koch, Paul Ehrlich and Alexander Fleming,* who saw the bridge that existed between the practice of clinical medicine and the physics of NMR and crossed it.

Each one of us sees the world differently. For each, events are seen through the lenses of past experience. The history of NMR teaches that, for NMR scanning to come to life, NMR had to be seen through the eyes of a physician. From the time of Bloch and Purcell's first report of the NMR phenomena in condensed matter in 1945, NMR had existed for 25 years in the hands of scientists with thousands of NMR spectroscopy machines in chemical laboratories around the world performing analytical spectra daily before someone saw that same test-tube analyzing NMR machine as a medical body scanner.

That someone was Raymond Damadian and this chapter is the amazing story of the medical doctor who perceived the test-tube NMR analyzer as a body scanner and the tortuous and even heroic course he traversed to build it. Raymond Damadian is, as Professor Henry Wallman has termed it, one of those "statistically very rare breeds" who could span the gulf between two such vastly different bodies of knowledge as the clinical practice of medicine and the physics of NMR and forge a connecting link between them.† This chapter is the story of the medical doctor and medical scientist who originated the idea of an NMR body scanner to detect disease, found the NMR signal that could achieve that purpose, and charted the course to the final construction of the first machine.

The research performed by Raymond Damadian during his first decade as a medical doctor places him in the category of a "medical scientist" engaged in "basic research." His work would not be performed at the bedside of a patient but rather at the side of a laboratory bench where, using the scientific method originally put forth four centuries earlier by Sir Francis Bacon, he labored to inductively uncover fundamental information about biological cells, how they maintain their chemical and electrical balance, and what happens to the integrity of those cells when they become cancerous.

The security provided by tenure would prove very valuable to Damadian as he began pursuing the risk-filled paths in which his

---

* Dr. Robert Koch, the medical scientist who discovered the tuberculosis bacillus, is considered, along with Pasteur, the founder of bacteriology. Dr. Paul Ehrlich, with his discovery of the "magic bullet," Salvarsan, for syphilis, opened the door to modern drug therapy of infectious disease (anti-microbial chemotherapy). Dr. Alexander Fleming is the discoverer of penicillin.

† Section referenced in Prologue.

research would lead him. It was in following those paths that Damadian would be led to his discovery of the greatest breakthrough in medical diagnosis since X-rays, and explains in part his appreciation for Robert Frost's poem, "The Road Not Taken," which concludes with the lines: "I took the one less traveled by, and that has made all the difference." Dr. Damadian's insistence on doing things his way hasn't always curried favor with those who have wanted him to conform to theirs, but it was that same independent spirit and focused tenacity that led to his invention of NMR scanning.

The following landmark steps in the development of NMR* scanning were provided by Dr. Damadian: 1) the scientific research and theory of the cell developed by Damadian that led him to consider NMR as a method for detecting cancer; 2) his discovery of the cancer NMR scanning signal in animal tissue together with the demonstration of the diversity of NMR relaxations among healthy tissues; 3) his filing of the original and foremost patent on NMR scanning; 4) his achievement of the first whole-body NMR scan of a human and the resultant image; and 5) his development of the world's first commercial NMR scanners.

It All Began With An Idea

Because new ideas are, by definition, an unconventional way of viewing reality, they often appear ridiculous to those with conventional perspectives. When Damadian first suggested using NMR to diagnose disease in the human body, his proposal was not taken seriously. Because NMR spectroscopists were used to spinning their test-tube samples to achieve better homogeneity, the very mention of using NMR to scan a patient prompted them to make light of the idea by asking Damadian, "How fast do you propose to spin the patient, Doctor?"

Today, however, with MRI universally recognized as the premier diagnostic imaging method, detecting disease more efficiently, more accurately and more safely than ever before, and with almost every MRI manufacturer adopting the architecture of Damadian's open-style magnets for their latest machines, the laughter has long since died away. If imitation is the sincerest form of flattery, Damadian's competitors have

---

* The acronym NMR, which stands for nuclear magnetic resonance, was eventually shortened to just MR when used in reference to medical imaging, primarily to avoid the misleading implication that the technology uses radioactive materials. Unlike X-rays or nuclear medicine, magnetic resonance scanning does not subject the patient to the danger associated with ionizing radiation.

become downright effusive in their praise. At the 1994 annual meeting of the Radiological Society of North America, virtually every MRI exhibitor had one or more new models using the open architecture, iron frame magnet designs originally created by Damadian.

Raymond Damadian was born in the Manhattan borough of New York City on March 16, 1936 to Vahan and Odette Damadian. Soon thereafter, the Damadian family moved to Elmhurst, Queens where Raymond's sister, Claudette, was born a year-and-a-half later. When Raymond was two, the family settled in the Forest Hills section of Queens where he ultimately was to acquire his considerable skills in tennis, sing in the children's choir of the community's Congregational church, play violin at church services and commute to the Juillard School of Music, becoming, at a young age, an accomplished violinist.

One of the powerful influences in Damadian's life was his maternal grandmother, Jeanne Pénot Yazedjian. During most of young Raymond's formative years, her loving, doting, disciplining ways were a potent combination in young Raymond's life that are still evident today when he speaks of her. "She was very kind, very French, and very strict. I remember that my grandmother as a young woman was a beautiful woman,"[1] Damadian recalled recently. It was more than outer beauty, however, that Grandmother Yazedjian possessed. It was her inner beauty and her spirit that caused Raymond to adore her in return and want to please her. "She would get me to sit up on her lap and teach me to read. She would get impatient when I didn't get it right, which was not so easy," he added with a chuckle, "because she couldn't speak English."[2]

When Raymond Damadian was 10 years old, his grandmother died of breast cancer. She and her husband, Haig, lived with their daughter's family on Austin Street in the Forest Hills section of Queens and when cancer struck his grandmother, it made a permanent impression on Raymond, as Odette Damadian, Raymond's mother, recalled.

> The last few months were very bad. She was in pain all the time. But she pleaded not to be put in the hospital. It was very hard. When you have your children run downstairs and say, "Mommy, do something for Grandma—she's suffering," that has to leave an impression on you. That happened frequently.[3]

Odette Damadian believes that her mother's death had a significant influence on her son's later desire to find a cure for cancer.

It was terrible [Raymond Damadian recalled]. . . . She had her own room on the second floor, and my mother had a hospital bed for her. During the last few months there was a full-time nurse. She had a terrible cancer of the breast. It was very swollen and red. It was gangrenous with a big cavity and malodorous. She just lay there for months and moaned. She would scream in pain in the middle of the night. She was getting pain medication, but still she moaned. . . .

For a long time, I didn't know she was going to die. It wasn't until I asked the nurse one day when Grandma was going to get well, and the nurse said she wasn't going to. Her suffering had a big impact. I had an early exposure to the ravages of the disease. I saw clearly what the horrid disease could do. For months after she died, I could still hear the moaning. Grandma was gone, but the moaning wouldn't stop. I kept hearing it as the nights passed on.[4]

Although it is difficult to separate one influence from another in one's life, his grandmother's death may well have affected the direction Damadian's medical research would take. "When I became a medical doctor," said Damadian, "cancer was the disease I always seemed to be focused on. It was ghastly [watching my grandmother die]. In my memory, it is still ghastly."[5]

The role of Damadian's parents in his development and motivation, however, should not be underestimated. "Nobody gave to his children like Raymond's father gave to him," said Joel Stutman, the computer scientist on Raymond Damadian's original team.

I had this conversation once with Raymond about his father [said Stutman], and I thought I came very close to understanding what makes Raymond run. I met him and his parents at a picnic and I had a long talk with his father. I told Raymond that his father seemed very, very sharp. I said I thought his mother reminded me of my mother—an authentic Jewish mother, the one who would really take charge in a family. He said that may be true, but he said it was his father who let him know he could do all these things. His father gave him the self-confidence.[6]

His father also gave him a lot of his time.

He rode the subway every day [said Raymond Damadian]. When he worked at the *World-Telegram*, he worked the night shift, 12 midnight to 8 a.m., and he did that for many years. So he was around a lot when I was growing up. When you woke up in the morning, he would be there through the day and that was nice for me.[7]

Every summer, when vacation time rolled around for Vahan Damadian, he and the family would climb into the family sedan and head north. An hour later and they had escaped the busyness of the city and were rolling through the small towns and rural environment of southwestern Connecticut. After following the course of the Connecticut River for three or four hours as it meandered north through Connecticut and Massachusetts, they eventually arrived at their destination, the Potter farm near Charlestown in southern New Hampshire, very close to that state's border with Vermont.

In the early 1950s, when Damadian attended Forest Hills High School, the school was becoming known for its excellent science program, outstripping even Bronx High School of Science in the number of Westinghouse Science Talent Search Awards won by its students. The teacher who made the biggest impression on Damadian was his mathematics instructor, Wally Manheim. "Manheim was terrific and I love math because of him [said Damadian]. You know, he was the kind of person that liked to challenge his students, so he would give me special problems to see if I could handle them. I really enjoyed it."[8]

Off to College

In the fall of 1952, Raymond Damadian matriculated at the University of Wisconsin in Madison. The year before, during his junior year at the age of 15, he had competed with some 10,000 or so other students for an advanced placement scholarship offered by the Ford Foundation and, after a winnowing-down process, had been one of 200 who were given the opportunity to attend, on the basis of a draft-like selection system, either Yale, Columbia, the University of Wisconsin or the University of Chicago. Damadian was drafted by the University of Wisconsin. To accept the offer would mean suspending his violin studies at the Juillard School of Music, where he had been accepted at age eight, and abandoning any prospects he had for a career as a concert violinist. To reject the Ford Scholarship, on the other hand, would mean passing up an opportunity for a free away-from-home education at a major university. Although he already knew which direction he was leaning, Damadian consulted with Andrew McKinley, his music instructor at Juillard, who helped him finalize his decision by pointing out the odds against making it as a soloist. "You can count the people on the concert stage on one hand," McKinley told him, "and the ones who are there versus the ones who aren't are not separated strictly on the basis of musical talent."[9]

The question was whether or not I would succeed on the concert stage with a career as a soloist [said Damadian]. The more usual thing is to be an orchestra player, which didn't really suit my temperament. I played in orchestras for a time and I can't really say that I loved it. I did like performing, however. Maybe if I did nothing but practice for eight hours a day like Heifetz, I could have made it, but that is a very tough row to hoe. It's much worse trying to make your living as a concert violinist than as a professional basketball player. There are approximately 20 teams today with 15 people each? That's 300 possibilities. You have fewer than four or five on the concert stage. The other thing I might have done was to have gone into composing. I'm still interested in that and may yet devote some time to musical composition.[10]

In the end, the decision wasn't that difficult. Considering that he did have other aspirations in science and medicine, it wasn't hard to forsake an uncertain shot at a career as a concert violinist in favor of the Ford offer. The latter was a bird-in-the-hand opportunity.

The economics of the scholarship were terribly persuasive [said Damadian]. Without a scholarship, I'm not sure I could have gone away to school. The schools I would have liked to have gone to in those days were Columbia, Yale, Princeton or Harvard and I couldn't afford to go to any of them without a scholarship, not even Columbia. The most persuasive thing was to have all my education paid for at a good school.[11]

As a member of the West Side Tennis Club, Damadian had also been playing championship tennis at the Junior Davis Cup level, putting him on target for a professional career in tennis. Forfeiting that option, however, came even easier for Damadian.

I don't think I ever wanted to be a career athlete [Damadian said]. I did well, but it just wasn't something I wanted to do with my life. Your productivity ends as a competitor when you are in your mid-30s. I beat some people who ended up with professional careers but what do you do after that? I saw that as a very short range professional career, even if I could make a living at it. In those days, it wasn't easy to make a living at professional tennis.

It's amusing that for my mere involvement teaching tennis in summers during medical school I was declared a pro. I couldn't be an amateur. One of my dreams was to play at Forest Hills and maybe at Wimbledon. I couldn't even consider that until I got myself reinstated as an amateur. After three or four years as a teaching pro to pay for medical school, I had to get reinstated formally by the USLTA as an amateur to reopen the possibilities of playing in either Wimbledon or Forest Hills. In those days, the much higher priority was to maintain your amateur status. As a pro, you got a marginal existence. Today, it's reversed.[12]

Other major changes have also occurred since Damadian entered college. Fall enrollment in 1952 at the University of Wisconsin in Madison totaled 13,571, of which 9,518 were men and 4,053 were women. Forty-two years later, not only had total enrollment nearly tripled to 40,305, the gender gap had virtually disappeared with 20,276 men and 20,029 women attending that school in the fall of 1994.

Located on scenic Lake Mendota near the state capitol and the narrow isthmus that separates Lake Mendota from Lake Monona, the University of Wisconsin has a long tradition of academic excellence. In the fall of 1952, however, it had a severe case of football fever. In fact, their winning season that fall would bring the Big Ten Wisconsin Badgers their first-ever invitation to play in Pasadena's Rose Bowl.* One of the players who helped lead the Badgers to victory and who was getting the attention of sportswriters and fans in the process was Alan Ameche, who would win the Heisman Trophy in 1954 and later be a star fullback for the Baltimore Colts.

Like Ameche, Damadian's presence on campus that fall was also noted in the school newspaper, but not as a BMOC—"Big Man on Campus." Instead, Damadian was greeted with a front-page article in the *Daily Cardinal* entitled "Percival Suckthumb Arrives." Profiling Damadian and the other young Ford Scholars descending on the campus, the article was accompanied by an illustration of the fictional Little Lord Fauntleroy, dressed in black velvet and sporting a lace collar beneath his prepubescent curls. What made the "welcome" even less welcome for Damadian

---

* On January 1, 1953, the Wisconsin Badgers played the University of Southern California Trojans. The Badgers lost 0-7.

was that the tongue-in-cheek characterization touched on a somewhat sensitive area, his youthful appearance.

> I was a little estranged when I first got there [he said] because I was small and very young looking. I guess I had a growth spurt at 14, so I had grown some, but I was still pretty young looking. I was always one of the smallest in my class. In fact, all through grade school I was number three in a lineup. We used to line up by height. David Goodrich and I always ended up next to each other near the short end of the line.[13]

Although the so-called "thick skin" Damadian developed in his youth may have appeared impervious to his often-heartless peers, the person underneath the skin was, in fact, very sensitive to the pointed barbs directed his way. "I sang soprano in boys choirs, played violin, played tennis, was chided for being an egghead and at an early age ended up as 'Little Lord Fauntleroy' in the *Daily Cardinal.* My preferences always seemed to leave me feeling different."[14]

To his credit, Alan Ameche was not among those who defined a man as one possessing a big body controlled by a small brain and, in spite of their odd-couple physical differences, he and Damadian, the Ford Scholar's "Percival," became friends.

Although Damadian never officially registered at Wisconsin in a premed program, he knew by the end of his second year that he wanted to go into medicine. With a major in mathematics, a minor in chemistry, and a number of other science courses mixed in, including biology and physics, by the time he graduated with a Bachelor of Science degree in 1956 he had the prerequisites needed for medical school. By that time, except for summer vacations, he had been away from home for four years, and had experienced living in a dormitory, a fraternity house and, finally, a rooming house. For his medical degree, Damadian preferred to live at home, in part to save money. That meant getting accepted by a medical school in New York City. Although he had applied to a number of medical schools across the country, he proceeded quickly with the admission process at the Albert Einstein College of Medicine as soon as he was notified of that school's acceptance of his application.

Medical School

In 1955, the year Albert Einstein died, the Albert Einstein College of Medicine was born, the first medical school in the United States under

Jewish auspices. When the school opened its doors that fall, a *New York Times* editorial predicted that, based on the reputation of the faculty it had been able to attract, the school was "assured . . . of a place in the ranks of the great medical schools of the world." It would also be one of the most selective when it came to students. Thirty-eight years after 20-year-old Raymond Damadian began his MD program at Einstein, one of four gentile students accepted for the program in 1956, some 9,000 applications were received by the school in 1994 to fill just 176 student slots.

Located on Eastchester Road at Morris Park Avenue in the Bronx, Albert Einstein College of Medicine is part of Yeshiva University, the main center of which is located in Washington Heights on Manhattan's Upper West Side. The roots of Yeshiva University, the oldest and largest Jewish-run university in the United States, go back to the Lower East Side where Yeshiva Eitz Chaim, the first Orthodox Jewish theological seminary in the United States, was founded in 1886. Twenty-nine years later, in 1915, it was absorbed by the Rabbi Isaac Elchanan Theological Seminary. In 1928, the name Yeshiva College was added and, in 1945, the institution became Yeshiva University.

Damadian is the first to admit that his performance in medical school was not all it could have been, a deficiency that he attributes to the type of learning that medical schools, perhaps of necessity, reward. "I think that probably what was tough was the massive memorization. It was just overwhelming. I always thought I had a good memory until I got into medical school."[15]

Because so much material must be assimilated in a relatively short period of time in medical school, there is often little opportunity for the student to filter and categorize the large amount of data. It's gorge now, digest later. For Damadian, only later as he began ruminating in the course of his research on the material he had once devoured with little discrimination, did he begin to see the benefit of some of the material he had learned in medical school.

It was when I was actually using the material where my knack for analytical things began to bear fruit. In fact, I would say that whatever education I had in analytical approaches was an interference in medical school. The material that had to be gorged was so massive that any analytical inclinations just slowed up the learning process.[16]

From the beginning, scientists at Albert Einstein have been on the leading edge of immunology, that branch of medicine which seeks to understand and thereby enhance the body's ability to ward off disease. Ironically, the same immune system in a body that mounts a healthy resistance to disease also resists the efforts of physicians to restore health to that body by replacing a diseased organ with a healthy one. The body, invested with its acute sense of self versus nonself, considers the transplanted organ as foreign tissue and just as dangerous to its health as a highly-infectious pathogen. Thus, the success of any organ-transplant procedure depends as much on the efficacy of the anti-rejection protocol used as it does on the skill of the surgeons who perform the transplant.

Although the first human heart transplant, performed by South Africa's Christiaan Barnard, would not occur until 1967, the possibility of transplanting major organs had been investigated for years. The first transplant operations, corneal grafting, carried out in the early 1900s, had been successful because the cornea has no blood supply and therefore no white blood cells and antibodies to reject a transplant. Kidney transplants had been shown to be technically feasible in the 1950s, but attempts to perform them had resulted in rejection as the drugs that would make transplantation possible, corticosteroids and cytotoxic agents, would not be developed until the 1960s.

In the late 1950s, however, Damadian found the possibility of such a feat captivating, its challenge inspiring. "I took an interest in transplant immunology," he said. "I became intrigued by the idea of transplanting organs. I dreamed up various schemes of immunizing animals so you could transplant organs. It seemed important to me. I was drawn to things that seemed important."[17]

Before he had been in medical school very long, Damadian decided he would focus on internal medicine. As an internist, he would be involved in the detective work of identifying and treating diseases of the internal organs, and it drew heavily upon the chemistry foundations he had laid as an undergraduate. Most significantly, it was internal medicine's puzzle-solving aspect that he found particularly appealing.

> It was the most analytical of the disciplines where chemistry came into play. It was the most fun. It was solving puzzles. The internist is the puzzle solver of medicine. The surgeon does his thing. The obstetrician delivers babies. But it's the internist who tries to solve the peculiar diagnostic problem. He's the "gum-shoe" of medicine.[18]

By the time he graduated, Damadian had decided that he would prefer to do his detective work in the research laboratory rather than the "doctor's office" of a clinician. It was a decision based on the premise that, if he was successful in his research, he would ultimately be able to help millions rather than the thousands to which a practitioner is limited in his or her daily practice. "It seemed to me that, given the proper diligence, a serious effort at experimental research could result in an important contribution to medicine," he said. "I didn't know if anything would come of research I might do, but I knew I wanted to try my hand at an effort to relieve patient suffering on a broader scale, through research, than would be possible as a practitioner."[19]

In 1956, to make ends meet while in medical school, Raymond Damadian took a summer job as a tennis pro at the Dune Deck Hotel in Westhampton, Long Island. In the course of a summer, he could make $2,500 or so by giving tennis pointers and exhibitions to the hotel's well-heeled clientele, which included the likes of U.S. Senator Jacob Javits. Coincidentally, Charlie Brukl, one of Damadian's childhood friends, frequent tennis rival, and fellow member of the West Side Tennis Club, had also gotten a summer job as a teaching pro at the nearby Westhampton Bath and Tennis Club. When they weren't teaching students or playing doubles against Senator Javits and his brother, as they did from time to time, Damadian and Brukl could sometimes be found tooling around in the 1947 Studebaker that they had purchased jointly at 40 dollars each or enjoying a cool refreshment down at the soda fountain of Speed's Pharmacy in Westhampton where a young woman by the name of Donna Terry was employed. Brukl dated Donna that first summer. The following summer, 1957, at Brukl's suggestion, Damadian asked her out and Donna consented.

Donna attended Houghton College, a Wesleyan Methodist college one hour's drive from Buffalo, New York. After two years, she transferred to Columbia University to obtain her RN (registered nurse) degree. In June 1960, one week after Raymond Damadian obtained his MD degree from Albert Einstein College of Medicine, Donna Terry became Donna Damadian. She received her degree from Columbia a year later.

> Donna was always a steadying influence and an unfailing supporter of extraordinary gentleness [said Damadian]. From her side, she endured enormous risks as her husband embarked on the course to build the first NMR body scanner, and risked the family finances to start the first MRI scanner company. In silence, she suffered the brickbats directed at her husband's pioneering and at his efforts to scan people in magnets. Even more frustrating was the knowledge

that there was little she could do herself to influence events. All she could do was pray. It was rare when her Bible was not close at hand and its pages tattered with the notes needed to provide her husband scriptural wisdom and support when she perceived the need.[20]

While Damadian would be the first to admit that "more things are wrought by prayer than man will ever know," as Tennyson put it, the point he makes about Donna is clear. Although it's the lightning rod that attracts the lightning, the ground wire that conducts the charge harmlessly into the ground plays just as significant a role. For Donna Damadian, it hasn't been easy being the ground wire for a lightning rod that has attracted more than its share of lightning bolts, but time and time again she has helped to keep him going with her prayer and encouragement and, in the process, protected both him and her household.

"Except that she was an extraordinary woman of faith," said Damadian, "we could not have stayed the course. She had to endure the anxieties and then raise the children alone. Few women could have endured that. Donna Damadian supplied the peace and understanding needed to fulfill the 'mission' and raise three children, Timothy, Jevan and Keira."[21] Timothy is an executive at FONAR Corporation, the MRI company founded by his father; Jevan is an electrical engineer at FONAR active in digital design; and Keira recently graduated from Geneva College, a Presbyterian college in Beaver Falls, Pennsylvania, a suburb of Pittsburgh, where she majored in Bible studies and obtained a minor in missions.

Internship and Residency

Damadian fulfilled both his internship and residency requirements at Downstate Medical Center in Brooklyn. (Internships are now referred to as first-year residencies.) Part of the State University of New York (SUNY) system, Downstate was one of two such facilities in New York— one in Brooklyn and one in Syracuse. It has since been renamed State University of New York Health Science Center at Brooklyn. Rising out of a cityscape in serious need of urban renewal, the towering, masonry-clad buildings of the medical complex that includes the Health Science Center, its teaching affiliate, Kings County Hospital, and the Kings County Psychiatric Center dominate the neighborhood's up-close horizon.

Fifty-three years before Damadian's arrival at Downstate, the surrounding area had served as an escape valve for the masses of immigrants who had flooded into the Lower East Side tenements of Manhattan around the turn of the century. David and Sheindel Rabi and their two children, Isidor and Gertrude, had been one of the many families who had crossed over the East River on the newly-built Williamsburg Bridge to find a less confined life in the "far reaches of Brooklyn," as I.I. Rabi later referred to the area. In fact, the first home of the Rabis in the Brownsville section of Brooklyn was located less than two miles east-northeast of Kings County Hospital. Their second home in the Eastern Parkway area of Brooklyn, where Rabi lived for a few years following his undergraduate work at Cornell University, was even closer to King's County and Downstate.

As a medical resident in the department of internal medicine, Damadian was very interested in the process by which the delicate balances of fluids and electrolytes are maintained by the human body. These electrolyte balances are fundamental to maintaining the electrical state of the human body, indeed, the electrical activity of the body can be viewed as the driving force that controls life itself. The role of the kidney in regulating these electrolyte balances is therefore central to the maintenance of a proper electrical state in the human body to support life.

Damadian chose to narrow his research focus and begin his investigative career into how the kidney worked and how it was always able to excrete exactly the right amount of electrolytes and water each day, retaining exactly what it needs and excreting the rest. Study of the kidney automatically directs one's attention to the kidney's intricate fluid filtration and reabsorption capabilities, made possible by the one million or so microscopic nephrons that comprise each of the two kidneys with which most humans are blessed.

Consisting of a glomerulus, which is a sort of in-line filter funnel, and a post-filter tubule, each nephron plays a tiny fractional but very significant role in the kidney's ability to eliminate waste and maintain chemical balance. After the initial gross filtration occurs, in which much of the body's water and usable minerals are removed from the blood along with the waste, the post-filter tubule determines if the excreted urine contains any fluids or salts which, on second thought, should be reabsorbed back into the body.

In other words, the glomerulus and the tubule play competitive roles. The glomerulus tends to throw as much away as possible by simple filtration while the tubule tends to be a conservative saver or "packrat," unwilling to throw away something that it thinks might come in handy. Picking through the material the glomerulus has discarded as unnecessary, the tubule reabsorbs those components with which it doesn't want to part. In a properly functioning nephron, it is the "duty" of the tubule to be discriminating while the glomerulus functions as a relatively non-discriminating passive filter. If conditions warrant, a very low intake of water, for example, very little urine will be discharged and water will be conserved. Two of the salts that the kidney's nephrons constantly seek to balance, among other minerals and fluids, are sodium and potassium, the primary contributors to biological electricity and basic, therefore, to life itself.

Damadian didn't realize it at the time, but the encouragement of the department chairman, Ludwig Eichna, for his medical officers and faculty to pursue research that probed the nature of the life process at the most "basic" level possible put him on a research track, right at the beginning of his medical career, that would eventually lead him, clue by clue, to the *seminal* and *fundamental* event in magnetic resonance scanning—his discovery that disease could be detected on the basis of NMR's T_1 and T_2 relaxation times.

The event would be *seminal* in that, although others had experimented with biological applications of NMR before, no one had discovered or realized that it could be used to detect disease and that body scanners based on NMR could be constructed to hunt the body for disease.

The event would be *fundamental* because no matter what the future would hold for diagnostic magnetic resonance as far as techniques were concerned, how the NMR signal would be displayed, whether as a line on an oscilloscope or as an image on a monitor, whether it would be collected by physically moving the patient in relationship to a "sweet spot" or by electronically addressing a spatial location in the patient defined by a magnetic gradient, whether the information would be gathered a line at a time or a plane at a time, one thing that would not change is that it is all made possible by the fact that different tissues, both normal and diseased, exhibit different T_1 and T_2 relaxation times. Just as X-rays would have no diagnostic benefit were it not for the fact that different tissues exhibit different degrees of X-ray attenuation, so NMR would have no diagnostic benefit—and there would be no NMR images—were it not for the fact that different tissues exhibit different T_1s and T_2s.

The analogy ends, of course, when it comes to signal or image contrast. As great a boon to medicine as Wilhelm Roentgen's X-rays became shortly after they were discovered in 1895, they would never, even when manipulated by computer techniques into CAT scans, be more than a shadow compared to the images constructed from the sharp contrasts that Raymond Damadian discovered in the NMR signals of the body's tissues. Only seventy-five years would elapse between Roentgen's X-rays and Damadian's diagnostic NMR signals, but the diagnostic benefits would be worlds apart.

Roentgen discovered X-rays and almost simultaneously discovered, once he recognized their properties, that they had medical benefits. He needed to be a physicist to discover the invisible light of material-penetrating X-rays but he didn't need to be a physician to discover their medical benefits. That the rays he dubbed "X," for lack of a better term, penetrated the human anatomy just like they did other materials and affected a photographic emulsion on the other side was discovered almost immediately and the concept quickly grabbed the imagination of the public. Indeed, the logical leap required to go from Roentgen's discovery that his light penetrated cardboard to the idea that maybe his light could pass through a hand was not a difficult step. It occurred very soon after Roentgen observed X-ray penetration of cardboard.

That was not the case with NMR. Thirty-three years would elapse between Rabi's first detection of nuclear magnetic resonance in 1937 and Damadian's discovery in 1970 that it could be used to detect disease. Other discoveries had to be made in the meantime—radiofrequency spectroscopy pioneered by Norman Ramsey, NMR in condensed matter by Edward Purcell and Felix Bloch, understanding of relaxation mechanisms by Nicolaas Bloembergen, discovery of spin echoes by Erwin Hahn and Fourier transformations of NMR by Richard Ernst. All of these scientists, with the exception of Ernst, were physicists. Ernst was a physical chemist. Unlike X-rays, the logical extension that NMR signals could be used to detect disease was not at all obvious. That discovery needed to be made by a physician who understood the "basic" chemical and physical processes at the cellular level, what happened when those mechanisms went berserk and became cancerous, and how the physics of NMR could be utilized to probe those processes. Raymond Damadian was that physician and his quest, unbeknownst to him at the time, began when Professor Ludwig Eichna of Downstate Medical Center set him on the course of "basic" research that led him to investigate ways to monitor water and salt levels in the human body.

Developing the Science Behind the NMR Scanner

In 1962, upon completion of his residency program at Downstate, Raymond and Donna Damadian moved a thousand miles west to St. Louis, Missouri where, for one year, Dr. Damadian worked with Dr. Neal S. Bricker as a postdoctoral Fellow in Nephrology in the Renal Division of the Department of Internal Medicine, Washington University School of Medicine. Today, Washington University is about six-and-a-half miles west of the 630-foot tall Gateway Arch, built to commemorate the 1803

Louisiana Purchase from France of nearly a million square miles of land, to honor President Thomas Jefferson, who initiated the purchase, and to remember the people who explored and settled the American West. When the Damadians arrived in St. Louis in 1962, via what was then the famous cross-country U.S. Route 66, construction of the Arch had just begun, with the contract awarded, appropriately it seems, to MacDonald Construction Company. Although each of the Arch's stainless-steel clad, triangular legs would be heading skyward by the time the Damadians left St. Louis in 1963—the first stainless-steel panel was set in place early that year—exterior completion of the unique structure designed by Finnish-American Eero Saarinen would not be accomplished until late 1965.

If Damadian had been involved in NMR in the early 1960s, he might have taken special note of the fact that an important early contributor to the science of NMR, George E. Pake, had just been appointed provost and executive vice chancellor at Washington University. From the fall of 1946 until the fall of 1947, George Pake and Nicolaas Bloembergen, Edward Purcell's first two graduate students, had occupied adjacent laboratories in the basement of Harvard University's Lyman Hall of Physics (see Chapter 5).

After getting his PhD in 1948, Pake had headed for St. Louis to become an assistant professor of physics at Washington University. Three years later, he became head of the department, but resigned in 1956, the year Damadian started medical school, to accept a position on the physics faculty of Stanford University, where he was a colleague of Felix Bloch. The reason Pake accepted the Stanford position, he said, was because it allowed him to teach and do research, both of which he preferred over the administrative duties of a department chairman. Six years later, however, when a close friend of Pake's became chancellor at Washington University, Pake was lured back to St. Louis to be the university's provost and executive vice-chancellor.[22]

Pake and Damadian have never met one another, but Pake, who had done research on photosynthesis in living cells using electron paramagnetic resonance during the 1950s, did take notice a few years later of Damadian's findings that relaxation times vary from tissue to tissue. In a recent article in *Physics Today*, in which he recapped the history of NMR in bulk matter, Pake observed:

The relaxation times T_1 and T_2 are significant for medical applications of NMR. . . . Perhaps the most useful distinctions come from the relaxation times—the T_1s and T_2s. . . . Unlike the universal gray scale in X-ray imaging, [magnetic resonance imaging] offers a contrast continuum corresponding to the variation of the interval between pulses in relation to the relaxation times. It takes advantage of a natural basis for image contrast: the fact that many diseased tissues tend to have longer relaxation times than do healthy tissues.[23]

Pake also points out in his article the importance of basic research and the absurdity of supposing that directed research, such as that used in the Manhattan Project, could have come up with a medical imaging technology to rival X-ray imaging. Under such a structured approach, how many scientists would have asked the right questions to lead them in the right direction?

How many [Pake queried] would have said, "Let us begin by trying to measure the strengths of the nuclear magnets within some atoms"? That surely sounds like a dumb, irrelevant idea—especially when you recall that all even-even nuclides (I guess about half of all the kinds of nuclides in nature) have zero spin.

Once the early Bloch and Purcell experiments were—by some miracle—done within this new Manhattan Project, who would then have said, "Let's learn how to measure and calculate T_1 and T_2 for various classes of bulk matter, such as liquids, crystals and biomolecules"?

Finally, who would have said, "Let's play games with pulses and see how many ways we can induce the nuclear magnetizations to dance to our radiofrequency tunes"? And while we were playing these esoteric and improbable games, of course, we would write quarterly research progress reports saying we do these things so we can build an instrument that we know will provide images that detect a multiple sclerotic brain, track the progress of a cerebral bleeding episode or diagnose a diseased liver.[24]

After concluding his series of highly improbable scenarios, Pake observed:

Magnetic resonance imaging could arise only out of the nondirected research, not focused upon ultimate applications, that gave rise to what we know today as NMR. The key was the series of basic quests to understand the magnetic moments of nuclear spins; to understand how these nuclear magnets interact in liquids, crystals and molecules; and to elucidate the structures of molecules of chemical interest. Out of these basic quests came the knowledge that enabled a vision of an imaging technique. Without the basic research, magnetic resonance imaging was unimaginable.[24]

The point Pake makes about the role of basic research or science versus applied science or technology is an important distinction and will be discussed in more detail later. It should be pointed out here, however, that the other "basic quest" not included in the list above but clearly qualifying for inclusion on the basis of Pake's earlier statements about the importance of relaxation times T_1 and T_2 for medical applications of NMR is the one Damadian began at Downstate and now continued at Washington University in St. Louis. After the series of basic quests by Rabi, Ramsey, Purcell, Bloch and Hahn, it was necessary that one more basic science quest be taken and that was the one Damadian provided regarding cell metabolism which led to his hypothesis that NMR could distinguish between healthy and cancerous tissue.

Amazingly, Damadian would not only provide the missing link of scientific knowledge that would open the door to NMR as a medically-useful diagnostic tool, he would also take the steps necessary to bring his idea from the laboratory to the marketplace by building the first whole-body scanner and introducing the first clinically-used commercial scanners. Over the years, he and his company would continue to contribute to the development of innovations that would further advance the technology of MRI, many of which would be patented. In 1962, Damadian still had a long way to go before his basic research would lead him to NMR, but he was on the right track.

Meet Me in St. Louis

In a sense, the situation in 1962 as seen against the discovery of diagnostic NMR by Damadian in 1970 can be compared to the construction of St. Louis' Gateway Arch. On one side, independent of Damadian, was the revolution that was taking place in chemistry with the growth and development of NMR spectroscopy.

The same year that Damadian moved to St. Louis to work with Professor Bricker, Richard R. Ernst in Switzerland completed the requirements for his PhD at the Swiss Federal Institute of Technology, the ETH. The field of NMR spectroscopy was still young, poised to explode and mature during the remainder of that decade. Ernst, however, finished his PhD thesis, he said, "with a feeling like an artist balancing on a high rope without any interested spectators."[25] Although Ernst had gained a great deal of knowledge in high resolution NMR during his graduate years which had led to improvements in NMR instrumentation, he felt that the imperatives of the marketplace might provide a more compelling stimulus for his work, so he would accept a job in 1963 at Varian Associates in Palo Alto, California. That move would prove fortuitous for there he would work for Weston Anderson, and together, their work would lead to the development of Fourier transform NMR as we know it today, resulting in further growth of NMR spectroscopy and the development of new pulsed NMR spectrometers that would eventually aid Damadian in his discovery of relaxation differences in biological tissue.

On his side of the diagnostic NMR arch, Damadian would spend the better part of the 1960s developing the basis for his hypothesis on the ionic theory of chemical transport in the cell. Although he was aware of NMR spectroscopy, Damadian would not make a solid connection between the basic biological research he was conducting on his side of the arch and the fast-growing developments taking place in NMR spectroscopy on the other side of the superstructure until 1969. Once the connection was made in his mind, however, he lost little time in testing his theories and seeing if they could indeed link the two structures which, for many to that date, appeared totally unrelated. The analogy should not be pushed too far, of course. Unlike the Gateway Arch, which was constructed with an overall plan to link the foundational structures high above the Mississippi River, neither side of the NMR scanning arch—neither the science done by Damadian nor the science done by the other NMR pioneers—was conducted with an eye toward ultimately linking them in the form of a new diagnostic modality that would largely replace X-rays. Had anyone attempted to achieve the technological ends of MRI without an appreciation of the prerequisite means—basic scientific research—the intended edifice would have been left without legs to stand on.

In June 1970, Damadian would test his theory. In March 1971, he would publish his theory in *Science* and, within days, other scientists would rush to confirm the validity of his findings. Although the response would be less dramatic than that which followed the discovery of nuclear fission, the analogy is not irrelevant. Just as the basic research of Lise Meitner, Otto Hahn and Fritz Strassmann, conducted on the shoulders of those who had made prerequisite discoveries, had led to the development of the atomic bomb, so the basic research of Raymond Damadian, conducted on the shoulders of biologists and medical researchers who had gone before as well as the shoulders of physicists and chemists who had brought NMR spectroscopy to where it was in

1969, would lead to the development of a new diagnostic modality called magnetic resonance imaging.

After the discovery of nuclear fission, others realized how close they had come to the same discovery without recognizing it; indeed, some had discovered it without realizing they had discovered it. In the case of diagnostic NMR, others were also quick to point out how close other research had come to achieving the discovery of Damadian; indeed, some even attempted to diminish the achievement of his discovery by equating it with anything that had been done previously with NMR in the area of biology. Those who did, however, were missing—either deliberately or otherwise—the essential point. Diagnostic medicine is not diagnostic unless it has a method for detecting serious pathology, and it is that component, more than any of the other comparisons, which makes Raymond Damadian the "father of diagnostic NMR."

He would also have more than his share of follow-on achievements, including the pioneer patent in NMR scanning, the first human whole-body NMR image, the first commercial NMR scanners and the first iron frame MRI magnets that have provided today's "open MRI" scanners and have also provided the much-needed pathway to low-cost MRI, but those would be finishing touches. The discovery that gave all of these follow-on developments purpose took place in June of 1970 when Raymond Damadian excised some tumors from some rats, compared their NMR relaxation rates with normal tissue from the same rats, and discovered that the NMR relaxations of cancerous tissues were substantially prolonged.

Had Damadian only noticed the prolonged relaxation rates, made no further statements about how this information could be used, and carried his work no further, a case could be made that he didn't go far enough, but such was not the case. Instead, as early as 1969, before he confirmed his hypothesis, he requested funds from the Health Research Council of the City of New York to purchase an NMR spectrometer on the premise that, as he wrote, "I am very much interested in the potential of NMR spectroscopy for early non-destructive detection of internal malignancies"[26] [underlining included in original letter]. Furthermore, Damadian's original 1971 NMR article in *Science* stated in the first paragraph, "In principle, nuclear magnetic resonance (NMR) techniques combine many of the desirable features of an external probe for the detection of internal cancer."[27] His patent would spell his ideas out further and, in fact, his patent techniques would be used exclusively in his prototype scanner and his first commercial scanners.

The finishing touches to the NMR scanning arch—the analogue of the Gateway Arch's stainless-steel-clad exterior—would come later, and they are still coming. Lauterbur would add the idea of displaying Damadian's tissue signals in image form. Mansfield would speed up Lauterbur's approach using pulsed gradients instead of steady gradients. Ernst, Kumar and Welti in Switzerland would develop two-dimensional Fourier transform for imaging and Edelstein, Hutchison and Mallard in Scotland would improve on their contributions. Thousands of other contributors and millions of patients would help refine the diagnostic approaches and today, at the brink of the 21st century, diagnostic magnetic resonance stands poised for a series of developments that will make the former ones appear as outdated as a 10-year-old personal computer.

A Focus for Research

As Damadian sees it, his time at Washington University actually sent him down a wrong but useful track for a few years, useful in that it eventually caused him to question the existence of a biochemical mechanism which, for most, was accepted as fact. It all started with a somewhat offhanded laboratory conversation that took place between Bricker, Damadian and a few others regarding the clear preference for potassium over sodium shown by nephrons and other living cells.

Although there is more potassium in the human body than sodium—approximately 5 ounces of potassium to 2 ounces of sodium*—an individual cell within that body is awash in a salty ocean in which sodium is 35 times more abundant than potassium. So where's the potassium? *Inside* the cell, where the ratio is exactly reversed. (The greater amount of potassium in the body is explained by the fact that the body is comprised of more intracellular than extracellular material.) The question is, how does the cell discriminate between the two, absorbing more potassium through the cell membrane than sodium? When the question was posed by someone in the group that day to Bricker, he responded, "Well, there's a sodium pump."[28]

The next question was, what was the evidence for the sodium pump; had it been isolated?

---

* According to the American Medical Association Encyclopedia of Medicine, the body of an "average-sized person contains about 5 ounces (140 grams) of potassium" and "about 2 ounces (55 grams) of sodium."
  —*The American Medical Association Encyclopedia of Medicine*, edited by Charles B. Clayman, MD, (New York: Random House, 1989), 812, 922.

"No," Bricker replied.

It was apparent to Damadian from his work with kidney nephrons at both Downstate and Washington University that here was something that was both important and challenging, and he grabbed onto the possibility of isolating this pump with the same zeal he had once demonstrated with tennis and the violin. Although he had heard of the sodium pump in passing back in medical school and was generally aware of its accepted role in evacuating unwanted sodium out of a cell, this was the first time he had ever heard that the pump had not been isolated. The idea of discovering through experimentation such an important mechanism which at that point was still only conjecture, intrigued him.

I could see that it was very important and I wanted to be working on something that was important. The reason it was important is that sodium is a positively charged ion, a cation. It's a dominant ion in the body, as is potassium which is also extremely positive. It is well known that these cations are critical to the maintenance of tissue electricity and therefore are fundamental to life itself. When life ceases, the body's electrical activity ceases simultaneously. EKGs, EEGs and tissue resting potentials go promptly to zero. The origin of the electricity that maintains life itself is rooted in the ability of cells and tissue to selectively move electric ions like potassium and sodium back and forth across their boundaries. I was interested in the origin of this physiological electricity. If the sodium pump was central to its genesis, I was interested in the sodium pump and how it operated.[29]

To the scientific community, the sodium pump had become much more than mere conjecture. Although the existence of a molecule situated on the membrane of a cell that pumped out unwanted sodium had originally been postulated in the 1940s by two scientists named Dean[30] and Krogh,[31] this pump became the next thing to fact when British scientists Alan Lloyd Hodgkin and Julian Huxley made use of it in their landmark research on the nature of nerve impulses.

Damadian knew that he would be unable to conduct the research necessary to isolate the sodium pump in Bricker's physiology laboratory. In St. Louis, Damadian had been working on an experiment in which he isolated non-urine forming nephrons in the diseased kidneys of dogs.[32] Isolating a single-molecule sodium pump situated on the outer membrane of a single cell would be a horse of an entirely different color.

Bricker's laboratory was not organized for the protein chemistry I needed to isolate the sodium pump. One of the places that was on the forefront of this type of basic research was A.K. Solomon's laboratory at Harvard. I wrote to him and he arranged an interview. In my interview with Dr. Solomon, I told him I was interested in isolating the sodium pump, and he said, "Well, the best place in the world to do that is in my lab." So I went to Harvard.[33]

Harvard

Damadian, now laden with the rather cumbersome title of United States Public Health Postdoctoral Research Fellow, moved to Massachusetts in 1963, where he reported in to Dr. Solomon in Boston at Harvard Medical School's Biophysics Laboratory on Shattuck Street. Like Rabi, Ramsey and Purcell, Arthur Kaskel Solomon was another bright alumnus of the MIT Radiation Laboratory, where he had been assigned during the war to Division 9, Airborne Systems. A physical chemist by training, Dr. Solomon had spent, Damadian recalled, at least a year or two of his Radiation Lab career working on radar in England. After the war, he started the biophysics laboratory, to which he brought a number of sophisticated technologies developed at the Rad Lab during the war. Skilled in instrument development, he was one of the first people to put these new technologies to use in evaluating biological samples and was a pioneer in the use of radioactivity and radioactive tracers for the purpose of studying biological phenomenon. Damadian would later credit Solomon with stimulating his own interest in instrument development.

Dr. Solomon taught that a lot of your ability to go forward in science is dependent to a considerable degree on the instruments you are able to make. The kind of precision that his laboratory was capable of in making instruments brought me the truth of that and when it came time for me to go ahead and get into NMR, I was not intimidated by the technology. I was eager to build instruments.[34]

Solomon, who was already doing research on sodium and potassium metabolism when Damadian contacted him, had also done some thinking about the sodium pump and, in fact, had an idea on how to go about isolating it, which he suggested to Damadian. "It would never have occurred to me [said Damadian], but Dr. Solomon had thought of a good idea for studying these pumps in single cells. He used bacteria. He had developed in his laboratory many methods and apparatus for studying and analyzing the electrolyte composition of bacteria."[35]

The first task Solomon put Damadian to work on was the measurement of the electrical potential across the membrane of the bacterium *E. coli*. Solomon had already published these measurements a couple years earlier in collaboration with Stanley Schultz,[36] also a former student of Ludwig Eichna, but Solomon wanted the results extended and wanted more detail on the parameters controlling the cellular electric potential of *E. coli*. Important as it was, the project seemed lackluster to Damadian. It wasn't getting him close enough to the sodium pump.

Dr. Solomon's next idea, however, delighted Damadian. Solomon proposed isolating the pump by developing a mutant *E. coli* bacteria that was deficient in the sodium-potassium transport mechanism.

The hypothesis [said Damadian], based on the "one gene-one enzyme" theory of the day, would lead to the enzyme (protein) responsible for sodium-potassium transport, Solomon reasoned. The pump was presumed by everybody to be a protein. If the pump was missing or ineffective in the mutant, then I should be able to isolate it. A one-by-one comparison of all the proteins of the mutant and parent strain was expected to uncover the defective mutant protein, ergo the "sodium pump." The first step was to isolate the mutant.[37]

Attempts had been made before to isolate potassium mutants in *E. coli* by Solomon and Schwartz in the biophysics department as well as by Professor Martin Lubin in the pharmacology department. Neither had met with total success. Lubin had decided that the pumps in his *E. coli* mutants weren't really missing, the cell was just leaky. Developing mutant bacteria is a laborious, time consuming and frustrating process. First the bacteria are exposed to a mutagenic agent which kills most of them. The hardier cells in the population, however, respond to the attack by mutating. The challenge is to identify the bacteria that have mutated and then to further identify those that have mutated in the desired manner, an elaborate and tedious process of elimination that combines the deductive powers of a Sherlock Holmes with the relentless persistence of a bloodhound.

Day after day, Damadian pursued the tiny, rod-shaped bacilli, searching for the survivors among them who had lost the ability of their long-since-divided ancestors to exchange sodium and potassium with the world outside their single cell.

Damadian's world in those days was centered around two foci. During the day, you could usually find him in the Biophysics Laboratory at Harvard Medical School, situated near the Fenway Park area of Boston at the center of a vast medical research and healthcare delivery complex that today includes, within a one-quarter square mile area, Beth Israel Hospital, New England Deaconness Hospital, Children's Hospital, Dana-Farber Cancer Institute, HCHP Hospital, New England Baptist Hospital, and Brigham & Women's Hospital. Assisting Damadian in his search was Margaret Ramsey, daughter of Professor Norman Ramsey.

In the evening or on weekends, you could often find Raymond and Donna Damadian on the other side of the Charles River, exploring the historic area which, during the time of the Puritan settlement in New England, was known as Charlestown, an area of special interest to Donna whose ancestors were among the earliest Puritan settlers of Long Island.* Raymond and Donna often spent their weekends eating Brigham's ice cream in Harvard Square, and browsing through the Square's many bookstores.

There are probably a dozen bookstores in the immediate environs of Harvard Square. We would go to Brighams for ice cream and a cup of coffee and after that we would just go through the bookstores and browse. The shopkeepers encouraged it because people bought a lot of books that way. They didn't have sofas where you could sit down like they do today. You had to stand up, but they were just chock full of books. That was a popular pastime for Donna and me. You could browse endlessly and it was a wonderful way to spend an evening. I got in the habit of doing that at Cambridge and once I left Cambridge I began doing that in libraries wherever I was. I'd go in a library, start looking around and just read books that caught my fancy. I do it to this day.[38]

During his time at Harvard, Damadian also audited the quantum physics course taught by Professor Edward Purcell. Here, for the first time, he was introduced by a pioneer of NMR to the topic of NMR spectroscopy, a field which, during Damadian's undergraduate years as a mathematics student at the University of Wisconsin, was virtually unknown. Damadian remembered Purcell drawing an NMR spectrum on the board one day and recalled recognizing that such an analytical

---

* The Terrys and Hallocks, Donna Damadian's paternal and maternal ancestors and the first settlers of Long Island, arrived at Southold, Long Island in 1640 aboard the ship *Abigail*.

approach might be useful in the work he was doing with sodium pumps in Solomon's laboratory but the concept was still new enough and Damadian's exposure to the topic limited enough that he didn't give it a great deal more thought. Although he did broach the topic to Professor Solomon, he pursued it no further when Dr. Solomon told him the machines were too expensive.

By 1965, Damadian had achieved Phase One of the Solomon sodium-pump plan, the development of mutant *E. coli* bacteria which lacked the ability to transport potassium across the cell membrane.[39] He probably would have gone on to Phase Two, attempting to isolate the pump itself, if he hadn't been called to active military duty.

On August 7, 1964, the U.S. Congress had passed the Tonkin Resolution, authorizing presidential action in Vietnam. In February 1965, President Lyndon Johnson ordered continuous bombing of North Vietnam below the 20th parallel. As a medical student at Albert Einstein, Damadian had been automatically deferred from the draft and, during his residency at Downstate, he was deferred under a military medical deferment program designed to supply the armed forces with the medical specialists it needed. The plan was called the Berry Plan. With the war heating up in Vietnam, Damadian received his orders from the U.S. Air Force to commence active duty. He was sent to Brooks Air Force Base, located about five miles southeast of the Alamo in San Antonio, Texas. Captain Damadian took his potassium-transport mutants along.

San Antonio

The USAF School of Aerospace Medicine, affiliated with the Aerospace Medical Division of Brooks Air Force Base, is a large campus-like facility. The Air Force sent Damadian to this facility to serve as a research scientist on topics important to the military. Fortunately, the Air Force, represented by Damadian's commanding officer, Lieutenant Colonel Lou Bitter, himself a scientist with a doctorate in physiology, agreed that Damadian should continue the work commenced at Harvard provided he also conducted the experiments on the liquid rocket propellant, hydrazine, needed by the Air Force. "I was able to conduct two years of concentrated research in the Air Force," said Damadian. "It was a fine research facility and it had a good library."[40] The library at Brooks AFB would prove to be a very important resource to Damadian before his return to civilian life two years later.

Damadian didn't have much success in Texas as far as isolating the protein molecule responsible for sodium and potassium transport in *E. coli* was concerned. He couldn't seem to find the specific protein in his mutant that was different from the normal and it became very frustrating for him. Eventually, his time ran out at Brooks Air Force Base, but in that period of time Damadian started looking through the library for explanations on why he was having trouble.

Damadian had decided there were three transport phenomena to explain. The first was, How does the cell build up such a large potassium gradient between the intracellular environment and the extracellular environment? The second was, By what mechanism was it able to distinguish between sodium and potassium on the outside of the cell and then opt for potassium? It not only had to be able to make the choice but it had to be able to make the choice against the odds since there was an abundance of sodium on the outside of the cell. The third thing Damadian had to explain was, What role did metabolism play in the phenomenon? He could see in his bacteria that the moment he added glucose to a culture of dormant bacteria, potassium would instantly enter the cell in large quantities. What was metabolism doing to potentiate the phenomenon? All three phenomena needed to be accounted for in any theory of transport.[41]

One day while Damadian was browsing through the School of Aerospace Medicine's library, he came across a book entitled *Ion Exchange*.[42] Published in 1962 and written by German-American Friedrich Helfferich, an employee of Shell Development Company who had lectured on the subject at the University of California at Berkeley, the book was a chemistry text that discussed ion exchange resins, one type of which are the beads found in household water softeners. Because of its rather esoteric nature, intended, one might suppose, for that "Culligan Man" who possessed a degree in chemistry, it wasn't the sort of book someone interested in the physiology of ion transport would normally pick up in casual browsing. By this time, however, Damadian's browse-and-read habit had become well-developed. He was soon rewarded for his effort with what he thought was a fascinating new insight.

Damadian knew that *E. coli* were able to internally accumulate 50 times more potassium per unit of cell volume than existed in an equivalent volume in their extracellular environment. All living cells shared this property. In fact, he had just pointed these phenomena out in the introduction to a recent paper, but had added: "These two qualities [of ion accumulation] convince us of its importance. Yet, despite its importance, we still lack a satisfying mechanism to explain it."[43] What he didn't know when he wrote those words was what he would learn from Helfferich, that similar phenomena were ubiquitous *throughout* nature.

Helfferich didn't catalog every natural occurrence of these phenomena—his book was written, after all, to provide a description of the wide range of synthetic materials which had been developed for that purpose by Shell Oil for the chemical industry—but Damadian had found the clue he needed to send him down another path of investigation in hopes of understanding the chemical transport mechanism of the cell. In his random prospecting at the library, he had uncovered what he felt at the time was a real nugget, the prospect that the cell was a living ion exchange resin. Whether it ultimately would have value or turn into "fool's gold" remained to be seen. One thing he knew, though, the majority were still favoring the sodium pump. As far as he was concerned, that prospect could be abandoned.

Those who still believe in the device in question and who disagree with Damadian's alternative explanation have not, in the intervening decades, isolated the object of their belief, nor has Damadian satisfactorily proven to many of them the merits of his concept. In other words, the jury is still out on the matter, but the point to be made in this context is that Damadian's search for the answer would lead him, step by step, to diagnostic NMR. His discovery, when it came, would be at the end of a continuous trail of evidence, followed over a period of nearly a decade, and not at the other end of a blind leap of faith.

Back to SUNY

By 1967, Damadian had fulfilled his military obligation and was ready to resume his civilian medical career, although, as already noted, his time at Brooks Air Force Base had proven very profitable. He had a number of offers from which to choose, but he went with the one from Ludwig Eichna, the chairman of the department of internal medicine at SUNY's Downstate Medical Center in Brooklyn under whom Damadian had completed his residency program and with whose encouragement and recommendation Damadian had pursued his work at Harvard.

Eichna, who dreamed of the day when researchers such as chemists and biophysicists would play a strategic role in bedside patient care, was a strong supporter of Damadian and recruited him for Downstate under a joint program in which he was hired principally by the Department of Internal Medicine, but in which he also taught biophysics in the graduate school, a separate division within the medical school that granted the PhD degree. Damadian's confidence in Eichna's support played an important role in his decision to return to SUNY. He knew he would need someone dedicated to truth and "basic research" as Eichna was if he was to flourish on a path of basic (and sometimes daring) original research.

At Brooks School of Aerospace Medicine, Damadian had collected many of the components for his new theory of the cell. It was there that his first concerns about the sodium pump began to take shape and it was there that he had found the book by Helfferich. In fact, the first published evidence of the new directions in which his research was moving was based on experiments performed at Brooks. In a paper entitled "Ion Metabolism in a Potassium Accumulation Mutant of *Escherichia coli B*," Damadian credited the important contribution provided by Helfferich. A footnote indicates that the present address of the author at the time the report was published was: Biophysical Laboratory, Department of Internal Medicine, State University of New York Downstate Medical Center, Brooklyn, N.Y. For the next 11 years, that address would be Damadian's academic home as he continued his research, taught graduate students, discovered the diagnostic basis of NMR scanning, and built the world's first whole-body NMR scanner.

Not long after his arrival at SUNY Downstate, Damadian acquired two graduate-student assistants who chose him as the thesis professor for their PhDs. As opposite as two poles of a magnet, and just as reactive to one another, Lawrence Minkoff was remote, spare in physique, and not given to many words; Michael Goldsmith was outgoing, massively built, and loquacious. Other students would also gather around Damadian in the coming years and contribute to the research coming out of his small laboratory located on the sixth floor of the biophysics building, but these two, Minkoff and Goldsmith, would figure more prominently than the other students in the building of "Indomitable," the world's first whole-body NMR scanner.

Atlantic City

April 1969 marks the entry point of Damadian's first substantive foray into the world of NMR spectroscopy and sets in motion the events that led to his June 1970 discovery of diagnostic NMR. It wasn't as though Damadian was totally oblivious, however, to NMR spectroscopy prior to April 1969. On the contrary, because his research into cellular composition and chemical transport had focused his attention on cell metabolism, he was aware of the ion imbalances associated with cancer and he had come to believe that there must be a quantitative way to tell a cancerous cell from a normal cell by direct chemical analysis and not just by its visual appearance under a microscope. His mental antennae were thus alert to any phenomena that might support or deny his new hypothesis.

What he found was additional confirmation in a standard chemistry textbook entitled *High-Resolution Nuclear Magnetic Resonance*. Authored by Pople, Schneider and Bernstein,[44] the resource was Damadian's first real exposure to the findings of Nicolaas Bloembergen on motional narrowing, the fact that, with a decrease in viscosity, there is a prolongation of NMR relaxation times T_1 and T_2 and an associated narrowing of NMR spectroscopic lines. Although Bloembergen had done his relaxation analyses of various substances two decades earlier, nothing had been done to compare relaxation times of biological tissues even though, as Damadian would later come to realize, Bloembergen's graphic representation of the relationship of T_1 and T_2 in glycerin actually revealed the same divergent relationship Damadian would later find exhibited by human tissue and by biologic tissue in general.

Damadian hadn't gotten that far in early 1969, however. The main thing he recognized then was that, with decreased viscosity came motional narrowing and prolonged relaxation, and that was sufficient for him to contemplate the use of NMR to compare signals between cancerous tissue and normal tissue. The value of NMR as a sensor of the motional freedom of water molecules would bear fruit when Damadian subsequently became aware that cancerous tissue had an abnormal alkali cation composition and that the alkali cations had an effect on the viscosity of water.

At the time, however, he didn't have ready access to an NMR spectrometer. The only one that was available was a continuous-wave (CW) machine at nearby Brooklyn College and, although it measured linewidths, it provided relaxation times only indirectly as the inverse of the spectral linewidth. Unfortunately, since the linewidth was only an *indirect* measure of the T_2 relaxation, it was altered by processes other than relaxation events. Thus, changes in the linewidth could not be unequivocally attributed to relaxation and were subject to change by a variety of factors having nothing to do with relaxation.

I remember making an attempt on the Brooklyn College machine [said Damadian] to see if the NMR response from cancer tissue was different from normal. I made a few irreproducible measurements and gave up. I remember being unhappy at the time that it didn't work.[45]

One of the studies that caught Damadian's attention during this period was contained in a book written by a Russian physical chemist by the name of O. Ya Samoilov. Translated into English, the title of the book was *The Structure of Aqueous Solutions.* Although Samoilov did not utilize NMR techniques in his research, his work paralleled Bloembergen's to some degree in that it compared the effect of different substances on the viscosity of water. Samoilov dissolved, for example, each of the following salts in water and then analyzed their structural effect: sodium chloride, potassium chloride, rubidium chloride, cesium chloride and lithium chloride.

These comparisons were of interest to Damadian because all of these chlorides were derived from the Group 1 elements he had been studying with respect to ion exchange and chemical transport in the living cell. What was especially interesting to Damadian, however, was Samoilov's concept of "structure breakers" and "structure makers." Samoilov wrote that if he put lithium or sodium in water, which were highest on the periodic table, that the viscosity of the solution tended to increase slightly. Samoilov concluded, as a result, that these elements were *creating* structure; in other words, that they tended to impose order when dissolved in water. He called them "structure makers." On the other hand, when he put potassium or cesium into water, the reverse happened. Viscosity decreased, water became freer and more mobile, and he classified this group of metals as "structure breakers." Damadian found Samoilov's results fascinating.

Another study that Damadian took note of was reported in a 25-year-old paper by L. Dunham, S. Nichols and A. Brunschwig[46] which reported cancer tissue as having elevated levels of potassium. This was the first evidence that Damadian had found that tied the cancer abnormality to abnormal electrolyte composition. He later would try to duplicate the findings of Dunham, et al. but found that the *sodium* content of cancer tissue was markedly elevated instead. He could not satisfy himself, from his own measurements, that a potassium elevation was general for cancer. The results for potassium were too inconsistent among various cancer tissues and the few that showed elevations showed only minimal elevations. The results were different for sodium. The sodium elevation in cancer tissue was marked and general.

The net effect on the course of Damadian's research was the same, however. The potassium elevation reported by Dunham, et al. directed Damadian's attention more intensely toward the science of nuclear magnetic resonance and the way in which it might help him probe cancerous tissue along the lines of his new hypothesis.

He would be invited to explore those possibilities for himself while attending a major conference, sponsored by the Federation of American Societies in Experimental Biology, scheduled for April 1969 in Atlantic City, New Jersey. Gilbert Ling, a physiologist and the author of an incisive treatise entitled *A Physical Theory of the Living State*, was also slated to attend.

The federation meetings were an annual affair [Damadian said] where thousands of biologists and chemists converged on Atlantic City in early April. All the boardwalk hotels were reserved for scientific seminars and symposia. At the meeting I met Gilbert Ling who invited me to attend a closed-circuit TV production on the physiology of water. He, Freeman Cope, Carlton Hazlewood and Swift were scheduled to debate the subject. After the filming, we headed for dinner at Zaberer's.

At dinner, Cope, who had made successful NMR measurements of sodium in brain, stated that he now wanted to measure potassium in biological tissue. He was concerned, however, that the weaker magnetic moment of potassium would make it difficult to detect in tissue. I volunteered that I might be able to secure some bacteria from the Dead Sea, *Halobacter Halobium*, that contained 20 times the normal complement of potassium and that might enhance the chances of detecting a signal. Dr. Cope was pleased with the idea and subsequently called and asked me to collaborate in the venture. Cope and I managed to borrow time on a machine at NMR Specialties, a small manufacturer of pulsed NMR spectrometers in New Kensington, Pennsylvania [near Pittsburgh].[47]

New Kensington, Fall of 1969

The spectrometer Cope and Damadian had obtained permission to use was one of NMR Specialties' new pulsed spectrometer models specially designed to take advantage of the contributions Erwin Hahn had brought to the science of NMR nearly two decades earlier when he used a pulsing technique and inadvertently discovered spin echoes and free induction decay (FID).

That's an important part of the story [said Damadian] because the machine that we elected to use for these experiments was completely different from the more commonly available CW spectrometers of the type I had used unsuccessfully at Brooklyn College. The machine the chemists were using at the time were of the Brooklyn College type. They were known as high-resolution spectrometers and measured the NMR signal entirely differently from the pulsed NMR machine we chose to use. While high-resolution spectrometers were abundant in analytic chemistry labs around the world, pulsed spectrometers were scarce. In the high-resolution, continuous-wave (CW) machines available in those days, the RF was applied continuously as the magnetic field was swept. As the field was swept, the sample eventually passed through resonance where the peak amplitude was recorded. The amplitude trailed off on either side of the resonance leaving an approximately gaussian-shaped line that diminished symmetrically on either side of the resonance peak.

In the high-resolution CW machine, the NMR signal was being measured as a function of magnetic field strength (or frequency). The signal was not being measured as a function of time. The method did not therefore permit *direct* access to relaxation times.

In the machine that we used, instead of the RF being turned on and left on (continuous wave), the RF was pulsed. Once the pulse was turned off, the experimenter could watch the signal decay over time, i.e. the relaxation process (relaxation times) could be *directly* observed and measured and did not have to be guessed at from indirect measurements of the CW linewidth, which were known to be affected by other things than the NMR relaxation itself, such as inhomogeneity of the magnetic field.[48]

A few weeks after the Atlantic City meeting, Cope and Damadian, each in their own cars, were heading west on the Pennsylvania Turnpike with Cope's car full of electronic equipment and Damadian's car loaded with carboys and a variety of other bacteria fermentation equipment. In the intervening period, Damadian, true to his promise, had secured the potassium-rich *halophiles* from Israel's Dead Sea. He also made contact with Stanley Schultz at the University of Pittsburgh and asked if he could grow the bacteria in Schultz's laboratory at Pitt. Schultz agreed. Once the bacteria were fully grown in Schultz's laboratory, Damadian spun them into a packed pellet in a centrifuge. The pellet of bacteria that these *halophiles* produced was pink, the same hue that appears over the Dead Sea at dusk. "Once a sufficient bacterial pellet was achieved," said Damadian, "I packed them on ice and sped over to the company to get them into the NMR quickly to minimize deterioration. Cope was waiting with the NMR calibrated and tested."[49]

For Damadian, that evening would be pivotal. Cope operated the controls. "We got a signal immediately," Damadian told the writer. "It was the first time potassium had been measured by NMR in a biological tissue."[50] In 1992, Damadian described the same event to the members of the Washington Patent Lawyers Club:

To our mutual delight, the potassium signal popped up on the oscilloscope screen the instant we put the bacteria into the machine. We were happy, but I was awed by something else. I observed with considerable excitement, "Good heavens, Freeman, this machine is doing chemistry entirely by 'wireless electronics,' " a terribly unsophisticated distillate of the distinguished practice of NMR. A few days later, still awed by the technology, I said to Freeman at breakfast, "If you could ever get this technology to provide the chemistry of the human body the way it does for the chemist on a test-tube of chloroform, you could spark an unprecedented revolution in medicine."[51]

For the better part of two decades, chemists had used NMR spectroscopy to analyze chemical compounds, revolutionizing chemical research in the process. Relatively little research, however, had been done biologically and nothing medically. Some of the early experimenters had poked their heads in magnet gaps to see what kind of a sensation or signal they would detect,* others had used NMR to characterize the gross signals obtained from biological tissue and fluids,[52-56] and two scientists at Los Alamos Scientific Laboratory had even built a "whole-body spectrometer" for a rat to acquire what they believed in 1967 to be "the first NMR signal ever obtained from a whole living animal."[57] The Los Alamos study demonstrates, however, two essential ingredients missing from these early biological experiments, 1) the *idea* of using NMR to detect disease in the live human body and 2) the *scientific basis* for such detection.

---

* Felix Bloch is said to have detected an NMR signal when he poked his finger into a magnet soon after his 1946 discovery of NMR in condensed matter. Edward Purcell and Norman Ramsey are reported to have constructed a tuned head coil and to have subjected themselves to the large magnetic field of the Harvard cyclotron and a radiofrequency field of the Larmor frequency when the cyclotron was down for repairs. They apparently experienced no ill effects and no signal. Later, Erwin Hahn and Sven Hartmann, Hahn's collaborator in double-resonance research, attempted to observe effects of physiological or emotional stimuli on gross free induction decay (FID) signals obtained from their own heads. "Unfortunately, because of the short T_2 and lack of enthusiasm for engineering a better nonadiabatic cut-off, we saw no signal," said Hahn in 1990.
—E.L. Hahn, "NMR and MRI in retrospect," *Phil. Trans. R. Soc. Lond. A* **333** (1990), 411.

Even at this early stage in his NMR career, Damadian was looking far beyond the chemical analysis of single-cell biological tissue. Although the detection of potassium in biological tissue by Cope and Damadian took place in the late summer of 1969 and another 10 months would pass before Damadian would detect prolonged relaxation rates in cancerous tissue, evidence that Damadian began thinking early on of using NMR for non-invasive, *in vivo* detection of cancer in humans is provided in a letter he sent 11 days after their successful potassium experiment to Dr. George Mirick of the Health Research Council of the City of New York, the agency that had named Damadian a career scientist.

After requesting $89,000 to purchase a pulsed NMR spectrometer for his Brooklyn laboratory so he could follow up this promising line of research, Damadian added the following postscript:

"I am enclosing a first draft of the manuscript we are submitting to *Science** for publication.[58] I want to mention that our findings have powerful application in anti-cancer technology. Malignant cells have marked alterations in the physical structure of their protoplasm. To the best of my knowledge, it is generally true that all malignant cells have been marked by elevated cell potassium values and depressed Ca^{++} levels. I am very much interested in the potential of NMR spectroscopy for early non-destructive detection of internal malignancies [underlining included in original letter]. To the extent that our primary research objectives will permit, I will make every effort myself and through collaborators, to establish that all tumors can be recognized by their potassium relaxation times or H_2O-proton spectra and proceed with the development of instrumentation and probes that can be used to *scan the body externally for early signs of malignancy.*"[59]

Discovery of the NMR Cancer Signal and Discovery of the Diversity of NMR Relaxations Among Healthy Tissues

As mentioned earlier, Damadian would come to have less confidence, after conducting his own experiments with cancer tissue, that Dunham, et al. were correct regarding the elevation of potassium in cancer tissue. When Damadian would later return to New Kensington to test whether or not NMR had the power to reveal cancer in tissue, he would compare the relaxation times of hydrogen protons rather than the relaxation times of potassium nuclei.

---

* The article ended up being published in *Nature*.

The opportunity came in June 1970. Damadian persuaded NMR Specialties president Paul Yajko to let him return to NMR Specialties for an attempt at the cancer measurements. In the intervening months, Damadian, by then obsessed with the idea of using NMR to explore the human body for cancer, had collected a menagerie of rats afflicted with Walker sarcoma tumors. At this point, Damadian picks up the story, telling it as he did to the Washington Patent Lawyers Club in 1992:

With a collection of tumor-bearing rats fixed securely in the trunk of my car, I made off for Pittsburgh and the NMR Specialties Company where Freeman and I had done the potassium-bacteria work. Paul Yajko, the company's president, had said I could have a few days on one of his NMR spectrometers that was en route to a customer, provided I worked on my own and didn't distract any company employees from their work. Mr. Yajko provided me with an operator's manual on how an NMR spectrometer worked and I was on my own.

Never having operated an NMR machine before (Freeman operated the NMR for the K^{39} experiment), the nest of coaxial cables, vacuum tube amplifiers and digital programmer units that constituted the electronics was very effective at intimidating beginners.

Eager not to wear out my welcome with Mr. Yajko, though, I kept my distance from company employees. I paged through the manual on my own until I came to a procedure I thought I could manage. It was called the T_1 Null measurement. I practiced T_1 measurements by this method for several days using distilled water samples until I could reproducibly get the published textbook values for T_1 of distilled water. I then tried the first rat tissues taken from the animals I had brought from Brooklyn.

After a few more days of measurements to be confident I was measuring T_1 in the different normal rat tissues reliably, I decided to attempt the cancer measurement. [The date was June 18, 1970.] To my mind, this was the measurement that would make or break my NMR body scanner idea. I needed that abnormal cancer signal if there was to be any hope of a human scanner that could hunt down cancer deposits in the body. I held my breath and made the first measurement. It was different—dramatically different!

Now I feared it was too good to be true and that I had made the measurement improperly. I repeated it and repeated it, each time getting the same result as I reexamined and tested my method on standard solutions to be certain of my method. Eventually, I concluded I wasn't [making the measurement improperly]. The T_1 of the rats' Walker sarcoma tumors was distinctly elevated when compared to normal. I concluded that if I could return to Brooklyn, grow up some more rats with a different tumor—in this case, the Novikoff hepatoma—come back to Pittsburgh and repeat the result, then I could trust the general NMR result of cancer versus normal and could consider generating a manuscript for reporting the findings to the scientific community.

After successfully repeating the T_1 measurements on the Novikoff tumor [on July 14, 1970], I soon had a manuscript on its way to *Science. Science* published the paper, "Tumor Detection by Nuclear Magnetic Resonance" in their March 19, 1971 issue.[60]

The possibilities that presented themselves to the euphoric Damadian were mind-boggling. If you could use NMR to detect cancer cells in a test tube, why couldn't you use it to detect cancer cells in a live human body if you had a big enough machine? And if NMR worked for cancer, maybe the same analytical power it brought to *in vivo* cancer could be used for *in vivo* detection of a wide range of diseases. Damadian's 1971 *Science* paper proposing the possibility of *in vivo* tumor detection with NMR was the first one ever to put forth the ground-breaking idea that disease could be externally detected in humans using NMR and that different tissues—both diseased and normal—exhibited different NMR relaxation rates.

Damadian made his revolutionary proposal gently to avoid offending reviewers who might reject the manuscript for publication if its conclusions were too bold. After reading a draft of the article, Damadian's department chairman, Ludwig Eichna, recommended additional changes to make the author's visionary ideas more palatable to the conservative scientific community. Damadian made the changes and incorporated them into the final manuscript. Even in its medical journal language, however, the message was clear. If Damadian's claim was valid, he had taken a major step forward in fathering a new diagnostic technology. During the 1970s and 1980s, Damadian's 1971 *Science* article

Table 1. Spin-lattice (T_1) and spin-spin (T_2) relaxation times (in seconds) of normal tissues.

Rat No.	Weight (g)	Rectus muscle		Liver		Stomach		Small intestine		Kidney		Brain	
		T_1	T_2	T_1	T_2	T_1	T_2	T_1	T_2	T_1	T_2	T_1	T_2
1	156	0.493	0.050	0.286	0.050	0.272		0.280		0.444		0.573	
2	150	.548	.050	.322	.060	.214		.225		.505		.573	
3	495	.541	.050	.241	.050	.260		.316		.423		.596	
4	233	.576 (0.600)*	.070	.306 (0.287)*	.048	.247 (0.159)*		.316 (0.280)*		.541 (0.530)*		.620 (0.614)*	
5	255	.531		.300		.360		.150		.489		.612	
		Mean and standard error											
		0.538 ± 0.015	0.055 ± 0.005	0.293 ± 0.010	0.052 ± 0.003	0.270 ± 0.016		0.257 ± 0.030		0.480 ± 0.026		0.595 ± 0.007	

* Spin-lattice relaxation time after the specimen stood overnight at room temperature.

Table 2. Spin-lattice (T_1) and spin-spin (T_2) relaxation times (in seconds) in tumors.

Rat No.	Weight (g)	T_1	T_2
Walker sarcoma			
6	156	0.700	0.100
7	150	.750	.100
8	495	.794 (0.794)*	.100
9	688		
10	255	.750	.100
Mean and S.E.		0.736 ± 0.022	.100
P		<.01†	
Naibelff hepatoma			
11	155	0.798	0.120
12	160	.852	.120
13	231	.827	.115
Mean and S.E.		0.826 ± 0.013	.118†
P		<.01†	
Fibroadenoma (benign)			
14		0.448	0.100
15		.537	
Mean		.492	
Distilled water			
		2.691	
		2.690	
		2.640	
Mean and S.E.		2.677 ± 0.021	

* Spin-lattice relaxation time after the specimen stood overnight at room temperature. † The P values are the probability of the significance of the difference in the mean of T_1 for the malignant tumor and for brain.

Figure 1. Original T_1 and T_2 Data Published by Dr. Damadian in the March 19, 1971 Issue of *Science*. Note the large range of NMR relaxations among the healthy tissues (compare oval-shaped, high-lighted healthy small intestine T_1 to oval-shaped, highlighted healthy brain T_1) as well as the striking elevations of NMR relaxation times for cancer tissue relative to normal (compare rectangular-shaped, highlighted healthy liver T_1 to rectangular-shaped, highlighted liver tumor T_1).

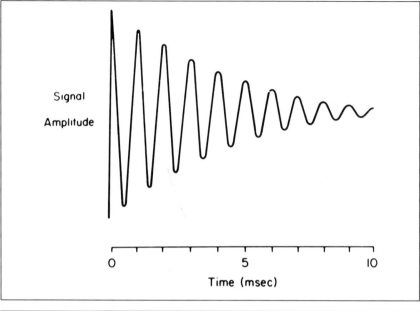

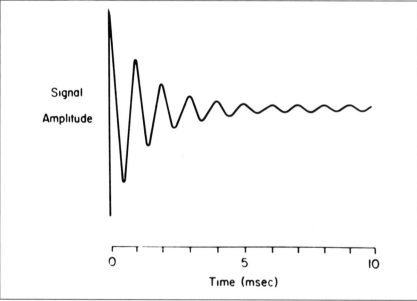

Figure 2. Schematic Illustration of the Decaying NMR Signal (Radio Signal) from Cancerous and Normal Tissue. Note the lengthened relaxation of the cancer tissue signal (upper signal) relative to normal (lower signal).

would be cited more times by other scientists than any other original publication* in the field of MR scanning and imaging. While waiting for the article to appear, Damadian forged ahead on a number of fronts, all intended to turn his new-found dream into reality, even though he was well aware of the risks.

> When the idea of the scanner and the measurements of cancerous tissue occurred to me [said Damadian], I thought that actually performing the experiments would be running off on a tangent. I had been proceeding nicely down a main highway of research in salt and water biophysics for almost eight years and here I was flirting with an idea that would detour directly into the unknown.[61]

As far as Damadian was concerned, however, once he took that detour, there was no turning back. He was committed. "Once you get a strong idea, you can become its prisoner," Damadian has said. "When the idea is compelling enough, it can be difficult to evade its allure. It seems to repeatedly force itself into consciousness to remind you of your failure to act."[62]

The MR Image Is Not a Photograph
(or Why Damadian's T_1 and T_2 Findings Were So Important)

Although an MRI image appears as if it were a photograph of the interior of the human body, it is *not* a photograph. The MR machine cannot, for example, produce a true-color image of the interior of the body. It has

---

* According to the Science Citation Index, the Damadian 1971 *Science* paper was the most widely cited publication in the field of MRI from 1970 to 1989, the years of the maximum rate of growth of MRI installations. Because of its exceptional citation frequency, it was designated a "Citation Classic" by the publishers of the Science Citation Index in 1987. The articles with the highest frequencies are listed below according to their citation frequencies (highest frequencies shown first). The number of citations is shown underlined and in bold following the reference. 1) RV Damadian, *Science* 171, (1971), **589**; 2) PC Lauterbur, *Nature* 242, (1973), **562**; 3) GM Bidder, *American Journal of Roentgenology* 139, (1982), **401**; 4) A Kumar, *Journal of Magnetic Resonance* 18, (1975), **356**; 5) LE Crooks, *Radiology* 143, (1982), **342**; 6) WA Edelstein, *Physics in Medicine and Biology* 25, (1980), **308**; 7) P Mansfield, *NMR Imaging in Biomedicine*, (1978), **278**; 8) IR Young, *Lancet* 2, (1981), **264**; 9) DI Hoult, *Journal of Magnetic Resonance* 24, (1976), **213**; 10) WS Hinshaw, *Journal of Applied Physics* 47, (1976), **204**; 11) PA Bottomley, *Medical Physics* 11, (1984), **188**; 12) AN Garroway, *Journal of Physics C: Solid State Physics* 7, (1974), **133**; 13) JMS Hutchison, *Journal of Physics E: Scientific Instruments* 13, (1980), **106**; 14) GN Holland, *Journal of Computer Assisted Tomography* 4, (1980), **101**; 15) ER Andrew, *Physics in Medicine and Biology* 22, (1977), **65**; 16) JR Mallard, *Philosophical Transactions of the Royal Society London* B 289, (1980), **52**; 17) WS Moore, *Journal of Computerized Tomography* 4, (1980), **38**.

no way to determine the actual color of the internal organs from the NMR signals of those organs and cannot therefore make a genuine photographic color image of the body's interior from its NMR signals. The MRI cannot, for example, tell that the NMR signal from the gallbladder is coming from a green organ or that the NMR signal from the liver is coming from a reddish-brown organ.

MRI can, however, determine the strength or intensity of each of the NMR signals collected by the MRI scanner and compile these signals into a matrix of "picture" elements or pixels whose brightness ("gray scale intensity") is set by the intensity of the signals, thus creating a black-and-white MR "image." A camera literally photographing the interior of the body would render a color photo or a black-and-white photo with almost equal ease. The MRI cannot because the MR image is not a photograph. It is a computer-generated map of the NMR signals acquired from the body.

The MR image, in other words, is a composite of tiny computer-generated squares, or pixels, similar to the half-tone dots of a newsprint image. During a typical MRI scan, 65,536 NMR signals* are collected from a cross-sectional "slice" of the body. The strength of each signal, its "S" value, is measured. The brightness of each image pixel is set proportional to the strength (S value) of the NMR signal collected from the region of anatomy represented by the pixel. A typical MR image is a square array of 256 by 256 pixels. Thus, a typical MR image is made up of 65,536 computer-generated pixels whose intensities (brightnesses) are set proportional to their S values.†

To display the image, the 65,536 S values are coded for brightness so that the individual S values can be displayed as 65,536 pixel brightnesses instead of as the numerical values that have actually been measured by the scan. They could, in fact, be displayed as numerical values since the numerical S values dictating the pixels' brightnesses are stored in the scanner's memory. The brightness assigned to each pixel is directly proportional to the S value. See Figure 3a on page 653 and Figure 3b on page 654.

A typical MR image, therefore, is a brightness display of 65,536 S values (signal intensity values) obtained from 65,536 NMR signals acquired from the body during a scan. The parameters that control the S values of

---

* In actual practice, 256 signals are collected and the Fourier transform converts those signals to 65,536 signal amplitudes or S values.

† Strictly speaking, the matrix of S values is scaled into a range suitable for display.

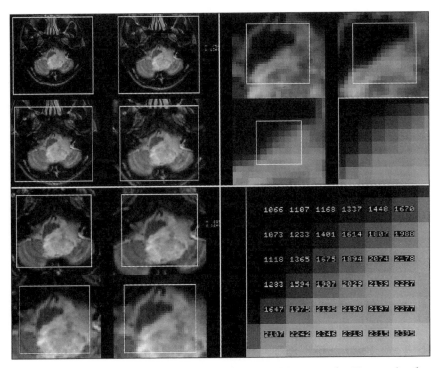

Figure 3a. A Stepwise Enlargement of an MRI Image of a Tumor in the Cerebellar Region of the Brain. The region being enlarged, the high contrast boundary between tumor and surrounding normal tissue, is marked by the inscribed inset. The final enlargement shows the pixels of this tumor-normal tissue interface together with the scaled S values from computer memory that were used to set the brightness of each pixel. Note that the highest S values accompany the brightest pixels, the lowest the darkest pixels, intermediate S values intermediate brightness, etc., demonstrating the direct correspondence between the image S values and their pixel brightness.

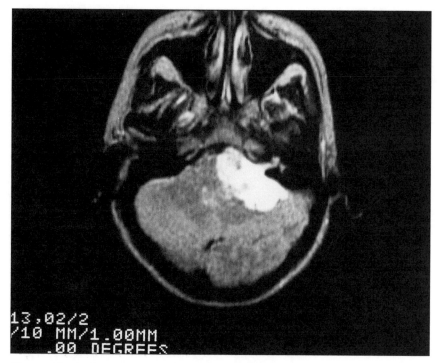

Figure 3b. An MRI Image of a Tumor of the Brain, an Acoustic Neuroma of the Auditory Nerve. The striking differences in pixel brightness that separate the tumor from surrounding normal tissue so that it can be detected on this T_2 MRI image are created by the marked differences in T_2 relaxation between tumors and normal tissue discovered by Damadian (see Figure 1, page 649, or Table 1, Appendix A8, following this chapter).

the collected NMR signals from the body, namely the NMR relaxations, therefore control the contrast visible between the body's tissues, the detail visible in the image, and the ability to detect lesions.

It is clear, for example, that if all the NMR signals acquired from the body had the same signal strength, or S values, then all the pixels of the MR image would have the same brightness, by their direct correspondence to the S value. The image would then be a blank, absent of all detail. The ability of the MR image to picture detail is therefore fundamentally dependent on the degree to which the S values of the NMR signals obtained from different tissues of the body differ. If they do not, then the MR image made up of pixels whose brightnesses are set by these S values will not distinguish them.

The missing link needed to go from the test-tube NMR of chemical solutions to the MRI of human tissues was supplied by Dr. Damadian. His 1971 paper in *Science* contained *two* key discoveries that were the missing link. First he showed that the NMR relaxations of cancerous tissue were markedly prolonged relative to healthy tissue. Second, in performing the relaxation measurements of the healthy tissues in order to provide the needed comparison with cancer tissue, he performed the first NMR relaxation measurements of a full spectrum of healthy tissues. For the first time, a diverse sampling of healthy tissues had their NMR relaxations measured at the same time, at the same frequency, and by direct pulsed NMR measurements of the relaxation instead of by indirect and inexact estimates obtained from the linewidth of frequency spectra. The measurements allowed direct comparisons of a full spectrum of healthy tissues to be made for the first time.

The marked variation of the NMR relaxations among healthy tissues, as reported by Damadian in his 1971 *Science* paper, is the reason MRI images reveal such exceptional anatomic detail. As the source of the extraordinary contrast range available in MRI, the diverse tissue relaxations enabled MRI to picture soft-tissue anatomy with far more detail than had ever before been possible in medical imaging.

Since the S value of the NMR signal, the basis for the marked variation in pixel brightness or contrast available in MRI images, is dependent upon T_1 and T_2 tissue relaxation, it follows that Dr. Damadian's discovery of these differences in relaxation provided the critical *raison d'être*—justification for existence—of MR images.

Felix Wehrli, former MRI imaging scientist and manager of the NMR Applications Division at General Electric, has acknowledged the fundamental importance of the discovery of the diversity of tissue relaxations. In a June 1992 article on NMR imaging in *Physics Today*, he stated:

"It was recognized early on that in most diseased tissues, such as tumors, the relaxation times are prolonged (R. Damadian 1971, *Science* **171**, 1151). This difference provides the basis for image contrast between normal and pathological tissues."[63]

Wehrli emphasized the key role the newly uncovered tissue relaxation differences play in creating the detail of MRI images when he pointed out that the few percent differences in proton density between tissues were too small to explain "the marked contrast found within soft tissue. . . . The clue," he stated, "is magnetic relaxation, a phenomenon which has no counterpart in X-ray CT."[64]

Dr. Paul Lauterbur also recognized the importance of the diverse tissue relaxations uncovered by Damadian and the impact it would have on scanning. Of his witnessing the successful repeat by Leon Saryan at NMR Specialties Corporation in September 1971 of the original Damadian relaxation measurements of healthy tissues, Lauterbur stated:

"Even normal tissues differed markedly among themselves in NMR relaxation times, and I wondered whether there might be some way to noninvasively map out such quantities within the body."[65]

A Comparison of X-ray and MRI Image Contrasts

A comparison of the image contrasts made possible by MRI with the contrasts achieved with the previous state-of-the-art modality, X-ray CT, makes clear the reason for Dr. Wehrli's conclusion. Table I, page 657, compares the T_1 relaxation values of normal and cancerous tissues published by Dr. Damadian in his 1971 *Science* paper with the published values of the X-ray attenuation coefficients of soft tissues in X-ray CT.

X-ray attenuation coefficients are a measure of the passage of an X-ray beam through a tissue. If the differences between tissues in their X-ray attenuation coefficients are small, then their respective ability to pass X-rays through to the target film differs very little. As a result, the exposure of the film corresponding to different soft tissue regions will be nearly equal, the brightness of different tissues will be very close, and image contrast, i.e. the ability to see detail, will be poor.

In the case of bone, for example, the difference between the attenuation coefficient of bone and surrounding soft tissue is large. Bones, therefore,

Table I. X-ray Attenuation Coefficients of Soft Tissues Compared to
T₁ Relaxation Data Published by Damadian in *Science*, 1971.

	X-Ray Attenuation Coefficient (cm^{-1})	T$_1$ Relaxation (msec)
H$_2$O	.2027	2650
Brain	.2079	595
Pancreas	.2157	—
Liver	.2167	293
Muscle	.2128	538
Kidney	—	480
Stomach	—	270
Small Intestine	—	257
Primary Brain Cancer	.2112	—
Liver Cancer	—	827
Maximum observable difference of **attenuation coefficients** between **healthy tissues**	**4.2 percent** (brain vs. liver)	
Max. observ. diff. of **attenuation coefficients** between **cancer and healthy tissue**, same type	**1.6 percent** (brain vs. brain cancer)	
Maximum observable difference of **T$_1$ relaxation times** between **healthy tissues**	**103.1 percent** (brain vs. liver) **131.5 percent** (brain vs. small intestine)	
Max. observ. diff. of **T$_1$ relaxations** between **cancer and healthy tissue** of same type	**182.3 percent** (liver vs. liver cancer)	

—Source for X-Ray attenuation data: M.E. Phelps, E.J. Hoffman, M.M. Ter-Pogossian, *Computed Tomography* **117**, (1975), 573.

are well visualized by X-ray. Bone, because of its high density, scatters the incident X-rays so they do not reach the target film whereas soft tissue passes them through to the film. The film region corresponding to bone is thus not exposed and shows up as a bright region on developed film. The film region corresponding, on the other hand, to soft tissue is exposed to X-rays and shows up as a dark region on developed film. The result is a sharp *contrast* of these two tissues, with bone clearly seen because of its comparative brightness to the darkness of the surrounding soft tissues.

If two tissues pass X-rays equally, i.e. if their attenuation coefficients are the same, the exposed target film will show equal brightness for both tissues and neither will be visibly distinct as there is no contrast between them. This is, in fact, the situation for X-ray imaging of the soft tissues. The differences of X-ray attenuation between the soft tissues are extremely small and soft tissues are thus poorly visualized by X-ray.

The differences in X-ray attenuation coefficients reported in Table I specify quantitatively the *differences* in the passage of the X-rays through various soft tissues, i.e. the *differences* in X-ray energy that the target X-ray film receives after the passage of the X-rays through different soft tissues. With the maximum observed differences for healthy tissues at 4.2 percent, it is clear that the differences of X-ray passage through the soft tissues of the body are very small. Only negligible contrast is therefore available from X-rays to visualize the body's soft tissue structures. By comparison, the full range of the soft tissues studied by Damadian with NMR exhibited a 132 percent variation with regard to T_1 relaxation. The brain vs. liver difference of T_1, for example, was 103.1 percent in the original Damadian data whereas the same tissues differ by only 4.2 percent when X-ray is applied. (See Table I, page 657.)

Indeed, were the soft tissue differences the only differences Roentgen observed in his original discovery of the medical uses of X-rays, little would probably have come of his observation. What was observed, however, was that the bones of the hand were distinct from the surrounding soft tissues, i.e., that the difference in the passage of X-rays through the bones of the hand was markedly different from their passage through the soft tissues of the hand even though the differences among the soft tissues themselves were negligible. In other words, the contrast between bone and soft tissue was large even though the contrast in the hand between the soft tissues themselves was small. The marked contrast between bone and soft tissue enabled the details of bone to be seen but did not enable any detail in the soft tissues to be visualized.

Deficiency with regard to contrast between soft tissues is intrinsic to the fundamental physical properties of X-rays themselves. From the outset of Roentgen's discovery, this deficiency was recognized as insurmountable. Furthermore, it was a serious shortcoming since the great majority of diseases occur within the soft tissues of the body. Dr. Damadian's discovery of the marked NMR relaxation differences of the soft tissues of the human body *remedied this 75-year-old deficiency in med-*

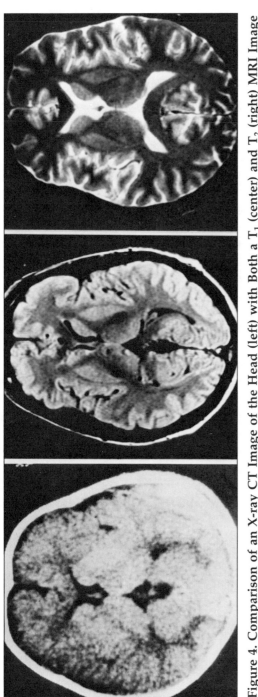

Figure 4. Comparison of an X-ray CT Image of the Head (left) with Both a T_1 (center) and T_2 (right) MRI Image Taken at the Same Level in the Brain. None of the images shown used contrast agents. The striking superiority of the two MRI images over the X-ray CT image arises from the marked differences in the tissue NMR relaxations, discovered by Damadian, that have no counterpart in X-ray CT. The relaxation differences create the sharp distinctions between gray matter, white matter, and cerebrospinal fluid that supply the exceptional image detail seen on these MRI images of the brain and on all MRI images. Note the marked differences in image contrast, achieved without injecting contrast agents, as commonly required in X-ray imaging, simply by changing the scanning parameters from T_1 dependence (center) to T_2 dependence (right). The differences in the X-ray attenuation coefficients of brain tissues and soft tissues in general (see Table I, page 657) are much too small to provide the contrast needed to visualize a corresponding level of detail in X-ray CT.

ical imaging. It is his discovery that has made possible detailed visualization of the soft tissues of the body, where the great bulk of disease occurs.
It is not only the T_1 relaxation differences discovered by Damadian,
however, that give MRI its powerful capability as the premier diagnostic
imaging modality; it is also the tissue T_2 differences he discovered. Taken
together, the T_1 and T_2 components provide a wealth of medical information never before available.

Setting the S Values for T_1 and T_2 Images—The S values finally displayed on the image screen can be altered to display different types of
image contrast for optimal lesion detection. In some instances, T_1 image
contrast is best for viewing the pathology. In other instances, T_2 contrast is
best. Altering the image so that its contrast is dominated by either T_1 or T_2
is achieved by altering the sequence of RF and gradient pulses to cause
the amplitude of the signal, i.e., its S value, to be dominated by whichev-
er tissue relaxation parameter, T_1 or T_2, is best suited to detect the pathology of interest. For example, the T_1 image is best for visualizing herniated
discs of the spine; the T_2 image is best for visualizing tumors of the spine.

In the T_1 spin echo image, the pulse sequence parameters are set so that
the S value depends directly on the T_1 value, i.e., $S = (K_1)(1 - e^{-TR/T_1})$.* Since
TR is a constant (K_2) throughout the scan and e is 2.718, the signal intensity or
S value can be rewritten as $S = (K_1)(1 - 2.718^{-K_2/T_1})$ where the direct dependence of the S value on T_1 in the T_1 image has been made more obvious.
TR is the repetition time that specifies the time interval after which the
imaging pulse sequence is repeated to complete the image. In a T_1 image,
the pixel intensity or brightness is set proportional to the S value in the
same way that it is in a T_2 image (see Figure 3b). The brightness of a pixel
seen on a T_1 image is thus directly determined by the T_1 value of the tissue. In this instance, S is proportional to $1 - 2.718^{-K_2/T_1}$. The only quantity
that varies in this expression is T_1. S can only change when T_1 changes.
Accordingly, the pixel brightness can only change when T_1 changes and
its brightness is therefore set by T_1.

Likewise, in the T_2 spin echo image, the pulse timing parameters are set
so that the S value is directly determined by the T_2 value of the tissue. In
this case, $S = (K_1) e^{-TE/T_2}$ where TE is a constant throughout the scan so
that $S = (K_1) 2.718^{-K_2/T_2}$. Indeed, in the case of the T_2 image, the S value is
directly proportional to $2.718^{-K_2/T_2}$ in which the only quantity that varies

---

* K_1 is the hydrogen density of the tissue. Since it varies by only a few percent[66] from tissue to tissue, its value is taken to be a constant.

in this proportion is the tissue T_2. Since the pixel brightness of a T_2 image is directly proportional to the S value of the pixel (see Figure 3b), the pixel brightness of a T_2 image is directly determined by the T_2 value of the tissue. TE is the echo time, the time after the stimulating RF when the Hahn echo of the body's NMR signal occurs.

The Hahn echo is particularly suited for obtaining T_1 and T_2 images since it allows the MRI scanner to adjust the echo time, TE, in concert with the repetition time, TR, to achieve independent T_1 and T_2 images. Since pixel brightness in T_1 and T_2 images is directly dependent, respectively, on the tissue T_1 and T_2 values, the sharp T_1 and T_2 differences discovered by Dr. Damadian to exist among the healthy tissues of the body and between cancers and healthy tissues have become the principal means by which the high degree of soft tissue detail seen on MRI images and the high sensitivity of MRI for visualizing pathologies such as cancers are made possible.

All MRI scanners today are equipped with pulse sequences that produce T_1 or T_2 scans which are referred to as T_1-weighted or T_2-weighted sequences. Ninety percent of all patients are scanned with either a T_1 scan or a T_2 scan or both. The purpose of these scans is to cause the contrast in the image to be dominated by either one or the other relaxation parameter, T_1 or T_2, the result of which are images with dramatically different contrasts.

Most commonly, both T_1 and T_2 images are obtained from the patient. In T_2 images, for example, the fluid-rich structures, e.g., spinal fluid, cysts, blood, tumors, etc. appear bright, or with high intensity, on the image with the result that the T_2 image is the mainstay of lesion detection. In T_1 images, the same structures generally appear dark, or with low intensity, relative to their surroundings.

Because of the marked differences in image contrast they provide, the two image types, T_1 and T_2, commonly serve as a diagnostic pair. Together, they add to the diagnostic sensitivity and specificity of MRI. In general, the T_1 image, because of its increased signal-to-noise, provides more anatomic detail for the evaluation of structures. The T_2 image, because of the high intensities with which lesions show up on these images, are best for detecting pathology. The two together permit the lesion first to be *detected* by the T_2 image and second to be *evaluated* on the T_1 image, thus supplying the details regarding its location and its impact on normal anatomy.

Often, the two together make key diagnostic distinctions between possible pathologies. For example, a bright mass appearing on a T_2 image of

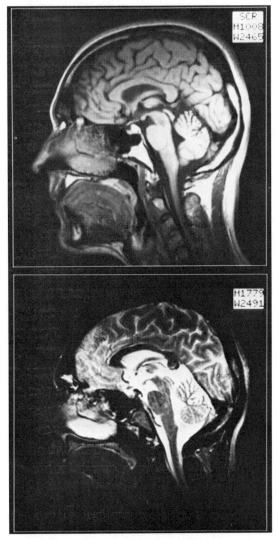

Figure 5. A T₁ Image (Top) and a T₂ Image (Bottom) of the Same Region of the Brain. The high levels of tissue contrast seen in these images were obtained without the injection of any contrast agents into the patient. The differences in the T_1 and T_2 NMR tissue relaxations uncovered by Damadian create these striking contrasts in image detail. The marked differences in tissue contrast obtained when one relaxation parameter (T_1) is used instead of the other (T_2) are dramatic and illustrate why the two, operating in concert as a diagnostic pair, have become the mainstay of diagnostic NMR imaging today.

the brain could be a subacute bleed or a tumor, an important medical distinction. If it appears on the T_1 image also as a high-intensity lesion, it *is* a bleed. If it appears, however, on the T_1 image to be a dark lesion, it is much more apt to be tumor. T_1 and T_2 thus function as contrast agents. As Pake has pointed out,[67] the T_1s and T_2s supply a *natural* basis for image contrast. Unlike X-ray, they do not have to be injected from the outside. Indeed, Damadian's discovery of the sensitivity of the magnetic relaxation to tissue pathology contributed internal contrast agents which are active participants in the dynamic chemistry of the living cell. Exceptionally sensitive indicators of tissue health, they are key to the use of MR imaging as a medical diagnostic tool.

Damadian's Method of Spatial Localization

Right from the start, even before filing his patent application, Damadian was quite open about his intentions; he planned to build a machine big enough to scan human beings. To accomplish that, however, would require a massive scale-up in size from the NMR spectrometers used for chemical analysis. Not only that, unlike a test-tube-full of uniformly-mixed chemicals, this spectrometer had to incorporate a method for spatial localization. To be diagnostically useful, it had to be capable of identifying and separating the cancer signal from all the other NMR signals transmitted by the body.

In the spring of 1971 (see page A4 of appendix to this chapter), six months before Lauterbur witnessed, on September 2, 1971, Saryan's successful repeat of Damadian's tissue NMR relaxation discovery and therefore six months before he entered the field (see pages B1 through B3 of appendix to Chapter 9), a second article appeared in the SUNY publication *Downstate Reporter*. (Dr. Damadian's Science article appeared in the March 1971 issue.) The article in the *Downstate Reporter* began as follows:

"Sometime in June, a truck will pull up at Downstate bearing a 14-foot-high machine for the biophysics laboratory of Dr. Raymond Damadian, Assistant Professor of Medicine and of Biophysics.

"The machine is a nuclear magnetic resonance instrument, which is more at home in physics or chemistry laboratories than in medical institutions. But to Dr. Damadian, the device is very much a medical instrument. He regards it as the prototype of a machine-to-be that could fulfill a long-standing dream of physicians: a quick, foolproof method of early cancer detection.

"Already, Dr. Damadian is planning to build a much larger nuclear magnetic resonance device, one that will be big enough to hold a human being. That machine, Dr. Damadian believes, will prove that nuclear magnetic resonance (NMR) is the tool that doctors have been looking for in their quest for a method of detecting cancer early, when treatment is most effective. . . ."[68]

Early on, Damadian knew he would have to come up with a spatial localization method. Until Ed Edelson, the writer of the article, interviewed Dr. Damadian in the beginning of 1971, Damadian had not really grappled with it. When Edelson asked him to clarify just how he would be able to detect the cancer signal when it was mixed in with the signals of the surrounding tissues, Damadian responded that a magnet moving back and forth across the patient's body would provide the necessary focus.

Later, he would call his focusing technique FONAR, an acronym taken from the first and second letters, alternately, of "Field fOcused Nuclear mAgnetic Resonance." Just as there was a method to Damadian's creation of an acronym, there was a solid basis for his magnetic focusing idea. Damadian knew that magnetic fields could be shaped in such a way as to create a small resonant window at a particular point of interest.

Perhaps the best way to visualize it is to imagine a magnetic field shaped like the surface of a saddle. The point of precise resonance, where the transmitted RF frequency matched the proton Larmor frequency, would be attained only at the saddle point, a precise point in the center of the saddle-shaped magnetic field where the point was a field minimum along one axis and a field maximum along the other. Only that part of the body situated at the saddle point or "sweet spot" would, by design, reside in the proper strength of field to achieve a resonant signal.

Damadian recognized that the resonant window or "sweet spot" approach was achievable because of his tissue experiments at NMR Specialties. His tissue measurements had taught him that NMR magnets in general had "sweet spots" usually situated in the magnetic center of the field. He learned early on that the tissue had to be placed at the magnet center to achieve a signal. Samples placed significantly "off-center" would not yield a signal because of the strong gradients outside the "sweet spot," hence Damadian's recognition that this "sweet spot" could be used to scan the human body.

Ordinary NMR magnets, Damadian recognized, had built-in "focusing" or "localizing" capability. As a first step in achieving an MR scan, the magnet only needed to be big enough to move the human body systematically back and forth across this signal-producing region, the "resonant window" or sweet spot, to accomplish a point-by-point scan.

In this regard, Damadian's point-by-point approach to the first human NMR scan is analogous to the approach taken by the early NMR spectroscopists in obtaining frequency spectra from their samples. Prior to pulsed Fourier spectroscopy, introduced by Anderson and Ernst, spectra were acquired using a point-by-point sweep of the magnetic field. The amplitude of the signal at each setting of the magnetic field was recorded sequentially to create the spectrum.

It wasn't until Damadian's interview with Edelson, however, that the approach took shape in his mind. "Not until Edelson pinned me down on how the needed spatial localization was to be achieved," he said, "did I think it through and find a solution."[69] Reporting what Damadian said, Edelson wrote in the *Downstate Reporter*:

"The proposed NMR device for detecting cancer in humans would not have to be highly elaborate, Dr. Damadian says. It would consist of a large coil to emit radio waves and a movable magnet to create the magnetic field required. The coil would be wrapped around the patient's chest, while the magnet passed back and forth across the body. A detector would pick up NMR emissions for analysis."[68] (See page A5 of appendix to this chapter.)

Six more years would go by before Damadian achieved the first whole-body human MR scan, six years of struggle, sacrifice, and discouragement, but eventually the sweet spot would bring him the sweet taste of victory when he performed the first human whole-body scan.

Meanwhile, On Other Fronts

After sending his article to *Science*, Damadian plunged directly into the follow-up research he knew was needed if NMR scanning was to be accepted as a viable modality in medicine's arsenal of diagnostic tools. Just as Roentgen had done three-quarters of a century earlier in exploring as many properties of X-rays as quickly as he could, so Damadian wanted to quickly determine what his new modality might be capable of achieving medically. Roentgen had found that his rays were not affected by electric or magnetic fields. Were there limitations to NMR as a diagnostic modality that would severely limit its usefulness? Or, on the positive side, did the possibility exist for the use of NMR for the treatment as well as the detection of disease?

Damadian's work during the next several years would take several directions. One of the first efforts his laboratory undertook was a much more comprehensive analysis of tissue types, based on their T_1 and T_2 relaxation times, than was originally provided by his first paper.[70-72] In addition to reinforcing what he had already announced to the world, the fact that cancer tissue displays dramatically prolonged relaxation times compared to normal tissue, Damadian was initially hopeful that he might find evidence that tumors displayed characteristic NMR signatures; in other words, that the relaxation time would help in *grading* a tumor's malignancy. As Damadian conducted more research—he and his assistants ran tests on many hundreds of human tumor samples obtained from University and Memorial Hospitals in Brooklyn and Sloan-Kettering Memorial Cancer Center in Manhattan—it soon became clear from his work and the work of others that this was not to be. Cancerous relaxations while different from *normal* overlapped other pathologies.

Damadian still hopes, however, to make more progress in the area of disease classification by NMR, to elevate what has often been more of a medical art into more of a medical science. He is not the only one to have expressed such a desire. In 1982, Peter Mansfield and Peter Morris stated that, in spite of their opinion that "it seems hardly reasonable to expect the relaxation processes to be identical in brain and muscle fiber, for instance, . . . our view is that all the NMR parameters, even though they are to a varying extent interrelated, may have some eventual role to play in tissue typing and diagnosis of disease states."[73]

Another focus of Damadian's research during this period was to analyze the diagnostic usefulness of NMR relaxation rates and spectroscopy with regard to other atomic nuclei. Because of the abundance of water in the human body, hydrogen is clearly the front-runner as a means of detecting disease. As water states within the body change, those changes are clearly evident on the basis of proton relaxation times, which was the focus of Damadian's original paper. Other chemical changes that take place in the body are also useful, however, as disease indicators and three of the best candidates in this regard are phosphorus-31, potassium-39 and sodium-23. Damadian and the people in his laboratory conducted extensive NMR testing on all three, analyzing both relaxation times and spectral signatures. All were found to be medically-useful and all were measured in cancer tissue by the professor and his students.

They found, for example, that the amplitude of the tumor sodium signal substantially exceeded the amplitude of the normal sodium signal and they found that phosphorus yielded relaxation times useful for detecting disease which were similar to that of water-based hydrogen. With regard to phosphorus, they found that "from our data, it appears that the phosphorus nucleus may prove to be a sensitive probe of malignancy, perhaps more sensitive than either protons or potassium."[74]

As the 21st century approaches, NMR spectroscopy promises to provide a great deal of medically-useful information, so much so that it may one day overshadow the ubiquitous and more user-friendly MR image. Already, television viewers are being exposed to NMR spectroscopy's potential when they see how it can be used in the analysis of brain function. MR researchers are studying the phosphorus-31 spectral changes that accompany muscle fatigue after exercise. The P^{31} changes after myocardial anoxia are also being established. Studies that once would have qualified as the stuff of science fiction are already being conducted at major research hospitals and eventually will become part of standard health-care practice.

Finally, the last area Damadian investigated to some extent was that of therapeutic treatment using NMR. The reasoning behind the concept was that if one could entice nuclei at a particular location to reveal their chemical makeup, which Damadian had proven was possible with biological tissue using the same chemical-shift principles that NMR spectroscopists had been using for years, perhaps it would be possible to deliver with pin-point accuracy a frequency-specific dose of elevated radio-wave energy to which only tumor cells exhibiting that frequency would react. In the process, mechanisms triggering runaway malignancy would be disrupted and the disease process halted.

To those who argued that it would be impractical to heat tissue sufficiently with the radio energy of a resonance to kill cancer cells, Damadian responded that—speaking only hypothetically, of course—it might not be necessary to heat the entire cancer tissue to its kill temperature to be effective. The same result might be achieved if an elevation of the spin temperature alone could be cascaded somehow into the degeneration of a molecule critical to cell survival such as DNA or RNA and thereby result in the death of the cell.

Such radiotherapy, Damadian knew, might well be delayed until the distant future, if it was possible at all. What he *was* convinced was achievable, however, based on his discovery of the cancer signal, was the use of NMR in scanning the human body for disease. To protect his idea and the investment of time and money that would be required to bring his idea to market, Damadian consulted with a patent attorney and, two days less than a year following publication of his *Science* article, he filed the "Pioneer Patent" of NMR scanning.

The "Pioneer Patent" of NMR Scanning

On March 17, 1972, one day after Raymond Damadian's 36th birthday, he filed the patent application for his "Apparatus and Method for Detecting Cancer in Tissue." Issued in 1974, U.S. Patent 3,789,832 was the first description ever of a device for scanning the human body by magnetic resonance. The patent establishes both the priority of Damadian's claim to the idea of NMR whole-body scanning as well as a workable method of using NMR scanning for diagnostic purposes, the same method he would use in achieving the world's first MR image of a human and the same method that would be used in his first commercial scanners.

The foundational nature of Damadian's patent is driven home by a visit to the United States Patent and Trademark Office in Washington, DC. Housed in four imposing buildings near Dulles International Airport, the Office today bears little resemblance to the tiny agency begun in 1790 under the direction of then-Secretary of State Thomas Jefferson, the "Father of the Patent Office," who would later become the nation's third president. Established on April 10, 1790 by act of Congress on the authority of Article 1, section 8 of the U.S. Constitution,* the U.S. Patent Office issued its first patent to Samuel Hopkins of Vermont on July 31, 1790 for his invention of a new method for making soap. Since then, more than five-and-a-half million patents have been issued, with information on all of them today accessible via high-speed computers. Patent examiners still use the terminology, however, inspired by the filing system Jefferson inaugurated to classify patents—the shoe box, or more precisely, the shoe drawer.

As each patent application was approved and granted a patent number by Jefferson, it was placed in a flat box or drawer originally intended for storing shoes. As the system quickly grew, new classifications required new boxes, which became known as "shoes." When Damadian submitted his 1972 patent application for a method and apparatus to detect cancer in humans, the patent examiner assigned to the application was initially bewildered. Damadian's idea didn't fit into any previously-established subclassification. When he inquired of his superiors where to put it, they responded, "You start a new shoe, of course." More than a decade later, the patent examiner told Damadian the story and said, "You know, Dr. Damadian, the lives of patent examiners are not too exciting, but your patent was responsible for one of the high moments of my career."[75]

---

* "Congress shall have power . . . to promote the progress of science and useful arts, by securing for limited times to authors and inventors the exclusive right to their respective writings and discoveries."
—United States Constitution, Article 1, section 8.

The new "shoe" that was created, a subclass of Class 128—General Surgery—was entitled "Magnetic Resonance Imaging or Spectroscopy," and given the subclass number of 653.2. Damadian's patent, given U.S. Patent No. 3,789,832[76] and issued on February 5, 1974, was the first patent to be placed in that shoe and, for the next nearly seven years, was the *only* patent to be placed in that shoe. It wasn't until December 23, 1980, 450,607 U.S. patents later, that Damadian's original MR Imaging and Spectroscopy patent, No. 3,789,832, was joined in the box by Patent No. 4,240,439.

By 1994, those two MRI patents had been joined by 740 others, including additional patents by Damadian and his associates. There is no question, therefore, which is the pioneering patent. It is No. 3,789,832, the one in which Damadian described his idea of using T_1 and T_2 relaxation times of atomic nuclei in biological tissue to detect *in vivo* cancer in the human body. It's the oldest patent in the first shoe box to be labeled 653.2 by the U.S. Patent Office. Created specifically for inventions relating to magnetic resonance imaging and spectroscopy, the 653.2 section continues to grow rapidly.

Visitors entering and leaving the premises of the U.S. Patent and Trademark Office pass through the National Inventors Hall of Fame in the building's massive marble-lined lobby. Established in 1973 to honor those inventors who have conceived the great advances fostered by the United States through its patent system, the Hall today recognizes (as of 1994) 113 inventors and their inventions. They go back as early as Eli Whitney and his cotton gin, for which a patent was granted by Thomas Jefferson. With more than five-and-a-half million patents issued since Samuel Hopkins' soap-making method and more than 50,000 additional patents issued every year, the chance of an idea earning its inventor recognition in this great hall is remote indeed. Inventors who are so recognized will share equal space with the likes of Thomas Alva Edison, Alexander Graham Bell, Henry Ford and the Wright Brothers. Of more recent vintage, Chester Carlson is recognized in the Hall for his invention of xerography, Edwin Land for the photographic development method used in Polaroid cameras, and John Bardeen, William Shockley, and Walter Brattain for the transistor.

In 1989, Raymond Damadian was inducted into the National Inventors Hall of Fame. He was inducted with John Deere (1804-1886), founder of the John Deere tractor company and inventor of the steel plow; Irving Langmuir (1881-1957), responsible for the creation of the high-vacuum electron tube and gas-filled incandescent light; and George Westinghouse (1846-1914), founder of Westinghouse Corp. and the inventor of the air brake. As part of the induction ceremonies, President George Bush acknowledged Damadian's efforts to strengthen the "spirit of invention" in the United States through Invent America!, a program designed to encourage inventiveness among the nation's youth. "I have seen Dr. Damadian at work," stated Bush, "captivating young imaginations with the fires of his own. I would not be surprised to see him joined in the Hall of Fame by some of those promising young minds. All it takes is imagination and encouragement, and he is an ideal source of both. He is living, reassuring proof that the spirit of invention continues to thrive in our great Nation."[77]

Dr. Damadian's induction into the Hall of Fame came less than a year after President Ronald Reagan honored the inventor by awarding him the National Medal of Technology. The award of the National Medal of Technology was shared by Damadian and the other MRI pioneer featured in this book, Paul C. Lauterbur. In making the award, the President cited both scientists "for their independent contributions in conceiving and developing the application of magnetic resonance technology to medical uses including whole-body scanning and diagnostic imaging."

Groundbreaking patents are known as "Pioneer Patents" and are by nature general. Separately recognized by U.S. courts, they set the foundation for new industries to occur as Damadian's patent did and, because of their pioneering status, are given special status by the legal system. Damadian's patented "sweet spot" method of spatial localization would later be set aside in favor of faster acquisition methods developed by scientists at the University of Aberdeen in Scotland and the University of Nottingham in England. Nonetheless, it was the "sweet spot" method of Damadian's original patent that provided a method simple enough to achieve the first MR scan and image of the live human body and to convince the world that medical MR scanning of the human body was, in fact, a reality.

More recently, support for Damadian's pioneering contributions to MR scanning have come in the form of a patent recently granted to John D. Larson III and assigned to Hewlett-Packard Company in Palo Alto, California for RF focusing methods for MR imaging. Issued February 9, 1993, patent no. 5,185,573 entitled, "Method for Focusing of Magnetic Resonance Images," harks back to concepts first expressed in Damadian's patent application 21 years earlier in which the "sweet spot" of the scanner's magnetic focus, together with the shaping of the RF beam in the manner commonly employed by today's MRI surface coils, provided the spatial localization needed for point-by-point scanning. As the Hewlett-Packard patent by Larson points out, the invention "uses RF focusing techniques together with nuclear magnetic resonance imaging in high magnetic fields to improve the signal-to-noise ratio per unit data acquisition time and to improve the spatial resolution" (Col. 1, line 8 of Larson patent).

As Peter Morris, biochemistry professor at Cambridge University, predicted in 1986, this adaptation of the original FONAR method is intended for imaging a particular region of interest, such as the cardiac region, and promises, according to Larson, to provide superior signal-to-noise, improved spatial resolution, spectroscopic sensitivity, and faster data throughput. Damadian originally chose his point-by-point scanning method as an analogue of the phosphor-refreshment raster scanning method of the television screen. In the early years following his achievement of the world's first whole-body scan on his prototype scanner dubbed "Indomitable," Damadian continued to adhere to this approach, stubbornly convinced that if high enough speeds could be attained by point-to-point methods, the costly computer processing of the gradient acquisition methods could be avoided. Instead of having to add the cost of sophisticated computer hardware to the scanner, he reasoned, the scan could be achieved by analog means in the same way that a television set constructs an image.

The ultimate potential for this type of scanner to operate as an analog display and escape the digital hardware costs was not lost on Hewlett-Packard, a manufacturer of medical equipment. John Larson and Hewlett-Packard therefore adopted the RF focusing approach of Damadian's point-by-point scanning method because of the promise it held for providing superior signal-to-noise, improved spatial resolution, spectroscopic sensitivity, and faster data throughput. Thus, an approach once dismissed as archaic may well provide an improved acquisition method in the future.

The Drama at New Kensington

Reaction to Damadian's *Science* article came quickly. Soon, research laboratories around the world were attempting to repeat Damadian's experiments. Two scientists who took an immediate interest were Donald Hollis, who had established an NMR laboratory at Johns Hopkins Medical School, and Leon Saryan, a graduate student in biochemistry at Hopkins. Because a pulsed spectrometer like the one Damadian had used was not available at Johns Hopkins, Hollis arranged to borrow time, as Damadian had done more than a year earlier, on one of the machines at NMR Specialties in New Kensington.

An interesting juxtaposition of notable players in the NMR drama now occurred on the small stage that was NMR Specialties. If printed in a playbill, the performance could be described as follows: Act 1, which takes place in August 1969, features Freeman Cope and Raymond Damadian and their successful detection of potassium in biological tissue. Act 2, a solo performance by Raymond Damadian, portrays his breakthrough discoveries that cancer tissues exhibit remarkably long relaxation times compared to normal tissues and that the normal tissues themselves possess a diversity of NMR relaxations, thus providing a basis for the use of NMR in disease detection. Act 3 takes place in the first few days of September 1971, and features two performers—Leon Saryan* and Paul Lauterbur. Saryan was there to repeat Damadian's experiments to see if the same or similar results would be obtained. Paul Lauterbur, a chemistry professor at the State University of New York at Stony Brook, was there in a role quite different from the one he normally played. Although he was still wearing the hat of a scientist, that summer he was also wearing the hat of a businessman. Playing supporting roles in the drama of Act 3 were four rats from Johns Hopkins Medical School, all afflicted with a somewhat slower-growing type of malignant tumor than the ones analyzed by Damadian the year before.

Lauterbur had previously resided in the Pittsburgh area where he had done NMR research on silicon and carbon-13 for Dow Corning. Eventually, he had become a member of the board of directors for NMR Specialties. In the early part of 1971, he was notified as a member of the board that the company was in imminent danger of bankruptcy. If NMR Specialties was to avoid immediate closure, it would have to prove intent to change its ways by appointing a new interim president. Faced with a crisis, the other members of the board turned to Paul Lauterbur and asked him to take over. Since academic duties at Stony Brook were not demanding his attention that summer, Lauterbur consented and thus began a series of long commutes between Long Island and Pittsburgh.

Had Paul Yajko rather than Paul Lauterbur been at NMR Specialties that September, chances are good that the history of MR scanning and imaging might have developed quite differently.

Although Lauterbur was aware of Damadian's work, he did not receive its full impact until he saw virtually the same experiment repeated by Leon Saryan that summer. As he watched the rats being sacrificed, their tumor specimens removed, and the NMR measurements made, the importance of the Damadian discovery struck home. Noting the consistent differences in relaxation times obtained from various normal and malignant tissues, he began to wonder about ways to map those differences in the human body.

---

* Hollis and his collaborators confirmed that "in a general way" the T_1s of the liver tumors they tested were "very different from that of normal liver" and also confirmed, they reported, "that the water of malignant tissue is in a significantly less ordered state than that of normal tissue judging by its significantly longer T_1."
—Donald P. Hollis, Leon A. Saryan and Harold P. Morris, "A nuclear magnetic resonance study of water in two Morris hepatomas," *Hopkins Medical Journal* **131**, (1972), 441.

Later on that evening—September 2, 1971—Lauterbur came up with the first step* in accomplishing that objective when he thought of superimposing on the strong, uniform magnetic field passing through a patient a weaker, non-uniform magnetic field. Different from the saddle-shaped, non-uniform field chosen by Damadian to achieve spatial localization, Lauterbur's non-uniform magnetic field was linear. Unlike the non-uniformity of Damadian's saddle-shaped field, which provided complete 3-dimensional resolution, Lauterbur's non-uniform field spanned the entire imaging volume in one dimension, leaving the ultimate 2-dimensional pixel resolution to be achieved by a series of gradients and back projection.

By varying the strength of the weaker "gradient" field from one side of the sample to the other, thus giving different parts of the sample different resonant frequencies, Lauterbur realized that, at least in a one-dimensional sample, spatial localization could be achieved. Excited about the idea he had come up with, Lauterbur immediately went out and purchased a notebook to record and validate it. As reported by Ros Herman in *New Scientist*, "He wrote out his proposal at the beginning of a notebook, together with a reference to Damadian's *Science* paper on cell differences to show its applications, dated all this, and asked a colleague to countersign it."[78] (See handwritten laboratory notes in pages B1 through B3 of appendix to Chapter 9.)

As for the idea of body scanning, Lauterbur would later claim that he was unaware that Damadian had plans for anything other than test-tube biopsies. Damadian had indicated, however, his intention to use NMR as a scanning device in the first paragraph of his *Science* article where he stated: "In principle, nuclear magnetic resonance (NMR) techniques combine many of the desirable features of an external probe for the detection of internal cancer."[79]

In the 1973 *Nature* article in which Lauterbur first published his idea, he proposed that "a possible application of considerable interest at this time would be to the *in vivo* study of malignant tumours, which have been shown to give proton nuclear magnetic resonance signals with much longer water spin-lattice relaxation times than those in the corresponding normal tissues."[80] Instead of citing the obvious, which was Damadian's 1971 *Science* article, Lauterbur cited a follow-up study to Damadian's[81] by I.D. Weisman, et al. which had been published in *Science* in 1972, and which had referenced Damadian's work. The omission irked Damadian.

---

* The second necessary step, the concept of using a series of gradients together with back projection reconstruction, came later. Lauterbur added this contribution on October 30, 1972.

Damadian's seminal contribution was publicly acknowledged by Lauterbur in 1986 in a reprint of the speech Lauterbur gave when he accepted the Charles F. Kettering Prize from General Motors for his contributions to cancer detection via zeugmatography. In that speech, Lauterbur stated:

"The attention of the medical community was first attracted by the report of Damadian that some animal tumors have remarkably long proton NMR relaxation times."[82]

Another acknowledgement by Lauterbur of the importance of Damadian's contribution came in October 1987 at a Consensus Development Conference sponsored by the National Institutes of Health. On that occasion, Lauterbur stated, "The observations on tissue specimens from animal tumors reported by Damadian [in 1971] generated a great deal of interest, and attempts by others to confirm and extend that work were soon underway . . . The concept of image formation by MRI evolved in 1971, stimulated by the tissue studies of Damadian and of the Hollis group, and was published in 1973."[83] The Hollis group including Saryan, as mentioned earlier, was the group that successfully repeated Damadian's results at New Kensington.

When Damadian was asked his opinion of the key steps in the development of MRI, he stated without hesitation that MRI was the result of a *series* of important contributions. He recalled that the initial steps were taken by himself, Lauterbur and Peter Mansfield who supplied, respectively, the tissue relaxations, the means of displaying them, and the pulsed-gradient sequence methods. He further pointed out that additional key steps were provided by the two-dimensional Fourier transform contributed by Ernst and the practical implementation of it, "spin warping," contributed by Hutchison, Edelstein and Mallard of Aberdeen.

Science vs. Technology:
Putting the Damadian-Lauterbur Contributions in Perspective

In spite of the honest differences of opinion that exist among scientists as to the respective roles played by Damadian and Lauterbur in the development of magnetic resonance scanning and imaging, there is no question that both have made major contributions. Without Damadian's relaxation discoveries that showed sharp discrimination between tissues and particularly a serious disease like cancer, there would have been no reason to entertain or even consider a method for displaying the relaxation differences so they could be visualized (the image). Moreover, except for the relaxation differences discovered by Damadian, there would be no reason to expect that such an image would show anything, i.e. that any tissue NMR contrast existed with which to make an image.

Lauterbur, on the other hand, came up with the first practical method for visualizing these differences (the image) using the gradient together with back projection. The discussion is not, therefore, equivalent to "which came first, the chicken or the egg." In the case of MRI, Damadian's relaxation discoveries came first. Lauterbur's imaging idea came second.

Making a distinction between science and technology thus seems critical to an accurate understanding of the related contributions of these two pioneers. Science and technology are distinctly different enterprises. Technology waits on science. It does not advance on its own. When the fund of new scientific knowledge is depleted, technology runs aground. Science is the branch of knowledge that is dedicated to compiling factual information and understanding natural phenomena. Scientific research is restricted to uncovering new truths and new understandings about phenomena as they occur normally in nature. Its obvious purpose is to understand the processes of nature as thoroughly as possible so that methods (technology) can be devised to cope with its adversities or benefit from its "know-how." Without the new knowledge of natural phenomena (science), new methods (technology) for exploiting and taking advantage of nature's secrets cannot be created. The new knowledge, i.e., new scientific information, is necessarily the first step. Modern electronics, for example, could not have come to pass but for the basic *scientific* breakthroughs on the fundamental nature of electricity achieved in the 19th-century electricity laboratories of Europe. Today's solid-state technologies could not have occurred without the modern *science* of the atom.

Just as Rabi, Ramsey, Purcell, Bloch, Bloembergen and Hahn provided the scientific discoveries that gave rise to the technology of NMR, Raymond Damadian, a physician-scientist, provided the scientific discovery that permitted the transition from NMR to MRI to take place. That key step required both a scientist who could envision exactly how the NMR signal, through its relaxation, could be used to detect critical diseases such as cancer as well as a physician who could recognize the valuable role an NMR body scanner could play in hunting down diseased tissue in the body. *Such a combination of attributes in one person represents "an individual of statistically rare occurrence," concluded the late Professor Henry Wallman, a member of the Royal Swedish Academy of Sciences for 25 years. As such, he was a principal reviewer of the technical publications of candidates on behalf of the Nobel Committees in physics, chemistry and economics and a participant for many years in the selection of the recipients of the Nobel Prize in these fields (see Prologue).*

After a comprehensive review of the documentary record of the origins of MRI, Professor Wallman, himself a professor of applied electronics who invented X-ray television, for which he was named an honorary doctor of medicine, stated in writing in letters recommending Dr. Damadian for important awards: "I am of the definite opinion that Dr. Damadian's contribution was both prior to and more fundamental than Dr. Lauterbur's" [underlining included in original].*

The late Professor Gelbart, chairman of the Gelbart Institute for Advanced Mathematics at Bar-Ilan University and collaborator with Albert Einstein at the Institute for Advanced Study at Princeton, independently arrived at a conclusion similar to that of Professor Wallman, his friend of almost 60 years:

> *"The key to the development of MRI was a physician-scientist who could bridge the disciplines of modern physics and medicine and see the connections to make it happen—a rare confluence of circumstances."*

Gelbart further recognized that Dr. Damadian is clearly unique among the pioneers in that he personally and tenaciously followed up his scientific discovery. He built a human-size MR scanner that produced the first MR image; he then personally followed up with the creation of the first commercial scanner so that his invention could benefit the general public. (It has, indisputably and without exaggeration, revolutionized diagnostic medicine.) Today, he and his company continue to make technological advances in MRI despite the fact that they have since been joined by, and must compete with, the giants of the medical industry. Professor Gelbart viewed Dr. Damadian as a devoted father who never left the side of his discovery.†

One test of the importance of a scientific advance relative to its application is the permanence of the scientific advance. The important relaxation differences among healthy tissues and the distinct deviation of the cancerous relaxation from normal is permanently true. Cancers will always exhibit lengthened relaxations relative to normal.

The technology that arose from this scientific advance, however, is continuously undergoing change. The methods of imaging have, for example, changed markedly from the method Lauterbur proposed. Phase encoding has been substituted for frequency encoding on one of the two principal read axes. Back-projection reconstruction has been abandoned altogether. The 2-dimensional Fourier transform (2DFT) has been substituted for the 1-dimensional Fourier transform. Pulsed gradients are now utilized in place of the steady-state gradients of the Lauterbur

---

* Section referenced in Prologue.
† Section referenced in Tribute to Abraham Gelbart.

method, and a pulsed gradient supplies slice selection where slice selection was not provided for at all in the Lauterbur method.

While this does not diminish the contribution of Lauterbur since change is the essence of technology, it does underscore the permanence of a contribution of science relative to a contribution in technology and the reason advances on the scientific front are given such importance. While today's imaging techniques have a considerable likelihood of eventually being totally replaced by better and faster methods, Damadian's basic contribution of the relaxation differences of tissue and its importance will remain, available indefinitely for scientists and technologists to draw on in the future.

The Building of Indomitable:
The First Whole-Body Magnetic Resonance Scanning Machine

The prototype machine Damadian built on the basis of his "Pioneer Patent," on permanent display in the Smithsonian Institution, might initially be judged by a layperson as a simple device, especially alongside one of FONAR Corporation's latest, state-of-the-art MRI scanners. Given a bit more explanation, however, about the building of the strange-looking structure and the challenges they had to overcome in its construction, the viewer's reaction will likely be one of astonishment at the audacity of Damadian in even beginning the project and admiration for his successful completion of it.

In his book, *Nuclear Magnetic Resonance Imaging in Medicine and Biology,* Cambridge biochemistry professor Peter Morris provides a diagram showing how Damadian achieved his focused-aperture "sweet spot" in producing "the first ever whole-body scan" and then continues: "The 53-inch bore superconducting magnet and associated dewar was constructed by Damadian and his colleagues who had no previous experience in superconducting technology—a truly remarkable feat."[84]

It's noteworthy that an I.I. Rabi dream—Brookhaven National Laboratory on Long Island—contributed indirectly to the making of the first magnetic resonance scanner. Nearly three decades after Rabi and Norman Ramsey played key roles in the founding of Brookhaven National Laboratory—Ramsey was the first director of its physics department—Damadian called upon that department for assistance. It seems he was planning to build in his cramped laboratory space at Downstate Medical Center what would be the ninth largest magnet in the world in terms of stored energy—the eight larger ones were all busy splitting atoms in nuclear accelerators. Although Damadian had never built a magnet before, much less a 5,000-gauss superconducting magnet with a 53-inch bore, the physics department at Brookhaven helped him out by putting him in touch with the people who were building their latest particle accelerator, dubbed "Isabelle." Aided by software code from Isabelle's creators for calculating magnetic fields together with some urgently needed last-minute financial gifts from Bill and Clark Akers, John Rich and Jim Stewart, all of Nashville, Tennessee, Damadian designed and built the first full-body human MR scanner. He would call his creation "Indomitable."

It was an apt name. Not only did the name signify the determination of its inventor to see a dream fulfilled, it also applied to the machine itself. It would not be dominated by anyone, including Damadian. They started building the machine in early 1976 and for the next year-and-a-half, the machine dictated their lives.

First came the design. Even with the aid of the MAGMAP program from Brookhaven, there were many unknowns that had to be figured out. It was not like building a Heathkit. Indomitable would be one of a kind.

Next came the assembly. This phase was also not a nuts-and-bolts or even, for that matter, a solder-gun type of operation. Certainly the electronic end of the machine required activities such as soldering, but much of the task was just plain heavy shop work. For a medical doctor who was used to hovering over microscopic E. coli for days on end, this was a totally different kind of work—more blue collar than white lab coat. It required welding, heavy lifting, jackhammers. The reason jackhammers were needed was because Indomitable needed a storage tank to sit astride each huge magnet-containing dewar to replenish their liquid helium levels. With a storage tank, however, each six-foot tall dewar became 10 feet tall, too high to permit the tanks to be filled from inside Damadian's laboratory. The tanks would have to be filled from the floor above through holes jackhammered into the ceiling.

The reason liquid helium was needed was to keep the huge magnet coils super-cooled to near absolute zero temperatures. Absolute zero is minus 273.15 degrees Celsius; the helium had to be kept below -269 degrees Celsius or it would boil off into a useless gas. That required a Thermos-bottle-like arrangement called a dewar to drastically slow down the three main types of heat transfer—conduction, convection and radiation. Damadian's magnet design called for the construction of three large doughnut-shaped, hollow metal rings, the smallest nested inside the next larger one, and those, in turn, nested inside the third—one set for each magnet.

First, however, the two magnets themselves had to be made, each comprised of 30 miles of niobium-titanium superconducting wire, tightly and
precisely wound into hoops. Wire of two different diameters was needed,
wound into 52 layers, each layer comprised of 76 to 91 turns. These hoops
were then placed inside the smallest doughnut, which was made of polished stainless steel. To reduce heat conduction, the magnet was prevented from touching its container with special stand-off supports made of
material which was a poor conductor of heat.

The second doughnut, to be filled with liquid nitrogen to help cool the
helium, was made of aluminum wrapped with 85 layers of super-insu-
lating aluminized Mylar to bounce off unwanted heat radiation.

The third and largest doughnut, made of half-inch-thick aluminum,
contained the other two doughnuts, which were isolated additionally
from the heat of the laboratory by a vacuum of 10^{-9} TORR.

The magnet was superconducting, which meant that once it was
assembled and electricity was circulating through its wires, a special
"persistent switch" could be used to disconnect the magnet from its outside electrical supply and connect all the windings in a continuous loop
which, because of the lack of electrical resistance in the helium-bathed
wires, would permit electrical current to continue indefinitely, at least
theoretically.

In the real world of Damadian's SUNY laboratory, however, the liquid
helium for the magnet had to be replenished daily. In the process,
Indomitable, not unlike the meat-eating flower in the movie *The Little
Shop of Horrors*, became an indomitable tyrant demanding a constant supply of liquid helium which, if denied, would cause the thirsty machine to
erupt in, horror of all horrors, a quench. If heat was allowed to get to the
helium or if a bad butt-weld in the continuous wire loop developed resistance, heat would quickly spread, the liquid helium would boil off, and
all Damadian and his assistants would have to show for the work they
had done would be a ruined magnet.

Unfortunately, the helium storage tanks leaked intolerably and many
weeks were lost in detecting and plugging the leaks in the porous skin of
the aluminum container with surface welds. Finally, Damadian made the
decision to go with half of a Helmholtz pair. He and Larry Minkoff were
unable to achieve the vacuum seal needed to activate the second magnet.
Although the magnet was built to operate at 5,000 gauss, they would
have to make do with much less operating wire and only 10 percent of the
planned field strength. The team would have to try producing a human
image at only 500 gauss.

Since the whole thing was Damadian's idea, he volunteered to be the first "guinea pig." The first attempt was made in May 1977. With a blood-pressure cuff affixed to his right arm, EKG wires attached to his chest, and a ready oxygen tank at hand, Damadian sat on the narrow board used to position him in the scanner's sweet spot and waited for the first signals to be received, while a cardiologist hovered nearby in case of an emergency. Nothing happened. There was no emergency and there was no signal. They finally decided that the sample was too large for the card-board vest that housed the receiver antenna and that it had become detuned. A thinner sample was needed.

They didn't need to look far. Larry Minkoff was definitely thinner, he would be perfect. Minkoff felt otherwise. As precious time slipped by and as Goldsmith worked diligently to make additional antennas that would work, Minkoff dealt with the ultimate issues of life and death and final-ly, weeks later, consented to be the new sample. At this point, Damadian continues with the story.

It was July 2, 1977, more than six weeks after the failed attempt on me. [Minkoff] said he had decided that "the time for NMR scanning had come" and that, moreover, in the intervening weeks since I had been scanned, he hadn't detected any undue deterioration.

With the good news of Larry's announcement, Mike and I worked feverishly through the day to get Indomitable up to speed before Larry changed his mind. We had to get a field on Indomitable's mag-net, verify the vacuum was holding on the seals, establish that her liquid helium level was adequate and not evaporating from some new heat leaks, and be sure that the maze of electronics we had assembled to operate Indomitable for the scan was functioning according to "spec." It took me the better part of 14 hours to run through the two pages and 50 or so items on my MR scan checklist before we were ready for countdown.

By midnight, July 2, Indomitable was ready. Larry took his upright sitting position on the movable scanning rail inside Indomitable. He was positioned in Indomitable's magnetic field so that the signal-pro-ducing "sweet spot" (pea-sized) was centered in his heart. Mike and I rushed to the controls to see if there was a signal. This was where things had come apart on my scan.

To our great delight, a generous signal from Larry's chest greet-ed us on the oscilloscope. At the same time, we had verified that Larry "had a heart" after all, something Mike had begun to question. The world's first human scan, after all these months, was finally underway.

If Larry had any thought of getting out of the scanner at this point, having fulfilled his plan to "get a signal," Mike and I hastened to pre-empt such a move by quickly advancing him to the next scanning location to proceed with the scan.

Within a few minutes, the "sweet spot" was moved into Larry's lung field, a gas-filled region lacking water and therefore a region where the hydrogen NMR signal should be absent. It was! The scan was working. The "sweet spot" was successfully focusing within Larry's chest.

We continued to scan, moving inch-wise along one scanning line until the line was completed and then moving the scanning rail backwards one inch to begin a new scanning line. We proceeded in this fashion until 4:45 a.m. the morning of July 3, 1977, by which time 106 scanning points, arranged in a rectangular grid, had been collected.

Mike and I drew a sketch of this first scan in Mike's lab book, marked the image with some jubilant exclamatory about achieving the world's first human scan and saved the data for Joel Stutman, our computer scientist, to computer-interpolate the raw data and to form, in color, the first human image. [See pages A20 and A21 of appendix to this chapter for the handwritten laboratory notes related to this first image.]

The success of the first scan, Mink 5,[85-86] as we called it, was followed immediately by scans using the same "sweet spot" technique on two patients with malignancies,[86, 101] both of the chest, and also by a scan of Larry's normal abdomen.[85, 102]

The cross-sectional image of Minkoff's chest created with the data from the first scan roughly delineated his body wall, his right and left lungs, and his heart (including the right atrium and one of its ventricles). The "jubilant exclamatory" penned in Goldsmith's notebook by an ecstatic Damadian triumphantly declared:

4:45 A.M. FANTASTIC SUCCESS!
First Human Image
Complete in Amazing Detail
Showing Heart
Lungs
Vertebra
Musculature

Damadian's "amazing detail" claim seems amusing when contrasted with the images his scanners produce today, but the first human body MR images ever were far ahead of the pictures generated by the first CT scanners only a few years earlier. The first CT pictures required specialists to explain to doctors and radiologists what they were viewing. Damadian expected far less than what actually showed up on the first scan. His 1977 cross-sectional view of the human thorax comprised only 106 picture elements, with the values for each element manually entered in a matrix hand-drawn in the laboratory notebook of his assistant, Michael Goldsmith. Today, Damadian's scanners can acquire, in just minutes, the data to portray pinpoint-sized anatomical structure on electronic grids comprised of 65,000 or more picture elements, or pixels. The difference between the two is somewhat comparable to the difference between a cross-sectional view of the chest constructed with 106 multicolored Legos® plastic building blocks versus a black-and-white photo of the chest printed as a high-resolution halftone.

Damadian's reaction, however, was based on his ecstasy at seeing any detail at all. Obtaining a cross-sectional image of a live mouse, as he had done the year before in a much smaller, commercially produced magnet was a much different proposition than obtaining a cross-sectional image of a human thorax in a superconducting magnet designed and built by three people who had never before constructed a magnet more elaborate than the kind built with six-volt batteries in a grade-school science project. Nor was the magnet the only unknown quantity. There was also the chest-sized receiver coil that six weeks earlier had produced nothing when Damadian had been the guinea pig and had climbed with trepidation into his own machine while a cardiologist stood by just in case the large magnetic field initiated cardiac arrest in the sample.

Looking back with hindsight, the precautions are seen as overkill. Of course, presoaking paraffin in a magnet for 10 hours, as Purcell did, to ensure that thermal equilibrium had occurred when it actually occurs in less than a second, was also overkill, as was Bloch's magnetic "cooking" of the water sample for his nuclear induction experiment to ensure thermal equilibrium had been reached. While waiting for the protons to thermally relax, Bloch relaxed on a ski trip to the Sierras. Looking silly, it seems, both before and after a breakthrough discovery, is one of the occupational hazards faced by those who make such discoveries. The risks associated with discovery, both real and imagined, are always taken by the inventor, not by the reverse engineer who traces his footsteps.

Nine Months After the First Whole-Body MR Image:
A Company to Build the First Commercial NMR Scanners

To follow his dream to conclusion so that MR scanners would quickly become available to the public and to enable himself to continue in the development of the medical uses of NMR to help alleviate as many diseases as possible, Damadian formed a company to manufacture MRI machines. Nine months after the first whole-body MR image was achieved, Damadian founded FONAR, named after the acronym he had used for his magnetic field focusing method. In June 1978, the fledgling company rented its first home, a 5,000-square-foot facility in Plainview, New York, near the border of Nassau and Suffolk counties on Long Island.

Even before launching his company, however, Damadian decided that for his first commercial scanner, he was going to go with a permanent magnet instead of a superconductor. Initially, the decision met with resistance. Why, after achieving success with a superconductor, would he drop what had already been proven to work and go with another kind of magnet? But Damadian was adamant. For him, the superconductor had proven too costly to be worthy of consideration commercially. What they saved in electricity, they more than made up for in helium costs. Hospitals would have to struggle to finance them. Patients and their insurance companies would find the high scan fees created by the high equipment costs a burden. His mind was made up; his next MRI scanner would have a permanent magnet.

But no one had ever built a permanent magnet MRI. Goldsmith doubted it could be done and was not convinced that the magnetic field homogeneity needed for imaging could be achieved with a permanent magnet. Damadian thought they could. He immediately began constructing model magnets using small permanent-magnet bricks and steel, and then wheeled over the NMR apparatus with a sample to get a signal. The first signals were feeble as Goldsmith had guessed, but within a few days Damadian had a magnet structure that would produce a robust signal. The anticipated homogeneity problem of the permanent magnet was solved. Damadian and his company had created the first permanent-magnet MRI machine. To Damadian's mind, a practical and cost-effective MRI scanner had at last been achieved.

The first MRI scanner was introduced to the world at the April 1980 annual meeting of the American Roentgen Ray Society and later that year at the annual meeting of the Radiological Society of North America (RSNA). It was also the first permanent-magnet MRI. For many of the radiologists roaming through the RSNA's technical exhibits in 1980, MRI wasn't even in their vocabulary. Those who, out of curiosity, ventured into the exhibit sponsored by FONAR saw a futuristic machine and a full array of MRI images which looked like nothing they had worked with in the past.

The first two scanners produced by the company were installed in the offices of Drs. Ross, Lie, Thompson and Associates, a radiology group in private practice in Cleveland, Ohio, and in the University of Mexico in Monterrey, Nuevo Leon, Mexico. Although Damadian would later adopt other scanning methods which would be faster and provide superior image quality, his first commercial scanners shipped in 1981 would prove beyond question the diagnostic validity of his original patented method. Before Damadian's first commercial scanners were retired from active service and replaced by later state-of-the-art machines, thousands of patients would be scanned using his "sweet spot" method.

A second model dropped the patented "sweet spot" technique and adopted, in part, Paul Lauterbur's gradient/back-projection imaging method. Two such scanners were shipped to users in Italy and Japan before Damadian abandoned further development of the Lauterbur back-projection approach and went to the greatly-improved method developed by the University of Aberdeen researchers that employed the 2-dimensional Fourier transform idea of Richard Ernst.

Interested next in the prospect of making MRI available to hospitals that could not afford the outright purchase of a scanner, he and his company took on the task of developing a new scanner that would be transportable on a truck and enable hospitals and their patients to share the services of an MRI scanner. Before this could be done, a third MRI magnet had to be created. The permanent magnet was too heavy. Retaining the iron frame of the permanent magnet, he and his company built the first iron-frame electromagnet for MRI. Water-cooled and much lighter in weight, these magnets are rapidly increasing in popularity as their versatility and ability to provide an "open" environment for the patient during scanning have become more widely appreciated.

The permanent magnet and water-cooled electromagnets Damadian and his company developed had another advantage. They overcame a significant problem encountered when the MRI was installed in a hospital setting, namely the large fringing magnetic field that interfered with hospital equipment and interacted with other metal in the hospital environment. The iron frame of Damadian's new MRI magnets contained the magnetic flux within the magnet and reduced the fringing magnetic field to a minimum. Overcoming this problem enabled his scanners to be used in conjunction with life-support equipment such as respirators and cardiac monitors, thus enabling emergency patients dependent on this equipment to be scanned, when they could not be scanned in supercon MRIs.

The vertical field of his new iron-frame permanent magnets and electromagnets had other advantages. It enabled him and his team to develop a new class of more versatile radiofrequency antennas, surface coils that could be individually wrapped around specific parts of the body for specialized scanning procedures. These "solenoidal" surface coils permitted high-quality images to be acquired from the knee, cervical spine, shoulder, temporomandibular joint and similar regions, together with motion-picture MRI images of these structures. The topical images made possible by the wide array of surface coils he and his company introduced and the anatomic detail they provide have made surface coils an indispensable part of modern-day MRI imaging.

In 1984, he and his company were able to advance MRI technology another step. Up to this point, MRI images were confined to the three right-angle planes, the so-called axial, sagittal and coronal planes. A small team of researchers within his company recognized that, by operating two slice-select gradients in concert, the slice could be tilted to any arbitrary angle. Oblique MRI imaging was born. A year later, the same team developed a technique that allowed the individual slices of a stack of slices to be individually angled. Oblique imaging and multi-angle oblique imaging, as the latter method was called, filled a common need in medical imaging, namely the ability to obtain accurate pictures of structures within the human anatomy that are oriented at arbitrary angles. The new method was quickly adopted and is in wide use today on MRI scanners around the world, particularly for showing herniation of vertebral discs.

The MRI Magnet: Damadian's Patents on the Superconducting Magnets, Iron Electromagnets and Permanent Magnets of MRI

Beginning with Indomitable, Dr. Damadian always perceived magnet capability as a principal limitation on which medical arenas MRI would be able to explore. As a result, of all the magnets in use today—the *"supercon"* magnet, the *permanent magnet* and *the iron frame electromagnet*—Damadian and his collaborators *pioneered and introduced all three.*

One of the disappointments Damadian has contended with since MR scanning became a commercial enterprise has been the high cost associated with magnetic resonance imaging. It had been his intention to see medical costs drop because of the usefulness of his invention in early detection and treatment of disease. He did not expect to see MRI costs become a burden to medicine. Most importantly, the high scan fee caused by the high scanner price has limited its use. Many valuable medical uses of MRI go unexplored because of the costliness of the MRI procedure. Earlier detection and treatment have, in fact, resulted from the availability of MRI. Almost everyone knows someone who has been helped because of MRI, if not by personal acquaintance, then certainly by news of public personalities who have had an MRI scan.

Unfortunately, costs did not go down. As Damadian had predicted, the high operating costs of superconducting MRI machines were being passed on in higher prices for the patient. He determined to find a way to change the trend.

Twenty-Five Years After the Cancer Signal: The Costs Must Come Down

June 1995 marked the 25th anniversary of Damadian's discovery of the abnormal relaxation times of cancer tissue. The way Damadian sees it, however, there is still so much more to be done. The cost of MRI must come down, he says, if MRI is to achieve the universal usage in medicine everyone foresees.

More Research

Substantially reducing the cost meant more research. Newer and more cost-efficient magnets, component designs and printed-circuit boards were in order. Damadian and his team dedicated themselves to research and development efforts to achieve substantial cost reduction. Their efforts to lighten the burden on the public purse were successful. In 1994, his company was able to introduce an MRI scanner with more capability than earlier models and at half the cost. The reduced cost of the scanner is expected to lower the scan price to the patient so that serious needs like MRI mammography, currently impeded by the high cost of an MRI scan, can be addressed. Damadian and his research teams have put a special emphasis on MRI mammography research where they believe MRI has a great deal to contribute to visualizing the soft tissue detail needed for accurate diagnosis of breast disease and where they believe X-ray imaging is at a disadvantage. The research to reduce scanner cost further continues.

From the beginning, unlike the superconducting MRI he put aside after the high operating costs he experienced with Indomitable, the MRI he and his team developed had a quiet environment and an open architecture so that patients could stretch out their arms. The open architecture and low fringe field of their designs have made them ideal for new MRI advancements.

The *openness* of the magnet design has enabled full-range-of-motion anatomical studies that cannot be undertaken in the confining cylindrical bore of the superconducting magnet. It has enabled him and his research group to develop dedicated, computer-automated fixtures to support joints such as the knee, shoulder, cervical spine and lumbar spine as they function. This "motion-picture" capability enables doctors to visualize the impact of surgery on function so they are not limited to evaluating surgical procedures from the static images provided by conventional imaging technology.

The second benefit derived from the open architecture iron-frame magnet designs he and his company pioneered has been the prospect of MRI-guided surgery. Damadian's most recent designs enable the patient to be approached from three sides, providing medical and surgical teams easy access to the patient while the patient is being scanned. Detailed visualizations of soft tissue anatomy via "on line" MRI imaging simultaneous with the performance of surgical procedures is expected to further advance the delicate art of surgery.

The new-found ability to visualize the soft tissue detail that MRI brings to the operating theater can be counted on in the future to greatly expand the number of operations that will be converted to "closed" techniques, such as laparoscopy, and to increase the precision with which they can be performed.

Over and over again, Damadian has been vindicated in his decisions regarding scanner design. To obtain the signal-to-noise ratios he thought necessary to obtain the first human scan, he built a superconducting magnet. When the costs of operating a "supercon" seemed clinically impractical, he abandoned it for a permanent magnet. Later, to reduce weight, he was the first to introduce a water-cooled, iron-frame, vertical-field electromagnet so that mobile MRI could be provided to hospitals that couldn't afford their own scanners.

For many years, MRI users have debated the benefits of high-field, superconducting, air-core solenoid magnets relative to the benefits of the mid-field iron frame magnets, both permanent and electromagnetic, pioneered by Dr. Damadian and his team. In recent years, the debate shows signs that it may be resolved in favor of the design Damadian considers best overall.

At a recent Radiological Society of North America (RSNA) show in December 1994, virtually every major MRI manufacturer introduced one of the 0.2 to 0.3 tesla iron-frame magnets, either a permanent magnet or an electromagnet—magnets and fields they once shunned—that Dr. Damadian and his company were the first to introduce and on which they hold the original patents.

As radiologist Dr. David Stark, author of the authoritative textbook of MRI, *Magnetic Resonance Imaging,* (Mosby) wrote in a recent editorial in *Applied Radiology,* the great field-strength debate is over.

The great field strength debate lasted one decade. . . . Increasing field strength was an obvious, and expensive, approach to improve image quality. Although it is unarguable that increasing field strength increases image quality by increasing image signal-to-noise ratios (SNR) achievable during a given scan time, over the past few years it has become apparent that increasing field yields only frac-tional gains in SNR, not the exponential bonanza touted in the 1980s. . . . The *Wall Street Journal* reported November 15, 1994 that applica-tions unique to MRI at high-field had failed to mature and that the market has turned toward modern mid-field and low-field systems offering improved image quality at lower cost. . . . The new-found prestige of mid-field systems is attributable to inexpensive perma-nent and resistive electromagnet technology (non-cryogenic) that offers the open architecture (non-claustrophobic) preferred by virtu-ally all patients.

Stark concluded his editorial by stating, "As we finish the century guided by cost and efficacy concerns, these efficient new MRI systems will allow more patients to benefit from comfortable, high-quality diag-nostic imaging."[88] Cost-effective MRI and open-access MRI, all made pos-sible by the iron-frame MRI magnets originally pioneered by Dr. Damadian and his company now appear to be the wave of the future in MRI and for a wide range of new MRI applications, a very bright future indeed.

Much has occurred in the century between Roentgen's 1895 discovery of the mysterious rays which enabled physicians, for the first time, to look beneath the surface of the human body and Stark's 1995 editorial. In 1939, Professor I.I. Rabi and his graduate student, Norman F. Ramsey, concluded the paper in which they announced their discovery of a new spectroscopy—NMR spectroscopy. "Our results," they wrote, "show that it is possible to apply exact spectroscopic principles and procedures to spectral regions which correspond to *ordinary radio waves* [italics added]. The accuracy to which the laws of quantum mechanics hold and the necessity of their application in a region of frequency in which one is accustomed to think classically we consider a striking confirmation of the theory."[89]

At the time, they could not foresee all of the method's potential, nor the major war that lay between them and further development of the method, a war in which the lives of thousands of physicists like themselves—including two by the names of Edward Purcell and Felix Bloch—would be disrupted by the duties of scientific combat. In fact, a decade would pass before Ramsey would develop the theory for chemical shifts, one of NMR spectroscopy's early finds that would revolutionize chemical analysis and two more decades would pass before a scientist by the name of Raymond Damadian would apply in 1970 the power of NMR to the detection of disease in biological tissue.

> In principle [wrote Damadian in late 1970], nuclear magnetic resonance (NMR) techniques combine many of the desirable features of an external probe for the detection of internal cancer. Magnetic resonance measurements cause no obvious deleterious effects on biologic tissue, the incident radiation consisting of *common radio frequencies* [italics added] at right angles to a static field. The detector is external to the sample, and the method permits one to resolve information emitted by the sample to atomic dimensions. Thus the spectroscopist has available for study a wide range of nuclei for evidence of deviant chemical behavior.[90]

Ramsey and Rabi and their associates, Jerome Kellogg and Jerrold Zacharias, said that their method used "ordinary radio waves." Damadian said his method used "common radio frequencies." But the medical results that emanated from the science of NMR would be anything but "ordinary" and "common."

For his pioneering contributions, Raymond Damadian has received: the National Engineers' Special Recognition Award (1985), the Lawrence Sperry Award (1984), the National Medal of Technology (1988), induction into the National Inventors' Hall of Fame (1989), and selection of the first human MRI scanner, Indomitable, for permanent exhibit in the Smithsonian Institution, Washington, DC (1986), among others.

A Vision for the Future

Early in his medical training, Damadian chose internal medicine because of its analytical nature. By the time he graduated, he decided to do his detective work in the research laboratory rather than the clinic because of the prospects that his research, if successful, might help millions of people rather than the thousands he could reach dispensing medical treatments. "I didn't know if anything would come of any research I might do, but I knew I wanted the chance to try to help many more than I could personally reach in a lifetime."[91]

Damadian, the First to Conceive of the NMR Whole-Body NMR Scanner (1969) and the First to Construct It (1977)

The *first step* across the vast terrain to be traversed from the practice of clinical medicine to the physics of NMR before the new medical scanner envisioned by Damadian could become reality came in *1969*, four years before Lauterbur's first paper appeared in *Nature* in *1973*. In a letter to the Health Research Council of the City of New York where Dr. Damadian had been chosen for the "Career Scientist" award, he wrote, "I am very much interested in the potential of NMR spectroscopy for early non-destructive detection [emphasis included in original document] of internal malignancies."[92] (See page A3 of appendix to this chapter.)

The *second step* towards the new scanner came in *March 1971*, two years before Lauterbur's March 1973 *Nature* paper, when Damadian proved the reality of his vision by showing that the NMR signal from cancer tissue was different from normal, that there were also marked differences among the healthy tissues, and that these differences could provide the basis for the new body scanner he envisioned. In this paper, published in *Science*, he wrote: "In principle, nuclear magnetic resonance (NMR) techniques combine many of the desirable features of an external probe for the detection of internal cancer."[93] (See page A7 of appendix to this chapter.)

The *third step* came very shortly thereafter in the *Spring 1971* issue of the *Downstate Reporter* (page A4 of appendix to this chapter), also two years before Lauterbur's first publication in *Nature*. In an article entitled, "Basic Research Leads to Radio Signals from Cancer Tissue," science reporter Ed Edelson spelled out Dr. Damadian's intentions to use that signal to build his new scanner:

"Already, Dr. Damadian is planning to build a much larger nuclear magnetic resonance device, one that will be big enough to hold a human being. That machine, Dr. Damadian believes, will prove that nuclear magnetic resonance (NMR) is the tool that doctors have been looking for in their quest for a method of detecting cancer early, when treatment is most effective."[94] (See page A4 of appendix to this chapter.)

The article also shows, two years before Lauterbur's first 1973 *Nature* paper,* Dr. Damadian taking the first step towards his "sweet spot" technique for achieving the spatial localization needed for scanning. It reported:

"The proposed NMR device for detecting cancer in humans would not have to be highly elaborate, Dr. Damadian says. It would consist of a large coil to emit radio waves and a movable magnet to create the magnetic field required. The coil would be wrapped around the patient's chest, while the magnet passed back and forth across the body. A detector would pick up NMR emissions for analysis."[95] [See page A5 of appendix to this chapter. See also the letter of G. Donald Vickers (pages A22-A23 of appendix to this chapter) who was the signatory witness for Lauterbur's conception of the gradient (pages B1 through B3 of appendix to Chapter 9).]

The *fourth step* toward fulfillment of Damadian's NMR body scanner vision came on *March 17, 1972*, one year before Lauterbur's publication appeared in *Nature*[96] on *March 16, 1973*, with the filing of his patent entitled "Apparatus and Method for Detecting Cancer in Tissue"[97] (page A13 of appendix to this chapter). Figure 2 of the patent depicts a man standing in an electromagnet, showing a mobile radiofrequency assembly to accompany the movement of the patient across the magnet's "sweet spot" for scanning. Shaping of the transmitted radiofrequency field is added in the patent to provide further spatial localization to the magnet's "sweet

---

* This *published* initial idea for the "sweet spot" approach to *3-dimensional* spatial localization by Damadian occurred six months before Lauterbur's initial idea, in his *notebook*, that a gradient can supply spatial localization for *one dimension* (pages B1 through B3 of appendix to Chapter 9). Lauterbur does not achieve a solution to the *2-dimensional* case needed for mapping a plane until a year later. As of the time of Lauterbur's notebook entry in September 1971, both scientists appear to be proceeding on the same path, Damadian referring to his spin localizing concept as NMR scanning and Lauterbur referring to his as mapping.

spot." The *complete* description of Damadian's "sweet spot" method of NMR scanning (pages A10 through A19 of appendix to this chapter) precedes Lauterbur's report of his *completed* scanning method by *seven months*. Lauterbur's manuscript describing his *completed* scanning method was received for the first time at the publishers on *October 30, 1972*.[98]

The *fifth step* in the final realization of Damadian's vision came in 1977 when he and his team constructed the first human scanner and used the "sweet spot" technique of his patent to accomplish the first human scan and prove to the world that whole-body NMR scanning was achievable.[99-100] Lauterbur did not take this step.

It is thus unambiguous that Damadian is the originator of the NMR body scanner concept, preceding Lauterbur's first conceptualization of an NMR scanner by years. Moreover, Damadian was the first to supply the tissue NMR signal differences that made the concept reality. While history has shown the Lauterbur method superior to the Damadian method in speed and efficiency, there is no doubt that Damadian is the originator of the NMR scanning concept and that he uncovered the tissue NMR signals that made it possible.

The contributions of *both* pioneers to the creation of MRI have been essential to its genesis. The President of the United States, for example, in a ceremony at the White House on July 15, 1988, awarded the nation's highest honor in technology, the National Medal of Technology, jointly to the two pioneers of MRI featured in this volume. He cited them "for their independent contributions in conceiving and developing the application of magnetic resonance technology to medical uses included whole-body scanning and diagnostic imaging" (page A24 of appendix to this chapter).

Today, because of Damadian, thousands of MR scanners around the world are producing millions of images that exquisitely depict both healthy and diseased tissue without the need for invasive procedures and without the ionizing radiation of X-rays. ■

REFERENCE NOTES:

1. R.V. Damadian, interview by James Mattson, 10 November 1994.
2. Ibid.
3. Sonny Kleinfield, *A Machine Called Indomitable*, (New York: Times Books, 1985), 45.
4. R.V. Damadian, interview by Mattson, 10 November 1994.
5. Ibid.
6. Kleinfield, *A Machine Called Indomitable*, 149-150.
7. R.V. Damadian, interview by Mattson, 10 November 1994.
8. Ibid.
9. Kleinfield, *A Machine Called Indomitable*, 47.
10. R.V Damadian, interview by Mattson, 11 November 1994.
11. Ibid.
12. Ibid.
13. Ibid.
14. Kleinfield, *A Machine Called Indomitable*, 147.
15. R.V. Damadian, interview by Mattson, 11 November 1994.
16. Ibid.
17. Kleinfield, *A Machine Called Indomitable*, 52.
18. Ibid.
19. R.V. Damadian, interview by Mattson, 11 November 1994.
20. R.V. Damadian, interview by Mattson, 18 November 1994.
21. Ibid.
22. George E. Pake, interview by James Mattson, 27 January 1993.
23. George E. Pake, "Nuclear magnetic resonance in bulk matter," *Physics Today*, October 1993, 49-50.
24. Ibid., 50.
25. Richard R. Ernst, autobiographical sketch, *Les Prix Nobel 1991*, (Stockholm: Nobel Foundation, 1982), 66.
26. R.V. Damadian, letter to George S. Mirick, MD, scientific director, The Health Research Council of the City of New York, 17 September 1969.
27. R.V. Damadian, "Tumor detection by nuclear magnetic resonance," *Science* **171**, (19 March 1971), 1151-1153.
28. Kleinfield, *A Machine Called Indomitable*, 9.
29. R.V. Damadian, interview by Mattson, 11 November 1994.
30. R. Dean, *Biol. Symp.* **3**, (1941), 331.
31. A. Krogh, *Proc. Roy. Soc. (London) Ser. B* **133**, (1946), 140.
32. Raymond V. Damadian, Edmond Shwayri and Neal S. Bricker, "On the existence of non-urine forming nephrons in the diseased kidney of the dog." *J. Lab. and Clin. Med.* **65**, (1965), 26-39.
33. R.V. Damadian, interview by Mattson, 11 November 1994.
34. Ibid.
35. Ibid.
36. S. Schultz and A.K. Solomon, "Cation transport in *Escherichia coli*. I. Intracellular Na and K concentrations and net cation movement," *J. Gen. Physiol.* **45**, (1961), 355.
37. R.V. Damadian, interview by Mattson, 11 November 1994.
38. R.V. Damadian, interview by Mattson, 10 December 1994.
39. R.V. Damadian and A.K. Solomon, "Bacterial mutant with impaired potassium transport and methionine biosynthesis," *Science* **145**, (1964), 1327-1328.
40. R.V. Damadian, interview by Mattson, 11 November 1994.
41. Ibid.

42. F. Hellferich, *Ion Exchange*, (New York: McGraw-Hill Book Co., 1962).

43. R.V. Damadian, "Abnormal phosphorus metabolism in a potassium transport mutant of *Escherichia coli*," *USAF Technical Report* **65**, (1967), 1-6.

44. J.A. Pople, W.G. Schneider and H.J. Bernstein, *High-Resolution Nuclear Magnetic Resonance*, (New York: McGraw-Hill, 1959).

45. R.V. Damadian, interview by Mattson, 11 November 1994.

46. L. Dunham, S. Nichols and A. Brunschwig, *Cancer Res.* **6**, (1946), 230.

47. R.V. Damadian, interview by Mattson, 11 November 1994.

48. Ibid.

49. Ibid.

50. Ibid.

51. R.V. Damadian, "The story of MRI," published reprint of speech given to Washington Patent Lawyers Club, Washington, DC, 10 February 1992.

52. E. Odeblad, B.N. Bohr and G. Lindstrom, "Proton magnetic resonance of human red blood cells in heavy water exchange experiments," *Arch. Biochem. Biophys.* **63**, (1956), 221-225.

53. E. Odeblad, "Micro-NMR in high permanent magnetic fields: theoretical and experimental investigations with an application to the secretions from single glandular units in the human uterine cervix," *Acta. Obstet. Gynecol. Scand.* (1966), Supplement 2, 45.

54. J.R. Singer, "Blood flow rates by NMR," *Science* **130**, (1959), 1652-1653.

55. C.B. Bratton, A.L. Hopkins and J.W. Weinberg, "Nuclear magnetic resonance studies of living muscle," *Science* **147**, (1965), 738-739.

56. T.R. Ligon, unpublished MS thesis, (1967), Oklahoma State University, Oklahoma.

57. Jasper A. Jackson and Wright H. Langham, "Whole-body NMR spectrometer," *Review of Scientific Instruments* **39**, (1967), 510-513.

58. F. Cope and R. Damadian, "Cell potassium by K^{39} spin echo nuclear magnetic resonance," *Nature* **228**, (1970), 76-77.

59. R.V. Damadian, letter to George S. Mirick, MD, scientific director, The Health Research Council of the City of New York, 17 September 1969.

60. R.V. Damadian, "The story of MRI," published reprint of speech given to Washington Patent Lawyers Club, Washington, DC, 10 February 1992.

61. R.V. Damadian, personal communication with James Mattson, 12 June 1995.

62. Ibid.

63. Felix W. Wehrli, "The origins and future of nuclear magnetic resonance imaging," *Physics Today*, June 1992, 38.

64. Felix W. Wehrli, "The significance of contrast in NMR images," back cover, *Radiology* **147**:12, (1983).

65. P.C. Lauterbur, "Cancer detection by nuclear magnetic resonance zeugmatographic imaging," *Cancer* **57**, (1986), 1899.

66. Felix W. Wehrli, "The significance of contrast in NMR images," back cover, *Radiology* **147**:12, (1983).

67. Pake, "Nuclear magnetic resonance in bulk matter," 49-50.

68. Ed Edelson, "Basic research leads to radio signals from cancer signals," *Downstate Reporter* **2**, (Spring 1971), 1.

69. R.V. Damadian, personal communication with Mattson, 12 June 1995.

70. R. Damadian, K. Zaner, D. Hor and T. DiMaio, "Human tumors by nuclear magnetic resonance," *Physiol. Chem. and Physics* **5**, (1973), 381-402.

71. R. Damadian, K. Zaner, D. Hor, T. DiMaio, L. Minkoff and M. Goldsmith, "Nuclear magnetic resonance as a new tool in cancer research: human tumors by NMR," International Conference on Electron Spin Resonance and Nuclear Magnetic Resonance in Biology and Medicine and Fifth International Conference on Magnetic Resonance in Biological Systems, *Annals of the New York Academy of Sciences* **222**, (1974), 1048-1076.

72. R. Damadian, K. Zaner, D. Hor and T. DiMaio, "Human tumors detected by nuclear magnetic resonance," *Proc. Nat. Acad. Sci. USA* 71, (1974), 1471-1473.

73. P. Mansfield and P.G. Morris, *NMR Imaging in Biomedicine*, Supplement 2 to *Advances in Magnetic Resonance*, edited by John S. Waugh, (New York: Academic Press, 1982), 21.

74. K.S. Zaner and R.V. Damadian, "Phosphorus-31 as a nuclear probe for malignant tumors," *Science* 189, (1975), 729-731.

75. R.V. Damadian, interview by James Mattson, 5 December 1994.

76. Raymond V. Damadian, U.S. Patent No. 3,789,832, "Apparatus and method for detecting cancer in tissue," filed 17 March 1972, issued 5 February 1974.

77. George W. Bush, President of the United States, in a letter written 10 February 1989 and read to the attendees of the 1989 induction ceremony of the National Inventors Hall of Fame.

78. Ros Herman, "A chemical clue to disease," *New Scientist*, 15 March 1979, 876.

79. R.V. Damadian, "Tumor detection by nuclear magnetic resonance," *Science* 171, (19 March 1971), 1151-1153.

80. P.C. Lauterbur, "Image formation by induced local interactions: examples employing nuclear magnetic resonance," *Nature* 242, (16 March 1973), 190.

81. Irwin Weisman, Lawrence H. Bennett, Louis R. Maxwell, Sr., Mark W. Woods and Dean Burk, "Recognition of cancer *in vivo* by nuclear magnetic resonance," *Science* 178, (1972), 1288.

82. P.C. Lauterbur, "Cancer detection by nuclear magnetic resonance zeugmatographic imaging," *Cancer* 57, (1986), 1899.

83. P.C. Lauterbur, "The first 20 years of MRI and *in vivo* spectroscopy," NIH Consensus Development Conference, National Institutes of Health, 26-28 October 1987.

84. Peter G. Morris, *Nuclear Magnetic Resonance Imaging in Medicine and Biology*, (Oxford: Clarendon Press, 1986), 79.

85. R. Damadian, M. Goldsmith and L. Minkoff, "NMR in cancer: XVI. FONAR image of the live human body," *Physiological Chemistry and Physics* 9, (1977), 97-108.

86. R. Damadian, "Field focusing n.m.r. (FONAR) and the formation of chemical images in man," *Phil. Trans. Royal Society London* B289, (1980), 489-500.

87. Raymond V. Damadian, "The story of MRI," reprint of a speech by Damadian delivered to the Washington Patent Lawyers Club on 10 February 1992.

88. David D. Stark, "The argument for mid-field MRI," *Applied Radiology*, (February 1995), 9.

89. J.M.B. Kellogg, I.I. Rabi, N.F. Ramsey and J.R. Zacharias, "The magnetic moments of the proton and the deuteron. The radiofrequency spectrum of H_2 in various magnetic fields," *Physical Review* 56, (1939), 728.

90. R.V. Damadian, "Tumor detection by nuclear magnetic resonance," *Science* 171, (19 March 1971), 1151-1153.

91. R.V. Damadian, interview by Mattson, 5 December 1994.

92. R.V. Damadian, letter to George S. Mirick, MD, scientific director, The Health Research Council of the City of New York, 17 September 1969.

93. R.V. Damadian, "Tumor detection by nuclear magnetic resonance," *Science* 171, (19 March 1971), 1151-1153.

94. Ed Edelson, "Basic research leads to radio signals from cancer signals," *Downstate Reporter* 2, (Spring 1971), 1.

95. Ibid., 4.

96. P.C. Lauterbur, "Image formation by induced local interactions: examples employing nuclear magnetic resonance," *Nature* 242, (16 March 1973), 190.

97. Raymond V. Damadian, U.S. Patent No. 3,789,832, "Apparatus and method for detecting cancer in tissue," filed 17 March 1972, issued 5 February 1974.

98. P.C. Lauterbur, "Image formation by induced local interactions: examples employing nuclear magnetic resonance," *Nature* 242, (16 March 1973), 191.

99. R. Damadian, M. Goldsmith and L. Minkoff, "NMR in cancer: XVI. FONAR image of the live human body," *Physiological Chemistry and Physics* **9**, (1977), 97-108.

100. R. Damadian, "Field focusing n.m.r. (FONAR) and the formation of chemical images in man," *Phil. Trans. Royal Society London* **B289**, (1980), 489-500.

101. R. Damadian, M. Goldsmith and L. Minkoff, "NMR in cancer: XX. FONAR scans of patients with cancer," *Physiological Chemistry and Physics* **10**, (1978), 285-290.

102. R. Damadian, L. Minkoff and M. Goldsmith, "NMR in cancer: XXI. FONAR scan of live human abdomen," *Physiological Chemistry and Physics* **10**, (1978), 561-563.

STATE UNIVERSITY
OF NEW YORK

DOWNSTATE MEDICAL CENTER

BIOPHYSICAL LABORATORY
• DEPARTMENT OF MEDICINE

· September 17, 1969

George S. Mirick, M.D.
Scientific Director
The Health Research Council
   of the City of New York
Department of Health
455 First Avenue
New York, New York 10016

Dear Dr. Mirick:

In accord with our telephone conversation of September 16, 1969, I am forwarding
a letter describing the success of our "Pittsburgh Experiment" and the request
for support it has inspired.

On August 21, 1969, Dr. Freeman Cope and I left for a small company (Nuclear
Magnetic Resonance Specialties Corporation) on the outskirts of Pittsburgh with
the remote hope that we could measure potassium by NMR spectroscopy and establish,
once and for all, that cell potassium is not free in solution as usually supposed
but organized in structured cell H_2O and complexed to fixed charges within the
cell. Our hopes were remote since K+ of any kind, cellular or inorganic, had never
been measured by NMR and most experts seemed to agree that our prospects were grim.
Grim, because out of all the nuclei on the atomic table, its resonance point was
among the lowest. Consequently, its signal was expected to be much weaker than
could be detected by existing equipment.

We banked our hopes on a superconducting magnet* that Nuclear Magnetic Resonance
Specialties Corporation had agreed to.make available to us for a few days use. If
we could generate large enough magnetic fields, we had a chance. The superconducting magnet was rated for 50,000 gauss (the best of the commercially available
electromagnets generate 25,000 gauss), which would permit us to receive the signal
at 10 megacycles instead of 2, thereby amplifying our sensitivity 25 times. Other
modifications such as the use of a signal pre-amplifier and a time averaging computer when taken together were estimated to produce an additional 10 fold amplification of signal.

*
Superconducting magnets make use of the absence of electrical resistivity of
certain alloys (e.g. niobium zirconium, niobium titanium, niobium tin, etc.) at
cryogenic temperatures (e.g. 4.3° Kelvin - achieved by immersion of the solenoid
in liquid helium). Zero electrical loss is the result and it is possible to produce magnetic fields with an efficiency that/approaches 100%. Conventional electromagnets dissipate most of the energy supplied to the windings as heat. Consequently
the fields that can be generated are limited by the heat tolerances of the windings.

George S. Mirick, M.D.   -2-   September 17, 1969

We completed the final assembly of the spectrometer and superconducting magnet in the early evening of August 30. At 2:30 A.M., we attempted to find the potassium signal in a saturated solution of K_2CO_3. Needless to say, we were jubilant when our first scan produced a resonance signal almost precisely where we expected to find it. The first NMR measurement of potassium of any kind had been made. (Attached below is a photograph of the K^+ resonance signal as it appeared on our oscilloscope - - an off-resonance beat pattern).

Additional measurements and some controls assured us that we had sufficient sensitivity to measure potassium in biological samples. Using Halobacterium Halobi---, selected for its high intracellular potassium content, the first NMR measure- r of biologic potassium were made the evening of September 6. Furthermore, the pu..ed techniques in our spin-echo spectrometer provided direct evidence (T_2 relaxation measurements) that potassium was complexed to fixed charge groups, and or, solvated by highly structured cell H_2O as we had originally suspected. It is decidedly not in free solution as usually supposed.

Since the superconducting magnet was now needed for other measurements, and we had exhausted the time allotted us, it was at this point that the experiment terminated.

Since no spectrometer-superconducting magnet systems of the type we assembled are available commercially and since no one to the best of our knowledge and the knowledge of Nuclear Magnetic Resonance Specialties Corporation in the continental United States or abroad possesses such an instrument, neither we nor anyone else can pursue our findings. The experiment will remain suspended until someone can assemble the equipment we have described. (See attached manuscript).

Our findings usher in a major revolution in biology and we have only scratched the surface. To suspend our momentum at this point would be unfortunate indeed. Accordingly, I am writing to ask the Health Research Council for the support to equip my laboratory at the State University of New York, Downstate Medical Center, with a High Field Spin Echo Nuclear Magnetic Resonance Spectrometer, so that we can resume work as soon as the spectrometer is constructed. The quoted price for the finished instrumentation by Nuclear Magnetic Resonance Specialties Corporation is $89,000. Although they would prefer to receive the full sum on delivery of the instrument, they have agreed that, if necessary, they will accept a 3-year leasing ar ement of $40,000 on delivery and $24,500 in the second and third year. A t / alternative would be equally divided payments of $26,666 over a three-year period. Furthermore, if these terms are still too encumbering, I feel fairly

George S. Mirick, M.D.   -3-   September 17, 1969

certain Nuclear Magnetic Resonance Specialties can be persuaded to accept a
longer term lease-purchase agreement.

Hopeful that the Health Research Council can help us expand the exciting success
of a project it has sponsored from infancy, I remain,

Sincerely yours,

Raymond Damadian

Raymond Damadian
Assistant Professor
Department of Internal Medicine

RD:aj
Enc.

P.S.   I am enclosing a first draft of the manuscript we are submitting to Science
for publication. I want to mention that our findings have powerful application
٦ anti-cancer technology. Malignant cells have marked alterations in the physical
ىtructure of their protoplasm. To the best of my knowledge, it is generally true
that all malignant cells have been marked by elevated cell potassium values and
depressed Ca^{++} levels. I am very much interested in the potential of NMR spectroscopy for early non-destructive detection of internal malignancies. To the extent
that our primary research objectives will permit, I will make every effort myself
and through collaborators, to establish that all tumors can be recognized by their
potassium relaxation times or H_2O-proton spectra and proceed with the development
of instrumentation and probes that can be used to scan the human body externally
for early signs of malignancy. Detection of internal tumors during the earliest
stages of their genesis should bring us very close to the total eradication of
this disease.

DownstateReporter ■

A quarterly publication   **Downstate Medical Center**

Vol. 2 No. 2   **Spring 1971**

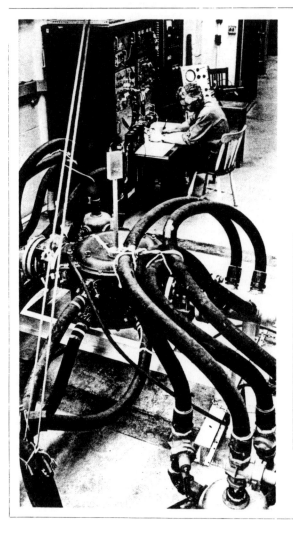

Basic Research Leads To Radio Signals From Cancer Tissue

Sometime in June, a truck will pull up at Downstate bearing a 14-foot-high machine for the biophysics laboratory of Dr. Raymond Damadian, Assistant Professor of Medicine and of Biophysics.

The machine is a nuclear magnetic resonance instrument, which is more at home in physics or chemistry laboratories than in medical institutions. But to Dr. Damadian, the device is very much a medical instrument. He regards it as the prototype of a machine-to-be that could fulfill a long-standing dream of physicians: a quick, foolproof method of early cancer detection.

Already, Dr. Damadian is planning to build a much larger nuclear magnetic resonance device, one that will be big enough to hold a human being. That machine, Dr. Damadian believes, will prove that nuclear magnetic resonance (NMR) is the tool that doctors have been looking for in their quest for a method of detecting cancer early, when treatment is most effective.

All that Dr. Damadian has to support his belief now is a series of tests in which NMR successfully distinguished cancerous cells from healthy tissue in the test tube. But several years of work with NMR, together with its proven power in chemistry, have convinced Dr. Damadian that the technique will work on something as complex as the human body. He hopes to start proving his belief by building and operating his planned larger machine in the next two years.

Dr. Raymond Damadian conducts research on cancer detection in the National Magnet Laboratory at the Massachusetts Institute of Technology. The heavy black hosing connected to the high field magnet in the foreground carries water from the Charles River to cool the magnet.

"By analyzing all these atoms with nuclear magnetic resonance, researchers could build a spectrum that would identify each cell in the same way that a fingerprint identifies a person."

Downstate Reporter, Vol. 2, No. 2, Spring 1971.

sembled at Downstate in June, when his new high field magnet arrives. At present, he is conducting his NMR experiments at the National Magnet Laboratory at the Massachusetts Institute of Technology, where the high field magnets necessary for his research are available.

The proposed NMR device for detecting cancer in humans would not have to be highly elaborate, Dr. Damadian says. It would consist of a large coil to emit radio waves and a movable magnet to create the magnetic field required. The coil would be wrapped around the patient's chest, while the magnet passed back and forth across the body. A detector would pick up NMR emissions for analysis.

Several kinds of analysis might be possible, Dr. Damadian says. For example, many different kinds of atoms could be studied in the same cells. By analyzing all these atoms with NMR, researchers could build a spectrum that would identify each cell in the same way that a fingerprint identifies a person. Analyzing these spectra could then enable a doctor not only to detect a cancer within the

Radio frequency signals are recorded on the oscilloscope for quantitative discrimination between tumor and normal tissue.

body, but also to pinpoint the cancer's location, Dr. Damadian believes. For that kind of analysis, he says, a computer would be needed, since the number of different spectra might be too great for any one man to handle. The computer would compare the signals coming from the patient's body with the spectra stored in its memory.

Dr. Damadian has begun to compile a catalogue of NMR responses from different tissues, both normal and cancerous. One of the first uses of this kind of catalogue, he hopes, will be quick identification of suspicious tissues removed by surgeons during exploratory operations.

Dr. Damadian also believes that NMR may give researchers a new insight into one of the most mysterious processes in biology: the transformation of a normal, controlled cell into the uncontrolled, malignant cancer cell.

To study the transformation, Dr. Damadian says, biologists can simply use some of the chemicals that are known cancer-causers to induce the cancerous transformation in the test tube. Then they can perform periodic (continued on page 16)

Jewish Ceremonial Art Subject of Doctor's Book

It's not unusual to hear that a doctor has written a book. Downstate has many authors on its staff. However, it is unusual to hear that the book has nothing to do with aches and pains, nothing to do with DNA and ACTH, and nothing to do with mental aberrations.

Dr. Abram Kanof, Professor of Pediatrics, has written a book entitled *Jewish Ceremonial Art and Religious Observance*. Of coffee-table size and arty price, the handsome book contains numerous color photographs of mosaics, jeweled wine cups, seder plates, coins, linens, and illustrated Hebrew manuscripts.

According to the author, the attractive appearance has a disadvantage, however. Dr. Kanof woefully points out, "My chief concern is that people will just want to look at the pictures and not read it. It's the written matter that I value most highly."

In its explanation of Jewish ceremonial objects, their use, and the ceremonies in which they are utilized, the book contains the history of many Jewish religious practices. Dr. Kanof explained that he had been working actively on the writing of the book for about four years. But his interest in ceremonial objects as art began about 20 years ago, when he became a member of the Board of the Jewish Museum and later its chairman.

"I started collecting ceremonial objects and I also became interested in the psychological importance of ceremony and the history of ceremonies. I was brought up to believe that all of the Jewish ceremonies were of Jewish origin," he states. "I realized as I read and studied that most religious ceremonies have a common source in the ancient heathen periods but that these practices have been revised and given a new meaning by the monotheistic religions of today."

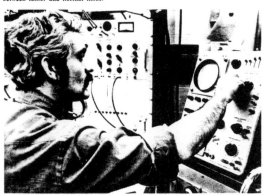

Ref rinted from
19 March 1971, Volume 171, pp. 1151-1153

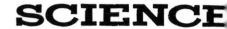

Tumor Detection by Nuclear Magnetic Resonance

Raymond Damadian

Tumor Detection by Nuclear Magnetic Resonance

Abstract. *Spin echo nuclear magnetic resonance measurements may be used as a method for discriminating between malignant tumors and normal tissue. Measurements of spin-lattice (T_1) and spin-spin (T_2) magnetic relaxation times were made in six normal tissues in the rat (muscle, kidney, stomach, intestine, brain, and liver) and in two malignant solid tumors, Walker sarcoma and Novikoff hepatoma. Relaxation times for the two malignant tumors were distinctly outside the range of values for the normal tissues studied, an indication that the malignant tissues were characterized by an increase in the motional freedom of tissue water molecules. The possibility of using magnetic relaxation methods for rapid discrimination between benign and malignant surgical specimens has also been considered. Spin-lattice relaxation times for two benign fibroadenomas were distinct from those for both malignant tissues and were the same as those of muscle.*

At present, early detection of internal neoplasms is hampered by the relatively high permeability of many tumors to x-rays. In principle, nuclear magnetic resonance (NMR) techniques combine many of the desirable features of an external probe for the detection of internal cancer. Magnetic resonance measurements cause no obvious deleterious effects on biologic tissue (*1*), the incident radiation consisting of common radio frequencies at right angles to a static magnetic field. The detector is external to the sample, and the method permits one to resolve information emitted by the sample to atomic dimensions. Thus the spectroscopist has available for study a wide range of nuclei for evidence of deviant chemical behavior.

The resonance technique selected for this particular application belongs to a group of techniques known as "transient" or induction methods. In this experimental arrangement the sample continues to emit a radio-frequency signal for a brief but measurable period after the incident radiation (pulse) has been removed. This method makes possible the direct measurement of spin-lattice (T_1) and spin-spin (T_2) relaxation times, thus avoiding the uncertainties of estimating them from the line width measurements of steady-state NMR spectra. In addition, it also makes possible the characterization of biologic tissues on the basis of the properties of their emitted radio frequency.

In order to determine whether neo-plastic tissues could be recognized from their NMR signals, I studied the proton resonance emissions from cell water. Recent NMR work of Cope (*2*), Hazlewood *et al.* (*3*), and Bratton *et al.* (*4*) has provided fresh insight into the physical nature of cell water. These authors have independently concluded that the decreased NMR relaxation times observed for cell water relative to distilled water (Tables 1 and 2) are due to the existence of a highly ordered fraction of cell water in which the protons of the water molecules have correlation times substantially less than the Larmor period. The reduction of the correlation times is presumably due to the adsorption of water molecules at macromolecular interfaces, findings that are consistent with the proposal by Ling (*5*) that intracellular water (endosolvent) exists as multiple polarized layers adsorbed onto cell proteins.

Two lines of evidence suggested that proton signals from the water in cancerous tissue would be distinct from the radio-frequency emissions of normal tissue. My own experiments with *Escherichia coli* (*6*) suggested that altered selectivity coefficients of alkali cations in biologic tissue, such as occur in neoplastic tissue (*5*), can indicate alterations in tissue water structure. In addition, Hazlewood and his co-workers have recently reported evidence from NMR measurements that growth and maturation of skeletal muscle in the newborn rat is accompanied by simultaneous changes in water structure and

Table 1. Spin-lattice (T_1) and spin-spin (T_2) relaxation times (in seconds) of normal tissues.

Rat No.	Weight (g)	Rectus muscle		Liver		Stomach T_1	Small intestine T_1	Kidney T_1	Brain T_1
		T_1	T_2	T_1	T_2				
1	156	0.493	0.050	0.286	0.050	0.272	0.280	0.444	0.573
2	150	.548	.050	.322	.060	.214	.225	.503	.573
3	495	.541	.050	.241	.050	.260	.316	.423	.596
4	233	.576 (0.600)*	.070	.306 (0.287)*	.048	.247 (0.159)*	.316 (0.280)*	.541 (0.530)*	.620 (0.614)*
5	255	.531			.300		.360	.150	.489	.612
						Mean and standard error			
		0.538 ± 0.015	0.055 ± 0.005	0.293 ± 0.010	0.052 ± 0.003	0.270 ± 0.016	0.257 ± 0.030	0.480 ± 0.026	0.595 ± 0.007

* Spin-lattice relaxation time after the specimen stood overnight at room temperature.

in the alkali cation composition of the muscle (7). These results suggest that dedifferentiation and anaplasia, commonly equated with neoplasia, may be associated with profound alterations in endosolvent structure. These data (7) suggest the nature of the alteration in H_2O structure that should be observed for dedifferentiated or neoplastic tissue. Substantially narrower line widths [the result of a decreased ordering of cell water (2, 3)] were observed for immature skeletal muscle than for mature muscle. On this basis undifferentiated neoplastic tissue can be expected to manifest increased relaxation times (narrow line widths).

The experiments were performed with Sprague-Dawley rats previously infected with either Walker sarcoma (solid form) or Novikoff hepatoma. The rats ranged in weight from 150 to 500 g and were selected at random in order to exclude variations in the age of the rat as a material consideration (8). The animals were killed by cervical fracture when tumor size reached approximately 1.5 ml in volume (4 to 5 days after inoculation in the case of animals with Novikoff hepatoma and 10 days in the case of animals with Walker sarcoma). The samples were excised and packed in cellulose nitrate tubes. In all cases the NMR measurements were obtained within 5 minutes after the death of the animal.

The experimental arrangement consisted of an electromagnet (Varian) 12 inches (30.5 cm) in diameter operating at approximately 5610 gauss, a pulse spectrometer (Nuclear Magnetic Resonance Specialties Corporation PS-60 AW), and a probe of cross-coil design operating at 24 Mhz.

Two types of NMR experiments were performed. Spin-lattice relaxation time was measured by the method of Carr and Purcell (9). In this method a sequence of two pulses is used with pulse widths for the two pulses set to produce a 180° nutation followed by a

90° nutation. With this sequence, one observes a free induction decay after the second pulse whose amplitude is given by

$$M(\tau) = M_0 (1 - 2e^{-\tau/T_1})$$

where M_0 is the equilibrium value of the pulse amplitude and τ is the interval between pulses. This equation implies that, if T_1 is multiplied by the natural logarithm of 2, the product is equal to the pulse interval that produces no free induction decay after the 90° pulse. In actual practice, once the two pulses were phased and pulse widths set for the proper nutation angle, an oscilloscope (Fairchild 766 H/F, 25 and 50 Mhz) was synchronized to trigger on the second pulse and the pulse interval was adjusted until the null free induction decay was obtained. The interval between the two pulses was obtained from a frequency counter (Com-

Table 2. Spin-lattice (T_1) and spin-spin (T_2) relaxation times (in seconds) in tumors.

Rat No.	Weight (g)	T_1	T_2
		Walker sarcoma	
6	156	0.700	0.100
7	150	.750	.100
8	495	.794 (0.794)*	.100
9	233	.688	
10	255	.750	
Mean and S.E.		0.736 ± 0.022	.100
P		< .01†	
		Novikoff hepatoma	
11	155	0.798	0.120
12	160	.852	.120
13	231	.827	.115
Mean and S.E.		0.826 ± 0.013	0.118 ±
P		< .01†	0.002
		Fibroadenoma (benign)	
14		0.448	
15		.537	
Mean		.492	
		Distilled water	
		2.691	
		2.690	
		2.640	
Mean and S.E.		2.677 ± 0.021	

* Spin-lattice relaxation time after the specimen stood overnight at room temperature.   † The P values are the probability estimates of the significance of the difference in the means of T_1 for the malignant tumor and for brain.

puter Measurement Company 200CN) interfaced with the output of the PS-60 spectrometer programmer.

I measured the spin-spin relaxation time by using a 90° to 180° pulse sequence and making use of the Carr-Purcell modification (9) to obtain the echo decay envelope. This method for measuring T_2 is free of diffusion effects and field inhomogeneities (9). Since the envelope height E is given by

$$E (2 n \tau) \propto e^{-2n\tau/T_2}$$

where n represents integral multiples of the pulse separation τ, T_2 was estimated from the oscilloscope trace as the time required for the envelope height to decay to $1/e$.

The spin echo resonance measurements are listed in Tables 1 and 2. The contrast between the relaxation rates of malignant Novikoff hepatoma and normal liver illustrates the degree of perturbation of endosolvent structure that can accompany malignant transformation. The considerable increase in relaxation times for the hepatoma (T_1, 0.826 second; T_2, 0.118 second) relative to normal liver (T_1, 0.293 second; T_2, 0.050 second) suggests a significant decrease in the degree of ordering of intracellular water (2) in malignant tissue. In addition, it is apparent from the prolonged relaxation times of the two malignant tumors reported in Table 2 that NMR techniques would make it possible for one to detect the presence of metastatic infiltrates in the liver from either Walker sarcoma or Novikoff hepatoma.

It was also found that the differences between the relaxation rates of malignant tumors and normal liver could be used to distinguish from all of the normal tissues studied [P values less than .01 (Table 2)]. The values of T_1 in Walker sarcoma (0.736 second) and Novikoff hepatoma (0.826 second) were significantly greater than the values of T_1 in any of the normal tissues (0.293 to 0.595 second). The values of T_2 in the malignant tumors (0.100 and 0.118 second) were about twice the values of T_2 in rectus muscle (0.055 second) and liver (0.052 second). Furthermore, replicate measurements of T_1 in the malignant tissues were found to be highly reproducible (standard error of the mean, < .02) and the normal tissues had a standard error of the mean of .03 or less despite deliberate scrambling of the ages and weights of the animals in the experimental colony.

On the whole, these results support the findings of Hazlewood and his co-workers (7) and are in general agreement with Szent-Györgyi's assertion that cancerous tissue has a lower degree of organization and less water structure than normal tissue (10). Furthermore, the data conformed to the results expected on the basis of a knowledge of the cation content of cancerous tissue. Dunham et al. have reported that with "few exceptions the potassium content of malignant neoplasms is increased" by comparison with that of normal cells (11). Ling has pointed out that the variations in alkali cation selectivity observed by Dunham et al. are readily explained by the association-induction hypothesis (5, p. 523). Nuclear magnetic resonance line width measurements in my laboratory (6) have demonstrated a correlation between narrowing of the line width of the cell water signal and potassium enrichment in bacteria (E. coli), which, in turn, is consistent with the aqueous properties of potassium as a "structure-breaking" agent (12). "Structure-breaking" by the alkali cations below Na in the periodic table (K, Rb, Cs), producing decreased ordering of the molecules in bulk water, results in narrowing of the NMR line width (6).

The measurements were also unaffected by any change in the elevation of the sample position in the probe, packing and repacking of the specimen, or the stepwise rotation of the sample tube in the probe through 360°. In fact T_1 proved to be even relatively unchanged after the specimens stood overnight at room temperature (Tables 1 and 2, parenthetical values for rats 4 and 8).

These studies indicate that NMR methods may be used to discriminate between two malignant tumors and a representative series of normal tissues. The results suggest that this technique may prove useful in the detection of malignant tumors.

The possibility that NMR might be used for rapid discrimination between benign and malignant surgical specimens was also considered. Relaxation times for two benign tumors (fibroadenomas) were distinct from those of the malignant tissues and were the same as those of muscle (Tables 1 and 2).

RAYMOND DAMADIAN*

Biophysical Laboratory, Department of Medicine, State University of New York, Brooklyn 11203

References and Notes

1. M. F. Barnothy, Ed., Biological Effects of Magnetic Fields (Plenum, New York, 1964), p. 17.
2. F. W. Cope, Biophys. J. 9, 303 (1969).
3. C. F. Hazlewood, B. L. Nichols, N. F. Chamberlain, Nature 222, 747 (1969).
4. C. B. Bratton, A. L. Hopkins, J. W. Weinberg, Science 147, 738 (1965).
5. G. N. Ling, A Physical Theory of the Living State (Blaisdell, Waltham, Mass., 1962).
6. R. Damadian, M. Goldsmith, K. S. Zaner, in preparation.
7. C. F. Hazlewood and B. L. Nichols, Physiologist 12, 251 (1969); ———, B. Brown, personal communication.
8. The rats with Walker sarcoma were prepared by J. Patti and were provided by Dr. B. Gardner's laboratory, Department of Surgery, State University of New York, Brooklyn. The animals with hepatoma came from Dr. A. Novikoff's laboratory, Albert Einstein College of Medicine, New York, and were provided by C. Davis and Dr. M. Beard.
9. H. Y. Carr and E. M. Purcell, Phys. Rev. 94, 630 (1954).
10. A. Szent-Györgyi, Bioenergetics (Academic Press, New York, 1957).
11. L. Dunham, S. Nichols, A. Brunschwig, Cancer Res. 6, 230 (1946).
12. O. Y. Samoilov, Structure of Aqueous Electrolyte Solutions and the Hydration of Ions (Consultants Bureau, New York, 1965).
13. I am grateful to P. Yajko, president of Nuclear Magnetic Resonance Specialties Corporation, for providing the Varian electromagnet used in these studies, and to F. Wyant and T. Hill for their assistance with instrumentation. I thank M. Goldsmith, graduate student in biophysics, for contributing the term "endosolvent" for intracellular water. Studies supported by grant 12-1804A from the New York Heart Association and grant 12-6065C from the Health Research Council of the City of New York.
* Career scientist of the Health Research Council of the City of New York.

12 October 1970; revised 18 November 1970

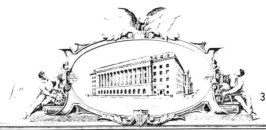

3789832

THE UNITED STATES OF AMERICA

TO ALL TO WHOM THESE PRESENTS SHALL COME:

𝔚𝔥𝔢𝔯𝔢𝔞𝔰, THERE HAS BEEN PRESENTED TO THE

Commissioner of Patents

A PETITION PRAYING FOR THE GRANT OF LETTERS PATENT FOR AN ALLEGED NEW AND USEFUL INVENTION THE TITLE AND DESCRIPTION OF WHICH ARE CONTAINED IN THE SPECIFICATION OF WHICH A COPY IS HEREUNTO ANNEXED AND MADE A PART HEREOF, AND THE VARIOUS REQUIREMENTS OF LAW IN SUCH CASES MADE AND PROVIDED HAVE BEEN COMPLIED WITH, AND THE TITLE THERETO IS, FROM THE RECORDS OF THE PATENT OFFICE IN THE CLAIMANT (S) INDICATED IN THE SAID COPY, AND WHEREAS, UPON DUE EXAMINATION MADE, THE SAID CLAIMANT (S) IS (ARE) ADJUDGED TO BE ENTITLED TO A PATENT UNDER THE LAW.

NOW, THEREFORE, THESE Letters Patent ARE TO GRANT UNTO THE SAID CLAIMANT (S) AND THE SUCCESSORS, HEIRS OR ASSIGNS OF THE SAID CLAIMANT (S) FOR THE TERM OF SEVENTEEN YEARS FROM THE DATE OF THIS GRANT, SUBJECT TO THE PAYMENT OF ISSUE FEES AS PROVIDED BY LAW, THE RIGHT TO EXCLUDE OTHERS FROM MAKING, USING OR SELLING THE SAID INVENTION THROUGHOUT THE UNITED STATES.

In testimony whereof, I have hereunto set my hand and caused the seal of the Patent Office to be affixed at the City of Washington this   fifth   *day of* February, *in the year of our Lord one thousand nine hundred and* seventy-four, *and of the Independence of the United States of America the one hundred and* ninety-eighth.

Attest:

Attesting Officer.

Acting Commissioner of Patents

3,789,832

SHEET 2 OF 2

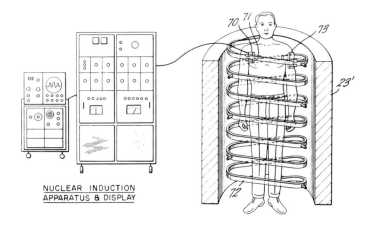

NUCLEAR INDUCTION
APPARATUS & DISPLAY

FIG. 2

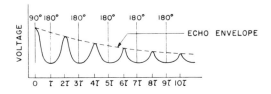

FIG. 3

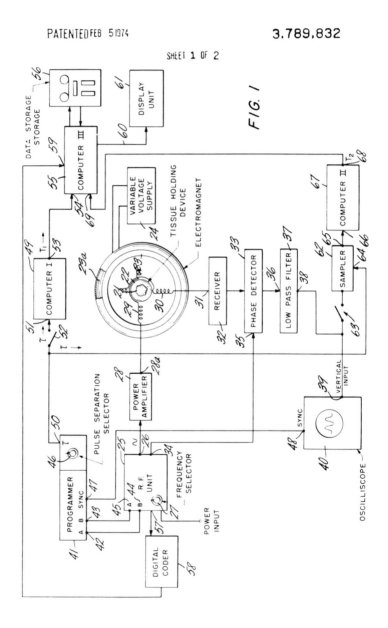

PATENTED FEB 5 1974   3,789,832

SHEET 1 OF 2

FIG. 1

United States Patent [19]

Damadian

[11] **3,789,832**

[45] **Feb. 5, 1974**

[54] **APPARATUS AND METHOD FOR DETECTING CANCER IN TISSUE**

[76] Inventor: **Raymond V. Damadian,** 64 Short Hill Rd., Forest Hill, N.Y. 11375

[22] Filed: **Mar. 17, 1972**

[21] Appl. No.: **235,624**

[52] U.S. Cl.............. **128/2 R,** 128/2 A, 324/.5 R
[51] Int. Cl... **A61b 5/05**
[58] Field of Search .... 128/2 R, 2 A, 1.3; 324/.5 A, 324/.5 B

[56]   **References Cited**
                  UNITED STATES PATENTS

3,691,455   9/1972   Moisio et al. .... 324/.5 R
3,557,777   1/1971   Cohen............................. 128/2 R
3,530,371   9/1970   Nelson et al. .... 324/.5 AC

                   OTHER PUBLICATIONS

Singer, J. R., Journ. of Applied Physics, Vol. 31, No.

1, Jan., 1960, pp. 125–127,

Primary Examiner—Kyle L. Howell
Attorney, Agent, or Firm—Brumbaugh, Graves, Donohue & Raymond

[57]   **ABSTRACT**

An apparatus and method in which a tissue sample is positioned in a nuclear induction apparatus whereby selected nuclei are energized from their equilibrium states to higher energy states through nuclear magnetic resonance. By measuring the spin-lattice relaxation time and the spin-spin relaxation time as the energized nuclei return to their equilibrium states, and then comparing these relaxation times with their respective values for known normal and malignant tissue, an indication of the presence and degree of malignancy of cancerous tissue can be obtained.

16 Claims, 3 Drawing Figures

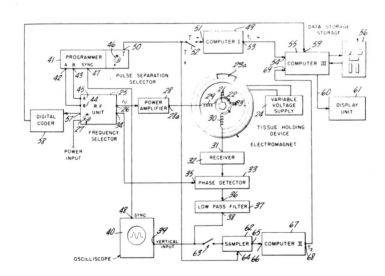

3,789,832

1

APPARATUS AND METHOD FOR DETECTING CANCER IN TISSUE

BACKGROUND OF THE INVENTION

This invention relates to an apparatus and method of detecting cancer in tissue and, more particularly, to the use of nuclear magnetic resonance techniques to detect alterations in the organization and structure of selected nuclei in the tissue which alterations are believed to be caused by cancer.

At present, early detection of internal cncerous tumors is hampered by the relatively high permeability of the many tumors to X-rays. Detection in these cases depends mainly on the indirect evidence provided by the displacement of normal radiopaque structures pushed aside by the tumor. Therefore, the present methods are directed to a qualitative analysis only and lack a quantitized aspect such that a firm basis for decision does not exist as to whether cancer is present and if so how malignant it is.

SUMMARY OF THE INVENTION

It is an object of this invention to provide apparatus and a method for the quantitative detection of cancer in tissue and in particular to provide apparatus for use by clinical and diagnostic laboratories and in the operating room for rapid screening of cancer in small samples of surgically removed tissue.

Furthermore, it is an object of this invention to provide criteria for determining the degree of malignancy of the cancerous tissue detected.

It is a further object of this invention to provide apparatus and method for the detection of cancer in humans which does not require tissue to be surgically removed and can be done with the probes entirely external to the body of the human who is being examined.

These and other objects are attained, in accordance with the invention, by measuring the degree of organization of selected nuclei in the tissue being analyzed.

It has now been found that certain molecules in cancerous cells are more disorganized and arranged with less structure than the same molecules in normal cells. It is known, for example, that the water molecules present in normal cells exist in multiple polarized layers absorbed onto cell protein chains. In cancerous tissue, however, the structure is broken down and the water molecules become disassociated from the protein chains, the result being that water molecules in cancerous tissue are not as compacted as they are in normal tissue.

It has now been found that, by measuring the degree of organization of these selected molecules in cells being studied and comparing this with the degree of organization in a known cancerous cell, cancer cells can be detected. Furthermore, it has now been found that the less the organization the greater the malignancy, therefore, a scale can be made to provide a standard for basing a decision on the degree of malignancy.

The present invention utilizes nuclear magnetic resonance (NMR) techniques to determine this degree of organization. Essentially, the tissue to be analyzed is placed in a tissue holder located in a nuclear induction apparatus and positioned to be exposed to two magnetic fields provided by two sources located in the induction apparatus. One source is an electromagnet in the preferred embodiment and provides a static mag-

2

netic field of known strength. The other source provides an oscillating magnetic field and is positioned so that the direction of its radiated field is orthogonal to the field provided by the electromagnet. The frequency of the oscillating magnetic field is adjusted to casue selected nuclei in the cells to be energized from their equilibrium states to higher energy states through NMR absorption. After a predetermined length of time, the oscillating source is turned off and measurements are made of the spin-lattice relaxation time and spin-spin relaxation time for the energized nuclei returning to their equilibrium states.

It is known that for any given nuclei, the relaxation times increase in proportion to the degree of motional freedom between the nuclei. For example, the relaxation times for hydrogen nuclei in distilled water is several orders of magnitude greater than the corresponding relaxation times for the hydrogen nuclei in ice.

In the present invention, the measurement of relaxation times for selected nuclei in the tissue cells being examined provide a way of measuring the degree of disorganization of the selected nuclei in these cells. By comparing the relaxation times for this tissue with relaxation times obtained for known normal tissue and known cancerous tissue, it can be determined whether cancer is present and if so the degree of malignancy.

In a second embodiment, apparatus is described which can be used to detect cancer in mammallian tissue and in particular humans without having to remove surgically a sample of the tissue to be analyzed. In this embodiment, the entire mammal or human being is placed in a magnetic field provided by an electromagnet sufficiently large to surround the mammal or human. The second magnetic field is directed to a unit which focuses the oscillating magnetic field radiation into a beam. Further apparatus is provided for scanning throughout the entire body during which time the relaxation times are measured for selected nuclei and compared with standards. In this way a determination can be made of the existence of cancer together with the location and degree of malignancy of the cancerous cells present.

For a better understanding of the invention, reference may be made to the following detailed description of the representative embodiments, taken in conjunction with the figures of the accompanying drawings in which:

FIG. 1 is a schematic diagram of suitable apparatus for detecting cancerous tissue in accordance with the invention;

FIG. 2 is a diagram of a particular application of this invention to the detection of cancer in humans; and

FIG. 3 is a diagram showing the signal output of the low pass filter used in the determination of the spin-spin relaxation time.

DESCRIPTION OF A PREFERRED EMBODIMENT

In the embodiment illustrated in FIG. 1, apparatus is shown for measuring the spin-lattice relaxation time and spin-spin relaxation time of a tissue sample 21 held by tissue holding means 22.

An electromagnet 23, having a wire coil 23a energized by a variable voltage supply 24, provides the necessary magnetic field for causing selected nuclei, generally protons, in the tissue sample 21 to separate into discrete energy levels. This separation is commonly known as nuclear Zeeman splitting.

3,789,832

3

Now if a second field is applied to the tissue sample in a direction orthogonal to the first with a frequency determined by inherent characteristics of the selected nuclei and the strength of the field provided by the electromagnet 23, the selected nuclei can be energized 5 from their equilibrium states to higher energy states through nuclear magnetic resonance (NMR) absorption.

In the present invention this second magnetic field is generated by a radio-frequency oscillator 25 which 10 provides a signal at its output terminal 26 having a frequency which can be adjusted manually by frequency selector 27.

The signal on output terminal 26 is directed to a power amplifier 28 whereby the amplitude of the signal 15 generated by the oscillator 25 is increased. The amplified signal appearing at the output terminal 28*a* is then directed to a coil transmitter probe 29 which radiates magnetic energy into the magnetic field space formed by the electromagnet 23. The orientation of the trans- 20 mitter probe 29, in the preferred embodiment, is adjusted to be orthogonal to the direction of the field formed by electromagnet 23.

In order to determine the spin-lattice relaxation time and the spin-spin relaxation time of the selected nuclei 25 returning to their equilibrium states from the higher energy states, a coil receiver probe 30 is provided for detecting signals generated by the decaying nuclei. This probe is positioned essentially at right angles with the transmitter probe 29 and also the direction of the field 30 provided by the electromagnet 23.

The signals detected by the receiver probe 30 are directed to the input terminal 31 of the receiver amplifier 32. The output of the receiver amplifier 32 is directed to a phase detector 33 which is commonly used in 35 NMR applications to determine when the frequency of the radio frequency source 25 has been properly adjusted to supply the conditions necessary for NMR absorption. A signal having the frequency of the radio frequency source 25 is supplied to the output terminal 34 40 of unit 25 and then supplied to the input terminal 25 of the phase detector 33.

The signal output of the phase detector 33 is in turn directed to the input terminal 36 of a low pass filter 37. This filter filters out the resonance frequencies and al- 45 lows the envelope responsive to the amplitude of the signal detected by the receiver probe 30 to appear at output terminal 38.

The signal appearing at 38 is directed to the vertical input 39 of oscilloscope 40 so that the signal can be dis- 50 played visually.

In the experiments described below, a programmer 41 (See FIG. 1) was used to provide a sequence of pulses necessary in NMR applications. By way of example, a Nuclear Magnetic Resonance Specialties, Model 55 P-102A Pulse Programmer, can be used. This Programmer is part of the Nuclear Magnetic Resonance Specialties, PS-60A NMR Spectrometer.

In programmer 41, an A pulse output terminal 42 and a B pulse output terminal 43 are provided and they are 60 connected with their respective input terminals 44 and 45 of radio frequency generator 25. Under operator control the programmer 41 through circuitry not shown signals the radio frequency generator 25 to produce pulse sequences necessary in measuring spin- 65 lattice and spin-spin relaxation times. These pulse sequences corresponding to the Carr-Purcell sequences

4

will be described in more detail below. The separation time between pulses is controlled manually by the pulse separation selector 46. The programmer 41 also provides a sync signal appearing on output terminal 47 which is directed to input terminal 48 of the oscilloscope 40 for synchronizing the oscilloscope with the pulse sequences.

Example I

Several experiments were performed using Sprague-Dawley rats. Five of the rats were normal, five had previously been infected with Walker sarcoma, three had been infected with Novikoff hepatoma and two of the rats had Fibroadenoma (benign tumors). The rats ranged in weight from 150 to 500 grams and were selected at random to exclude variations in the age of the rat as a material consideration.

The animals were killed by cervical fracture. The infected rats were killed when tumor size reached approximately 1.5 ml in volume. This was 4 to 5 days after inoculation in the case of animals with Novikoff hepatoma and 10 days after inoculation in the case of animals with Walker sarcoma. The samples were excised and packaged in cellulose nitrate tubes. In all cases, NMR measurements were obtained within 5 minutes after the death of the animal.

NMR measurements were taken with an apparatus comprising a Varian electromagnet, 12 inches in diameter operating at approximately 5,610 gauss, a pulse spectrometer model PS-60 AW, made by Nuclear Magnetic Resonance Specialties Corporation, together with a probe of cross-coil design operation at 24 Mhz.

Two types of NMR measurements were taken for each tissue sample. The first measurement was the so-called spin-lattice relaxation time (T_1) and was measured by the method of Carr and Purcell, *Phys. Rev.* 94, 630 (1954). In accordance with this method, a sequence of two pulses is used with pulse widths for the two pulses set to produce a 180° nutation followed by a 90° nutation.

With this sequence, one observes a free induction decay after the second pulse whose amplitude is given by

$$M(\tau) = M_0(1 - 2e^{-\tau/T_1})$$

where M_0 is the equilibrium value of the pulse amplitude and τ is the interval between pulses. This equation implies that, if T_1 is multiplied by the natural logarithm of 2, the product is equal to the pulse interval that produces no free induction decay after the 90° pulse. In actual practice, once the two pulses were phased and pulse widths set for the proper nutation angle, an oscilloscope 40, Fairchild 766 H/F, 25 and 50 Mhz, was synchronized to trigger on the second pulse and the pulse interval was adjusted until the null free induction decay was obtained. The interval between the two pulses was obtained from a frequency counter, Computer Measurement Company 200 CN, interfaced with the output of the PS-60 spectrometer programmer 41.

The second NMR measurement taken was the so-called spin-spin relaxation time. This was accomplished by using a 90° to 180° pulse sequence, making use of the Carr-Purcell modification identified in the reference noted above to obtain the echo decay envelope. This method for measuring T_2 is free of diffusion effects and field inhomogeneities. Since the envelope height E is given by

3,789,832

5

$$E(2n\tau) \quad \propto e^{-2n\tau} \quad /T_2$$

where n represents integral multiples of the pulse separation τ, T_2 was estimated from the oscilloscope trace as the time required for the envelope height to decay to $1/e$.

Five normal rats were sacrificed, and various types of normal tissue were subject to NMR measurements. The results of these tests are summarized in Table 1 below.

6

static infiltrates of the liver from either Walker sarcoma or Novikoff hepatoma.

The differences between the relaxation rates of malignant tumors and normal liver may be used to distinguish the two malignancies from all of the normal tissues studied [P values less than 0.01 (Table 2)]. The values of T_1 in Walker sarcoma (0.736 second) and Novikoff hepatoma (0.826 second) were significantly greater than the values of T_1 in any of the normal tis-

TABLE 1
Spin-lattice (T_1) and spin-spin (T_2) relaxation times (in seconds) of normal tissues

Rat No.	Weight (g.)	Rectus muscle T_1	T_2	Liver T_1	T_2	Stomach T_1	Small intestine T_1	Kidney T_1	Brain T_1
....	156	0.493	0.050	0.286	0.050	0.272	0.280	0.444	0.573
....	150	.518	.050	.322	.060	.214	.563	.563	.573
....	495	.541	.050	.241	.050	.290	.316	.423	.596
....	233	.576(*0.600)	.070	.306(*0.287)	.048	.247(*0.150)	.316(*0.260)	.541(*0.530)	.620(*0.614)
....	255	.531	.....	.306	.300	.....	.360	.150	.180	.612
Mean and standard error									
....		0.538±0.015	0.055±0.005	0.283±0.010	0.052±0.003	0.270±0.016	0.257±0.030	0.480±0.026	0.595±0.007

*Spin-lattice relaxation time after the specimen stood overnight at room temperature.

In addition, tumor tissue from a number of infected rats was subjected to NMR measurements and the results of these tests are given in Table 2. As a standard comparison the NMR T_1 values for distilled water are also given.

TABLE 2

Spin-lattice (T_1) and spin-spin (T_2) relaxation times (in seconds) in tumors

Rat No.	Weight (g)	T_1	T_2
		Walker sarcoma	
6	156	0.700	0.100
7	150	.750	0.100
8	495	.794(0.794)*	0.100
9	233	.688	
10	255	.750	
	Mean and S.E.	0.736±0.022	0.100
	P	<.01*	
		Novikoff hepatoma	
11	155	0.798	0.120
12	160	0.852	0.120
13	231	0.827	0.115
	Mean and S.E.	0.826±0.013	0.118±0.002
	P	<.01*	
		Fibroadenoma (benign)	
14		0.448	
15		.537	
	Mean	.492	
		Distilled water	
		2.691	
		2.690	
		2.640	
	Mean and S.E.	2.677±0.021	

*Spin-lattice relaxation time after the specimen stood overnight at room temperature.
†The P values are the probability estimates of the significance of the difference in the means of T_1 for the malignant tumor and for brain.

The contrast between the relaxation rates of malignant Novikoff hepatoma and normal liver illustrates the degree of perturbation of endosolvent structure that can accompany malignant transformation. The considerable increase in relaxation times for the hepatoma T_1, 0.826 second; T_2, 0.118 second) relative to normal liver (T_1, 0.293 second; T_2, 0.050 second) suggests a significant decrease in the degree of ordering of intracellular water in malignant tissue. In addition, it is apparent from the prolonged relaxation times of the two malignant tumors reported in Table 2 that NMR values make it possible to one to detect the presence of meta-

sues (0.293 to 0.595 second). The values of T_2 in the malignant tumors (0.100 and 0.118 second) were about twice the values of T_2 in rectus muscle (0.055 second) and liver (0.052 second). Furthermore, replicate measurements of T_1 in the malignant tissues were found to be highly reproducible (standard error of the mean, <0.02) and the normal tissues had a standard error of the mean of 0.03 or less despite deliberate scrambling of the ages and weights of the animals in the experimental colony.

The measurements were also unaffected by any change in the elevation of the sample position in the probe, packing and repacking of the specimen, or stepwise rotation of the sample tube in the probe through 360°. In fact T_1 proved to be even relatively unchanged after the specimens stood overnight at room temperature (Tables 1 and 2, parenthetical values for rats **4** and **8**).

The above experiments were conducted without the aid of equipment which could automatically compute T_1 and T_2 and automatically compare these values with their respective standards for the detection of cancerous tissue. However, a computer **49** could be provided to calculate $T_1 = \tau null/\ln 2$ where τ is the time interval between the 180° pulse and the 90° pulse in the Carr-Purcell method described above that produces no free induction decay after the 90° pulse. This value of $\tau null$ is the value τ selected manually on the pulse separation selector **46** to produce the above condition. An electrical signal responsive to the setting of τ on selector **46** is provided by the programmer **41** and appears at output terminal **50**. The signal is directed to an input terminal **51** of computer **49** through a switch **52** which is closed when it is desired to compute and compare values of T_1 with a standard.

The value of T_1 appearing as a signal at an output **53** of computer **49** is directed to an input terminal **54** of a computer **55**. This computer compares the value of T_1 at input terminal **54** with a table of standard values for non-cancerous and cancerous tissues stored on a data storage unit **56**. This comparison provides an indication whether cancer is present and if so its degree of malignancy. The comparison is made for the particular nuclei selected, each type of nuclei having a separate

3,789,832

7

table of standards. For a given field strength provided by electromagnet 23 the frequency of the radio frequency generator 25 determines which nuclei are selected. Thus, the selected nuclei are known from the setting of the frequency selector 27. An electrical signal responsive to the setting of the frequency selector 27 appears at output terminal 57 of the radio frequency generator 25. This signal is converted into a digital code by a digital coder 58 and supplied to an input terminal 59 of computer 55.

After comparing the values of T_1 for the sample 21 with the standards on a data storage unit 56, the computer 55 supplies a signal via line 60 to a display unit 61. This signal is converted by display unit 61 into a visual signal indicating whether cancer is present in tissue sample 21 and if so the degree of malignancy.

For automatically calculating values of T_2 for comparing with a standard, a sampler 62 is provided for sampling the signal appearing at terminal 38 of the low pass filter when the switch 63 is closed. The sampler 62 samples the signal at terminal 38 at times 0, 2τ, 4τ, 6τ, etc., where τ is again the time interval between the 180° pulse and the 90° pulse generated by the programmer 41 for determining T_2. A signal responsive to the τ selected on selector 46 appears at output terminal 50 of programmer 41 and is supplied to input terminal 64 of sampler 62. To better understand the technique used to determine T_2, reference is made to FIG. 3 wherein a plot of the signal appearing at terminal 38 is shown. This plot shows the signal when the programmer 41 has been set to supply a 90° pulse and a train of 180° pulses pursuant to the Carr-Purcell method of measuring T_2. The 90° pulse is applied at time 0, and a 180° pulse is applied at times τ, 3τ, 5τ, 7τ, etc. The sampler 62 samples the signal at times 0, 2τ, 4τ, 6τ, etc., thus obtaining values of the signal which lie on the echo envelope.

The sampled values detected by sampler 62 appear on an output terminal 65 of sampler 62 and are directed to an input terminal 66 of computer 67. The sampled values appearing on input terminal 66 are stored on a real time basis in the computer 67 as is well known in the art.

A computer program could be designed according to the art to label the stored sampled values giving them the labels V(0), V(1), V(2) ... V(I) where I is one less than the total number of samples stored (one less because the count started with zero). The computer could then be programmed to compute T_2 by performing the following steps:

```
    START
    READ V(0)
    COMPUTE A = 1/e V(0)
    N = 1
2
    READ V(N)
    IF V(N) < A GO TO 3
    N = N + 1
    GO TO 2
3
    T₂ = V(N)
    END
```

In this manner an approximate value of T_2 can be computed. Further refinements can be made by determining the best curve connecting the sampled values V(0), V(1), V(2), etc. and then determining the point at which the curve intersects the Y value of 1/e V(0) as is well known in the art. The program set forth above

8

is only an example of a method for determining approximate values of T_2.

The output of computer 67 is T_2 and appears on output terminal 68. This signal is directed to input terminal 69 of computer 55 where it is compared with a table of standards for the selected nuclei stored on data storage unit 56 in the same manner as T_1 is compared with its respective standards. Again the computer 55 supplies a signal via line 60 to the display unit 61 where the signal is converted into a visual signal indicating whether cancer is present in tissue sample 21 and if so the degree of malignancy.

In another embodiment of this invention illustrated in FIG. 2, apparatus is shown for detecting cancerous cells in mammals and particularly human beings.

The only modification of the apparatus in FIG. 2 with the apparatus shown in FIG. 1 is the design of the electromagnet 23, the tissue holder 22 and the transmitter and receiver probes 29 and 30.

In FIG. 2 an electromagnet 23' shown in cross-section is designed to have sufficiently large dimensions to hold a mammal or human being to be examined. A transmitter probe 70 is provided with a beam focusing mechanism 71 for focusing the radiated magnetic energy from the radio frequency generator 25 into a beam having a narrow cross-section. This probe is slidably mounted on a helical track 72 and positioned so that the radiated beam is orthogonal to the direction of the field provided by electromagnet 23. The transmitter probe 70 is moved on the track 72 by means not shown so that the probe 70 may scan the entire body to be examined. Also mounted on track 72 is a receiver probe 73 of the same design as transmitter probe 70 which detects a beam having the same cross-sectional width as the beam radiated by probe 70. The probe 73 is positioned to detect only beams which are orthogonal to both the direction of the field provided by electromagnet 23' and the direction of the beam radiated by probe 70. As the probe 70 scans the body being examined, the probe 73 moves correspondingly by means not shown to maintain the orthogonal relationship during the scanning process.

In a preferred embodiment the electromagnet 23' is cylindrically shaped so that the field generated has a maximum along the axis of the electromagnet 23' and the transmitter probe 70 is focused to direct its radiated beam to intersect this axis. Further, the receiver probe 73 is focused to receive a beam emanating from the region of impingement of the transmitted beam with the axis of electromagnet 23'.

Since the field strength a particular frequency is required for NMR absorption of selected nuclei and since the maximum field strength of the field generated by electromagnet 23' lies along its axis which is uniquely defined for the cylindrical space encompassed by the electromagnet 23', it is possible to select a frequency determined by the maximum field strength provided by electromagnet 23' and the nuclei selected so that a small area defined by the impingement of the beam radiated by transmitter probe 70 and the axis of the electromagnet 23' can be examined. By moving probes 70 and 73 move along the track 72 the entire area of the body lying on the axis of the electromagnet 23' is examined. By repositioning the body with respect to the axis of the electromagnet 23' and rescanning the axis, the entire body can be examined.

The apparatus and method described above has

3,789,832

9

10

many desirable features including the ability to detect internal cancer with an external probe. Thus by using this apparatus and method it is unnecessary to surgically remove a tissue sample for examination.

In determining relaxation times for tissue cells within the body being examined, it is necessary to have quite high magnetic field strengths to penetrate the body. There have been some recent studies by NASA on the effect of high strength magnetic fields on humans. A study of their conclusions indicates that the strength of the magnetic fields contemplated here would not be deleterious to the tissue under examination.

Since NMR analysis is directed to the atomic level, the operator of this system has available for study a wide range of nuclei in determining deviant chemical behavior. In the experiments noted above the hydrogen nuclei of water were selected for studying the organization of water molecules in tissue cells. It can be appreciated that there may be other nuclei which may be subjected to NMR analysis for cancer detection. For example, it is generally known that the cancerous change is uniformly associated with derangements in the cells chromosomes. Since DNA is the main constituent of chromosomes and further since phosphorus is a main element in the polymer backbone of DNA, chromosome derangements are reflected in the chemistry of the phosphorus nucleus and hence, in the NMR spectra of cellular phosphorus.

From the foregoing it will be seen that the present invention provides a much needed method and apparatus for detecting the presence of cancer and providing a quantitative analysis of the malignancy of any cancer cells detected. It will be understood that many modifications of the structure of the preferred embodiments will occur to those skilled in the art, and it is understood that this invention is to be limited only by the scope of the following claims.

I claim:

1. A method for detecting cancer comprising:
 a. measuring and establishing standard NMR spin-lattice relaxation times and spin-spin relaxation times for both normal and cancerous tissue of the type under analysis using as an indicator nuclei at least one nuclei which exhibits deviant behavior in cancerous tissue;
 b. measuring the NMR spin-lattice relaxation times and spin-spin relaxation times for the suspected tissue to determine the extent of deviant behavior of the indicator nuclei; and
 c. comparing the values obtained in (b) against the standards obtained in (a).

2. The method of claim 1, wherein the indicator nuclei are cell water protons.

3. A method for distinguishing cancerous tissue from normal, healthy tissue which comprises:
 a. positioning a tissue sample in a nuclear induction apparatus having two sources of magnetic energy;
 b. actuating the first source to expose the sample to a magnetic field;
 c. actuating the second source to expose the sample to oscillating magnetic radiation having a frequency selected to permit the absorption by selected nuclei of energy from the oscillating field through nuclear magnetic resonance absorption, thereby inducing transistors between equilibrium states and higher energy states;

d. terminating the radiation from the second source after a predetermined duration;
 e. measuring the spin-lattice relaxation time and spin-spin relaxation time as the energized nuclei return to their equilibrium states; and
 f. comparing the relaxation times with respective predetermined standards for normal and cancerous tissue, said comparisons indicating the presence and degree of malignancy of cancerous tissue.

4. The method according to claim 3, wherein the first source of magnetic energy is actuated to provide a static magnetic field orthogonal to the second magnetic field.

5. A method according to claim 4, wherein the selected nuclei comprise water protons.

6. A method according to claim 2, wherein the selected nuclei are phosphorus.

7. A method of detecting cancerous mammalian tissue comprising:
 a. providing a magnetic field space having a locus therein of equal field strength;
 b. positioning a mammal within said space;
 c. directing a beam of magnetic radiation having a predetermined frequency to impinge on said locus in a direction orthogonal to the direction of the magnetic field, the frequency being selected to permit absorption by selected nuclei in the region of impingement of energy from the beam through nuclear magnetic resonance absorption, thereby inducing transitions in the selected nuclei between equilibrium states and higher energy states;
 d. terminating the beam after a predetermined duration;
 e. measuring the spin-lattice relaxation time and the spin-spin relaxation time values as the energized nuclei return to their equilibrium states; and
 f. comparing the values obtained in (e) with predetermined like values for normal and for cancerous tissue, said comparison indicating the existence and degree of malignancy.

8. A method according to claim 7 further comprising scanning the beam of magnetic radiation across the locus.

9. A method according to claim 8, wherein the magnetic field is formed within a hollow, cylindrical superconducting solenoid, and the locus comprises the axis of the superconducting solenoid along which axis the field strength is a maximum.

10. A method according to claim 7, wherein the selected nuclei comprise water protons.

11. The method of claim 7, wherein the selected nuclei is phosphorus.

12. Apparatus for determining whether a tissue sample is cancerous comprising:
 a. nuclear induction apparatus including a magnetic field source means for forming a magnetic field space of a predetermined field strength and an oscillator source means for selectively supplying oscillating magnetic energy to the magnetic field space together with means for adjusting the frequency of the oscillator to satisfy nuclear magnetic resonance conditions for selected nuclei in the tissue sample;
 b. a tissue holding means for holding the tissue sample in the magnetic field space;
 c. means for determining the spin-lattice relaxation time of the selected nuclei in the tissue sample;

3,789,832

11

d. means for determining the spin-spin relaxation time of the selected nuclei in the tissue sample;

e. means for storing reference tables comprising the standard spin-lattice relaxation times and spin-spin relaxation times for the selected nuclei;

f. means for comparing the spin-lattice relaxation time and the spin-spin relaxation time of the selected nuclei in the tissue sample with the respective standards for normal tissue for the selected nuclei, and means for indicating that the tissue sample is cancerous if the relaxation times are greater than the respective standards.

13. The apparatus according to claim 12, wherein the frequency adjusting means is adjusted so that the oscillator provides a magnetic field having a frequency which satisfies the nuclear magnetic resonance conditions of water protons.

14. The apparatus according to claim 12, wherein the frequency adjusting means is adjusted so that the oscillator provides a magnetic field having a frequency which satisfies the nuclear magnetic resonance conditions of phosphorus nuclei.

15. Apparatus for detecting cancerous cells in mammalian tissue comprising:

a. nuclear induction apparatus including a magnetic field source means for forming a magnetic field space and an oscillator source means for selectively supplying oscillating magnetic energy to the magnetic field space together with means for adjusting the frequency of the oscillator to satisfy nuclear magnetic resonance conditions for selected nuclei;

b. means for selecting a locus in the field space of

12

equal field strength;

c. means adapted for holding the mammal in the magnetic field space;

d. means for focusing the oscillating magnetic energy into a beam;

e. means for directing the beam to impinge on said locus in a direction orthogonal to the direction of the magnetic field;

f. means for determining the spin-lattice relaxation time of the selected nuclei in tissue cells of the mammal when said mammal is located in the region of impingement;

g. means for determining the spin-spin relaxation time of the selected nuclei in tissue cells of the mammal when said mammal is located in the region of impingement;

h. means for storing reference tables comprising standard spin-lattice relaxation times and spin-spin relaxation times for the selected nuclei;

i. means for comparing the spin-lattice relaxation time and the spin-spin relaxation time of the selected nuclei in the region of impingement with their respective standards for normal tissue for the selected nuclei, and means for indicating that said mammal contains cancerous cells in the region of impingement if the relaxation times are greater than the respective standards.

16. Apparatus according to claim 13 further including means for scanning the beam across the locus.

* * * * *

7/2/77   **71**

Oscar II in 5" Lung
Human Attempt 11:03 PM   7/2/77
X = 18 ,   15 = Z ,   Y = 6½
Beam   2¼" from bottom surface of
beam to magnet Dewar surface

$\mathcal{F}$ANTASTIC SUCCESS !
1:45AM. First Human Image
Complete in Amazing Detail
Showing Heart
           Lungs
           Vertebra
           Musculature

Image taken at Minkoff
    nipple level

START TIME 11:45 PM ½ hour out for break
FINISH TIME 4:35 PM. LAWRENCE IMAGE [2 min 11 seconds per point]

$y = 6.5$

at level C13

$z =$	10	11	12	13	14	<u>15</u>	16	17	18	19	20	21	22

$x = 10$

106 points

at 2 min 11 sec
= 3.86 hours of data accum time

4.50
3.86   38
.64 hr minutes

Points written in black were taken after Larry got end of coil in a ½ hour break.

.64 hr = 38 minutes spent off data collection

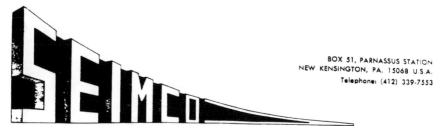

BOX 51, PARNASSUS STATION
NEW KENSINGTON, PA. 15068 U.S.A.
Telephone: (412) 339-7553

SCIENTIFIC ELECTRONIC INSTRUMENT and MANUFACTURING CO. INCORPORATED

January 7, 1987

Dr. Raymond Damadian, President
Fonar Corporation
110 Marcus Drive
Melville, LI, NY 11733

Dear Dr. Damadian:

As I promised during our conversation yesterday, I read through your patent number 3,789,832. My knowledge and beliefs regarding the origins of Magnetic Resonance Imaging based upon my recollections and upon the information contained in your patent are as follows:

1. You expressed to me your intent to use NMR to differentiate between normal and cancerous tissue.

2. When you conducted a series of experiments with rats at NMR Specialties you observed a longer longitudinal relaxation time in cancerous tissue than in normal tissue.

3. You expressed to me your intent to "build an NMR instrument capable of containing a human body and to use that instrument for in-vivo diagnosis of pathology; especially, detecting and localizing cancer."

4. All of these events took place prior to Paul Yajko's departure from NMR Specialties which was in June of 1971. At the time of Paul Yajko's departure, your work and intentions were common knowledge at NMR Specialties and were openly discussed.

Dr. Raymond Damadian, President
Fonar Corporation
Melville, LI, NY 11733
January 7, 1987
Page 2

    5. During your visit to NMR Specialties in June of 1971 you
gave me a copy of the Downstate Reporter that provided the
first means I had ever seen for spatially localizing NMR
information to produce a point by point scan. In 1977 you
sent me a photograph of the first human image obtained by
that method.

After Paul Yajko's departure from NMR Specialties, during the
summer of 1971, and therefore after all of the above enumerated
events, Paul Lauterbur, who succeeded Paul Yajko as president of
NMR Specialties, discussed with me a plan for using an NMR
spectrometer and field gradients for making pictures.

In summary, relative to current MRI scanning technology, I believe
that you were the first to conceive of using the NMR technique in
a manner that would permit a scan of NMR signals from the entire
human body and the first to provide a method for spatially
localizing that information to produce a point by point scan.

Sincerely,

G. D. Vickers
President

cc: Dr. Lawrence Minkoff

1988
National Medal of Technology
Jointly to
Raymond Damadian
and
Paul Lauterbur

"For their independent contributions in
conceiving and developing the application
of magnetic resonance technology to
medical uses including whole-body
scanning and diagnostic imaging."

President Reagan
White House
July 15, 1988

I would like to see students get to the point where they begin to understand a science enough to be secure. Now they take enough to feel insecure. It's like being taken into a restaurant and only getting some olives.

—I.I. Rabi

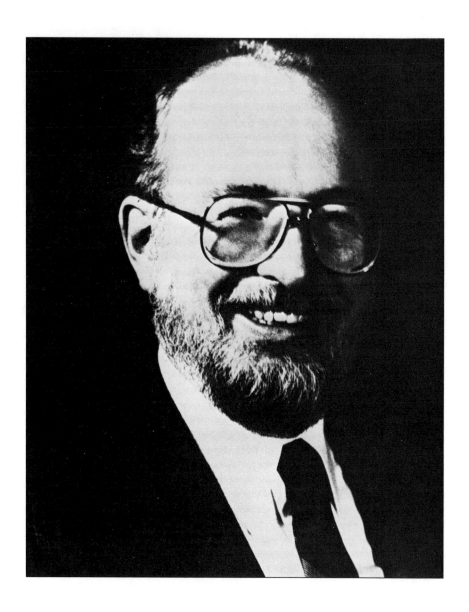

9

PAUL C. LAUTERBUR

Originator of a Method for Spatially Localizing NMR
Relaxation Information from a Sample and
Displaying It as a Pictorial Map

THE SAME MONTH that Edward M. Purcell graduated from Mattoon High School in Illinois, Paul Christian Lauterbur was born in Sidney, Ohio, about 250 miles due east. Sidney, Ohio is a growing community. Located midway between Lima and Dayton, it serves a prosperous farming region that raises primarily winter wheat, corn and oats. Just a few miles to the northwest, underground deposits of natural gas and crude oil also contribute to the area's prosperity. With a 1990 population of 18,710, up a healthy six percent from the 1980 census, it has a better chance of remaining physically healthy these days because of the relatively new diagnostic modality called MRI.

In 1980, the first commercial scanner ever sold in the United States, a FONAR QED 80 permanent magnet scanner, was placed in a diagnostic imaging center in Cleveland, Ohio, 200 miles away. For the first half of that decade, placement of such scanners was largely limited to major cities, but today Sidney, typical of thousands of communities across the United States, also has local access to an MRI scanner. On Thursdays and Saturdays, a mobile MRI scanner owned by Mid-America Imaging pulls up to the docking area outside of the 112-bed Wilson Hospital and processes the current list of patients scheduled for scans.

They come for a wide variety of anatomical studies, ranging from cross-sectional views of the brain to shoulders to spines to knees, all of them depicting the inside of the body—including soft tissue—with the precision of an anatomical atlas. MRI is becoming well-known in Sidney, a household acronym whose benefits are touted by word of mouth. "I'm getting an MRI" and "Maybe you should ask your doctor to prescribe an MRI" are two statements that are being heard more and more in Sidney these days as its residents see for themselves its amazing ability to reveal anatomical structure with detail far superior to X-rays. Ironically, there may still be MRI beneficiaries in Sidney who don't realize that the idea of converting NMR signals into pictures was the brainchild of one of their own native sons, Paul C. Lauterbur.

Paul Lauterbur's father, Edward Joseph Lauterbur, was the youngest of six children born to Paul and Margaret (Hillan) Lauterbur. In 1898, Paul and Margaret Lauterbur moved to Sidney, Ohio from Fort Loramie, a wide spot in the road about 15 miles northeast of Sidney. Edward was born the following year. In 1926, Edward Lauterbur married Gertrude Wagner of Tiffin, Ohio, who was also born in 1899. The couple would have three sons: Thomas Edward, born September 26, 1927, Paul Christian, born May 6, 1929, and Edward Joseph II, born in 1932. Their youngest child, a daughter, Margaret, was born in 1935. Their oldest son, Thomas, would live only two days.

Paul Lauterbur's grandfather, who was also named Paul, had three sons who, like him, were all mechanically inclined. For a time, the elder Paul had worked in sales for two threshing machine manufacturers, Altman Company and Reeves and Company. Frank, his oldest son, who had been in sales with him at Reeves, organized, together with his brothers, the Lauterbur Machine Company in 1909. In 1913, Frank Lauterbur helped organize Peerless Bread Machine Company, where he served as general manager. Frank's brother Edward and his father Paul also worked at Peerless, Paul until his retirement in 1927, Edward until his departure for Troy, Ohio in 1947.

Edward Lauterbur, the father of Paul C. Lauterbur, was educated as a mechanical engineer and would work for all of young Paul's growing-up years as an employee of Peerless Bread Machine Company. Frank Lauterbur died in 1932 at the age of 45, the victim of complications from a tonsilectomy. In the 1927 Sidney city directory, Edward is listed as a factory manager at Peerless and in the 1939-40 directory as an engineer for the same firm.

In 1929, the year Paul C. Lauterbur was born, the economy started out on a positive note in the United States. President Herbert Hoover took office on March 4 of that year, at a time when the nation was in a period of rapidly-growing prosperity. With flourishing trade, industrial expansion, hefty corporate profits and stockholder dividends, and the national treasury posting a surplus even with reduced taxes, it was a period of general optimism. Convinced that the "bull market" of rising stock prices would last forever, in spite of warnings from a few stockbrokers and economists to the contrary, many people from all walks of life were putting themselves in serious financial jeopardy in the hope of "getting rich quick."

In contrast to the frenzied pace on Wall Street, rural America—places like Sidney, Ohio, for instance—lay in sheltered quiet. About six months later, however, on October 6—"Black Thursday" as it has come to be known—the bottom would fall out of the stock market and the effect would soon be felt across the United States, even in Sidney. Because he was so young when the Depression hit, it would be a few years before Paul Lauterbur would even be aware of its existence. The economic slump would leave many with an obsessive concern about financial security, an almost debilitating incapacity to take risks, but it appears to have had little or no detrimental effect on young Paul Lauterbur's curious, inquisitive nature.

He had a love for science. As a boy he took an interest in a number of sciences including biology, chemistry, physics and astronomy. He also had a mild interest in mathematics, particularly as it related to the orbital revolutions of planets and other celestial bodies.

He didn't spend all of his time in books, however. Like many children who grow up in a semi-rural area, Lauterbur enjoyed what city kids often only dream about—riding and caring for horses; walking in the quiet, beautiful and serene outdoors with a gun or a fishing pole; and having pets, including snakes and a skunk.

Although he was not negatively molded by the Depression, neither was he unaware of the difficulties others had in trying to make ends meet during those hard times. No stranger to physical labor, young Lauterbur sometimes worked during the summer for a local share-cropper who gave a portion of the harvest to the landlord in lieu of rent and then tried to exist the rest of the year on what he could earn from the leftovers.

In high school, although Lauterbur's academic performance tended to fluctuate, he acquired a taste for scientific experimentation, a description some may have termed over-generous after witnessing the strange concoctions and ruined glassware generated by Lauterbur in his home laboratory. A leader and organizer, he formed a high school science club and in 1945, at the age of 16, gave lectures on the atomic bomb to science classes. The news event to which the lectures were connected was still very fresh in the minds of his listeners. Just before school started that year, atomic bombs had been dropped on the Japanese cities of Hiroshima and Nagasaki.

If Lauterbur's academic performance was less than stellar, a test given by the National Honor Society in his senior year indicated that he wasn't lacking in ability. In Ohio District 11, also known as the Miami District, Lauterbur came in fourth in physics and seventh overall. For the entire state of Ohio, he was in eleventh place.

Lauterbur was a reader of science fiction and an astronomy buff. Like Neil Armstrong, the future astronaut, who was close to his age and who lived just a few miles to the north, Lauterbur might have dreamed of rocket travel to the moon or distant planets as he built solid-fuel model rockets and launched them into the Ohio sky. But he was keeping his options open. Using a home-made microtome, he also made a collection of microscope slides that enabled him to see images from another world, a hidden world which, although it is all around us, is often closed to our limited, unassisted view.

Case School of Applied Science/Case Institute of Technology

When Paul Lauterbur finished high school in the spring of 1947, he made plans to attend Case School of Applied Science in Cleveland that fall. By the time he matriculated there, however, the school had changed its name to Case Institute of Technology, the name it would keep until its 1967 amalgamation with Western Reserve University into Case Western Reserve University.

For Lauterbur, the big decision was whether to go for a major in chemistry or physics. He had an interest in both and it was basically a flip of the coin as to which one came out on top. It turned out to be chemistry. Four years later, he would graduate with a Bachelor of Science in Industrial Chemistry.

Before finishing his freshman year at college, however, he and his family would experience a tragic loss. Shortly before Paul graduated from high school, his father Edward accepted a new job at Hobart Company, a manufacturer of food scales, in Troy, Ohio, 25 miles south of Sidney. When Paul entered college in Cleveland, his brother Edward, known as Joe, age 16, enrolled as a junior at Troy High School. On the morning of February 19, 1948, Joe was driving a 1946 Plymouth to school when he struck the side of a steam locomotive operated by the Baltimore and Ohio Railroad. As a result of the impact, the car ricocheted toward a nearby service station where it struck a gas pump, throwing Lauterbur from the car. Taken to a local hospital, the youth, a member of the high school football team in Troy, died a few hours later. An account of the accident in the *Sidney Daily News* observed:

The tragic accident brought widespread sorrow in Sidney; until the Lauterbur family moved to their present home on Stringtown road, north of Troy, they were prominent in local circles. The youthful victim was popular with Sidney high school students where he was a student and at Holy Angels school where he had studied during elementary classes. . . . The youth is survived by his parents, Mr. and Mrs. Edward J. Lauterbur, a sister, Margaret, 13, who attends St. Patrick School, and a brother, Paul C., student in Case School of Applied Science, Cleveland.[1]

Edward, Sr. would remain an employee of Hobart Manufacturing until his retirement in 1964. Three years later, at the age of 68, Edward would die in Crowley, Texas, a suburb of Dallas, just a few days after he and his wife Gertrude had arrived in that city to make their home in St. Francis Village, a retirement community operated by the Third Order of St. Francis [of Assisi]. Paul's mother, age 96, now lives in Ohio.

During his undergraduate years at Case Institute, Lauterbur had two prevailing scientific interests—biology and organosilicon chemistry. Stimulated somewhat by his readings in science fiction, he wondered whether there could be a biology based, either entirely or in part, on silicon, rather than carbon. (Early attempts at answering that question were responsible for some of the broken glass in his basement laboratory back in Sidney.)

Magnetism also attracted him. During his junior year, Lauterbur built an apparatus for measuring magnetic susceptibility. In this regard, he was following in the footsteps of I.I. Rabi and E.M. Purcell. Rabi had measured the magnetic susceptibility of Tutton salts about two decades earlier for his PhD dissertation, devising a greatly improved method in the process, and Purcell, collaborating as a Harvard graduate student with Malcolm Hebb and Professor John Van Vleck in 1937, had published a paper on adiabatic demagnetization which sought to explain certain anomalies in specific heats and magnetic susceptibilities that experimenters had noted at temperatures within one degree of absolute zero. For Lauterbur's senior thesis, he worked on synthesizing hexaphenylsilaethane.

It is interesting to note that Lauterbur didn't have much patience for classroom lectures. He basically found them boring and even slept through some of them. He much preferred to spend his time in a laboratory doing experiments rather than sitting in a classroom taking notes. He would be the first to admit later on, however, that some things he did learn at such lectures would later be critical to the formulation and practical implementation of his ideas.

Mellon Institute, Phase One

Upon graduation in 1951, Lauterbur accepted a position as a research assistant with Mellon Institute in Pittsburgh. Supported by Dow Corning, the Institute was engaged at the time in synthesizing and testing organosilicon compounds and polymers, a natural extension of Lauterbur's own research interests.

Lauterbur's decision to go directly into industry and hold off on enrolling in graduate school was made primarily because of his reluctance to listen to more classroom lectures and his desire to spend time in the laboratory. A tuition-free PhD program offered by Mellon in concert with the University of Pittsburgh soon lured him, however, into straddling both worlds—industrial and academic. For much of the next decade, except for a stint in the military, Lauterbur would split his time between Mellon Institute and "Pitt," until receiving his PhD degree in chemistry in 1962.

Lauterbur's initial research at Mellon Institute was on silicone elastomers, silicon-based polymers which possess the elastic properties of natural rubber. Basically, he was trying to understand the cross-linking reactions involving the silicon and hydrogen groups and also the sources of the "filler effect," the reinforcement of silicone rubber with small particles such as fumed silica. (In carbon-based rubbers, carbon black plays an equivalent reinforcing role.) The cross-linking reaction Lauterbur was studying led to his investigation of the role that free radicals play in the process which, in turn, led him to electron spin resonance, also called EPR, the acronym for electron paramagnetic resonance.

Magnetic resonance of the electron was first discovered by a Soviet physicist, E.K. Zavoisky, in 1944, more than a year before Edward Purcell and Felix Bloch detected magnetic resonance in atomic nuclei. Because the electron has smaller mass and therefore a larger gyromagnetic ratio than the proton, in a given magnetic field it precesses much more rapidly. Because the electron's Larmor precession frequency is higher, the wavelength of the emitted radiation is shorter and is therefore detected in a magnetic resonance apparatus with microwave techniques. Otherwise, the process operates on the same principle as nuclear magnetic resonance.

In the same way that nuclear magnetic resonance in bulk matter would be undetectable if there were exactly the same number of parallel spins as antiparallel, EPR is of no use in analyzing substances in which the atomic electrons are all paired, because the "magnetism" of each electron is canceled. In the case of substances with unpaired electrons, EPR can play an important analytical role.

More exciting has been the discovery [wrote George Pake* in 1958] that electron resonance can be used to investigate free radicals, the transitory molecular fragments that play a crucial role in many chemical processes . . . At first thought one might suppose that the resonance spectrum of the unpaired electron in a free radical should always be the same—one free radical indistinguishable from another. But this is not the case. The electron is affected by the magnetic field of the nuclei in whose neighborhood it happens to be, and as the free electron wanders about in the molecular environment, it is subjected to varying magnetic fields. As a result its resonance may be split into a "hyperfine structure." From the splitting we may learn where the electron spends its time and at what rate the free radical is likely to enter into chemical reactions. . . . [Electron] magnetic resonance also looks promising as a tool for investigating the free radicals that catalyze the synthesis of high polymers such as rubber and polyethylene.[2]

Lauterbur's continued interest in elastomeric chemical interactions drew his attention further into the atom, toward the nucleus and nuclear magnetic resonance. This time, his interest was stimulated by the dramatic effects that non-covalent interactions between particles and polymer chains have on the elasticity and tear resistance of rubber. A report that he gave in a physical chemistry seminar during this period on a paper that had recently been published about NMR relaxation times in such systems also served to spark his interest in the relatively young science. NMR gained further public recognition in December 1952 when the Nobel Prize in physics was awarded to Edward Purcell and Felix Bloch for their late 1945 and early 1946 discoveries of NMR in condensed matter.

It is noteworthy that Lauterbur also gave a seminar report on the chemistry of interstellar molecules, a subject area related to the 21-

---

* As discussed in Chapter 5, George Pake was a PhD candidate under Edward Purcell at Harvard from 1946 to 1948. For part of that time, he was a fellow graduate student with Nicolaas Bloembergen.

centimeter hydrogen line discovered in 1951 by Purcell and his graduate student, Harold Ewen. The topic is also related to interstellar dust, another area in which Purcell would later conduct extensive research.

During the 1952-53 academic year, Lauterbur would make a third and very significant contact in the field of NMR when he attended a seminar at the University of Pittsburgh given by Herb Gutowsky from the chemistry department at the University of Illinois. The reader may recall that Gutowsky, while a graduate student at Harvard, had collaborated with Edward Purcell, George Pake and George Kistiakowsky in an NMR investigation of crystal structure.[3] About the time Erwin Hahn, then a graduate student at the University of Illinois who had not yet discovered spin echoes, visited Purcell and Robert Pound at Harvard in 1948, Gutowsky moved west to accept a faculty position at Illinois. Later, after Hahn had moved even further west to Stanford to work with Felix Bloch as a postdoctoral fellow, Hahn and graduate student Don Maxwell would be investigating a mysterious echo envelope modulation using pulses about the same time that Gutowsky and Charles Slichter were investigating steady-state manifestations of a similar phenomenon. This work had placed Gutowsky on the cutting edge of research on chemical shifts. Ramsey and Purcell would later provide the theoretical explanation for this particular chemical shift. Hahn-Maxwell and Gutowsky-Slichter would publish their experimental findings in the same 1951 issue of *Physical Review*.[4]

The seminar Gutowsky gave at the University of Pittsburgh, which was attended by Paul Lauterbur, was on the proton NMR chemical shifts of substituted methanes and their use in deducing electron densities. Lauterbur recognized immediately that nuclear magnetic resonance would be the ideal tool to investigate the differences between silicon and carbon chemistry, an interest of his since his undergraduate days at Case Institute. Rushing up to Gutowsky after the meeting, Lauterbur proposed sending him a variety of samples of substituted silanes, which were not readily available commercially, and asked the Illinois professor if it would be possible to work together in interpreting the comparative NMR data. To Lauterbur's delight, Gutowsky agreed. Lauterbur still had to convince his supervisor back at Mellon Institute, however, to let him synthesize the necessary compounds.

His boss complied with his request. Unfortunately, the Korean War was then in full swing and the U.S. Army wanted Lauterbur's services. As it turned out, however, Lauterbur would have opportunity to further pursue his interest in NMR while serving his stint in the military.

You're in the Army Now

The Korean War had started in 1950 when North Korea invaded South Korea with 60,000 troops on June 25. A multinational force led by the United States, with United Nations approval, responded. By November of that year, the UN forces had reached the border between North Korea and China, but were driven back when 200,000 Chinese troops crossed the Yalu River into North Korea. By mid-1951, the opposing forces were back near the original line of demarcation between North and South Korea where they would remain, fighting a war of attrition, until an armistice was signed on July 27, 1953. It didn't come soon enough, however, to keep Lauterbur, by then a research associate at Mellon Institute, from being drafted into the U.S. Army.

Because of his education and background, Lauterbur was spared from service on the battlefield and was appropriately assigned, at least from the Army's point of view, to where he could do the war effort and the Army the most good—the Army Chemical Center in Edgewood, Maryland. When word got out that Lauterbur had an interest and some "experience" in NMR, he was transferred to the NMR lab and assigned to help set up an NMR machine the Army had acquired for supporting chemical warfare research. Although not the kind of work Lauterbur would have chosen to do, this was war and he was "in the Army now." As it turned out, his specific assignment was to conduct NMR surveys of such materials as phosphorus compounds and exotic boron compounds,[5] relatively innocuous endeavors considering the range of possible assignments he might have been given. "So we weren't really doing Army work in the sense that we weren't putting hand grenades containing toxic gases into our machine,"[6] Lauterbur said. He was able, however, to learn more about NMR and even had a few papers published.

Return to Mellon Institute

Following his discharge from the Army in 1955, Lauterbur knew he wanted to continue his NMR work, having come to recognize what other chemists would come to recognize in the next decade, that NMR spectroscopy was indispensable for analyzing chemical compounds.

"The problem in chemistry," he said, "is you take one flask of a substance and mix it with a second flask of a substance and create a third substance. How do you know what you've got? What is the structure of what you've done? These are the questions you ask every day in the chemistry lab."[7]

He had two options, either join Herb Gutowsky as a graduate student at the University of Illinois, or return to Mellon Institute. Unwilling now to work without an NMR machine, he told Mellon Institute that he would return there on one condition, that they provide him with an NMR spectrometer. The Institute did not accede to his request, but Dow Corning, which was providing funding for the Institute, did, in part because of Lauterbur's claim that he would be able to obtain silicon-29 spectra for them with the machine. When Lauterbur checked with the manufacturer, Varian Associates in Palo Alto, California, he was able to confirm that silicon-29 spectra could, in fact, be obtained, but after returning to Mellon Institute, Lauterbur's research interest would soon be refocused on carbon-13.

Resonances from carbon-13 nuclei would not be easy to observe, for two reasons. First, there is comparatively very little of it, only 1.1 percent of all carbon atoms are carbon-13 atoms. Second, the magnetic moment of carbon-13 is very small, its resonance signal about 6,000 times weaker than hydrogen.[8]

Lauterbur's techniques, however, were successful. His initial publication on carbon-13 was the first ever to describe its spectra. He followed up that publication with a series of papers that were not only foundational in carbon-13 spectroscopy but which also opened new areas of NMR study in organic and inorganic chemistry.[9] With the introduction of Fourier transform techniques by Richard Ernst and others, together with more powerful magnets, carbon-13 NMR spectroscopy would eventually come to be widely used.

Lauterbur had a number of other accomplishments during his eight-year stay at Mellon Institute. He made the first observation of a chemical shift anisotropy in a single crystal, published the first NMR spectra for tin, and resolved a controversy concerning the signs of proton-proton coupling constants.[10]

During his second stint at Mellon Institute, Lauterbur returned to his course work at the University of Pittsburgh. Although he hadn't changed his personal point of view about the value of the lecture format for learning, he did manage to pick up what would turn out to be a couple of extremely valuable techniques. He learned, for example, that there were iterative methods that were being used successfully in quantum chemistry. He also learned about single-center expansions for molecular wave functions.

For his PhD thesis, Lauterbur chose to research nitrogen-14 using nuclear quadrupole resonance spectroscopy under the mentorship of a physics professor. Nothing much came of it. For one thing, the two of them didn't get along very well, apparently a case of irreconcilable research styles. When his advisor left the university to take a job working on a weather satellite project, Lauterbur decided to drop the research he had begun.

The exercise turned out not to be a total loss, however, as Lauterbur was able to sharpen his electronics skills. After regrouping, he decided to do his thesis research on carbon-13 instead, this time with neither the benefit nor the obstacle of an advisor. In 1962, he received his PhD in chemistry, more than 10 years after completing his bachelors degree, with most of that time spent at Mellon Institute. With 20 published papers already to his credit and now in possession of a PhD, Lauterbur decided it was time to look elsewhere for employment.

Eventually, four options presented themselves: Dow Corning in Midland, Michigan; the National Bureau of Standards; Brookhaven National Laboratory on Long Island; and the State University of New York at Stony Brook, also located on Long Island. Oddly enough, Lauterbur, who had more than once found classrooms a convenient place to take a nap, decided he would take the associate professorship he was offered by Stony Brook. Although Stony Brook was not, at first glance, the most promising of the offers available for consideration, Lauterbur recognized one particular benefit which Stony Brook offered and the rest did not, the freedom to do whatever he chose to do, even if it might seem crazy. From Lauterbur's perspective, that was an offer he couldn't refuse, and he agreed to start in February 1963.

Stony Brook

Soon after his arrival at Stony Brook, Lauterbur began setting up an NMR program in the chemistry department. Specifically, he continued his work on chemical shift anisotropies by measuring the first hydrogen and lead shielding tensors in single crystals; wrote a series of papers on intramolecular and solvent isotope effects on chemical shifts; and continued his work on carbon-13 with studies of organometallic compounds.

The 1969-70 academic year, however, would be his seventh at Stony Brook, his sabbatical year, and he intended to use it as a time for refocusing. "That's what academic sabbaticals are for, to get away from the mess on your desk to look at some new perspectives,"[11] Lauterbur said. For a professor involved in NMR, for that's what he now was, a full professor as of 1969, Lauterbur made an appropriate pilgrimage for his sabbatical. He went to Stanford University, the home of Felix Bloch and other NMR notables, where he would be a Visiting Scholar on Sabbatical Leave in the Department of Chemistry.

Stanford Sabbatical

At Stanford, Lauterbur was officially associated with John Baldeschwieler's group, but worked primarily with Thomas Link in George Stark's laboratory in the Stanford Medical Center where he spent most of the year doing carbon-13 labeling of proteins. He also worked with Syntex on tritium, a rare isotope of hydrogen used for biological tracing. With a 100 MHz RF unit borrowed from Varian Associates, the researchers were able to see tritium signals from labeled steroids. As a result of this work, Lauterbur would later set up a resource for further research in this area at Stony Brook, sponsored by the National Institutes of Health.

The protein labeling project, although successful from the standpoint of providing the first carbon-13 NMR spectrum of a protein, was unsuccessful with regard to labeling due to an equipment malfunction. When the temperature control unit went down during an overnight acquisition of data in which they were doing $^{13}CH_3I$ labeling of the fours methionines of ribonuclease A, Lauterbur's entire sample was ruined. It was impossible to interpret the spectrum of a material that had become a yellow gum.

Another phase of the protein labeling project, carbon-13 iodoacetate labeling, was scheduled to be done just before Lauterbur's sabbatical ended, but had to be canceled when a supplier shipped the wrong material. With no time to make up for the mistake by having the supplier send a replacement, Lauterbur had to content himself with packing his bags and heading back to Long Island. His sabbatical was over. He had made progress, however, in getting a program in isotopic labeling underway and had gotten his foot in the door with regard to pursuing other biological applications.

Learning of a Crucial Fundamental Discovery

One of the biological applications Lauterbur pursued after his return to Stony Brook was some biopolymer work that included research in which he planned to study enzymes by replacing calcium with cadmium. In 1971, plans were underway to purchase a superconducting NMR spectrometer from NMR Specialties, a company of about 30 employees that manufactured pulsed NMR spectrometers and other NMR equipment in New Kensington, Pennsylvania.

Lauterbur was no stranger to NMR Specialties. Going back to the days when he was at Mellon Institute, the double-resonance experiments he was doing in carbon-13 called for a "spin decoupler." Unfortunately for Lauterbur, Varian Associates in Palo Alto, California, the company from

whom he expected to acquire the equipment, had discontinued their production of the item. Consequently, Lauterbur decided to pitch in and help
a start-up company, NMR Specialties, get on its feet in the hope that the
new enterprise would be able to provide the badly-needed decoupler.
Since that time, Lauterbur had earned himself a reputation in the field of
NMR and in 1971 was on NMR Specialties' board of directors.

As a board member of NMR Specialties who was ordering a machine
from that company for the University at Stony Brook, Lauterbur had
taken pains to secure all the necessary approvals to avoid any charges of
conflicts of interest and in May 1971 was looking forward to getting his
machine when a strange series of events was set in motion. At a hastily-
called board meeting of NMR Specialties, it was revealed by the company's attorney (also a member of the board) that the company was finan-
cially on the ropes. With the company president forced out, the bank was
threatening to shut the company down that day and start bankruptcy
proceedings unless someone else could be found to take charge while
getting things back on track. The directors asked Lauterbur to take the
position.

Lauterbur weighed the pluses and the minuses. On the positive side,
classes were over; he had no grant money to spend right then; he had no
summer salary coming from the University; and he might be able to save
the superconducting NMR spectrometer he had ordered.

On the negative side, the commute from Long Island to Western
Pennsylvania was a 10- to 12-hour haul, and the prospect of taking the
helm of a nearly-sunken ship was not particularly appealing.

After mulling over the pros and cons, however, Lauterbur decided to
take the challenge and assumed the position of president and chairman
of NMR Specialties. That's how he found himself at New Kensington in
September 1971 when researchers were there to confirm* the results

---

* The collaborators in the study were Donald P. Hollis and Leon A. Saryan, both of the
Department of Physiological Chemistry at Johns Hopkins University School of Medicine,
and Harold P. Morris, of the Department of Biochemistry at Howard University College of
Medicine. In the introduction to their paper, Hollis, et al. briefly reported Damadian's
results and stated that their study extended the earlier research to two Morris hepatomas,
one a faster-growing tumor and the other displaying slow or intermediate growth rates. In
the follow-up discussion, they wrote: "The results shown in Table I confirm in a general way
the results reported earlier by Damadian and by Hazlewood, et al. for Walker sarcoma,
Novikoff hepatoma and malignant mouse mammary tissues in the sense that the T_1's of
both tumors are very different from that of normal liver."
—Donald P. Hollis, Leon A. Saryan and Harold P. Morris, "A nuclear magnetic resonance study of water in two Morris
hepatomas," *Johns Hopkins Medical Journal* **131**, (1972), 441-444,

Raymond Damadian had obtained in his 1970 experiments and which he had published in *Science* in March 1971.[12]

In 1986, *Cancer* magazine published a speech by Lauterbur in which he recalled that:

> "the attention of the medical community was first attracted by the report of Damadian that some animal tumors have remarkably long proton NMR relaxation times. Efforts to reproduce these results and to explore their significance were soon underway in other laboratories."[13]

One of those efforts took place right before Lauterbur's eyes at NMR Specialties, with the experiments conducted by Leon A. Saryan, a graduate student in biochemistry from Johns Hopkins University. "It was measurements that I observed Saryan carrying out in September of 1971 that caught my attention,"[14] said Lauterbur.

Lauterbur's Idea for Visualizing the Different T₁s and T₂s of Normal and Cancerous Tissue

Saryan did his research at NMR Specialties because he was not in a position to duplicate the experiments on his own NMR machine at Johns Hopkins University.[15] When Lauterbur watched Saryan successfully repeat the Damadian experiments, he viewed the procedure with great interest and was impressed by the results. He stated:

> "Even normal tissues differed markedly among themselves in NMR relaxation times, and I wondered whether there might be some way to noninvasively map out such quantities within the body."[16]

If there was a way to tell exactly which locations these NMR signals were coming from within an intact complex object like the human body, there might be a way to devise a map using the information-packed tissue signals Damadian had uncovered.

That evening Lauterbur went to a local fast-food restaurant, the "Eat 'N Run," sat down with his hamburger and intensely pondered the intriguing and difficult problem. In the case of hydrogen proton imaging of a living object, it was clear that the intact object contains a host of hydrogen protons. With every one of them simultaneously emitting NMR signals that contain information about the structure in which they reside, how could one determine what information is coming from where when all you have to work with is one composite, garbled NMR signal? Was there a way to somehow encode the NMR signals emitted from each part of an object so that they would disclose their spatial location? Before Lauterbur finished his meal, he came up with the key to a technique that would help do just that.

Having worked with NMR spectrometers for years, Lauterbur was very familiar with both magnet homogeneities and inhomogeneities—the former preferred, the latter despised. From this, he realized that inhomogeneous magnetic fields actually labeled NMR signals according to their spatial coordinates! By deliberately imposing an ordered system of magnetic inhomogeneities on the magnetic field, he could use these inhomogeneities to extract valuable NMR tissue information otherwise lost in the composite NMR cacophony. This idea would be the basis upon which Lauterbur would develop his technique to spatially encode NMR signals and create images.

Spatial Encoding

Basically, the NMR signals emitted by hydrogen protons in a homogeneous magnetic field are all of the same frequency, the Larmor frequency for hydrogen corresponding precisely to the strength of the magnetic field. Although the intensity of the emitted NMR signals may vary from location to location, depending on such factors as proton density, for example, the frequencies of all the hydrogen NMR responses are identical. However, if there is a certain spot in the field where the strength of the magnetic field is different, i.e. where there is an inhomogeneity at that location, the frequency of the NMR signals emitted by hydrogen protons residing in that spot is different from the frequency of those in the properly-calibrated region. More specifically, if the strength of the field in that region is lower than that of the homogeneous region, the frequency of the NMR signal from that spot will be lower, too, and vice versa.

The following are Lauterbur's recollections of his thoughts that evening while sitting in a Pennsylvania diner.

"I got to thinking that magnetic field gradients provide a general solution to the problem. The reason you couldn't tell the different tissues in a normal NMR machine is that you make a magnetic field that's the same everywhere. If you have a magnetic field that is different on one side of the sample from the other side, then the frequencies of the spectra are different, too. In a uniform field, if you have a little bit of tissue here and a little bit of tissue there, then the signal is the same. If you plot that out, the signals would be right on top of each other and you couldn't distinguish one from the other. Now, if you have a smoothly varying field, then you would have different frequencies and so you could study the signals and distinguish the differences.

"Now this is 1-dimensional. We're dealing with a 3-dimensional object. So the question was, 'Could you extend this idea to resolve completely the 3-dimensional object?' I thought if you could . . . you should be able to go all the way."[17]

The next day Lauterbur went out and bought himself a notebook in which to record his idea for making NMR images.

On *September 2, 1971,* Lauterbur wrote the following in his notebook under the title of "Spatially Resolved Nuclear Magnetic Resonance Experiments:"

"The distribution of magnetic nuclei, such as protons, and their relaxation times and diffusion coefficients, may be obtained by imposing magnetic field gradients (ideally, a complete set of orthogonal spherical harmonics) on a sample, such as an organism or a manufactured object, and measuring the intensities and relaxation behavior of the resonance as functions of the applied magnetic field. Additional spatial discrimination may be achieved by the application of time-dependent gradient patterns so as to distinguish, for example, protons that lie at the intersection of the zero-field (relative to the main magnetic field) lines of three linear gradients.

"The experiments proposed above can be done most conveniently and accurately by measurements of the Fourier transform of the pulse response of the system. They should be capable of providing a detailed three-dimensional map of the distributions of particular classes of nuclei (classified by nuclear species and relaxation times) within a living organism. For example, the distribution of mobile protons in tissues, and the differences in relaxation times that appear to be characteristic of malignant tumors [R. Damadian, *Science,* **171,** (1971), 1151], should be measurable in an intact organism."[18] (See pages B1 through B3 of appendix to this chapter.)

Lauterbur discussed his ideas with G.D. Vickers, then Vice President of Applications at NMR Specialties, and, as scientists do to protect their ideas, had Vickers witness his three-page entry in the notebook by signing his name and entering the date—*September 3, 1971*—at the bottom of each page.[19] (See pages B1 through B3 of appendix to this chapter.)

The Gradient and the Fourier Transform

Using gradients to provide spatial discrimination in one dimension had been described a couple of decades earlier, back when Lauterbur was still finishing up his undergraduate work at Case Institute of Technology. Robert Gabillard in France and Herman Carr* and Edward Purcell at Harvard had all described and used such a concept. One of those researchers, Professor Herman Carr of Rutgers University, writing in a letter to the editor of *Physics Today* in 1993, stated:

"A radically new component *was* introduced in the 1970s, but it was not the basic concept of spatial localization and spin maps, which had already been introduced for one (spatial) dimension in the early days of NMR. . . .

"To the best of my knowledge the idea for superimposing a magnetic field gradient onto the main homogeneous magnetic field had its origin in the self-diffusion effects Erwin L. Hahn observed on his spin-echo envelopes as nuclei diffused through the small residual inhomogeneity of his main magnetic field. Based on this clue, Edward M. Purcell and I intentionally superimposed a strong magnetic field gradient onto the main field, giving a linear dependence of the resonant frequency on the spatial position of the diffusing nucleus. The enhanced diffusion effect then enabled us to make accurate quantitative measurements of the self-diffusion coefficient for suitable fluids. . . .

"The new component of the 1970s is perhaps best described as the vision that a useful spin map as complicated as an interior medical image was in principle obtainable and was a goal worth pursuing."[20]

That it was a goal worth pursuing was proven by the discovery that cancers could be detected with NMR. That a useful spin map could be achieved had been perceived by both Damadian and Lauterbur with their respective NMR scanning and mapping spin localizing methods. (See A5, A10 through A19 of appendix to Chapter 8; see pages B1 through B3 of appendix to this chapter.)

---

* Carr was completing his doctoral thesis in NMR physics under Professor Edward Purcell at the time.

For Lauterbur's part, the mapping would be expressed as a combination of the magnetic gradient, the idea of which was first expressed in 1950, and back projection, a concept that had made possible computed axial tomography in the early 1970s. He has disclaimed these influences in his conception of NMR imaging. He did, nevertheless, combine these two useful approaches to achieve the needed visualization of these disease-discriminating signals.

Although Lauterbur already had a key to the NMR map he was seeking—encoding with a gradient—he had more or less made a "leap of faith" that a 2-dimensional map could somehow be extracted with 1-dimensional encoding of the composite NMR signals. As of September 1971, Lauterbur was not sure how it could be done, only confident that it could be done.

The problem was that a linear gradient of the type Lauterbur envisioned and the type Carr used with Purcell in 1950 would identify the position of the atom in only one dimension. To be useful medically, the spatial position of the atom (or spin) being mapped must be known in three dimensions. The solution to the problem of using these linear gradients in combination to achieve full 3-dimensional resolution was not immediately apparent to Lauterbur in September 1971.

The obvious approach, for example, of applying two gradients at right angles simultaneously to determine two coordinates of the atom (or spin) being mapped, or three gradients simultaneously at right angles to specify all three spatial coordinates of the atom (spin) doesn't work. Two magnetic field gradients applied simultaneously produce only one gradient, a new gradient that is the resultant of the two gradient magnetic fields, with a new direction that is intermediate between the two gradients. The resulting gradient still only specifies one spatial coordinate of the needed three. The problem is the same for three gradients applied simultaneously. They specify only a single new gradient that is the vector sum of all three gradients and therefore still only locate a spin in one dimension, even though three gradients have been applied.

Lauterbur's confidence was based primarily on 1) the expectation that some sort of iterative method would work, a technique he had learned about in some of the university classes he had dutifully attended years earlier; and 2) his knowledge that shim coils such as those used on NMR spectrometers were able to shape magnetic fields.

Although the gradient performed the function of encoding, complete decoding would require a computer-performed mathematical process known as the Fourier transform. The Fourier transform discloses the strength of the signals at each of the component frequencies that comprise the composite NMR signal. In other words, starting with a time-dependent signal such as an emitted NMR signal, the Fourier transform determines the frequencies that comprise the composite signal along with their respective intensities. The frequencies, in turn, yield spatial location information.

Another example of a complex, time-dependent signal is the sound made by an orchestra which is a composite of many acoustic frequencies. The human ear is capable of distinguishing individual notes or tones. One can, for example, discriminate the tones of the first violin and the cello, or distinguish the flute from the bassoon. In other words, the ear is capable of performing a Fourier analysis. By contrast, the eye is not capable of analyzing visible light. White appears as white rather than its composite rainbow of colors. In this case, a simple Fourier analyzer would be a prism which decomposes the light according to its specific frequencies and corresponding wavelengths.[21]

Lauterbur's method used a one-dimensional Fourier transform. The two-dimensional Fourier transform method would later be provided by Richard R. Ernst from the Swiss Federal Institute of Technology in Zürich together with refinements by W.A. Edelstein, J.M.S. Hutchison and J. Mallard at the University of Aberdeen in Scotland.

The idea of the gradient for spatial encoding had been conceived. What remained unresolved as of September 2 and 3, 1971 (see appendix to this chapter) was the means for obtaining a 2-dimensional map from a 1-dimensional gradient. The solution was not yet complete and Lauterbur would produce the solution for the 2-dimensional case until a year later.

Upon his return to Stony Brook University, Lauterbur modified his NMR equipment so it could produce a usable spatial-encoding gradient. He also went to work on the method needed to reconstruct an image from a set of gradients. It took time. In fact, it wasn't until October 1972 when Lauterbur submitted the first draft of his "zeugmatography" paper to *Nature* that he produced a practical solution for the 2-dimensional case.[22]

The solution was to impose successive gradients from different radial directions. He calculated some simple examples by hand and discovered, to his delight, that his method was relatively easy to perform and worked well. In the process, he came up with the well-known reconstruction method known as "back projection."

Lauterbur later learned that several methods for reconstruction from projections had already been invented, including the one he had developed. "Only after [the calculations] had been done was my attention called to a report by Gordon and Herman[23] containing an essentially identical algorithm."[24] For example, X-ray-based CAT (computed axial tomography) scanners, which were beginning to be widely used at the time, used the back projection method.

The Back Projection Technique

The application of a single gradient is not sufficient to reconstruct a two-dimensional image. More specifically, one elicited NMR signal provides just one "projection," i.e. it does spatial encoding in only one direction. Although it is necessary information, in and of itself it is not sufficient to remove all spatial ambiguities. However, if more projections are collected, each with a different angular orientation of the gradient, an image can, by application of mathematical algorithms to the collection of the projections, be accurately reconstructed.

Consider someone standing outside a house at night trying to determine the position of two people standing inside a lighted room solely by observing their silhouettes on the shades at the windows. Viewing the silhouette at only one window is clearly insufficient to make a definitive, non-ambiguous determination. From this one "projection," the viewer can only determine how far the two are standing apart from one another in one direction, but the viewer cannot determine how far apart they are from one another in any other direction. However, with a sufficient number of different projections (i.e. silhouettes at different windows), the viewer can accurately deduce, or reconstruct, the exact locations of the two people in the room.

Although Lauterbur's method for image reconstruction is not currently used on clinical MRI scanners, the employment of gradients for the purpose of spatial localization, the distinctive feature of Lauterbur's approach, has remained widely used.

The Idea Published

Nature rejected Lauterbur's paper at first because "it was not of sufficiently wide significance for inclusion in *Nature*." In consideration of the eventual impact of Lauterbur's idea on the field of medicine, such an evaluation, in retrospect, is surprising, to say the least. These things do happen, however. *Nature* had also rejected the first paper describing the Krebs cycle![25]

The editors were looking for an application of his technique. According to Ros Herman, writing in the *New Scientist* in 1979, the referees at *Nature* "couldn't work out from the first paper what the technique could possibly be used for, so to ensure publication he was forced to add a note about the possibility that it could be used to diagnose cancer."[26] Lauterbur wrote a lengthy rejoinder to this judgment and acquiesced to their concerns by rewriting his manuscript in a more exuberant style.[27] *Nature* accepted the revisions and agreed to publish his paper. The paper, "Image Formation by Induced Local Interactions: Examples Employing Nuclear Magnetic Resonance," appeared in the March 16, 1973 issue.[28]

In the paper, Lauterbur introduced his imaging method as *zeugmatography* derived from the Greek word *zeugma* meaning "that which is used for joining." The name, although it never really caught on, was suitable because the method required the joining together of two magnetic fields to make the image—the main magnetic field and the smaller superimposed field, the gradient. He gave two examples of its use in the paper.

In the first example, the test object was a pair of glass capillaries filled with pure water that were immersed in a larger tube filled with D_2O. With the use of a single gradient, he obtained, by rotating the test object, four projections from which a crude yet impressive 2-dimensional, cross-sectional image of the two 1-millimeter capillary tubes was reconstructed.

In the second example, one of the capillaries contained pure water and the other contained a 0.19 mM solution of $MnSO_4$ in H_2O—the latter with a shorter T_1 value than that of the water. By changing the power levels of the radiofrequency transmitter, Lauterbur also showed that the different relaxation times would produce dramatic effects on the images. This means that diseased tissues which have abnormal relaxation times (Figures 1, 3a and 3b of Chapter 8 and Table I of Chapter 8) would be readily recognized on the images.

In both examples, the maps of the capillary tubes displayed with Lauterbur's zeugmatography method were resolved in only two dimensions, the two dimensions of the cross-sectional image plane as in CT. The third dimension at right angles to the image plane, namely the thickness of the slice plane, was not resolved. The third dimension is important for medical imaging since the thickness of the slice without the third dimension resolved would be the length of the human body. The 3-dimensional solution needed for medical imaging had another step to go. Lauterbur continued to pursue the 3-dimensional generalization of his back-projection method that followed naturally from his 2-dimensional success, but in the end the final solution took a different form.

As the technology progressed, the problem of the fusion of two gradients into a single gradient with an intermediate direction was overcome by applying the gradients in sequence instead of simultaneously, and pulsing them instead of applying them steadily so that they could be sequenced. Additionally, the duration of the transmitted radiofrequency pulse was used to control the bandwidth of the transmitted RF so that the width of the slice could be selected and varied.

With regard to possible applications of his methods, Lauterbur drew the following conclusions:

"Applications of this technique to the study of various inhomogeneous objects, not necessarily restricted in size to those commonly studied by magnetic resonance spectroscopy, may be anticipated. The experiments outlined above demonstrate the ability of the technique to generate pictures of the distributions of stable isotopes, such as H and D, within an object. In the second experiment, relative intensities in an image were made to depend upon relative nuclear relaxation times. The variations in water content and proton relaxation times among biological tissues should permit the generation, with field gradients large compared to internal magnetic inhomogeneities, of useful zeugmatographic images from the rather sharp water resonances of organisms, selectively picturing the various soft structures and tissues. A possible application of considerable interest at this time would be the *in vivo* study of malignant tumors, which have been shown to give proton nuclear magnetic resonance signals with much longer water spin-lattice relaxation times than those in the corresponding normal tissues."[29]

The reference Lauterbur used at this point in his paper was to a December 1972 paper in *Science* authored collaboratively by Irwin D. Weisman and Lawrence H. Bennett of the National Bureau of Standards, by Louis Maxwell, Sr. of Chevy Chase, Maryland, and by Mark W. Wood and Dean Burk of the National Cancer Institute in Bethesda, Maryland. Entitled "Recognition of Cancer *In Vivo* by Nuclear Magnetic Resonance," the paper reported on an experiment in which pulsed NMR had been used by the authors to differentiate *in vivo* between normal mouse tail tissue and a malignant transplanted melanoma, located on the tail of the mouse. The opening paragraph of the Weisman paper, citing Damadian's 1971 article in *Science,* stated: "Measurements of the proton nuclear spin-lattice relaxation time T_1 have been shown by Damadian and subsequently by others to have different values in some normal biological tissues, benign tumors, and malignant tumors observed *in vitro.*"[30]

Lauterbur did not, however, cite Damadian's paper upon which the Weisman study had been predicated. Unfortunately, this omission would create estrangement between Lauterbur and Damadian for years to come. In 1986, Lauterbur indirectly acknowledged Damadian's role when he stated that "the attention of the medical community was first attracted by the report of Damadian that some animal tumors have remarkably long water proton NMR relaxation times."[31]

Damadian, when asked, is complimentary of Lauterbur. "I don't believe I ever give a talk," he said, "where I don't say that, once I succeeded in showing the relaxation differences that got NMR scanning up off the ground, Lauterbur took the key next step by providing a practical method for acquiring and visualizing the tissue differences and Mansfield followed with the gradient pulse sequence technique that completed the physical part of the NMR scanning puzzle."

As to potential uses, Lauterbur stated in his 1973 paper:

"The basic zeugmatographic principle may be employed in many different ways, using a scanning technique, as described above, or transient methods. Variations on the experiment, to be described later, permit the generation of two- or three-dimensional images displaying chemical compositions, diffusion coefficients and other properties of objects measurable by spectroscopic techniques. Although applications employing nuclear magnetic resonance in liquid or liquid-like systems are simple and attractive because of the ease with which field gradients large enough to shift narrow resonances by many line widths may be generated, NMR zeugmatography of solids, electron spin resonance zeugmatography and analogous experiments in other regions of the spectrum should also be possible. Zeugmatographic techniques should find many useful applications in studies of the internal structures, states, and compositions of microscopic objects."[32]

Thus, Lauterbur had published the first NMR image of two 1-millimeter tubes of water. While working out the zeugmatographic method for combining gradients to produce an image, a couple of other items remained unresolved in Lauterbur's mind. First, he wondered if a sufficient signal-to-noise ratio could be derived from large objects in low magnetic fields in order to achieve a useful level of image resolution. Using Abragam's book as a reference, some simple calculations showed him that the laws of physics would work in his favor, promising ample signal-to-noise.

Having been as close to an engineering degree as one can get without actually achieving it—his BS degree would have been in Chemical Engineering had he not taken a graduate chemistry course instead of the required engineering lab—Lauterbur had gained the confidence that whatever physics allowed, engineers could somehow achieve.

Second, he wondered if large enough magnets with sufficiently good homogeneity could be built. In reviewing the literature, he not only found examples of fairly large, homogeneous resistive magnets, but he also found papers describing how easily they could be designed and built. It was becoming increasingly more evident to Lauterbur that his leap of faith was a sound one after all.

With these two issues resolved in his mind, the only remaining concern he had, ironically, was how useful such images of the body would prove to be in the practice of medicine. This concern was understandable because, at the time, Lauterbur knew little about medical science or clinical medicine. In an effort to remedy that deficiency so that he would be able to discuss with doctors the potential uses of NMR imaging in medicine, Lauterbur skimmed through a host of books and journals at the medical school library in Stony Brook to pick up some of the vocabulary and maybe even identify some possible applications.

Before long, he felt comfortable with the direction in which he was headed and was beginning to recognize the enormous potential of his imaging idea, even if others didn't. He dreamed of a human-sized scanner. In 1972, he started doing experiments and giving talks at the University and at Brookhaven National Laboratory a few miles down the road. He also spoke at the American Physical Society meeting in January of 1973. He started writing papers and grant proposals, most of which were rejected, although he did obtain a grant from the National Cancer Institute which allowed him to buy an NMR spectrometer and to assemble a research team.

Taking to the scientific meeting circuit in the United States and abroad, Lauterbur shared the good news of NMR imaging with all who would listen. Not everyone who listened agreed with his ideas, but Lauterbur forged ahead, somehow managing to cope with the nay-sayers, waiting for the world to see the light.

Meanwhile . . .

A year minus one day before Lauterbur published his ideas on zeugmatography in *Nature*, Raymond Damadian filed a patent application for a human scanner.[33] Damadian's acquisition method provided the means for full 3-dimensional signal acquisition, making it possible, in other words, to collect data from a precise point in space which was dimensionally limited in length, width and height. The major drawback of Damadian's acquisition method was the speed at which data could be collected since it required physical positioning and repositioning of the fixed "sweet spot" within the sample which, in the case of humans, required physically moving the patient across the "sweet spot" to complete a scan.

Lauterbur's method, on the other hand, once the technology had progressed to the point that the 2-dimensional limitation of his original method had been overcome, provided faster data acquisition for the whole-body application.

The idea of imaging itself and a method for achieving that goal in two dimensions by combining the linear magnetic gradient method and the back projection method would thus be Lauterbur's unique pioneering contributions to the early history of magnetic resonance in medicine. Both methods of data acquisition—Damadian's and Lauterbur's—would be used in the early stages of MRI and both would later be superseded.

The drawbacks to Lauterbur's method would be worked out by other contributors to the field in the months and years that followed. Soon after Lauterbur's original zeugmatography publication, four methods of NMR imaging would be demonstrated by four geographically disparate groups.[34-37] The contributions of one man—Peter Mansfield—are particularly noteworthy. Mansfield's first paper dealing with imaging was published in 1974.[38] Mansfield came up with the way for NMR to "home in" on particular slices of the sample by sequencing and pulsing the gradients.

Although magnetic resonance imaging would come about initially because of the contributions of two men—Damadian and Lauterbur—its evolution into the state-of-the-art technology with which we are familiar today would occur as a host of others climbed onboard and added their ideas. As the others climbed aboard, Damadian and Lauterbur did not disembark. Both would continue to make contributions to the fast-growing technology.

Lauterbur the Person

Lauterbur is the classic professorial type. A man of broad interests, both inside and outside of the sciences, Lauterbur was once described by R. Robert Schneider, associate vice provost at Stony Brook, as having musical tastes "ranging from the country to the classical, with a little Kingston Trio in between. In fact, at one time Lauterbur enjoyed folk singing with a campus group in a little inn just off the campus." As a result of being well-read in a wide variety of subjects, Lauterbur has developed an extensive vocabulary. He is precise in language, sometimes pausing between his carefully-weighed and deliberate phrases.[39]

"As a teacher," Schneider continued, "Lauterbur is a superb one-to-one teacher with graduate students. In fact, they don't always recognize immediately how much they have learned from him."[40]

There is a lighter side to the Lauterbur persona as well. Schneider recalled a New Year's Eve costume party: "Paul Lauterbur was sensational—dressed as a huge worm in a fabric costume with a dozen hoops." Dr. Sei Sujishi, dean of physical sciences and mathematics, enjoyed Lauterbur's sense of humor—"Not high humor, just easy wit."[41]

Lauterbur is and always has been an idea man, a thinker, always dreaming up new methods and schemes, searching for solutions to problems or looking for new areas for exploration. When it comes to agendas, however, he can be contrary and independent. On the other hand, his contrary independence can be seen as an asset in his dedication to the development of MRI.

Like many pioneers, Lauterbur has always been totally and energetically committed to his work. When he wasn't on the lecture circuit, he would spend long hours at the laboratory. His family, like those of many a pioneer, would suffer from his absence. Waylan House, a one-time associate of Lauterbur's, recalled, "One night I asked him why he worked so hard. He had a wife, some kids. And he said, 'Well, I guess one does it for the approbation of one's peers.'"[42]

The Patent

Lauterbur tried to convince others—individuals and institutions—that his idea was patent-worthy. Securing a lawyer who had worked with NMR Specialties, he tried to get the patent wheels turning on his idea. When proceedings got under way, the lawyer, worried that any further work by Lauterbur on the idea at Stony Brook might somehow weaken the claim, counseled him to discontinue all testing. In the meantime, Lauterbur figured he would use his time most profitably by getting a head start on the next logical step—approaching entrepreneurs about forming a company to build human-size NMR scanners.

He spoke to several of them. They were looking for return-on-investment figures, market potential and production schedules. Lauterbur offered only what they saw as a very interesting idea. Although he firmly believed his idea would be a smashing commercial success, it simply wasn't enough to make the entrepreneurs reach into their pockets. Before the patent process had gotten very far, friction had developed between Lauterbur and his lawyer over matters having to do with NMR Specialties. At the same time, Lauterbur was getting impatient—he wanted to get back to his experiments. Consequently, he decided to drop the commercial patent application.[43]

Instead, Lauterbur turned to Research Corporation, which acted as an agent for Stony Brook University, as it did for other universities, in securing patents on their behalf. He fared no better there. The following is an excerpt from a February 20, 1974 letter to Lauterbur from an associate in Research Corporation's Patent Programs regarding their decision not to seek patenting and licensing of Lauterbur's idea:

> At our meeting I explained our inability to identify a potential market of sufficient size to justify our undertaking the patenting and licensing of this invention. In response you reviewed some of the uses you believed to be promising. I stated that, as a group, the applications you mentioned, although interesting technically and scientifically, did not appear to be sufficient to excite the interest of industry in investing in the development, manufacture and marketing of imaging systems based on this concept.
>
> The difficulty as we see it is that your invention is still at such an early stage of development that its true usefulness and superiority over other already established imaging techniques, such as ultrasonics, radioactive tracers, x-ray, etc., is still unknown. As a specific example, we discussed the case of the EMI radioactive scanner which uses an image reconstruction technique similar to that which you employ in your invention. I said that we were not able to see how your invention could possibly compete with the EMI device in the specific problem of head tumor imaging.
>
> In summary, in light of the yet to be demonstrated distinct advantages of your scanning invention and our inability at this point to visualize any reasonable possibility of being able to license it successfully, we have regretfully decided not to accept it for administration under our Agreement with the State University of New York Research Foundation.

Today, MRI is a billion-dollar industry; thousands of MRI scanners are helping people the world over. Now considered the premier diagnostic imaging modality, MRI not only competes with CAT scanners but many diagnosticians believe that MRI will eventually replace CAT scanners.

While the gross misjudgment of Research Corporation may cause the reader to smile in amazement, this incident does not mark the first time that decision makers missed by a mile, nor will it be the last. With the decision by Research Corporation not to pursue the patent, Lauterbur received the right from the University to try to secure the patent on his own. He decided to drop the matter.

Meanwhile, the inexorable march toward the first human-sized scanner was under way. In order to do biomedical NMR, apparatus that was originally constructed for the study of small chemical samples had to be modified. With only 5 millimeters of space available, Lauterbur was having a difficult time coming up with a suitably-sized creature. Sharyn, his nine-year-old daughter, was therefore drafted into service and she came up with a 4 millimeter clam that she found near their home in Setauket Harbor on Long Island. Tinier than Lauterbur thought existed, this clam would be the first animal to be imaged using an NMR machine. The image of its soft body within the shell was reconstructed using four projections. After imaging the clam, Lauterbur went on to do images of nuts and tree branches.[44]

Lauterbur, typical of a scientific pioneer just starting out, had to "make do" with the equipment he had available, at least until he acquired the financial support he needed to pursue his dream further. "The equipment was being used for real chemical work during the day," he told his hometown paper in Sidney, Ohio, "so in the evenings, I'd put bits of plants, earthworms, clams, fruit, you name it, into the spectrometer and just look at the MRI signals."[45]

Although in the beginning Lauterbur worked alone, he eventually received funding from the National Cancer Institute to build his apparatus and to acquire some help.[46] After obtaining larger spectrometers, Lauterbur began imaging larger objects, up to 3 centimeters in diameter, including a live mouse. A transmitter coil wrapped around the mouse's body for irradiation and a smaller receiver coil, sensitive only to the region in its plane, were used to stimulate and pick up the NMR signal. Image reconstruction using projections in two dimensions, but undefined in the third dimension, produced an image of a live mouse.

Lauterbur's "mouse-sized" machine would, for the next two years, be used to attempt the imaging of malignant tumors in living animals, to make further improvements on his imaging techniques and to develop an intermittent CW technique for the measurement of T_1, the spin-lattice relaxation time.[47]

In England, Peter Mansfield had also begun imaging. Starting with imaging of dead chicken legs in 1974, he worked his way up to scanning human fingers.[48] In 1976, Mansfield, along with A.A. Maudsley, published a paper showing a very respectable image of a human finger—the world's first human NMR image.[49] He would later order a resistive magnet large enough for a human, in which he would image small animals such as rabbits, rats, guinea pigs, cats and a human cadaver.[50-52]

Other groups also jumped onto the imaging bandwagon, including another University of Nottingham group led by Waldo Hinshaw and E. Raymond Andrew, and a group from the University of Aberdeen in Scotland headed by John Mallard from the department of biomedical physics and biomedical engineering. Even EMI, the British firm that introduced the CAT scanner, had an eye on the ultimate goal, an NMR machine that could scan the whole human body.[53] Lauterbur, too, was looking to build a human-sized NMR machine. Nothing panned out.

On July 3, 1977, Damadian, using the 53-inch superconducting magnet he and his students built from the ground up, produced its first human image, a cross-sectional slice of a live human through the heart and lungs, using the point-by-point, "sweet spot" technique described in his patent. The scan took 4 hours and 45 minutes. In 1978, Mansfield produced the world's second whole-body image, that of his abdomen, which took only 40 minutes.[54]

Throughout the 1970s until the mid-1980s, Lauterbur's laboratory also conducted research in other areas of NMR imaging, not just the scanning of larger and larger living creatures. These studies included chemical shift imaging of proton signals in 1975[55] and the introduction of paramagnetic contrast agents in 1978.[56] In the period from 1977 to 1981, Lauterbur worked on 3-dimensional projection reconstruction[57-60] for the generation of isotropic NMR images of entire objects for 3-dimensional display, and from 1981 to 1984 in their applications,[61] including: surface coil imaging; an off-resonance saturation technique; electrocardiogram-synchronized heart imaging; NMR imaging of gases for the study of lung ventilation; rapid 3-D human imaging and 3-D image display; and a whole-body 3-D system constructed for 3-D imaging in which cancer specimens that had been removed from surgery were studied.[62]

Lauterbur had approximately 80 papers published during his tenure at the State University of New York at Stony Brook. He was named Research Professor of Radiology in 1978, Leading Professor in Chemistry in 1982 and University Professor in 1984, one of only two professors in the University to hold that rank.[63]

In 1984, Lauterbur was working on such things as microscopic imaging and some new mathematical algorithms, also for imaging. Beset by inadequate research funds at the time and still using some of the same magnets he had used nearly 10 years earlier, Lauterbur decided it was time for another move.

In 1985, he joined the University of Illinois where, from the very beginning, honors were lavishly bestowed upon him. He was appointed to three professorships: one in the Department of Medical Information Science at the College of Medicine at Urbana-Champaign, another in the Department of Chemistry at Urbana-Champaign, and the third at the College of Medicine in Chicago. On the basis of Lauterbur's past accomplishments, he was also named a Senior University Scholar for a three-year period. In the ensuing years, he would be appointed Director of the Biomedical Magnetic Resonance Laboratory, Professor of Physiology in the Biophysics Division of the Department of Physiology and Biophysics, Professor in the Neuroscience and Bioengineering Programs and in the Beckman Institute and Professor in the Center for Advanced Study, the highest honor for a faculty member on the Urbana-Champaign campus. Finally, Lauterbur would hold the rank of Distinguished Professor in the College of Medicine in Chicago.[64]

For his pioneering contributions, Paul Lauterbur has received the Albert Lasker Clinical Research Award (1984), the Charles F. Kettering Prize from General Motors Cancer Research Foundation (1985), the National Medal of Technology (1988), the Bower Award and Prize (1990) and the Dickson Prize for Science from Carnegie-Mellon University (1993), among others.

Lauterbur has two children from his first marriage: Daniel, age 34, and Sharyn, age 32. In 1984, he married M. Joan Dawson, a faculty member at Stony Brook. Dr. Dawson received her BS from Columbia University in 1964 and her PhD from the University of Pennsylvania in 1972. While at Stony Brook, Dr. Dawson was a research physiologist studying magnetic resonance.[65] Drs. Lauterbur and Dawson both hold positions at the University of Illinois.[66] They have a daughter, Mary, age 10.

Lauterbur has continued to make substantial contributions in his field since his move to the University of Illinois. They include: an entirely new approach to spectroscopic localization for *in vivo* NMR, dubbed SLIM for Spectral Localization by Imaging; the continuing development of standard NMR microscopy to reach new levels of resolution; the development of microscopic receiver coils and signal enhancement techniques for increased resolution; electron paramagnetic resonance imaging; magnetic labeling of cells; and the development of new magnetic contrast agents including ones that are sensitive to electric fields. More recently, Lauterbur has been performing NMR studies of microscopic anatomy, flow, perfusion, blood oxygenation and *in vivo* spectroscopy as part of an overall effort in making detailed anatomical and functional mappings of the brain. Such studies, it is hoped, will lead to a fuller understanding of the nature of the neural maps and circuits involved in various activities of the brain, including cognition, sensory processing and motor activity.[67]

It would be difficult to overstate the impact that magnetic resonance imaging has had on the medical field and the contributions of pioneer Paul Lauterbur to MRI should not be underestimated. Although it is true that gradients, Fourier transforms and methods of back projection were known, it was Paul Lauterbur who used them to originate a method for spatially localizing NMR relaxation information from a sample and to display it as a pictorial map, thus helping to open the way to MRI. ■

❋ ❋ ❋

Because of the contributrions of Dr. Raymond Damadian and Dr. Paul Lauterbur, magnetic resonance imaging has become the most powerful and reliable diagnostic tool in medicine. Without using harmful X-rays, MRI depicts anatomy in exquisite detail, particularly in the soft tissues of the body. Because of MRI, abnormalities and diseases can now be detected safely, comfortably and noninvasively.

The future of MRI is extremely bright. New applications of MRI are anticipated and its complete or, at least, partial displacement of other imaging modalities, such as CAT scanning, is expected. Millions of people the world over enjoy a higher quality of life and many lives have been saved, thanks to the contributions of Damadian and Lauterbur.

NMR scanning resulted from *two* essential steps. They were taken by the two great MRI pioneers of this volume, Dr. Raymond Damadian and Dr. Paul Lauterbur. Dr. Damadian provided the first step, the discovery of tissue NMR signal differences from which the image is made and the first concept of an NMR body scanner that would utilize these signal differences to detect disease in the live human body. Dr. Lauterbur provided the next step of visualizing these signal differences as an image and supplied the first method for acquiring these signals at practical speeds. It does not seem likely that MRI could have come to pass without the key steps contributed by both scientists.

Without Damadian's discovery, it could not be known that serious diseases like cancer could be detected by an NMR scanner or that tissue NMR signals possessed sufficient contrast to create medically useful images. Without Lauterbur's contribution, development of a practical method for visualizing these signal differences as an image might have occurred much less efficiently. The image required the tissue signal differences in order to make the image and the tissue signal differences required a practical method for acquiring and displaying them.

Recognizing their contributions, the President of the United States awarded the nation's highest honor in technology, the National Medal of Technology, jointly to Dr. Damadian and Dr. Lauterbur for the development of MRI. In presenting the award on July 15, 1988 in a ceremony at the White House, President Ronald Reagan cited both scientists "for their independent contributions in conceiving and developing the application of magnetic resonance technology to medical uses including whole-body scanning and diagnostic imaging." ■

REFERENCE NOTES:

1. *Sidney Daily News*, 20 February 1948.
2. George E. Pake, "Magnetic resonance," *Scientific American* **199**, (1958), 58-65.
3. H.S. Gutowsky, G.B. Kistiakowsky, G.E. Pake and E.M. Purcell, "Structural investigations by means of nuclear magnetism," *J. Chem. Phys.* **17**, (1949), 972-981.
4. E.L. Hahn and D.E. Maxwell, "Chemical shift and field independent frequency modulation of the spin echo envelope," *Physical Review* **84**, (1951), 1246; H. Gutowsky, S.L. McCall, C. Slichter and E.B. McNeil, *Physical Review* **84**, (1951), 1246.
5. S. Kleinfield, *A Machine Called Indomitable*, (New York: Times Books, 1985), 56.
6. Ibid.
7. Ibid., 57.
8. Pavia, Lampman and Kriz, *Saunders Golden Sunburst Series*, (Holt, Rinehart and Winston, PA: Saunders Publishing, 1979), 165.
9. P.C. Lauterbur, "Academic history and scientific accomplishments," unpublished, 28 September 1993.
10. Ibid.
11. Kleinfield, *A Machine Called Indomitable*, 57.
12. R. Damadian, "Tumor detection by nuclear magnetic resonance," *Science* **171**, (1971), 1151-1153.
13. P.C. Lauterbur, "Cancer detection by nuclear magnetic resonance zeugmatographic imaging," speech given at award of Charles F. Kettering Prize by General Motors Cancer Research Foundation, reprinted in *Cancer* **57**, (15 May 1986), 1899.
14. Ibid.
15. Kleinfield, *A Machine Called Indomitable*, 54.
16. Lauterbur, "Cancer detection by nuclear magnetic resonance zeugmatographic imaging," *Cancer* **57**, (15 May 1986), 1899.
17. Kleinfield, *A Machine Called Indomitable*, 59.
18. P.C. Lauterbur, "Spatially Resolved Nuclear Magnetic Resonance Experiments," handwritten by Lauterbur in laboratory notebook on 2 September 1971, countersigned by G.D. Vickers on 3 September 1971.
19. Kleinfield, *A Machine Called Indomitable*, 59-60.
20. Herman Y. Carr, letter to the editor, *Physics Today*, January 1993, 94.
21. "NMR: A Perspective on Imaging," General Electric.
22. Lauterbur, "Image formation by induced local interactions: Examples employing nuclear magnetic resonance," *Nature* **242**, (1973), 190-191.
23. R. Gordon and G.T. Herman, "Reconstruction of pictures from their projections," *Comm. ACM* **14**, (1971), 759-768.
24. Lauterbur, "Cancer detection by nuclear magnetic resonance zeugmatographic imaging," *Cancer* **57**, (15 May 1986), 1900.
25. R. Manuel Mourino, "From Thales to Lauterbur, or from the Lodestone to MR imaging: Magnetism and medicine," *Radiology* **180**, (1991), 611.
26. Ros Herman, "A chemical clue to disease," *New Scientist*, 15 March 1979, 876.
27. Mourino, "From Thales to Lauterbur, or from the Lodestone to MR imaging: Magnetism and medicine," 611.
28. Lauterbur, "Image formation by induced local interactions: Examples employing nuclear magnetic resonance," *Nature* **242**, (1973), 190-191.
29. Ibid.
30. Irwin D. Weisman, Lawrence H. Bennett, Louis R. Maxwell, Sr., Mark W. Woods and Dean Burk, "Recognition of cancer *in vivo* by nuclear magnetic resonance," *Science* **178**, (1972), 1288-1290.

31. Lauterbur, "Cancer detection by nuclear magnetic resonance zeugmatographic imaging," *Cancer* **57,** (15 May 1986), 1899.

32. Lauterbur, "Image formation by induced local interactions: Examples employing nuclear magnetic resonance," *Nature* **242,** (1973), 190-191.

33. R.V. Damadian, "Apparatus and method for detecting cancer in tissue," filed with U.S. Patent Office on 17 March 1972, application no. 235,624, granted U.S. Patent 3,789,832 on 5 February 1974.

34. A.N. Garroway, P.K. Grannell and P. Mansfield, "Image formation in NMR by a selective irradiative process," *J. Phys. C: Solid State Phys.* **7,** (1974), L457-L462.

35. J.M.S. Hutchison, J.R. Mallard and C.C. Goll, "Magnetic resonance and related phenomena," Proceedings of the 18th Ampère Congress, Nottingham, 9-14 September 1974, Vol. 1, Amsterdam: North-Holland, 1974, ed. by P.S. Allen, E.R. Andrew, C.A. Bates, 283-284.

36. W.S. Hinshaw, "Spin mapping: the application of moving gradients to NMR," *Phys. Lett.* **48A,** (1974), 87-88.

37. A. Kumar, D. Welti and R.R. Ernst, "Imaging of macroscopic objects by NMR Fourier zeugmatography," *Naturwissenschaften* **62,** (1975), 34.

38. A.N. Garroway, P.K. Grannell and P. Mansfield, "Image formation in NMR by a selective irradiative process," *J. Phys. C: Solid State Phys.* **7,** (1974), L457-L462.

39. *Stony Brook News,* 18 November 1984.

40. Ibid.

41. Ibid.

42. Kleinfield, *A Machine Called Indomitable,* 139.

43. Ibid., 65-66.

44. Ibid., 64.

45. *Sidney Daily News,* 18 June 1985.

46. Ibid.

47. Lauterbur, "Cancer detection by nuclear magnetic resonance zeugmatographic imaging," *Cancer* **57,** (15 May 1986), 1901.

48. Kleinfield, *A Machine Called Indomitable,* 100.

49. P. Mansfield and A.A. Maudsley, "Planar and line-scan spin imaging by NMR," *Proc. XIXth Congress Ampère,* Heidelberg (1976), 247-252.

50. P. Mansfield, H. Pykett II and P.G. Morris, "Human whole body line-scan imaging by NMR," *Br. J. Radiol.* **51,** (1978), 921-922.

51. E.R. Andrew, P.A. Bottomley, W.S. Hinshaw, G.N. Holland, W.S. Moore and C. Simaroj, "NMR images by the multiple sensitive point method: Application to larger biological specimens," *Phys. Med. Biol.* **22,** (1977), 971.

52. Kleinfield, *A Machine Called Indomitable,* 100.

53. Ibid.

54. Ibid., 196.

55. P.C. Lauterbur, D.M. Kramer, W.V. House, Jr. and C.N. Chen, "Zeugmatographic high-resolution nuclear magnetic resonance spectroscopy of chemical inhomogeneity within macroscopic objects," *J. Am. Chem. Soc.* **97,** (1975), 6866-6868.

56. P.C. Lauterbur, M.H. Mendonca Dias and A.M. Rudin, "Augmentation of tissue water proton spin-lattice relaxation rates by *in vivo* addition of paramagnetic ions," in *Frontiers of Biological Energetics,* edited by P.O. Dutton, J.S. Leigh and A. Scarpa, (New York: Academic Press, 1978), 752-759.

57. C.N. Chen, "1: Direct three-dimensional image reconstructions from plane integrals and their applications in nuclear magnetic resonance zeugmatography. 2: Silicon-29 nuclear magnetic resonance zeugmatography," PhD dissertation, Department of Chemistry, State University of New York at Stony Brook, New York, 1980.

58. P.C. Lauterbur and C.M. Lai, "Zeugmatography by reconstruction from projection," *IEEE Trans. Nucl. Sci.* **NS-27,** (1980), 1227-1231.

59. C.M. Lai and P.C. Lauterbur, "True three-dimensional image reconstruction by nuclear magnetic resonance zeugmatography," *Phys. Med. Biol.* **26**, (1981), 851-856.

60. R.B. Marr, C.N. Chen and P.C. Lauterbur, "On two approaches to 3D reconstruction in NMR zeugmatography," ed. by G.T. Herman and F. Natterer, *Mathematical Aspects of Computerized Tomography,* Vol. 8, *Lecture Notes in Medical Informatics,* ed. by D.A.B. Lindberg and P.L. Reichertz, (Berlin: Springer-Verlag, 1981), **21**:239-241.

61. D.M. Kramer, J.S. Schneider, A.M. Rudin and P.C. Lauterbur, "True three-dimensional capabilities," Application of Optical Instrumentation in Medicine IX. *Proc. Soc. Photo-Optical Instrumentation Engineers* **273**, (1981), 41-49.

62. Lauterbur, "Cancer detection by nuclear magnetic resonance zeugmatographic imaging," *Cancer* **57**, (15 May 1986), 1902.

63. Lauterbur, "Academic history and scientific accomplishments," unpublished, 28 September 1993.

64. Ibid.

65. *Sidney Daily News,* 18 June 1985.

66. Ibid.

67. Lauterbur, "Academic history and scientific accomplishments," unpublished, 28 September 1993.

APPENDIX, CHAPTER 9

1

Spatially Resolved Nuclear Magnetic
Resonance Experiments.

    The distribution of magnetic nuclei,
such as protons, and their relaxation times
and diffusion coefficients, may be obtained
by imposing magnetic field gradients
(ideally, a complete set of orthogonal
spherical harmonics) on a sample, such
as an organism or a manufactured object,
and measuring the intensities and relaxation
behavior of the resonances as functions
of the applied magnetic field. Additional
spatial discrimination may be achieved
by the application of time-dependent
gradient patterns so as to distinguish,

Paul C. Lauterbur

Sept. 2, 1971
Sept. 3, 1971

2

for example, protons that lie at the intersection of the zero-field (relative to the main static field) lines of three linear gradients.

    The experiments proposed above can be done most conveniently and accurately by measurements of the Fourier transform of the pulse response of the system. They should be capable of providing a detailed three-dimensional map of the distributions of particular classes of nuclei (classified by nuclear species and relaxation times) within a living organism. For example, the distribution of mobile protons in

Paul C. Lauterbur

Sept. 2, 1971
Sept 3, 1971

3

tissues, and the differences in relaxation times that appear to be characteristic of malignant tumors [R. Damadian, Science, 171, 1151 (1971)], should be measurable in an intact organism.

Paul C. Lauterbur

Sept. 2, 1971
Sept. 3, 1971

A P P E N D I X

The Holocaust, 1939-1945

The following are estimates of the number of Jewish men, women and children put to death between 1939 and 1945, by national origin (not place of death). Taken from Alan Bullock, *Hitler and Stalin: Parallel Lives* (New York, Alfred A. Knopf, 1991), Appendix 3, who quoted the statistics from Jeremy Noakes and Geoffrey Pridham, *Nazism, 1919-1945*, Vol. III: *Foreign Policy, War and Racial Extermination* (Exeter: 1988), 918.

Country	Estimated Previous Number of Jews	Losses Lowest Estimate	Losses Highest Estimate	Percent
Poland	3,300,000	2,350,000	2,900,000	88%
USSR*	4,700,000	2,200,000	2,200,000	46%
Romania	850,000	200,000	420,000	49%
Czechoslovakia	360,000	233,000	300,000	83%
Germany	240,000	160,000	200,000	83%
Hungary	403,000	180,000	200,000	50%
Lithuania	155,000	—	135,000	87%
France	300,000	60,000	130,000	43%
Holland	150,000	104,000	120,000	80%
Latvia	95,000	—	85,000	89%
Yugoslavia	75,000	55,000	65,000	87%
Greece	75,000	57,000	60,000	80%
Austria	60,000	—	40,000	67%
Belgium	100,000	25,000	40,000	48%
Italy	75,000	8,500	15,000	26%
Bulgaria	50,000	—	7,000	14%
Luxembourg	—	3,000	3,000	—
Norway	—	700	1,000	—
Denmark	—	fewer than 100	—	—
TOTAL	11,000,000	5,636,000	6,921,000	64%

* NOTE:
Alan Bullock, author of *Hitler and Stalin: Parallel Lives*, indicates that he used the higher estimates for the number of Jews in the Soviet Union in the summer of 1941 (4.7 million in place of the earlier estimate of 2.1 million) and for the number killed by the Germans and their allies (2.2 million in place of 700,000) which were the result of further research by K. Krausnick and H.H. Wilhelm, *Die Truppe der Weltanschauungskrieger: Die Einsatzgruppen der Sicherheitspolizei und der SD 1938-1942* (Stuttgart: 1981), pp. 618ff. Bullock therefore has added the same figure of 2.2 million killed in Russia to each of the two columns giving the lower and higher estimate of losses.

Professionals in Mathematics, Science and Medicine who Emigrated to the United States from Europe Between 1930 and 1941—A partial list compiled primarily from Laura Fermi's book, *Illustrious Immigrants,* Second Edition, (Chicago: University of Chicago Press, 1971).

Anker, Herbert S. (Biochemist, Germany, 1912)

Artin, Emil (Mathematician, Austria, 1898-1963)

Artom, Camillo (Biochemist, Italy, 1893)

Auger, Pierre V. (Physicist, France, 1899)

Baer, Reinhold (Mathematician, Germany, 1902)

Baumann, Franz (Dermatologist, Germany, 1896)

Beck, Paul (Metallurgist. Hungary, 1908)

Becker, William (Orthopedist, humanitarian, Germany, 1896-1963)

Bergman, Stefan (Mathematician, Poland, 1903)

Bergmann, Max (Chemist. Germany, 1886-1944)

Bergmann, Peter Gabriel (Mathematician, Germany, 1915)

Bers, Lipman (Mathematician, Latvia, 1914)

Bethe, Hans Albrecht (Physicist, France, 1906)

Biot, Maurice (Physicist, Belgium, 1905)

Birnbaum, William Z. (Mathematician, Poland, 1903)

Bloch, Felix (Physicist, Switzerland, 1905)

Bloch, Konrad E. (Biochemist, Germany, 1912)

Bochner, Salomon (Mathematician, Poland, 1899)

Bohr, Niels H.D. (Physicist, Denmark, 1885-1962)

Born, Max (Physicist, Germany)

Brauer, Alfred (Mathematician, Germany, 1894)

Brauer, Richard Dagobert (Mathematician, Germany, 1901)

Brillouin, Leon N. (Physicist, France, 1889-1969)

Castiglioni, Arturo (Historian of medicine, Italy, 1874-1952)

Chain, Boris (Medicine, Germany)

Chargaff, Erwin (Biochemist, Austria, 1905)

Chevalley, Claude S. (Mathematician, South Africa, 1909)

Clausen, Jens (Botanist, Denmark, 1891)

Courant, Richard (Mathematician, Poland, 1888)

Dam, C.P. Hendrik (Biochemist, Denmark, 1895)

De Benedetti, Sergio (Physicist, Italy, 1912)

Debye, Peter (Chemist. Holland, 1884-1966)

de Hevesy, George (Chemist, Hungary)

Dehn, Max (Mathematician, Germany, 1878-?)

Delbruck, Max (Biophysicist, Germany, 1906)

de Santillana, Giorgio D. (Science historian, Italy, 1902)

Edelstein, Ludwig (Classical philologist, historian of medicine, Germany, 1902)

Eilenberg, Samuel (Mathematician, Poland, 1913)

Einstein, Albert (Physicist, Germany, 1879)

Ekstein, Hans (Physicist, Russia, 1908)

Erdos, Paul (Mathematician, Hungary, 1913)

Fajans, Kasimir (Physical chemist, Poland, 1887)

Fankhauser, Gerhard (Biologist, Switzerland, 1901)

Fano, Ugo (Physicist, Italy, 1912)

Feller, William (Mathematician, Yugoslavia, 1906)

Fermi, Enrico (Physicist, Italy, 1901)

Fraenkel-Conrat, Heinz (Biochemist, Germany, 1910)

Franck, James (Chemist, Germany, 1882)

Frank, Philipp G. (Physicist-philosopher, Austria, 1884)

Friedrichs, Kurt Otto (Mathematician, Germany, 1901)

Fubini, Eugene G. (Electronic engineer, Italy, 1913)

Fubini, Guido (Mathematician, Italy, 1879)

Gabor, Dennis (Physicist, Hungary)

Gamow, George (Physicist, Russia, 1904)

Gero, Alexander (Chemist, Hungary, 1907)

Godel, Kurt (Mathematician, Czechoslovakia, 1906)

Goldfeder, Anna (Cancer researcher, Poland, 1897)

Goldstein, Kurt (Neurologist, Poland, 1878)

Gomori, George (Physician, Hungary, 1904)

Grosse, Aristid V. (Chemist, Russia, 1905)

Gumpert, Martin (Physician-writer, Germany, 1897)

Gyorgy, Paul (Pediatrician, Hungary, 1893)

Haagen-Smit, Arie Jan (Biochemist, Holland, 1900)

Haber, Fritz (Chemist, Germany)

Hadamard, Jacques (Mathematician, France, 1865)

Hertz, Gustav (Physicist, Germany)

Herzberg, Gerhard (Chemist, Germany)

Hess, Victor Francis (Physicist, Austria, 1883)

Horner, Imre (Physician, Hungary, 1901)

Hurewicz, Witold (Mathematician, Poland, 1904)

Infeld, Leopold (Physicist, Poland, 1898)

John, Fritz (Mathematician, Germany, 1910)

Kac, Mark (Mathematician, Poland, 1914)

Kalckar, Herman M. (Physiologist-biochemist, Denmark, 1908)

Kolin, Alexander (Biophysicist, Russia, 1910)

Koyre, Alexander (Science historian, Russia, 1912)
Krebs, Hans A. (Medicine, Germany)
Lanczos, Cornelius (Mathematician, Hungary, 1893)
Lattes, Raffaele (Pathologist, Italy, 1910)
Lewy, Hans (Mathematician, Germany, 1904)
Lipmann, Fritz (Biochemist, Germany, 1899)
Loewi, Otto (Physiologist-pharmacologist, Germany, 1873)
Loewner, Charles (Mathematician, Czechoslovakia, 1893)
London, Fritz Wolfgang (Physicist, Germany, 1900)
Lorente de No, Rafael (Physiologist, Spain, 1902)
Luisada, Aldo (Cardiologist, Italy, 1901)
Luria, Salvador E. (Virologist, Italy, 1912)
Mandelbrojt, Szolem (Mathematician, Poland, 1899)
Mayer, Maria Goeppert (Physicist, Poland, 1906)
Menger, Karl (Mathematician, Austria, 1902)
Meyer, Karl (Biochemist, Germany, 1809)
Meyerhof, Otto (Biochemist, Germany, 1884)
Nachmansohn, David (Neurologist, Russia, 1907)
Neurath, Hans (Biochemist, Austria, 1909)
Neyman, Jerzy (Mathematician, Rumania, 1894)
Noether, Emmy (Mathematician, Germany)
Ochoa, Severo (Biochemist, Spain, 1905)
Pauli, Wolfgang (Physicist, Austria, 1900)
Perrin, Francis Henri (Physicist, France, 1901)
Pirani, Conrad L. (Pathologist, Italy, 1914)
Placzek, George (Physicist, Czechoslovakia, 1905)
Polya, George (Mathematician, Hungary, 1887)
Prager, William (Applied mathematician, Germany, 1903)
Pringsheim, Peter (Physicist, Germany, 1881)
Rabinowitch, Eugene (Chemist, biologist. Russia, 1901)
Racker, Efraim (Biochemist, Poland, 1913)
Rademacher, Hans (Mathematician, Germany, 1892)
Rado, Tibor (Mathematician, Hungary, 1895)
Rasetti, Franco (Physicist, Italy, 1901)
Reichenbach, Hans (Philosopher of science, Germany, 1891)
Rossi, Bruno (Physicist, Italy, 1905)
Rothman, Stephen (Dermatologist, Hungary, 1894)
Schein, Marcel (Physicist, Czechoslovakia, 1902)
Schindler, Rudolf (Gastroenterologist, Germany, 1888)
Schoenheimer, Rudolf (Biochemist, Germany, 1898)

Schroedinger, Erwin (Physicist, Austria)
Schwartz, Philipp (Pathologist, Hungary, 1894)
Segre, Emilio (Physicist, Italy, 1905)
Siegel, Carl Ludwig (Mathematician, Germany, 1896)
Sigerist, Henry Ernest (Historian of medicine, France, 1891)
Staub, Hans (Physicist, Switzerland, 1908)
Stern, Curt (Geneticist, Germany, 1902)
Stern, Otto (Physicist, Germany, 1888)
Stucklen, Hildegard (Physicist, Germany, 1891)
Swings, Pol (Astrophysicist, Belgium, 1906)
Szasz, Otto (Mathematician, Hungary, 1884)
Szego, Gabor (Mathematician, Hungary, 1895)
Szilard, Leo (Physicist, Hungary, 1898)
Tarski, Alfred (Mathematician, Poland, 1902)
Teller, Edward (Physicist, Hungary, 1908)
Ulam, Stanislaw Marcin (Mathematician. Poland, 1909)
von Karman, Theodore (Aeronautical engineer, Hungary, 1881)
von Mises, Richard (Mathematician, Austria, 1883)
von Neumann, John (Mathematician, Hungary, 1903)
Wald, Abraham (Statistician, Rumania, 1902)
Wasow, Wolfgang (Mathematician, Switzerland, 1909)
Weil, Andre (Mathematician, France, 1906)
Weiss, Paul Alfred (Biologist, Austria, 1898)
Weisskopf, Victor Frederick (Physicist, Austria, 1908)
Weyl, Hermann (Mathematician, Germany, 1885)
Wigner, Eugene Paul (Physicist, Hungary, 1902)
Wintner, Aurel (Mathematician, Austria, 1903)
Wolf, Frantisek (Mathematician, Czechoslovakia, 1904)
Wundheiler, Alexander (Mathematician, Poland, 1902)
Zachariasen, William (Physicist, Norway, 1906)
Zygmund, Antoni (Mathematician, Poland, 1900)

List of Publications: I.I. RABI (Selected)

1. I.I. Rabi, "On the principal magnetic susceptibilities of crystals," *Phys. Rev.* **29,** (1927), 174-85.
2. I.I. Rabi, "Refraction of beams of molecules," *Nature* **123,** (1929), 163-64.
3. I.I. Rabi, "Zur Methode der Ablenkung von Molekularstrahlen," *Z. Phys.* **54,** (1929), 190-97.
4. Breit and I.I. Rabi, "The measurement of nuclear spin," *Phys. Rev.* **38,** (1931), 2082-83.
5. I.I. Rabi, "The nuclear spin of caesium by the method of molecular beams," *Phys. Rev.* **39,** (1932), 864.
6. I.I. Rabi and V.W. Cohen, "The nuclear spin of sodium," *Phys. Rev.* **43,** (1933), 582-583.
7. I.I. Rabi, J.M.B. Kellogg and J.R. Zacharias, "The magnetic moment of the proton," *Phys. Rev.* **46,** (1933), 157-63.
8. I.I. Rabi, J.M.B. Kellogg and J.R. Zacharias, "The magnetic moment of the deuton," *Phys. Rev.* **46,** (1933), 163-65.
9. I.I. Rabi and M. Fox, "On the nuclear moments of lithium, potassium and sodium," *Phys. Rev.* **48,** (1935), 746.
10. I.I. Rabi, "On the process of space quantization," *Phys. Rev.* **49,** (1936), 324-28.
11. J.M.B. Kellogg, I.I. Rabi and J.R. Zacharias, "The gyromagnetic properties of the hydrogens," *Phys. Rev.* **50,** (1936), 472-81.
12. I.I. Rabi, "Space quantization in a gyrating magnetic field," *Phys. Rev.* **51,** (1937), 652-54.
13. I.I. Rabi, J.R. Zacharias, S. Millman and P. Kusch, "A new method of measuring nuclear magnetic moments," *Phys. Rev.* **53,** (1937), 318.
14. I.I. Rabi, J.R. Zacharias, S. Millman and P. Kusch, "The molecular beam resonance method for measuring nuclear magnetic moment: The magnetic moments of $_3\text{Li}^6$, $_3\text{Li}^7$ and $_9\text{F}^{19}$," *Phys. Rev.* **55,** (1939), 526-35.
15. J.M.B. Kellogg, N.F. Ramsey, Jr., J.R. Zacharias and I.I. Rabi, "An electrical quadrupole moment of the deuteron," *Phys. Rev.* **55,** (1939), 318-319.
16. I.I. Rabi, J.M.B. Kellogg, N.F. Ramsey, Jr. and J.R. Zacharias, "The magnetic moments of the proton and the deuteron: The radiofrequency spectrum of H_2 in various magnetic fields," *Phys. Rev.* **56,** (1939), 728-43.
17. J.M.B. Kellogg, I.I. Rabi, N.F. Ramsey, Jr. and J.R. Zacharias, "An electrical quadrupole moment of the deuteron: The radiofrequency spectra of HD and D_2 molecules in a magnetic field," *Phys. Rev.* **57,** (1940), 677-95.
18. P. Kusch, S. Millman and I.I. Rabi, " The radiofrequency spectra of atoms: Hyperfine structure and Zeeman effect in the ground states of Li^6, Li^7, K^{39} and K^{41}," *Phys. Rev.* **57,** (1940), 765-80.
19. I.I. Rabi, "Radiofrequency spectroscopy (Richtmeyer lecture)," *Phys. Rev.* **67,** (1945), 199.
20. I.I. Rabi, "The physicist returns from the war," *The Atlantic* (October 1947), 107.
21. I.I. Rabi, J.E. Nafe and E.B. Nelson, "The hyperfine structure of atomic hydrogen and deuterium," *Phys. Rev.* **71,** (1947), 914-15.
22. I.I. Rabi, W.W. Havens, Jr. and L.J. Rainwater, "Interaction of neutrons with electrons in lead," *Phys. Rev.* **72,** (1947), 636-40.
23. I.I. Rabi, "International cooperation in science," *Columbia Alumni News* **47** (12), (1955), 9-12.
24. I.I. Rabi, "Peaceful uses of atomic energy," *Proc. Int. Conf. Peaceful Uses At. Energy* **16,** (1956), 9.
25. I.I. Rabi, "UNESCO Resolution," In *UNESCO—Purpose, Progress, Prospects*, eds., H.C. Laws and C.A. Thompson, (Bloomington, Indiana: Indiana University Press, 1957).
26. I.I. Rabi, *My Life and Times as a Physicist*, (Claremont, California: Claremont College Press, 1960).
27. I.I. Rabi, *Science the Center of Culture*, (New York: World Publishing, 1970).
28. I.I. Rabi, "Testimony," In *The Matter of J. Robert Oppenheimer*, (Cambridge: Massachusetts Institute of Technology Press, 1970), 452-68.
29. I.I. Rabi, "Opening remarks," *Peaceful Uses At. Energy* **1,** (1972), 79.

30. I.I. Rabi, "Government, sicence and technology—twilight of the gods," *I.A.E.A. Bulletin* **21 (2/3),** (1979), 3-10.

31. I.I. Rabi, "The President and his scientific advisors," *Technol. Soc.* **2,** (1980), 16-20.

32. I.I. Rabi and N.F. Ramsey, *Cosmos Club Bulletin,* (November 1980).

33. I.I. Rabi as told to John S. Rigden, "Otto Stern and the discovery of space quantization," *Z. Phys.* **D10,** (1988), 119.

List of Publications: NORMAN F. RAMSEY

1. J.M.B. Kellogg and Norman F. Ramsey, "On the magnetic moments of neon and argon," *Phys. Rev.* **53,** (1938), 331(A).
2. J.M.B. Kellogg, I.I. Rabi, N.F. Ramsey and J.R. Zacharias, "Magnetic moments of proton and deuteron," *Phys. Rev.* **55,** (1939), 595(A).
3. J.M.B. Kellogg, I.I. Rabi, N.F. Ramsey and J.R. Zacharias, "An electrical quadrupole moment of the deuteron," *Phys. Rev.* **55,** (1939), 318(L).
4. I.I. Rabi, J.R. Zacharias, N.F. Ramsey and J.M.B. Kellogg, "Magnetic resonances experiments on H_2 and D_2 molecules," *Phys. Rev.* **55,** (1939), 595(A).
5. N.F. Ramsey, "Rotational magnetic moment measurements on H_2 and D_2," *Phys. Rev.* **55,** (1939), 595(A).
6. J.M.B. Kellogg, I.I. Rabi, N.F. Ramsey and J.R. Zacharias, "The radiofrequency spectrum of the HD molecules in magnetic fields," *Phys. Rev.* **56,** (1939), 213(A).
7. J.M.B. Kellogg, I.I. Rabi, N.F. Ramsey and J.R. Zacharias, "Magnetic moments of the proton and the deuteron. The radiofrequency spectrum of H_2 in various magnetic fields," *Phys. Rev.* **56,** (1939), 728.
8. J.M.B. Kellogg, I.I. Rabi, N.F. Ramsey and J.R. Zacharias, "Electrical quadrupole moment of the deuteron. Radiofrequency spectra of HD and D_2 molecules in a magnetic field," *Phys. Rev.* **57,** (1940), 677.
9. J.A. Van Allen and N.F. Ramsey, "A technique of counting high energy protons in the presence of fast neutrons," *Phys. Rev.* **57,** (1940), 1069(A).
10. E.O. Salant and N.F. Ramsey, "Fast neutron collision cross sections of C and H," *Phys. Rev.* **57,** (1940), 1075(A).
11. N.P. Heydenburg and N.F. Ramsey, "Scattering of one to three MeV protons by helium," *Phys. Rev.* **57,** (1940), 1077(A).
12. N.F. Ramsey, "The diamagnetism and the quadrupole moment of hydorgen molecules," *Phys. Rev.* **58,** (1940), 190(A).
13. N.F. Ramsey, "Rotational magnetic moments of H_2, D_2 and HD molecules," *Phys. Rev.* **58,** (1940), 226.
14. N.P. Heydenburg and N.F. Ramsey, "Scattering of 1 MeV to 3 MeV protons by He," *Physical Review* **60,** (1941), 42.
15. N.F. Ramsey, S. Roberts and R.M. Alexander, "Radar system at three centimeter wavelength," U.S. Library of Congress Publication Board, *PB-6829,* (May 20, 1941).
16. N.F. Ramsey, S.J. Simmons and J. Halpern, "Airborne three centimeter radar," U.S. Library of Congress Publication Board, *PB-3750,* (May 22, 1942).
17. N.F. Ramsey, H.F. Balmer and E.A. Luebke, "Indicator photographs of three centimeter airborne radar over water and land," U.S. Library of Congress Publication Board, *PB-3724,* (October 27, 1942).
18. Numerous classified technical reports, 1941-1946.
19. S.B. Brody, W.A. Nierenberg and N.F. Ramsey, "Nuclear moments of the bromine isotopes," *Phys. Rev.* **72,** (1947), 258(L).
20. W.A. Nierenberg, N.F. Ramsey and S.B. Brody, "Measurements of nuclear quadrupole moment interactions," *Phys. Rev.* **70,** (1946), 773(L).
21. W.A. Nierenberg, N.F. Ramsey and S.B. Brody, "Measurements of nuclear quadrupole interactions," *Phys. Rev.* **71,** (1947), 466(A).
22. W.A. Nierenberg and N.F. Ramsey, "The radiofrequency spectra of the sodium halides," *Phys. Rev.* **72,** (1947), 1075.
23. N.F. Ramsey, "Large quadrupole interactions in nuclear radiofrequency spectra," *Phys. Rev.* **73,** (1948), 1243(A).
24. N.F. Ramsey, "Effect of large quadrupole interactions on nuclear radiofrequency spectra at twice Larmor frequency," *Phys. Rev.* **74,** (1948), 286.

25. N.F. Ramsey, "New molecular beam magnetic resonance method," *Phys. Rev.* **75,** (1949), 1326(A); *Phys. Rev.* **76,** (1949), 996(L).

26. N.F. Ramsey, "The internal diamagnetic field correction in measurements of the proton magnetic moment," *Phys. Rev.* **77,** (1950), 567(L); *Phys. Rev.* **78,** (1950), 339(A).

27. N.F. Ramsey, "Quadrupole moment of the electron distribution in hydrogen molecules," *Phys. Rev.* **78,** (1950), 221.

28. N.F. Ramsey, "Molecular beam resonance method with separated oscillating fields," *Phys. Rev.* **78,** (1950), 695.

29. N.F. Ramsey, "Magnetic shielding of nuclei in molecules," *Phys. Rev.* **78,** (1950), 699.

30. E.M. Purcell and N.F. Ramsey, "On the possibility of electric dipole moments for elementary particles and nuclei," *Phys. Rev.* **78,** (1950), 807(L).

31. H.G. Kolsky, T.E. Phipps, N.F. Ramsey and H.B. Silsbee, "Radiofrequency spectrum of H_2 in a magnetic field," *Phys. Rev.* **79,** (1950), 883(L).

32. N.F. Ramsey, "Nuclear magnetic moment of scandium[45]," *Phys. Rev.* **79,** (1950), 1010(L).

33. H.G. Kolsky, T.E. Phipps, N.F. Ramsey and H.B. Silsbee, "Radiofrequency spectrum of D_2 in a magnetic field," *Phys. Rev.* **80,** (1950), 483(L).

34. N.F. Ramsey, "Atomic and nuclear moments," *Collier's Encyclopedia,* (1950).

35. W.G. Cross and N.F. Ramsey, "The conservation of energy and momentum in compton scattering," *Phys. Rev.* **80,** (1950), 929.

36. N.F. Ramsey, L.L. Davenport, et al. "Design construction and operation of the Harvard University 95" cyclotron," Harvard University, Cambridge Mass., (1950).

37. N.F. Ramsey and R.V. Pound, "Nuclear audiofrequency spectroscopy by resonant heating of the nuclear spin system," *Phys. Rev.* **81,** (1951), 278(L).

38. H.G. Kolsky, T.E. Phipps, N.F. Ramsey and H.B. Silsbee, "Deuteron quadrupole moment and the radiofrequency spectra of H_2 and D_2 in low magnetic fields," *Phys. Rev.* **81,** (1951), 1061(L); *Phys. Rev.* **82,** (1951), 322(A).

39. U.E. Kruse and N.F. Ramsey, "The integral $_0 y^3 \exp (-y^2 + ix/y) dy$," *Journ. Math. Phys.* **30,** (1951), 40.

40. N.F. Ramsey, "Nuclear magnetic resonance experiments," *Phys. Rev.* **82,** (1951), 342.

41. D. Bodansky and N.F. Ramsey, "Neutron energy distributions in proton bombardment of Be and C at 100 MeV," *Phys. Rev.* **82,** (1951), 831.

42. N.F. Ramsey, "Radiofrequency spectra of H_2 and D_2 by a new molecular beam resonance method," *Physics* **17,** (1951), 388.

43. N.F. Ramsey, "Magnetic shielding of nuclei in molecules," *Physics* **17,** (1951), 303.

44. L.L. Davenport, L. Lavetelli, R.A. Mack, A.J. Pote and N.F. Ramsey, "A. Dee biasing system for a frequency modulated cyclotron," *Rev. Sci. Inst.* **22,** (1951), 601.

45. U.E. Kruse, R.A. Mack and N.F. Ramsey, "Trochoidal orbits in synchrocyclotrons," *Rev. Sci. Inst.* **22,** (1951), 839(L).

46. R.W. Brige, U.E. Kruse and N.F. Ramsey, "Proton-proton scattering at 105 MeV and 75 MeV," *Phys. Rev.* **83,** (1951), 274.

47. N.F. Ramsey, "Dependence of magnetic shielding of nuclei upon molecular orientation," *Phys. Rev.* **83,** (1951), 540.

48. N.F. Ramsey, "Measurement of nuclear polarizabilities by nuclear scattering experiments," *Physical Review* **8,** (1951), 659(L).

49. N.F. Ramsey, "Diatomic homonuclear molecules in magnetic fields," *Physical Review* **83,** (1951), 881(A).

50. N.F. Ramsey and H.B. Silsbee, "Phase shifts in the molecular beam method of separated oscillating fields," *Phys. Rev.* **84,** (1951), 506.

51. U. Liddel and N.F. Ramsey, "Temperature dependent magnetic shielding in ethyl alcohol," *J. Chem. Phys.* **19,** (1951), 1608(L).

52. N.F. Ramsey, "Theory of molecular hydrogen and deuterium in magnetic fields," *Phys. Rev.* **85,** (1952), 60.

53. N.F. Ramsey and E.M. Purcell, "Interactions between nuclear spins in molecules," *Phys. Rev.* **85**, (1952), 143(L).

54. N.F. Ramsey, "Use of HD for experiments on the proton-deuteron magnetic moment ratio," *Phys. Rev.* **85**, (1952), 688(L).

55. N.F. Ramsey, "Nuclear moments," *Annual Review of Nuclear Science,* Vol. 1, (National Academy of Science, 1952), 97.

56. N.F. Ramsey, "Long range proton-proton tensor force," *Phys. Rev.* **85**, (1952), 937(L).

57. N.F. Ramsey, "Chemical effects in nuclear magnetic resonance and in diamagnetic susceptibility," *Phys. Rev.* **86**, (1952), 243.

58. H.G. Kolsky, T.E. Phipps, N.F. Ramsey and H.B. Silsbee, "Nuclear radiofrequency spectra of H_2 and D_2 in high and low magnetic fields," *Phys. Rev.* **87**, (1952), 395.

59. N.F. Ramsey, "Vibrational and centrifugal effects on nuclear interactions and rotational moments in molecules," *Phys. Rev.* **87**, (1952), 1075.

60. N.M. Hintz and N.F. Ramsey, "Excitation Functions to 100 MeV," *Phys. Rev.* **88**, (1952), 19.

61. N.J. Harrick and N.F. Ramsey, "Rotational magnetic moment, magnetic susceptibilities and electron distribution in H_2," *Phys. Rev.* **88**, (1952), 228.

62. N.F. Ramsey, "Pseudo-quadrupole effect for nuclei in molecules," *Phys. Rev.* **89**, (1953), 527(L).

63. U.E. Kruse, N.F. Ramsey and B.J. Malenka, "Electric scattering of deuterons," *Phys. Rev.* **89**, (1953), 655(L).

64. N.F. Ramsey, "Nuclear moments and statistics," *Experimental Nuclear Physics,* Part III, (New York: John Wiley and Sons, Inc., 1953).

65. N.F. Ramsey, "Elements of nuclear structure and nuclear two-body problems," *Experimental Nuclear Physics,* Part IV, (New York: John Wiley and Sons, Inc., 1953).

66. N.F. Ramsey, "Electron distribution in molecular hydrogen," *Science* **117**, (1953), 470(A).

67. N.F. Ramsey, "Spin interactions of accelerated nuclei in molecules," *Phys. Rev.* **90**, (1953), 232.

68. N.J. Harrick, R.G. Barnes, P.J. Bray and N.F. Ramsey, "Nuclear radiofrequency spectra of D_2 and H_2 in intermediate and strong magnetic fields," *Phys. Rev.* **90**, (1953), 260.

69. B.J. Malenka, U.E. Kruse and N.F. Ramsey, "Polarizability of the deuteron," *Phys. Rev.* **90**, (1953), 365(A).

70. N.F. Ramsey, "Spin interactions of accelerated nuclei in molecules," *Phys. Rev.* **90**, (1953), 382(A).

71. N.F. Ramsey, "Electron coupled interactions between nuclear spins in molecules," *Physical Review* **91**, (1953), 303.

72. N.F. Ramsey, B.J. Mulenka and U.E. Kruse, "Polarizability of the deuteron," *Phys. Rev.* **91**, (1953), 1162.

73. B.J. Malenka, U.E. Kruse, and N.F. Ramsey, "Electric scattering of the polarizable deuteron," *Phys. Rev.* **91**, (1953), 1165.

74. N.F. Ramsey, *Nuclear Moments,* (New York: John Wiley and Sons, Inc., 1953).

75. M.S. Livingston, N.F. Ramsey, R.Q. Twiss, et al., "Design study for a 15-BeV accelerator," Massachusetts Institute of Technology Laboratory for Nuclear Science, *Report No. 60,* (1953).

76. V.W. Cohen, N.R. Corngold and N.F. Ramsey, "Experiment for measurement of magnetic moment of neutron," *Phys. Rev.* **93**, (1954), 941(A).

77. R.G. Barnes, P.J. Bray and N.F. Ramsey, "Variations of hydrogen rotational magnetic moments with rotational quantum number and isotopic mass," *Phys. Rev.* **94**, (1954), 893.

78. U.E. Kruse, J.M. Teem and N.F. Ramsey, "Proton-proton scattering from 40-95 MeV," *Phys. Rev.* **94**, (1954), 1795(L).

79. I.I. Rabi, N.F. Ramsey and J. Schwinger, "Use of rotating coordinates in magnetic resonance problems," *Revs. Mod. Phys.* **26**, (1954), 167.

80. P. Hillman, R.H. Stahl and N.F. Ramsey, "Total cross section of liquified gases for high energy neutrons," *Phys. Rev.* **96**, (1954), 115.

81. P. Hillman, V. Culler and N.F. Ramsey, "Polarization in high-energy p-n-n double scattering," *Phys. Rev.* **95,** (1954), 462.

82. R.H. Stahl and N.F. Ramsey, "Neutron-proton scattering at 91 MeV," *Phys. Rev.* **96,** (1954), 1310.

83. N.F. Ramsey, "Collision alignment of molecules, atoms and nuclei," *Phys. Rev.* **98,** (1955), 1853(L).

84. N.F. Ramsey, "Resonance transitions induced by perturbations at two or more different frequencies," *Phys. Rev.* **100,** (1955), 1191.

85. N.F. Ramsey, "Negative absolute temperatures," *Ordnance XL* **215,** (March-April, 1956), 898.

86. U.E. Kruse, J.M. Teem and N.F. Ramsey, "Proton-proton scattering from 40-95 MeV," *Phys. Rev.* **101,** (1956), 1079.

87. N.F. Ramsey, "Neutron physics," *Advances in Science,* (New York: Interscience Publishers, 1956), 197-211.

88. N.F. Ramsey, "Thermodynamics and statistical mechanics at negative absolute temperatures," *Phys. Rev.* **103,** (1956), 20.

89. N.F. Ramsey, *Molecular Beams,* (England: Oxford University Press, 1956).

90. V.M. Cohen, N.R. Corngold and N.F. Ramsey, "Magnetic moment of the neutron," *Phys. Rev.* **104,** (1956), 283.

91. N.F. Ramsey, "Resonance experiments in successive oscillatory fields," *Rev. Sci. Instr.* **28,** (1957), 57(L).

92. W.E. Quinn, J.M. Baker, J.T. LaTourrette and N.F. Ramsey, "Radiofrequency spectrum of hydrogen deuteride," *Bull. Am. Phys. Soc.* **2,** (1957), 200(A).

93. N.F. Ramsey, "Theoretical shapes of molecular beam resonances," *Bull. Am. Phys. Soc.* **2,** (1957), 200(A).

94. I.A. Pless, N.F. Ramsey, et al., "Angular distributions of low energy positrons from μ^+ - e^+ decays," *Bull. Am. Phys. Soc.* **2,** (1957), 205(A).

95. H.R. Lewis, A. Pery, W. Quinn and N.F. Ramsey, "Distortions of magnetic resonances by additional and excessive oscillatory fields," *Phys. Rev.* **107,** (1957), 446.

96. J.T. LaTourrette, W.E. Quinn and N.F. Ramsey, "Magnetic moment of Ne^{21}," *Phys. Rev.* **107,** (1957), 1202.

97. J.H. Smith, E.M. Purcell and N.F. Ramsey, "Experimental limit to the electric dipole moment of the neutron," *Phys. Rev.* **108,** (1957), 120.

98. Norman F. Ramsey and Henry R. Lewis, "Theory of hydrogen deuteride in magnetic fields," *Phys. Rev.* **108,** (1957), 1246.

99. N.F. Ramsey, "Time reversal, charge conjugation, magnetic pole conjugation, and parity," *Phys. Rev.* **109,** (1958), 225.

100. J.N. Palmieri, A. Cormack, N.F. Ramsey and R. Wilson, "Small angle polarized proton scattering," *Bull. Am. Phys. Soc.* **3,** (1958), 204.

101. N.F. Ramsey, "Molecular beam resonances in oscillatory fields of nonuniform amplitudes and phases," *Phys. Rev.* **109,** (1958), 822.

102. Daniel Kleppner, Norman F. Ramsey and Paul Fjelstadt, "Broken atomic beam resonance experiment," *Phys. Rev. Letters* **1,** (1958), 232.

103. J.N. Palmieri, A.M. Cormack, N.F. Ramsey and Richard Wilson, "Proton-proton scattering at energies from 46 to 147 MeV," *Annals of Physics* **5,** (1958), 299.

104. W.E. Quinn, A. Pery, J.M. Baker, H.R. Lewis, N.F. Ramsey and J.T. LaTourrette, "Electron-bombardment detection of noncondensable molecular beams," *Rev. Sci. Instr.* **29,** (1958), 935.

105. N.F. Ramsey, "Resonances dans des champs oscillante successifs," *Jour. Phys. et Radium* **19,** (1958), 809.

106. W.E. Quinn, J.M. Baker, J.T. LaTourrette and N.F. Ramsey, "Radiofrequency spectra of hydrogen deuteride in strong magnetic fields," *Phys. Rev.* **112,** (1958), 1929.

107. Norman F. Ramsey, "Hyperfine structure and atomic beam methods," *Handbook of Physics*, (New York: McGraw-Hill Book Co. 1958), Section 7, page 58.

108. Norman F. Ramsey, "Nuclear Moments," *Handbook of Physics*, (New York: McGraw-Hill Book Co., 1958), Section 9, page 63.

109. C.F. Hwang, T.R. Ophel, E.H. Thorndyke, Richard Wilson and N.F. Ramsey, "p-p triple scattering at 143 MeV," *Phys. Rev. Letters* **2**, (1959), 310; *Bull. Am. Phys. Soc.* **4**, (1959), 61.

110. Norman. F. Ramsey, "Shapes of molecular beam resonaces," *Recent Research in Molecular Beams*, (New York: Academic Press, 1959).

111. A.M. Cormack, N.N. Palmieri, N.F. Ramsey and Richard Wilson, "Elastic scattering and polarization of protons by helium at 147 and 66 MeV," *Phys. Rev.* **115**, (1959), 599.

112. W.H. Furry and N.F. Ramsey, "On the significance of potentials in quantum thoery," *Bull. Am. Phys. Soc.* **5**, (1960), 66; *Phys. Rev.* **118**, (1960), 623.

113. M.R. Baker and N.F. Ramsey, "Nuclear magnetic interaction in hydrogen fluoride," *Bull. Am. Phys. Soc.* **5**, (1960), 344.

114. C.H. Anderson and N.F. Ramsey, "Radiofrequency spectrum of $C_2 H_2$ and $C_2 D_2$," *Bull. Am. Phys. Soc.* **5**, (1960), 344.

115. H.M. Goldenberg, D. Kleppner and N.F. Ramsey, "Effect of surface collisions on the hyperfine state of Cs^{133}," *Bull. Am. Phys. Soc.* **5**, (1960), 344.

116. H.M. Goldenberg, D. Kleppner and N.F. Ramsey, "Atomic hydrogen maser," *Phys. Rev. Letters* **8**, (1960), 361.

117. M. Baker, C. Anderson, J. Pinkerton and N.F. Ramsey, "Rotational magnetic moments of HF, DF, and CH_4," *Bull. Am. Phys. Soc.* **6**, (1961), 19.

118. A.M. Cormack, J.N. Palmieri, H. Postma, N.F. Ramsey and Richard Wilson, "Elastic (p,α) and (p,d) scattering at 147 and 66 MeV, "*Nuclear Forces and the Two Body Problem*, (Pergamon Press, 1960).

119. D. Kleppner, H.M. Goldenberg, N. Fortson and N.F. Ramsey, "Preliminary experiments with atomic hydrogen maser," *Bull. Am. Phys. Soc.* **6**, (1961), 68.

120. M.R. Baker, H.M. Nelson, J.A. Leavitt and N.F. Ramsey, "Nuclear magnetic interactions of hydrogen flouride," *Bull. Am. Phys. Soc.* **5**, (1960), 344; *Phys. Rev.* **121**, (1961), 807.

121. H.M. Nelson, J.A. Leavitt, M.R. Baker and N.F. Ramsey, "Nuclear interactions in deuterium fluoride," *Phys. Rev.* **122**, (1961), 856.

122. T.R. Lawrence, C.A. Anderson and N.F. Ramsey, "Rotational magnetic moments of LiH and LiD," *Bull. Am. Phys. Soc.* **6**, (1961), 271.

123. N.F. Ramsey, "Thermodynamics and statistical mechanics at negative absolute temperatures," *Fourth Symposium on Temperature* **1**, (1961), 4.

124. H.M. Goldenberg, D. Kleppner and N.F. Ramsey, "Atomic beam experiments with stored beams," *Phys. Rev.* **123**, (1961), 530.

125. Norman F. Ramsey, "Nuclear interactions in molecules," *American Scientist* **49**, (1961), 509.

126. J.A. Leavitt, M.R. Baker, H.M. Nelson and N.F. Ramsey, "Proton radiofrequency spectrum of HCl," *Phys. Rev.* **124**, (1961), 1482.

127. D. Kleppner, H.M. Goldenberg and N.F. Ramsey, "Properties of the hydrogen maser," *Applied Optics* **1**, (1962), 55.

128. R. Fox and N.F. Ramsey, "Low energy proton production by 160 MeV protons," *Phys. Rev.* **125**, (1962), 1609.

129. D. Kleppner, H.M. Goldenberg and N.F. Ramsey, "Theory of the hydrogen maser," *Phys. Rev.* **126**, (1962), 603.

130. N.F. Ramsey, "The hydrogen maser," *Inst. of Radio Engineers, Transactions on Instrumentation* **I-II**, (1962), 178.

131. N.F. Ramsey, "Thermodynamics and statistical mechanics at negative absolute temperatures," *Temperature – Its Measurement and Control* **3(1)**, (Reinhold Publishing Company, 1962), 15.

132. N.F. Ramsey, "The hydrogen maser," *Microwave Journal* **VI(4)**, (March 1963), 89.

133. N.F. Ramsey, "Nuclear interactions in molecules," *Science in Progress* **13**, (Yale University Press, 1963), 59.

134. R.A. Brooks, C.H. Anderson and N.F. Ramsey, "Rotational magnetic moments of diatomic alkalis," *Phys. Rev. Letters* **10**, (1963), 441.

135. "High energy accelerator physics," Report by the panel of the President's Science Advisory Committee and the General Advisory Committee of the Atomic Energy Commission, *Report TID-18636*, (1963).

136. J.W. Cederberg, C.H. Anderson, and N.F. Ramsey, "Measurements of rotational magnetic moments of molecules," *Bull. Am. Phys. Soc.* **8**, (1963), 327.

137. "Science and the Policies of Governments," Report by Advisory Group on Science Policy, Organization for Economic Cooperation and Development, Paris, France, (1963).

138. H.C. Berg, D. Kleppner and N.F. Ramsey, "Spin exchange and chemical relaxation in atomic hydrogen maser," *Bull. Am. Phys. Soc.* **8**, (1963), 379.

139. T.R. Lawrence, C.H. Anderson and N.F. Ramsey, "Rotational magnetic moments of lithium hydride and deuteride," *Phys. Rev.* **130**, (1963), 1865.

140. J.R. Dunning, Jr., K.W. Chen, N.F. Ramsey, J.R. Rees, W. Shlaer, J.K. Walker and Richard Wilson, "Electron-proton elastic scattering at 1 and 4 BeV," *Phys. Rev.* **10**, (1963), 500.

141. S.B. Crampton, D. Kleppner and N.F. Ramsey, "Hyperfine structure of ground state of atomic hydrogen," *Phys. Rev. Letters* **11**, (1963), 338.

142. K.W. Chen, A.A. Cone, J.R. Dunning, Jr., S.G.F. Frank, N.F. Ramsey, J.K. Walker and Richard Wilson, "Electron-proton scattering at high momentum transfers," *Phys. Rev. Letters* **11**, (1963), 561.

143. A.A. Cone, K.W. Chen, J.R. Dunning, Jr., N.F. Ramsey, J.K. Walker, Richard Wilson and Guenther Hartwig, "Inelastic electron proton scattering at high momentum transfers," *Bull. Am. Phys. Soc.* **9**, (1964), 379.

144. N.F. Ramsey, "Rotational magnetic moments in molecules," *Bull. Am. Phys. Soc.* **9**, (1964), 89.

145. M.R. Baker, C.H. Anderson and N.F. Ramsey, "Nuclear magnetic anti-shielding in molecules; Nuclear magnetic moments of F^{19}, N^{14} and N^{15}," *Phys. Rev.* **133**, (1964), A1533.

146. N.F. Ramsey, "The atomic hydrogen maser," *Quantum Electonics* **III**, (Columbia University Press, 1964), 333.

147. J.W. Cederberg and N.F. Ramsey, "Magnetic resonance with large angular momenta," *Phys. Rev.* **135**, (1964), A39.

148. N.F. Ramsey and D. Kleppner, "Le maser à hydrogene atomique comme étalon de fréquence et de temps," Comité International des Poids et Mesures, (1964).

149. E.N. Fortson, D. Kleppner and N.F. Ramsey, "Stark shift of the hydrogen hyperfine separation," *Phys. Rev. Letters* **13**, (1964), 22.

150. *Electron-Proton Scattering at Large Momentum Transfer, Nucleon Structure*, ed. by Hofstadter and Schiff, (Stanford University Press, 1964).

151. "Electromagnetic interactions," Proceedings 1964 International Conference on High Energy Physics, Dubna, USSR, (1964).

152. J.W. Cederberg, C.H. Anderson and N.F. Ramsey, "Rotational magnetic moments," *Phys. Rev.* **136**, (1964), A960.

153. I. Ozier, L.M. Crapo, J.W. Cederberg and N.F. Ramsey, "Nuclear interactions and rotational moment of F_2," *Phys. Rev. Letters* **13**, (1964), 482.

154. R.A. Brooks, C.H. Anderson and N.F. Ramsey, "Rotational magnetic moments of the alkali molecules," *Phys. Rev.* **136**, (1964), A62.

155. S.I. Chan, R.R. Baker and N.F. Ramsey, "Molecular beam magnetic resonace studies of the nitrogen molecule," *Phys. Rev.* **136**, (1964), A1224.

156. J.R.Dunning, Jr., K.W. Chen, A.A. Cone, G. Hartwig, N.F. Ramsey, J.K. Walker and Richard Wilson, "Electromagnetic structure of the neutron and proton," *Phys. Rev. Letters* **13**, (1964), 631.

157. *Quick Calculus*, (New York, New York: J.Wiley and Sons, Inc., 1965).

158. N.F. Ramsey, "The atomic hydrogen maser," *Metrologia* **1**, (1965), 7.

159. C.H. Anderson, M. Baker and N.F. Ramsey, "Multiple molecular beams," *Rev. Sci. Instr.* **36**, (1965), 57.

160. A.A. Cone, K.W. Chen, J.R. Dunning, Jr., G. Hartwig, N.F. Ramsey, J.K. Walker and Richard Wilson, "Baryon spectroscopy by inelastic electron-proton scattering," *Phys. Rev. Letters* **14**, (1965), 326.

161. D. Kleppner, H.C. Berg, S.B. Crampton, N.F. Ramsey, R.F.C. Vessot, H.E. Peters and J. Vanier, "Hydrogen maser principles and techniques," *Phys. Rev.* **138**, (1965), A972.

162. N.F. Ramsey, "The atomic hydrogen maser," *Progress in Radio Science* **VII**, (1965), 111.

163. N.F. Ramsey and D. Kleppner, "Atomic hydrogen maser," U.S. Patent No. 3,255,423 (June 7, 1966).

164. F. Mehran, R.A. Brooks and N.F. Ramsey, "Rotational magnetic moments of alkali-halide molecules," *Phys. Rev.* **141**, (1966), 93.

165. N.F. Ramsey, "Early history of Associated Universities and Brookhaven National Laboratory," BNL 922, T-421, (1966).

166. K.W. Chen, J.R. Dunning, Jr., A.A. Cone, N.F. Ramsey, J.K. Walker and Richard Wilson, "Measurement of proton electromagnetic form factors at high momentum transfer," *Phys. Rev.* **141**, (1966), 1267.

167. J.R. Dunning, Jr., K.W. Chen, A.A. Cone, G. Hartwig, N.F. Ramsey, J.K. Walker and Richard Wilson, "Quasi-elastic electron-deuteron scattering and neutron form factors," *Phys. Rev.* **141**, (1966), 1286.

168. L.H. Chen, K.W. Chen, J.R. Dunning, Jr., N.F. Ramsey, J.K. Walker and Richard Wilson, "Nucleon form factors and their interpretation," *Phys. Rev.* **141**, (1966), 1298.

169. R. Budnitz, J.R. Dunning, Jr., M. Goitein, N.F. Ramsey, J.K. Walker and Richard Wilson, "Unsuccessful search for an excited electron," *Phys. Rev.* **141**, (1966), 1313.

170. T. Myint, D. Kleppner, N.F. Ramsey and H.G. Robinson, "Absolute value of the proton g factor," *Phys. Rev. Lett.* **17**, (1966), 405.

171. C.H. Anderson and N.F. Ramsey, "Magnetic resonance molecular beam spectra of methane," *Phys. Rev.* **149**, (1966), 14.

172. W. Dress, P.D. Miller, N.F. Ramsey and J.K. Baird, "Experiment to detect and measure an electric dipole moment of the neutron," *Bull. Am. Phys. Soc.* **11**, (1966), 740.

173. I. Ozier and N.F. Ramsey, "Molecular beam spectrum of F_2 in low field," *Bull. Am. Phys. Soc.* **11**, No. 1, (1966), 23.

174. T. Myint, D. Kleppner and H.G. Robinson, "Electron-proton g factor ration in hydrogen," *Bull. Am. Phys. Soc.* **11**, (1966), 327.

175. B.S. Mathur, S.B. Crampton and D. Kleppner, "Hyperfine frequency of tritium," *Bull. Am. Phys. Soc.* **11**, (1966), 328.

176. I. Ozier, "Nuclear interactions in spherical top molecules," *Bull. Am. Phys. Soc.* **12**, (1967), 8.

177. I. Ozier, "Scaler electron coupled spin spin interaction in HD," *Am. Phys. Soc.* **12**, No. 1, (1967), 132.

178. I. Ozier, P.N. Yi, A. Khosla and N.F. Ramsey, "Signs and magnitude of the rotational moment of $C^{12}0^{16}$," *Journ. Chem. Phys.* **46**, (1967), 1530.

179. A.A. Cone, K.W. Chen, J.R. Donning, Jr., G. Hartwig, N.F. Ramsey, J.K. Walker and R. Wilson, "Inelastic scattering of electrons by protons," *Phys. Rev.* **156**, (1967), 1490.

180. N.F. Ramsey, "Support of high energy physics," Proceedings of Sixth International Conference on High Energy Accelerated (CEAL-2000), (1967), 1.

181. B.S. Mather, S.B. Crampton, D. Kleppner and N.F. Ramsey, "Hyperfine separation of tritium," *Phys. Rev.* **158**, (1967), 14.

182. P.D. Miller, N.F. Ramsey, J.K. Baird and W.B. Dress, "New upper limit for electric dipole moment of the neutron," *Bull. Am. Phys. Soc.* **12**, (1967), 419.

183. P.N. Yi, I. Ozier and N.F. Ramsey, "Hyperfine structure of CH_4," *Am. Phys. Soc.* **12**, (1967), 509.

184. W. Dress, P.D. Miller, J.K. Baird and N.F. Ramsey, "Search for neutron electric dipole moment," *Bull. Am. Phys. Soc.* **12**, (1967), 651 and 1073.

185. P.D. Miller, W.B. Dress, J.K. Baird and N.F. Ramsey, "Limit to the electric dipole moment of the neutron," *Phys. Rev. Letters* **19**, (1967), 381.

186. N.F. Ramsey, "Hyperfine structure and atomic beam methods," *Handbook of Physics*, (New York: McGraw-Hill Book Co., 1967), Section 7, page 66.

187. N.F. Ramsey, "Nuclear moments," *Handbook of Physics*, (New York: McGraw-Hill Book Co., 1967), Section 9, page 89.

188. N.F. Ramsey, "Neutron electric dipole moment experiments," *Bull. Am. Phys. Soc.* **12**, (1967), 1125.

189. N.F. Ramsey, ed., "Research at 200 BeV," Universities Research Association, URA-1, (1967).

190. N.F. Ramsey, "Atomic hydrogen maser with enlarged atom storage container," U.S. Patent No. 3,388,342 (June 11, 1968).

191. N.F. Ramsey, "Search for neutron electric dipole moment by a magnetic resonance experiment," *Bull. Am. Phys. Soc.* **13**, (1968), 50.

192. I. Ozier, L.M. Crapo and N.F. Ramsey, "Spin-rotation constant and rotational magnetic moment of $C^{13}O^{16}$," *Bull. Am. Phys. Soc.* **13**, (1968), 423.

193. T.L. Follett, I. Ozier, L.M. Crapo and N.F. Ramsey, "Spin-rotation interactions in C3v molecules," *Bull. Am. Phys. Soc.* **13**, (1968), 595.

194. E.E. Uzgiris and N.F. Ramsey, "Large storage box hydrogen maser," *Proceedings of Symposium on Frequency Control* **22**, (1968), 452.

195. V.W. Cohen, R. Nathans, H. Silsbee, E. Lipworth and N.F. Ramsey, "Electric dipole moment of the neutron," *Bull Am. Phys. Soc.* **13**, (1968), 872.

196. W.B. Dress, J.K. Baird, P.D. Miller and N.F. Ramsey, "An improved upper limit for the neutron electric dipole moment," *Bull. Am. Phys. Soc.* **13**, (1968), 1380.

197. W.B. Dress, J.K. Baird, P.D. Miller and N.F. Ramsey, "Upper limit for the electric dipole moment of the neutron," *Phys. Rev.* **170**, (1968), 1200.

198. R.F. Code, A. Khosla, I. Ozier, N.F. Ramsey and P.N. Yi, "Nuclear magnetic hyperfine spectra of HCl^{35} and HCl^{37}," *Journ. Chem. Phys.* **49**, (1968), 1895.

199. N.F. Ramsey, "Early history of Associated Universities and Brookhaven National Laboratory," *Vistas in Research* **2**, (Gordon and Breach Science Publishers, 1968), 181.

200. N.F. Ramsey, "The atomic hydrogen maser," *American Scientist* **56**, (1968), 420.

201. E. Uzgiris and N.F. Ramsey, "Large storage box hydrogen maser," *IEEE Journal of Quantum Electronics* **2E-4**, (1968), 563.

202. I. Ozier, L.M. Crapo and N.F. Ramsey, "Spin rotation constant and rotational magnetic moment of $^{13}C^{16}O$," *Journ. Chem. Phys.* **49**, (1968), 2314.

203. J.K. Baird, P.D. Miller, W. Dress and N.F. Ramsey, "Improved upper limit to the electric dipole moment of the neutron," *Phys. Rev.* **179**, (1969).

204. E.E. Uzgiris and N.F. Ramsey, "Large storage box hydrogen maser," *Polarization Matiere et Rayonnement* **1**, (Presses Universitaires de France, 1969), 493.

205. V.W. Cohen, R. Nathans, E. Lipworth, H.B. Silsbee and N.F. Ramsey, "Electric dipole moment of the neutron," *Phys. Rev.* **177**, (1969), 1942.

206. P.A. Valberg and N.F. Ramsey, "Measurement of atomic magnetic moments with the hydrogen maser," *Bull. Am. Phys. Soc.* **14**, (1969), 943.

207. N.F. Ramsey, *Science as an Art*, (Middlebury College Press, April 1969).

208. T.F. Gallagher, R.C. Hilborn and N.F. Ramsey, "A simple graphical method for the calculation of atomic and molecular beam intensities: Design example and experimental results," *Bull. Am. Phys. Soc.* **14**, (1969), 943.

209. P.W. Zitzewitz and N.F. Ramsey, "Temperature dependence of the wall shift of the hydrogen maser," *Bull. Am. Phys. Soc.* **14**, (1969), 943.

210. R.F. Code and N.F. Ramsey, "Low temperature molecular beams," *Bull. Am. Phys. Soc.* **14,** (1969), 943.

211. D.J. Larson, P.A. Valberg and N.F. Ramsey, "Measurement of the hydrogen-deuterium atomic magnetic moment ratio and of the deuterium hyperfine frequency," *Phys. Rev. Letters* **23,** (1969), 1369.

212. N.F. Ramsey, "Hunting the neutron electric dipole moment," *Physics of One and Two Electron Atoms,*"(Amsterdam: North Holland Publishing Co., 1969), 170.

213. N.F. Ramsey, "Atomic hydrogen hyperfine structure," *Physics of One and Two Electron Atoms,* (Amsterdam: North Holland Publishing Co., 1969), 218.

214. P.W. Zitzewiz, E. Uzgiris and N.F. Ramsey, "Wall shift of FEP Teflon in the hydrogen maser," *Rev. Sci. Instr.* **41,** (1970), 81.

215. S.B. Crampton, H.C. Berg, H. Robinson and N.F. Ramsey, "Determination of the quadrupole coupling constant in the N^{14} atomic ground state," *Phys. Rev. Letters* **24,** (1970), 195.

216. I. Ozier, P.N. Yi, A. Khosla and N.F. Ramsey, "Direct observation of the ortho-para transitions in methane," *Phys. Rev. Letters* **24,** (1970), 642.

217. R.F.C. Vessot and N.F. Ramsey, "An orbiting clock experiment to determine the gravitational red shift," *Astrophysics and Space Science* **6,** (1970), 13.

218. E.E. Uzgiris and N.F. Ramsey, "Multiple region hydrogen maser with reduced wall shift," *Phys. Rev.* **A1,** (1970), 429.

219. N.F. Ramsey, "Possibility of field dependent nuclear magnetic shielding," *Phys. Rev.* **A1,** (1970), 1320.

220. N.F. Ramsey, et al., *Teaching of Physics in Liberal Arts Colleges,* (Middlebury, Vermont: Middlebury College, 1970).

221. N.F. Ramsey, "We need a pollution tax," *Bulletin of the Atomic Scientists* (April 1970), 3.

222. N.F. Ramsey, "Spin temperature and negative absolute temperatures," *A Critical Review of Thermodynamics,* (Baltimore: Mono Book Corporation, 1970).

223. N.F. Ramsey, "Electric dipole moment of the neutron," *A Tribute to I.I. Rabi,* (Columbia University Press, 1970).

224. P.W. Zitzewitz and N.F. Ramsey, "Studies of the wall shift in the hydrogen maser," *Phys. Rev.* **A3,** (1971), 51.

225. P.A. Valberg and N.F. Ramsey, "Hydrogen maser measurements of atomic magnetic moments," *Phys. Rev.* **A3,** (1971), 554.

226. N.F. Ramsey, "U.S. physics at the graduate level," *Physics in India, Proceedings of Conference on Physics Education and Research,* (Delhi, India: University Grants Commission, 1971), 216.

227. N.F. Ramsey, "Some problems in U.S. higher education," *Physics in India, Proceedings of Conference on Physics Education and Research,* (Delhi, India: University Grants Commission, 1971), 212.

228. R.F. Code and N.F. Ramsey, "A low temperature molecular beam source," *Rev. Sci. Instr.* **42,** (1971), 896.

229. N.F. Ramsey, "History of atomic and molecular control of frequency and time," *Proceedings Annual Symposium on Frequency Control* **25,** (Washington, DC: Electronics Industries Association, 1971), 46.

230. T.F. Gallagher and N.F. Ramsey, "The hyperfine spectrum of $Li^7 Cl^{35}$," *Bull. Am. Phys. Soc.* **16,** (1971), 86.

231. N.F. Ramsey, "Fine and hyperfine structure of atomic hydrogen," *Precision Measurement and Fundamental Constants, Bureau of Standards Special Publications* **343,** (1971), 317.

232. R.F.C. Vessot, M.W. Levine, P.W. Zitzewitz, P. Debely and N.F. Ramsey, "Recent developments affecting the hydrogen maser as a frequency standard," *Precision Measurement and Fundamental Constants, National Bureau of Standards Special Publication* **343,** (1971), 27.

233. N.F. Ramsey, "Thomas precession," *Journal of Physics Education* **1**, Dehli: National Council of Science Education (1971), 46.

234. P.N. Yi, I. Ozier and N.F. Ramsey, "Low field spectrum of CH_4," *Journal of Chemical Physics* **55**, (1971), 5215.

235. R.F. Code and N.F. Ramsey, "Molecular beam magnetic resonance studies of HD and D_2," *Phys. Rev.* **A4**, (1971), 1945.

236. P.C. Gibbons and N.F. Ramsey, "Electric field dependence of the atomic hydrogen hyperfine separation," *Phys. Rev.* **A5**, (1972), 73.

237. R.C. Hilborn, T.F. Gallagher and N.F. Ramsey, "Hyperfine structure of $Li^7Br^{79,81}$ by molecular beam electric resonance," *Journal of Chemical Physics* **56**, (1972), 855.

238. D.J. Wineland and N.F. Ramsey, "Atomic deuterium maser," *Phys. Rev.* **A5**, (1972), 821.

239. N.F. Ramsey, "Concentration in physics," *Perspectives on Concentrations* **96**, (Harvard College, 1972).

240. N.F. Ramsey, "History of atomic and molecular standards of frequency and time," *IEEE Transactions on Instrumentation and Measurement* **IM-21**, No. 2, (1972), 90.

241. R.A. Brooks, C.H. Anderson and N.F. Ramsey, "Molecular beam measurements on K, Na and LiNa," *Journal of Chemical Physics* **56**, (1972), 5193.

242. I. Ozier, J.A. Vitkevich and N.F. Ramsey, "Carbon-13 spin rotation constant of $C^{13}H^1$," Symposium on Molecular Structure and Spectroscopy, Columbus, Ohio, (1972).

243. T.F. Gallagher, R.C. Hilborn and N.F. Ramsey, "Hyperfine spectra of Li^7Cl^{35} and Li^7 and Cl^{37}," *Journal of Chemical Physics* **56**, (1972), 5972.

244. K.B. MacAdam and N.F. Ramsey, "Molecular beam magnetic resonance measurement of the anisotropies of the electric polarizabilities of H_2 and D_2," *Phys. Rev.* **A6**, (1972), 898.

245. J.L. Cecchi and N.F. Ramsey, "The molecular beam spectrum of LiBr by molecular beam electric resonance," *Bull. Am. Phys. Soc.* **18**, (1973), 62.

246. W.B. Dress, P.D. Miller and N.F. Ramsey, "Improved upper limit for the electric dipole moment of the neutron," *Phys. Rev.* **D7**, (1973), 3147.

247. N.F. Ramsey, "Hydrogen maser research," *Fundamental and Applied Laser Physics* **437**, (1973).

248. R. Freeman and N.F. Ramsey, "Measurement of the deuterium quadrupole moment in LiD," *Bull. Am. Phys. Soc.* **18**, (1973), 1500.

249. K. Docken, R. Freeman and N.F. Ramsey, "Vibrational averaged field gradient at deuterium in LiD," *Bull. Am. Phys. Soc.* **18**, (1973), 1500.

250. J.L. Cecchi and N.F. Ramsey, *Molecular Zeeman Spectra of* $^{6,7}Li$ $^{79,81}Br$.

251. N.F. Ramsey, "Spin temperature and negative absolute temperature," *Modern Developments in Thermodynamics*, ed. by B. Gal-Or, (Jerusalem: Israel Universities Press; New York: John Wiley and Sons, 1974).

252. D.J. Larson and N.F. Ramsey, "Measurement of the hydrogen-tritium g-factor ratio," *Phys. Rev.* **A9**, (1974), 1543.

253. Richard R. Freeman, David W. Johnson, Abram R. Jacobson and Norman F. Ramsey, "The molecular Zeeman spectra of LiH and LiD," *Bull. Am. Phys. Soc.* **19**, (1974), 447.

254. N.F. Ramsey, "Beams of molecules, atoms and nucleons," *Bull. Am. Phys. Soc.* **19**, (1974), 540.

255. J.M. Hirsch, G.H. Zimmerman, III, D.J. Larson and N.F. Ramsey, "Precision determination of the dipolar and quadrupolar hyperfine interactions, and $g_J(N)/g_J(H)$ of atomic nitrogen (14)," *Bull. Am. Phys. Soc.* **19**, (1974), 1177.

256. Richard R. Freeman, David W. Johnson and Norman F. Ramsey, "Molecular beam electric resonance study of the Zeeman spectrum of lithium chloride," *Journal of Chemical Physics* **61**, (1974), 3471.

257. N.F. Ramsey, "Technology and economic growth," Statement at Hearings Before the Subcommittee on Economic Growth of the Joint Economic Committee, Congress of the United States, July 16, 1975, (U.S. Government Printing Office, 1976).

258. Richard R. Freeman, Abram R. Jacobson, David W. Johnson and Norman F. Ramsey, "The molecular Zeeman and hyperfine spectra of LiH and LiD by molecular beam high resolution electric resonance," *Journal of Chemical Physics* **63**, (1975), 2597.

259. Norman F. Ramsey, "Time and the atom," *The Sciences* **15**, No. 9, (The New York Academy of Sciences, 1975), 20.

260. Norman F. Ramsey, "The electric and magnetic dipole moments of the neutron," *Neutrino 1975 IUPAP Conference Proceedings*, Vol. I, (Hungarian Physical Society, 1976), 307.

261. Norman F. Ramsey, "The electric and magnetic dipole moments of the neutron," *Bull. Am. Phys. Soc.* **21**, (1976), 61.

262. Abram R. Jacobson and Norman F. Ramsey, "The hyperfine structure of LiI by molecular beam techniques," *Journal of Chemical Physics* **65**, (1976), 1211.

263. Norman F. Ramsey, "Molecular and atomic beams," *Bol'shaia Sovetskaia Entsiklopedia*, Moscow, USSR.

264. I. Ozier, S.S. Lee and N.F. Ramsey, "Rotational magnetic moments of a series of tetrahedral molecules," *Journal of Chemical Physics* **65**, (1976), 3985.

265. I. Ozier, P.N. Yi and N.F. Ramsey, "Rotational magnetic moment spectrum of SF_6," *Journal of Chemical Physics* **66**, (1977), 143.

266. W.B. Dress, P.D. Miller, J.M. Pendlebury, P. Perrin and N.F. Ramsey, "Search for an electric dipole moment of the neutron," *Phys. Rev.* **D15**, (1977), 9.

267. Norman F. Ramsey, "The atomic hydrogen maser," *Proceedings Eighth Annual Precise Time and Time Interval, (PTTI) Applications and Planning Meeting*, (Maryland: Goddard Space Flight Center, 1977), 183-196.

268. Norman F. Ramsey, "Quantum science and its impact on metrology," *Science and Technology in America*, (Washington, D.C.: U.S. National Bureau of Standards, 1977), 11-21.

269. David W. Johnson and Norman F. Ramsey, "Stark hyperfine structure of hydrogen bromide," *Journal of Chemical Physics* **67**, (1977), 941.

270. J.M. Hirsch, G.H. Zimmerman, III, D.J. Larson and N.F. Ramsey, "Precision measurement of the hyperfine structure and g_J factor of atomic nitrogen 14," *Phys. Rev.* **A16**, (1977), 484.

271. Norman F. Ramsey, "Atomic and molecular standards of time and frequency," *Science Technology and the Modern Navy*, (Arlington, Virginia: Office of Naval Research, 1977), 19-39.

272. Norman F. Ramsey, "Future experiments on properties of the neutron," *Proceedings of Conference on Fundamental Physics with Reactor Neutrons and Neutrinos* (Grenoble, France: Institute Laue-Langevin, 1977), 2.8-1-17.

273. Norman F. Ramsey, "The electric and magnetic moments of the neutron," *Transactions of the New York Academy of Sciences* **II38**, (1977), 148.

274. G.L. Greene, N.F. Ramsey, W. Mampe, J.M. Pendlebury, K. Smith, W.B. Dress, P.D. Miller and P. Perrin, "A new measurement of the magnetic moment of the neutron," *Physics Letters* **71B**, (1977), 297.

275. J.G. Stuart, D.J. Larson and N.F. Ramsey, "Stark effect in the hydrogen hyperfine frequency," *Bull. Am. Phys. Soc.* **23**, (1978), 563.

276. Norman F. Ramsey, "Dipole moments and spin rotations of the neutron," *Physics Reports* **43**, (1978), 410.

277. Norman F. Ramsey, "Future experiments on the properties of free neutrons," *Int. Phys. Conf. Series* **42**, (1978), 61.

278. Norman F. Ramsey, "Dipole moments and spin rotatiions of the neutron," *Bull. Am. Phys. Soc.* **24**, (1979), 39.

279. W.M. Itano and N.F. Ramsey, "Hyperfine structure of tetrahedral molecules," *Bull. Am. Phys. Soc.* **24**, (1979), 17.

280. Norman F. Ramsey, "The state of the APS and of physics in 1978," *Physics Today* (April 1979), 25.

281. L.A. Cohen, J.H. Martin, and N.F. Ramsey, "Signs of rotational g-factors," *Phys. Rev.* **A19,** (1979), 433.

282. Norman F. Ramsey, "The role of basic science in national development," *New Physics* **18,** (Korean Physical Society, 1978), 183.

283. Norman F. Ramsey, "Address of the retiring president of the American Physical Society," *Bull. Am. Phys. Soc.* **24,** (1979), 38.

284. Norman F. Ramsey, "The electric and magnetic dipole moment of the neutron," *Journal of the Korean Physical Society* **12,** (1979), 17.

285. Norman F. Ramsey, "The tensor force between two protons at long range," *Physica* **96A,** (1979), 285.

286. G.L. Greene, N.F. Ramsey, W. Mampe, J.M. Pendlebury, K. Smith, W.B. Dress, P.D. Miller and P. Perrin, "Measurement of the neutron magnetic moment," *Phys. Rev.* **D20,** (1979), 2139.

287. N.F. Ramsey, "Neutron electric dipole moment," *Bull. Am. Phys. Soc.* **25,** (1980), 9.

288. M. Forte, B. Heckel, N.F. Ramsey, K. Green, G. Greene, M. Pendlebury, T. Sumner, P.D. Miller and W.B. Dress, "A first measurement of parity violating neutron spin precession," *Bull. Am. Phys. Soc.* **25,** (1980), 526.

289. Wayne M. Itano and Norman F. Ramsey, "Avoided-crossing molecular beam spectroscopy of SiH_4 and GeH_4," *Journal of Chemical Physics* **72,** (1980), 4941.

290. Norman F. Ramsey, "Negative absolute temperatures," *Encyclopedia of Science and Technology,* (New York: McGraw-Hill, 1980).

291. N.F. Ramsey, "Experiments on time reversal symmetry and parity," *Bull. Canadian Assoc. of Physicists* **36,** (1980), 31.

292. N.F. Ramsey, "The method of successive oscillatory fields," *Physics Today* **33, 7,** (July 1980), 25.

293. N.F. Ramsey, "The Eastman Professorship," *The American Oxonian* **LXVII, 2,** (1980), 98.

294. I.I. Rabi and N.F. Ramsey, *Cosmos Club Bulletin* (November 1980).

295. N.F. Ramsey, "Precession," *Encyclopedia of Physics,* (Addison-Wesley Publishing Co., 1980).

296. James G. Stuart, Daniel J. Larson and Norman F. Ramsey, "Differential stark shifts in the hydrogen maser," *Phys. Rev.* **A22,** (1980), 2092.

297. M. Forte, B.R. Heckel, N.F. Ramsey, K. Green and G.L. Greene, "First measurement of parity-nonconserving neutron spin rotation: The tin isotopes," *Phys. Rev. Lett.* **45,** (1980), 2088.

298. G.L. Greene, N.F. Ramsey, W. Mampe, J.M. Pendlebury, K. Smith, W.B. Dress, P.D. Miller and P. Perrin, "Determination of the neutron magnetic moment," *Precision Measurements and Fundamental Constants* (National Bureau of Standards, June 1981).

299. N.F. Ramsey, "Dipole moments and parity violating spin rotations of the neutron," Summer Institute of Particle Physics Conf. – 800782, *SLAC-239* (T/E) UC-34d, (National Technical Information Service, 1981), 559.

300. N.F. Ramsey, "Physics in 1981 ± 50," *Bull. Am. Phys. Soc.* **26,** (1981), 24.

301. N.F. Ramsey, "Experiments on time reversal symmetry and parity," *Atomic Physics 7,* (Plenum Press, 1981), 65.

302. N.F. Ramsey, "Physics in 1981 ± 50," *Physics Today* **34,** No. 11, (1981), 26.

303. Norman F. Ramsey, "Electric dipole moment of the neutron," *Comments Nucl. Part. Phys.* **10,** (1981)., 227.

304. L.W. Alvarez, H. Chernoff, R.H. Dicke, J.I. Elkind, J.C. Feggeler, R.L. Garwin, P. Horowitz, A. Johnson, R.A. Phinney, C. Rader and F.W. Sarles, "Report of the Committee on Ballistic Acoustics (John F. Kennedy Assassination)," N.F. Ramsey, Chairman, (National Academy Press, 1982).

305. N.F. Ramsey, "Electric dipole moments of elementary particles," *Reports on Progress in Physics* **48,** (1982), 95.

306. N.F. Ramsey, et al., "Reexamination of acoustic evidence in the Kennedy assassination," *Science* **218,** (1982), 127.

307. Norman F. Ramsey, "August 1945: The B-29 flight logs," *The Bulletin of Atomic Science* (December 1982), 33.

308. Norman F. Ramsey, "Electric dipole moments of particles," *Ann. Rev. Nucl. Part. Sci.* **32**, (1982), 211.

309. B. Heckel, N.F. Ramsey, et al., "A measurement of parity non-conversing neutron spin rotation in lead and tin," *Phys. Lett.* **119B**, (1982), 298.

310. G.L. Greene, N.F. Ramsey, W. Mampe, J.M. Pendlebury, K. Smith, W.B. Dress, P.D. Miller and P. Perrin, "An improved derived value for the neutron magnetic moment in nuclear magnetons," *Metrologia* **18**, (1982), 93.

311. N.F. Ramsey, "Negative temperature," *Encyclopedia of Science and Technology*, (McGraw-Hill, 1982), 63.

312. Norman F. Ramsey, "Inner space: Physics at short distances," The Murdock Lectures, Leverett House, Harvard University VI, (1982), 1.

313. Norman F. Ramsey, "Particle properties of the neutron," *Bul. Am. Phys. Soc.* **27**, (1982), 725.

314. Norman F. Ramsey, "Particle properties of the neutron," *Inst. Phys. Conf Ser.* **64**, Sect. 2, (1983), 5.

315. N.F. Ramsey, "Origins of radiofrequency spectroscopy, separated oscillatory fields and hydrogen maser," *NASA Conference Publications* **2265**, (1982), 635.

316. Norman F. Ramsey, "Neutron magnetic resonance," *Bull. of Magn. Resonance* **5**, (1983), 112.

317. Norman F. Ramsey, "History of atomic frequency standards," *Proceedings of the Annual Frequency Control Symposium* **37**, (1983), 5.

318. Norman F. Ramsey, "History of atomic atomic clocks," *Journal of Res. of NBS* **88**, (1983), 301.

319. John S. Rigden, "Molecular beam experiments on the hydrogens during the 1930's," *Historical Studies in the Physical Sciences* **13** (2), (1983), 335-373.

320. Norman F. Ramsey, "Neutron magnetic resonance," *Bull. Magn. Resonace* **5**, (1983), 113.

321. D.A. Wilkening, N.F. Ramsey and D.J. Larson, "Search for P and T violations in the hyperfine structure of thallium flouride," *Phys. Rev.* **A29**, (1984), 425.

322. N.F. Ramsey, "Ten years of congressional fellows," *Bull. Am. Phys. Soc.* **29**, (1984), 621.

323. Norman F. Ramsey, "Magnetic shielding of nuclei in molecules," *Citation Classic in Current Contents* **24**, No. 18, **18**, (April 30, 1984).

324. J.M. Pendlebury, et al., "Search for a neutron electric dipole moment," *Phys. Letters*, **136B**, (1984)., 327.

325. N.F. Ramsey, "Reactor based fundamental physics," *Journal de Physique* **45**, (1984), C3-285.

326. B. Heckel, et al., "Parity non-conserving neutron spin rotation," *Journal de Physique* **45**, (1984), C3-89.

327. N.F. Ramsey, "Low energy tests of conservation laws in particle physics," *AIP Conference Proceedings* **33**, (1984), 308.

328. B. Heckel, et al., "Measurement of parity non-conserving neutron spin rotation in lanthanum," *Phys. Rev.* **C29**, (1984), 2489.

329. Norman F. Ramsey, "High sensitivity tests of conservation laws," *AIP Conference Proceedings* **114**, (1984), 308.

330. Norman F. Ramsey, "Feasibility of a ^{3}He magnetometer for neutron electric dipole moment experiments," *Acta Physical Hungarica* **55**, (1984), 117.

331. Norman F. Ramsey, "Reactor based fundamental physics," *Journal de Physique* **45**, (1984), C3-285.

332. Norman F. Ramsey, "Early history of magnetic resonance," *Bull. of Magn. Resonance* **7**, (1985), 94.

333. Norman F. Ramsey, "Inner space: physics at short distances," *The School Science Review* **51**, (September 1985).

334. Norman F. Ramsey and Carol Davis, "Education of physicists for professional work in physics," *AAPT Topical Conference Series*, (1985), 87.

335. Norman F. Ramsey, "Neutron magentic resonance," *Ann. Phys. Fr.* **10**, (1985), 945.

336. Norman F. Ramsey, "Molecular beam experiments with successive oscillatory fields," Symposium on Molecular Beams, X (Cannes, France International, 1985).

337. Norman F. Ramsey, "Seventy-five years of molecular beams," *Bull. Am. Phys. Soc.* **30**, (1985), 857.

338. Norman F. Ramsey, "Particle properties of the neutron," *NBS Publication* **711**, (1986), 1.

339. Norman F. Ramsey, "Neutron magnetic resonance experiments," *Physica* **137B**, (1986), 223.

340. Norman F. Ramsey, "Oscillations in the history of molecular beams," *Electronic and Atomic Collisions* **3**, (Elsevier Publications, 1986).

341. Norman F. Ramsey, "The successive oscillatory field method," *Proceeding of the 40th frequency control symposium, IEEE Colloquiua* **86**, (1986), Ch. 2330-9; Library of Congress No. 58-60781.

342. Norman F. Ramsey, "Search for a neutron electric dipole moment," *Proceedings of Heidelberg International Symposium on Weak and Electromagnetic Interactions* **1**, (Springer Verlag, 1986), 861.

343. Norman F. Ramsey, "Advice on science for the U.S. government," *The Presidency and Science Advising*, (Boston: University Press of America, 1986), 39-61.

344. Norman F. Ramsey, "Quantum mechanics and precision measurements," *IEEE Transactions on Instrumentation and Measurement* **IM36**, (1987), 155.

345. Norman F. Ramsey, "Experiments on time reversal symmetry and parity," *New Directions in Physics*, (Academic Press, 1987), 115-.

346. Norman F. Ramsey, "The neutron magnetic moment," *Discovering Alvarez*, ed. by W.P. Trower, (University of Chicago Press, 1987), 30.

347. Norman F. Ramsey, "Early history of URA and Fermilab," *Fermilab 1987, Annual Report* **20**, (1988), 157.

348. Norman F. Ramsey, "I.I. Rabi and research with atoms and molecules," *Commets on Atomic and Molecular Physics XIII*, (1988), 87.

349. Norman F. Ramsey, "New teaching technologies and research with molecular beams," *Am. Journ of Physics* **56**, (1988), 875.

350. Norman F. Ramsey, "Molecular beams: Our legacy from Otto Stern," *Zeits Phys.* **D10**, (1988), 121.

351. Norman F. Ramsey, "Obituary: I.I. Rabi," *Physics Today* **41/10**, (1988), 82.

352. Norman F. Ramsey, "Atoms, molecules and I.I. Rabi," *Atomic Physics* **11**, (Singapore: World Scientific, 1988), 5.

353. Norman F. Ramsey, "Precise measurements of time," *American Scientist* **76**, (1988), 42.

354. Norman F. Ramsey, "The electric dipole moment of the neutron," *Physica Scripts* **T22**, (1988), 140.

355. Norman F. Ramsey, "Molecular beams, federal support of research and Brookhaven National Laboratory," Proceedings of International Conference of the restructuring of Physical Sciences in Europe and the United States 1945-46, (Singapore: World Scientific Publishers, 1989).

356. Norman F. Ramsey, "Alvarez: The war years," *Bull. Am. Phys. Soc.* **34**, (1989), 1147.

357. Norman F. Ramsey with K.F. Smith, M. Pendlebury, et al., "A search for the electric dipole moment of the neutron," *Physics Letters* **B234**, (1990), 191.

358. N.F. Ramsey, "The Rabi school," *Eur. Journ. Physics* **11**, (1990), 137.

359. Norman F. Ramsey, "Experiments with separated oscillatory fields and hydrogen masers," *Les Prix Nobel*, (Nobel Foundation, 1989).

360. Norman F. Ramsey, "Experiments with separated oscillatory fields and hydrogen masers," *Science* **248,** (June 28, 1990), 1612; *Angewandte Chemie* **29,** (1990), 725; *Rev. Mod. Phys.* **62,** (1990), 541.

361. Norman F. Ramsey, "Experiments with separated oscillatory fields and hydrogen masers," *Frequency Controll Symposium* **44,** (1990, 3; CH2818-3/90/0000-003 IEEE and IEEE Transactions of Instruments and Measurements* **40,** No. 2, (1991), 70.

362. Norman F. Ramsey, "Electric dipole moment of the neutron," *Ann. Rev. Nucl. Part. Scil.* **40,** (1990), 1.

363. Norman F. Ramsey, "Atomic hydrogen hyperfine structure experiments," *Quantum Electrodynamics,* ed. by T. Kinoshita, (Singapore: World Scientific Publishers, 1990) , Vol. 7, pg. 674 in Directions in High Energy Physics,.

364. Norman F. Ramsey, "Past and future of atomic time," *Proceedings of 4th European Frequency and Time forum* **4,** (Switzerland: Neuchatel University, 1990), 9.

365. N.F. Ramsey, "Measurements with separated oscillatory fields and hydrogen masers," *Atomic Phsics.* **12,** (1990), 1; AIP Conf. Proceedings 233.

366. N.F. Ramsey, "Precession," *Encylopedia of Physics,* (McGraw-Hill, 1990), 960.

367. N.F. Ramsey, "Experiments in time reversal symmetry and parity," *European Physical Society* **8,** (1990), 160.

368. N.F. Ramsey, "The past, present and future of atomic time and frequency," *Proceedings of IEEE* **79,** (1991), 921.

369. N.F. Ramsey, "Time and the physical universe," *Australian and New Zealand Physicist* **28,** No. 1/2, (1991), 6.

370. N.F. Ramsey, "Some implications of Radiation Laboratory developments," *Microwave Journal* **34,** No. 8, (1991), 74.

371. N. F. Ramsey, "Summary talk on discrete symmetries and atomic or neutron systems," *Moriond Conference Proceedings* **11,** (Gif Sur Yvette, France: Editions Frontieres, 1991), 439.

372. N.F. Ramsey, "Past, present and future of atomic time keeping," *Precision Time and Frequency Handbook* **8,** (1991), 13.3.

373. N.F. Ramsey, "Quantum mechanics and precision measurements," *International Measurements Confederation (IMEKO)* **12,** (Beijing, China, Chinese Society for Measurement, 1991), I-1.

374. N.F. Ramsey, "Early history of molecular beams," *International Conference on Molecular Beam Proceedings XIII,* (Madrid: Universidad Computense, 1991), 1.1.

375. N.F. Ramsey, "Experiments on time reversl symmetry and parity," *BNL Summer Study of CP Violation* **1,** (Singapore: Edit a Soni, Wold Scientific, 1991), 75.

376. K.T. Bainbride, E.M. Purcell, N.F. Ramsey and K. Strauch, *Jabez Curry Street, Memorial Minute,* (Faculty of Arts and Sciences, Harvard University, May 19, 1992).

377. N.F. Ramsey, "APS should not police physics," *APS News* **1,** No. 5, (1992), 15.

378. N.F. Ramsey, "Atomic and nuclear moments," *Collier Encyclopedia* **1,** (1992), 181.

379. N.F. Ramsey, "Beams of atoms and molecules," *Proc. Intl. School for Physics CXVIII,* (Laser Manipulation of Atoms and Ions, Italian Physical Society, 1992), 1.

380. N.F. Ramsey, "Quantum mechanics and the science of measurements," *J. Phys. II, France* **2,** (1992), 573.

381. N.F. Ramsey, "Early years of molecular beam resonances," *A Festschrift for Vernon Hughes,* ed. M.E. Zeller, (Singapore: World Scientific, 1992).

382. N.F. Ramsey, "Earliest criticisms of assumed P and T symmetries, " *Time Reversal – The Arthur Rich Memorial Symposium, AIP Conference Proceedings* **270,** (1993), 179.

383. N.F. Ramsey, "Fifty-five years of molecular beams," *Bull. Am. Phys. Soc.* **38,** (1993), 1112.

384. W.M. Itano and N.F. Ramsey, "Accurate measurement of time," *Scientific American* **269** (1), (1993), 56.

385. N.F. Ramsey, "Complementarity with two path neutron interference and separated oscillatory fields," *Phys. Rev.* **A48,** (1993), 80.

Publication List: EDWARD M. PURCELL

1. With K.Lark-Howovitz and H.J. Yearian, "Electron diffraction from vacuum-sublimated layers," *Phys. Rev.* **45** (1934), 123.
2. With K. Lark-Horovitz and J.D. Howe, "Method of making extremely thin films," *Rev. Sci. Inst.* **6,** (1935), 401-403.
3. "A model for the one-dimensional Schrödinger equation," *Phys. Rev.* **49,** (1936), 875.
4. With M.H. Hebb, "A theoretical study of magnetic cooling experiments," *J. Chem. Phys.*, 5 (1937), 338-350.
5. "The focusing of charged particles by a spherical condenser," *Phys. Rev.* **54,** (1938), 818-825.
6. With H.C. Torrey and R.V. Pound, "Resonance absorption by nuclear magnetic moments in a solid," *Phys. Rev.* **69,** (1946), 37-38.
7. "The radar equation," Chapter 2 in *Radar System Engineering*, ed. by L.N. Ridenour, (McGraw-Hill, 1947).
8. "Limitations of pulse radar," Chapter 4 in *Radar System Engineering*, ed. by L.N. Ridenour, (McGraw-Hill), 1947.
9. With J.H. Van Vleck and H. Goldstein, "Atmospheric attenuation," Chapter 8 in *Propagation of Short Radio Waves*, ed. by Donald E. Kerr, (McGraw-Hill, 1951).
10. With C.G. Montgomery and R.H. Dicke, *Principles of Microwave Circuits*, (McGraw-Hill, 1948).
11. With R.V. Pound and H.C. Torrey, "Measurement of magnetic resonance absorption by nuclear moments in a solid," *Phys. Rev.* **69,** (1946), 681.
12. With H.C. Torrey and R.V. Pound, "Theory of magnetic resonance absorption by nuclear moments in a solid," *Phys. Rev.* **69,** (1946), 680.
13. "Spontaneous transition probabilities in radio-frequency spectroscopy," *Phys. Rev.* **69,** (1946), 681.
14. With R.V. Pound and N. Bloembergen, "Nuclear magnetic resonance absorption in hydrogen gas," *Phys. Rev.* **70,** (1946), 986-987.
15. With N. Bloembergen and R.V. Pound, "Resonance absorption by nuclear magnetic moments in single crystal of CaF_2," *Phys. Rev.* **70,** (1946), 988.
16. With N. Bloembergen and R.V. Pound, "Nuclear magnetic relaxation," *Nature* **160,** (1947), 475.
17. With N. Bloembergen and R.V. Pound, "Relaxation effects in nuclear magnetic resonance absorption," *Phys. Rev.* **73,** (1948), 679-712.
18. "Nuclear magnetism in relation to problems of liquid and solid states," *Science* **107,** (1948), 433-440.
19. With G.E. Pake, "Line shapes in nuclear paramagnetism," *Phys. Rev.* **74,** (1948), 1184-1188.
20. With R.M. Brown, "Nuclear magnetic resonance in weak fields," *Phys. Rev.* **75,** (1949), 1262.
21. With J.H. Gardner, "A precise determination of the proton magnetic moment in Bohr magnetons," *Phys. Rev.* **76,** (1949), 1262-63.
22. With H.S. Gutowsky, G.B. Kistiakowsky and G.E. Pake, "Structural investigations by means of nuclear magnetism, I. rigid crystal lattices," *J. Chem. Phys.* **17,** (1949), 972-981.
23. With N.F. Ramsey, "On the possibility of electric dipole moments for elementary particles and nuclei," *Phys. Rev.* **78,** (1950), 807.
24. With H.I. Ewen, "Observation of a line in the galactic radio spectrum," *Nature* **168,** (1951), 356.
25. With W.H. Furry and J.C. Street, *Physics*, (Blakiston, 1952).
26. With R.V. Pound, "A nuclear spin system of negative temperature," *Phys. Rev.* **81,** (1951), 279-280.
27. "Nuclear resonance in crystals," *Physica* **17,** (1951), 282-302.
28. With N.F. Ramsey, "Interactions between nuclear spins in molecules," *Phys. Rev.* **85,** (1952), 143-144.

29. With D.K. Bailey, R. Bateman, L.V. Berkner, H.G. Booker, G.F. Montgomery, W.W. Salisbury and J.B. Wiesner, "A new kind of radio propagaton at very high frequencies observable over long distances," *Phys. Rev.* **86,** (1952), 141-145.

30. With H.Y. Carr, "Interaction between nuclear spins in HD gas," *Phys. Rev.* **88,** (1952), 415-416.

31. "The lifetime of the $2^2S_{1/2}$ state of hydrogen in an ionized atmosphere," *Astrophysical Journal* **116,** (1952), 457-436.

32. "Research in nuclear magnetism," *Les Prix Nobel en 1952* **97-109,** (Stockholm, 1953); *Science* **118,** (1953), 431-436.

33. "Kernmagnetische forschung," *Physikalische Blätter* **9,** (1953), 442-463.

34. With S.J. Smith, "Visible light from localized surface charges moving across a grating," *Phys. Rev.* **92,** (1953), 1069.

35. With F. Reif, "Nuclear magnetic resonance in solid hydrogen," *Phys. Rev.* **91,** (1953), 631-641.

36. "Line spectra in radio astronomy," *Proc. Am. Acad. Arts & Sciences* **82,** (1953).

37. With G.B. Benedek, "Nuclear magnetic resonance in liquids under high pressure," *J. Chem. Phys.* **22,** (1954), 2003-2012.

38. With H.Y. Carr, "Effects of diffusion on free precession in nuclear magnetic resonance experiments," *Phys. Rev.* **94,** (1954), 630-38.

39. "Nuclear Magnetism," *Am. J. Phys.* **22,** (1954), 1-8.

40. "Resonance nucleaire et mouvements des molecules dans les fluides," *J. Phys. et radium,* **15,** (1954).

41. With G.B. Field, "Influence of collisions upon populaton of hyperfine states in hydrogen," *Astrophysical Journal* **124,** (1956), 542-549.

42. "The question of correlation between photons in coherent light rays," *Nature* **178,** (1956), 1449-50.

43. "Nuclear magnetism and nuclear relaxation," *Nuovo Cimento Suppl,* **6,** (1957), 961-92.

44. "Gravitation torsion balance," Am. J. Phys. **25,** (1957), 393-94.

45. With J.H. Smith and N.F. Ramsey, "Experimental limit to the electric dipole moments, of the neutron,"*Phys. Rev.* **108,** (1957), 120-22.

46. "Nuclear spin relaxation and nuclear electric dipole moments," *Phys. Rev.* **117,** (1960), 828-31.

47. "Nuclear magnetism and molecular motion," Conference Proceedings 1958, (Welch Foundation).

48. "Radio astronomy and communicaton through space," *Brookhaven Lecture Series BNL* **658,** (1960), T214; Reprinted in *Interstellar Communication,* ed. by A.G.W. Cameron, (W.A. Benjamin, Inc., 1963).

49. "Identification of a high-energy particle by multiple measurements of its collision loss," Brookhaven National Laboratory Report PD-31 (1961).

50. "The case for the 'Needles' experiment," *New Scientist* **13,** (1962), 245-247.

51. *Parts and Wholes,* ed. by Daniel Lerner, (The Free Press of Glencoe, Inc., 1963), 11-39.

52. "Nuclear physics without the neutron: clues and contradictions," *Proceedings of the 10th International Congress on the History of Science,* (Hermann, Paris, 1964), 121-132.

53. With G.B. Collins, J. Hornbostel, T. Fujii, and F. Turkot, "Search for the Dirac monopole with 30-BeV protons," *Phys. Rev.* **129,** (1963), 2326-36.

54. *Electricity and Magnetism,* Berkeley Physics Course, Vol. II, (McGraw-Hill, 1965).

55. With H.C. Berg and W.W. Stewart, "A method for separating according to mass a mixture of macromolecules or small particles suspended in a fluid," *Proc. Nat. Acad. Sci.* **58,** (1967), 862-869; 1286-1291; 1821-1828.

56. "On the alignment of interstellar dust," *Physica* **41,** (1969), 100-127.

57. "On the absorption and emission of light by interstellar grains," *Astrophysical Journal* **158,** (1969), 100-127.

58. With H.C. Berg, U.S. Patent No. 3523610, (August 11, 1970).

59. With L. Spitzer, Jr., "Orientation of rotating grains," *Astrophysical Journal* **167**, (1971), 31-62.

60. With P. Annestad, "Interstellar grains," *Annual Review of Astronomy and Astrophysics*,11, (1973), 309-372.

61. With C.R. Pennypacker, "Scattering and absorption of light by nonspherical dielectric grains," *Astrophysical Journal* **186**, (1973), 705-714.

62. "Interstellar grains as pinwheels," *The Dusty Universe*, Published for the Smithsonian Astrophysical Observatory, (Neal Watson Academic Publications, Inc., 1975), 155-168.

63. "Temperature fluctuations in very small interstellar grains," *Astrophysical Journal* **206**, (1976), 685-690.

64. "Production of synchrotron radiation by Wiggler magnets," Stanford Synchroton Radiation Report No. 77/05, (1977).

65. "Life at low Reynolds number," *American Journal of Physics* **45**, (1977), 3-11.

66. With P.R. Shapiro, "A model for the optical behavior of grains with resonant impurities," *Astrophysical Journal* **214**, (1977), 92-105.

67. With H.C. Berg, "Physics of chemoreception," *Biophysical Journal* **20**, (1977), 193-219.

68. "The effects of fluid motions on the absorption of molecules by suspended particles," *J. Fluid Mech.* **84**, (1978), 551-559.

69. "Suprathermal rotation of interstellar grains," *Astrophysical Journal* **231**, (1979), 404-416.

70. Comments on "Special relativity theory in engineering," *Einstein Centennial Symposium*, ed. by H. Woolf, (Addison-Wesley, 1980), 106-108.

71. "New practical physics, APPT pathways," *Proceedings of the Fiftieth Anniversary of the APPT*, (1981), 31-36; 43-44. (Latter is text of Oersted Medal Response given in 1967).

72. With S. Dimopoulos, S.L. Glashow, and F. Wilczek, "Is there a local source of magnetic monopoles?" *Nature* **298**, (1982), 284.

73. "Monopoles and the galactic magnetic field," *Magnetic Monopoles*, ed. by R.A. Carrigan and W.P. Trower, (Plenum Press, 1983), 141-149.

74. "The back of the envelope," *American Journal of Physics* **51**, (1983), 11, 107, 205, 299, 391, 494, 586, 685, 780, 874, 970, 1068; *American Journal of Physics* **52**, (1984), 8, 107, 203, 301, 394, 490, 589, 681; *American Journal of Physics* **55**, (1987), 680, 778, 876, 972, 1066; *American Journal of Physics* **56**, (1988), 12, 108, 202, 298, 392, 490.

75. *Electricity and Magnetism*, Berkeley Physics Course, Vol. II, (McGraw-Hill, 1965; Second Edition, McGraw-Hill, 1985).

76. *Solutions Manual for Electricity and Magnetism*, (McGraw-Hill, 1965; Second Edition, McGraw-Hill, 1985).

77. Foreword, *Magnetic Resonance Imaging*, 2nd Edition, ed. by Partain, Price, Patton, Kulkarni, and James, (W.R. Sanders & Co., 1988).

78. "Helmholtz coils revisited," *Am. Jour. Phys.* **57**, (1989), 1.

79. With M.J. Schnitzer, S.M. Block, and H.C. Berg, "Strategies for chemotaxis," *General Microbiology Symposium*, Vol. 46, (Cambridge University Press, 1990), 15-34.

80. "Helmholtz coils re-revisited," *Am. Jour. Phys.* **58**, (1990), 296.

Publication List: FELIX BLOCH

1. "Radiation damping in quantum mechanics," *Phys. Zeits.* **29**, (1928), 58.
2. "Quantum mechanics of electrons in crystal lattices," *Zeits. f. Physik* **52**.7-8, (1928), 555.
3. "Susceptibility and change of resistance of metals in a magnetic field," *Zeits, f. Physik* **53**.3-4, (1929), 216.
4. "Electronic theory of ferromagnetism and electric conductivity," *Zeits. f. Physik* **57**.7-8, (1929), 545.
5. "Temperature variation of electrical resistance at low temperatures," *Zeits. F. Physik* **59**.3-4, (1930), 208.
6. "Theory of ferromagnetism," *Zeits. f. Physik* **61**.3-4, (1930), 206.
7. With G. Gentile, "Anisotropy of magnetisation of ferromagnetic single crystals," *Zeits. f. Physik* **70**.5-6, (1931), 395.
8. "Conduction and photoelectric effects," *Phys. Zeits.* **32**, (1931), 881.
9. "Theory of the exchange problem and of residual ferromagnetism," *Zeits, f. Physik* **74**.5-6, (1932), 295.
10. "Stopping power of matter for swiftly moving charged particles," *Ann. d. Physik* **16**.3, (1933), 285.
11. "Stopping power of atoms with several electrons," *Zeits. f. Physik* **81**.5-6, (1933), 363.
12. "Conservation theorem of the metallic state," *J. de Physique et le Radium* **4**, (1933), 486.
13. "Physical significance of multiple times in quantum electrodynamics," *Phys. Zeits. d'Sowjetunion* **5**.2, (1934), 301.
14. "Incoherent scattering of x-rays," *Helv. Phys. Acta* **7**.4, (1934), 385.
15. "Theory of the Compton line," *Phys. Rev.* **46**, (1934), 674.
16. "Molecular theory of magnetism," *Handbook of Radiology*, Vol. VI/2, 2nd Edition.
17. With P.A. Ross, "Radiative auger effect," *Phys. Rev.* **47**, (1935), 884.
18. "Double electron transitions in x-ray spectra," *Phys. Rev.* **48**, (1935), 187.
19. With N.E. Bradbury, "Mechanism of unimolecular electron capture," *Phys. Rev.* **48**, (1935), 689.
20. "On the scattering of neutrons," *Phys. Rev.* **50**, (1936), 259.
21. With G. Gamow, "On the probability of gamma-ray emission," *Phys. Rev.* **50**, (1936), 260.
22. "Continuous gamma radiation accompanying beta decay," *Phys. Rev.* **50**, (1936), 272.
23. "On the scattering of neutrons. II," *Phys. Rev.* **51**, (1937), 994.
24. With A. Nordsieck, "Radiation field of the electron," *Phys. Rev.* **52**, (1937), 54.
25. With Bradbury, Tatel and Ross, "Scattering and absorption cross section of neutrons in cobalt," *Phys. Rev.* **52**, (1937), 256, 1023.
26. "On the temperature dependence of the scattering of slow neutrons in ferromagnetics," *Phys. Rev.* **55**, (1939), 1118.
27. With L.W. Alvarez,"Quantitative determination of the neutron moment in absolute nuclear magnetons," *Phys. Rev.* **57**, (1940), 111, 352.
28. With A. Siegert, "Magnetic resonance for non-rotating fields," *Phys. Rev.* **57**, (1940), 522.
29. "Theory of resonance scattering of protons and neutrons on He," *Phys. Rev.* **58**, (1940), 829.
30. With M. Hamermesh, "Further results on magnetic scattering of neutrons," *Phys. Rev.* **61**, (1942), 203.
31. "Reduction of the problem of arbitrary spin to that of spin 1/2," *Phys. Rev.* **62**, (1942), 305.
32. With M. Hamermesh and H. Staub, "Neutron polarization and ferromagnetic saturation," *Phys. Rev.* **62**, (1942), 303; *Phys. Rev.* **64**, (1943), 47.
33. With I.I. Rabi, "Atoms in variable magnetic fields," *Rev. Mod. Phys.* **17**, (1945), 237.
34. With W.W. Hansen and M. Packard, "Nuclear induction," *Phys. Rev.* **69**, (1946), 127, 680.
35. "Nuclear induction," *Phys. Rev.* **70**, (1946), 460.
36. With W.W. Hansen and M. Packard, "The nuclear induction experiment," *Phys. Rev.* **70**, (1946), 474.

37. With R.I. Condit and H.H. Staub, "Neutron polarization and ferromagnetic saturation," *Phys. Rev.* **70,** (1946), 972.

38. "Radar reflections from long conductors," *J. Appl. Phys.* **17,** (1946), 1015.

39. With J.H. VanVleck and M. Hamermesh, "Theory of radar reflection from wires or thin metallic strips," *J. Appl. Phys.* **18,** (1947), 274.

40. With Graves, Packard and Spence, "Spin and magnetic moment of tritium," *Phys. Rev.* **71,** (1947), 373.

41. With Graves, Packard and Spence, "Relative moments of H_1 and H_3," *Phys. Rev.* **71,** (1947), 551.

42. With E.C. Levinthal and M.E. Packard, "Relative nuclear moments of H^1 and H^2," *Phys. Rev.* **72,** (1947), 1125.

43. With D. Nicodemus and H.H. Staub, "A quantitative determination of the magnetic moment of the neutron in units of the proton moment," *Phys. Rev.* **74,** (1948), 1025.

44. With D.H. Garber, "Nuclear induction proton signals below noise level from gases at one atmosphere," *Phys. Rev.* **76,** (1949), 585.

45. With R.K. Wangsness, "The differential equations of nuclear induction," *Phys. Rev.* **78,** (1950), 82.

46. With W.E. Meyerhof and D.B. Nicodemus, "Polarization effects of scattered neutrons," *Phys. Rev.* **80,** (1950), 132.

47. With C.D. Jeffries, "A direct determination of the magnetic moment of the proton in nuclear magnetons," *Phys. Rev.* **80,** (1950), 305.

48. "Nuclear induction," *Physica* **17,** (1951), 272.

49. "Magnetic moments of even-odd nuclei," *Phys. Rev.* **83,** (1951), 839.

50. "Nuclear relaxation in gases by surface catalysis," *Phys. Rev.* **83,** (1951), 1062.

51. With R.K. Wangsness, "Dynamical theory of nuclear induction," *Phys. Rev.* **89,** (1953), 728.

52. "The principle of nuclear induction," *Science* **118,** (1953), 425.

53. "Recent developments in nuclear induction," *Phys. Rev.* **93,** (1954), 944.

54. "Line-narrowing by macroscopic motion," *Phys. Rev.* **94,** (1954), 496.

55. "Dynamical theory of nuclear induction II," *Phys. Rev.* **102,** (1956), 104.

56. "Generalized theory of relaxation," *Phys. Rev.* **105,** (1957), 1206.

57. "Theory of line-narrowing by double-frequency irradiation," *Phys. Rev.* **111,** (1958), 841.

58. "Zur wirkung aeusserer elektromagnetischer felder auf kleine systeme," Sonderdruck aus Werner Heisenberg und die Physk unserer Zeit Verlag Friedr. Vieweg und Sohn, Brunschweig (1961).

59. With H.E. Rorschach, "Energetic stability of persistent currents in a long hollow cylinder," *Phys. Rev.* **128,** (1962), 1697.

60. "Off-diagonal long-range order and persistent currents in a hollow cylinder," *Phys. Rev.* **137,** (1965), A787.

61. "Some remarks on the theory of superconductivity," *Physics Today* **19,** (1966).

62. "Flux quantization and dimensionality," *Phys. Rev.* **166,** No. 2, (1968), 415.

63. "Simple interpretation of the Josephson effect," *Phys. Rev. Letters* **21,** (1968), 1241.

64. "Josephson effect in a superconducting ring," *Phys. Rev.* **B 2,** (1970), 109.

65. "Superfluidity in a ring," *Phys. Rev.* **A 7,** (1973), 2187.

Publication List: NICOLAAS BLOEMBERGEN

1. With G.A.W. Rutgers and J.C. Kluyver, "On the straggling of po-a-particles in solid matter," *Physica* **7**, (1940), 669-72.
2. "Note on the internal secondary emission," *Physics* **11**, (1945), 343-44.
3. With J.M.W. Milatz, "The development of an a.c. fotoelectric amplifier with a.c. galvanometer," *Physics* **11**, (1946), 449-64.
4. With E.M. Purcell and R.V. Pound, "Nuclear magnetic resonance in hydrogen gas," *Phys. Rev.* **70**, (1946), 986-87.
5. With E.M. Purcell and R.V. Pound, "Resonance absorption by nuclear magnetic moments in a single crystal of CaF_2," *Phys. Rev.* **70**, (1946), 988.
6. With R.V. Pound and E.M. Purcell, "Nuclear magnetic relaxation," *Nature* **160**, (1947), 475-76.
7. With E.M. Purcell and R.V. Pound, "Relaxation effects in nuclear magnetic absorption," *Phys. Rev.* **73**, (1948), 679-712.
8. *Nuclear Magnetic Relaxation*, Ph.D. thesis, Leiden, (1948); republished by W.A. Benjamin, Inc. , (1961), monograph.
9. "On the interaction of nuclear spins in a crystalline lattice," *Physica* **15**, (1949), 386-426.
10. "Nuclear magnetic relaxation in metallic copper," *Physics* **15**, (1949), 588-92.
11. "Fine structure of the magnetic resonance line of protons in $CuSo_4 \cdot 5H_2O$," *Phys. Rev.* **75**, (1949), 1326, abstract.
12. "Fine structure of the magnetic resonance line of protons in $CuSo_4 \cdot 5H_2O$," *Physica* **16**, (1950), 95-112.
13. With N.J. Poulis, "On the nuclear magnetic resonance in an antiferromagnetic crystal," *Physica* **16**, (1950, 915-19.
14. "On the ferromagnetic resonance in nickel and supermalloy," *Phys. Rev.* **78**, (1950) 572-80.
15. With W.C. Dickinson, "On the shift of the nuclear magnetic resonance in paramagnetic solutions," *Phys. Rev.* **79**, (1950), 179-180.
16. With W. Kohn, "Remarks on nuclear resonance shift in metallic lithium," *Phys. Rev.* **80**, (1950), 913; *Erratum Phys.*, **82**, (1951), 283.
17. With P.J. van Heerden, "The range and straggling of protons between 35 and 120 MeV," *Phys. Rev.* **83**, (1951), 561-64.
18. With M.S. Raben, "Determination of radioactivity by solution in a liquid scintillator," *Science* **114**, (1951), 363-64.
19. With R.W. Damon, "Relaxation effects in ferromagnetic resonance," *Phys. Rev.* **85**, (1952), 699.
20. With S. Wang, "The influence of anisotropy on ferromagnetic relaxation," *Phys. Rev.* **87**, (1952), 392-3.
21. "On the magnetic resonance absorption in conductors," *J. of Ap. Phys.* **23**, (1952), 1383-89.
22. With G. Temmer, "Nuclear magnetic resonance of aligned radioactive nuclei," *Phys. Rev.* **89**, (1953), 883.
23. With F.K. Willenbrock, "Paramagnetic resonance in N- and P-type silicon," *Phys. Rev.* **91**, (1953), 1281.
24. With T.J. Rowland, "On the nuclear magnetic resonance in metals and alloys," *Acta Metallurgica* **1**, (1953), 731-46.
25. "Magnetic relaxation in solids," *Proceedings of the International Conference on Theoretical Physics*, Kyoto, Japan, (1953), 757-772.
26. With S. Wang, "Relaxation effects in para- and ferromagnetic resonance," *Phys. Rev.* **93**, (1954), 72-83.
27. With R.V. Pound, "Radiation damping in magnetic resonance experiments," *Phys. Rev.* **95**, (1954), 8-12.
28. "Nuclear magnetic relaxation in semiconductors," *Physica* **20**, (1954), 130-33.

29. "Nuclear magnetic resonance in imperfect crystals," *Bristol Conference on defects in crystaline solids*, ed. by N.F. Mott, Phys. Soc. London, (1954), 1-32.

30. With T.J. Rowland, "Nuclear spin exchange in solids," *Phys. Rev.* **97**, (1956), 1679-98.

31. With I. Solomon, "Nuclear magnetic interactions in the HF molecule," *J. Chem. Phys.* **25**, (1956), 261-66.

32. "Magnetic resonance in ferrites," *Proc. I.R.E.* **44**, (1956), 1259-69.

33. "Proposal for a new type solid state maser," *Phys. Rev.* **104**, (1956), 324-27.

34. With T. Kushida and G.B. Benedek, "The dependence of the pure quadrupole resonance frequency on pressure and temperature," *Phys. Rev.* **104**, (1956), 1364-77.

35. "Nuclear magnetic resonance and electronic structure of conductors," *Can. J. of Phys.* **34**, (1956), 1299-1314.

36. "Spin relaxation processes in a two-proton system," *Phys. Rev.* **104**, (1956), 1542-47.

37. "Proton relaxation times in paramagnetic solutions," *J. Chem. Phys.* **27**, (1957), 572-73.

38. Comments on "Proton relaxation times in paramagnetic solutions," *J. Chem. Phys.* **27**, (1957), 595-96.

39. With W.M. Walsh, Jr., "Paramagnetic resonance of nickel fluosilicate under high hydrostatic pressure," *Phys. Rev.* **107**, (1957), 904-5.

40. With J.O. Artman and S. Shapiro, "Operation of a three-level solid state maser at 21 centimeters," *Phys. Rev.* **109**, (1957), 904-5.

41. "Electron spin and phonon equilibrium in masers," *Phys. Rev.* **109**, (1958), 2209-10.

42. "Higher order transitions in double nuclear resonance experiments in solids," *J. Phys. Soc. Japan* **13**, (1958), 660.

43. With P.P. Sorokin, "Nuclear magnetic resonance in the cesium halides," *Phys. Rev.* **110**, (1958), 865-875.

44. With R.S. Codrington, "Overhauser effect in manganese solutions in low magnetic fields," *J. Chem. Phys* **29**, (1958), 600-4.

45. With S. Shapiro, P.S. Persham, and J.O. Artman, "Cross relaxation in spin systems," *Phys. Rev.* **120**, (1959).

46. With E.F. Taylor, "Nuclear spin saturation by ultrasonics in sodium chloride," *Phys. Rev.* **113**, (1959), 431-38.

47. "Solid-state infrared quantum counters," *Phys. Rev. Letters* **2**, (1959), 84-85.

48. With S. Shapiro, "Relaxation effects in a maser material, K_3 (CoCr) $(CN)_6$," *Phys. Rev.* **116**, (1959), 1453-1458.

49. With D.L. Weinberg, "Nuclear resonance study of electronic magnetism in copper-nickel," *J. Chem. Solids* **13**, (1960), 240-248.

50. With L. Rimai, "Nuclear magnetic resonance in alkali alloy systems, NaK and NaRb," *J. Phys. Chem. Solids* **13**, (1960), 257-270.

51. "The zero-field solid state maser as a possible time standard," *1st conference on quantum electronics*, (New York: Columbia University Press, 1960), 160-166.

52. With P.S. Pershan and L.R. Wilcox, "Microwave modulation of light in paramagnetic crystals," *Phys. Rev.* **120**, (1960), 2014-2023.

53. "Cross-relaxation effects in magnetic resonance," *Extrait du bulletin Ampere*, 9ᵉ annee, fasc. special, (1960).

54. With L.O. Morgan, "Proton relaxation time in paramagnetic solutions: Effects of electron spin relaxation," *J. Chem. Phys.* **34**, ((1961), 842-850.

55. "Theory of the variation of the nuclear quadrupole interaction in covalent bonds with applied electric field," *J. Chem. Phys.* **35**, (1961), 1131-1132.

56. *Solid-State Masers, Progress in Low Temperature Physics*, Vol. III., ed. by C.J. Gorter, (Amsterdam: North Holland Publ. Co., 1961), 396-429.

57. With J. Armstrong and D. Gill, "Linear effect of electric field on the C quadrupole interaction in paradichlorobenzene,"*J. Chem. Phys.* **35**, (1961), 1132-1133.

58. With P.S. Pershan, "Microwave modulation of light," *Advances in Quantum Electronics*, ed. by J.R. Singer, (New York: Columbia University Press, 1961), 187-199.

59. With J. Armstrong and D. Gill, "Linear effect of applied electric field on nuclear quadrupole resonance," *Phys. Rev. Letters* **7**, (1961), 11-14.

60. "Linear effect of applied electric field on magnetic hyperfine interaction," *Phys. Rev. Letters* **7**, (1961), 90-92.

61. With P.S. Pershan, "Electrically induced shift of the F^{19} resonance frequency in MnF_2," *Phys. Rev. Letters* **7**, (1961), 165-167.

62. With P.S. Pershan, "Cross-relaxation in masers," *Advances in Quantum Electronics*, ed. by J.R. Singer, (Columbia University Press, 1961), 373-387.

63. "Linear stark effect in magnetic resonance spectra," *Science* **133**, (1961), 1363.

64. "Masers," Chapter 4 in *Foundations of Future Electronics*, ed. by R.V. Langmuir and W.D. Hershberger, (New York: McGraw-Hill, 1961), 85-112.

65. "Relaxation and temperature in magnetic spin systems," *Proceedings of the Seventh International Conference on Low Temperature Physics*, (University of Toronto Press, 1961), 36-50.

66. "Nuclear magnetic resonance in alloys," *J. Phys. and Radium* **23**, (1962), 658-664.

67. With J.A. Armstrong, J. Ducuing and P.S. Pershan, "Interactions between light waves in a nonlinear dielectric," *Phys. Rev.* **127**, (1962), 1918-1939.

68. With P.S. Pershan, "Light waves at the boundary of nonlinear media," *Phys. Rev.* **128**, (1962), 606-622.

69. "Spin resonance in high fields," *High Magnetic Fields*, ed. by H. Kolm, B. Lax, F. Bitter and R. Mills, (New York: MIT Press and Wiley & Sons, 1962), 454-463.

70. "Cross relaxation in nuclear and electron spin magnetic resonance," *Physical Sciences: Some Recent Advances in France and the United States*, (New York University Press, 1962), 83-92.

71. With E.B. Royce, "Electric shift of the Cr^{3+}," *Low Symposium on Paramagnetic Resonance* **2**, (New York: Academic Press, Inc., 1963), 607-619.

72. "Topics in quantum electronics," *Lectures in Theoretical Physics* **5**, (New York: Interscience Publishers, A division of John Wiley & Sons, 1963), 217-157.

73. "Wave propagation in nonlinear electromagnetic media," *Proceedings IEEE* **51**, (1963), 124-131.

74. With S.-Y. Feng, "Relaxation time measurements in ruby by a dc magnetization technique," *Phys. Rev.* **130**, (1963), 531-535.

75. With D. Gill, "Linear stark splitting of nuclear spin levels in GaAs," *Phys. Rev.* **129**, (1963), 2398-2403.

76. "Electric shifts in magnetic resonance: magnetic and electric resonance and relaxation," *Proceedings of the XIth Colloque Ampère*, ed. by J. Smidt, (Amsterdam: North-Holland Publishing, 1963), 39-57.

77. "Some theoretical problems in quantum electronics," *Proceedings of the Symposium on Optical Masers*, (Polytechnic Institute of Brooklyn, 1963), 13-22.

78. With E.B. Royce, "Linear electric shifts in the paramagnetic resonance of Al_2O_3:Cr and MgO:Cr.," *Phys. Rev.* **131**, (1963), 1912-1923.

79. With P.S. Pershan, "Frequency response of the photomixing process," *Applied Phys. Letters* **2**, (1963), 117-119.

80. "Magnetic resonance and its applications," *Materials Science*, ed. by P. Leurgans, Benjamin, Inc., New York, (1963), 51-74.

81. With Y.R. Shen, "Quantum-theoretical comparison of non-linear susceptibilities in parametric media, lasers and Raman lasers," *Phys. Rev.* **133** (1964), A37-A49.

82. With Y.R. Shen, "Theory of light modulation by the diamagnetic Faraday effect," *J. Opt. Soc. Amer.* **54**, (1964), 551-552.

83. With R.K. Chang, J. Ducuing and P. Lallemand, "Non-linearites optiques de quelques composes III-V," *Proceedings of the 7th Inst. Conf. on the Physics of Semiconductors, Dunod, Paris*, (1964), 121-127.

84. With J.P. van der Ziel, "Temperature dependence of optical harmonic generation in KH_2PO_4 ferroelectrics," *Phys. Rev.* **135**, (1964), A1662-A1669.

85. With F.A. Collins, "Stark effects on the nuclear quadrupole coupling of ^{35}Cl in sodium chlorate," *J. Chem. Phys.* **40**, (1964), 3479-3492.

86. With M.G. Cohen, "Magnetic and electric-field effects of the B_1 and B_2 absorptiion lines in ruby," *Phys. Rev.* **135**, (1964).

87. With R.W. Dixon, "Linear electric shifts in the nuclear quadrupole interaction in Al_2O_3," *Phys. Rev.* **135** (1964), A1669-A1675.

88. With R.W. Dixon, "Electrically induced perturbations of halogen nuclear quadrupole interactions in polycrystalline compounds: I. Phenomenological theory and experimental results," *J. Chem. Phys.* **41**, (1964), 1720-1738.

89. With R.W. Dixon, "Electrically induced perturbations of halogen nuclear quadrupole interactions in polycrystalline compounds: II. Microscopic theory," *J. Chem. Phys.* **41**, (1964), 1739-1747.

90. With Y.R. Shen, "Multimode effects in stimulated Raman emission," *Phys. Rev. Letters* **13**, (1964), 720-724.

91. "Optique Non-lineaire," *Proceedings of the 3rd International Conference of Quantum Electronics*, ed. by P. Grivet and N. Bloembergen, (New York: Dunod, Paris and Columbia University Press, 1964), 1501-1512.

92. "Nonlinear optics, quantum optics and electronics," *Les Houches Summer School Lectures*, (New York: Gordon and Breach, 1964), 411-522.

93. With P. Grivet, *Quantum Electronics*, Volumes I & II, Proceedings from the Third International Conference, (New York: Columbia University Press; Dunod Editeur Paris, 1964).

94. With Y.R. Shen, "Theory of stimulated Brillouin and Raman scattering," *Phys. Rev.* **137**, (1965), A1787-A1805.

95. "Nonlinear optics," *Estratto da Rendiconti della Scuola Internazionale di Fisica, E. Fermi, XXXI Corso*, ed. by P.A. Miles, (New York: Academic Press, 1965), 247-272.

96. With J.P. van der Ziel, "Optically induced magnetization in ruby," *Phys. Rev.* **138**, (1965), A1287-A1292.

97. With S.L. Hou, "Paramagnetoelectric effects in $NiSO_4$, $6H_2O$," *Phys. Rev.* **138**, (1965), A1218-A1226.

98. With P. Lallemand, "Multimode effects in the gain of Raman amplifiers and oscillators, I. Oscillators," *Applied Phys. Letters* **6**, (1965), 210-212.

99. With P. Lallemand, "Multimode effects in the gain of Raman amplifiers and oscillators, II. Amplifiers," *Applied Phys. Letters* **6**, (1965), 212-213.

100. With R.K. Chang and J. Ducuing, "Relative phase measurement between fundamental and second-harmonic light," *Phys. Rev. Letters* **15**, (1965), 6-8.

101. With Y.R. Shen, "Faraday rotation of rare-earth ions in CaF_2," *Phys. Rev.* **133**, (1964), A515-520.

102. With J. Ducuing, "Statistical fluctuations in nonlinear optical processes," *Phys. Rev.* **133**, (1964), A1493-1502.

103. "Changing identity of electrical engineering education," *Editorial in the Proc. IEEE* **53**, (1965), 562-563.

104. With R.D. Chang and J. Ducuing, "Dispersion of the optical nonlinearity in semiconductors," *Phys. Rev. Letters* **15**, (1965), 415-418.

105. With P. Lallemand, "Light waves with exponential gain," *Proceedings of the International Conference of the Physics of Quantum Electronics*, ed. by B. Lax and P.M. Kelley, (New York: McGraw-Hill, 1965), 137-154.

106. With R.K. Chang and J. Ducuing, "Dispersion of the optical nonlinearity suscepti-bility," ibid., 67-79.

107. With Y.R. Shen, "Coupling of light with phonons, magnons and plasmons," ibid., 119-128.

108. With R. K. Chang, "Second harmonic generation of light from surface layers of media with inversion symmetry," ibid., 80-85.

109. "Light," *Encyclopedia of Physics*, ed. by R.M. Besancon, (New York: Reinhold Publishing Co.), 370-372.

110. With W.M. Walsh and J. Jeener, "Temperature dependent crystal field and hyperfine interactions," *Phys. Rev.* **139**, (1965), A1338-1350.

111. *Nonlinear Optics*, (New York: W.A. Benjamin, Inc., 1965), 3rd printing 1976; Republished as "Advanced Book Classic," (Addison-Wesley, 1992), monograph.

112. With P. Lallemand, "Self-focusing of laser beams and stimulated Raman gain in liquids," *Phys. Rev. Letters* **16**, (1966), 1010-1012.

113. With P. Lallemand, "Complex intensity-dependent index of refraction, frequency broadening of stimulated Raman lines and stimulated Rayleigh scattering," *Phys. Rev. Letters* **16**, (1966), 81-84.

114. With Y.R. Shen, "Optical nonlinearities of plasma," *Phys. Rev.* **141**, (1966), 298-305.

115. With Y.R. Shen, "Interaction between light waves and spin waves," *Phys. Rev.* **143**, (1966), 372-384.

116. With M. Hanabusa, "Nuclear magnetic relaxation in liquid metals, alloys and salts," *J. Chem. Phys. Solids* **27**, (1966), 363-375.

117. With R.K. Chang, "Experimental verification of the laws for the reflected intensity of second harmonic light," *Phys. Rev.* **144**, (1966), 775-780.

118. With R.K. Chang and C.H. Lee, "Second harmonic generation of light in reflection from media with inversion symmetry, "*Phys. Rev. Letters* **16**, (1966).

119. "Second harmonic reflected light," *Optica Acta* **13**, (1966), 311-322.

120. With P. Lallemand and A. Pines, "The influence of self-focusing on the stimulated Brillouin, Raman and Rayleigh effects," *IEEE Journal of Quantum Electronics* **2**, (1966), 246-249.

121. With G. Bret P. Lallemand, A. Pine and P. Simova, "Controlled stimulated Raman amplification and oscillation in hydrogen gas," *IEEE Journal of Quantum Electronics* **3**, (1967), 197-201.

122. With C.H. Lee and R.K. Chang, "Nonlinear electroreflectance in silicon and silver," *Phys. Rev. Letters* **18**, (1967), 167-170.

123. "The stimulated Raman effect," *American Journal of Physics* **11**, (1967), 989-1023.

124. With C.H. Lee, "Total reflection in second harmonic generation," *Phys. Rev. Letters* **19**, (1967), 835-837.

125. "Interactions between light waves in media with inversion symmetry," *Proceedings of the Symposium of Modern Optics*, Vol. 17, (Polytechnic Institute of Brooklyn, 1967), 287-298.

126. "New horizons in quantum electronics," *IEEE Spectrum* **4**, (1967), 82-86.

127. With S.S. Jha, "Nonlinear optical susceptibilities in group IV and III-V semiconductors," *Phys. Rev.* **171**, (1968), 891-898.

128. With H.J. Simon, "Second harmonic light generation in crystals with natural optical activity," *Phys. Rev.* **171**, (1968), 1104-1114.

129. With R.K. Chang, S.S. Jha and C.H. Lee, "Optical second harmonic generation in reflection from media with inversion symmetry," *Phys. Rev.* **174**, (1968), 813-822.

130. "Picosecond laser pulses," *Comments on Solid State Physics* **1**, (1968), 37-42.

131. "Tunable parametric light oscillators," *Comment on Solid State Physics* **1**, (1968), 75-80.

132. "Nonlinear optics," in *Topics in Nonlinear Physics*, ed. by J. Zabusey, (Berlin: Springer Press, 1968), 425-484.

133. With S.S. Jha, "Nonlinear optical coefficients in group IV and III-V semiconductors," *IEEE J. of Quantum Electronics* **4**, (1968). 670-673.

134. "Conservation of angular momentum for optical processes in crystals," *Polarization, Matiere et Rayonnement*, ed. by Cohen-Tannoudji, (Paris: Presses Universitaires, 1969), 109-119.

135. With H.J. Simon and C.H. Lee, "Total reflection phenomena in second harmonic generation of light," *Phys. Rev.* **181**, (1969), 1261-1271.

136. "Some remarks on the symmetry properties of nonlinear optical susceptibilities," in *Physics of the Solid State*, ed. by Balakrishna, Krishnamurthy and Ramchandra Rao, (London: Academic Press, 1969), 277-288.

137. With H. Shih, "Conical refraction in nonlinear optics," *Optics Communications* **1**, (1969), 70-73.

138. With H. Shih, "Conical refraction in second harmonic generation," *Phys. Rev.* **184**, (1969), 895-904.

139. "Laser light diffraction as a spectroscopic tool for excitations in solids and liquids," *Comments on Solid State Physics* **2**, (1969), 119.

140. "Optical nonlinear susceptibilities," *Comments on Solid State Physics* **2**, (1969), 161.

141. With W.K. Burns and M. Matsuoka, "Reflected third harmonic generated by picosecond laser pulses," *Optics Communications* **1**, (1969), 195-198.

142. With R.L. Carman, M.E. Mack and F. Shimizu, "Forward picosecond Stokes pulse generation in transient stimulated Raman scattering," *Phys. Rev. Letters* **23**, (1969), 1327-1330.

143. With J.J. Wynne, "Measurement of the lowest order nonlinear susceptibility in III-V semiconductors by second harmonic generation with a CO_2 laser," *Phys. Rev.* **188**, (1969), 1211-1220.

144. "Review of nonlinear optical phenomena in condensed matter," *Proceedings of the 1969 Scottish Universities Summer School, Quantum Optics*, ed. by S.M. Kay and A. Maitland, (Academic Press, 1970), 355-394.

145. With M.E. Mack, R.L. Carman, J. Reintjes, "Transient stimulated rotational and vibrational Raman scattering in gases," *Appl. Phys. Letters* **16**, (1970), 209-211.

146. "Fundamentals of damage in laser glass," Chairman of committee report, *NMAB-271*, (Washington, D.C.: National Academy of Sciences, 1970).

147. With R.L. Carman, F. Shimizu, C.S. Wang, "Theory of Stokes pulse shapes in transient simulated Raman scattering," *Phys. Rev.* **2**, (1970), 60—72.

148. With W.H. Lowdermilk and C.S. Wang, "Observation of simulated concentration scattering in a mixture of SF_6 and He," *Phys. Rev. Letters* **25**, (1970), 1476-1478.

149. With A.J. Sievers, "Nonlinear optical properties of periodic laminar structures," *Appl. Phys. Letters* **17**, (1970), 483-486.

150. "Nonlinear optics, scientific past and technological future," *Laser Interaction and Related Phenomena*, ed. by H.J. Schwarts and H. Hora, (Plenum Press, 1971), 477-482.

151. With H. Shih, "Phase-matched critical total reflection and the Goos-Haenchen shift in second harmonic generation," *Phys. Rev.* **3**, (1971), 412-420.

152. With W.H. Lowdermild, M. Matsuoka and C.S. Wang, "Theory of stimulated concentration scattering," *Phys. Rev.* **3**, (1971), 404-412.

153. With E. Yablonovitch and J.J. Wynne, "Dispersion of the nonlinear optical susceptibility in n-InSB," *Phys. Rev.* **3**, (1971), 2060-2062.

154. With W.S. Gornall, C.S. Wang and C.C. Yang, "Coupling between Rayleigh and Brillouin scattering in a disparate mass gas mixture," *Phys. Rev. Letters* **26**, (1971), 1094-1097.

155. With W.K. Burns and C.L. Tang, "Symmetry of nonlinear optical susceptibilities in absorbing media and conservation of angular momentum," *International Journal for Quantum Chemistry* **5**, (1971.), 555-562.

156. With W.K. Burns, "Third harmonic generation in media of cubic or isotropic symmetry," *Phys. Rev.* **B4**, (1971.), 3437-3450.

157. With W.H. Lowdermilk, "Stimulated concentration scattering in the binary gas mixtures Xe-He and Sf_6-He," *Phys. Rev.* **A5**, (1972), 1423-1443.

158. "Picosecond nonlinear optics," *Proceedings of the Esfahan Symposium on Fundamental and Applied Laser Physics*, ed. by N.S. Field, A. Javan, S. Kurnit, (New York: Wiley, 1973), 21-50.

159. With M.J. Colles, J. Reintjes and C.S. Wang, "Transient spontaneous and stimulated Raman scattering," *Indian Journal of Pure and Applied Physics* **9**, (1971), 874-876.

160. With E. Yablonovitch, "Avalanche ionization and the limiting diameter of filaments induced by light pulses in transparent media," *Phys. Rev. Letters* **29**, (1972), 907-910.

161. "High-power infrared-laser windows," Chairman of committee report, *NMAB-292*, (Washington, D.C.: National Academy of Sciences, 1972).

162. With M.D. Levenson and C. Flytzanis, "Interference of resonant and nonresonant three-wave mixing in diamond," *Phys. Rev.* **B6**, (1972), 3962-3965.

163. With E. Yablonovitch and C. Flytzanis, "Anisotropic interference of three-wave and double two-wave frequency mixing in GaAs," *Phys. Rev. Lett.* **29**, (1972), 865-868.

164. "The concept of temperature in magnetism," *Am. Journal of Physics* **41**, (1973), 325-331. Translated from the Dutch, *Ned. Tydschrift voor Natuurk* **38**, (1972), 198-201.

165. "Role of cracks, pores and absorbing inclusions on laser-induced damage threshold at surfaces of transparent dielectrics," *Applied Optics* **12**, (1973), 661-664.

166. With D. Bedeaux, "On the relation between macroscopic and microscopic nonlinear susceptibilities,"*Physica* **69**, North Holand Publ., (1973), 57-66.

167. "Natuurkundig perspectief," Inaugural Address, Lorentz Guest-Professor, (Leiden University Press, 1973).

168. "The influence of electron plasma formation on superbroadening in light filaments," *Optics Comm.* **8**, (1973), 285-288.

169. With D.W. Fradin and J.P. Letellier, "Dependence of laser-induced breakdown field strength on pulse duration," Appl. Phys. Lett. **22**, (1974), 635-637.

170. With M.D. Levenson, "Dispersion of nonlinear optical susceptibilities of organic liquids and solutions," *J. Chem. Phys.* **60**, (1974), 1323-1327.

171. With S.D. Kramer and F.G. Parsons, "Interference of third-order light mixing and second-harmonic excitation generation in CuCl," *Phys. Rev.* **B9**, (1974), 1853-1856.

172. "Laser-induced electric breakdown in solids," *IEEE Journal of Quantum E1* **10**, (1974), 375-386.

173. With M.D. Levenson, "Observation of two-photon absorption without Doppler broadening on the 3S-5S transition in sodium vapor," *Phys. Rev. Lett.* **32**, (1974), 645-648.

174. With M.D. Levenson and M.M. Salour, "Zeeman effect in the two-photon 3S-5S transition in sodium vapor," *Phys. Rev. Lett.* **32**, (1974), 876-869.

175. With S.L. Hou, "Paramagnetoelectric effect in crystals," *Int. J. Magnetism* **5**, (1974), 327-336.

176. With M.D. Levenson, "Feasibility of measuring the nonlinear index of refraction by third-order frequency mixing," *IEEE J. of Quantum Electronics* **QE-10**, (1975), 110-115.

177. With M.D. Levenson and M.M. Salour, "Fine and hyperfine structure in highly excited states of sodium," *Physics Lett.* **48A**, (1974), 332-332.

178. With R.T. Lynch and M.D. Levenson, "Experimental test for deviation from Kleinman's Symmetry in the third-order susceptibility tensor," *Physics Lett.* **50A**, (1974), 61-62.

179. With M.D. Levenson, "Dispersion of the nonlinear optical susceptibility tensor in centrosymmetric media," *Phys. Rev.* **B10**, (1974), 4446-4463).

180. "Lasers, a renaissance in optics research," *American Scientist* **63**, (1975), 16-22.

181. With J.H. Bechtel and W.L. Smith "Four-photon photoemission from tungsten," *Optics Comm.* **13**, (1975), 56-59.

182. With W.L. Smith and J.H. Bechtel, "Dielectric breakdown threshold and nonlinear refractive index measurements with picosecond laser pulses," *Phys. Rev.* **B12**, (1975), 706-714.

183. With M.D. Levenson and R.T. Lynch, Jr., "Nonlinear spectroscopy in transparent crystals," *Optical Properties of Highly Transparent Solids*, ed. by S.S. Mitra and B. Bendow, (New York: Plenum, 1975), 329-337.

184. With W.L. Smith and J.H. Bechtel, "Picosecond laser-induced damage in transparent media," ibid., 381-392.

185. With S.D. Kramer, "Nonlinear spectroscopy of excitons in CuCl," ibid., 365-371.

186.   With Chr. Flytzanis, "Infrared dispersion of third-order susceptibilities in dielectrics," *Progress in Quantum Electronics*, Vol. 4, Part 3, ed. by J.H. Sanders and S. Stenhold, (New York: Pergamon, 1976), 271—300.

187.   "General Introduction, Quantum Electronics Vol. I, Part A.," *Nonlinear Optics*, ed. by H. Rabin and C.L. Tang, (New York: Academic Press, 1975) 1-6.

188.   "Nonlinear laser spectroscopy," Third Conference on the Laser, ed. by L. Goldman, *Ann. New York Acad. of Sc.* **267**, (1976), 51-60.

189.   "Comments on the dissociation of polyatomic molecules by 10.6 µm radiation," *Optics Comm.* **15**, (1975), 416-418.

190.   With R.T. Lynch, Jr., S.D. Kramer and H. Lotem, "Double resonance interference in third-order light mixing," *Optics Comm.* **16**, (1976), 372-375.

191.   With M.D. Levenson, "Doppler-free two-photon spectroscopy," *Topics in Applied Physics, Vol. 13, High Resolution Laser Spectroscopy*, ed. by K. Shimoda, (Berlin: Springer-Verlag, 1976) 315-369.

192.   With D.M. Larsen, "Excitation of polyatomic molecules by radiation," *Optics Comm.* **17**, (1976), 254-258.

193.   "Nonlinear spectroscopy," *Proceedings of E. Fermi Course* **59**, ed. by N. Bloembergen, (Amsterdam: North-Holland Publ., 1976), 1-16.

194.   With C.D. Cantrell and D.M. Larsen, "Collisionless dissociation of polyatomic molecules by infrared radiation," *Tunable Lasers and Application*, ed. by A. Mooradian et al., (Berlin: Springer-Verlag 1976), 162-176.

195.   "Nonlinear spectroscopy," *Laser Spectroscopy*, ed. by S. Haroche et al., (Berlin: Springer-Verlag, 1975), 31-38.

196.   With S.D. Kramer, "Third-order nonlinear optical spectroscopy in CuCl," *Phys. Rev.* **B14**, (1976), 4654-4669.

197.   With W.L. Smith and J.H. Bechtel, "Picosecond breakdown studies: Threshold and nonlinear refractive index measurements and damage morphology," *Laser-Induced Damage in Optical Materials: 1975, National Bureau of Standards Special Publication #435*, ed. by A.J. Glass and A.H. Guenther, (Washington, D.C.: U.S. Government Printing Office, 1976), 321.

198.   With W.L. Smith and J.H. Bechtel, "Picosecond laser-induced damage morphology: Spatially resolved microscopic plasma sites," *Optics Comm.* **18**, (1976), 592-596.

199.   With H. Lotem and R.T. Lynch, Jr., "Interference between Raman resonances in four-wave difference mixing," *Phys. Rev.* **A14**, (1976), 1748-1755.

200.   With A.J. Schell, "Second harmonic conical refraction," *Optics Comm.* **21**, (1977), 150-153.

201.   With W.L. Smith and J.H. Bechtel, "Picosecond laser-induced breakdown at 5321 and 3547 angstroms: Observation of frequency-dependent behavior," *Phys. Rev.* **B15**, (1977), 4039-4055.

202.   "Citation of classics: remarks on 'Relaxation effects in nuclear magnetic absorption,'" *Physical Review,* **73**, (1948), 679-712; *Current Contents* **17**, No. 18, (1977), 7.

203.   With R.T. Lynch, Jr. and H. Lotem, "Coherent anti-Stokes Raman scattering near a one-photon resonance," *J. Chem. Phys.* **66**, (1977), 4250-4251.

204.   With J.H. Bechtel and W.L. Smith, "Two-photon photoemission from metals induced by picosecond laser pulses," *Phys. Rev.* **B15**, (1977), 4557-4563.

205.   With J.G. Black, E. Yablonovitch and S. Mukamel, "Collisionless multiphoton dissociation of SF$_6$: a statistical thermodynamic process," *Phys. Rev. Let.* **38**, (1977), 1131-1134.

206.   With W.L. Smith and P. Liu, "Superbroadening in H$_2$0 and D$_2$0 by self-focused picosecond pulses from a YAIG:Nd laser," *Phys. Rev.* **A15**, (1977), 2396-2403.

207.   *Nonlinear Spectroscopy*, Proceedings of the International School of Physics "Enrico Fermi" Course LXIV, Italian Physical Society, (Amsterdam, New York, Oxford: North-Holland Publishing Co., 1977).

208.   With H. Lotem and R.T. Lynch, Jr., "Lineshapes in coherent resonant Raman scattering," *Indian. J. Pure and Applied Physics* **16**, (1978), 151-158.

209. With P. Liu, W.L. Smith, H. Lotem and J.H. Bechtel, "Absolute two-photon absorption coefficients at 355 and 266 nm," *Phys. Rev.* **B17**, (1978), 4620-4632.

210. With A.J. Schell, "Laser studies of internal conical diffraction: I. Quantitative comparison of experimental and theoretical conical intensity distributions in argonite," *J. Opt. Soc. Am.* **68**, (1978), 1093-1098.

211. With A.J. Schell, "Laser studies of internal conical diffraction: II. Intensity patterns in an optically active crystal, α-iodic acid," *J. Opt. Soc. Am.* **68**, (1978), 1098-1106.

212. With A.J. Schell, "Laser studies of internal conical diffraction: III. Second harmonic conical refraction in α-iodic acid," *Phys. Rev.* **A18**, (1978), 2592-2602.

213. With E. Yablonovitch, "Infrared laser induced unimolecular reactions," *Physics Today* **31**, (May 1978), 23.

214. With P. Liu and R. Yen, "Dielectric breakdown threshold, two-photon absorption and other optical damage mechanisms in diamond," *IEEE J. Quantum Electron* **QE-14**, (1978), 574-576.

215. "Stimulated Raman effect and coherent Raman scattering," *Proceedings of the 6th International Conference on Raman Spectroscopy, Bangore, India, 4-9 September, 1978*, ed. by E.D. Schmid, R.S. Krishnan, W. Kiefer and H.W. Schrotter, (London-Philadelphia-Rheine, Heyden, 1978) Vol. 1, 335-344.

216. "Interference effects in three- and four-wave light mixing," Actas del Primer Seminario Latinoamercano Sobre El laser y sus Aplicaciones a La Fiscia y a La Quimica, La Plata - Republica Argentina, (August, 1978), 21-26.

217. "Infrared laser-induced unimolecular reactions," Actas del Primer Seminario Latinoamercano Sobre El laser y sus Aplicaciones a La Fiscia y a La Quimica, La Plata - Republica Argentina, (August, 1978), 21-26.

218. "Nonlinear optical response of atoms, ions and molecules: a survey, in nonlinear behaviour of molecules, atoms and ions in electric, magnetic or electromagnetic fields," *Proc. 31st Int. Mtg. Societe de Chimie Physique, Abbaye de Fontevreau, September 1978*, ed. by Louis Neel, (Amsterdam: Elsevier, 1979), 1-20.

219. With E. Yablonovitch, "Laser-induced unimolecular reactions," Laser-Induced Processes in Molecules, Proc. European Physical Society Conference, Edinburgh, September 1978, ed. by K.L. Kompa and S.D. Smith, *Springer Series in Chemical Physics* **6**, (New York, Heidelberg, Berlin: Springer-Verlag, 1979), 117-120.

220. Acceptance speech on receiving the Lorentz Medal [in Dutch], Minutes of the Special Meeting of the Royal Dutch Academy of Sciences, (Amsterdam, September 30, 1978).

221. With J.G. Black, P. Kolodner, M.J. Shultz and E. Yablonovitch, "Collisionless multiphoton energy deposition and dissociation of SF," *Phys. Rev.* **A19**, (1979), 704-716.

222. With P. Liu and R. Yen, "Two-photon absorption coefficients in UV window and coating materials," *Appl. Optics* **18**, (1979), 1015-1018.

223. With P. Liu, R. Yen and R.T. Hodgson, "Picosecond laser-induced melting and resolidification morphology on Si," *Appl. Phys. Lett.* **34**, (1979), 864-866.

224. "Fundamentals of laser-solid interactions," Conference on Laser Solid Interactions and Laser Processing, Boston, November 1978, AIP Conference Proceedings, New York, 1979; also in *Applications of Lasers in Materials Processing*, ed. by E.A. Metzbower, Materials/Metalworking Technology Series (Metals Park, Ohio: American Society for Metals, 1979), 1-11.

225. "Recent progress in four-wave mixing spectroscopy in crystals," *Light Scattering in Solids*, ed. by J.L. Birman, H.Z. Cummins and K.K. Rebane, (New York: Plenum, 1979), 423-435.

226. "Recent progress in four-wave mixing spectroscopy," *Laser Spectroscopy IV*, ed. by H. Wather and K.W. Rothe, Springer Series in Optical Sciences 21, (New York, Heidelberg, Berlin: Springer-Verlag, 1979), 340-348.

227. With R. Yen, P. Liu and M. Dagenais, "Incident angle and polarization dependence of four-photon photoemission from tungsten," *Optics Comm.* **31**, (1979), 334-339.

228. "Reflections on light," Gandhi Memorial Lecture, Indian Academy of Sciences, Bangalore, 1979.

229. "Citation classic: Nonlinear Optics," *Current Contents* **10**, No. 39, (1979), 12.

230. "Stimiulated Raman and two-photon absorption processes in molecules," *Spectroscopy in Chemistry and Physics: Modern Trends*, ed. by E.J. Comes, A. Muller and W.J. Orville-Thomas, (Amsterdam: Elsevier, 1980), 331-338.

231. Chapter on physics, *Science in Contemporary China*, ed. by L.A. Orleans, (Stanford University Press, 1981), 85-109.

232. With R. Yen and J. Liu, "Thermally assisted multiphoton photoelectric emission from tungsten," *Optics Comm.* **35**, (1980), 227-282.

233. With H.S. Kwok and E. Yablonovitch, "Study of collisionless multiphoton absorption in SF_6 using picosecond CO_2 laser pulses," *Phys. Rev.* **A23**, (1981), 3094-3106.

234. "Conservation laws in nonlinear optics," *J. Opt. Soc. Am.* **70**, (1980), 1429-1436.

235. With J.M. Liu, R. Yen, E.P. Donovan and R.T. Hodgson, "Lack of importance of ambient gases on pico-second laser-induced phase transitions of silicon," *Appl. Phys. Lett.* **38**, (1981), 617-619.

236. With A.R. Bogdan and Y. Prior, "Pressure-induced degenerate frequency resonance in four-wave light mixing," *Optics Lett.* **6**, (1981), 82-84.

237. With M. Dagenais, M. Downer and R. Neumann, "Two-photon absorption as a new test of the Judd-Ofelt theory," *Phys. Rev. Lett.* **46**, (1981), 561-565.

238. With Y. Prior, A.R. Bogdan and M. Dagenais, "Pressure-induced extra resonances in four-wave mixing," *Phys. Rev. Lett.* **46**, (1981), 111-114.

239. With T.B. Simpson, "Collisionless infrared energy deposition in OCS," *Optics Comm.* **37**, (1981), 256-260.

240. With J.Y. Tsao and I. Burak, "Origin of the infrared multiphoton induced luminescence of chromyl chloride," *J. Chem. Phys.* **75**, (1981), 1-8.

241. With A.R. Bogdan and M. Downer, "Quantitative characteristics of pressure induced four-wave mixing signals observed with c.w. laser beams," *Phys. Rev.* **A24**, (1981), 623-626.

242. With A.R. Bogdan and M.W. Downer, "Quantitiative characteristics of pressure induced degenerate frequency resonance in four-wave mixing with c.w. laser beams," *Optics Lett.* **6**, (1981), 348-350.

243. With M. Dagenais, R. Neumann and M. Downer, "c.w. intraconfigurational (4f-4f) two-photon observation of Ge^{3+} ions in a LaF_3 crystal," *J. Opt. Soc. Am.* **70**, (1980), 1392 and 593.

244. With M. Dagenais, M.W. Downer and R. Neumann, "On the validity of the Judd-Ofelt theory for two-photon absorption in the rare earths," *Laser Spectroscopy V*, ed. by A.R.W. McKellar, T. Oka and B.P. Stoicheff, (Berlin, Heidelberg: Springer-Verlag, 1981), 264-267.

245. With A.R. Bogdan and M.W. Downer, "Collision-induced coherence in four-wave light mixing," *Laser Spectroscopy V*, ed. by A.R.W. McKellar, T. Oka and B.P. Stoicheff, (Berlin, Heidelberg: Springer-Verlag 1981), 157-165.

246. With J.M. Liu, R. Yen and H. Kurz, "Phase transformation and charged particle emission from a silicon crystal surface," *Appl. Lett.* **39**, (1981), 755-757.

247. With R.C. Sharp and E. Yablonovitch, "Picosecond infrared double resonance studies on SF_6," *J. Chem. Phys.* **74**, (1981), 5357-5365.

248. With R. Yen, J.M. Liu and H. Kurz, "Space-time resolved reflectivity measurements of picosecond laser-pulse induced phase transitions in <111> silicon surface layers," *Appl. Phys.* **A27** (1982), 153-160.

249. With R. Yen, J.M. Liu, T.K. Yee, J.G. Fujimoto and M.M. Salour, "Picosecond laser interaction with metallic zirconium," *Appl. Phys. Lett.* **40**, (1982), 185-187.

250. With R.C. Sharp and E. Yablonovitch, "Picosecond infrared double resonance studies on pentafluorobenzene," *Chem. Phys.* **76**, (1982), 2147-2154.

251. With H. Kurz, J.M. Liu and R. Yen, "Fundamentals of energy transfer during picosecond irradiation of silicon," *Proc. Materials Research Society Symposium on Laser and Electric Beam Interactions with Solids*, ed. by B.R. Appleton and G.K. Geller, (New York: Elsevier North-Holland, 1982), 3-11.

252. With J.M. Liu and H. Kurz, "Emission of charged particles from laser irradiated silicon," ibid., 29-35.

253. With R. Yen, J.M. Liu and H. Kurz, "Space-time resolved reflectivity measurements of picosecond laser induced phase transitions in <111> silicon," ibid., 37-42.

254. With M.C. Downer and A. Bivas, "Selection rule violation, anisotropy and anomalous intensity of two-photon absorption lines in Gd^{3+} :LaF_3," *Optics Commun.* **41**, (1982), 335-340.

255. "Nonlinear optics and spectroscopy," Nobel Lecture, 8 December 1981, in *Les Prix Nobel, 1981*, (Stockholm: Nobel Foundation, 1982); Also in *Rev. Mod. Phys.* **54**, (1982), 685-695; *Science* **216**, (1982), 1057-1064; *Czechoslovak Journal of Physics A; Wuli* **11**, 7 (Beijing: Institute of Physics of Chinese Academy of Sciences, 1982), 385-393.

256. With J.Y. Tsao, T.B. Simpson and I. Burak, "The dynamics of the infrared multiphoton pumping of optically excited $N0_2$ molecules," *J. Chem. Phys.* **77**, (1982), 1274-1285.

257. With T. Simpson, J.Y. Tsao and I. Burak, "The dynamics of the multiphoton pumping of excited $N0_2$ molecules," Proc. of 12th International Quantum Electronics Conference, Munich, 22-25 June 1982, *Appl. Phys.* **B28**, (1982), 181-182.

258. With M.C. Downer and A. Bivas, "New third-order contributions to two-photon absorption line strengths in Gd^{3+} :LaF_3," Proc. of 12th International Quantum Electronics Conference, Munich, 22-25 June 1982, *Appl. Phys.* **B28**, (1982), 281-282.

259. With J.M. Liu and H. Kurz, "Picosecond time-resolved plasma and temperature-induced changes of reflectivity and transmission in silicon," Appl. Phys. Lett. **41**, (1982), 643-646.

260. "Topic in Nonlinear Optics," A Reprint Volume, Indian Academy of Sciences, Bangalore, (1982), monograph.

261. With T. B. Simpson, E. Mazur, K.K. Lehmann and I. Burak, "Infrared multiphoton excitation and photochemistry of DN_3," *J. Chem. Phys.* **79**, (1983), 3373-3381.

262. With J.M. Liu and H. Kurz, "Picosecond time-resolved detection of plasma formation and phase transition in silicon," *Picosecond Phenomena III, Proc. Third Int. Conf. on Picosecond Phenomena, Gramische-Partenkirchen, June 1982*, ed. by K.B. Eisenthal, R.M. Hochsstrasser, W. Kaiser and A. Laubereau, (Berlin, Heidelberg: Springer-Verlag, 1982), 332-335.

263. With M.C. Downer and L.J. Rothberg, "Doppler narrowing and collision-induced Zeeman coherence in four-wave light mixing," *Atomic Physics 8, Proc. 8th Int. Conference on Atomic Spectroscopy, Goteborg, Sweden, August 1982*, ed. by I. Lindgren and S. Svanberg (New York: Plenum, 1983), 71-81.

264. With J.M. Liu and H. Kurz, "Picosecond time-resolved detection of plasma formation and phase transitions in silicon," in *Laser-Solid Interactions and transient Thermal Processing of Materials*, ed. by W.L. Brown, R.A. Lemons and J. Narayan, Mat. Res. Soc. Symp. Proc., Vol. 13, (New York: Elsevier N-H, 1983), 3-13.

265. With L.A. Lompre, J.M. Liu and H. Kurz, "Time-resolved temperature measurement of picosecond laser irradiated silicon," *Appl. Phys. Lett.* **43**, (1983), 168-170.

266. With R.C. Sharp and E. Yablonovitch, "Infrared double resonance studies of intramolecular energy transfer," *Appl. Phys.* **B28**, (1982), 314; title only, of paper presented at the 3rd Topical Meeting on Picosecond Phenomena, Garmisch-Partenkirchen, June 1982.

267. With T.B. Simpson, "Infrared multiphoton excitation of $S0_2$ to fluorescent states," *Chem. Phys. Lett.* **100**, (1983), 325-328.

268. With H. Kurz, L.A. Lompre and J.M. Liu, "Fundamentals of pulses laser irradiation of silicon," Proc. of 1st Materials Research Society of Materials, May 1983, Strasbourg, France, *J.De Physique* **44**, Colloque C5, (1983), C5-23-36.

269. With L.J. Rothberg, "Collision-induced coherence in Na atoms," *Proc. of 5th Rochester Conference on Coherence and Quantum Optics, June 1983*, ed. by L. Mandel and E. Wolf, (New York: Plenum, 1984), 775-780.

270. With L.J. Rothberg, "Collision-induced population gratings and Zeeman coherences in the 3^2S ground state of socium" *Laser spectroscopy VI. Proc. of 6th International Conference on Laser Spectroscopy, Interlaken, June 1983*, ed. by H.P. Weber and W. Luthy, Springer Series in Optical Sciences, (Springer, Berlin, Heidelberg, New York, 1983), 178-182.

271. With I. Burak and T.B. Simpson, "Infrared multiphoton excitation of small molecules," *J. Molecular Structure* **113**, (1984), 69-82.

272. With H.M. van Driel and L.A. Lompre, "Picosecond time-resolved reflectivity and transmission at 1.9 and 2.8 μm of laser-generated plasmas in silicon and germanium," *Appl. Phys. Lett.* **44**, (1984), 282-287.

273. With J.G. Fujimoto, J.M. Liu and E.P. Ippen, "Femotosecond laser interaction with metallic tungsten and nonequilibrium electron and lattice temperatures," *Phys. Rev. Lett.* **53**, (1984), 1837-1840.

274. With L.A. Lompre, J.M. Liu and H. Kurz, "Picosecond time-resolved optical studies of plasma formation and lattice heating in silicon," *Energy Beam-Solid Interactions and Transient Thermal Processing*, ed. by J.C.C. Fan and N.M. Johnson, Mat. Res. Soc. Symp. Proc. Boston, 1983, Vol. 23, (New York: Elsevier, 1984), 57-62.

275. With A.M. Malvezzi and J.M. Liu, "Photoelectric emission studies from crystalline silicon at 266 nm," *Energy Beam-Solid Interactions and Transient Thermal Processing*, ed. by J.C.C. Fan and N.M. Johnson, Mat. Res. Soc. Symp. Proc. Boston, 1983, Vol. 23, (New York: Elsevier, 1984), 135-139.

276. With L.A. Lompre, J.M. Liu and H. Kurz, "Optical heating of electron-hold plasma in silicon by picosecond pulses," *Appl. Phys. Lett.* **44**, (1984), 3-5.

277. With I. Burak, E. Mazur and T.B. Simpson, "Infrared multiphoton excitation of small molecules," *Israel J. Chem.* **24**, (1984), 179-186.

278. With E. Mazur and I. Burak, "Collisionless vibrational energy redistribution between infrared and Raman active modes in SF_6," *Chem. Phys. Lett.* **105**, (1984), 258-262.

279. With J.M. Liu, L.A. Lompre and H. Kurz, "Phenomenology of picosecond heating and evaporation of silicon surfaces coated with SiO_2 layers," *Appl. Phys.* **A34**, (1984), 25-29.

280. "Onderzoek," *Nederlands Tijdschrift voor Natuurkunde-A* **50**, (1984),3.

281. "Nonlinear optics—past, present and future," *IEEE J. Quantum Electron* **QE-20**, (1984), 556-558.

282. With L.J. Rothberg, "High-resolution four-wave light-mixing studies of collision-induced coherence in Na vapor," *Phys. Rev.* **A30**, (1984), 820-830.

283. With L.J. Rothberg, "Collision-induced coherence and population gratings in four-wave light mixing in sodium vapor," *Spectral Line Shapes*, Vol. 3, (Berlin, New York: Walder de Gruyter, 1985), 265-286.

284. With C.D. Cordero-Montalvo, "Two-photon transition from ^3H to $^1S_0$ of Pr^{3+} in LaF_3," *Phys. Rev.* **B30**, (1984), 438-440.

285. With R.S. Rana and C.D. Cordero-Montalvo, "The $^1S_0$ level of Pr^{3+} in $LaCl_3$," *J. Chem. Phys.* **81**, (1984), 1951-1952.

286. With A.M. Malvezzi and J.M. Liu, "Second harmonic generation in reflection from crystalline GaAs under intense picosecond laser irradiation," *Appl. Phys. Lett.* **45**, (1984), 1019-1021.

287. With A.M. Malvezzi and J.M. Liu, "Ultrafast phase transition of GaAs surfaces irradiated by picosecond laser pulses," *Mat. Res. Soc. Symp. Proc.* **35**, (1985), 138-142.

288. With A.M. Malvezzi and H. Kurz, "Picosecond photoemission studies of laser-induced phase transitions in silicon," *Proc. Opt. Soc. Amer. Topical Meeting on Ultrafast Phenomena, Monterey, California, 12-15 June 1984*, (Springer, Berlin, Heidelberg, New York, 1985), 118-121.

289. With L.A. Lompre, J.M. Liu and H. Kurz, "Dynamics of dense electron-hole plasma and heating of silicon lattice under picosecond laser irradiation," *Proc. Opt. Soc. Am. Topical Meeting on Ultrafast Phenomena, Monterey, California*, 12-15 June 1984, (Springer, 1985), 122-125.

290. With H. Kurz, "Physics of laser annealing of semiconductors," Paper presented at XIII International Conference on Quantum Electronics, Anaheim, California, 18-21 June 1984; summary in *J. Opt. Soc. Amer.; Optical Physics*, **1**, (1984), 446.

291. With J.G. Fujimoto, J.M. Liu and E.P. Ippen, "Femtosecond laser interaction with metallic tungsten and nonequilibrium electron and lattice temperatures," *Phys. Rev. Lett.* **53**, (1984), 1837-1840.

292. "The solved puzzle of two-photon rare earth spectra in solids," *J. Luminescence* **31 & 32**, (1984), 23-28.

293. With A.M. Malvezzi and J.M. Liu, "Ultrafast phase transition of GaAs surfaces irradiated by picosecond laser pulses," *Mat. Res. Soc. Symp. Proc.* **35**, (1985), 137-142.

294. With A.M. Malvezzi and H. Kurz, "Picosecond photoemission studies of the laser-induced phase transition in silicon," *Mat. Res. Soc. Symp. Proc.* **35**, (1985), 75-80.

295. With H. Kurz, "Picosecond photon-solid interaction," *Mat. Res. Soc. Symp. Proc.* **35**, (1985), 3-13.

296. With A.H. Zewail, "Energy redistribution in isolated molecules and the question of mode-selective laser chemistry revisited," *J. Physical Chemistry* **88**, (1985), 5459-5465.

297. With Y.H. Zou and L.J. Rothberg, "Collision-induced Hanle resonances of kilohertz width in phase-conjugate four-wave light mixing," *Phys. Rev. Lett.* **54**, (1985), 186-188.

298. "Collision-induced Hanle resonances in four-wave light mixing," *Ann. Phys. Fr.* **10**, (1985), 681-693.

299. With A.M. Malvezzi and H. Kurz, "Nonlinear photoemission from picosecond irradiated silicon," *Appl. Phys.* **A36**, (1985), 143-146.

300. With T.B. Simpson, J.G. Black, I. Burak and E. Yablonovitch, "Infrared multiphoton excitation of polyatomic molecules," *J. Chem. Phys.* **83**, (1985), 628-640.

301. With G.-Z. Yang, "Effective mass in picosecond-laser produced high-density plasma in silicon," *IEEE J. Quant. Electron* **1**, QE-22, (1986), 195-196.

302. With Y.H. Zou, "The relationship between collision-assisted Zeeman and Hanle resonances and transverse optical pumping," *Optical Sciences, Laser Spectroscopy VII*, ed. by T.W. Hansch and Y.R. Shen, Springer Series, (1985), 186-191.

303. With Y.H. Zou, "Collision-enhanced Hanle resonances and transverse optical pumping in four-wave light mixing in Na vapor," *Phys. Rev.* **A33**, (1986), 1730-1742.

304. "Pulsed laser interactions with condensed matter," *Mat. Res. Soc. Symp. Proc.* **51**, (1986), 3-13.

305. With J.M. Liu and A.M. Malvezzi, "Time-resolved optical studies of picosecond laser interactions with GaAs Surfaces," *Mat. Res. Soc. Symp. Proc.* **51**, (1986), 225-229.

306. With C.Y. Huang, A.M. Malvezzi and J.M. Keu, "Time-resolved piosecond optical study of laser-excited graphite," *Mat. Res. Soc. Symp. Proc.* **51**, (1986), 245-249.

307. With A.M. Malvezzi and C.Y. Huang, "Time-resolved picosecond optical measurements of laser-excited graphite," *Phys. Rev. Lett.* **57**, (1986), 146-149.

308. With Y.H. Zou, "Collision and stochastic-fluctuation-induced Hanle resonances in four-wave light mixing in samarium," *Phys. Rev.* **34**, (1986), 2968-2976.

309. With J.M. Liu and A.M. Malvezzi, "Picosecond laser melting and evaporation of GaAs surfaces," *Appl. Phys. Lett.* **49**, (1986), 622-624.

310. With A.M. Malvezzi, C.Y. Huang and H. Kurz, "Time-resolved spectroscopy of plasma resonances in highly excited silicon and germanium," ed. by H. Kurz, G.L. Olson and J.M. Poate, *Res. Soc. Symp. Proc.* **51**, (1986), 201-212.

311. "A quarter century of stimulated Raman scattering," *Int. Journal of Mod. Phys.* **B1**, (1987); Also in *Pure and Applied Chemistry* **59**, (1987), 1229-1236.

312. "Science and technology of directed energy weapons," Report of the American Physical Society Study Group, N. Bloembergen and C.K.N. Patel, co-chairmen, *Reviews of Modern Physics* **59**, (1987), S1-S202.

313. With C.K.N. Patel, "Strategic defense and directed-energy weapons," *Sci. Am.* **257**, (1987), 39-45.

314. With C.Y. Huang, A.M. Malvezzi and F.J. di Salvo, "Time-resolved picosecond reflectivity study of laser-excited layer compounds," *Mat. Res. Soc. Proc.* **74**, (1987), 269-274.

315. "Collision-induced coherences in nonlinear optics," *Nuovo Cimento* **D10**, (1988), 483-488.

316. With A.M. Malvezzi, G. Reverberi, "Optical properties of picosecond laser irradiated graphite," *Mat. Res. Soc. Symp. Proc.* **100**, (1988), 483-488.

317. "A laser commercial: NICOLS after-dinner talk," *Laser Spectroscopy IX, Proc. of the Ninth International Conference on Laser Spectroscopy*, ed. M.S. Feld, J.E. Thomas and A. Mooradian, (Boston: Academic Press, 1989).

318. "Time reversal and spatial inversion in magnetoelectric and nonlinear optical phenomena," in Proc. of Symp. on Space-Time Symmetries, *Journal of Nuclear Physics B* **6**, Proc. Suppl., (1989), 283-289.

319. With K.-H. Chen, C-Z. Lu and E. Mazur, "Multiplex pure rotational coherent anti-Stokes Raman spectroscopy in a molecular beam," *Journal of Raman Spectroscopy* **21**, (1990), 819-825.

320. "The science and technology of directed-energy weapons," *Interdisciplinary Science Review* **14**, No. 4, (1989), 362-364.

321. With P. Saeta, J.-K. Wang, Y. Siegal and E. Mazur, "Ultrafast electronic disordering during femtosecond laser melting of GaAs," *Phys. Rev. Lett.* **67**, No. 8, (1991), 1023-1026.

322. "Citation clasics; light waves interacts," *Phys. Rev.* **128**, (1962), 606-622; *Current Contents* **22**, No. 6, (Feb. 11, 1991).

323. *Nonlinear Optics—A Historical Perspective in Huygens' Principle, 1690-1990: Theory and Applications*, ed. by H. Block, H.A. Ferwerda, H.K. Kuiken, (B.V.: Elsevier Science Publishers, 1992), 383-394.

324. "First Light on fluid carbon," *Nature* **356**, (March 11, 1991), 110-11.

325. "Nonlinear optics: past, present and future," *Guided Wave Nonlinear Optics*, ed. by D.B. Ostrowsky and R. Reinisch (Dordrecht: Kluwer Academic Publishers, 1992), 1-9.

326. "Physics 1992: perceptions and perspectives," Retiring presidential address, *APS News* **1**, (August 1992), 26-31.

327. "Laser-material interactions; fundamentals and applications," in Proc. of the Second Int. Conference on Laser Advanced Materials Processing, Nagaoka, Japan, (1992).

328. "Science and society in the 21st century; prospects and problems," *1992 Hania World Dialogues*, ed. by E.D. Haidenmenakis, (1992).

329. "Optical materials, then and now," *Annual Review of Materials Science* **23**, (1993).

330. "Recollections about multiphoton processes," Proc. of 6th International Conference on Multiphoton Processes, Quebec City, Canada, (1993).

331. "Physical review records birth of laser era," *Physics Today*, (October, 1993), 28-31.

Publication List: ERWIN L. HAHN

1. E.L. Hahn, "An accurate nuclear magnetic resonance method for measuring spin-lattice relaxation times," *Phys. Rev.* **76,** (1949), 145.

2. E.L. Hahn, "Nuclear induction due to free Larmor precession," *Phys. Rev.* **77,** (1950), 297.

3. E.L. Hahn, "Spin echoes," *Bull. Amer. Phys. Soc.* **24** (7), (1949), 13. Abs. G9. Also in *Phys. Rev.* **77,** (1950), 746.

4. E.L. Hahn, "Spin echoes," *Phys. Rev.* **80,** (1950), 580.

5. E.L. Hahn and D.E. Maxwell, "Chemical shift and field independent frequency modulation of the spin echo envelope," *Phys. Rev.* **84,** (1951), 1246.

6. H.W. Knoebel and E.L. Hahn, "A transitron nuclear magnetic resonance detector," *Rev. Sci. Instrum.* **22,** (1951), 904.

7. E.L. Hahn and D.E. Maxwell, "Spin echo measurements of nuclear spin coupling molecules," *Phys. Rev.* **88,** (1952), 1070.

8. E.L. Hahn, "Free nuclear induction," *Physics Today* **6,** (1953), 4.

9. E.L. Hahn and B. Herzog, "Anisotropic relaxation of quadrupole spin echoes,"*Phys. Rev.* **93,** (1954), 639.

10. A.G. Anderson, R.L. Garwin, E.L. Hahn, J.W. Horton, G.L. Tucker and R.M. Walker, "Spin echo serial storage memory," *J. Appl. Phys.* **26,** (1955), 1324.

11. M. Bloom, E.L. Hahn and B. Herzog, "Free magnetic induction in nuclear quadrupole resonance," *Phys. Rev.* **97,** (1955), 1966.

12. B. Herzog and E.L. Hahn, "Relaxation time modification by double nuclear resonance," *Phys. Rev.* **98,** (1955), 226.

13. E.L. Hahn and B. Herzog, "A diffusion model for nuclear precession in solids," *Phys. Rev.* **98,** (1955), 265.

14. E.L. Hahn, "Spin echo technique and apparatus," US Patent #2,705,790; issued 5 April 1955.

15. A.G. Anderson and E.L. Hahn, "Spin echo storage technique," US Patent #2,714,714; issued 2 August, 1955.

16. B. Herzog and E.L. Hahn, "Transient nuclear induction and double nuclear resonance in solids," *Phys. Rev.* **103,** (1956), 148.

17. K.E. Kaplan and E.L. Hahn, "Experiences de double irradiation en resonance magnetique par la methode d'impulsions," *J. Phys. Radium* **19,** (1958), 821.

18. T.P. Das and E.L. Hahn, "Nuclear quadrupole resonance spectroscopy," *Solid state physics,* Supplement 1. ed. F. Seitz and D. Turnbull, (New York: Academic Press, 1958).

19. E.L. Hahn, "Pulsed nuclear induction spin echo technique," US Patent #2,887,673; issued 9 May 1959.

20. E.M. Emshwiller, E.L. Hahn and D. Kaplan, "Pulsed nuclear resonance spectroscopy," *Phys. Rev.* **118,** (1960), 414.

21. E.G. Wikner, W.E. Blumberg and E.L. Hahn, "Nuclear quadrupole spin-lattice relaxation in alkali halides," *Phys. Rev.* **118,** (1960), 631.

22. E.L. Hahn, "Detection of sea-water motion by nuclear precession," *J. Geophys. Res.* **65,** (1960), 776.

23. M.J. Weber and E.L. Hahn, "Selective spin excitation and relaxation in nuclear quadrupole resonance," *Phys. Rev.* **120,** (1960), 365.

24. C. Froidevaux, E.L. Hahn and R. Walstedt, "Nuclear spin thermometry and relaxation below 1 K," In *Proceedings of VIIth International Conference on Low Temperature Physics,* Toronto, September 1960, eds. G.M. Graham and A.C. Hollis Hallett, (Canada/North-Holland, Amsterdam: University of Toronto Press, (1961).

25. M. Weger, E.L. Hahn and A.M. Portis, "Transient excitation of nuclei in ferromagnetic metals," *J. Appl. Phys.* **32,** (1961), Suppl. 124S.

26. S.R. Hartmann and E.L. Hahn, "Nuclear double resonance in the rotating frame,"*Phys. Rev.* **128,** (1962), 2042.

27. E.L. Hahn and S.R. Hartmann, "Nuclear double resonance in the rotating frame," in *Fluctuation, Relaxation and Resonance in Magnetic Systems*, ed. D. ter Harr, (Edinburgh : Oliver and Boyd,1962).

28. R.E. Walstedt, M.W. Dowley, E.L. Hahn and C. Froidevaux, "Nuclear magnetic resonance in platinum," *Phys. Rev. Lett.* **8**, (1962), 406.

29. R.E. Walstedt, C. Froidevaux and E.L. Hahn, "Nuclear magnetic resonance in platinum metal," also S.R. Hartmann and E.L. Hahn, "Nuclear double resonance in the rotating frame," (1962). International Conference on Magnetic and Electric Resonance and Relaxation, XI Eindhoven Conference, July 1962. In *Compte rendu du IIe Colloque Ampere: Eindhoven*, ed. J. Smidt, (North-Holland, Amsterdam, (1962).

30. R.L. Strombotne and E.L. Hahn, "Longitudinal nuclear spin-spin relaxation," *Phys. Rev.* **133**, (1964), A1616.

31. R.E. Slusher and E.L. Hahn, "Sensitive detection of pure quadrupole spectra of nuclei (10^{15} to 10^{18} cm^{-3}) near impurities in NaCl," *Phys. Rev. Lett.* **12**, (1964), 246.

32. E.L. Hahn, "Double resonance and cross relaxation-detection of nuclear moment interactions," (1965), *Leuven Conference Report, XIII Colloque Ampère.* September 1964. In *Nuclear Magnetic Resonance and Relaxation in Solids*, ed. L. Van Gerven, (North-Holland, Amsterdam).

33. D.E. MacLaughlin and E.L. Hahn, "Zero field nuclear spin-spin relaxation in normal and superconducting aluminium," *Bull. Amer. Phys. Soc.* **10**, (1965), 1206, Abs. R2.

34. L.G. Rowan, E.L. Hahn and W.B. Mims, "Electron-spin-echo envelope modulation," *Phys. Rev.* **137**, (1965), A61.

35. R.E. Walstedt, E.L. Hahn, C. Froidevaux and E. Geissler, "Nuclear spin thermometry below 1 K," *Proc. Roy. Soc.* **284**, (1965), 499.

36. R.E. Walstedt, D.A. McArthur and E.L. Hahn "Nuclear double resonance of Ca^{43} in CaF$_2$," *Phys. Lett.* **15**, (1965), 7.

37. L.W. Riley, M. Bass and E.L. Hahn, "Stimulated emission from 4.3% abundant Cr^{50} ions in ruby," *Appl. Phys. Lett.* **7**, (1965), 88.

38. R.E. Walstedt, D.A. McArthur and E.L. Hahn, "Measurement of T_1 and T_2 of Ca^{43} in CaF$_2$," *Bull. Amer. Phys. Soc.* **11**, (1966), 907. Abs. Q14.

39. G.W. Leppelmeier and E.L. Hahn, "Nuclear dipole field quenching of integer spins," *Phys. Rev.* **141**, (1966), 724.

40. G.W. Leppelmeier and E.L. Hahn, "Zero field nuclear quadrupole spin-lattice relaxation in the rotating frame," *Phys. Rev.* **142**, (1966), 179.

41. R.E.J. Sears and E.L. Hahn, "Upper limits to electric field induced nuclear magnetic dipole-dipole couplings in polar liquids," *J. Chem. Phys.* **45**, (1966), 2753.

42. D.E. MacLaughlin and E.L. Hahn, "Zero-field nuclear spin relaxation and resonance absorption in superconducting aluminum," *Phys. Rev.* **159**, (1967), 359.

43. S.L. McCall and E.L. Hahn "Self-induced transparency by pulsed coherent light," *Phys. Rev. Lett.* **18**, (1967), 908.

44. R.E.J. Sears and E.L. Hahn, "Erratum: upper limits to electric-field-induced nuclear magnetic dipole-dipole couplings in polar liquids," *J. Chem. Phys.* **47**, (1967), 348.

45. E.L. Hahn, "Developments in nuclear double resonance spectroscopy," (1968), in *Magnetic Resonance and Relaxation*, ed. R. Blinc, Proceedings of the XIV Colloque Ampère, Ljubljana, (North-Holland, Amsterdam, Sept. 1966).

46. J.W. Shaner, S.A. Miller and E.L. Hahn, "Zero field precession measurements of the hyperfine interaction in cesium vapor," *Bull. Amer. Phys. Soc.* **13**, (1968), 358. Abs. AD11.

47. R. Slusher and E.L. Hahn, "Sensitive detection of nuclear quadrupole interactions in solids," *Phys. Rev.* **166**, (1968), 326.

48. S.L. McCall and E.L. Hahn, "Self-induced transparency," *Phys. Rev.* **183**, (1969), 457.

49. D.A. McArthur and E.L. Hahn, "Rotating-frame nuclear-double-resonance dynamics: dipolar fluctuation spectrum in CaF$_2$," *Phys. Rev.* **188**, (1969), 609.

50. E.L. Hahn, "The ebb and flow of atomic chaos—the physicist as King Canute," *Proc. R. Inst.* **44**, (1970), 26.

51. J.W. Shaner and E.L. Hahn, "Cyclotron echoes in a weakly ionized caesium plasma" *J. Appl. Phys.* **41**, (1970), 839.

52. M. Schwab and E.L. Hahn, "Scheme for sensitive nuclear double-resonance detection: deuterium and ^{13}C," *J. Chem. Phys.* **52**, (1970), 3152.

53. S.L. McCall and E.L. Hahn, "Pulse-area-pulse-energy description of a traveling wave laser amplifier," *Phys. Rev. A* **2**, (1970), 861.

54. E.L. Hahn, N.S. Shiren and S.L. McCall, "Application of the area theorem to photon echoes," *Phys. Lett.* **37A**, (1971), 265.

55. T.M. Pierce and E.L. Hahn, "Self induced transparency in purely homogeneously broadened systems," *Bull. Amer. Phys. Soc.* **17**, (1972), 47. Abs. BJ1.

56. P.E. Nordal and E.L. Hahn, "Nuclear double resonance study of K^{39} in ferroelectric KH_2PO_4," *Bull. Amer. Phys. Soc.* **17**, (1972), 129, Abs. J17.

57. Y. Hsieh, J.C. Koo and E.L. Hahn "Pure nuclear quadrupole resonance of naturally abundant 0^{17} in organic solids," *Chem. Phys. Lett.* **13**, (1972), 563.

58. E.L. Hahn, "Macroscopic optical coherence phenomena," *Pure Appl. Chem.* **32**, (1972), 171.

59. R.G. Brewer and E.L. Hahn, "Coherent Raman beats," *Phys. Rev. A* **8**, (1973), 464.

60. J.C. Diels, E.L. Hahn, "Carrier-frequency distance dependence of a pulse propagating in a two-level system," *Phys. Rev. A* **8**, (1973), 1084.

61. E.L. Hahn and S.L. McCall, "Method and apparatus for propagating travelling wave energy through resonant media," US Patent #3,714,438; issued 30 January, 1973.

62. E.L. Hahn and J.C. Diels, "Off-resonance pulse propagation in a two level system—distance dependence of the carrier frequency," In *Proceedings of the Laser Spectroscopy Conference,* Vail, Colorado, June 1973, ed. R.G. Brewer and A. Mooradian, (New York: Plenum Press, 1974), 323-32.

63. S.B. Grossman and E.L. Hahn, "Microwave pulse propagation in a paramagnetic spin system," In Proceedings of the First Specialized 'Colloque Ampère,' Krakow, Poland. 1973, *Radzikowskilys* **15**, ed. J.W. Hennel, (Krakow, Poland: Institute of Nuclear Physics, 1973), 63.

64. J.C. Diels and E.L. Hahn, "Phase-modulation propagation effects in ruby," *Phys. Rev. A* **10**, (1974), 2501.

65. E.L. Hahn, "Optics (nonlinear): a review of recent advances in self-induced transparency," In *Yearbook of Science and Technology,* (New York: McGraw-Hill, 1974).

66. R.G. Brewer and E.L. Hahn, "Coherent two-photon process: transient and steady state cases," *Phys. Rev. A* **11**, (1975), 1641.

67. J.C. Diels and E.L. Hahn, "Pulse propagation stability in absorbing and amplifying media," *IEEE J. Quantum Elect.* **QE-12**, (1976), 411.

68. E.L. Hahn, "Macroscopic dipole coherence phenomena," In *Introductory Essays, NMR: Basic Principles and Progress,* ed. M. Pinter, (Berlin: Springer, 1976.)

69. S.B. Grossman and E.L. Hahn, "Microwave EPR self-induced transparency," *Phys. Rev. A* **14**, (1976), 2206.

70. E.L. Hahn and R. Wilson, "Coherent emission of phonons by spatially phased spins," In *Proceedings of XIX Congress Ampère,* Heidelberg, 1976: *Magnetic Resonance and Related Phenomena,* eds. H. Brunner, K.H. Hausser and D. Schweitzer, (Heidelberg: Groupement Ampère, 1976), 27.

71. T.L. Andrade and E.L. Hahn, "Principles of NQR double resonance—application to deuterium. In *Magnetic resonance in Condensed Matter—Recent Developments; Proceedings of the 4th Ampère International Summer School,* Pula, Yugoslavia, 1976, eds. R. Bloinc and G. Lehajnar, (J. Stefan Institute, Ljubljana, 1976), 181-95.

72. D.G. Gold and E.L. Hahn, "Mascroscopic resonance dynamics of three-level systems," In *Magnetic Resonance in Condensed Matter—Recent Developments; Proceedings of the 4th*

Ampère International Summer School, Pula, Yugoslavia, 1976, eds. R. Blinc and G. Lahajnar, (J. Stefan Institute, Ljubljana, 1976), 197-203.

73. Y. Prior and E.L. Hahn, "Optical rotary saturation," *Phys. Rev. Lett.* **39**, (1977), 1329.

74. D.G. Gold and E.L. Hahn, "Two-photon transient phenomena," *Phys. Rev. A* **16**, (1977), 324.

75. Y. Prior, J.A. Kash and E.L. Hahn, "Optical rotary saturation in a gas," *Phys Rev. A* **18**, (1978), 2603.

76. E.L. Hahn, "Spin echoes, designated Citation Classic of the Month," In *Current Contents* **19**, (39), (1979), 12.

77. E.L. Hahn, "Pulsed nuclear magnetic resonance in solids: a survey," *Disc. Faraday Soc.* **13**, (1979), 8.

78. D.W. Dolfi and E.L. Hahn, "Study of soliton interactions in sodium vapor," *Phys. Rev. A* **21**, (1980), 1272.

79. E.L. Hahn, "Heritage of the Bloch equations in quantum optics," In *Felix Bloch and 20th Century Physics, a Festschrift*, Rice University Studies, Vol. 66. No. 3. (Texas: Rice University Press, 1980).

80. J.A. Kash and E.L. Hahn, "Coherent optical transient effects of the spin-rotation interaction in $^{13}CH_3F$," *Phys. Rev. Lett.* **47**, (1981), 167.

81. J.A. Kash, S. Tao-Heng and E.L. Hahn, "Spin rotation coupling in a laser experiment," In *Proceedings Conference on Diagnostic Methods of High Frequency Spectroscopy*, Nov. 1981, (G.D.R.: Schloss Reinhardsbrunn, 1981), 2-6.

82. R.J. Wilson and E.L. Hahn, "Off-resonance transient response of a three-level system," *Phys. Rev. A* **26**, (1982), 3404.

83. J.A. Kash, S. Tao-Heng and E.L. Hahn, "Optical mixed state transient effects by Stark switching," *Phys. Rev. A* **26**, (1982), 2682.

84. R.J. Wilson and E.L. Hahn, "Local-field-induced multiple-pulse free-induction decay," *Phys. Rev. B* **27**, (1983), 4129.

85. E.L. Hahn, "Non-adiabatic laser induced spin coupling phenomena," *Bulletin of Magnetic Resonance* **6**, No. 2, (2), (1984), 20.

86. R.G. Brewer and E.L. Hahn, "Atomic memory,"*Sci. Am.* **251**, (6), (1984), 50-7.

87. T.-H. Sun, M.-K. Kim and E.L. Hahn, "Rotary echo measurements of dipole transition matrix elements," In *Proceedings of the Conference on Lasers and Electro-Optics*, Baltimore, Maryland. Abs WN5, Laser and Electro-optics Branch of the IEEE and the Optical Society of America (1985).

88. S. Tao-Heng, J.A. Kash and E.L. Hahn, "The calculation and observation of optical rotary echoes," *Acta. Phys. Sin.* **34**, No. 3 (1985).

89. F.W. Otto, M. Lukac and E.L. Hahn, "Spin-spin reservoir cross-relaxation of Pr^{+3}: LaF_3 via optical pumping," In *Laser spectroscopy VII from the Proceedings of the Seventh International Conference (SEICOLS)*, Hawaii, 24-28 June 1985, eds. T.W. Hansch and Y.R. Shen, (New York: Springer, 1985), 274-8.

90. C. Hilbert, J. Clarke, T. Sleator and E.L. Hahn, "Applications of a DC squid to RF amplification: NQR," *Proceedings of the 3rd International Conference on SQUIDs*, West Berlin, 1985. In *Superconducting Quantum Interference Devices and Their Applications*. (Berlin: De Gruyter, 1985),.

91. C. Hilbert, J. Clarke, T. Sleator and E.L. Hahn, "Nuclear quadrupole resonance detected at 30 MHz with a DC superconducting quantum interference device," *Appl. Phys. Lett.* **47**, (6), (1985), 637.

92. T. Sleator, E.L. Hahn, C. Hilbert and J. Clarke, "Nuclear-spin noise," *Phys. Rev. Lett.* **55**, (1985), 1742.

93. E.L. Hahn, "Felix Bloch and magnetic resonance," Presented at the Felix Bloch Memorial Symposium American Physical Society, Washington D.C. April 25, 1984 and published in *Bulletin of Magnetic Resonance* **7**, (2/3), (1985), 82-9.

94. E.L. Hahn and T. Sleator, "Spin noise," In *Proceedings of the Beijing Conference and Exhibition on Instrumental Analysis,* Beijing, Nov. 1985, (1985).

95. F.W. Otto, F.X. D'Amato, M. Lukac and E.L. Hahn, "Spin-spin cross-relaxation of optically-excited rare-earth ions in crystals," In *Proceedings of the Fritz-Haber Conference on Lasers:* Dead Sea. Israel, Dec. 1985. *Methods of Laser Spectroscopy,* eds. Y. Prior, A. Ben-Reuven and M. Rosenbluh, (New York: Plenum, 1986).

96. F.W. Otto, M. Lukac and E.L. Hahn, "Spin Hamiltonian spectroscopy and spin-spin cross relaxation of otical pumping of Pr^{+3}: LaF_3," *J. Luminesc.* **35,** (1986), 321-7.

97. T. Sleator, E.L. Hahn, M.B. Heaney, C. Hilbert and J. Clarke, "Nuclear electric quadrupole induction of atomic polarization," *Phys. Rev. Lett.* **57,** (1986), 2756.

98. T. Sleator, E.L. Hahn, C. Hilbert and J. Clarke, "Nuclear-spin noise and spontaneous emission," *Phys. Rev. B.* **36,** (1987), 1969.

99. C.J. Grayce, R.A. Harris and E.L. Hahn, "The nuclear quadrupole-induced dipole moment of HD," *Chem. Phys. Lett.* **147,** (1988), 443.

100. T. Sleator and E.L. Hahn, "Nuclear-quadrupole induction of atomic polarization," *Phys. Rev. B* **38,** (1988), 8609.

101. M. Lukac and E.L. Hahn, "External reflection and transmission spectroscopy of Pr^{3+}:LaF_3 by Stark modulated optical pumping," *J. Luminesc.* **42,** (1988), 257.

102. J. Clarke, C. Hilbert, E.L. Hahn and T. Sleator, "Josephson junction Q-spoiler," US Patent #4,733,182; issued 22 March, 1988,.

103. M. Lukac, F.W. Otto and E.L. Hahn, "Spin-spin cross relaxation and spin-Hamiltonian spectroscopy by optical pumping of Pr^{+3}: LaF_3," *Phys. Rev. A* **39,** (1989), 1123.

104. M. Lukac and E.L. Hahn, "Spectroscopy of symmetry broken optical doublets in Pr^{+3}:LaF_3," *Opt. Commun.* **70,** (1989), 195.

105. J. Chang, C. Connor, E.L. Hahn, H. Huber and A. Pines, "Direct detection of aluminum-27 resonance with SQUID spectrometer," *Journal of Magnetic Resonance* **82,** (1989), 387.

106. N.Q. Fan, M.B. Heaney, J. Clarke, D. Newitt, L. Wald, E.L. Hahn, A. Bielecki and A. Pines, "Nuclear magnetic resonance with D.C. SQUID preamplifiers," *IEEE Trans. Mag.* **25,** (1989), 1193.

107. E.L. Hahn, J. Clarke, T. Sleator, C. Hilbert and M.B. Heaney, "Apparatus and method for measuring electrostatic polarization," US Patent #4,833,392; issued 23 May, 1989,.

108. M. Lukac and E.L. Hahn, "Optical pumping measurements of nuclear cross relaxation and electric doublets," In *Advances in Magnetic Resonance,* ed. W.S. Warren, (New York: Academic Press, 1990), 75.

109. E.L. Hahn, "Felix Bloch reminiscences," *Internatl. J. Mod. Phys.* **B4,** (1990), 1283. Also in Little W.A., ed., *Conductivity and Magnetism: The Legacy of Felix Bloch,* (New Jersey: World Scientific, 1990).

110. E.L. Hahn "NMR and MRI in retrospect," *Phil. Trans. Roy. Soc. Lond.* **A333,** (1990), 403.

111. N.Q. Fan, B. Heaney, J. Clarke, D. Newitt, L.L. Wald and E.L. Hahn, "Nuclear magnetic resonance with D.C. SQUID preamplifiers," In *Proceedings of the 24th Ampère Congress 1988. Magnetic Resonance and Related Phenomena,* ed. J. Stankowski, (Poland: Polish Academy of Sciences, 1988).

112. E.L. Hahn, "The ebb and flow of atomic chaos," In *Proceedings of the Binational Colloquium for Humboldt Awardees,* Stanford, USA, 1983, ed. H. Hanle, Alexander von Humboldt Siftung, (Bad Godesburg, Germany , 1984).

113. L.L. Wald, E.L. Hahn and M. Lukac, "Flourine spin diffusion barrier in Pr^{3+}:LaF_3 observed by cross-relaxation," In *Persistent Spectral Hole-burning: Science and Applications,* 1991. The Technical Digest Series, Vol. 16., (Washington D.C., USA: Optical Society of America, 1991).

114. L.L. Wald, E.L. Hahn and M. Lukac, "Optical pumping detection of anomalous NQR spectra of Pr^{3+} in Pr^{3+}:LaF_3," In *Persistent Spectral Hole-burning: Science and Applications,* 1991. The Technical Digest Series, Vol. 16. (Washington, D.C., USA: Optical Society of America, 1991).

Publication List: RICHARD R. ERNST

1. R.R. Ernst, O.A. Stamm and Hch. Zollinger, "Kinetischer isotopeneffekt und isomerenverhältnis bei der kupplung von deuterierter I-naphtol-3-sulfosäure," *Helv. Chem. Acta* **41**, (1958), 2274.

2. H. Primas, R. Arndt and R. Ernst, "Group contributions to the chemical shift in proton magnetic resonance of organic compounds," International Meeting of Mol. Spectrosc., Bologna, Sept. 1959; *Advances in Molecular Spectroscopy*, (London: Pergamon Press, 1962), 1246.

3. H. Primas, R. Arndt and R. Ernst, "Die konstruktion von kernresonanz-spektrographen hoher auflösung," *Z. Instrumentenkunde* **67**, (1959), 293.

4. H. Primas, R. Arndt and R. Ernst, "Die konstruktion von kernresonanz-spektrographen hoher auflösung," *Z. Instrumentenkunde* **68**, (1960), 8.

5. H. Primas, R. Arndt and R. Ernst, "Die konstruktion von kernresonanz-spektrographen hoher auflösung," *Z. Instrumentenkunde* **68**, (1960), 21.

6. H. Primas, R. Arndt and R. Ernst, "Die konstruktion von kernresonanz-spektrographen hoher auflösung," *Z. Instrumentenkunde* **68**, (1960), 55.

7. R. Ernst and H. Primas, "High-resolution NMR-instrumentation: recent advances and prospects," Offprinted from the "Discussions of The Faraday Society," (1962), 43.

8. R. Ernst, "Kernresonanz-spektroskopie mit stochastischen hochfrequenzfeldern, II. Zur konstruktion eines optimalen kernresonanz-messkopfes," Diss. Eth Zürich, 1962.

9. R.R. Ernst and H. Primas, "Nuclear magnetic resonance with stochastic high-frequency fields," *Helv. Phys. Acta* **36**, (1963), 583.

10. R.R. Ernst and H. Primas, "Gegenwärtiger stand und entwicklungstendenzen in der instrumentierung hochauflösender kernresonanz-spektrometer," *Ber. Bunsenges. für Phys. Chemie* **67**, (1963), 261.

11. R.R. Ernst and J.M. Anderson, "Symmetry properties of double-resonance spectra. II. Additional comments and errata," *J. Chem. Phys.* **40**, (1964), 3737.

12. R.R. Ernst, "Sensitivity enhancement in magnetic resonance. I. Analysis of the method of time averaging," *Rev. Sci. Instrum.* **36**, (1965), 1689.

13. R.R. Ernst and W.A. Anderson, "Sensitivity enhancement in magnetic resonance. II. Investigation of intermediate passage conditions," *Rev. Sci. Instrum.* **36**, (1965), 1696. 13A. Errata of Number 13.

14. R.R. Ernst and W.A. Anderson, "Application of Fourier transform spectroscopy to magnetic resonance," *Rev. Sci. Instrum.* **37**, (1966), 93.

15. R.R. Ernst, "Nuclear magnetic double resonance with an incoherent radio-frequency field," *J. Chem. Phys.* **45**, (1966), 3845.

16. R.R. Ernst, "Sensitivity enhancement in magnetic resonance," *Adv. In Magn. Resonance*, Vol. 2, (New York: Academic Press, 1966).

17. R. Freeman, R.R. Ernst and W.A. Anderson, "Line profiles in nuclear magnetic double resonance," *J. Chem. Phys.* **46**, (1967), 1125.

18. R.R. Ernst, "Recent applications of computer techniques in nuclear magnetic resonance," unpublished (Palo Alto, CA: Varian Associates, Analytical Instrument Division, 1967).

19. R.R. Ernst, R. Freeman, Bo Gestblom and T.R. Lusebrink, "Detection of very small NMR spin coupling constants by resolution enhancement," *Mol. Phys.* **13**, (1967), 283.

20. R.R. Ernst, "Measurement and control of magnetic field homogeneity," *Rev. Sci. Instrum.* **39**, (1968), 998.

21. R.R. Ernst, "Numerical Hilbert transform and automatic phase correction in magnetic resonance spectroscopy," *J. Magn. Resonan.* **1**, (1969), 7.

22. R.R. Ernst, "NMR studies of ^{19}F chemical shifts and coupling constants in cyclobutane derivatives. An example of the application of noise decoupling," *Mol. Phys.* **16**, (1969), 241.

23. R.R. Ernst, "Methoden breitbandiger Simultanerregung in der hochauflösenden Kernresonanz-Spektroskopie," Int. Konferenz über Hochfrequenz-Spektroskopie, Leipzig, 1969.

24. R. Freeman, S. Wittekoek and R.R. Ernst, "High-resolution NMR study of relaxation mechanisms in a two-spin system," *J. Chem. Phys.* **52**, (1970), 1529.

25. R.R. Ernst, "Magnetic resonance with stochastic excitation," *J. Magn. Reson.* **3**, (1970), 10.

26. M. El Moghazi, R.R. Ernst and Hs. H. Günthard, "Anisotropic NMR spectra of 1,3,5-trichlorobenzene substituted in an (α)-sulfur single crystal," *J. Magn. Reson.* **3**, (1970), 480.

27. R.R. Ernst and H. Benz, "Optimum line shape analysis by least-square approximation and linear transformation processes," *IEEE Transact. on Audio & Electroacoustics* **AU-18**, (1970), 380.

28. R.R. Ernst, "Fourier difference spectroscopy," *J. Magn. Reson.* **4**, (1971), 280.

29. R.R. Ernst, "Difference frequency spectroscopy with analog Fourier analyzer," *J. Magn. Reson.* **5**, (1971), 398.

30. R.R. Ernst, "Fourier transform spectroscopy," in *The Applications of Computer Techniques in Chemical Research*, The Institute of Petroleum, London, 1972.

31. R.R. Ernst, "Die Anwendung von Digitalrechnern zur Steuerung und Datenverarbeitung im spektroskopischen Laboratorium," *Chimia* **26**, (1972), 53.

32. R.R. Ernst, 'Comment on "Systems limitations on the Fourier transform relationship between NMR free induction decay and cw line shape,"' *J. Chem. Phys* **59**, (1973), 989.

33. R.R. Ernst and R.E. Morgan, "Saturation effects in Fourier spectroscopy," *Mol. Phys.* **26**, (1973), 49.

34. E. Bartholdi and R.R. Ernst, "Fourier spectroscopy and the causality principle," *J. Magn. Reson.* **11**, (1973), 9.

35. R.R. Ernst, "Recent developments in Fourier spectroscopy," *First Specialized 'Colloque Ampère,'* (Krakow, Poland, 1973), 38.

36. S. Schäublin, A. Höhener and R.R. Ernst, "Fourier spectroscopy on nonequilibrium states, application to CIDNP, Overhauser experiments and relaxation time measurements," *J. Magn. Reson.* **13**, (1974), 196.

37. R. Kaiser, E. Bartholdi and R.R. Ernst, "Diffusion and field-gradient effects in NMR Fourier spectroscopy," *J. Chem. Phys.* **60**, (1974), 2966.

38. R.R. Ernst, W.P. Aue, E. Bartholdi, A. Höhener and S. Schäublin, "Equivalence of Fourier spectroscopy and slow passage in nuclear magnetic resonance," *Pure and Appl. Chem.* **37**, (1974), 47.

39. L. Müller, A. Kumar, Th. Baumann and R.R. Ernst, "Transient oscillations in NMR cross-polarization experiments in solids," *Phys. Rev. Lett.* **32**, (1974), 1402.

40. A. Höhener, G. Bodenhausen and R.R. Ernst, "Determination of relaxation parameters in coupled nuclear spin systems by complete sets of Overhauser experiments," *18th Congress Ampere, Nottingham (1974)*, 469.

41. L. Müller, A. Kumar, Th. Baumann and R.R. Ernst, "Transient oscillations in NMR cross-polarization experiments in solids," *18th Congress Ampere, Nottingham, 1974*, 557.

42. A. Kumar, D. Welti and R.R. Ernst, "Imaging of macroscopic objects by NMR Fourier zeugmatography," *Naturwissenschaften* **62**, (1975), 34.

43. R.R. Ernst, "Two-dimensional spectroscopy," *Chimia* **29**, (1975), 179.

44. A. Kumar, D. Welti and R.R. Ernst, "NMR Fourier zeugmatography," *J. Magn. Reson.* **18**, (1975), 69.

45. L. Müller, A. Kumar and R.R. Ernst, "Two-dimensional carbon-13 NMR spectroscopy," *J. Chem. Phys.* **63**, (1975), 5490.

46. A. Kumar and R.R. Ernst, "Carbon-13 spin echo modulations in liquids caused by heteronuclear spin coupling," *Chem. Phys. Lett.* **37**, (1976), 162.

47. W.P. Aue, E. Bartholdi and R.R. Ernst, "Two-dimensional spectroscopy. Application to nuclear magnetic resonance," *J. Chem. Phys.* **64**, (1976), 2229.

48. W.P. Aue, J. Karhan and R.R. Ernst, "Homonuclear broad band decoupling and two-dimensional J-resolved NMR spectroscopy," *J. Chem. Phy.* **64**, (1976), 4226.

49. S. Schäublin, A. Wokaun and R.R. Ernst, "The creation of off-diagonal elements in chemically induced dynamic nuclear polarization experiments," *Chem. Phys.* **14,** (1976), 285.

50. Anil Kumar and R.R. Ernst, "Influence of nonresonant nuclei on NMR spin echoes in liquids and in solids," *J. Magn. Reson.* **24,** (1976), 425.

51. E. Bartholdi, A. Wokaun and R.R. Ernst, "Theory of stochastic NMR spectroscopy. Application of the Itô and Stratonovich calculus," *Chem. Phys.* **18,** (1976), 57.

52. L. Müller, Anil Kumar and R.R. Ernst, "Two-dimensional carbon-13 spin-echo spectroscopy," *J. Magn. Reson.* **25,** (1977), 383.

53. Anil Kumar, W.P. Aue, P. Bachmann, J. Karhan, L. Müller and R.R. Ernst, "Two-dimensional spin-echo spectroscopy; a means to resolve proton and carbon NMR spectra," *XIXth Congress Ampere,* Heidelberg, 1976, 473.

54. J.A. Ferretti and R.R. Ernst, "Interference effects in NMR correlation spectroscopy of coupled spin systems," *J. Chem. Phys.* **65,** (1976), 4283.

55. A. Frey and R.R. Ernst, "Deformation and orientation of solute molecules in nematic phases," *Chem. Phys. Lett.* **49,** (1977), 75.

56. S. Schäublin, A. Wokaun and R.R. Ernst, "Pulse techniques applied to chemically induced dynamic nuclear polarization," *J. Magn. Reson.* **27,** (1977), 273.

57. A. Wokaun and R.R. Ernst, "Selective excitation and detection in multilevel spin systems: application of single transition operators," *J. Chem. Phys.* **67,** (1977), 1752.

58. A.A. Maudsley and R.R. Ernst, "Indirect detection of magnetic resonance by heteronuclear two-dimensional spectroscopy," *Chem. Phys. Lett.* **50,** (1977), 368.

59. K. Nagayama, K. Wüthrich, P. Bachmann and R.R. Ernst, "Two-dimensional J-resolved ^{1}H NMR spectroscopy for studies of biological macromolecules," *Biochem. Biophys. Res. Commun.* **78,** (1977), 99.

60. P. Bachmann, W.P. Aue, L. Müller and R.R. Ernst, "Phase separation in two-dimensional spectroscopy," *J. Magn. Reson.* **38,** (1977), 29.

61. K. Nagayama, K. Wüthrich, P. Bachmann and R.R. Ernst, "Two-dimensional NMR spectroscopy. A powerful tool for the investigation of biopolymers in solution," *Naturwissenschaften* **64,** (1977), 581.

62. A. Wokaun and R.R. Ernst, "Selective detection of multiple quantum transitions in NMR by two-dimensional spectroscopy," *Chem. Phys. Lett.* **52,** (1977), 407.

63. R.R. Ernst, W.P. Aue, P. Bachmann, J. Karhan, Anil Kumar and L. Müller, "Two-dimensional NMR spectroscopy," in Magnetic Resonance in Condensed Matter–Recent Developments, ed. by R. Blinc and G. Lahajnar, *Proceedings of the IVth Ampere International Summer School,* Pula, Yugoslavia, 1976, 89.

64. D.H. Welti, M. Linder and R.R. Ernst, "Comparison of molecular geometries determined by paramagnetic nuclear magnetic resonance relaxation and shift reagents in solution," *J. Am. Chem. Soc.* **100,** (1978), 403.

65. A.A. Maudsley, L. Müller and R.R. Ernst, "Cross-correlation of spin-decoupled NMR spectra by heteronuclear two-dimensional spectroscopy," *J. Magn. Reson.* **28,** (1977), 463.

66. A.A. Maudsley, A. Wokaun and R.R. Ernst, "Coherence transfer echoes," *Chem. Phys. Lett.* **55,** (1978), 9.

67. W.P. Aue, P. Bachmann, A. Wokaun and R.R. Ernst, "Sensitivity of two-dimensional NMR spectroscopy," *J. Magn. Reson.* **29,** (1978), 523.

68. K. Nagayama, P. Bachmann, K. Wüthrich and R.R. Ernst, "The use of cross-sections and of projections in two-dimensional NMR spectroscopy," *J. Magn. Reson.* **31,** (1978), 133.

69. A. Wokaun and R.R. Ernst, "The use of multiple quantum transitions for relaxation studies in coupled spin systems," *Mol. Phys.* **36,** (1978), 317.

70. R.R. Ernst, L. Müller, K. Nagayama and K. Wüthrich, "Décrypter la structure des molécules complexes," *La Recherche,* No. 95, Vol. 9 (1978), 1124.

71. W.P. Aue and R.R. Ernst, "Scaling of heteronuclear spin coupling by multipulse techniques," *J. Magn. Reson.* **31,** (1978), 533.

72. K. Nagayama, P. Bachmann, R.R. Ernst and K. Wüthrich, "Selective spin decoupling in the J-resolved two-dimensional ^{1}H NMR spectra of proteins," *Biochem. Biophys. Res. Commun.* **86,** (1979), 218.

73. R.O. Kühne, T. Schaffhauser, A. Wokaun and R.R. Ernst, "Study of transient chemical reactions by NMR. Fast stopped-flow Fourier transform experiments," *J. Magn. Reson.* **35,** (1979), 39.

74. K. Wüthrich, K. Nagayama and R.R. Ernst, "Two-dimensional NMR spectroscopy," *Trends Biochem. Sci.* **4,** (1979), N178.

75. P. Brunner and R.R. Ernst, "Sensitivity and performance time in NMR imaging," *J. Magn. Reson.* **33,** (1979), 83.

76. K. Nagayama, K. Wüthrich and R.R. Ernst, "Two-dimensional spin echo correlated spectroscopy (SECSY) for ^{1}H NMR studies of biological macromolecules," *Biochem. Biophys. Res. Commun.* **90,** (1979), 305.

77. L. Müller and R.R. Ernst, "Coherence transfer in the rotating frame. Application to heteronuclear cross-correlation spectroscopy," *Mol. Phys.* **38,** (1979), 963.

78. A. Höhener, L. Müller and R.R. Ernst, "Dipole-coupled carbon-13 spectra, a source of structural information on liquid crystals," *Mol. Phys.* **38,** (1979), 909.

79. R.R. Ernst, W.P. Aue, P. Bachmann, A. Höhener, M. Linder, B. Meier, L. Müller and A. Wokaun, "Application of two-dimensional spectroscopy to problems of physical, chemical and biological relevance," *XXth Congress Ampere,* Tallinn, 1978, 15.

80. M. Linder, A. Höhener and R.R. Ernst, "Proton-enhanced carbon-13 resonance in helium-cooled probe; chemical shielding tensor of benzene," *J. Magn. Reson.* **35,** (1979), 379.

81. B.H. Meier and R.R. Ernst, "Elucidation of chemical exchange networks by two-dimensional NMR spectroscopy: The heptamethylbenzenonium ion," *J.Am. Chem. Soc.* **101,** (1979), 6441.

82. A. Wokaun and R.R. Ernst, "Multiple quantum double resonance," *Mol. Phys.* **38,** (1979), 1579.

83. J. Jeener, B.H. Meier, P. Bachmann and R.R. Ernst, "Investigation of exchange processes by two-dimensional NMR spectroscopy," *J. Chem. Phys.* **71,** (1979), 4546.

84. W.P. Aue, D.P. Burum and R.R. Ernst, "Scaling of heteronuclear spin interactions by multipulse sequences. Practical guidelines," *J. Magn. Reson.* **38,** (1980), 375.

85. Anil Kumar, R.R. Ernst and K. Wüthrich, "A two-dimensional nuclear Overhauser enhancement (2D NOE) experiment for the elucidation of complete proton-proton cross-relaxation networks in biological macromolecules," *Biochem. Biophys. Res. Commun.* **95,** (1980), 1.

86. D.P. Burum and R.R. Ernst, "Net polarization transfer via a J-ordered state for signal enhancement of low-sensitivity nuclei," *J. Magn. Reson.* **39,** (1980), 163.

87. K. Nagayama, Anil Kumar, K. Wüthrich and R.R. Ernst, "Experimental techniques of two-dimensional correlated spectroscopy," *J. Magn. Reson.* **40,** (1980), 321.

88. A. Minoretti, W.P. Aue, M. Reinhold and R.R. Ernst, "Coherence transfer by radiofrequency pulses for heteronuclear detection of multiple-quantum transitions," *J. Magn. Reson.* **40,** (1980), 175.

89. P. Brunner, M. Reinhold and R.R. Ernst, "Double quantum cross polarization. Heteronuclear excitation and detection of NMR double quantum transitions in solids," *J. Chem. Phys.* **73,** (1980), 1086.

90. Anil Kumar, G. Wagner, R.R. Ernst and K. Wüthrich, "Studies of J-connectivities and selective ^{1}H–^{1}H Overhauser effects in H_2O solutions of biological macromolecules by two–dimensional NMR experiments," *Biochem. Biophys. Res. Commun.* **96,** (1980), 1156.

91. S. Macura and R.R. Ernst, "Elucidation of cross relaxation in liquids by two-dimensional NMR spectroscopy," *Mol. Phys.* **41,** (1980), 95.

92. M. Linder, A. Höhener and R.R. Ernst, "Orientation of tensorial interactions determined from two-dimensional NMR powder spectra," *J. Chem. Phys.* **73,** (1980), 4959.

93. Ch. Bösch, Anil Kumar, R. Baumann, R.R. Ernst and K. Wüthrich, "Comparison of selective proton-proton Overhauser effects in biological macromolecules observed by one-dimensional and two-dimensional NMR experiments," *J. Magn. Reson.* **42**, (1981), 159.

94. M. Reinhold, P. Brunner and R.R. Ernst, "Double quantum cross polarization via dipolar order," *J. Chem. Phys.* **74**, (1981), 184.

95. G. Wider, R. Baumann, K. Nagayama, R.R. Ernst and K. Wüthrich, "Strong spin-spin coupling in the two-dimensional J-resolved 360-MHz ^{1}H NMR spectra of the common amino acids," *J. Magn. Reson.* **42**, (1981), 73.

96. S. Macura, Y. Huang, D. Suter and R.R. Ernst, "Two-dimensional chemical exchange and cross-relaxation spectroscopy of coupled nuclear spins," *J. Magn. Reson.* **43**, (1981), 259.

97. D.P. Burum, M. Linder and R.R. Ernst, "A new 'tune-up' NMR pulse cycle for mini-mizing and characterizing phase transients," *J. Magn. Reson.* **43**, (1981), 463.

98. Anil Kumar, G. Wagner, R.R. Ernst and K. Wüthrich, "Buildup rates of the nuclear Overhauser effect measured by two-dimensional proton magnetic resonance spectroscopy: implications for studies of protein conformation," *J. Am. Chem. Soc.* **103**, (1981), 3654.

99. S. Macura and R.R. Ernst, "The study of solvent-solute interactions by two-dimen-sional NMR spectroscopy," *Periodicum Biologorum* **83**, (1981), 87.

100. T. Schaffhauser, R.R. Ernst, B. Hilti and C.W. Mayer, "Magnetic resonance study of the quasi one-dimensional conductor bis-(tetrathiotetracene)-triiodide $TTT_2(I_3)_{1+\delta}$ and ist selenium analogon $TSeT_2I$," *Chemica Scripta* **17**, (1981), 27.

101. R. Baumann, Anil Kumar, R.R. Ernst and K. Wüthrich, "Improvement of 2D NOE and 2D correlated spectra by triangular multiplication," *J. Magn. Reson.* **44**, (1981), 76.

102. D.P. Burum, M. Linder and R.R. Ernst, "Low-power multipulse line narrowing in solid-state NMR," *J. Magn. Reson.* **44**, (1981), 173.

103. R. Baumann, G. Wider, R.R. Ernst and K. Wüthrich, "Improvement of 2D NOE and 2D correlated spectra by symmetrization," *J. Magn. Reson.* **44**, (1981), 402.

104. T. Schaffhauser, R.R. Ernst, B. Hilti and C.W. Mayer, "Dynamics of the conduction electrons in the one-dimensional conductor bis-tetrathiotetracene-tri-iodide: a proton NMR relaxation study," *Phys. Rev.* **B 24**, (1981), 76.

105. Y. Huang, S. Macura and R.R. Ernst, "Carbon-13 exchange maps for the elucidation of chemical exchange networks," *J. Am. Chem. Soc.* **103**, (1981), 5327.

106. F. Graf, R. Meyer, T.-K. Ha and R.R. Ernst, "Dynamics of hydrogen bond exchange in carboxylic acid dimers," *J. Chem. Phys.* **75**, (1981), 2914.

107. G. Bodenhausen and R.R. Ernst, "The Accordion experiment, a simple approach to three-dimensional NMR spectroscopy," *J. Magn. Reson.* **45**, (1981), 367.

108. M. Reinhold, P. Brunner and R.R. Ernst, "Double-quantum cross-polarization, appli-cation to ^{14}N spectroscopy," *Bull. Magn. Reson.* **2**, (1981), 91.

109. F. Graf, B.H. Meier and R.R. Ernst, "Dynamics of hydrogen bonds in molecular solids," *Bull. Magn. Reson.* **2**, (1981), 116.

110. M. Linder and R.R. Ernst, "Orientation of tensorial interactions determined from two-dimensional NMR powder spectra," *Bull. Magn. Reson* **2**, (1981), 128.

111. S. Marcura, R.R. Ernst, Anil Kumar and K. Wüthrich, "Study of cross-relaxation and nuclear Overhauser effects by two-dimensional NMR spectroscopy," *Bull. Magn. Reson.* **2**, (1981), 293.

112. D.P Burum, M. Linder and R.R. Ernst, "Windowless multipulse sequences," *Bull. Magn. Reson.* **2**, (1981), 413.

113. S. Macura, Y. Huang and R.R. Ernst, "Two-dimensional chemical exchange spec-troscopy," *Bull. Magn. Reson.* **2**, (1981), 316.

114. Y. Huang, G. Bodenhausen and R.R. Ernst, "Use of spy nuclei for relaxation studies in nuclear magnetic resonance," *J. Am. Chem. Soc.* **103**, (1981), 6988.

115. S. Macura, K. Wüthrich and R.R. Ernst, "Separation and suppression of coherent transfer effects in two-dimensional NOE and chemical exchange spectroscopy," *J. Magn. Reson.* **46**, (1982), 269.

116. B.H. Meier, F. Graf and R.R. Ernst, "Structure and dynamics of intramolecular hydrogen bonds in carboxylic acid dimers: a solid state NMR study," *J. Chem. Phys.* **76**, (1982), 767.

117. S. Macura, K. Wüthrich and R.R. Ernst, "The relevance of J cross-peaks in two-dimensional NOE experiments of macromolecules," *J. Magn. Reson.* **47**, (1982), 351.

118. G. Bodenhausen and R.R. Ernst, "Direct determination of rate constants of slow dynamic processes by two-dimensional 'Accordion' spectroscopy in nuclear magnetic resonance," *J. Am. Chem. Soc.* **104**, (1982), 1304.

119. G. Bodenhausen, P. Caravatti, J. Deli and R.R. Ernst, "Optical alignment in magic-angle NMR," *J. Magn. Reson.* **48**, (1982), 143.

120. P. Caravatti, G. Bodenhausen and R.R. Ernst, "Heteronuclear solid-state correlation spectroscopy," *Chem. Phys. Lett.* **89**, (1982), 363.

121. R.R. Ernst, "The information content of two-dimensional Fourier spectroscopy," *ACS Symposium Series, No. 191, NMR Spectroscopy: New Methods and Applications,* ed. by G.C. Levy, (1982), 47.

122. D. Suter and R.R. Ernst, "Spectral spin diffusion in the presence of an extraneous dipolar reservoir," *Phys. Rev.* **B 25**, (1982), 6038.

123. G. Eich, G. Bodenhausen and R.R. Ernst, "Exploring nuclear spin systems by relayed magnetization transfer," *J. Am. Chem. Soc.* **104**, (1982), 3731.

124. G. Bodenhausen and R.R. Ernst, "Two-dimensional exchange difference spectroscopy. Applications to indirect observation of quadrupolar relaxation," *Mol. Phys.* **47**, (1982), 319.

125. P. Caravatti, J.A. Deli, G. Bodenhausen and R.R. Ernst, "Direct evidence of microscopic homogeneity in disordered solids," *J. Am. Chem. Soc.* **104**, (1982), 5506.

126. M. Hintermann, L. Braunschweiler, G. Bodenhausen and R.R. Ernst, "Design of a digital phase shifter for multiple-quantum NMR," *J. Magn. Reson.* **50**, (1982), 316.

127. U. Piantini, O.W. Sorensen and R.R. Ernst, "Multiple quantum filters for elucidating NMR coupling networks," *J.Am. Chem. Soc.* **104**, (1982), 6800.

128. M.H. Levitt, O.W. Sorensen and R.R. Ernst, "Multiplet-separated heteronuclear two-dimensional NMR spectroscopy," *Chem. Phys. Lett.* **94**, (1983), 540.

129. L. Braunschweiler, G. Bodenhausen and R.R. Ernst, "Analysis of networks of coupled spins by multiple quantum NMR," *Mol. Phys.* **48**, (1983), 535.

130. O..W. Sorensen and R.R. Ernst, "Elimination of spectral distortion in polarization transfer experiments. Improvements and comparison of techniques," *J. Magn. Reson.* **51**, (1983), 477.

131. A. Wokaum, H.-P. Lutz, A.P. King, U.P. Wild and R.R. Ernst, "Energy transfer in surface enhanced luminescence," *J. Chem. Phys.* **79**, (1983), 509.

132. M.H. Levitt, G. Bodenhausen and R.R. Ernst, "The illusions of spin decoupling," *J. Magn. Reson.* **53**, (1983), 443.

133. L. Braunschweiler and R.R. Ernst, "Coherence transfer by isotropic mixing: application to proton correlation spectroscopy," *J. Magn. Reson.* **53**, (1983), 521.

134. R.V. Hosur, R.R. Ernst and K. Wüthrich, "A simple two-dimensional measurement of the decoupler power during continuous homonuclear irradiation for the correction of Bloch-Siegert shifts," *J. Magn. Reson.* **54**, (1983), 142.

135. O.W. Sorensen and R.R. Ernst, "Sign determination of ^{13}C-^{13}C coupling constants by sign-labeled polarization transfer," *J. Magn. Reson.* **54**, (1983), 122.

136. M. Rudin, J.M. Fauth, A. Schweiger, R.R. Ernst, L. Zoller and J.H. Ammeter, "Spin density distribution in cobaltocene. A proton ENDOR study on $CO(cp)_2$ diluted in $Mn(cp)(CO)_3$ single crystals," *Mol. Phys.* **49**, (1983), 1257.

137. M.H. Levitt and R.R. Ernst, "Spin-pattern recognition in high-resolution proton NMR spectroscopy," *Chem. Phys. Lett.* **100**, (1983), 119.

138. P. Caravatti, L. Braunschweiler and R.R. Ernst, "Heteronuclear correlation spectroscopy in rotating solids," *Chem. Phys. Lett.* **100**, (1983), 305.

139. P. Caravatti, G. Bodenhausen and R.R. Ernst, "Selective pulse experiments in high-resolution solid state NMR," *J. Magn. Reson.* **55**, (1983), 88.

140. H. Kogler, O.W. Sorensen, G. Bodenhausen and R.R. Ernst, "Low-pass J filters. Suppression of neighbor peaks in heteronuclear relayed correlation spectra," *J. Magn. Reson.* **55**, (1983), 157.

141. O.W. Sorensen, M.H. Levitt and R.R. Ernst, "Uniform excitation of multiple-quantum coherence: application to multiple quantum filtering," *J. Magn. Reson.* **55**, (1983), 104.

142. O.W. Sorensen, G.W. Eich, M.H. Levitt, G. Bodenhausen and R.R. Ernst, "Product operator formalism for the description of NMR pulse experiments," *Progr. in NMR Spectrosc.* **16**, (1983), 163.

143. H. Kessler, H. Oschkinat, O.W. Sorensen, H. Kogler and R.R. Ernst, "Multiple-quantum-filtered homonuclear J,δ spectra," *J. Magn. Reson.* **55**, (1983), 329.

144. M.H. Levitt and R.R. Ernst, "Composite pulses constructed by a recursive expansion procedure," *J. Magn. Reson.* **55**, (1983), 247

145. O.W. Sorensen and R.R. Ernst, "Remote heteronuclear correlation via pseudo multiple-quantum spectroscopy," *J. Magn. Reson.* **55**, (1983), 338.

146. M.H. Levitt and R.R. Ernst, "Improvement of pulse performance in NMR coherence transfer experiments. A compensated INADEQUATE experiment," *Mol. Phys.* **50**, (1983), 1109.

147. H. Kessler, M. Bernd, H. Kogler, J. Zarbock, O.W. Sorensen, G. Bodenhausen and R.R. Ernst, "Peptide conformations. 28. Relayed heteronuclear correlation spectroscopy and conformational analysis of cyclic hexapeptides containing the active sequence of somatostatin," *J. Am. Chem. Soc.* **105**, (1983), 6944.

148. M. Rance, O.W. Sorensen, G. Bodenhausen, G. Wagner, R.R. Ernst and K. Wüthrich, "Improved spectral resolution in COSY ^{1}H NMR spectra of proteins via double quantum filtering," *Biochem. Biophys. Res. Commun.* **117**, (1983), 479.

149. G. Wider, S. Macura, Anil Kumar, R.R. Ernst and K. Wüthrich, "Homonuclear two-dimensional ^{1}H NMR of proteins. Experimental procedures," *J. Magn. Reson.* **56**, (1984), 207.

150. O.W. Sorensen, M. Rance and R.R. Ernst, "Z-filters for purging phase–or multiplet-distorted spectra," *J. Magn. Reson.* **56**, (1984), 527.

151. M.H. Levitt, D. Suter and R.R. Ernst, "Composite pulse excitation in three-level systems," *J. Chem. Phys.* **80**, (1984), 3064.

152. G. Bodenhausen, H. Kogler and R.R. Ernst, "Selection of coherence-transfer pathways in NMR pulse experiments," *J. Magn. Reson.* **58**, (1984), 370.

153. M.H. Levitt, G. Bodenhausen and R.R. Ernst, "Sensitivity of two-dimensional spectra," *J. Magn. Reson.* **58**, (1984), 462.

154. B.H. Meier, R. Meyer, R.R. Ernst, P. Zolliker, A. Furrer and W. Hälg, "Neutron scattering study of dynamically disordered hydrogen bonds: terephthalic acid," *Chem. Phys. Lett.* **103**. (1983), 169.

155. B.H. Meier, R. Meyer, R.R. Ernst, A. Stöckli, A. Furrer, W. Hälg and I. Anderson, "The mechanism of proton dynamics in solid carboxylic acids. Reply to the comment by K. Furic," *Chem. Phys. Lett.* **108**, (1984), 522.

156. M. Rance, G. Wagner, O.W. Sorensen, K. Wüthrich and R.R. Ernst, "Application of ω₁-decoupled 2D correlations spectra to the study of proteins," *J. Magn. Reson.* **59**, (1984), 250.

157. G. Bodenhausen, G. Wagner, M. Rance, O.W. Sorensen, K. Wüthrich and R.R. Ernst, "Longitudinal two-spin order in 2D exchange spectroscopy (NOESY)" *J. Magn. Reson.* **59**, (1984), 542.

158. P. Caravatti, P. Neuenschwander and R.R. Ernst, "Characterization of heterogeneous polymer blends by two-dimensional proton spin diffusion spectroscopy," *Macromolecules* **18**, (1985), 119.

159. M. Rance, O.W. Sorensen, W. Leupin, H. Kogler, K. Wüthrich and R.R. Ernst, "Uniform excitation of multiple-quantum coherence. Application to two-dimensional double-quantum spectroscopy," *J. Magn. Reson.* **61,** (1985), 67.

160. M.H. Levitt, C. Radloff and R.R. Ernst, "Coherence transfer selection rules induced by symmetry: application to NMR correlation spectroscopy," *Chem. Phys. Lett.* **114,** (1985), 435.

161. R.R. Ernst, "Elucidation of nuclear spin systems by coherence transfer techniques," Plenary lecture of RAMIS-83, Proceedings of the Conference RAMIS-83, Poznan, Poland, Adam Mickiewicz University, 1985.

162. A. Schweiger, L. Braunschweiler, J.-M. Fauth and R.R. Ernst, "Coherent and incoherent echo spectroscopy with extended-time excitation," *Phys. Rev. Lett.* **54,** (1985), 1241.

163. M. Rance, G. Bodenhausen, G. Wagner, K. Wüthrich and R.R. Ernst, "A systematic approach to the suppression of J cross peaks in 2D exchange and 2D NOE spectroscopy," *J. Magn. Reson.* **62,** (1985), 497.

164. C. Counsell, M.H. Levitt and R.R. Ernst, "Analytical theory of composite pulses," *J. Magn. Reson.* **63,** (1985), 133.

165. O.W. Sorensen and R.R. Ernst, "Design of pulse sequences sensitive to relative signs of J coupling constants. Corrections to the SLAP experiment," *J. Magn. Reson.* **63,** (1985), 219.

166. R. Kreis, D. Suter and R.R. Ernst, "Time-domain zero-field magnetic resonance with field pulse excitation," *Chem. phys. Lett.* **118,** (1985), 120.

167. L. Braunschweiler, A. Schweiger, J.-M. Fauth and R.R. Ernst, "Selective excitation in electron spin-echo modulation experiments," *J. Magn. Reson.* **64,** (1985), 160.

168. M.H. Levitt and R.R. Ernst, "Multiple-quantum excitation and spin topology filtration in high-resolution NMR," *J. Chem. Phys.* **83,** (1985), 3297.

169. C.J.R. Counsell, M.H. Levitt and R.R. Ernst, "The selection of coherence-transfer pathways by inhomogeneous z pulses," *J. Magn. Reson.* **64,** (1985), 470.

170. P. Pfändler, G. Bodenhausen, B.U. Meier and R.R. Ernst, "Toward automated assignment of nuclear magnetic resonance spectra: pattern recognition in two-dimensional correlation spectra," *Anal. Chem.* **57,** (1985), 2510.

171. C. Griesinger, O.W. Sorensen and R.R. Ernst, "Two-dimensional correlation of connected NMR transitions," *J. Am. Chem. Soc.* **107,** (1985), 6394.

172. G. Wagner, G. Bodenhausen, N. Müller, M. Rance, O.W. Sorensen, R.R. Ernst and K. Wüthrich, "Exchange of two-spin order in nuclear magnetic resonance: separation of exchange and cross-relaxation processes," *J. Am. Chem. Soc.* **107,** (1985), 6440.

173. D. Suter and R.R. Ernst, "Spin diffusion in resolved solid-state NMR spectra," *Phys. Rev.* **B 32,** (1985), 5608.

174. O.W. Sorensen, C. Griesinger and R.R. Ernst, "Time reversal of the evolution under scalar spin-spin interactions in NMR. Application for ω_1 decoupling in two-dimensional NOE spectroscopy," *J. Am. Chem. Soc.* **107,** (1985), 7778.

175. M.H. Frey, G. Wagner, M. Vasák, O.W. Sorensen, D. Neuhaus, E. Wörgötter, J.H.R. Kägi, R.R. Ernst and K. Wüthrich, "Polypeptide-metal cluster connectivities in metallothionein 2 by novel ^{1}H-^{113}Cd heteronuclear two-dimensional NMR experiments," *J. Am. Chem. Soc.* **107,** (1985), 6847.

176. N. Müller, G. Bodenhausen, K. Wüthrich and R.R. Ernst, "The appearance of forbidden cross-peaks in two-dimensional nuclear magnetic resonance spectra due to multi-exponential T_2 relaxation," *J. Magn. Reson.* **65,** (1985), 531.

177. Monograph by R.R. Ernst, G. Bodenhausen and A. Wokaun, "Principles of nuclear magnetic resonance in one and two dimensions," (London: Oxford University Press, 1986).

178. M.H. Levitt, D. Suter and R.R. Ernst, "Spin dynamics and thermodynamics in solid-state NMR cross-polarization," *J. Chem. Phys.* **84,** (1986), 4243.

179. P. Caravatti, M.H. Levitt and R.R. Ernst, "Selective excitation in solid state NMR in the presence of multiple pulse line narrowing," *J. Magn. Reson.* **68,** (1986), 323.

180. P. Caravatti, P. Neuenschwander and R.R. Ernst, "Characterization of polymer blends by selective proton spin diffusion NMR measurements," *Macromolecules* **19**, (1986), 1889.

181. R. Kreis, D. Suter and R.R. Ernst, "Radiofrequency-pulse excitation in time-domain zero-field magnetic resonance," *Chem. Phys. Lett.* **123**, (1986), 154.

182. B.H. Meier and R.R. Ernst, "Structure and dynamics of terephthalic acid from 2 to 300 K. II. The temperature dependence of the disorder: a solid state NMR study," *J. Solid State Chem.* **61**, (1986), 126.

183. J.-M. Fauth, A. Schweiger, L. Braunschweiler, J. Forrer and R.R. Ernst, "Elimination of unwanted echoes and reduction of dead time in three-pulse electron spin-echo spectroscopy," *J. Magn. Reson.* **66**, (1986), 74.

184. P. Fischer, P. Zolliker, B.H. Meier, R.R. Ernst, A.W. Hewat, J.D. Jorgensen and F.J. Rotella, "Structure and dynamics of terephthalic acid from 2 to 300 K. I. High-resolution neutron diffraction evidence for a temperature-dependent order-disorder transition: a comparison of reactor and pulsed neutron source powder techniques," *J. Solid State Chem.* **61**, (1986), 109.

185. M.H. Frey, W. Leupin, O.W. Sorensen, W.A. Denny, R.R. Ernst and K. Wüthrich, "Sequence-specific assignment of the backbone ^{1}H- and ^{31}P-NMR lines in a short DNA duplex with homo- and heteronuclear correlated spectroscopy," *Biopolymers* **24**, (1985), 2371.

186. A. Stöckli, A. Furrer, Ch. Schönenberger, B.H. Meier, R.R. Ernst and I. Anderson, "Dynamics of hydrogen bonds in carboxylic acids," *Physica* **136B**, (1986), 161.

187. N. Müller, R.R. Ernst and K. Wüthrich, "Multiple-quantum-filtered two-dimensional correlated NMR spectroscopy of proteins," *J. Am. Chem. Soc.* **108**, (1986), 6482.

188. C. Griesinger, O.W. Sorensen and R.R. Ernst, "Correlation of connected transitions by two-dimensional NMR spectroscopy," *J. Chem. Phys.* **85**, (1986), 6837.

189. H. Kessler, C. Griensinger, R. Kerssebaum, K. Wagner and R.R. Ernst, "Separation of cross-relaxation and J cross-peaks in 2D rotating-frame NMR spectroscopy," *J. Am. Chem. Soc.* **109**, (1987), 607.

190. R. Meyer and R.R. Ernst, "Hydrogen transfer in double minimum potential: kinetic properties derived from quantum dynamics," *J. Chem. Phys.* **86**, (1987), 784.

191. O.W. Sorensen, C. Griesinger and R.R. Ernst, "Antisymmetric two-dimensional NMR spectra," *Chem. Phys. Lett.* **135**, (1987), 313.

192. M.H. Levitt, C. Radloff and R.R. Ernst, "Simplification of 2D spectra by (a) topology-selective multiple-quantum filtration or (b) by bilinear mixing," in *Advanced Magnetic Resonance Techniques in Systems of High Molecular Complexity*, Vol. 2, (Birkhäuser Boston, Inc., 1986), 49.

193. L. Braunschweiler, A. Schweiger, J.-M. Fauth and R.R. Ernst, "Extended-time excitation electron spin echo spectroscopy," in *Advanced Magnetic Resonance Techniques in Systems of High Molecular Complexity*, Vol. 2, (Birkhäuser Boston, Inc., 1986), 307.

194. L. Braunschweiler, A. Schweiger, J.-M. Fauth and R.R. Ernst, "Determination of the microwave field strength by microwave-induced transitory oscillations in pulsed electron spin resonance," *J. Magn. Reson.* **72**, (1987), 579.

195. Z. Mádi, B.U. Meier and R.R. Ernst, "Detection of cross peaks in two-dimensional NMR by cluster analysis," *J. Magn. Reson.* **72**, (1987), 584.

196. R. Brüschweiler, J.C. Madsen, C. Griesinger, O.W. Sorensen and R.R. Ernst, "Two-dimensional NMR spectroscopy with soft pulses," *J. Magn. Reson.* **73**, (1987), 380.

197. C. Griesinger, O.W. Sorensen and R.R. Ernst, "A practical approach to three-dimensional NMR spectroscopy," *J. Magn. Reson.* **73**, (1987), 574.

198. R.R. Ernst, "Methodology of magnetic resonance imaging," *Quart. Rev. Biophys.* **19**, (1987), 183.

199. R.R. Ernst, "Two-dimensional NMR spectroscopy: A powerful tool for the investigation of molecular structure and dynamics," *Chimia* **41**, (1987), 323.

200. C. Griesinger, C. Gemperle, O.W. Sorensen and R.R. Ernst, "Symmetry in coherence transfer. Application to two-dimensional NMR," *Mol. Phys.* **62**, (1987), 295.

201. C. Griesinger, O.W. Sorensen and R.R. Ernst, "Novel three-dimensional NMR techniques for studies of peptides and biological macromolecules," *J. Am. Chem. Soc.* **109**, (1987), 7227.

202. B.U. Meier, Z.L. Mádi and R.R. Ernst, "Computer analysis of nuclear spin systems based on local symmetry in 2D spectra," *J. Magn. Reson.* **74**, (1987), 565.

203. R.R. Ernst, "Advanced NMR methods for liquids and solids: two-dimensional spectroscopy," *Ber. Bunsenges. Phys. Chemie* **91**, (1987), 1087.

204. C. Griesinger and R.R. Ernst, "Frequency offset effects and their elimination in NMR rotating-frame cross-relaxation spectroscopy," *J. Magn. Reson.* **75**, (1987), 261.

205. N. Müller, G. Bodenhausen and R.R. Ernst, "Relaxation-induced violations of coherence transfer selection rules in nuclear magnetic resonance," *J. Magn. Reson.* **75**, (1987), 297.

206. C. Griesinger, O.W. Sorensen and R.R. Ernst, "Practical aspects of the E.COSY technique. Measurement of scalar spin-spin coupling constants in peptides," *J. Magn. Reson.* **75**, (1987), 474.

207. H. Hauser, C. Radloff, R.R. Ernst, S. Sundell and I. Pascher, "The ^{31}P chemical shielding tensor in phospholipids," *J. Am. Chem. Soc.* **110**, (1988), 1054.

208. C. Gemperle, A. Schweiger and R.R. Ernst, "ESR-detected nuclear transient nutations: detection schemes and applications," *Chem. Phys. Lett.* **145**, (1988), 1.

209. M.G. Colombo, B.H. Meier and R.R. Ernst, "Rotor-driven spin diffusion in natural-abundance ^{13}C spin systems," *Chem. Phys. Lett.* **146**, (1989), 189.

210. A. Schweiger and R.R. Ernst, "Pulsed ESR with longitudinal detection. A novel recording technique," *J. Magn. Reson.* **77**, (1988), 512.

211. R.R. Ernst, "A brief account of two-dimensional NMR spectroscopy," *Physics of NMR Spectroscopy in Biology and Medicine, 1988,* ed. by Soc. Italiana di Fisica, Bologna, Italia, 158-185.

212. R. Brüschweiler, C. Griesinger, O.W. Sorensen and R.R. Ernst, "Combined use of hard and soft pulses for ω_1 decoupling in two-dimensional NMR spectroscopy," *J. Magn. Reson.* **78**, (1988), 178.

213. Z.L. Mádi and R.R. Ernst, "Computer analysis of two-dimensional NMR spectra. Estimation of spectral parameters by least-squares approximation," *J. Magn. Reson.* **79**, (1988), 513.

214. B.U. Meier and R.R. Ernst, "Cross-peak analysis in 2D NMR spectroscopy by recursive multiplet contraction," *J. Magn. Reson.* **79**, (1988), 540.

215. S. Pfenninger, A. Schweiger, J. Forrer and R.R. Ernst, "Echo-detected ESR spectroscopy with magnetic field vector jumps: a novel approach for improving the spectral resolution in disordered systems," *Chem. Phys. Lett.* **151**, (1988), 199.

216. C. Griesinger and R.R. Ernst, "Cross-relaxation in time-dependent nuclear spin systems: invariant trajectory approach," *Chem. Phys. Lett.* **152**, (1988), 239.

217. C. Griesinger, G. Otting, K. Wüthrich and R.R. Ernst, "Clean TOCSY for ^{1}H spin system identification in macromolecules," *J. Am. Chem. Soc.* **110**, (1988), 7870.

218. R. Kreis, A. Thomas, W. Studer and R.R. Ernst, "Low frequency pulse excitation in zero field magnetic resonance," *J. Chem. Phys.* **89**, (1988), 6623.

219. H. Oschkinat, C. Griesinger, P.J. Kraulis, O.W. Sorensen, R.R. Ernst, A.M. Gronenborn and G.M. Clore, "Three-dimensional NMR spectroscopy of a protein in solution," *Nature* **332**, (1988), 374.

220. C. Bühlmann, A. Schweiger and R.R. Ernst, "Hyperfine-selective ENDOR," *Chem. Phys. Lett.* **154**, (1989), 285.

221. C. Radloff and R.R. Ernst, "Spin topology filtration in NMR," *Mol. Phys.* **66**, (1989), 161.

222. J.-M. Fauth, A. Schweiger and R.R. Ernst, "Recovery of broad hyperfine lines in electron spin-echo envelope modulation spectroscopy of disordered systems," *J. Magn. Reson.* **81**, (1989), 262.

223. M.A. McCoy and R.R. Ernst, "Nuclear spin noise at room temperature," *Chem. Phys. Lett.* **159**, (1989), 587.

224. C. Griesinger, O.W. Sorensen and R.R. Ernst, "Three-dimensional Fourier spectroscopy. Application to high-resolution NMR," *J. Magn. Reson.* **84**, (1989), 14.

225. H. Cho, S. Pfenninger, C. Gemperle, A. Schweiger and R.R. Ernst, "Zero deadtime pulsed ESR by remote echo detection," *Chem. Phys. Lett.* **160**, (1989), 391.

226. B.H. Meier, M. Colombo, T. Burmeister and R.R. Ernst, "Speeding-up and slowing-down spin dynamics and spin diffusion in high-resolution solid state NMR," *24th Congress Ampere, Poznan, Poland*, 1988, 825.

227. R. Brüschweiler, C. Griesinger and R.R. Ernst, "Correlated motion monitored by NMR relaxation in the rotating frame. A source of structural and dynamic information on macromolecules," *J. Am. Chem. Soc.* **111**, (1989), 8034.

228. P. Robyr, B.H. Meier and R.R. Ernst, "Radiofrequency-driven nuclear spin diffusion in solids," *Chem. Phys. Lett.* **162**, (1989), 417.

229. S. Boentges, B.U. Meier, C. Griesinger and R.R. Ernst, "Local symmetry in 2D and 3D NMR spectra," *J. Magn. Reson.* **85**, (1989), 337.

230. A. Schweiger, C. Gemperle and R.R. Ernst, "Soft pulse electron-spin-echo-envelope modulation spectroscopy (soft ESEEM)," *J. Magn. Reson.* **86**, (1990), 70.

231. Z.L. Mádi, C. Griesinger and R.R. Ernst, "Conformational dynamics of proline residues in antamanide. J coupling analysis of strongly coupled spin systems based on E.COSY spectra," *J. Am. Chem. Soc.* **112**, (1990), 2908.

232. C. Gemperle, O.W. Sorensen, A. Schweiger and R.R. Ernst, "Optimized polarization transfer in pulse ENDOR experiments," *J. Magn. Reson.* **87**, (1990), 502.

233. C. Gemperle, G. Aebli, A. Schweiger and R.R. Ernst, "Phase cycling in pulse EPR," *J. Magn. Reson.* **88**, (1990), 241.

234. C. Griesinger, R. Brüschweiler, Z.L. Mádi., O.W. Sorensen and R.R. Ernst, "Recent achievements in multidimensional NMR," *Makromol. Chem., Macromol. Symp.* **34**, (1990), 17.

235. A. Stöckli, B.H. Meier, R. Kreis, R. Meyer and R.R. Ernst, "Hydrogen bond dynamics in isotopically substituted benzoic acid dimers," *J. Chem. Phys.* **93**, (1990), 1502.

236. R. Meyer and R.R. Ernst, "Transitions induced in a double minimum system by interaction with a quantum mechanical heat bath," *J. Chem. Phys.* **93**, (1990), 5518.

237. B. Roux, R. Brüschweiler and R.R. Ernst, "The structure of gramicidin A in dimethylsulfoxide/acetone," *Eur. J. Biochem.* **194**, (1990), 57.

238. C. Gemperle, A. Schweiger and R.R. Ernst, "Novel analytical treatments of electron spin-echo envelope modulation with short and extended pulses," *J. Magn. Reson.* **91**, (1991), 273.

239. T. Schulte-Herbrüggen, Z.L. Mádi, O.W. Sorensen and R.R. Ernst, "Reduction of multiplet complexity in COSY-type NMR spectra. The bilinear and planar COSY experiments," *Mol. Phys.* **72**, (1991), 847.

240. C. Gemperle, A. Schweiger and R.R. Ernst, "Electron-spin-echo envelope modulation with improved modulation depth," *Chem. Phys. Lett.* **178**, (1991), 565.

241. R. Brüschweiler, M. Blackledge and R.R. Ernst, "Multi-conformational peptide dynamics derived from NMR data: a new search algorithm and its application to antamanide," *J. Bio NMR* **1**, (1991), 3.

242. G.A. Sierra, A. Schweiger and R.R. Ernst, "Electron-Zeeman-resolved EPR," *Chem. Phys. Lett.* **184**, (1991), 363.

243. J. Briand and R.R. Ernst, "Computer-optimized homonuclear TOCSY experiments with suppression of cross relaxation," *Chem. Phys. Lett.* **185**, (1991), 276.

244. M. Ernst, C. Griesinger, R.R. Ernst and W. Bermel, "Optimized heteronuclear cross polarization in liquids," *Mol. Phys.* **74**, (1991), 219.

245. P. Robyr, B. H. Meier and R. R. Ernst, "Tensor correlation by 2D spin-diffusion powder NMR spectroscopy: determination of the asymmetry of the hydrogen-bond potential in benzoic acid," *Chem. Phys. Lett.* **187**, (1991), 471.

246. R. R. Ernst, "Without computers - no modern NMR," *Computational Aspects of the Study of Biological Macromolecules by Nuclear Magnetic Resonance Spectroscopy*, by ed. J. C. Hoch et al., (New York: Plenum Press, 1991), 1.

247. R. R. Ernst, M. Blackledge, S. Boentges, J. Briand, R. Brüschweiler, M. Ernst, C. Griesinger, Z. L. Mádi, T. Schulte-Herbrüggen and O. W. Sorensen, "Molecular dynamics of peptides and proteins investigated by NMR," *Proteins: Structure, Dynamics, Design*, by eds. V. Renugopalakrishnan et al., (Escom, Leiden, 1991), 11.

248. R. Brüschweiler and R. R. Ernst, "Molecular dynamics monitored by cross-correlated cross relaxation of spins quantized along orthogonal axes," *J. Chem. Phys.* **96**, (1992), 1758.

249. R. R. Ernst, "Nuclear Magnetic resonance Fourier transform spectroscopy" (Nobel lucture, *Angew. Chem. Int. Ed. Engl.* **31**, (1991), 805.

250. R. R. Ernst, "Kernresonanz-Fourier-Transformations-Spektroskopie" (Nobel Vortrag), *Angew. Chem.* **104**, (1992), 817.

251. R. R. Ernst, "Nuclear Magnetic resonance Fourier transform spectroscopy" (Nobel lecture), *Bioscience Reports* **12**, (1992), 143.

252. R. Brüschweiler, B. Roux, M. Blackledge, C. Griesinger, M. Karplus and R. R. Ernst, "Influence of rapids intramolecular motion on NMR cross-relaxation rates. A molecular dynamics study of antamanide in solution," *J. Am. Chem. Soc.* **114**, (1992), 2289.

253. E. J. Hustedt, A. Schweiger and R. R. Ernst, "Stimulated soft electron spin echo envelope modulation spectroscopy," *J. Chem. Phys.* **96**, (1992), 4954.

254. R. R. Ernst, "The multidimensional importance of time domain magnetic resonance," in: *Pulsed Magnetic Resonance: NMR, ESR and Optics*, a recognition of E. L. Hahn, ed. D.M.S. Bagguley, (Oxford: Clarendon Press, 1992), 95.

255. Shanmin Zhang, B. H. Meier and R. R. Ernst, "Polarization echoes in NMR," *Phys. Rev. Lett.* **69**, (1992), 2149.

256. Shanmin Zhang, B. H. Meier, S. Appelt, M. Mehring and R. R. Ernst, "Transient oscillations in phase-switched cross-polarization experiments," *J. Magn. Reson.* **A 101**, (1993), 60.

257. D. Suter, M. Ernst and R. R. Ernst, "Quantum time-translation machine. An experimental realization," *Mol. Phys.* **78**, (1993), 95.

258. Shanmin Zhang, B. H. Meier and R. R. Ernst, "Local monitoring of proton spin diffusion in static and rotating samples via spy detection," *Solid State NMR* **1**, (1992), 313.

259. M. Tomaselli, B. H. Meier, P. Robyr, U. W. Suter and R. R. Ernst, "Probing microheterogeneity in polymer systems via two-dimensional ^{129}xenon NMR spy detection. A heterogeneous model blend system," *Chem. Phys. Lett.* **205**, (1993), 145.

260. R. R. Ernst, "Why just NMR?" *Israel J. Chem.* **32**, (1992), 135.

261. R. R. Ernst, "Nuclear magnetic resonance Fourier transform spectroscopy," (Nobel Lecture), Les Prix Nobel, 1991, The Nobel Foundation, 1992.

262. R. M. Brunne, W. F. van Gunsteren, R. Brüschweiler and R. R. Ernst, "Molecular dynamics simulation of the proline conformational equilibrium and dynamics in antamanide using the GROMOS force field," *J. Am. Chem. Soc.* **115**, (1993), 4764.

263. J. Briand and R. R. Ernst, "Sensitivity comparison of two-dimensional correlation spectroscopy in the laboratory frame and in the rotating frame," *J. Magn. Reson.* **A 104**, (1993), 54.

264. J. M. Schmidt, R. Brüschweiler, R. R. Ernst, R. L. Dunbrack, Jr., D. Joseph and M. Karplus, "Molecular dynamics simulation of the proline conformational equilibrium and dynamics in antamanide using the CHARMM force field," *J. Am. Chem. Soc.* **115**, (1993), 8747.

265. S. Hediger, B. H. Meier and R. R. Ernst, "Cross polarization under fast magic angle sample spinning using the amplitude-modulated spin-lock sequences," *Chem. Phys. Lett.* **213**, (1993), 627.

266. M. J. Blackledge, R. Brüschweiler, C. Griesinger, J. M. Schmidt, Ping Xu and R. R. Ernst, "Conformational backbone dynamics of the cyclic decapeptide antamanide. Application of a new multiconformational search algorithm based on NMR data," *Biochem.* **32**, (1993), 10960.

267. M. Tomaselli, B. H. Meier, P. Robyr, U. W. Suter and R. R. Ernst, "Direct measurement of xenon exchange between gas and liquid phase by 2D NMR," *Chem. Phys. Lett.* **214,** (1993), 1.

268. S. A. Smith, T. O. Levante, B. H. Meier and R. R. Ernst, "Computer-simulations in magnetic resonance. An object-oriented programming approach," *J. Magn. Reson.* **A 106,** (1994), 75.

269. Shanmin Zhang, B. H. Meier and R. R. Ernst, "Mismatch-compensated cross polarization. W-MOIST, an improved pulse scheme," *J. Magn. Reson.* **A 108,** (1994), 30.

270. S. Hediger, B. H. Meier, Narayanan D. Kurur, Geoffrey Bodenhausen, R. R. Ernst, "NMR cross polarization by adiabatic passage through the Hartmann-Hahn condition (APHH)," *Chem. Phys. Lett.* **223,** (1994), 283.

271. Jürgen M. Schmidt, Ole W. Sorensen and Richard R. Ernst, "Measurement of homonuclear long-range J couplings by relayed E.COSY," *J. Magn. Reson.* **A 109,** (1994), 80.

272. P. Robyr, B. H. Meier, P. Fischer and R. R. Ernst, "A combined structural study using NMR chemical-shielding-tensor correlation and neutron diffraction in polycrystalline methanol," *J. Am. Chem. Soc.* **116,** (1994), 5315.

273. Richard R. Ernst, "ENC, a motor of progress in NMR," *Concepts in Magn. Reson.* **6,** (1994), 201.

274. M. Tomaselli, B. H. Meier, M. Baldus, J. Eisenegger and R. R. Ernst, "An rf-driven nuclear spin-diffusion experiment using zero-angle sample spinning,"*Chem. Phys. Lett.* **225,** (1994), 131.

275. Richard R. Ernst, "Recent development in NMR methodology for the study of molecular structure and dynamics," *Pure and Appl. Chem.* **66,** (1994), 1583.

276. Tobias Bremi, Matthias Ernst and Richard R. Ernst, "Side-chain motion with two degrees of freedom in peptides. An NMR study of phenylalanine side chains in antamanide." *J. Phys. Chem.* **98,** (1994), 9322.

277. Richard R. Ernst, "The study of intramolecular dynamics by nuclear magnetic resonance," *Pure & Appl. Chem.* **66,** (1994), 1955.

278. Matthias Ernst and Richard R. Ernst, "Heteronuclear dipolar cross-correlated cross relaxation for the investigation of side-chain motions," *J. Magn. Reson.* **A 110,** (1994), 202.

279. Shanmin Zhang, Ping Xu, Ole W. Sorensen and Richard R. Ernst, "Absence of conservation laws and the reciprocity relation in polarization-transfer experiments," *Concepts in Magn. Reson.* **6,** (1994), 275.

280. Richard R. Ernst, "Nuclear magnetic resonance Fourier transform spectroscopy (Nobel Lecture," *Bull. Magn. Reson.* **16,** (1994), 5.

281. M. Baldus, M. Tomaselli, B. H. Meier and R. R. Ernst, "Broadband polarization-transfer experiments for rotating solids," *Chem. Phys. Lett.* **230,** (1994), 329.

282. R.R. Ernst, S. Boentges and J.M. Schmidt, "Basic aspects of NMR spectroscopy in multiple dimensions," *Proc. Indian Acad. Sci. Chem. Sci.* **106,** (1994), 1427.

283. S. Hediger, B.H. Meier and R.R. Ernst, "Rotor-synchronized amplitude-modulated nuclear magnetic resonance spin-lock sequences for improved cross polarization under fast magic angle sample spinning," *J. Chem. Phys.* **102,** (1995), 4000.

284. P. Robyr, M. Tomaselli, J. Straka, C. Grob-Pisano, U.W. Suter, B.H. Meier and R.R. Ernst, "Rf-driven and proton-driven NMR polarization transfer for investigating local order. An application to solid polymers," *Mol. Phys.* **84,** (1995), 995.

285. M. Baldus, B.H. Meier, R.R. Ernst, A.P.M. Kentgens, H. Meyer zu Altenschildesche and R. Nesper, "Structure investigation on anhydrous disodium hydrogen phosphate using solid-state NMR and X-ray techniques," *J. Am. Chem. Soc.* **117,** (1995), 5141.

Publication List: RAYMOND V. DAMADIAN

1. R. Damadian and A. K. Solomon, "Bacterial mutant with impaired potassium transport and methionine biosynthesis," *Science* **145**, (1964), 1327-1328.

2. R. Damadian, E. Shwayri and N.S. Bricker, "Non-urine forming nephrons in the diseased kidney of the dog," *J. Lab. Clin. Med.* **65**, (1965), 26-39.

3. R. Damadian, "Potassium transport mutant of *E. coli,*" *USAF Technical Report* **66-19**, (1966), 1-14.

4. R. Damadian, "Non-urine forming nephrons in the diseased kidney of the dog," *Urology Digest* **5**, (1966), 79, abstract.

5. R. Damadian and D.L. Trout, "Potassium transport mutant of *E. coli B,*" *Fed. Proc.* **25**, (1966), 632, abstract.

6. R. Damadian, "Abnormal phosphorus metabolism in a potassium transport mutant of *E. coli,*" *USAF Technical Report* **65-10**, (1967), 1-6.

7. R. Damadian, "Abnormal phosphorus metabolism in a potassium transport mutant of *E. coli,*" *Biochim. Biophys. Acta,* **135** (1967), 378-380.

8. R. Damadian, "Abnormal phosphorus metabolism in a potassium transport mutant of *E. coli B,*" *Biophysical J.* **7**, (1967), 61, abstract.

9. R. Damadian, C.V. Payne and D.L. Trout, "Irregularities of phosphorus metabolism in a potassium transport mutant of *E. coli B,*" *Fed. Proc.* **26**, (1967), abstract.

10. R. Damadian, "Ion metabolism in a potassim accumulation mutant of *Escherichia coli B.* I. potassium metabolism," *J. Bacteriol.* **95**, (1968), 113-122.

11. R. Damadian, "Potassium binding proteins of *Escherichia coli B,*" Annual meeting of the Biophysical Society, Oxford, England, (1968), abstract.

12. R. Damadian, "Ion exchange in *Escherichia coli*: Potassium binding proteins," *Science* **165**, (1969), 79-81.

13. R. Damadian, in *Membrane Proteins,* (Rockefeller University Press, 1969), 110.

14. F. Cope and R. Damadian, "Cell potassium by K^{39} spin echo nuclear magnetic resonance," *Nature* **228**, (1970), 76-77.

15. F. Cope and R. Damadian, "Cell potassium by K^{39} spin echo nuclear magnetic resonance," Fourth International Congress on Magnetic Resonance in Biological Systems, Oxford, England, (1970), abstract.

16. R. Damadian, "Tumor detection by nuclear magnetic resonance," *Science* **171**, (1971), 1151-1153.

17. R. Damadian, "Biological ion exchanger resins. I. Quantitative electrostatic correspondence of fixed charge and mobile counter ion." *Biophysical Journal* **11**, (1971), 739-760.

18. Ed Edelson, "Basic research leads to radio signals from cancer tissue," *Downstate Reporter,* **2**, (Spring 1971), 2. {State University of New York, Downstate Medical Center - First full description by Dr. Damadian (one year prior to his patent) of his concept of the whole-body NMR scanner.}

19. R. Damadian, M. Goldsmith and K.S. Zaner, "Biological ion exchanger resins. II. Cell water and ion exchange selectivity," *Biophysical Journal* **11**, (1971), 761-772.

20. R. Damadian, "Biological ion exchanger resins. III. Molecular interpretation of cellular ion exchange," *Biophysical Journal* **11**, (1971), 773-785.

21. R. Damadian and L. Minkoff, "Caloric requirements of bacterial ion exchange," *American Society of Biological Chemists, Federation Proceedings* **30**, #3, Part II, (1971), abstract.

22. R. Damadian, Chairman of Session, "Ion exchange and absorption in physical and biological systems," at the International Conference on the Physico-Chemical State of Ions and Water in Living Tissues and Model Systems, New York Academy of Sciences, New York, (1972), abstract.

23. L. Minkoff and R. Damadian, "Energy requirements of bacterial ion exchange," International Conference on Physico-Chemical State of Ions and Water in Living Tissues and Model Systems, New York Academy of Sciences, (1972), abstract.

24. R. Damadian, "Tumor detection by nuclear magnetic resonance," in *Nuclear Medicine, Yearbook of Cancer 1972* **286**, (Chicago: Yearbook Medical Publishers, 1972), abstract.

25. R. Damadian, K.S. Zaner and L. Minkoff, "Nuclear magnetic resonance as a new tool in cancer research," International Conference on Electron Spin Resonance and Nuclear Magnetic Resonance in Biology and Medicine; and Fifth International Conference on Magnetic Resonance in Biological Systems, New York Academy of Sciences, (1972), abstract.

26. R. Damadian, "Apparatus and method for detecting cancer in tissue," U.S. Patent 3,789,832, filed 17 March 1972, world's first patent for MR scanning.

27. R. Damadian, "Biological ion exchanger resins," International Conference on Physico-Chemical State of Ions and Water in Living Tissues and Model Systems, New York Academy of Sciences, January 10-12, 1972, *Annals of the New York Academy of Sciences* **204**, (1973), 211-248.

28. L. Minkoff and R. Damadian, "Energy requirements of bacterial ion exchange," International Conference on Physico-Chemical State of Ions and Water in Living Tissue and Model Systems, New York Academy of Sciences, January 10-12, 1972. *Annals of the New York Academy of Sciences* **204**, (1973), 249-260.

29. R. Damadian, "Introduction to part III." International Conference on Physico-Chemical State of Ions and Water in Living Tissues and Model Systems, New York Academy of Sciences, January 10-12, 1972. *Annals of the New York Academy of Sciences* **204**, (1973), 210.

30. L. Minkoff and R. Damadian, "Caloric catastrophe," *Biophysical Journal* **13**, (1973), 167-178.

31. R. Damadian, R. Zaner, D. Hor and T. DiMaio, "Human tumors detected by nuclear magnetic resonance," *Physiol. Chem. and Physics* **5**, (1973), 381-402.

32. R. Damadian, "Cation transport in bacteria," In *Critical Reviews in Microbiology*, (CRC Press, March, 1973), 377-422.

33. R. Damadian, F. Cope, "Potassium NMR relaxations in muscle and in normal *E. coli* and a potassium transport mutant, *Physiol. Chem. and Physics* **5**, (1973), 511-514.

34. R. Damadian, K. Zaner, D. Hor, T. DiMaio, L. Minkoff and M. Goldsmith, "Nuclear magnetic resonance as a new tool in cancer research: Human tumors by NMR," International Conference on Electron Spin Resonance and Nuclear Magnetic Resonance in Biology and Medicine and Fifth International Conference on Magnetic Resonance in Biological Systems Conference," *Annals of the New York Academy of Sciences* **222**, (1974), 1048-1076.

35. L. Minkoff and R. Damadian, "Reply to letters of caloric catastrophe," *Biophysical Journal* **14**, (1974), 69-72.

36. R. Damadian, K. Zaner, D. Hor and T. DiMaio, "Human tumors detected by nuclear magnetic resonance," *Proc. Nat. Acad. Sci, USA* **71**, (1974), 1471-1473.

37. F. Cope and R. Damadian, "Biological ion exchanger resins. IV. Evidence for potassium association with fixed charges in muscle and brain by pulsed nuclear magnetic resonance of K^{39}," *Physiol. Chem. and Physics* **6**, (1974), 17-30.

38. M. Goldsmith and R. Damdian, "Biological ion exchanger resins. V. The invalidity of the Donnan equation," *Physiol. Chem. and Physics* **6**, (1974), 51-65.

39. R. Damadian and F. Cope, "NMR in cancer. V. Electronic diagnosis of cancer by potassium (K^{39}) nuclear resonance: Spin signatures and T_1 beat patterns," *Physiol. Chem. and Physics* **6**, (1974), 309-322.

40. M. Goldsmith, D. Hor and R. Damadian, "Biological ion exchanger resins. VI. Determination of the Donnan potentials of single ion exchange beads with microelectrodes," *J. Physical Chemistry* **79**, (1975), 342-344.

41. K.S. Zaner and R. Damadian, "P^{31} as a nuclear probe for malignant tumors," *Science* **189**, (1975), 729-731.

42. M. Goldsmith, D. Hor and R. Damadian, "Biological ion exchanger resins. VII. Counter-ion activity coefficients in solutions of biological polyelectrolytes," *Physiol. Chem. and Physics* **7**, (1975), 225-234.

43. M. Goldsmith and R. Damadian, "NMR in cancer. VII. Sodium-23 magnetic resonance of normal and cancerous tissues," *Physiol. Chem. and Physics* **7**, (1975), 263-270.

44. L. Minkoff and R. Damadian, "Biological ion exchanger resins. VIII. A preliminary report on actin-like protein in *E. coli* and the cytotonus concept," *Physiol. Chem. and Physics* **7**, (1975).

45. K.S. Zaner and R. Damadian, "NMR in cancer. IX. The concept of cancer treatment by NMR: A preliminary report of high resolution NMR of phosphorus in normal and malignant tissues," *Physiol. Chem. and Physics* **7**, (1975), 437-451.

46. R. Damadian, L. Minkoff, M. Goldsmith, M. Stanford and J. Koutcher, "Tumor imaging in a live animal by field focusing NMR, (FONAR)," *Physiol. Chem. and Physics* **8**, (1975), 61-65.

47. R. Damadian, "The nuclear resonance effect in cancer," presented at 10th meeting of Federation of European Biochemical Societies, Paris, France, July 1975, abstract 1635.

48. R. Damadian, "The nuclear resonance effect in cancer," presented at 5th International Biophysics Congress, Copenhagen, Denmark, August 1975, abstract P-583.

49. M. Goldsmith, D. Hor and R. Damadian, "Sodium-23 nuclear magnetic resonance of resins and mixed solvent systems," *J. Chem. Physics* **65**, (1976), 1708-1710.

50. L. Minkoff, J. Abramowitz and R. Damadian, "Biological ion exchanger resins. IX. Isolation and partial identification of a potassium sensitive contractile-like protein from *E. coli*," *Physiol. Chem. and Physics* **8**, (1976), 167-173.

51. L. Minkoff and R. Damadian, "Biological ion exchanger resins. X. The cytotonus hypothesis: Biological contractility and the total regulation of cellular physiology through quantitative control of cell water," *Physiol. Chem. and Physics* **8**, (1976), 349-387.

52. L. Minkoff and R. Damadian, "Actin-like proteins from *E. coli*: The link between cell metabolism and the biological ion exchanger resin," *J. Bacteriol.* **125**, (1976), 353-365.

53. R. Damadian, L. Minkoff, M. Goldsmith, M. Stanford and J. Koutcher, "Field focusing nuclear magnetic resonance (FONAR): Visualization of a tumor in a live animal," *Science* **194**, (1976), 1430-1432.

54. M. Goldsmith and R. Damadian, "Sodium-23 magnetic resonance of biological and non-biological ion exchanger systems," *Biophysical Journal* **16**, (1976), 67a, abstract.

55. R. Damadian, L. Minkoff, M. Goldsmith, M. Stanford and J. Koutcher, "Tumor imaging in a live animal by field focusing NMR (FONAR)," *Abstracts*, XIXth Congress Ampère (1976), 97.

56. R. Damadian, L. Minkoff, M. Goldsmith, M. Stanford and J. Koutcher, "Field focusing NMR (FONAR): Visualization of a tumor in a live animal," *Proceedings of the X1Xth Congress on Magnetic Resonance and Related Phenomena*, (1976), 253-256.

57. R. Damadian, "Nuclear magnetic resonance: A noninvasive approach to cancer," *Hosp. Prac.* **12**, (1977), 63-70.

58. R. Damadian, M. Goldsmith and L. Minkoff, "NMR in cancer XVI: FONAR Image of the live human body," *Physiol. Chem. and Physics* **9**, (1977), 97-100.

59. L. Minkoff, R. Damadian, T.E. Thomas, N. Hu, M. Goldsmith, "NMR in cancer XVII: Dewar for a 53-inch superconducting NMR magnet," *Physiol. Chem. and Physics* **9**, (1977), 101-104.

60. M. Goldsmith, R. Damadian, M. Stanford and M. Lipkowitz, "NMR in cancer XVIII: A superconductive NMR magnet for a human sample," *Physiol. Chem. and Physics* **9**, (1977), 105-107.

61. M. Goldsmith, J. Koutcher and R. Damadian, "NMR in cancer XII: Application of the NMR malignancy index to human lung tumors," *Brit. J. of Cancer* **36**, (1977), 235.

62. J.A. Koutcher and R. Damadian, "Spectral differences in the P^{31} NMR of normal and malignant tissue," *Physiol. Chem. and Physics* **9**, (1977), 181-187.

63. L. Minkoff and R. Damadian, "Biological ion exchanger resins. XI. Actin in *Escherichia coli*," *Physiol. Chem. and Physics*.

64. K.S. Zaner and R. Damadian, "NMR in Cancer VIII: Phosphorus-31 as a nuclear probe for malignant tumors," *Physiol. Chem. and Physics* **9**, (1977), 473-483.

65. M. Goldsmith, J. Koutcher and R. Damadian, "The NMR detection of malignancy in specimens of human tissue," *Biophysical Journal* **17**, (1977), 303a, abstract.

66. J. Koutcher, M. Goldsmith and R. Damadian, "NMR in cancer X: A malignancy index to discriminate normal and cancerous tissue," *Cancer* **41**, No. 1, (1978), 174-182.

67. M. Goldsmith, J. Koutcher and R. Damadian, "NMR in cancer XI: Application of the NMR malignancy index to human gastrointestinal tumors," *Cancer* **41**, No. 1, (1978), 183-191.

68. R. Fruchter, M. Goldsmith, J. Boyce, A. Nicastri, J. Koutcher and R. Damadian, "NMR in Cancer XIV: Application of the NMR malignancy index to human gynecological tumors," *Oncology* **6**, (1978), 243-255.

69. R. Damadian, L. Minkoff, M. Goldsmith and J. Koutcher, "Field focusing nuclear magnetic resonance (FONAR) and the formation of chemical scans in man," *Naturwissenschaften* **65**, (1978), 250-252.

70. R. Damadian, M. Goldsmith and L. Minkoff, "NMR in cancer XX: FONAR scans of patients with cancer," *Physiol. Chem. Physics* **10**, (1978), 285-286.

71. R. Damadian, L. Mindoff and M. Goldsmith, "NMR in cancer XXI: FONAR scan of live human abdomen," *Physiol. Chem. Physics* **10**, (1978), 561-563.

72. R. Damadian, "Field focusing NMR (FONAR) and the formation of chemical images in man," *Phil. Trans. R. Soc. London Biol.* **289** 1037,(1980), 489-500.

73. R. Damadian, editor, *NMR in Medicine*, (Heidelberg, Germany: Springer-Verlag).

74. R. Damadian, "Apparatus and method for nuclear magnetic resonance scanning and mapping," U.S. Patent 4,354,499, filed 8 August 1982.

75. R Damadian, "Apparatus and method for nuclear magnetic scanning and mapping," U.S. Patent 4,411,270, filed 25 October 1983.

76. Gordon T. Danby, R. Damadian and Lawrence A. Minkoff, "Nuclear magnetic resonance apparatus including permanent magnet configuration," U.S. Patent 4,675,609, filed 20 March 1986.

77. Rajendra K. Shenoy, Robert B. Wolf, Terry Morrone and R. Damadian, "Method for obtaining T_1-weighted and T_2-weighted NMR images for a plurality of selected planes in the course," U.S. Patent 4,734,646, filed 16 September 1986.

78. Gordon T. Danby, Jan V. Votruba, R. Damadian and Guo-Ping Zhang, "Apparatus and method for processing an electrical signal and increasing a signal-to-noise ratio thereof," U.S. Patent 4,737,713, filed 26 November 1986.

79. Gordon T. Danby, Hank Hsieh, John W. Jackson and R. Damadian, "Nuclear magnetic resonance scanners," U.S. Patent 4,766,378, filed 28 November 1986.

80. R. Damadian, Anthony Giambalvo, Rajendra K. Shenoy and Jan V. Votruba, "Apparatus and method for processing an electrical signal and increasing the S/N ratio thereof," U.S. Patent 4,737,713, filed 12 April 1988.

81. Gregory Eydelman, Anthony Giambalvo and R. Damadian, "MRI antennas with spiral coils and imaging methods employing the same," U.S. Patent 5,050,605, filed 24 October 1991.

List of Publications: PAUL C. LAUTERBUR

1. E.L. Warrick and P.C. Lauterbur, "Filler phenomena in silicone rubber," *Ind. Eng. Chem.* **47**, (1955), 485.
2. G.R. Holzman, P.C. Lauterbur, J.H. Anderson and W. Koth, "Nuclear magnetic resonance field shifts of Si^{29} in various materials," *J. Chem. Phys.* **25**, (1956), 172.
3. N. Muller, P.C. Lauterbur and J. Goldenson, "Nuclear magnetic resonance spectra of phosphorous compounds," *J. Am. Chem. Soc.* **78**, (1956), 3557.
4. P.C. Lauterbur, , "C^{13} nuclear magnetic resonance spectra," *J. Chem. Phys.* **26**, (1957), 217.
5. N. Muller, P.C. Lauterbur and G.F. Svatos, "Nuclear magnetic resonance spectra of some perfluoroalkyl derivatives of sulfur hexafluoride," *J. Am. Chem. Soc.* **79**, (1957), 1043.
6. N. Muller, P.C. Lauterbur and G.F. Svatos, "Nuclear magnetic resonance spectra of some fluorocarbon derivatives," *J. Am. Chem. Soc.* **79**, (1957), 1807.
7. W.S. Koski, J.J. Kaufman and P.C. Lauterbur, "Nuclear magnetic resonance study of the B_2D_6-B_5H_9 exchange reaction," *J. Am. Chem. Soc.* **79**, (1957), 2382.
8. P.C. Lauterbur, "Some applications of C^{13} nuclear magnetic resonance spectra to organic chemistry," *Ann. N.Y. Acad. Sci.* **70**, 4, (1958), 841.
9. P.C. Lauterbur, "Anisotropy of the C^{13} chemical shift in calcite," *Phys. Rev. Letters* **1**, (1958), 343.
10. R. Ettinger, P. Blume, A. Patterson, Jr. and P.C. Lauterbur, "C^{13} chemical shifts in CO and CO_2," *J. Chem. Phys.* **33**, (1960), 1597.
11. J.J. Burke and P.C. Lauterbur, "Sn^{119} nuclear magnetic resonance spectra," *J. Am. Chem. Soc.* **83**, (1961), 326.
12. P.C. Lauterbur, "C^{13} nuclear magnetic resonance spectroscopy. I. Aromatic hydrocarbons," *J. Am. Chem. Soc.* **83**, (1961), 1838.
13. P.C. Lauterbur, "C^{13} nuclear magnetic resonance spectroscopy. II. Phenols, anisole and dimethoxybenzenes," *J. Am. Chem. Soc.* **83**, (1961), 1846.
14. J.G. Pritchard and P.C. Lauterbur, "Proton magnetic resonance, structure and stereoisomerism in cyclic sulfites," *J. Am. Chem. Soc.* **83**, (1961), 2105.
15. P.C. Lauterbur, "Magnetic shielding and the electronic structures of aromatic molecules," *Tetrahedron Letters* (1961), 274.
16. P.C. Lauterbur, "Nuclear magnetic resonance spectra of elements other than hydrogen and fluorine," *Determination of Organic Structures by Physical Methods*, Vol. 2, ed. by F.C. Nachod and W.D. Phillips, (New York, NY: Academic Press, 1962), Chpt. 7.
17. G.V.D. Tiers and P.C. Lauterbur, "Fluorine NMR spectroscopy. X. Analysis of carbon-13 satellites in the spectra of Cis- and Trans-CFC1=CFC1. Assignment of coupling constants for fluorinated olefins," *J. Chem. Phys.* **36**, (1962), 1110.
18. P.C. Lauterbur and R.J. Kurland, "On the signs of CH and HH coupling constants," *J. Am. Chem. Soc.* **84**, (1962), 3405.
19. P.C. Lauterbur, "C^{13} nuclear magnetic resonance spectroscopy. III. Iodobenzene and Methyliodobenzenes," *J. Chem. Phys.* **38**, (1963), 1406.
20. P.C. Lauterbur, "C^{13} nuclear magnetic resonance spectroscopy. IV. Aniline, N, N-dimethylaniline and their methyl derivatives. Steric inhibition of conjugation," *J. Chem. Phys.* **38**, (1963), 1415.
21. P.C. Lauterbur, "C^{13} nuclear magnetic resonance spectroscopy. V. Nitrobenzene and methylnitrobenzenes: Steric inhibition of conjugation," *J. Chem. Phys.* **38**, (1963), 1432.
22. P.C. Lauterbur, J.G. Prichard and R.L. Vollmer, "The isomeric pentane-2, 4-diol cyclic sulphites," *J. Chem. Soc.* (1963), 5307.
23. J.J. Burke and P.C. Lauterbur, "C^{13} and H^1 nuclear magnetic resonance spectra of cycloalkanes," *J. Am. Chem. Soc.* **86**, (1964), 1870.
24. J.B. Stothers and P.C. Lauterbur, "C^{13} chemical shifts in organic carbonyl compounds," *Canadian J. Chem.* **42**, (1964), 1563.

25. P.C. Lauterbur and J.J. Burke, "Anisotropic ^{207}Pb magnetic shielding in a single crystal of wulfenite, PbMoO$_4$," *J. Chem. Phys.* **42,** (1965), 439.

26. P.C. Lauterbur, "Isotope effects on ^{59}Co magnetic shielding in K$_3$Co(CN)$_6$," *J. Chem. Phys.* **42,** (1965), 799.

27. P.C. Lauterbur and R.B. King, "C^{13} nuclear magnetic resonance spectra of transition metal cyclopentadienyl and carbonyl derivatives," *J. Am. Chem. Soc.* **87,** (1965), 3266.

28. P.C. Lauterbur, "C^{13} nuclear magnetic resonance spectroscopy. VI. Azines and methyl azines," *J. Chem. Phys.* **43,** (1965), 360.

29. G.G. Emerson, K. Ehrlich, W.P. Giering and P.C. Lauterbur, "Trimethylenemethaneiron tricarbonyl," *J. Am. Chem. Soc.* **88,** (1966), 3172.

30. D.N. Ford, P.R. Wells and P.C. Lauterbur, "The ^{1}H nuclear magnetic resonance spectra of methylmercury compounds," *Chem. Commun.* (1967), 616.

31. A. Loewenstein, J. Shporer, P.C. Lauterbur and J.E. Ramierez, "Solvent isotope effects on chemical shifts of ions in aqueous solutions," Chem. Commun., (1968), 214.

32. P.C. Lauterbur, R.C. Hopkins, R.W. King, O.V. Ziebarth and C.W. Heitsch, "The nuclear magnetic resonance spectra of aluminum borohydride-trimethylamine," *Inorganic Chemistry* **7,** (1968), 1025.

33. P.C. Lauterbur and F. Ramirez, "Pseudorotation in trigonal-bipyramidal molecules," *J. Am. Chem. Soc.* **90,** (1968), 6722.

34. D.C. Haddix and P.C. Lauterbur, "Nuclear magnetic resonance studies of single crystals of trichloroacetic acid," *Molecular Dynamics and Structure of Solids,* ed. by R.S. Carter and J.J. Rush, NBS Special Publ. 301, (1969), 403.

35. P.C. Lauterbur, "^{13}C nuclear magnetic resonance spectra of proteins," *Applied. Spectrosc.* **24,** (1970), 450.

36. P.C. Lauterbur, E.J. Runde and B.L. Blitzer, "^{13}C NMR spectroscopy of biopolymers," *Magnetic Resonances in Biological Research,* ed. by C. Franconi, (London: Gordon and Breach, 1971).

37. P.C. Lauterbur, "Image formation by induced local interactions: Examples employing nuclear magnetic resonance," *Nature* **242,** (1973), 190-191.

38. P.C. Lauterbur, "Stable isotope distributions by NMR zeugmatography," *Proc. First International Conf. on Stable Isotopes in Chemistry, Biology and Medicine,* U.S.A.E.C. CONF-730525, (1973), 255.

39. P.C. Lauterbur, "Magnetic resonance zeugmatography," *Pure Appl. Chem.* **40,** (1974), 149.

40. P.C. Lauterbur, "Reconstruction in zeugmatography—the spatial resolution of magnetic resonance signals," *Techniques of Three-Dimensional Reconstruction: Proceedings of an International Workshop,* July 16-19, 1974, Brookhaven National Laboratory, ed. by R.B. Marr, Pub. BNL 20425, 20-22.

41. P.C. Lauterbur, C.S. Dulcey, Jr., C.-M. Lai, M.A. Feiler, W.V. House, Jr., D.M. Kramer, C.-N. Chen and R. Dias, "Magnetic resonance zeugmatography," Vol. 1, *Magnetic Resonance and Related Phenomena, Proceedings of the 18th Ampere Congress,* Nottingham, 9-14 Sept. 1974, ed. by P.S. Allen, E.R. Andrew and C.A. Bates, (North-Holland, Amsterdam, 1975), 27.

42. P.C. Lauterbur, W.V. House, Jr., D.M. Kramer, C.-N. Chen, F.W. Porretto and C.S. Dulcey, Jr., "Reconstruction from selectively-excited signals in nuclear magnetic resonance zeugmatography," in Image Processing for 2-D and 3-D Reconstruction from Projections: Theory and Practice in Medicine and the Physical Sciences, *Opt. Soc. Am.,* (1975) MA10-1.

43. P.C. Lauterbur, D.M. Kramer, W.V. House, Jr. and C.-N. Chen, "Zeugmatographic high resolution nuclear magnetic resonance resonance spectroscopy. Images of chemical inhomogeneity within microscopic objects," *J. Am. Chem. Soc.* **97,** (1975), 6866-6868.

44. P.C. Lauterbur, C.-M. Lai, J.A. Frank, C.S. Dulcey, Jr., "*In vivo* zeugmatographic imaging of tumors," *Physics in Canada* **32,** Special July Issue: *Digest of the Fourth International Conference on Medical Physics,* Abstract 33.11, (1976).

45. P.C. Lauterbur, J.A. Frank and M.J. Jacobson, "Water proton spin-lattice relaxation times in normal and edematous dog lungs," *Physics in Canada* **32**, Special July Issue: *Digest of the Fourth International Conference on Medical Physics*, Abstract 33.9, (1976).

46. J.A. Frank, M.A. Feiler, W.V. House, Jr., P.C. Lauterbur and M.J. Jacobson, "Measurement of proton nuclear magnetic longitudinal relaxation times and water content in infarcted canine myocardium and induced pulmonary injury," *Clinical Research* **24**, (1976), 217A.

47. P.C. Lauterbur, "Spatially-resolved studies of whole tissues, organs and organisms by NMR zeugmatography," *NMR in Biology*, ed. by R.A. Dwek, I.D. Campbell, R.E. Richards and R.J.P. Williams, (London: Academic Press, 1977), 323-335.

48. N. Lee, M. Inouye and P.C. Lauterbur, "^{19}F- and ^{13}C-NMR studies of a specifically-labelled lipoprotein in the *Escherichia coli* membrane," *Biochem. Biophys. Res. Comm.* **78**, (1977), 1211-1218.

49. P.C. Lauterbur and C.-M. Lai, "Feasibility study of nuclear magnetic resonance zeugmatography for use in detecting atherosclerosis," *Proc. of the NHLBI Division of Heart and Vascular Diseases*, Devices and Technology Branch Annual Contractors Meeting 1977, 158-159.

50. P.C. Lauterbur, B.V. Kaufman and M.K. Crawford, "NMR studies of the protein-solvent interface," *Biomolecular Structure and Function*, ed. by P.F. Agris, (New York, NY: Academic Press, 1978), 329-351.

51. C.-M. Lai, W.V. House, Jr. and P.C. Lauterbur, "Nuclear magnetic resonance zeugmatography for medical imaging," *Proc. of IEEE Electro/78 Conference*, Session 30, "Technology for non-invasive monitoring of physiological phenomena," May 25, 1978, paper 2.

52. P.C. Lauterbur, M.H. Mendonca Dias and A.M. Rudin, "Augmentation of tissue water proton spin-lattice relaxation rates by *in vivo* addition of paramagnetic ions," *Frontiers of Biological Energetics*, ed. by P.O. Dutton, J. Leigh and A. Scarpa, (New York, NY: Academic Press, 1978), 752-759.

53. P.C. Lauterbur, "Feasibility of NMR zeugmatographic imaging of the heart and lungs," *Medical Imaging Techniques: A Comparison*, (Plenum Press, 1979), 209-218.

54. C.-M. Lai, J.W. Shook and P.C. Lauterbur, "Microprocessor-controlled reorientation of magnetic field gradients for NMR zeugmatographic imaging," *Chem. Biomed. Environ. Instr.* **9**, (1979), 1-27.

55. D.I. Hoult and P.C. Lauterbur, "The sensitivity of the zeugmatographic experiment involving human samples," *J. Magn. Reson.* **34**, (1979), 425-433.

56. D.M. Krammer and P.C. Lauterbur, "On the problem of reconstructing images of non-scalar parameters from projections. Application to vector fields," *IEEE Trans. Nucl. Sci.*, Vol. NS-26, Part 2, April 1979, 2674-2677.

57. P.C. Lauterbur, "Medical imaging by nuclear magnetic resonance zeugmatography," *IEEE Trans. Nucl. Sci.*, Vol. NS-26, No. 2, Part 2, April 1979, 2808-2811.

58. W.V. House and P.C. Lauterbur, "Nuclear magnetic resonance zeugmatographic imaging," *Application of Optical Instrumentation in Medicine VII*, Proc. Soc. Photo-Opt. Instr. Eng. **173**, (1979), 356-359.

59. P.C. Lauterbur, W.V. House, Jr., H.E. Simon, M.H. Mendonca Dias, M.J. Jacobson, C.-M. Lai, P. Bendel and A.M. Rudin, "NMR zeugmatographic imaging of organs and organisms," *Stereodynamics of Molecular Systems*, ed. R.H. Sarma, (Oxford, New York, Frankfurt, Paris: Pergamon Press, 1979), 453-456.

60. P. Bendel, C.-M. Lai and P.C. Lauterbur, "^{31}P spectroscopic zeugmatography of phosphorus metabolites," *J. Magn. Reson.* **38**, (1980), 343-356.

61. P.C. Lauterbur and C.-M. Lai, "Zeugmatography by reconstruction from projections," *IEEE Trans. Nucl. Sci.* Vol. NS-27, No. 3, (June 1980), 1227-1231.

62. P.C. Lauterbur, "Progress in n.m.r. zeugmatographic imaging," *Phil. Trans. R. Soc. Lond.* **B289**, (1980), 483-487.

63. C.-M. Lai and P.C. Lauterbur, "A gradient control device for complete three-dimensional nuclear magnetic resonance zeugmatographic imaging," *J. Phys. E: Sci. Instrum.* **13**, (1980), 747-750.

64. C.-M. Lai and P.C. Lauterbur, "Automatic correction of nuclear magnetic resonance zeugmatographic projection," *J. Phys. E: Sci. Instrum.* **14**, (1981), 874-879.

65. R.B. Marr, C.-N. Chen and P.C. Lauterbur, "On two approaches to 3D reconstruction in NMR zeugmatography," *Mathematical Aspects of Computed Tomography*, Vol. 8, Ed. by G.T. Herman and F. Natterer, (Springer-Verlag, 1981), 225-240.

66. R. Klimek, P.C. Lauterbur and M.H. Mendonca Dias, "A discussion of nuclear magnetic resonance (NMR) relaxation times of tumors in terms of their interpretation as self-organizing dissipative structures and of their study *in vivo* by NMR zeugmatographic imaging," *Gin. Pol.* **52, 6**, (1981), 493-402.

67. G.T. Herman, J.K. Udupa, D.M. Kramer, P.C. Lauterbur, A.M. Rudin and J.S. Schneider, "Three-dimensional display of nuclear magnetic resonance images," *Application of Optical Instrumentation in Medicine IX*, Proc. Soc. Photo-Opt. Instr. Eng. **273**, (1981), 35-40.

68. D.M. Kramer, J.S. Schneider, A.M. Rudin and P.C. Luterbur, "True three-dimensional nuclear magnetic resonance zeugmatographic images of a human brain," *Neuroradiology* **21**, (1981), 239-244.

69. C.-M. Lai and P.C. Lauterbur, "True three-dimensional image reconstruction by nuclear magnetic resonance zeugmatography," *Phys. Med. Biol.* **26**, 5, (1981), 851-856.

70. P.C. Lauterbur, "NMR zeugmatographic imaging in medicine," *Proc. 15th Annual Hawaiian Intnl. Conf. on Syst. Sci.*, Vol. II, (1982), 435-439.

71. G.L. Brownell, T.F. Budinger, P.C. Lauterbur and P.L. McGeer, "Position tomography and nuclear magnetic resonance imaging," *Science* **215**, (1982), 619-626.

72. M.A. Heneghan, T.M. Bincaniello, E. Heidelberger, S.B. Petersen, M.J. Marsh and P.C. Lauterbur, "Nuclear magnetic resonance zeugmatographic imaging of the heart: Application to the study of ventricular septal defect," *Radiology* **143**, (1982), 183-186.

73. P.C. Lauterbur, "NMR in medicine: A brief historical review and prospectus," *Medical Image Technology and Information Display* **14**, (1982), 586-592.

74. M.L. Bernardo, Jr., A.J. Cohen and P.C. Lauterbur, "Radiofrequency coil designs for nuclear magnetic resonance zeugmatographic imaging," *Proc. Intnl. Workshop on Phys. and Eng. in Medical Imaging*, (IEEE Compt. Soc., 1982), 277-284.

75. M.H. Mendonca Dias, W.J. Mann, J. Chumas, M.L. Bernardo, Jr. and P.C. Lauterbur, "Three-dimensional nuclear magnetic resonance zeugmatographic imaging of surgical specimens," *Bioscience Reports* **2**, (1982), 713-717.

76. R. Klimek, P.C. Lauterbur, M.H. Mendonca Dias, F. DeBlase and W. Doroszkiewicz, "Nuclear magnetic resonance relaxation time as a proof of the presence of plasmid in *Escherichia coli*," *Przeglad Lekarski* **39**, (1982), 533-534.

77. G.T. Herman, J.K. Udupa, D.M. Kramer, P.C. Lauterbur, A.M. Rudin and J.S. Schneider, "Three-dimensional display of nuclear magnetic resonance images," *Opt. Eng.* **21**, (1982), 923-926.

78. M.J. Marsh, M.L. Bernardo, Jr., R.N. Muller and P.C. Lauterbur, "Limb imaging by contrast enhanced NMR zeugmatography: Potential application to three-dimensional investigation of joint and muscular diseases," *Abstracts*, First Annual Meeting of the Society of Magnetic Resonance in Medicine, Boston, (1982), 100-101.

79. E. Heidelberger, S.B. Petersen and P.C. Lauterbur, "3D synchronized proton NMR imaging of the beating heart," *Abstracts*, First Annual Meeting of the Society of Magnetic Resonance in Medicine, Boston, (1982), 72-73.

80. E. Heidelberger and P.C. Lauterbur, "Gas phase ^{19}F NMR zeugmatography: A new approach to lung ventilation imaging," *Abstracts*, First Annual Meeting of the Society of Magnetic Resonance in Medicine, Boston, (1982), 70-71.

81. M.H. Mendonca Dias, P.C. Lauterbur and A.M. Rudin, "The use of paramagnetic contrast agents in NMR imaging. I. Preliminary *in vitro* studies," *Abstracts*, First Annual Meeting of the Society of Magnetic Resonance in Medicine, Boston, (1982), 103-104.

82. M.H. Mendonca Dias, P.C. Lauterbur and E.J. Brown, Jr., "The use of paramagnetic contrast agents in NMR imaging. II. *In vivo* studies," *Abstracts*, First Annual Meeting of the Society of Magnetic Resonance in Medicine, Boston, (1982,) 105-106.

83. S.K. Mun, M.H. Mendonca Dias, P.C. Lauterbur, R. Heidelberger, C.J. Chrzan, "Multicomponent water proton T_1 analysis in organs and tissues from animals injected with manganese," *Abstracts*, First Annual Meeting of the Society of Magnetic Resonance in Medicine, Boston, (1982), 111.

84. C.-N. Chen, R.B. Marr and P.C. Lauterbur, "A comparative study on three 3D reconstruction methods in NMR zeugmatography," *Abstracts*, First Annual Meeting of the Society of Magnetic Resonance in Medicine, Boston, (1982), 41-42.

85. P.C. Lauterbur, "NMR zeugmatographic imaging in medicine," *J. Med. Syst.* **6**, No. 6, (1982), 591-597.

86. M.H. Mendonca Dias, M.L. Bernardo, Jr., T.M. Biancaniello, S.E. Harms, E. Heidelberger, M.A. Heneghan, P.C. Lauterbur, W.J. Mann, M.J. Marsh, R.N. Muller, S.B. Petersen and A.M. Rudin, "Clinical results and preliminary studies at Stony Brook," *Abstracts*, Third World Congress of Nuclear Medicine and Biology, Paris, France, (1982), 2657-2662.

87. P.C. Lauterbur, "Nuclear magnetic resonance and positron emission tomography," *Cerebrovascular Diseases*, ed. by M. Reivich and H.I. Hurtig, (New York: Raven Press, 1983), 1-5.

88. M.L. Bernardo and P.C. Lauterbur, "Rapid medium-resolution 3-D NMR zeugmatographic imaging of the head," *Europ. J. Radioil.* **3**, (1983), 257-263.

89. E. Heidelberger, S.B. Petersen and P.C. Lauterbur, "Aspects of cardiac diagnosis using synchronized NMR imaging," *Europ. J. Radiol.* **3**, (1983), 281-285.

90. R.N. Muller, M.J. Marsh, M.L. Bernardo and P.C. Lauterbur, "True 3-D imaging of limbs by NMR zeugmatography with off-resonance irradiation," *Europ. J. Radiol.* **3**, (1983), 286-290.

91. M.H. Mendonca Dias, E. Gaggelli and P.C. Lauterbur, "Paramagnetic contrast agents in NMR medical imaging," *Seminars in Nuclear Medicine*, Vol. XIII, No. 4, (1983), 364-376.

92. P.C. Lauterbur, D.N. Levin and R.B. Marr, "Chemical shift NMR imaging with unswitched gradients," *Radiology* **149**, (1983), 255.

93. W.J. Mann, M.H. Mendonca Dias, P.C. Lauterbur, R. Klimek, M.L. Stone, M.L. Bernardo, Jr., J. Chumas, R. Heidelberger, V. Acuff and A. Taylor, "Preliminary *in vitro* studies of nuclear magnetic resonance spin-lattice relaxation times and three-dimensional nuclear magnetic resonance imaging in gynecologic oncology," *Am. J. Obstet. Gynecol.* **148**, (1984), 91-95.

94. P.C. Lauterbur, "New directions in NMR imaging," *IEEE Trans. Nucl. Sci.* **31, 4**, (1984), 1010.

95. T.F. Budinger and P.C. Lauterbur, "NMR technology for medical studies," *Science* **226**, (1984), 288-298.

96. P.C. Lauterbur, D.N. Levin and R.B. Marr, "Theory and simulation of NMR spectroscopic imaging and field plotting by projection reconstruction involving an intrinsic frequency dimension," *J. Magn. Reson.* **59**, (1984), 536-541.

97. M.L. Bernardo, Jr., P.C. Lauterbur and L.K. Hedges, "Experimental example of NMR spectroscopic imaging by projection reconstruction involving an intrinsic frequency dimension," *J. Magn. Reson.* **61**, (1985), 168-174.

98. P.C. Lauterbur, "New techniques in NMR zeugmatographic imaging," *Biomedical Imaging: Proceedings of the Third Takeda Science Foundation Symposium on Bioscience—1984*, ed. by O. Hayaishi and K. Torizuka, (Orlando: Academic Press, 1986), 97-106.

99. M.H. Mendonca Dias, M.L. Bernardo, Jr., R.N. Muller, V. Acuff and P.C. Lauterbur, "Ferromagnetic particles as contrast agents for magnetic resonance imaging," *Abstracts,* Fourth Annual Meeting of the Society of Magnetic Resonance in Medicine, London, (1985), 887.

100. X.-R. Liu, P.C. Lauterbur and R.B. Marr, "Reconstruction by back transformation: Application to the case of continuously rotating gradients," *Abstracts,* Fourth Annual Meeting of the Society of Magnetic Resonance in Medicine, London, (1985), 1017-1018.

101. M. Bernardo, Jr., D. Chaudhuri, X-R. Liu and P.C. Lauterbur, "Hadamard zeugmatography using 3-D projection reconstruction," *Abstracts,* Fourth Annual Meeting of the Society of Magnetic Resonance in Medicine, London, (1985), 944-945

102. D.-Q. Chen, R.E. Marr and P.C. Lauterbur, "Reconstruction from data acquired with imaging gradients having arbitrary time dependence," *Abstracts,* Fourth Annual Meeting of the Society of Magnetic Resonance in Medicine, London, (1985), 950-951.

103. A.E. Stillman, D.N. Levin, D.B. Yang, R.B. Marr and P.C. Lauterbur, "Method for reduction of number of projections required for projection reconstruction of magnetic resonance spectroscopic images," *Abstracts,* Fourth Annual Meeting of the Society of Magnetic Resonance in Medicine, London, (1985), 182-183.

104. P.C. Lauterbur and M.L. Bernardo, Jr., "Spectroscopic imaging of microscopic objects," *Abstracts,* Fourth Annual Meeting of the Society of Magnetic Resonance in Medicine, London, (1985), 742

105. A.E. Stillman, D.N. Levin, D.B. Yang, R.B. Marr and P.C. Lauterbur, "Back projection reconstruction of spectroscopic NMR images from incomplete sets of projections," *J. Magn. Reson.* **69,** (1986), 168-175.

106. M.H. Mendonca Dias and P.C. Lauterbur, "Contrast agents for nuclear magnetic resonance imaging," *Biological Trace Element Research* **13,** (1987), 229-239.

107. M.H. Mendonca Dias and P.C. Lauterbur, "Ferromagnetic particles as contrast agents for magnetic resonance imaging of liver and spleen," *Magn. Reson. in Med.* **3,** (1986), 328-330.

108. P.C. Lauterbur, "New directions in NMR zeugmatographic imaging," *NMR in Biology and Medicine,* ed. by S. Chien and C. Ho, (New York: Raven Press, 1986), 135-140.

109. P.C. Lauterbur, "Cancer detection by nuclear magnetic resonance zeugmatographic imaging," *Accomplishments in Cancer Research, 1985 Prize Year, General Motors Cancer Research Foundation,* (Philadelphia: J.B. Lippincott Co., 1986), *Cancer* **57,** (May 1986), 1899-1904.

110. Peter A. Rinck, S.B. Peterson, E. Heidelberger, Virgil Acuff, Johan Reinders, M.L. Bernardo, Jr., Lewis K. Hedges, P.C. Lauterbur, "NMR lung ventilation imaging," Scientific Program from the 69th Scientific Assembly and Annual Meeting of the Radiological Society of North America, Chicago, November 13-18, (1983); *Radiology* **149,** Special Edition, (Nov. 1983).

111. P.A. Rinck, S.B. Peterson and P.C. Lauterbur, "NMR-imaging von fluorhaltigen substanzen," (NMR imaging of fluorine-containing substances.), *Rontgenstr.* **140, 3,** (1984), 239-243.

112. P.A. Rinck, S.B. Peterson, E. Heidelberger, V. Acuff, J. Reinders, M.L. Bernardo, L.K. Hedges and P.C. Lauterbur, "NMR ventilation imaging of the lungs using perfluorinated gases," *Abstracts,* Second Annual Meeting of the Society of Magnetic Resonance in Medicine; *Magn. Reson. Med.* **1,** (1984), 237.

113. P.C. Lauterbur and L. Kyle Hedges, "Microscopic NMR Imaging," *Abstracts,* XXIII Congress Ampere on Magnetic Resonance, Rome, Italy, (1986), 24-27.

114. D.-Q. Chen, R.B. Marr and P.C. Lauterbur, "Reconstruction from NMR data acquired with imaging gradients having arbitrary time dependence," *IEEE Trans. on Med. Imaging,* Vol. MI-5, No. 3, (1986), 162-164.

115. P.C. Lauterbur, M.L. Bernardo, Jr., M.H. Mendonca Dias and L.K. Hedges, "Microscopic NMR imaging of the magnetic fields around magnetite particles," *Works in Progress Abstract,* Fifth Annual Meeting of the Society of Magnetic Resonance in Medicine, Montreal, Canada, (1986), 229-230.

116. D.N. Levin, X. Hu, P.C. Lauterbur, "Localization of spectra using structural information from non-spectroscopic imaging," *Abstracts,* 1987 European Workshop on Magnetic Resonance in Medicine, London, (1987), 27-28.

117. X. Hu, D.N. Levin, P.C. Lauterbur and T. Spraggins, "Localization of spectra using structural information from non-spectroscopic imaging," *Abstracts,* Sixth Annual Meeting of the Society of Magnetic Resonance in Medicine, New York, NY, (1987), 941.

118. P.C. Lauterbur, "NMR imaging in biomedicine," *Cell Biophysics* **9**, 1-2, (1986), 211-214.

119. R.K. Woods, G. Bacic, H.M. Swartz and P.C. Lauterbur, "Three dimensional electron spin resonance imaging," R.K. Woods, G. Bacic, H.M. Swartz and P.C. Lauterbur, *Biophysical Journ.* **53**, No. 2, Part 2, (1988), 202a.

120. P.C. Lauterbur, "Microscopic NMR imaging and particulate contrast agents," *Biophysical Journ.* **53**, No.2, Part 2, (1988), 445a.

121. G. Bacic, T. Walczak, P. Morse II, F. Demsar, R. Woods, M. Nilges, J. Dobrucki, P. Lauterbur and H. Swartz, "ESR imaging microscopy of biological samples at 9 GHz (X-BAND)," *Biophysical Journ.* **53**, No. 2, Part 2, (1988), 626a.

122. X. Hu, D.N. Levin, P.C. Lauterbur and T. Spraggins, "SLIM: Spectral localization by imaging," *Magn. Reson. Med.* **8**, (1988), 314-322.

123. X. Hu, D.N. Levin, P.C. Lauterbur and T.A. Spraggins, "*In vivo* applications of spectroscopic localization by imaging (SLIM)," *Abstracts,* 74th Scientific Assembly of the RSNA, Chicago, IL, (1988), 157.

124. X. Hu, D.N. Levin, P.C. Lauterbur and T.A. Spraggins, "*In vivo* applications of spectroscopic localization by imaging (SLIM)," *Abstracts,* Seventh Annual Meeting of the Society of Magnetic Resonance in Medicine, San Francisco, CA, (1988), 926.

125. Haakil Lee and Paul C. Lauterbur, "*In vivo* localized phosphorus NMR spectroscopy in regions of arbitrary shape by the *SLIM* method," *Bioiphysical Journ.* **55**, No. 2, Part 2, (1989), 452a.

126. R.K. Woods, G. Bacic, P.C. Lauterbur and H.M. Swartz, "Three-dimensional electron spin resonance imaging," *J. Magn. Reson.* **84**, (1989), 247-254.

127. Xiaohong Zhou, Clinton S. Potter, Paul C. Lauterbur and Brian Voth, "3D microscopic NMR imaging with $(6.37\mu m)^3$ isotropic resolution," *Abstracts,* Eighth Annual Meeting of the Society of Magnetic Resonance in Medicine, Amsterdam, The Netherlands, (1989), 286.

128. Haakil Lee and Paul C. Lauterbur, "Application of the SLIM (Spectral Localization by Imaging) technique with surface coil," Eighth Annual Meeting of the Society of Magnetic Resonance in Medicine, Amsterdam, The Netherlands, 1989, 651.

129. P.C. Lauterbur, "Nuclear magnetic resonance microscopy," *Proceedings of the 47th Annual Meeting of the Electron Microscopy Society of America,* (San Francisco Press, 1989), 828-829.

130. Haakil Lee and Paul C. Lauterbur, "SLIM, spectral localization by imaging with water suppression," *Works in Progress Abstracts,* Eighth Annual Meeting of the Society of Magnetic Resonance in Medicine, Amsterdam, The Netherlands, (1989), 1117.

131. X. Zhou, J.C. Alameda, Jr. R.L. Magin and P.C. Lauterbur, "3-D microscopy of rat spleen at 4.7T: Improved contrast using dextran magnetite," *Works in Progress Abstracts,* Eighth Annual Meeting of the Society of Magnetic Resonance in Medicine, Amsterdam, The Netherlands, (1989), 1121.

132. Xiachong Zhou, Clinton S. Potter, Brian Voth, J.C. Alameda, Jr., Richard L. Magin and P.C. Lauterbur, "3-D Nuclear magnetic resonance microscopy," *Abstract,* Tenth Meeting of the International Society of Magnetic Resonance, Morzine, France, (1989), S1.

133. P.C. Lauterbur and Haakil Lee, "Extensions of the SLIM (Spectral Location by Imaging with Water Suppression) localization technique," *Abstract,* Tenth Meeting of the International Society of Magnetic Resonance, Morzine, France, (1989), P11-14.

134. Schachar Frank, Ingrid Stuermer and Paul C. Lauterbur, "Iron oxide particles as contrast enhancing agents in magnetic resonance imaging," *Nuclear Medicine Quantitative Analysis in Imaging and Function,* ed. by H.A.E. Schmidt and J. Chambron, (New York: NY: Schattauer-Verlag, 1990), 48-50.

135. Shachar Frank, Ingrid Stuermer and Paul C. Lauterbur, "Iron oxide particles as contrast enhancing agents in magnetic resonance imaging," Abstracts of the European Association of Nuclear Medicine Congress, No. 115, (Strasbourg, France 1989); *Europ. J. Nucl. Med.* **15**, (1989), 427.

136. R.K. Woods, W.B. Hyslop, R.B. Marr and P.C. Lauterbur, "Image Reconstruction," *EPR Imaging and In Vivo EPR,* ed. by G.R. Eaton, S.S. Eaton and K. Ohno, (Boca Raton, FL: CRC Press, Inc. 1991), 91-117.

137. Z.-P. Liang, Haakil Lee and P.C. Lauterbur, "On errors of the SLIM technique," *Abstracts,* Ninth Annual Meeting of the Society of Magnetic Resonance in Medicine, New York, NY, (1990), 1077.

138. W.B. Hyslop and P.C. Lauterbur, "Effects of restricted diffusion in NMR microscopy," *Abstracts,* Ninth Annual Meeting of the Society of Magnetic Resonance in Medicine, New York, NY, (1990), 393.

139. Haakil Lee and P.C. Lauterbur, "Frequency-encoded SLIM," *Abstracts,* Ninth Annual Meeting of the Society of Magnetic Resonance in Medicine, New York, NY, (1990), 1086.

140. Haakil Lee and P.C. Lauterbur, "SLIM with an adiabatic half-passage pulse," *Abstracts,* Ninth Annual Meeting of the Society of Magnetic Resonance in Medicine, New York, NY (1990), 1078.

141. T.L. Peck, R.L. Magin and P.C. Lauterbur, "Microdomain magnetic resonance imaging," *Abstracts,* Ninth Annual Meeting of the Society of Magnetic Resonance in Medicine, New York, NY, (1990), 207.

142. E.S. Fletcher, C.D. Gregory, H. Lee, W.T. Greenough, P.C. Lauterbur and M.J. Dawson, "Simultaneous, 3D-localized, ^{31}P spectroscopy of brain and muscle in the intact head of the living rat using the SLIM technique," *Works-in-Progress Abstracts,* Ninth Annual Meeting of the Society of Magnetic Resonance in Medicine, New York, NY, (1990), 1332.

143. Z.-P. Liang and P.C. Lauterbur, "GSLIM: A general spectral localization method that unifies SLIM and CSI," *Works-in-Progress Abstracts,* Ninth Annual Meeting of the Society of Magnetic Resonance in Medicine, New York, NY, (1990), 1129.

144. E.Wiener and P.C. Lauterbur, "Relaxivity and stabilities of metal complexes of starburst dendrimers: A new class of MRI contrast agents," *Works-in-Progress Abstracts,* Ninth Annual Meeting of the Society of Magnetic Resonance in Medicine, New York, NY, (1990), 1106.

145. P. Ghosh, N. Hawrylak, J. Broadus, W.T. Greenough and P.C. Lauterbur, "NMR imaging of transplated iron oxide-labelled cells in the rat brain," *Works-in-Progress Abstracts,* Ninth Annual Meeting of the Society of Magnetic resonance in Medicine, New York, NY, (1990), 1193.

146. E.S. Fletcher, C.D. Gregory, H. Lee, W.T. Greenough, M.J. Dawson and P.C. Lauterbur, "Localized *in vivo* [31]P spectra of the rat brain using spectral localization by imaging (SLIM): A better method for studies of brain development," *Soc. Neurosci. Abstr.,* Vol. 16, Part 1, (1990), 573.

147. N. Hawrylak, P. Ghosh, J. Broadus, W.T. Greenough and P.C. Lauterbur, "Nuclear magnetic resonance (NMR) imaging of fetal brain grafts," *Soc. Neurosci. Abstr.,* Vol. 16, Part 2, (1990), 1285.

148. Paul C. Lauterbur, "Technical aspects and methods in ultrahigh resolution imaging," *Abstracts,* Ninth Annual Meeting of the Society of Magnetic Resonance in Medicine, New York, NY, (1990), 253.

149. P. Ghosh, H. Lee, N. Hawrylak, W.T. Greenough and P.C. Lauterur, "*In vivo* NMR imaging of magnetically labelled brain cells," *Biophysical Journ.* **59**, (1991), 164a.

150. C. Gregory, E.S. Fletcher, H. Lee, M.J. Dawson, D.N. Levin, W.T. Greenough and P.C. Lauterbur, "3D-localized ^{31}P NMR spectroscopy of brain and muscle using the SLIM technique—simultaneous acquisition of multiple regions of interest," *Biophysical Journ.* **59**, (1991), 163a.

151. Z.-P. Liang and P.C. Lauterbur, "A generalized series approach to MR spectroscopic imaging," *IEEE Trans. Med. Imaging*, Vol. 10, No. 2, (1991), 132-137.

152. W.B. Hyslop and P.C. Lauterbur, "Effects of restricted diffusion on microscopic NMR imaging," *J. Magn. Reson.* **94**, (1991), 501-510.

153. H. Lee, H.D. Morris and P.C. Lauterbur, "NMR imaging of flow velocity by phase tagging," *Abstracts*, Experimental NMR Conference (ENC) St. Louis, MO, (1991), 188.

154. X. Zhou, C.S. Potter and P.C. Lauterbur, "An echo artifact in NMR microscopy," *Abstracts*, Tenth Annual Meeting of the Society of Magnetic Resonance in Medicine, San Francisco, CA, (1991), 345.

155. X. Zhou and P.C. Lauterbur, "3D microscopy using surface coils," Abstracts, Tenth Annual Meeting of the Society of Magnetic Resonance in Medicine, San Francisco, CA, (1991), 878.

156. Haakil Lee and P.C. Lauterbur, "^{13}C MRS by the SLIM localization technique," *Abstracts*, Tenth Annual Meeting of the Society of Magnetic Resonance in Medicine, San Francisco, CA, (1991), 457.

157. H.Lee, D.H. Morris, S. Chandra and P.C. Lauterbur, "Encoding velocity information in NMR images by phase tagging," *Abstracts*, Tenth Annual Meeting of the Society of Magnetic Resonance in Medicine, San Francisco, CA, (1991), 812.

158. W.B. Hyslop and P.C. Lauterbur, "Effects of bounded diffusion on MR microscopy," *Abstracts*, International Conference on NMR Microscopy, Heidelberg, Germany, (1991), 109.

159. R. Ruan, X. Zhou, J.B. Litchfield and P.C. Lauterbur, "Three-dimensional NMR microscopy of corn kernels using fast interleaved projection reconstruction," *Abstracts*, International Conference on NMR Microscopy, Heidelberg, Germany, (1991), 133.

160. X. Zhou, C.S. Potter and P.C. Lauterbur, "A comparison of 3D NMR microscopy and subsequent optical microscopy of thin sections of fixed human brain tissue," *Abstracts*, International Conference on NMR Microscopy, Heidelberg, Germany, (1991), 127.

161. X. Zhou and P.C. Lauterbur, "Sensitivity and resolution on NMR microscopy using surface coils," *Abstracts*, International Conference on NMR Microscopy, Heidelberg, Germany, (1991), 87.

162. X. Zhou and P.C. Lauterbur, "Diffusion limited resolution for different pulse sequences in NMR microscopy," *Abstracts*, International Conference on NMR Microscopy, Heidelberg, Germany, (1991), 88.

163. Z.-P. Liang C. Gregory, M.J. Dawson and P.C. Lauterbur, "Utilizing the data in the phase-encoding 'dead-time' by modified SLIM processing," *Works-in-Progress Abtracts*, Tenth Annual Meeting of the Society of Magnetic Resonance in Medicine, San Francisco, CA, 1991, p. 1168.

164. Z.-P Liang and P.C. Lauterbur, "Effective use of anatomical information for spectroscopic imaging by GSLIM," *Works-in-Progress Abstracts*, Tenth Annual Meeting of the Society of Magnetic Resonance in Medicine, San Francisco, CA, (1991), 1004.

165. Z.-P. Liang, C. Gregory, M.J. Dawson and P.C. Lauterbur, "An improved linear prediction method for correction of phase and baseline artifacts," *Works-in-Progress Abstracts*, Tenth Annual Meeting of the Society of Magnetic Resonance in Medicine, San Francisco, CA, (1991), 1169.

166. P. Ghosh, X. Zhou, W. Lin, A.S. Feng, E. Groman and P.C. Lauterbur, "Neuronal tracing with magnetic labels," *Works-in-Progress Abstracts*, Tenth Annual Meeting of the Society of Magnetic Resonance in Medicine, San Francisco, CA, (1991), 1042.

167. C. Gregory, I. Connolly, S. Xu, Y. Yang, P.C. Lauterbur, Z.-P. Liang and M.J. Dawson, "Regional variation of phosphorus metabolite levels in the human brain: A ^{31}P NMR spec-

troscopy study using SLIM," *Abstracts,* Fourth Annual Cell & Molecular Biology/Molecular Biophysics Research Symposium, Urbana, IL, (1991).

168. X. Zhou and P.C. Lauterbur, "NMR microscopy using projection reconstruction," *Magnetic Resonance Microscopy: Methods and Applications in Materials Science, Agriculture and Biomedicine,* eds. B. Blümich and W. Kuhn, (New York: VCH Publications, 1991), 3-27.

169. P.C. Lauterbur, "Advances in MRI," *Abstracts,* 10th Annual Meeting of the Society of Magnetic Resonance Imaging, New York, NY, (1992), 33.

170. A. Webb, Z.-P. Liang, R.L. Magin and P.C. Lauterbur, "Application of a generalized series reconstruction algorithm to biological MRI," *Works-in-Progress Abstracts,* 10th Annual Meeting of the Society for Magnetic Resonance Imaging, New York, NY, (1992), S26.

171. Z.-P. Liang and P.C. Lauterbur, "Improved temporal/spatial resolution in functional imaging through generalized series reconstruction," *Works-In-Progress Abstracts,* 10th Annual Meeting of the Society for Magnetic Resonance Imaging, New York, NY, (1992), S15.

172. P. Ghosh, X. Zhou, M. Miller, M. Hashimoto, S. Siddique and P.C. Lauterbur, "MR microscopy of magnetically labelled embryonic cells," *Works-in-Progress Abstracts,* 10th Annual Meeting of the Society for Magnetic Resonance Imaging, New York, NY (1992), S21.

173. E.C. Wiener, R.L. Magin, O.A. Gansow, M.W. Brechbiel, D.A. Tomalia and P.C. Lauterbur, "*In vivo* use of starburst dendrimer based MRI contrast agents," *Works-In-Progress Abstracts,* 10th Annual Meeting of the Society for Magnetic Resonance Imaging, New York, NY (1992), S8.

174. S. Chandra, H. Lee and P.C. Lauterbur, "Double-grid double DANTE," *Abstracts,* 33rd Experimental NMR Conference (ENC), Pacific Grove, CA, (1992), 254.

175. P. Ghosh, H.D. Morris, A. Webb, T. Peck, R. Magin and P.C. Lauterbur, "FLASH imaging using a parallel conductor gradient coil with very fast rise times," *Abstracts,* 33rd Experimental NMR Conference (ENC), Pacific Grove, CA, (1992), 236.

176. P. Ghosh, T. Peck, R. Magin and P.C. Lauterbur, "Multi-mode, electronically switched, easy to wrap gradient coil assembly for nuclear magnetic resonance immaging," *Abstracts,* 33rd Experimental NMR Conference (ENC), Pacific Grove, CA, (1992), 144.

177. W.B. Hyslop, R.K. Woods and P.C. Lauterbur, "Four-dimensional projection reconstruction imaging," *Proceedings from Biomedical Image Processing and Three-Dimensional Microscopy,* SPIE, San Jose, CA., Vol. 1660, (1992), 44-49.

178. Y. Cao, G.J. So, D.N. Levin, C.D. Gregory, M.J. Dawson, T. Raidy, P.C. Lauterbur and C.A. Pelizzari, "Integrated 3D display of gyral anatomy and MR spectra on the brain surface," *Abstracts,* 10th Annual Meeting of the Society for Magnetic Resonance Imaging, New York, NY, (1992), 159.

179. Z.-P. Liang, F.E. Boada, R.T. Constable, E.M. Haacke, P.C. Lauterbur and M.R. Smith, "Constrained reconstruction methods in MR imaging," *Rev. of Mag. Res. in Med.* **4,** (1992), 67-185.

180. E.S. Fletcher, I. Syed, S. Pae, C.D. Gregory, W.T. Greenough, P.C. Lauterbur and M.J. Dawson, "An *in vivo* study of brain biochemistry in differentially reared rats using ^{31}P spectral localization by imaging (SLIM)," *Abstracts,* 11th Annual Meeting of the Society of Magnetic Resonance in Medicine, Berlin, Germany, (1992), 2124.

181. E.C. Wiener, R.L. Magin and P.C. Lauterbur, "*In vivo* use of Starburst™ dendrimer-based contrast agents: applications as marcromolecular MR contrast agents," *Abstracts,* 11th Annual Meeting of the Society of Magnetic Resonance in Medicine, Berlin, Germany, (1992), 863.

182. Z.-P. Liang and P.C. Lauterbur, "Efficient time-sequential imaging through generalized series modeling: a simulation analysis," *Works-In-Progress Abstracts,* 11th Annual Meeting of the Society of Magnetic Resonance in Medicine, Berlin, Germany, (1992), 4266.

183. C.D. Gregory, Y. Yang, J. Shimony, S. Xu, H.D. Morris, Z.-P. Liang, M.J. Dawson and P.C. Lauterbur, "Toward quantitative three-dimensional analysis of functional regions of the human brain using SLIM and GSLIM," *Works-In-Progress Abstracts,* 11th Annual Meeting of the Society of Magnetic Resonance in Medicine, Berlin, Germany, (1992), 3830.

184. David N. Levin, Xiaoping Hu, Paul C. Lauterbur and Thomas Spraggins, "Method for calculating localized magnetic resonance spectra from a small number of spatially-encoded spectroscopic signals," US Patent No. 5,081,992, (Jan. 1992).

185. S. Chandra, H.D. Morris, Z.-P. Liang and P.C. Lauterbur, "Efficient perfusion imaging using generalized series reconstruction," *Works-In-Prgress Abstracts*, 11th Annual Meeting of the Society of Magnetic Resonance in Medicine, Berlin, Germany, 1992, 1141.

186. Z.-P. Liang and P.C. Lauterbur, "A theoretical analysis of the SLIM technique," *J. Magn. Reson.* Series B, **102**, (1993), 54-60.

187. P.C. Lauterbur, W.B. Hyslop and H.D. Morris, "NMR microscopy: Old resolutions and new desires," *XI International Society of Magnetic Resonance Conference*, Vancouver, B.C. Canada, (1992), 124.

188. T.L. Peck, A.G. Webb, R.L. Magin and P.C. Lauterbur, "Sensitivity and noise analysis of solenoidal coils for nuclear magnetic resonance microscopy," *Abstracts*, 3rd Annual Workshop on Magnetic Resonance Microscopy and Materials Imaging, Charlestown, MA (1992), 8.

189.N. Hawylak, P. Ghosh, J. Broadus, C. Schlueter, W.T. Greenough and P.C. Lauterbur, "Nuclear magnetic resonance (NMR) imaging of iron oxide-labelled neural transplants," *Experimental Neurology* **121**, (1993), 181-192.

190. S. Frank and P.C. Lauterbur, "Voltage-sensitive magnetic gels as magnetic resonance monitoring agents," *Nature* **363**, (1993), 334-336.

191. Y. Yang and P.C. Lauterbur, "Spatially localized 2D correlation spectroscopy with COSY SLIM," *Works-In-Progress Abstracts*, 11th Annual Meeting of the Society for Magnetic Resonance Imaging, San Francisco, CA, (1993), S39.

192. S. Chandra, A. Webb and P.C. Lauterbur, "Use of constrained image reconstruction in fast T^1 mapping," *Abstracts*, 11th Annual Meeting of the Society for Magnetic Resonance Imaging, San Francisco, CA, (1993), 141.

193. H. Douglas Morris, Z.-P. Liang, C. Potter, Y. Cao and P.C. Lauterbur, "Efficient functional imaging with RIGR on a clinical system," *Abstracts*, 12th Annual Meeting of Magnetic Resonance in Medicine, New York, NY, (1993), 1393.

194. N.J. Cohen, M.T. Banich, A.F. Kramer, H.D. Morris, P.C. Lauterbur, C.S. Potter, Y. Cao and D.N. Levin, "Assessing test-retest reliability of functional MRI data," *Abstracts*, 12th Annual Meeting of the Society of Magnetic Resonance in Medicine, New York, NY (1993), 1410.

195. C.P. Hess, B. Bridges, Z.-P. Liang, C. Gregory, M.J. Dawson and P.C. Lauterbur, "A new method for automatic correction of phase and baseline artifacts in MR spectroscopic imaging data," *Abstracts*, 12th Annual Meeting of the Society of Magnetic Resonance in Medicine, New York, NY (1993), 687.

196. Z.-P. Liang and P.C. Lauterbur, "(k, t)-space sampling considerations for image of time-varying functions," *Abstracts*, 12th Annual Meeting of the Society of Magnetic Resonance in Medicine, New York, NY (1993), 710.

197. Z.-P. Liang and P.C. Lauterbur, "Efficient dynamic imaging using concentric scanning," *Abstracts*, 12th Annual Meeting of the Society of Magnetic Resonance in Medicine, New York, NY (1993), 477.

198. S. Chandra, Z.-P. Liang and P.C. Lauterbur, "Application of RIGR to efficient BOLD imaging," *Abstracts*, 12th Annual Meeting of the Society of Magnetic Resonance in Medicine, New York, NY (1993), 699.

199. J.M. Hanson, Z.-P. Liang and P.C. Lauterbur, "A new method for fast dynamic imaging using wavelet transforms," *Abstracts*, 12th Annual Meeting of the Society of Magnetic Resonance in Medicine, New York, NY (1993), 712.

200. T.L. Peck, R.L. Magin, L. LaValle, I. Adesida and P.C. Lauterbur, "RF microcoils with micron-scale feature sizes for NMR microscopy," *Abstracts*, 12th Annual Meeting of the Society of Magnetic Resonance in Medicine, New York, NY (1993), 296.

201. A.K. Marumoto, C.L. Minor, D.N. Calvert and P.C. Lauterbur, "The synthesis and relaxometry of Gd(3+)-DTPA bisamide macrocycles," *Abstracts*, 12th Annual Meeting of the Society of Magnetic Resonance in Medicine, New York, NY (1993), 760.

202. X. Zhou, Z.-P. Liang, G.P. Cofer, S.L. Gewalt, P.C. Lauterbur and G.A. Johnson, "An FSE pulse sequence with circular sampling for MR microscopy," *Abstracts*, 12th Annual Meeting of the Society of Magnetic Resonance in Medicine, New York, NY (1993), 297.

203. E.C. Wiener, F.P. Auteri, R.L. Belford, R.B. Clarkson and P.C. Lauterbur, "Molecular dynamics of paramagnetic ions attached to Starburst™ dendrimer," *Abstracts*, 12th Annual Meeting of the Society of Magnetic Resonance in Medicine, New York, NY, (1993), 241.

204. Y. Yang, C.D. Gregory and P.C. Lauterbur, "A Bloch equation-based simulation analysis of SLIM," *Abstracts*, 12th Annual Meeting of the Society of Magnetic Resonance in Medicine, New York, NY, (1993), 910.

205. X. Zhou, R.L. Magin, J.C. Alameda, Jr., H.A. Reynolds and P.C. Lauterbur, "Three-dimensional NMR microscopy of rat spleen and liver," *Mag. Res. in Med.* **30**, (1993), 92-96.

206. T.L. Peck, L. LaValle, R.L. Magin, I. Adesida, B.C. Wheeler and P.C. Lauterbur, "RF microcoils patterned using microlithographic techniques for use as microsensors in NMR," *Proc. of the 15th Annual International Conference of IEEE Engineering in Medicine and Biology Society*, San Diego, CA, (1993), 174-175.

207. C.S. Potter, M. Banich, N. Cohen, A. Kramer, P.C. Lauterbur and H.D. Morris, "NEU-ROVISION: A software tool for functional MRI neuroimaging analysis," *Abstracts*, SMRM/SMRI Functional MRI of the Brain Workshop, Arlington, VA, (1993), 243.

208. Paul C. Lauterbur, W. Brian Hyslop and H. Douglas Morris, "Toward ultra-resolution NMR microscopy," *Abstracts*, 2nd International Conference on Magnetic Resonance Microscopy, Heidelberg, Germany, (1993), 17.

209. T.L. Peck, L. LaValle, R.L. Magin, I. Adesida and P.C. Lauterbur, "Planar microcoils sensors for NMR microscopy," *Abstracts*, 2nd International Conference on Magnetic Resonance Microscopy, Heidelberg, Germany, (1993), 90.

210. Paul C. Lauterbur and Shachar Frank, "Voltage sensitive magnetic gels as MRI agents," US Patent No. 051,965, (filed April 1993), Pending.

211. E.C. Wiener, M.W. Brechbiel, H. Brothers, R.L. Magin, O.A. Gansow, D.A. Tomalia and P.C. Lauterbur, "Dendrimer-based metal chelates: A new class of MRI contrast agents," *Mag. Res. in Med.* **31**, (1994), 1-8.

212. A.G. Webb, Z.-P. Liang, R.L. Magin and P.C. Lauterbur, "Applications of reduced-encoding MR Imaging with generalized-series reconstruction (RIGR), *JMRI* **3:6**, (1993) 925-928.

213. Z.-P. Liang and P.C. Lauterbur, "An efficient method for dynamic magnetic resonance imaging," *IEEE Trans. on Med. Imaging*, **13:4**, (1994), 677-686.

214. H.D. Morris, B.K. Hyslop, J. Lee and P.C. Lauterbur, "Scanning magnetic resonance microscopy with diffusional amplification," *Abstracts*, 35th Annual ENC Conference, Pacific Grove, CA, (1994), 212.

215. S. Agahi, E. Meisami and P.C. Lauterbur, "Magnetic resonance imaging of olfactory bulb and cavities in the rat," *Abstracts*, Society for Neuroscience Meeting, Miami Beach, FL, Vol. 20, (1994), 328.

216. R.A. Swain, A.B. Harris, E.C. Wiener, H.D. Morris, C.R. Swain, P.C. Lauterbur and W.T. Greenough, "MRI of rat motor cortex following physical exercise," *Abstracts*, Society for Neuroscience Meeting, Miami Beach, FL, Vol. 20, (1994), 147.

217. H.D. Morris, W.B. Hyslop and P.C. Lauterbur, "Diffusion-enhanced NMR microscopy," *Proceedings of the Society of Magnetic Resonance*, Second Meeting, San Francisco, CA, Vol. 1, (1994), 37.

218. Z.-P. Liang, J.M. Hanson, C.S. Potter and P.C. Lauterbur, "Efficient high-resolution dynamic imaging with explicit boundary constraints," *Proceedings of the Society of Magnetic Resonance*, Second Meeting, San Francisco, CA, Vol. 1, (1994), 53.

219. C.S. Potter, C.D. Gregory, H.D. Morris, Z.-P. Liang and P.C. Lauterbur, "The NEU-ROSCOPE: An interactive system for real-time functional MRI of the brain," *Proceedings of the Society of Magnetic Resonance,* Second Meeting, San Francisco, CA, Vol. 2, (1994), 835.

220. Y. Yang and P.C. Lauterbur, "Flip angle mapping by optimized multiple echo imaging and its application to localized spectroscopy," *Proceedings of the Society of Magnetic Resonance,* Second Meeting, San Francisco, CA, Vol. 2, (1994), 847.

221. Y. Yang, J.S. Shimony, S. Xu, V. Gulani, M.J. Dawson and P.C. Lauterbur, "A sequence for measurement of anisotropic diffusion by projection reconstruction imaging and its application to skeletal and smooth muscle," *Proceedings of the Society of Magnetic Resonance,* Second Meeting, San Francisco, CA, Vol. 2, (1994), 1036.

222. V. Gulani, Y. Yang, J.S. Shimony, S. Chandra and P.C. Lauterbur, "Determination of orientation and diffusion anisotropy of parallel fibers using four diffusion measurements," *Proceedings of the Society of Magnetic Resonance,* Second Meeting, San Francisco, CA, Vol. 2, (1994), 1040.

223. A.K. Marumoto, J.A. Kopale, C.L. Minor, J.E. Vogel. and P.C. Lauterbur, "MR imaging and physical studies of Gd(3+)-DTPA bisamide macrocycle complexes," *Proceedings of the Society of Magnetic Resonance,* Second Meeting, San Francisco, CA, Vol. 2, (1994), 912.

224. Y. Yang, S. Xu, M.J. Dawson and P.C. Lauterbur, "Localized diffusion measurement in phantoms and tissues by SLIM," *Proceedings of the Society of Magnetic Resonance,* Second Meeting, San Francisco, CA, Vol. 2, (1994), 1058.

225. C.S. Potter, Z.-P. Liang, C.D. Gregory, H.D. Morris and P.C. Lauterbur, "Toward a neuroscope: A real-time imaging system for evaluation of brain function," *IEEE International Conference on Image Processing,* Austin, TX, Vol. III, (1994), 25-29.

226. W.B. Hyslop, R.K. Woods and P.C. Lauterbur, "Four-dimensional spectral-spatial imaging using projection reconstruction," *IEEE Trans. in Med. Imaging,* (1995).

227. P.C. Lauterbur, "Learning from frogs and TV: How to use K-space for efficient redundancy minimization of imaging techniques (KERMIT)," *Abstracts,* 36th Annual ENC Conference, Boston, MA (1995), 47.

228. H.D. Morris, W.B. Hyslop, J.J. Lee, P. Gorkov, N. Yang, K.-T. Yung and P.C. Lauterbur, "DESIRE: A novel approach to ultra-microscopic NMR imaging using scanning magnetic resonance microscopy with diffusional amplification," *Abstracts,* 36th Annual ENC Conference, Boston, MA, (1995), 264.

229. T.L. Peck, R.L. Magin, P.C. Lauterbur, "Design and analysis of microcoils for NMR microscopy," *J. Magn. Reson.* Series B, (1995).

INDEX